EDITION 10

Fundamental Nursing Skills and Concepts

BARBARA KUHN TIMBY, RN, BC, BSN, MA
Professor Emeritus
Glen Oaks Community College
Centreville, Michigan

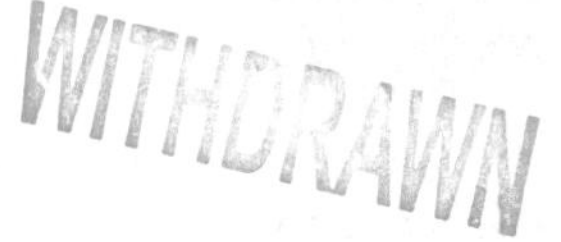

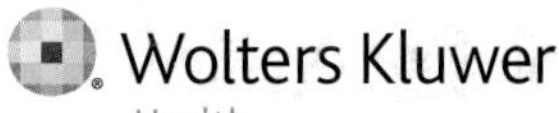

Lippincott Williams & Wilkins
Philadelphia • Baltimore • New York • London
Buenos Aires • Hong Kong • Sydney • Tokyo

Acquisitions Editor: Elizabeth Nieginski
Product Manager: Annette Ferran
Editorial Assistant: Zack Shapiro
Design Coordinator: Joan Wendt
Illustration Coordinator: Brett MacNaughton
Manufacturing Coordinator: Karin Duffield
Prepress Vendor: Aptara, Inc.

Tenth Edition

9 8 7 6 5 4 3 2 1

Printed in the U.S.A.

Library of Congress Cataloging-in-Publication Data

Timby, Barbara Kuhn.
Fundamental nursing skills and concepts / Barbara Kuhn Timby. — 10th ed.
p. ; cm.
Includes bibliographical references and index.
ISBN 978-1-60831-787-5 (alk. paper)
I. Title.
[DNLM: 1. Nursing Care. WY 100.1]
610.73—dc23

2011048255

LWW.COM

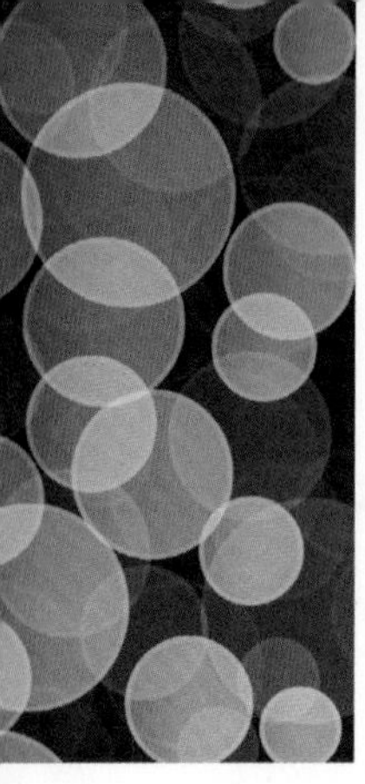

*This edition of **Fundamental Nursing Skills and Concepts** is dedicated to all student nurses who will join the ranks of practicing nurses to meet the nation's health care needs during this time of the nursing shortage.*

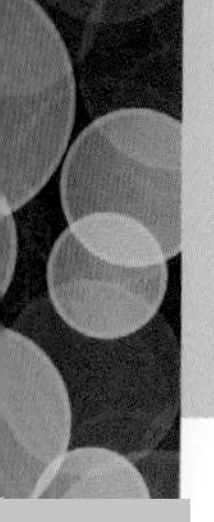

Contributor & Reviewers

Contributor

Susan G. Dudek, RN, CDN, BS
Nursing Instructor, Dietetic Technology Program
Erie Community College
Williamsville, New York

Reviewers

Michelle Bennet, RN
Nursing Instructor
Nunez Community College
Chalmette, Louisiana

Pat Clowers, MSN
Director of Nursing and Allied Health
East Mississippi Community College
Mayhew, Mississippi

Elizabeth DeMarsh-Smith, RN, BA
Curriculum Chairperson
Robert T. White LPN School
Canton, Ohio

Theresa Fontaine
Practical Nursing Instructor
Arkansas Tech University – Ozark Campus
Ozark, Arkansas

Marion Goodman, BSN
Coordinator of Vocational Nursing
Lone Star College – CyFair
Cypress, Texas

Cynthia Hotaling, RN, MSN
Associate Professor
Owens Community College
Findlay, Ohio

Connie Hyde, RN, BSN
Practical Nursing Instructor
Louisiana Technical College – Lafayette Campus
Lafayette, Louisiana

Tammy McKinney, MSN, FNP-C, RNC
Associate Professor of Nursing
Danville Community College
Danville, Virginia

Peggy Penn
San Jacinto College – Central Campus
Pasadena, Texas

Rebecca Romagna, RN, MSN
Practical Nursing Instructor
Greater Altoona Career & Technology Center
Altoona, Pennsylvania

Deborah Shaw, RN, BSN
Instructor, Vocational Nursing
Schreiner University
Kerrville, Texas

Becky Shuttlesworth, RN, BSN
Skills Lab Coordinator
San Jacinto College South
Houston, Texas

Pattie Sunderhaus, RN, MSN, EdD
Director of Faculty Development
Brown Mackie College
Cincinnati, Ohio

Collene Thaxton, RN, MSN
Associate Professor of Nursing
Mount Wachusett Community College
Gardner, Massachusetts

Olma Weaver, RN
Vocational Nursing Instructor
Coastal Bend College – Beeville
Beeville, Texas

Muriel Zraunig, RN, MSN
Practical Nursing Program Director
McCann Technical School
North Adams, Massachusetts

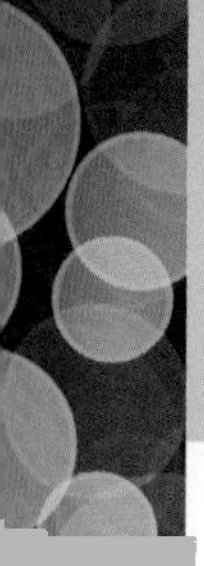

Preface

Fundamental Nursing Skills and Concepts is designed to assist beginning nursing students in acquiring a foundation of basic nursing theory and developing clinical skills. In addition, its content can serve as a ready reference for updating the skills of currently employed nurses or those returning to work after a period of inactive practice.

PHILOSOPHICAL FOUNDATIONS OF THE TEXT

Several philosophical concepts are the bases for this text:

- The human experience is a composite of physiologic, emotional, social, and spiritual aspects that affect health and healing.
- Caring is the essence of nursing and is extended to every client.
- Each client is unique, and nurses must adapt their care to meet the individual needs of every person without compromising safety or achievement of desired outcomes.
- A supportive network of health care providers, family, and friends promotes health restoration and health promotion. Therefore, it is essential to include the client's significant others in teaching, formal discussions, and provision of services.
- Licensed and student nurses are accountable for their actions and clinical decisions; consequently, each must be aware of legislation as it affects nursing practice.

In today's changing health care environment, nurses face many challenges and opportunities. The tenth edition of *Fundamental Nursing Skills and Concepts* was written to help nurses meet these challenges and take advantage of expanding opportunities.

NEW TO THIS EDITION

- **Integration of Gerontologic, Pharmacologic, and Nutritional Considerations.** Information that focuses on gerontologic, pharmacologic, and nutritional considerations is integrated within the text of each chapter where they are more applicable to the immediate content rather than appearing at the end of each chapter. Their location is identified by unique, recurring icons.
- **Brand-new NANDA diagnoses and terminology.** The NANDA diagnoses labels and definitions found in the Nursing Implications and accompanying Nursing Care Plans throughout the text have been updated according to the latest NANDA-I publication, *Nursing Diagnoses 2012–2014.*
- **New Content.** The entire text has been revised and updated to reflect current medical and nursing practice. Additionally, several skills and sections contain brand new content. The following are some highlights:
  - Chapter 1, "Nursing Foundations," reflects changes to *Nursing: A Social Policy Statement,* 3rd edition (2010), in which the American Nurses Association (ANA) provides a current definition of nursing. This chapter introduces the term *evidence-based practice* and relates its significance to current nursing practice. Based on data provided by the US Bureau of Labor Statistics, this chapter reinforces the projected increase in the demand for licensed practical nurses in a variety of healthcare settings. Because LPNs, as well as RNs, work with unlicensed assistive personnel (UAPs), Chapter 1 expands the criteria for appropriate delegation. Updated statistics on enrollments and numbers of licensed nurses in various nursing programs demonstrate a continuing shortage of nurses as well as trends toward a demand for higher levels of nursing education, specialty certifications, and continuing education. The content reiterates the crises in health care and how efforts to extend the Nurse Reinvestment Act or create similar federal legislation would somewhat help relieve the shortage of nurses in the United States.
  - Chapter 4, "Health and Illness," includes information on Healthy People 2020, the newest goals of the national health-promotion effort, which include achieving health equity among the nation's citizens. The chapter also includes a discussion of recent Medicare changes.
  - Chapter 6, "Culture and Ethnicity," updates the demographic information on the various ethnic groups that make up the population of the United States, based on the 2010 census data, and discusses the effects these changes might have on nursing. The chapter also discusses technological advances for communicating with deaf clients, clients who do not speak English, or those who speak English as a second language.
  - Chapter 7, "The Nurse–Client Relationship," expands its discussion of special techniques to be used in communicating with deaf clients and with those who are verbally impaired or have Alzheimer's disease.
  - Chapter 8, "Client Teaching," includes new coverage of the benefits of client teaching, to the client as well as the nurse, and insights into the concept of "health literacy."
  - Chapter 9, "Recording and Reporting," updates the criteria of the Joint Commission, formerly known as the The

Joint Commission on Accreditation of Healthcare Organizations (JCAHO), for record-keeping.

- Chapter 10, "Asepsis" discusses the latest guidelines on hand-washing and alcohol-based hand rubs, the agents used to achieve surgical asepsis, and the use of protective gear.
- Chapter 12, "Vital Signs," contains new sections on temporal artery thermometry, including a new Nursing Guidelines feature for using the temporal artery thermometer.
- Chapter 13, "Physical Assessment," discusses the newest guidelines for breast self-examination, and the impact these guidelines have on client teaching.
- Chapter 15, "Nutrition," has been thoroughly updated to reflect the recent changes recommended by the American Dietary Association, including the new MyPlate nutrition guidelines that replace "MyPyramid."
- Chapter 16, "Fluid and Chemical Balance," contains new information about oxygen therapeutics and perfluorocarbons.
- Chapter 18, "Comfort, Rest, and Sleep," contains a new box outlining the components of phototherapy.
- Chapter 19, "Safety," includes a new table outlining the latest National Patient Safety Goals, updated in 2009–2010.
- Chapter 22, "Infection Control," contains the new advice on "cough etiquette," including an illustration. The chapter also discusses the new Standard Precautions recommendations and new safe injection practices and infection control practices in lumbar puncture.
- Chapter 23, "Body Mechanics, Positioning, and Moving," explains the newest policies proposed in Congress to protect the safety of nurses and clients.
- Chapter 32, "Oral Medications," includes discussion of the new technology of barcode medication administration systems.
- Chapter 37, "Resuscitation," reflects the American Heart Association's (AHA's) International Cardiopulmonary Resuscitation (CPR) and Emergency Cardiovascular Care (ECC) Guidelines of 2010 for performing basic life support techniques.
- Chapter 38, "End-of-Life Care," includes new discussion of multicultural considerations for the nurse caring for clients and their families and they approach the client's death.

- **Art and Photography Program.** Contemporary nursing practice is illustrated by the many full-color photos and line drawings. These illustrations assist visual learners to become familiar with the latest equipment, techniques, and practices in today's health care environment.

FEATURES AND LEARNING TOOLS

Many of the features that long-time users of Timby love are found in the tenth edition as well:

- **Table of Contents.** Based on market feedback, Section I in the tenth edition provides chapters that relate to Fundamental Nursing Concepts. Section II, "Fundamental Nursing Skills," begins with Chapter 10, "Asepsis," to underscore the importance of hand hygiene and other aseptic practices when providing nursing care.
- **Words to Know.** These key terms are listed at the beginning of each chapter and set in boldface type within the text where they appear with or near their definition. Additional technical terms are italicized throughout the text.
- **Learning Objectives.** These student-oriented objectives appear at the beginning of each chapter to serve as guidelines for acquiring specific information. They are now numbered, so that the corresponding student and intructors resources can be easily matched.
- **Nursing Process Focus.** The focus on the Nursing Process continues to be strong. The concepts and paradigm for the nursing process appear in Chapter 2. The premise is that early familiarity with its components will reinforce its use in the Skills and sample Nursing Care Plans throughout the text. Each skill chapter has the most recent Applicable Nursing Diagnoses that correlate with the types of problems recipients of the respective skills may have.
- **Nursing Care Plans.** The diagnostic statements contain three parts for actual diagnoses and two parts for potential diagnoses. A double-column format lists interventions on one side and corresponding rationales on the other. The evaluation step is reinforced by evidence indicating expected outcome achievement.
- **Skills.** The Skills continue to be clustered at the end of each chapter for ease of access and to avoid interrupting the narrative and distancing related Tables and Boxes to locations where they previously seemed out of context. In addition, each illustration within the skills has been closely reviewed to ensure that it complies with Standard Precautions, infection control guidelines from the Centers for Disease Control and Prevention.
- **Nursing Guidelines.** These mini-procedures provide directions for performing various kinds of nursing care or suggestions for managing client care problems.
- **Client and Family Teaching** boxes. These specially numbered boxes found throughout chapters highlight essential education points for nurses to communicate to clients and their families.
- **Critical Thinking Exercises.** More critical thinking questions have been added at the end of each chapter to facilitate application of the material, using clinical situations or rhetorical questions.
- **NCLEX-PN Style Questions.** Additional questions have been added to help students apply their acquired knowledge by answering questions that reflect the formats within the 2011 NCLEX-PN Test plan.
- **End of Unit Exercises.** Found at the end of each unit, these challenging groups of activities consolidate information found in previous chapters to assist students to review and master critical material. The problems build from simple to complex, with special sections designed to help readers apply their knowledge and prepare for the NCLEX-PN. Answers are provided on the Instructor CD-ROM and on thePoint.

- **Glossary.** Found at the back of the book, this is a quick reference of definitions for Words to Know that are used throughout the text.
- **Bibliography.** A comprehensive listing of references and suggested readings, including general recommendations as well as unit-specific citations, provides a streamlined guide to current literature about topics discussed in the text.
- **Detailed Table of Contents.** Located at the beginning of the textbook, this provides an outline of each unit's and chapter's subject matter.

USE WITH *INTRODUCTORY MEDICAL-SURGICAL NURSING*

Fundamental Nursing Skills and Concepts may be adopted as a single text for students in a nursing program. Additionally, the book may be adopted with *Introductory Medical–Surgical Nursing* by Timby and Smith. The content, designs, features, and styles of these two texts have been coordinated closely to facilitate understanding and to present a consistent approach to learning.

TEACHING—LEARNING PACKAGE

The tenth edition of *Fundamental Nursing Skills and Concepts* features a compelling and comprehensive complement of additional resources to help students learn and instructors teach.

RESOURCES FOR STUDENTS

Valuable learning tools for students are available on thePoint:

- **Concepts in Action** animations and **Watch and Learn** video clips demonstrate important concepts related to various topics explored in the accompanying text.
- NCLEX-style review questions that correspond with each book chapter help students review important concepts and practice for the NCLEX.
- A Spanish-English glossary lists words commonly encountered or needed in the nurse's practice.
- Journal Articles about relevant topics enable students to stay aware of the latest research and information available in the current literature.
- Case Studies help students apply their learning about nursing concepts and skills to client-oriented scenarios.
- Answer Keys for the Stop, Think, and Respond boxes, NCLEX-Style Review Questions, Critical Thinking Exercises, and End of Unit Exercises allow students to check their comprehension of textbook presentations as desired.

RESOURCES FOR INSTRUCTORS

The above student-oriented materials are available for instructors on thePoint. Additionally, instructors have access to the following tools to assist with teaching:

- An extensive collection of materials is provided for each book chapter:
  - **Pre-Lecture Quizzes and Answers** are quick, knowledge-based assessments that allow instructors to check students' reading and comprehension.
  - **PowerPoint presentations** provide an easy way to integrate the textbook with students' classroom experience, either via computerized slide shows or handouts.
  - **Guided Lecture Notes** walk instructors through the chapters, objective by objective, and provide corresponding PowerPoint slide numbers.
  - **Discussion Topics (and suggested answers)** are organized by learning objective and can be used as classroom conversation starters.
  - **Assignments (and suggested answers)**, also organized by learning objective, include group, written, clinical, and web-based activities.
- An **Image Bank** provides the photographs and illustrations from this textbook to be used as best suits instructor needs, including in PowerPoint slides.
- A sample syllabus provides guidance for structuring an LPN/LVN course.
- The Test Generator lets teachers assemble exclusive new tests from a bank containing more than 900 questions to help assess students' understanding of the material. These questions are formatted to match the NCLEX, so students can practice preparing for this important examination.

STUDENT WORKBOOK

The *Workbook for Fundamental Nursing Skills and Concepts, 10th edition,* is available for purchase and provides an engaging review of important material. Featuring **images** from the text, **review exercises, application activities,** and more **NCLEX-PN practice questions,** the Workbook complements this textbook and provides dynamic reinforcement of everything students need to learn from it. Answers to the exercises in the Workbook are available to instructors through thePoint.

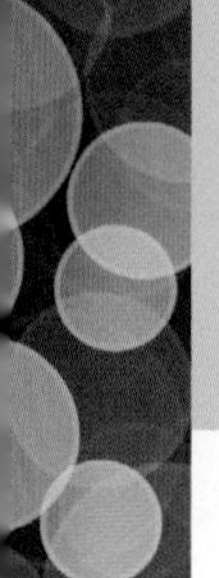

Acknowledgments

It is my belief that this text and its ancillary package will facilitate learning and produce safe, effective practitioners, capable of providing quality care for diverse clients in a variety of settings. Thanks go to the following people at Lippincott Williams & Wilkins for their help in preparing this book and for supporting the revision and new ideas and organization of the text material:

- Elizabeth Nieginski, Executive Editor
- Annette Ferran, Product Manager

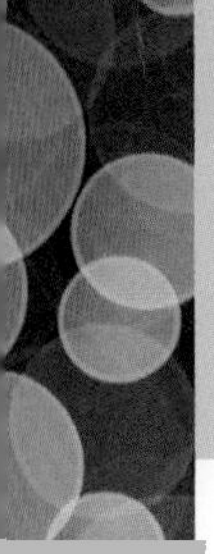

Contents

UNIT 1

Exploring Contemporary Nursing 1

UNIT 2

Integrating Basic Concepts 33

UNIT 4

Performing Basic Client Care 139

UNIT 5

Assisting With Basic Needs 283

UNIT 9

Medication Administration 735

UNIT 10

Intervening in Emergency Situations 809

UNIT 11

Caring for the Terminally Ill 841

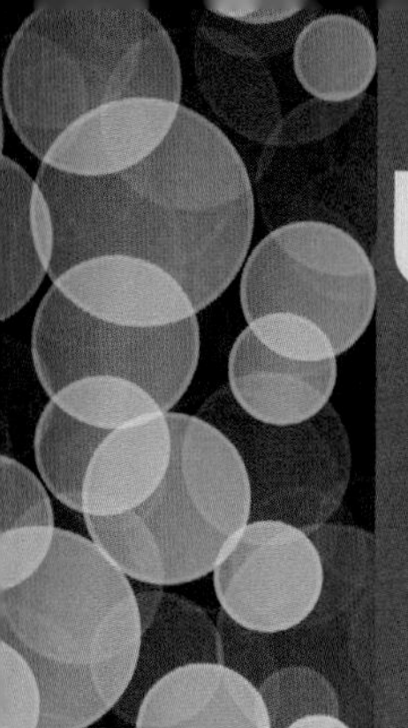

UNIT 1
Exploring Contemporary Nursing

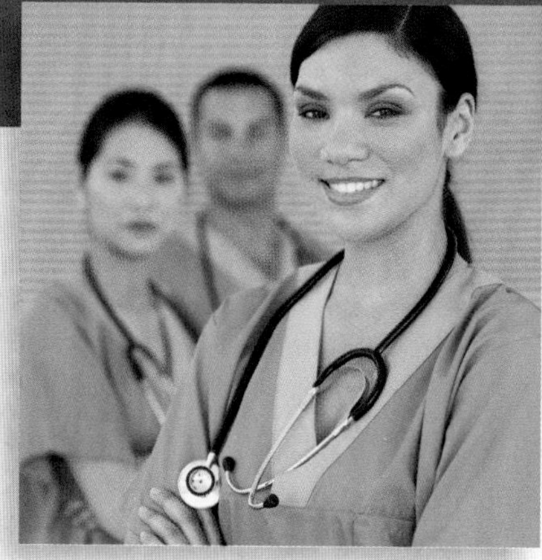

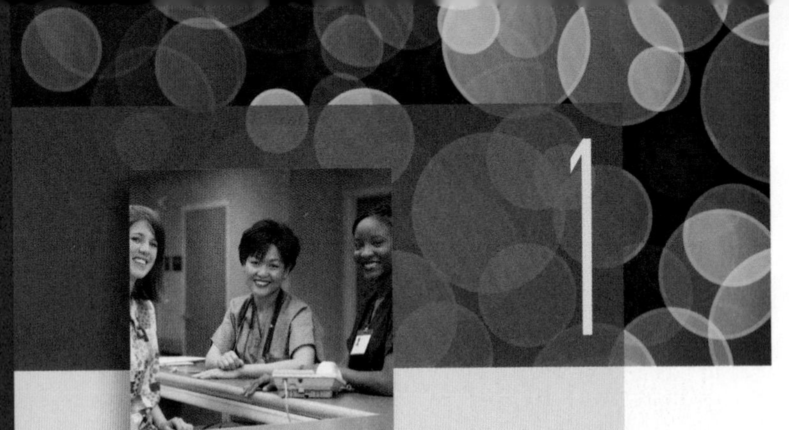

1

Nursing Foundations

Words To Know

active listening
activities of daily living
advanced practice
art
assessment skills
capitation
caring skills
clinical pathways
comforting skills
counseling skills
cross-trained
discharge planning
empathy
evidence-based practice
managed care practices
multicultural diversity
nursing skills
nursing theory
primary care
quality assurance
science
sympathy
theory

Learning Objectives

On completion of this chapter, the reader should be able to:

1. Name one historical event that led to the demise of nursing in England before the time of Florence Nightingale.
2. Identify four reforms for which Florence Nightingale is responsible.
3. Describe at least five ways in which early US training schools deviated from those established under the direction of Florence Nightingale.
4. Name three ways that nurses used their skills in the early history of US nursing.
5. Explain how art, science, and nursing theory have been incorporated into contemporary nursing practice.
6. Discuss the evolution of definitions of nursing.
7. List four types of educational programs that prepare students for beginning levels of nursing practice.
8. Identify at least five factors that influence choice of educational nursing program.
9. State three reasons that support the need for continuing education in nursing.
10. List examples of current trends affecting nursing and health care.
11. Discuss the shortage of nurses and methods to reduce the crisis.
12. Describe four skills that all nurses use in clinical practice.

This chapter traces the historical development of nursing from its unorganized beginning to current sophisticated practice. Nurses in the 21st century owe a debt of gratitude to their pioneering counterparts who served clients on battlefields, in urban settlement houses, in Boston's harbor on a floating "children's hospital," and on horseback in the Appalachian frontier. Ironically, nursing is returning to its original community-based practice model.

NURSING ORIGINS

Nursing is one of the youngest professions but one of the oldest arts. It evolved from the familial roles of nurturing and caretaking. Early responsibilities included assisting women during childbirth, suckling healthy newborns, and ministering to the ill, aged, and helpless within households and surrounding communities. Its hallmark was caring more than curing.

During the Middle Ages in Europe, religious groups assumed many of the roles of nursing. Christian nuns, priests, and brothers

BOX 1-1 Rules of Employment for Nursing Attendants—1789

- No dirt, rags, or bones may be thrown from the windows.
- Nurses are to punctually shift the bed and body linen of patients, viz., once in a fortnight (2 weeks), their shirts once in 4 days, their drawers and stockings once a week or oftener, if found necessary.
- All nurses who disobey orders, get drunk, neglect their patients, quarrel with men shall be immediately discharged.

From Goodnow, M. (1933). *Outlines of nursing history* (5th ed., pp. 57–58). Philadelphia, PA: W.B. Saunders.

combined their efforts to save souls with a commitment to care for the sick. Despite their zeal, they were overworked and overwhelmed because of their limited numbers, especially during periods when plagues and pestilence spread quickly in communities. Consequently, some convents and monasteries engaged conscientious penitent and disadvantaged lay people to assist with the burden of physical care.

In England, the character and quality of nursing care changed dramatically when religious groups were exiled to Western Europe during the schism between King Henry VIII and the Catholic Church. The management of parochial hospitals and the ill within them fell to the state. Hospitals became poorhouses, which some characterized more accurately as "pest houses." The English state recruited the hospital labor force from the ranks of criminals, widows, and orphans, who repaid the Crown for their meager food and shelter by tending to the unfortunate sick. An example of the menial requirements for employment appears in Box 1-1. Generally, nursing attendants were ignorant, uncouth, and apathetic to the needs of their charges. Without supervision, they rarely performed even minimal duties. Infections, pressure sores, and malnutrition were a testimony to their neglect.

THE NIGHTINGALE REFORMATION

In the midst of deplorable health care conditions, Florence Nightingale, an Englishwoman born of wealthy parents, announced that God had called her to become a nurse. Despite her family's protests, she worked with nursing deaconesses, a Protestant order of women who cared for the sick in Kaiserswerth, Germany. After becoming suitably prepared through her nursing apprenticeship, Nightingale embarked on the next phase of her career.

The Crimean War

While Nightingale was providing nursing care for residents at the Institution for the Care of Sick Gentlewomen in Distressed Circumstances, England found itself allied with Turkey, France, and Sardinia in defending the Crimea, a peninsula on the north shore of the Black Sea (1854 to 1856). The British military suffered terribly, and

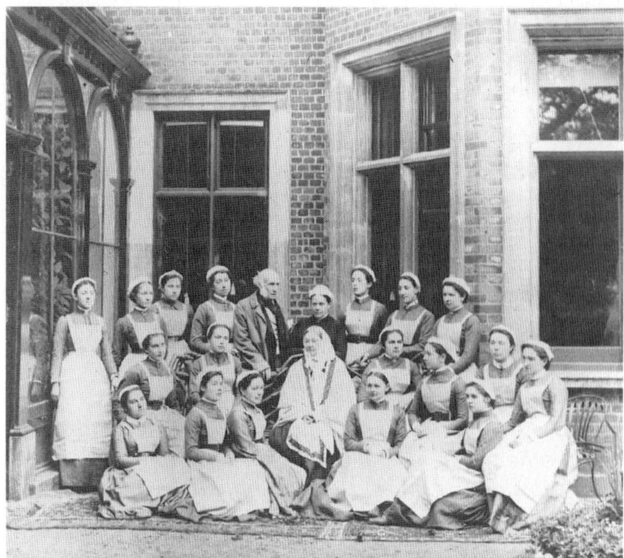

FIGURE 1-1 Florence Nightingale (*center*), her brother-in-law, Sir Harry Verney, and Miss Crossland, the nurse in charge of the Nightingale Training School at St. Thomas Hospital, with a class of student nurses. (Courtesy of The Florence Nightingale Museum Trust, London, England.)

war correspondents at the front lines made public the dire circumstances of the soldiers. Reports of high death rates and complications among the war casualties caused outrage among the British people. As a result, the government became the object of national criticism.

It was then that Florence Nightingale offered a strategic plan to Sidney Herbert, Britain's Secretary of War and an old family friend. She proposed that the sick and injured British soldiers at Scutari, a military barracks in Turkey, would fare better if a team of women trained in nursing skills could care for them (Fig. 1-1). With Herbert's approval, Nightingale selected women with reputations beyond reproach. She realized intuitively that only people with devotion and idealism could accept the discipline and hard work necessary for the looming task.

To the British medical staff at Scutari, the arrival of this group of women implied that they were incapable of providing adequate care. Jealousy and rivalry caused them to refuse any help from Nightingale and her 38 volunteers. When it became clear that the daily death rate, which averaged about 60%, was not subsiding, the medical staff allowed Nightingale's nurses to work. Under Nightingale's supervision, the women cleaned the filth, eliminated the vermin, and improved ventilation, nutrition, and sanitation. They helped control infection and gangrene and lowered the death rate to 1%.

Servicemen and their families alike were grateful, and England adored Nightingale. To show their appreciation, many donated funds to sustain her great work. Nightingale used this money to start the first training school for nurses at St. Thomas Hospital in England. This school became the model for others in Europe and the United States.

Nightingale's Contributions

Nightingale changed the negative image of nursing to a positive one. She is credited with the following:

- Training women for future work
- Selecting only those with upstanding characters as potential nurses
- Improving sanitary conditions for the sick and injured
- Significantly reducing the death rate of British soldiers
- Providing classroom education and clinical teaching
- Advocating that nursing education should be lifelong

Stop, Think, and Respond Box 1-1

How did Florence Nightingale convince the English and others that formal education of people who cared for the sick and injured was essential?

NURSING IN THE UNITED STATES

The American Civil War occurred around the same time as the Nightingale reformation. Like England, the United States found itself involved in a war with a lack of an organized trained nursing staff to care for the sick and wounded. The military had to rely on untrained corpsmen and civilian volunteers, who were often the mothers, wives, and sisters of soldiers.

The Union government appointed Dorothea Lynde Dix, a social worker who had proved her worth by reforming health conditions for the mentally ill, to select and organize women volunteers to care for the troops. In 1862, Dix followed Nightingale's advice and established the following selection criteria. Applicants were to be

- Thirty-five to fifty years old
- Matronly and plain-looking
- Educated
- Neat, orderly, sober, and industrious, with a serious disposition

Applicants also had to submit two letters of recommendation attesting to their moral character, integrity, and capacity to care for the sick. Once selected, a volunteer nurse was to dress plainly in brown, gray, or black and had to agree to serve for at least 6 months (Donahue, 1985).

US Nursing Schools

After the Civil War, US training schools for nurses began to be established. Unfortunately, however, the standards of these schools deviated substantially from those of the Nightingale paradigm (Table 1-1). While planned and consistent formal education was the priority in Nightingale's schools, the training of US nurses was like an unsubsidized apprenticeship. Eventually, the curricula and content of US training schools became more organized and uniform. Training periods lengthened from 6 months to 3 full years. Graduate nurses received a diploma attesting to their successful completion of training.

Expanding Horizons of Practice

Diplomas in hand, US nurses began the 20th century by distinguishing themselves in caring for the sick and disadvantaged outside of hospitals (Fig. 1-2). Some nurses moved into communities and established "settlement houses" where they lived and worked among poor immigrants. Others provided midwifery services, especially in rural Appalachia. The success of their public health efforts in administering prenatal and obstetric care, teaching child care, and immunizing children is well documented.

Like previous counterparts, nurses continued to volunteer during wars. They offered their services to fight yellow fever, typhoid, malaria, and dysentery during the Spanish-American War. They replenished the nursing staff in military hospitals during World Wars I and II (Fig. 1-3). They worked alongside physicians in Mobile Army Surgical Hospitals (MASH) during the Korean War, acquiring knowledge about trauma care that later would help reduce the mortality

TABLE 1-1 Differences in Nightingale Schools and US Training Schools

NIGHTINGALE SCHOOLS	US TRAINING SCHOOLS
• Training schools were affiliated with a few select hospitals. • Training hospitals relied on employees to provide client care. • Education costs were borne by students or endowed from the Nightingale Trust Fund. • Training of nurses provided no financial advantages to the hospital. • Class schedules were planned separately from practical experiences. • Curricular content was uniform. • A previously trained nurse provided formal instruction, focusing on nursing care. • The number of clinical hours during training was restricted. • At the end of training, graduates became paid employees or were hired to train others.	• Any hospital, rural or urban, could establish a training school. • Students staffed the hospital. • Students worked without pay in return for training, which usually consisted of chores. • Hospitals profited by eliminating the need to pay employees. • No formal classes were held; training was an outcome of work. • Curricular content was unplanned and varied according to current cases. • Instruction was usually informal, at the bedside, and from a physician's perspective. • Students were expected to work 12 hours a day and to live in or adjacent to the hospital in case they were needed unexpectedly. • At the end of training, students were discharged and new students took their places. Most graduates sought private-duty positions.

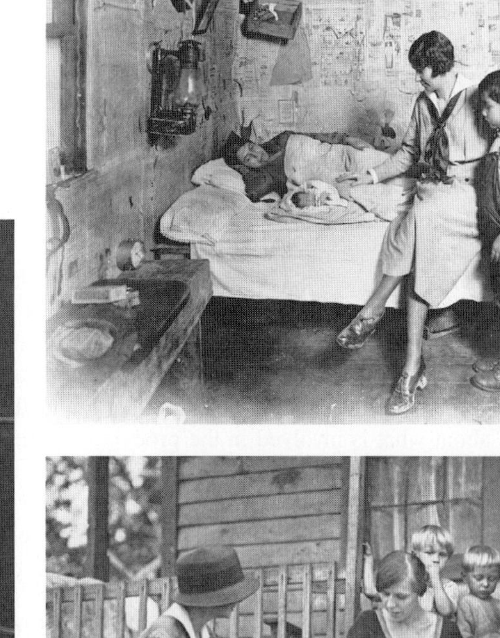

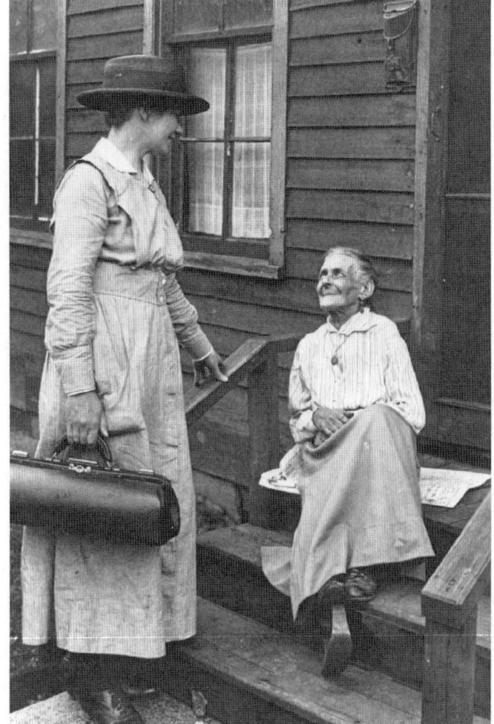

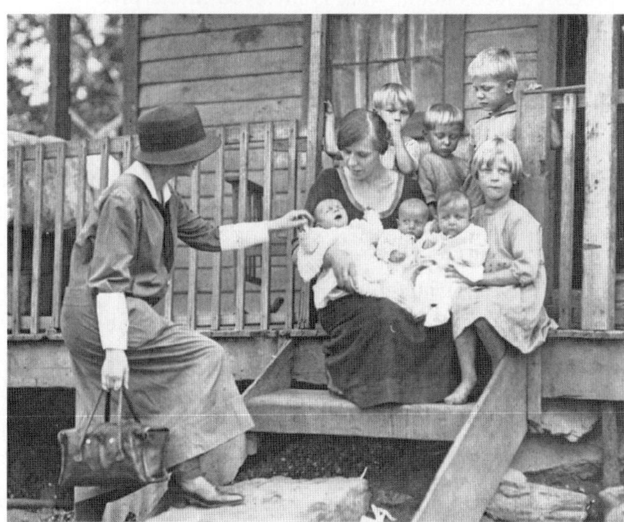

FIGURE 1-2 Community health nurses circa late 1800s to early 1900s. (Courtesy of Visiting Nurse Association, Inc., Detroit, MI.)

rate of US soldiers in Vietnam. More recently, nurses again answered the call during the conflicts in Iraq and Afghanistan. Whenever and wherever there has been a need, nurses have put their own lives on the line.

CONTEMPORARY NURSING

Combining Nursing Art With Science

At first, the training of nurses consisted of learning the **art** (ability to perform an act skillfully) of nursing. Students learned this art by watching and imitating the techniques performed by other, more experienced nurses. In this way, mentors informally passed skills on to students.

Contemporary nursing practice has added another dimension: science. The English word "science" comes from the Latin word *scio*, which means, "to know." A **science** (body of knowledge unique to a particular subject) develops from observing and studying the relationship of one phenomenon to another. By developing an accumulating body

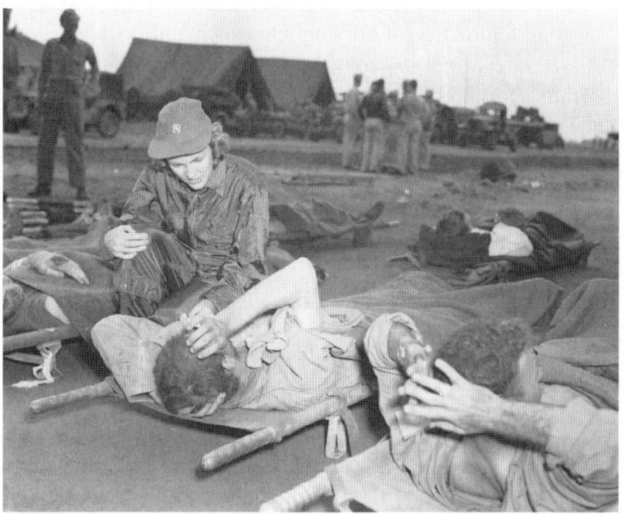

FIGURE 1-3 A military nurse comforts a soldier during World War II. (Courtesy of the National Archives, Washington, DC.)

of unique scientific knowledge, it is now possible to predict which nursing interventions are most likely to produce desired outcomes, a process referred to as **evidence-based practice**.

Integrating Nursing Theory

The word **theory** (opinion, belief, or view) comes from a Greek word that means vision. For example, a scientist may study the relation between sunlight and plants and derive a theory of photosynthesis that explains how plants grow. Others who believe in the theorist's view may then apply the theory for their own practical use.

Nursing has undergone a similar scientific review. Florence Nightingale and others have examined the relationships among humans, health, the environment, and nursing. The outcome of such analysis becomes the basis for **nursing theory** (proposed ideas about what is involved in the process called nursing). Nursing programs then adopt a theory to serve as the conceptual framework or model for their philosophy, curriculum, and most importantly, approach to clients. Similarly, psychologists have adopted and used Freud's psychoanalytic theory or Skinner's behavioral theory, for example, as a model for diagnostic and therapeutic interventions with clients.

Table 1-2 summarizes some nursing theories and how each has been applied to nursing practice. These are only a few of many; additional information can be found in current nursing literature and academic courses in nursing theory.

Defining Nursing

To clarify for the public, and nurses themselves, what nursing encompasses, various working definitions have been proposed. Nightingale is credited with the earliest modern definition: "putting individuals in the best possible condition for nature to restore and preserve health."

Other definitions have been offered by nurses who are recognized as authorities, and therefore qualified spokespersons, on the practice of nursing. One such authority was Virginia Henderson (1897 to 1996). Her definition, adopted by the International Council of Nurses, broadened the description of nursing to include health promotion, not just illness care. As stated in 1966:

> The unique function of the nurse is to assist the individual, sick or well, in the performance of those activities contributing to health or its recovery (or to a peaceful death) that he could perform unaided if he had the necessary strength, will or knowledge. And to do this in such a way as to help him gain independence as rapidly as possible.

Henderson proposed that nursing is more than carrying out medical orders. It involves a special relationship and service between the nurse and the client (and his or her family). According to Henderson, the nurse acts as a temporary proxy, meeting the client's health needs with knowledge and skills that neither the client nor family members can provide.

In *Nursing's Social Policy Statement,* 3rd edition (2010), the American Nurses Association (ANA) defines nursing as follows:

- Protection, promotion, and optimization of health and abilities
- Prevention of illness and injury
- Alleviation of suffering through the diagnosis and treatment of human response
- Advocacy in the care of individuals, families, communities, and populations

The ANA (2010) further attests that six essential features characterize nursing: (1) provision of a caring relationship that facilitates health and healing, (2) attention to the range of human experiences and responses to health and illness within the physical and social environments, (3) integration of objective data with knowledge gained from an appreciation of the client's or group's subjective experience, (4) application of scientific knowledge to the processes of diagnosis and treatment through the use of judgment and critical thinking, (5) advancement of professional nursing knowledge through scholarly inquiry, and (6) influence on social and public policy to promote social justice.

Based on statements from the ANA, clearly nursing has an independent area of practice in addition to traditional dependent and interdependent functions involving physicians. As the role of the nurse evolves, the definition of nursing and the scope of nursing practice will undergo further revisions.

THE EDUCATIONAL LADDER

Two basic educational options are available to those interested in a nursing career: practical (vocational) nursing and registered nursing. Several types of programs prepare graduates in registered nursing. Each educational track provides the knowledge and skills for a particular entry level of practice. The following factors influence the choice of a nursing program:

- Career goals
- Geographic location of schools
- Costs involved
- Length of programs
- Reputation and success of graduates
- Flexibility in course scheduling
- Opportunity for part-time versus full-time enrollment
- Ease of movement into the next level of education

Practical/Vocational Nursing

During World War II, many registered nurses enlisted in the military. As a result, civilian hospitals, clinics, schools, and other health care agencies faced an acute shortage of trained nurses. To fill the void expeditiously, abbreviated programs

TABLE 1-2 Nursing Theories and Applications

THEORIST	THEORY	EXPLANATION
Florence Nightingale 1820–1910	**Environmental Theory**	
	Man	An individual whose natural defenses are influenced by a healthy or unhealthy environment
	Health	A state in which the environment is optimal for the natural body processes to achieve reparative outcomes
	Environment	All the external conditions capable of preventing, suppressing, or contributing to disease or death
	Nursing	Putting the client in the best condition for nature to act
	Synopsis of theory	External conditions such as ventilation, light, odor, and cleanliness can prevent, suppress, or contribute to disease or death
	Application to nursing practice	Nurses modify unhealthy aspects of the environment to put the client in the best condition for nature to act
Virginia Henderson 1897–1996	**Basic Needs Theory**	
	Man	An individual with human needs that have unique meaning and value
	Health	The ability to independently satisfy human needs composed of 14 basic physical, psychological, and social elements
	Environment	The setting in which a person learns unique patterns for living
	Nursing	Temporarily assisting a person who lacks the necessary strength, will, and knowledge to satisfy one or more of 14 basic needs
	Synopsis of theory	People have basic needs that are components of health. The significance and value of these needs are unique to each person
	Application to nursing practice	Nurses assist in performing those activities that the client would perform if he or she had the strength, will, and knowledge
Dorothea Orem 1914–2007	**Self-Care Theory**	
	Man	An individual who uses self-care to sustain life and health, to recover from disease or injury, or to cope with its effects
	Health	The result of practices that people have learned to carry out on their own behalf to maintain life and well-being
	Environment	External elements with which people interact in the struggle to maintain self-care
	Nursing	A human service that assists people to progressively maximize their self-care potential
	Synopsis of theory	People learn behaviors that they perform on their own behalf to maintain life, health, and well-being
	Application to nursing practice	Nurses assist clients with self-care to improve or to maintain health
Sister Callista Roy 1939–	**Adaptation Theory**	
	Man	A social, mental, spiritual, and physical being affected by stimuli in the internal and external environments
	Health	A person's ability to adapt to changes in the environment
	Environment	Internal and external forces in a continuous state of change
	Nursing	A humanitarian art and expanding science that manipulates and modifies stimuli to promote and to facilitate humans' ability to adapt
	Synopsis of theory	Humans are biopsychosocial beings; a change in one component results in adaptive changes in the others
	Application to nursing practice	Nurses assess biologic, psychological, and social factors interfering with health; alter the stimuli causing the maladaptation; and evaluate the effectiveness of the action taken

in practical nursing were developed across the country to teach essential nursing skills. The goal was to prepare graduates to care for the health needs of infants, children, and adults who were mildly or chronically ill or convalescing so that registered nurses who remained stateside could be used effectively to care for acutely ill clients.

After the war, many registered nurses opted for part-time employment or resigned to become full-time housewives. Thus, the need for practical nurses persisted. It became obvious that the role of practical nurses would not be temporary. Consequently, leaders in practical nursing programs organized to form the National Association for Practical Nurse Education and Service, Inc. This group worked to standardize practical nurse education and to facilitate the licensure of graduates. By 1945, eight states had approved practical nurse programs (Mitchell & Grippando, 1993); the current number has grown to 1,500 state-approved schools (Bureau of Labor Statistics, 2007). Career centers, vocational schools, hospitals, independent agencies, and community colleges generally offer practical nursing programs and arrange clinical experiences at local community hospitals, clinics, and nursing homes. The length of a practical

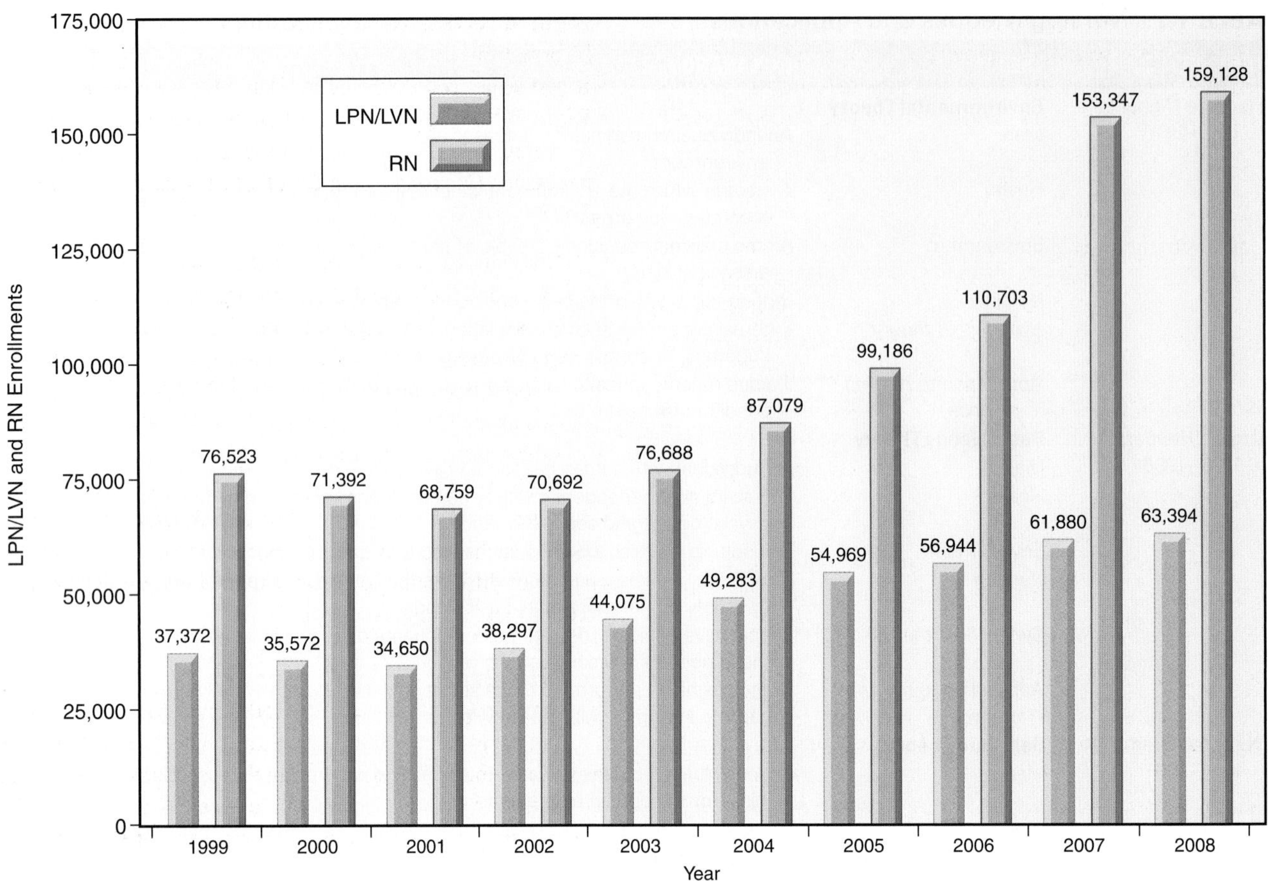

FIGURE 1-4 Trends in licensed practical nurses/licensed vocational nurses (LPN/LVN) and registered nurses (RN) enrollments, 1999 to 2008. Numbers are based on US candidates taking the National Council Licensure Examination (NCLEX) for the first time in respective years, as reported by the National Council of State Boards of Nursing.

nursing program averages from 12 to 18 months, after which graduates are qualified to take their licensing examination. Because this nursing preparatory program is the shortest, many consider it the most economical.

After a low ebb in 2001, enrollments in practical and vocational schools continued to rise yearly (Fig. 1-4). In 2008, a total of 63,394 US educated candidates passed the National Council Licensure Examination-Practical Nurse (NCLEX-PN) on their first attempt (National Council of State Boards of Nursing, 2009). Job security for licensed practical nurses (LPNs) is supported by the Bureau of Labor Statistics' prediction (2007) that job opportunities in practical nursing will increase to a projected 854,000 by 2016, an increase of 14%. However, hospitals will not be the primary employers. Licensed practical nurses will most likely secure positions in nursing homes, physicians' offices, home health agencies, outpatient centers, residential care facilities, correctional institutions, and government agencies (Larson, 2008).

Licensed practical nurses are a vital link between the registered nurse and the unlicensed assistive personnel (UAP). They work under the supervision of a registered nurse, physician, or dentist, but their role may be expanded to include supervision of UAPs in circumstances like long-term care (National Council of State Boards of Nursing, 2005). LPNs or licensed vocational nurses (LVNs) provide nursing care to clients with common health needs that have a predictable outcome. Their scope of practice is described in the nurse practice act in the state in which the nurse is licensed. Each state interprets the limits of practice differently. For example, in one state, an LPN may monitor and hang intravenous solutions, discontinue the infusion, and dress the site. The same may not be true in another state. An LPN also may delegate tasks to UAPs, who may or may not have acquired state certification. The LPN, therefore, must know the extent to which nursing assistants can function and the outcomes of their actions (see guidelines for delegation under "Registered Nursing"). Because of the geographic disparities in LPN practice, educational programs, and state regulations, the National Council of State Boards of Nursing is researching and pursuing strategies to promote more consistency (Practical Nurse Scope of Practice White Paper, 2005). Additional information on nursing practice standards for the licensed practical/vocational nurse can be obtained from the National Federation of Licensed Practical Nurses Web site.

Opportunities for post-licensure certifications in pharmacology and long-term care are available through the National Association for Practical Nurse Education and Services, Inc. Achieving certification via testing demonstrates knowledge above minimum standards. To provide career mobility, many schools of practical nursing have developed "articulation agreements" to help graduates enroll in another school that offers a path to registered nursing through associate or baccalaureate degrees.

Registered Nursing

Registered nurses (RNs) work under the direction of a physician or dentist in various health care settings ranging from preventive to acute care. They manage or provide direct care to clients who are stable but may have complex health needs, or who are unstable with unpredictable outcomes. In addition to managing client care, RNs educate clients and the public about various medical conditions and provide emotional support to clients and their family members (Bureau of Labor Statistics, 2007). RNs delegate client care to LPNs and UAPs when appropriate.

Regardless of whether it is an RN delegating to an LPN or a UAP or an LPN delegating to an UAP, delegation requires adhering to the following six guidelines:

- **Right task:** matching the client's needs with the caregiver's skills
- **Right circumstance:** ensuring that the situation is appropriate
- **Right person:** knowing the unique competencies of the caregiver
- **Right direction (communication):** providing sufficient information
- **Right supervision:** being available for assistance
- **Right follow-up:** validating that the task was completed, obtaining the results, and analyzing if further actions are necessary (National Council of State Boards of Nursing, 2005)

Students can choose one of the three paths to become an RN: a hospital-based diploma program, a program that awards an associate degree in nursing, or a baccalaureate nursing program. All three meet the requirements for taking the national licensing examination (NCLEX-RN). A person licensed as an RN may work directly at the bedside or supervise others in managing the care of groups of clients.

Table 1-3 describes how educational programs prepare graduates to assume separate but coordinated responsibilities. When hiring new graduates, however, many employers do not differentiate between these educational programs, arguing that "a nurse is a nurse."

Hospital-Based Diploma Programs

Diploma programs were the traditional route for nurses through the middle of the 20th century. Their decline became obvious in the 1970s, and the number of diploma programs continues to be lowest in relation to other basic nursing educational programs (Fig. 1-5). The reasons for their decline

TABLE 1-3 Levels of Responsibilities for the Nursing Process[a]

	PRACTICAL/VOCATIONAL NURSE	ASSOCIATE DEGREE NURSE	BACCALAUREATE NURSE
Assessing	Gathers data by interviewing, observing, and performing a basic physical examination of people with common health problems with predictable outcomes	Collects data from people with complex health problems with unpredictable outcomes, their family, medical records, and other health team members	Identifies the information needed from individuals or groups to provide an appropriate nursing database
Diagnosing	Contributes to the development of nursing diagnoses by reporting abnormal assessment data	Uses a classification list to write a nursing diagnostic statement, including the problem, its etiology, and signs and symptoms Identifies problems that require collaboration with the physician	Conducts clinical testing of approved nursing diagnoses Proposes new diagnostic categories for consideration and approval
Planning	Assists in setting realistic and measurable goals Suggests nursing actions that can prevent, reduce, or eliminate health problems with predictable outcomes Assists in developing a written plan of care	Sets realistic, measurable goals Develops a written individualized plan of care with specific nursing orders that reflects the standards for nursing practice	Develops written standards for nursing practice Plans care for healthy or sick individuals or groups in structured health care agencies or the community
Implementing	Performs basic nursing care under the direction of a registered nurse	Identifies priorities Directs others to carry out nursing orders	Applies nursing theory to the approaches used for resolving actual and potential health problems of individuals or groups
Evaluating	Shares observations on the progress of the client in reaching established goals Contributes to the revision of the plan of care	Evaluates the outcomes of nursing care routinely Revises the plan of care	Conducts research on nursing activities that may be improved with further study

[a]Note that each more advanced practitioner can perform the responsibilities of those identified previously.

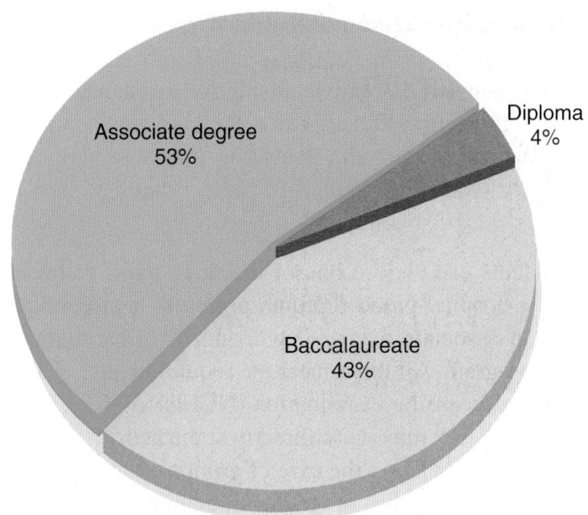

FIGURE 1-5 Enrollments in basic RN programs by program type, 2008. (From National League for Nursing [2010]. Nursing Data Review Academic Year 2007 to 2008: Baccalaureate, Associate Degree, and Diploma Programs. Retrieved from http://www.nln.org/research/slides/ndr_0708.pdf.)

are twofold. First, there has been a movement to increase professionalism in nursing by encouraging education in colleges and universities. Second, hospitals can no longer financially subsidize schools of nursing.

Diploma nurses were, and are, well trained. Because of their vast clinical experience (compared with students from other types of programs), they are often characterized as more self-confident and more easily socialized into the role requirements of a graduate nurse.

A hospital-based diploma program generally lasts 3 years. Many hospital schools of nursing collaborate with nearby colleges to provide basic science and humanities courses; graduates can transfer these credits if they choose to pursue associate or baccalaureate degrees later.

Associate Degree Programs

During World War II, when qualified nurses were being used for the military effort, hospital-based schools accelerated the education of some RN students through the Cadet Nurse Corps. After the end of the war, Mildred Montag, a doctoral nursing student at the time, began to question whether it was necessary for students in RN programs to spend 3 years acquiring a basic education. She believed that nursing education could be shortened to 2 years and relocated to vocational schools or junior or community colleges. The graduate from this type of program would acquire an associate degree in nursing, would be referred to as a technical nurse, and would not be expected to work in a management position.

This type of nursing preparation has proved extremely popular and now commands the highest enrollment among all RN programs. Despite the condensed curriculum, graduates of associate degree programs have demonstrated a high level of competence in passing the NCLEX-RN.

Baccalaureate Programs

Although collegiate nursing programs were established at the beginning of the 20th century, until recently they did not attract many students. Their popularity has been increasing at a progressive rate, perhaps because of proposals by the ANA and the National League for Nursing to establish baccalaureate education as the entry level into nursing practice. The deadline for implementation of this goal, once set for 1985, has been postponed for three reasons:

- The date coincided with a national shortage of nurses.
- There was tremendous opposition from nurses without degrees, who believed that their titles and positions would be jeopardized.
- Employers feared that paying higher salaries to personnel with degrees would escalate budgets beyond their financial limits.

Consequently, the adoption of a unified entry level into practice remains in limbo.

Although this preparatory program is the longest and most expensive, baccalaureate-prepared nurses have the greatest flexibility in qualifying for nursing positions, both staff and managerial. Nurses with a baccalaureate degree usually are preferred in areas requiring substantial independent decision making, such as public health and home health nursing.

Currently, many nurses are returning to school to earn baccalaureate degrees. Articulation has been difficult for some because of problems transferring credits for courses they took during their diploma or associate degree programs. To increase enrollment, some collegiate programs are offering nurses an opportunity to obtain credit by passing "challenge examinations." In addition, many colleges and universities provide satellite or outreach programs to accommodate nurses who cannot go to school full-time or travel long distances. Despite a renewed interest in acquiring a nursing education, approximately 99,000 (26%) qualified applicants for admission were rejected in 2007 to 2008 (National League for Nursing, 2008; Fig. 1-6). Qualified applicants are being rejected or waitlisted because (1) very few nursing faculty are available to teach required courses, (2) there is a lack of clinical placements, (3) there is a lack of space, and (4) there is intense competition for selective admissions.

Graduate Nursing Programs

Graduate nursing programs are available at both the master's and the doctoral levels. Master's-prepared nurses fill roles as clinical specialists, nurse practitioners, administrators, and educators. Unfortunately, too few are pursuing advanced degrees in sufficient numbers to fill the positions vacated by retiring faculty, 75% of whom will be eligible to retire by 2019 (Health Resources and Services Administration, 2005). Nurses with doctoral degrees conduct research and advise, administer, and instruct nurses pursuing undergraduate and graduate degrees. Although a graduate degree in nursing is preferred, some nurses pursue advanced education in fields outside of nursing, such as business, leadership, and education, to enhance their nursing career.

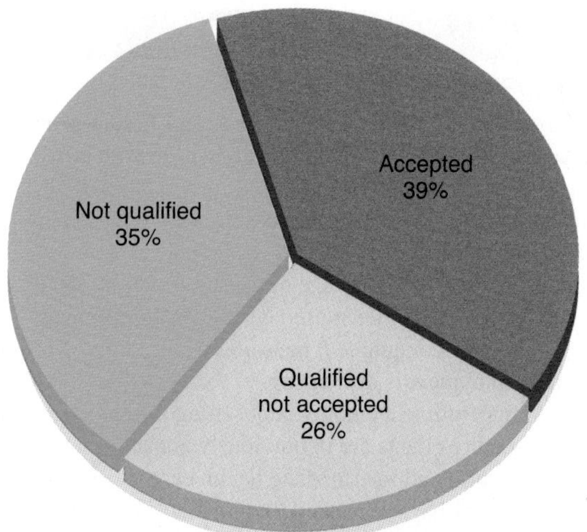

FIGURE 1-6 Disposition of applications to basic RN programs by program type, 2007 to 2008. (From National League for Nursing [2010]. Nursing Data Review Academic Year 2007 to 2008: Baccalaureate, Associate Degree, and Diploma Programs. Retrieved from http://www.nln.org/research/slides/ndr_0708.pdf.)

Continuing Education

Continuing education in nursing is any planned learning experience beyond the basic nursing program. Nightingale is credited with having said, "to stand still is to move backwards." The principle that learning is a lifelong process still applies. Box 1-2 lists reasons why nurses, in particular, pursue continuing education. Many states now require nurses to show proof of continuing education to renew their nursing license.

FUTURE TRENDS

Two major issues dominate nursing today. The first concerns methods of eliminating the shortage of nurses. The second involves strategies for responding to a growing aging population with chronic health problems.

BOX 1-2 Rationales for Acquiring Continuing Education

- No basic program provides all the knowledge and skills needed for a lifetime career.
- Current advances in technology make previous methods of practice obsolete.
- Assuming responsibility for self-learning demonstrates personal accountability.
- To ensure the public's confidence, nurses must demonstrate evidence of current competence.
- Practicing according to current nursing standards helps to ensure that care is legally safe.
- Renewal of state licensure often is contingent on evidence of continuing education.

Health care officials hope that enrollment in all nursing programs and continuing education will reduce the current and projected critical shortage of nurses. However, the future looks alarming. The nursing shortage is projected to reach a deficit of one million nurses by 2020 (Health Resources and Services Administration, 2005). Besides a retirement rate of nurses that exceeds their replacement and the attrition of aging faculty, which restricts the numbers of student applicants, some factors contributing to the nursing shortage include the following:

- Increased aging population requiring health care
- Disappointing salaries for nurses with longevity employment
- Job dissatisfaction as a result of stress and the unrelenting rigor of working in health care
- Heavier workloads and sicker clients
- Publicity about mandatory overtime
- Downsizing nursing staff from dwindling revenues and managed care policies
- Negative stereotypes for traditionally female occupations like nursing

Governmental Responses

The federal government has addressed the shortage of nurses by approving the American Recovery and Reinvestment Act in 2009. This legislation authorizes the following:

1. Loan repayment programs and scholarships for nursing students
2. Funding for public service announcements to encourage more people to enter nursing
3. Career ladder programs to facilitate advancement to higher levels of nursing practice
4. Establishment of nurse retention and client safety enhancement grants
5. Grants to incorporate gerontology into nursing curricula
6. Loan repayment programs for nursing students who agree to teach after graduation (American Association of Colleges of Nursing, 2009)

Proactive Strategies

Rather than taking a "wait-and-see" position about the nursing shortage and the ramifications of the Nurse Reinvestment Act, many nurses are proactively responding to the trends affecting their role in health care (Box 1-3). Nurses are dealing with the unique challenges of the 21st century by:

- Switching from part-time to full-time positions.
- Delaying retirement.
- Pursuing post-licensure education.
- Training for **advanced practice** roles (nurse practitioner, nurse midwifery) to provide cost-effective health care in areas in which numbers of primary care physicians are inadequate.

BOX 1-3 Trends in Health Care and Nursing

Health Care

- The most underserved health care populations include older adults, ethnic minorities, and the poor, who delay seeking early treatment because they cannot afford it.
- The number of uninsured rose from 37 million in 1995 to 41.2 million in 2002. This figure now exceeds 50 million in 2009.
- Medicare and Medicaid benefits are being modified and reduced.
- Chronic illness is the major health problem.
- Disease and injury prevention and health promotion are priorities.
- Medicine tends to focus on high technology, which improves outcomes for a select few.
- Hospitals are downsizing and hiring unlicensed personnel to perform procedures once in the exclusive domain of licensed nurses for cost containment.
- There are fewer primary care physicians in rural areas.
- Changes in reimbursement practices have created a shift in decision making from hospitals, nurses, and physicians to insurance companies.
- Health care costs continue to increase despite **managed care practices** (cost-containment strategies used to plan and coordinate a client's care to avoid delays, unnecessary services, or overuse of expensive resources).
- **Capitation** (strategy for controlling health care costs by paying a fixed amount per member) encourages health providers to limit tests and services to increase profits.
- Hospitals, practitioners, and health insurance companies are being required to measure, monitor, and manage quality of care.

Nursing

- Enrollments and numbers of graduates from LPN/LVN and RN educational programs are not keeping pace with projected shortages.
- More licensed nurses are earning master's and doctoral degrees.
- There continues to be a shortage of nurses in various health care settings because of decreased enrollments, retirement, attrition, and cost-containment measures.
- Hospital employment is decreasing.
- Client-to-nurse ratios in employment settings are higher.
- More high-acuity clients are in previously nonacute settings such as long-term and intermediate health care facilities.
- Job opportunities have expanded to outpatient services, home health care, hospice programs, and community health, and mental health agencies.

- Becoming **cross-trained** (able to assume non-nursing jobs, depending on the census or levels of client acuity on any given day). For example, nurses may be trained to provide respiratory treatments and to obtain electrocardiograms, duties that non-nursing health care workers previously performed.
- Learning more about **multicultural diversity** (unique characteristics of ethnic groups) as it affects health beliefs and values, food preferences, language, communication, roles, and relationships.
- Supporting legislative efforts toward national health insurance and other health care reforms that involve nurses in **primary care** (the first health care worker to assess a person with a health need).
- Promoting wellness through home health and community-based programs.
- Helping clients with chronic diseases learn techniques for living healthier and, consequently, longer lives.
- Referring clients with health problems for early treatment, a practice that requires the fewest resources and thus minimizes expenses.
- Coordinating nursing services across health care settings—that is, **discharge planning** (managing transitional needs and ensuring continuity).
- Providing older adults can receive a variety of nursing services such as physical assessment during periods of illness, teaching, and managing medications, in assisted-living facilities at less cost than care in nursing homes.
- Developing and implementing **clinical pathways**, standardized multidisciplinary plans for a specific diagnosis or procedure that identify aspects of care to be performed during a designated length of stay (Fig. 1-7).
- Participating in **quality assurance** (process of identifying and evaluating outcomes).
- Concentrating on the knowledge and skills to manage the health needs of older Americans, whose numbers will reach 70 million by 2030 (National Center for Chronic Disease Prevention and Health Promotion, 2005).

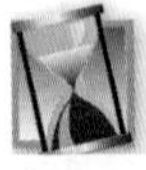

Gerontologic Considerations

■ Currently, 30% or more older adults in nursing homes return to community settings, necessitating an increase in the need for home care services (Miller, 2009).

DRG 209: (81.51) **RECOVERY PATHWAY TOTAL HIP** ADDRESSOGRAPH

Exp. LOS: 6 days

M.D.: ____________

(Recovery Pathways do not represent a standard of care. They are guidelines for consideration which may be modified according to the individual patient's need.)

	DATE: Pre-Admit	DAY OF WK:	DAY OF WK:	DAY OF WK:	DAY OF WK:	DAY OF WK:	DAY OF WK:
		DATE:	DATE:	DATE:	DATE:	DATE:	DATE:
		DAY 1 (OR Day)	DAY 2- 1st PostOp	DAY 3- 2nd PostOp	DAY 4- 3rd PostOp	DAY 5- 4th PostOp	DAY 6- 5th PostOp
Diagnostic Studies	Auto Blood Y N Pre-op Lab, EKG, CXR	X-ray Joint PACU Y N	CBC Y N PT/PTT (INR) Y N	CBC Y N ________	________	________	________
Treatments		- Waffle - Foley - TED Hose - in OR Y N - SCD in OR Y N - Drain Y N - IS	- TED Hose Y N - SCD Y N - Drain Y N - IS - Foley (consider D/C) Y N	——→ - SCD Y N - IS (pt doing own) Y N - Drain D/C Y N - Foley D/C 0700 Y N	——→ - SCD Y N - IS - Consider IV out Y N	——→	——→
Therapy PT (one time/day unless specified)	Pre-Op teaching Y N OT safety checklist	Total Hip protocol WB per M.D. (PT & OT) (Evaluation & Treatment) Y N	- Gait training 10-20' ______ Y N - Total Hip precautions given Y N - OT - Precaution instruction Y N	- Gait training 20-25' as tol. ____ Y N - THR exercise x 10 rep with min Asst Y N - Understand total hip precautions Y N - Supine→sit w/__asst Y N - Sit→stand w/__asst Y N - OT: Pt participation as tol with LE dressing/bathing with equipment Y N	- Gait training 25-40' as tol ____ Y N - Transfer sit ⇆ stand minimal asst Y N - Exercise 10-15 reps Y N - Begin ↕ stairs Y N - OT: Transfer training - tub/ toilet/auto Y N	- Gait training 40-50' as tol ____ Y N - Transfer sit ⇆ stand Y N - in ⇆ OOB independently Y N - Exercise 15-20 reps Y N - ↕ stairs Y N - OT: Refining/ reviewing prior instruction with home safety, task simplification Y N	- Gait training 50-60' as tol____ Y N - ↕steps independently YN - Independent with 15-20 reps of exercise Y N - Discharge Instructions
Multi-disciplinary Consults	SW Screen Medical Evaluation	Other MD consults			Consider Home Health Assessment Y N		
Medications	Physician preference	Antibiotics Analgesics	Antibiotics Analgesics	Antibiotics D/C Y N Analgesics (push po) Y N	Analgesics (po) Y N	Analgesics (po) Y N	Rx Written Analgesics
Nutrition	NPO after midnight	Clear liquids → DAT	Clear liquids → DAT	DAT GI function Y N	DAT	DAT	DAT

FIGURE 1-7 Example of recovery pathway in managed care. (Courtesy of Elkhart General Hospital, Elkhart, IN.)

(continues)

	DATE: Pre-Admit	DAY OF WK: DATE: DAY 1 (OR Day)	DAY OF WK: DATE: DAY 2- 1st PostOp	DAY OF WK: DATE: DAY 3- 2nd PostOp	DAY OF WK: DATE: DAY 4- 3rd PostOp	DAY OF WK: DATE: DAY 5- 4th PostOp	DAY OF WK: DATE: DAY 6- 5th PostOp
Activity	Pre-Op Teaching	- BR w/position ▵ q2° - Maintain Abduction Y N - Dorsiplantar Flex q2° Y N - DB Y N - If early a.m. surgery - ↑ chair Y N	- Chair Y N - Dorsiplantar Flex q4° Y N - DB Y N	- Chair/Up in room, Hall as tol Y N - Dorsiplantar Flex q4° Y N - DB Y N	- Chair/up in room/hall Y N - Dorsiplantar Flex q4° Y N - DB Y N	- Chair/Up in room/Hall Independent Y N - Dorsiplantar Flex q4° Y N - DB Y N	- Chair/Up in room/Hall Independent Y N - Dorsiplantar flex q4° Y N - DB Y N
Teaching	- Video Education - Pain Mgmt - Lt supper/ suppository	- Reinforce pre-op education Y N - Hip Precautions Y N - Pain Scale (0-10) Y N	Continue to reinforce	Continue to reinforce: - Ted Hose Y N - Gait training/transfers Y N - Hip Precautions Y N	Continue to reinforce	- Coumadin (if going home on) Y N - Continue to reinforce	Discharge Instructions Follow-up appointments
Discharge Planning	Patient to bring pre-op instuctions with them	SS- meet with family - Develop initial plan Y N	SS - Monitor progress	- Assess rehab potential vs. ECF Y N	- Assess rehab potential vs. ECF Y N - Identify equipment needs (for home) Y N - Clarify plan with patient/ family Y N	- Assess rehab potential vs. ECF Y N - Order Equipment Y N - Clarify plan with patient/ family Y N - Coordinate discharge home (home health/ equipment needs) Y N	DC to home or ECF Home Health liaison to finalize HH involvement Y N
Expected Patient Outcomes	Patient states his responsibility/role in recovery Y N	Patient understands treatment rationale Y N	- Patient actively participates in care Y N - Verbalizes understanding of care Y N	- Verbalize hip precautions Y N	Verbalizes/ Demonstrates: - hip precautions Y N - discharge plans Y N - Discharge to Rehab Y N	- Patient/family demonstrates independence w/ADLs Y N Discharge to - ECF Y N - rehab Y N - Home Y N	Patient/family understands discharge instructions and is confident in ability to care for self. Y N - Discharge to home Y N

Signatures: ______

MR-　　　Page 2　　　Rev. 3/1/94

FIGURE 1-7 *(Continued).*

In addition to strategies that are being pursued by nurses themselves, there are suggestions for workplace reforms that are believed to attract and promote the retention of more nurses. Some of these include: (1) developing nontraditional and flexible work schedules, (2) offering on-site child care facilities, (3) supporting refresher courses for inactive nurses, (4) abandoning mandatory overtime policies, (5) eliminating understaffing, and (6) improving the salary scale (Oncology Nursing Society, 2007).

UNIQUE NURSING SKILLS

Although employment locations and how they carry out **nursing skills** (activities unique to the practice of nursing) differ according to educational preparation, all nurses share the same philosophy. In keeping with Nightingale's traditions, contemporary nursing practice continues to include assessment skills, caring skills, counseling skills, and comforting skills.

Assessment Skills

Before the nurse can determine what care a person requires, he or she must determine the client's needs and problems. This requires the use of **assessment skills** (acts that involve collecting data), which include interviewing, observing, and examining the client, and in some cases, the client's family (*family* is used loosely to refer to the people with whom the client lives and associates). Although the client and the family are the primary sources of information, the nurse also reviews the client's medical record and talks with other health care workers to obtain facts. Assessment skills are discussed in more detail in Unit 4.

Caring Skills

Caring skills (nursing interventions that restore or maintain a person's health) may involve actions as simple as assisting with **activities of daily living** (ADLs), the acts that people normally do every day, for example, bathing, grooming, dressing, toileting, and eating. Increasingly, however, the nurse's role is expanding to include the safe care of clients who require invasive or highly technical equipment. This textbook introduces beginning nurses to the concepts and skills needed to provide care for clients whose disorders have fairly predictable outcomes. After this foundation has been established, students may add to their initial knowledge base.

Traditionally, nurses always have been providers of physical care for people unable to meet their own health needs independently. But caring also involves the concern and attachment that result from the close relationship of one human being with another. Nevertheless, the nurse ultimately wants clients to become self-reliant. The nurse who assumes too much care for clients, like a parent who continues to tie a child's shoes, often delays their independence.

Counseling Skills

A counselor is one who listens to a client's needs, responds with information based on his or her area of expertise, and facilitates the outcome that a client desires. Nurses implement **counseling skills** (interventions that include communicating with clients, actively listening during exchanges of information, offering pertinent health teaching, and providing emotional support) in relationships with clients.

To understand the client's perspective, the nurse uses therapeutic communication techniques to encourage verbal expression (see Chap. 7). The use of **active listening** (demonstrating full attention to what is being said, hearing both the content being communicated and the unspoken message) facilitates therapeutic interactions. Giving clients the opportunity to be heard helps them organize their thoughts and to evaluate their situation more realistically.

When the client's perspective is clear, the nurse provides pertinent health information without offering specific advice. By reserving personal opinions, nurses promote the right of every person to make his or her own decisions and choices on matters affecting health and illness care. The role of the nurse is to share information about potential alternatives, to allow clients the freedom to choose, and to support the final decision.

While giving care, the nurse finds many opportunities to teach clients how to promote healing processes, stay well, prevent illness, and carry out ADLs in the best possible way. People know much more about health and health care today, and they expect nurses to share accurate information with them.

Because clients do not always communicate their feelings to strangers, nurses use **empathy** (intuitive awareness of what the client is experiencing) to perceive the client's emotional state and need for support. This skill differs from **sympathy** (feeling as emotionally distraught as the client). Empathy helps the nurse become effective at providing for the client's needs while remaining compassionately detached.

Comforting Skills

Nightingale's presence and the light from her lamp communicated comfort to the frightened British soldiers in the 19th century. As a result of that heritage, contemporary nurses understand that illness often causes feelings of insecurity that may threaten the client's or family's ability to cope; they may feel very vulnerable. At this point, the nurse uses **comforting skills** (interventions that provide stability and security during a health-related crisis) (Fig. 1-8). The nurse becomes the client's guide, companion, and interpreter. This supportive relationship generally increases trust and reduces fear and worry.

As a result of one woman's efforts, modern nursing was born. It has continued to mature and flourish ever since. The skills that Nightingale performed on a very grand scale are repeated today during each and every nurse–client relationship.

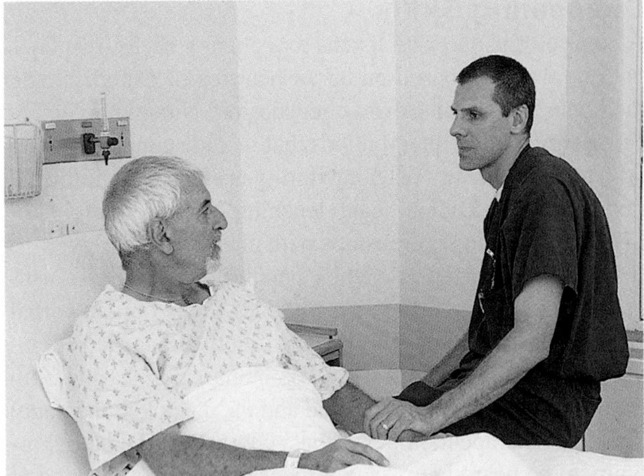

FIGURE 1-8 This nurse offers comfort and emotional support. (Photo by B. Proud.)

Stop, Think, and Respond Box 1-2

Identify which of the following nursing actions is an assessment skill, a caring skill, a counseling skill, and a comforting skill: (a) the nurse discusses with a family the progress of a client undergoing surgery; (b) the nurse provides information on advanced directives, which allows a client to identify his or her end-of-life decisions; (c) the nurse asks a client to identify his or her current health problems; (d) the nurse provides medication for a client in pain.

CRITICAL THINKING EXERCISES

1. Describe some outcomes that may result if the nursing shortage is not reduced or resolved.

2. There are four major categories of questions on the NCLEX-PN: Safe and Effective Care Environment, Health Promotion and Maintenance, Psychosocial Integrity, and Physiological Integrity (refer to National Council of State Boards of Nursing, 2011 NCLEX-PN Detailed Test Plan). Based on your personal experiences during wellness or illness care, identify nursing skills (other than those in Stop, Think, and Respond Box 1-2) that would be examples of each of the four NCLEX-PN categories.

3. How might the shortage of registered nurses affect LPNs both positively and negatively?

4. If Florence Nightingale were alive today, how might she view the current education and practice of nursing?

NCLEX-STYLE REVIEW QUESTIONS

1. Before delegating the task of assessing a client's blood sugar to a UAP, what should the LPN do first?
   1. Review the client's trends in blood sugar measurements
   2. Check the diabetic medications prescribed for the client
   3. Determine whether the UAP is qualified to check the blood sugar
   4. Assess what the client knows about controlling blood sugar

2. After receiving an assignment from the RN in charge, which client should the LPN assess first?
   1. Client A, who will be discharged in the morning
   2. Client B, who returned from surgery an hour ago
   3. Client C, who received recent pain medication
   4. Client D, who has not urinated in 4 hours

3. What information is most important for an LPN to receive when obtaining a report on an assigned postoperative client?
   1. The client's age
   2. The client's occupation
   3. The client's last consumption of food
   4. The client's most recent blood pressure

4. After an LPN delegates the assessment of a client's blood pressure to a UAP, what is the most important action to take next?
   1. Check the results of the delegated task
   2. Recheck the client's blood pressure
   3. Teach the client about controlling blood pressure
   4. Assess the client's family history for heart disease

5. When an RN determines an LPN's assignment, which client assignment is most reasonable for the LPN to question?
   1. Client A, who has unrelieved chest pain
   2. Client B, whose fractured leg is in traction
   3. Client C, who is recovering after an appendectomy
   4. Client D, whose white blood cell count is elevated

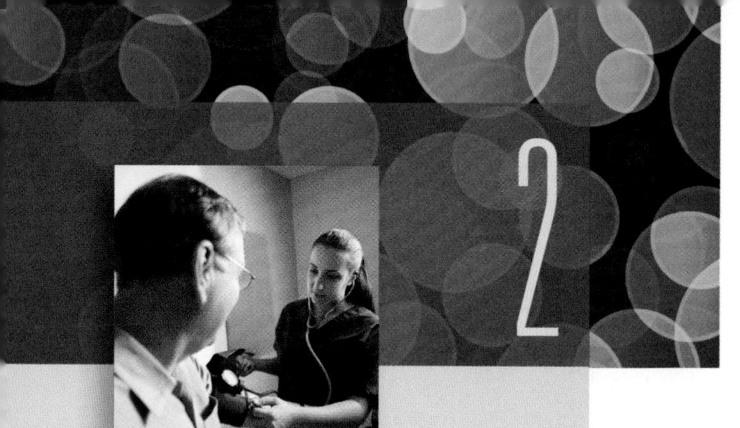

2 Nursing Process

Words To Know
actual diagnosis
assessment
collaborative problems
concept mapping
critical thinking
database assessment
diagnosis
evaluation
focus assessment
functional assessment
goal
implementation
long-term goals
nursing diagnosis
nursing orders
nursing process
objective data
planning
possible diagnosis
risk diagnosis
short-term goals
signs
standards for care
subjective data
symptoms
syndrome diagnosis
wellness diagnosis

Learning Objectives

On completion of this chapter, the reader should be able to:

1. Define the term nursing process.
2. Describe seven characteristics of the nursing process.
3. List five steps in the nursing process.
4. Identify four sources of assessment data.
5. Differentiate between data base, focus, and functional assessments.
6. Distinguish between a nursing diagnosis and a collaborative problem.
7. List three parts of a nursing diagnostic statement.
8. Describe the rationale for setting priorities.
9. Discuss appropriate circumstances for short-term and long-term goals.
10. Identify four ways to document a plan of care.
11. Describe the information that is documented in a plan of care.
12. Discuss three outcomes that result from an evaluation.
13. Describe the process of concept mapping as an alternative learning strategy for student clinical experiences.

In the past, nursing practice consisted of actions based mostly on common sense and the examples set by older, more experienced nurses. The actual care of clients tended to be limited to the physician's medical orders. Although nurses today continue to work interdependently with physicians and other health care practitioners, they now plan and implement client care more independently. In even stronger terms, nurses are held responsible and accountable for providing client care that is safe and appropriate and reflects currently accepted standards for nursing practice.

DEFINITION OF THE NURSING PROCESS

A process is a set of actions leading to a particular goal. The **nursing process** is an organized sequence of problem-solving steps used to identify and manage the health problems of clients (Fig. 2-1). It is the accepted standard for clinical practice established by the American Nurses Association (ANA) (Box 2-1).

The nursing process is the framework for nursing care in all health care settings. When nursing practice follows the nursing process, clients receive quality care in minimal time with maximal efficiency.

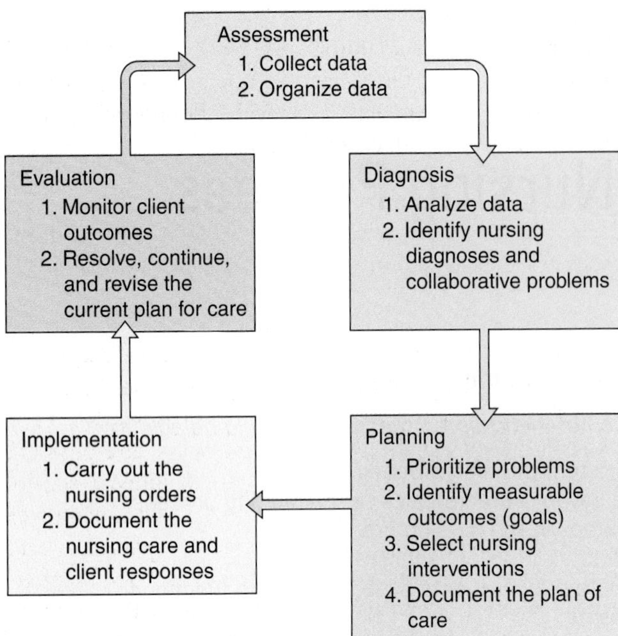

FIGURE 2-1 The steps in the nursing process.

CHARACTERISTICS OF THE NURSING PROCESS

The nursing process has seven distinct characteristics:

- *Within the legal scope of nursing.* Most state nurse practice acts define nursing as an independent problem-solving role that involves the diagnosis and treatment of human responses to actual or potential health problems.
- *Based on knowledge.* The ability to identify and resolve client problems requires **critical thinking**, which is a process of objective reasoning or analyzing facts to reach a valid conclusion. Critical thinking enables nurses to determine which problems necessitate collaboration with the physician and which fall within the independent domain of nursing. Critical thinking helps nurses select appropriate evidence-based nursing interventions for achieving predictable outcomes.
- *Planned.* The steps of the nursing process are organized and systematic. One step leads to the next in an orderly fashion.
- *Client-centered.* The nursing process makes it easier to formulate a comprehensive and unique plan of care for each client. Clients are expected, whenever possible, to actively participate in their care.
- *Goal-directed.* The nursing process involves a united effort between the client and the nursing team to achieve desired outcomes.
- *Prioritized.* The nursing process provides a focused way to resolve the problems that represent the greatest threat to health.
- *Dynamic.* Because the health status of any client is constantly changing, the nursing process acts like a continuous loop. Evaluation, the last step in the nursing process, involves data collection, beginning the process again.

BOX 2-1 Standards of Clinical Nursing Practice

Standard I — Assessment
The nurse collects patient health data.

Standard II — Diagnosis
The nurse analyzes the assessment data to determine diagnoses.

Standard III — Outcome Identification
The nurse identifies expected outcomes individualized to the patient.

Standard IV — Planning
The nurse develops a plan of care that prescribes interventions to attain expected outcomes.

Standard V — Implementation
The nurse implements the interventions identified in the plan of care.

Standard VI — Evaluation
The nurse evaluates the patient's progress toward attainment of outcomes.

Reprinted with permission from American Nurses Association. (1998). *Standards of clinical nursing practice* (2nd ed.). Washington, DC: American Nurses Association.

STEPS OF THE NURSING PROCESS

The steps of the nursing process, each of which is discussed in detail throughout this chapter, are as follows:

1. Assessment
2. Diagnosis
3. Planning
4. Implementation
5. Evaluation

Licensed practical nurses (LPNs) and registered nurses (RNs) have different responsibilities related to the nursing process. For example, RNs may delegate some parts of an initial assessment to an LPN, but the RN is still responsible for ensuring that data collection is complete. After obtaining the assessment data, the RN develops the initial plan of care. Differences exist in various locales as to whether the LPN makes changes to the plan of care independently or collaboratively with the RN (National Council of State Boards of Nursing, 2005, Practical Nurse Scope of Practice White Paper). Also refer to Table 1-3.

Assessment

Assessment, the first step in the nursing process, is the systematic collection of facts or data. Assessment begins with the nurse's first contact with a client and continues as

BOX 2-2 Examples of Objective and Subjective Data

OBJECTIVE DATA	SUBJECTIVE DATA
Weight	Pain
Temperature	Nausea
Skin color	Depression
Blood cell count	Fatigue
Vomiting	Anxiety
Bleeding	Loneliness

long as a need for health care exists. During assessment, the nurse collects information to determine areas of abnormal function, risk factors that contribute to health problems, and client strengths (Alfaro-LeFevre, 2009).

Types of Data

Data are either objective or subjective (Box 2-2). **Objective data** are observable and measurable facts and are referred to as **signs** of a disorder. An example is a client's blood pressure measurement. **Subjective data** consist of information that only the client feels and can describe, and are called **symptoms**. An example is pain.

Stop, Think, and Respond Box 2-1

Which of the following represent objective data?

1. *A client rates his pain as 8 on a scale of 0 to 10, with 10 being the most pain he has ever experienced.*
2. *A client has an incisional scar in the right lower quadrant of the abdomen.*
3. *A client says she slept very well and feels rested.*
4. *A client's blood pressure is 165/86 mm Hg.*
5. *A client's heart rate is irregular.*

Sources for Data

The primary source of information is the client. Secondary sources include the client's family, reports, test results, information in current and past medical records, and discussions with other health care workers.

Types of Assessments

There are three types of assessments: database assessment, focus assessment, and functional assessment (Table 2-1).

Database Assessment

A **database assessment** (initial information about the client's physical, emotional, social, and spiritual health) is lengthy and comprehensive. The nurse obtains data base information during the admission interview and physical examination (see Chap. 13). Health care facilities generally provide a form that is printed or available on a computer for use as a guide (Fig. 2-2). Information obtained during a database assessment serves as a reference for comparing all future data and provides the evidence used to identify the client's initial problems. Comparisons of ongoing assessments with baseline data help determine whether the client's health is improving, deteriorating, or remaining unchanged.

Focus Assessment

A **focus assessment** is information that provides more details about specific problems and expands the original database. For instance, if during the initial interview the client tells the nurse that constipation is the rule rather than the exception, more questions follow. The nurse obtains data about the client's dietary habits, level of activity, fluid intake, current medications, frequency of bowel elimination, and stool characteristics. The nurse may ask the client to save a stool for inspection.

TABLE 2-1 Comparison of Data Base, Focus, and Functional Assessments

DATABASE ASSESSMENT	FOCUS ASSESSMENT	FUNCTIONAL ASSESSMENT
Obtained on admission	Compiled throughout subsequent care	Completed within the first 14 days of admission
Consists of predetermined questions and systematic head-to-toe examination	Consists of unstructured questions and a collection of physical assessments	Can follow various assessment tools, one of which is standardized minimum data set (MDS)
Performed once	Repeated each shift or more often	Repeated at least every 12 months or immediately after a significant change in physical or mental status; reviewed every 3 months
Suggests possible problems	Rules out or confirms problems	Identifies physical, psychological, and social factors that affect self-care
Findings documented on an admission assessment form	Findings documented on a checklist or in progress notes	Findings documented on various assessment tools, one of which is standardized MDS
Time-consuming; may take 1 hour or more	Completed in a brief amount of time (about 15 minutes)	Labor intensive; may involve a multidisciplinary team with final completion by an RN
Supplies a broad, comprehensive volume of data	Collects limited data	Comprehensive evaluation of current strengths and the potential for avoidable decline
Provides breadth for future comparisons	Adds depth to the initial database	Provides comparative data
Reflects the client's condition on entering the health care system	Provides comparative trends for evaluating the client's response to treatment	Data may also be used as a facility's quality indicator

Community Health Center of Branch County

ADMISSION ASSESSMENT RECORD

RESPIRATION

[ ] PROBLEM
[ ] POTENTIAL FOR REFERRAL

HISTORY OF: [ ] CHEST PAIN [ ] PNEUMONIA [ ] BRONCHITIS [ ] ASTHMA [ ] EMPHYSEMA

SHORTNESS OF BREATH: [ ] YES [ ] NO [ ] WITH EXERCISE [ ] WITHOUT EXERCISE

COUGH: [ ] YES [ ] NO [ ] PRODUCTIVE [ ] NON-PRODUCTIVE [ ] SPUTUM COLOR

BREATH SOUNDS (DESCRIBE)

RATE	RHYTHM	QUALITY	SKIN COLOR
		[ ] LABORED [ ] SHALLOW	[ ] PINK [ ] PALE [ ] CYANOTIC

ACCESSORY MUSCLES

COMMENTS

CIRCULATION

[ ] PROBLEM
[ ] POTENTIAL FOR REFERRAL

HISTORY OF: [ ] BLOOD CLOTS [ ] EDEMA [ ] ABNORMAL EKG [ ] NUMBNESS [ ] TINGLING [ ] POOR CIRCULATION [ ] FATIGUE [ ] HYPERTENSION

APICAL RATE	APICAL RATE	RHYTHM
	[ ] REGULAR [ ] IRREGULAR	

NECK VEIN DISTENSION: [ ] PRESENT [ ] ABSENT

NAIL BEDS: [ ] PINK [ ] PALE [ ] CYANOTIC

PEDAL EDEMA: [ ] PRESENT [ ] ABSENT

PEDAL PULSES:
LEFT [ ] PRESENT [ ] WEAK [ ] ABSENT
RIGHT [ ] PRESENT [ ] WEAK [ ] ABSENT

COMMENTS

NUTRITIONAL/METABOLIC

[ ] PROBLEM
[ ] POTENTIAL FOR REFERRAL

HISTORY OF: [ ] DIABETES [ ] HYPOGLYCEMIA [ ] THYROID PROBLEMS

NUTRITIONAL STATUS: [ ] WELL NOURISHED [ ] EMACIATED [ ] OBESE

MEALS PER DAY	DIET AT HOME	DIET PREFERENCE	LAST MEAL	RECENT WEIGHT CHANGES
			[ ] A.M. [ ] P.M.	

NUTRITIONAL DISTURBANCES: [ ] VOMITING [ ] NAUSEA [ ] ANOREXIA [ ] CHEWING PROBLEMS [ ] OTHER (DESCRIBE)

JAUNDICE PRESENT	DENTAL HYGIENE (DESCRIBE)	TEETH	TONGUE CONDITION	ORAL MUCOSA	COLOR
[ ] YES [ ] NO		[ ] OWN [ ] DENTURES	[ ] DRY [ ] COATED [ ] MOIST [ ] SWOLLEN	[ ] DRY [ ] MOIST	

COMMENTS

ELIMINATION

[ ] PROBLEM
[ ] POTENTIAL FOR REFERRAL

BOWEL HABITS: STOOLS PER DAY ______ COLOR [ ] SOFT FORMED [ ] DIARRHEA [ ] CONSTIPATED [ ] USE LAXATIVE — LAST BOWEL MOVEMENT

BLADDER: [ ] DYSURIA [ ] URGENCY [ ] NOCTURIA [ ] CALCULI [ ] FREQUENCY [ ] HEMATURIA [ ] PROSTATE PROBLEM

BOWEL SOUNDS [ ] PRESENT [ ] ABSENT
OSTOMIES OR TUBES (DESCRIBE)

ABDOMEN: [ ] TENDER [ ] SOFT [ ] FIRM [ ] DISTENDED [ ] NOT DISTENDED

URINARY DEVICES (DESCRIBE)

COMMENTS

COGNITIVE/PERCEPTUAL

[ ] PROBLEM
[ ] POTENTIAL FOR REFERRAL

HISTORY OF: [ ] SEIZURES [ ] FREQUENT [ ] INFREQUENT; [ ] HEADACHES [ ] FREQUENT [ ] INFREQUENT

LIMITATION OR RESTRICTION RELATED TO
[ ] HEARING - IMPAIRED [ ] YES [ ] NO
[ ] VISION - IMPAIRED [ ] YES [ ] NO

LEVEL OF CONSCIOUSNESS: [ ] ALERT [ ] LETHARGIC [ ] CONFUSED [ ] LISTLESS [ ] RESPONDS TO PAIN [ ] UNRESPONSIVE

ORIENTED TO: [ ] TIME [ ] PLACE [ ] PERSON

AFFECT: [ ] CALM [ ] WITHDRAWN [ ] APPREHENSIVE [ ] OTHER (DESCRIBE)

BEHAVIOR: [ ] COOPERATIVE [ ] UNCOOPERATIVE

PUPILS: [ ] EQUAL [ ] REACTIVE [ ] OTHER (DESCRIBE)

COMMUNICATION: [ ] SPEAKS ENGLISH [ ] ABLE TO READ [ ] ABLE TO WRITE [ ] COMMUNICATES ADEQUATELY

AWARENESS: [ ] NO PROBLEM WITH MEMORY [ ] PROBLEM WITH MEMORY

DISCOMFORT/PAIN	WHERE	TYPE	PAIN MANAGEMENT	POTENTIAL RISK OF FALLS
[ ] YES [ ] NO				[ ] YES [ ] NO

COMMENTS

FIGURE 2-2 One page of a multipage admission assessment form is shown. (Courtesy of the Community Health Center of Branch County, Coldwater, MI.)

BOX 2-3 Functional Assessment as It Applies to Bathing

5: Unable to assist in any way
4: Able to cooperate, but cannot assist
3: Able to wash hands, face, and chest with supervision; needs help with completing the bath
2: Able to wash face, chest, arms, and upper legs; needs help with completing the bath
1: Bathes self, but requires devices (e.g., long-handled sponge)
0: Bathes self independently

Focus assessments generally are repeated frequently or on a scheduled basis to determine trends in a client's condition and responses to therapeutic interventions. Examples include conducting postoperative surgical assessments (see Chap. 27), monitoring the client's level of pain before and after administering medications, and checking the neurologic status of a client with a head injury.

Functional Assessment

A **functional assessment** is a comprehensive evaluation of a client's physical strengths and weaknesses in areas such as (1) the performance of activities of daily living (see Box 2-3 for an example that relates to bathing), (2) cognitive abilities, and (3) social functioning. The results of the functional assessment help formulate an individualized plan for care that identifies specific interventions for achieving the maximum possible functioning to ensure a better quality of life. Currently, the performance of a functional assessment is being promoted by the Joint Commission in all general health care settings.

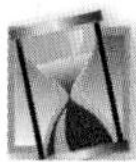

Gerontologic Considerations

Since 1987, all Medicare- and Medicaid-funded nursing homes must complete a Resident Assessment Instrument (RAI) to document a client's functional assessment. It includes a form known as the minimum data set (MDS) for Resident Assessment and Care Screening. When used on a cyclical basis, a functional assessment indicates changes—in both improvement and deterioration—experienced by aging clients over time.

Organization of Data

Interpreting data is easier if information is organized. Organization involves grouping related information. For example, consider the following list of words: apple, wheels, orchard, pedals, tree, and handlebars. At first glance, they appear to be a jumble of terms. If asked to cluster the related terms, however, most people would correctly group apple, tree, and orchard together, and wheels, pedals, and handlebars together.

Nurses organize assessment data similarly. Using knowledge and past experiences, they cluster related data (Box 2-4). Data organized into small groups are easier to analyze and they take on more significance than when the nurse considers each fact separately or examines the entire group at once.

BOX 2-4 Organization of Data

Assessment Findings
Lassitude; distended abdomen; dry, hard stool passed with difficulty; fever; weak cough; thick sputum

Related Clusters
Lassitude, fever
Weak cough, thick sputum
Distended abdomen; dry, hard stool passed with difficulty

Stop, Think, and Respond Box 2-2

Organize the following data into two related clusters: cough, dry skin, infrequent urination, fever, nasal congestion, thirst.

Diagnosis

Diagnosis, the second step in the nursing process, is the identification of health-related problems. Diagnosis results from analyzing the collected data and determining whether they suggest normal or abnormal findings.

Nursing Diagnoses

Nurses analyze data to identify one or more nursing diagnoses. A **nursing diagnosis** is a health issue that can be prevented, reduced, resolved, or enhanced through independent nursing measures. It is an exclusive nursing responsibility. Nursing diagnoses are categorized into five groups: actual, risk, possible, syndrome, and wellness (Table 2-2).

TABLE 2-2 Categories of Nursing Diagnoses

TYPE	EXPLANATION AND EXAMPLE
Actual diagnosis	A problem that currently exists *Impaired Physical Mobility related to pain as evidenced by limited range of motion, reluctance to move*
Risk diagnosis	A problem the client is uniquely at risk for developing *Risk for Deficient Fluid Volume related to persistent vomiting*
Possible diagnosis	A problem may be present, but requires more data collection to rule out or confirm its existence *Possible Parental Role Conflict related to impending divorce*
Syndrome diagnosis	Cluster of problems predicted to be present because of an event or situation (Carpenito-Moyet, 2009) *Rape Trauma Syndrome and Disuse Syndrome*
Wellness diagnosis	A health-related problem with which a healthy person obtains nursing assistance to maintain or perform at a higher level *Potential for Enhanced Breastfeeding*

BOX 2-5 Parts of a Nursing Diagnostic Statement

1. Disturbed Sleep Pattern = problem
2. Related to excessive intake of coffee = etiology
3. As manifested by difficulty in falling asleep, feeling tired during the day, and irritability with others = signs and symptoms

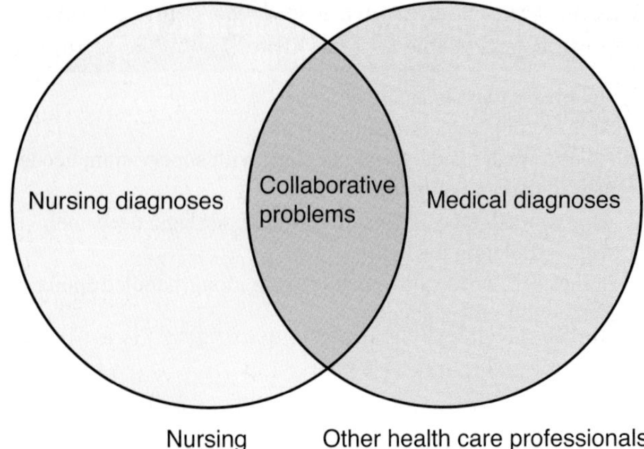

FIGURE 2-3 These two overlapping circles illustrate that the nurse independently treats nursing diagnoses. Doctors, other health professionals, and nurses work together on collaborative problems.

The NANDA List

The ANA has designated NANDA International (NANDA-I; formerly the North American Nursing Diagnosis Association) as the authoritative organization for developing and approving nursing diagnoses. NANDA is the clearinghouse for proposals suggesting diagnoses that fall within the independent domain of nursing practice. NANDA reviews the proposals for appropriateness. While research is ongoing, NANDA incorporates its findings into a list published for clinical use. The most recent index, which is revised every 2 years, is provided on the inside back cover of this book.

Although entries in the NANDA list change, most authorities believe that nurses should use the language of the approved diagnoses whenever possible. When a client's problem does not fit into any of the NANDA-approved categories, the nurse can use his or her own terminology when stating the nursing diagnosis.

Diagnostic Statements

An actual nursing diagnostic statement contains three parts:

1. Name of the health-related issue or problem as identified in the NANDA list
2. Etiology (its cause)
3. Signs and symptoms

The name of the nursing diagnosis is linked to the etiology with the phrase "related to," and the signs and symptoms are identified with the phrase "as manifested (or evidenced) by" (Box 2-5).

Different types of diagnoses have different stems. **Risk diagnoses** are prefaced with the term "risk for," as in Risk for Impaired Skin Integrity related to inactivity. The word "possible" is used in a diagnostic statement to indicate uncertainty; for example, Possible Sexual Dysfunction related to anxiety. Wellness diagnoses are prefaced with the phrase "potential for enhanced."

Risk and possible nursing diagnoses do not include the third part of the statement. In risk nursing diagnoses, the signs or symptoms have not yet manifested; in possible nursing diagnoses, the data are incomplete. The factors that place the client at risk or make the nurse suspect such a diagnosis, however, are identified in the nursing assessment documentation. Syndrome diagnoses and wellness diagnoses are one-part statements; they are not linked with an etiology or signs and symptoms.

Collaborative Problems

Collaborative problems are physiologic complications that require both nurse- and physician-prescribed interventions. They represent an interdependent domain of nursing practice (Fig. 2-3). The nurse is specifically responsible and accountable for the following:

- Correlating medical diagnoses or medical treatment measures with the risk for unique complications.
- Documenting the complications for which clients are at risk.

TABLE 2-3 Correlation of Collaborative Problems

MEDICAL DIAGNOSIS OR MEDICAL TREATMENT	POSSIBLE CONSEQUENCE	COLLABORATIVE PROBLEM
Myocardial infarction (heart attack)	Abnormal heart rhythm	PC: Dysrhythmias
Heart failure	Fluid in the lungs	PC: Pulmonary edema
Severe burns	Serum moves into tissue, depleting blood volume	PC: Hypovolemic shock
HIV positive (infected with AIDS virus)	Decreased blood cells that fight infection	PC: Immunodeficiency
Gastric decompression (suctioning stomach fluid)	Removes acid and electrolytes	PC: Alkalosis PC: Electrolyte imbalance
Cardiac catheterization (inserting a catheter into the heart)	Arterial bleeding	PC: Hemorrhage

- Making pertinent assessments to detect complications.
- Reporting trends that suggest development of complications.
- Managing the emerging problem with nurse- and physician-prescribed measures.
- Evaluating the outcomes.

Collaborative problems are identified on a client's plan for care with the abbreviation PC, which stands for potential complication (Table 2-3). Because a collaborative problem requires the nurse to use diagnostic processes, some nursing leaders are proposing the use of the term "collaborative diagnosis" instead (Alfaro-LeFevre, 2009).

Stop, Think, and Respond Box 2-3

Which of the following nursing diagnostic statements is written correctly based on the data and the information in this chapter?

Data: The client eats only bites of the food served. She has lost 15 lb in the last 3 weeks and currently weighs 130 lb, which is more than 10% underweight for her height. She has been experiencing chronic vomiting after eating for the last 3 weeks and is physically weak.

1. *Risk for Imbalanced Nutrition: Less than Body Requirements related to vomiting*
2. *Imbalanced Nutrition: Less than Body Requirements related to inadequate intake of food secondary to vomiting as manifested by caloric intake below daily requirements, recent weight loss of 15 lb, and current weakness*
3. *Weight Loss related to vomiting as evidenced by reduced intake of food*
4. *Possible Malnutrition due to inadequate consumption of nutrients*

Planning

The third step in the nursing process is **planning**, or the process of prioritizing nursing diagnoses and collaborative problems, identifying measurable goals or outcomes, selecting appropriate interventions, and documenting the plan of care. Whenever possible, the nurse consults the client while developing and revising the plan.

Setting Priorities

Not all clients' problems can be resolved in a brief time. Therefore, it is important to determine which problems require the most immediate attention. This is done by setting priorities. Prioritization involves ranking, from those that are most serious or immediate to those of lesser importance.

There is more than one way to determine priorities. One method nurses frequently use is Maslow's Hierarchy of Human Needs (see Chap. 4). Problems interfering with physiologic needs have priority over those affecting other levels of needs (Table 2-4). The ranking can change as problems are resolved or new problems develop.

TABLE 2-4 Prioritizing Nursing Diagnoses

HUMAN NEED	EXAMPLES OF NURSING DIAGNOSES
Physiologic	Imbalanced nutrition: less than body requirements Ineffective breathing pattern Pain Impaired swallowing Urinary retention
Safety and security	Risk for injury Impaired verbal communication Disturbed thought processes Anxiety Fear
Love and belonging	Social isolation Impaired social interactions Interrupted family processes Parental role conflict
Esteem and self-esteem	Disturbed body image Powerlessness Caregiver role strain Ineffective breastfeeding
Self-actualization	Delayed growth and development Spiritual distress

Establishing Goals

A **goal** (expected or desired outcome) helps the nursing team know whether the nursing care has been appropriate for managing the client's nursing diagnoses and collaborative problems. Therefore, a written goal accompanies each one. Although the terms "goal" and "outcome" are sometimes used interchangeably, outcomes are generally more specific (Box 2-6). What is important is that the goal statement or outcome contains the criteria or objective evidence for verifying that the client has improved. Depending on the agency, nurses may identify short-term goals, long-term goals, or both.

Short-Term Goals

Nurses use **short-term goals** (outcomes achievable in a few days to 1 week) more often in acute care settings because most hospital stays are no longer than 1 week. Short-term goals have the following characteristics (Box 2-7):

- *Developed from the problem portion of the diagnostic statement*
- *Client-centered*, reflecting what the client will accomplish, not the nurse
- *Measurable*, identifying specific criteria that provide evidence of goal achievement
- *Realistic*, to avoid setting unattainable goals, which can be self-defeating and frustrating
- *Accompanied by a target date* for accomplishment, the predicted time when the goal will be met; identifying a target date establishes a time line for evaluation.

Long-Term Goals

Nurses generally identify **long-term goals** (desirable outcomes that take weeks or months to accomplish) for clients with chronic health problems that require extended care in a nursing home or who receive community health or home

BOX 2-6 Goals Versus Outcomes

Goal
The client will be well hydrated by 8/23.

Outcome
The client will have adequate hydration as evidenced by an oral intake between 2,000 and 3,000 mL/24 hours and a urine output plus or minus 500 mL of the intake amount by 8/23.

health services. An example of a long-term goal for the client with a cerebrovascular accident (stroke) is the return of full or partial function to a paralyzed limb. The client is unlikely to have achieved this goal by discharge. If a client achieves short-term goals in the hospital, however, he or she is more likely to achieve long-term goals during care at home or in other community settings.

Goals for Collaborative Problems

Goals for collaborative problems are written from a nursing rather than from a client perspective. They focus on what the nurse will monitor, report, record, or do to promote early detection and treatment (Alfaro-LeFevre, 2009).

The format for writing a nursing goal is, "The nurse will manage and minimize (identify complication) by (insert evidence of assessment, communication, and treatment activities)," or "(identify complication) will be managed and minimized by (evidence)." For example, if the nurse identifies gastrointestinal bleeding as a PC, he or she may state the goal, "The nurse will examine emesis and stools for blood and report positive test findings, changes in vital signs, and decreased red blood cell counts to the physician" or "Gastrointestinal bleeding will be managed and minimized as evidenced by negative Hemoccult tests, red blood cell count greater than 2.5 million/dL, and vital signs within normal ranges."

Selecting Nursing Interventions

Planning the measures that the client and nurse will use to accomplish identified goals involves critical thinking. Nursing interventions are directed at eliminating the etiologies. The nurse selects strategies based on evidence-based knowledge that certain nursing actions produce desired effects. Whatever interventions are planned, they must be safe, within the legal scope of nursing practice, and compatible with medical orders.

Initial interventions generally are limited to selected measures with the potential for success. Nurses should reserve some interventions in case a client does not accomplish the goal.

BOX 2-7 Components of Short-Term Goals

Nursing Diagnostic Statement
Constipation related to decreased fluid intake, lack of dietary fiber, and lack of exercise as manifested by no normal bowel movement for the past 3 days, abdominal cramping, and straining to pass stool

Short-Term Goal

The client will	*client-centered*
have a bowel movement	identifies *measurable* criteria that reflect the *problem portion* of the diagnostic statement
in 2 days (specify date)	identifies a *target date* for achievement within a *realistic* time frame

Documenting the Plan of Care

Plans of care can be written by hand (Fig. 2-4), standardized on printed forms, computer generated, or based on an agency's written standards or clinical pathways. Whatever method is used, The Joint Commission requires that every client's medical record provide evidence of the planned nursing interventions for meeting the client's needs (Carpenito-Moyet, 2009).

Nursing orders (directions for a client's care) identify the what, when, where, and how for performing nursing interventions. They provide specific instructions so that all health team members understand exactly what to do for the client (Box 2-8). Nursing orders are also signed to indicate accountability.

Standardized care plans are preprinted. Both computer-generated and standardized plans provide general suggestions for managing the nursing care of clients with a particular problem. It is up to the nurse to transform the generalized interventions into specific nursing orders and to eliminate whatever is inappropriate or unnecessary.

Agency-specific **standards for care** (policies that indicate which activities will be provided to ensure quality client care) and clinical pathways (see Chap. 1) relieve the nurse from writing time-consuming plans. Both tools help nurses use their time efficiently and ensure consistent client care.

Communicating the Plan of Care

Clients need consistency and continuity of care to achieve goals. Therefore, the nurse shares the plan of care with nursing team members, the client, and the client's family. In some agencies, the client signs the plan of care.

BOX 2-8 Nursing Orders

Nursing Order
Encourage fluids

Weaknesses
Lacks specificity
Likely to be interpreted differently
May result in inconsistent or less than adequate care

Improvement
Provide 100 mL of oral fluid every hour while awake

Name: Mrs. Rita Williard Age: 68 Date of Admission: 11/10

Diagnosis on admission: CVA c̄ left-sided weakness

Nursing diagnosis: Impaired Physical Mobility, High Risk for Injury, Situational Low Self-esteem

Long-term goals: Independent mobility using walker or quad cane, record of personal safety, positive self-regard

DATE	PROBLEM	GOAL	TARGET DATE	NURSING ORDERS
11/10	#1 Impaired Physical Mobility related to left sided weakness as manifested by decreased muscle strength in left leg and arm, slowed gait, dragging foot	The client will stand and pivot from bed to wheelchair or commode.	11/24	1) Passive ROM t.i.d. to left arm and leg 2) Physical therapy b.i.d. for practice at parallel bars 3) Apply left leg brace and sling to left arm when up 4) Assist to balance on right leg at bedside before and after physical therapy daily C. Meyer, RN
11/10	#2 Risk for Injury related to motor deficit	The client will transfer from bed to wheelchair without injury	12/1	1) Keep side rails up and trapeze over bed 2) Use shoe c̄ nonskid sole on right foot (leg brace on left) before transfer 3) Dangle for 5 minutes before attempting to stand 4) Lock wheels on wheelchair before transfer 5) Obtain help of second assistant 6) Block left foot to avoid slipping during pivot 7) Place signal light on right side within reach at all times C. Meyer, RN
12/2	#3 Situational Low Self-Esteem related to dependence on others as manifested by statements, "I need as much help as a baby; I feel so useless; How embarrassing to be so dependent"	The client will identify one or more positive feelings regarding improved mobility and self-care	12/18	1.) Allow to express feelings without disagreeing or interrupting. 2.) Reinforce concept that the right side of body is unaffected. 3.) Help to set and accomplish one realistic goal daily. S. Moore, RN

FIGURE 2-4 Sample nursing care plan.

The plan of care is a permanent part of the client's medical record. It is placed in the client's chart, kept separately at the client's bedside, or located in a temporary folder at the nurses' station for easy access. Wherever it is located, each nurse assigned to the client refers to it daily, reviews it for appropriateness, and revises it according to changes in the client's condition.

Implementation

Implementation, the fourth step in the nursing process, means carrying out the plan of care. The nurse implements medical orders as well as nursing orders, which should complement each other. Implementing the plan involves the client and one or more members of the health care team. A wide circle of care providers with assorted roles may be called on

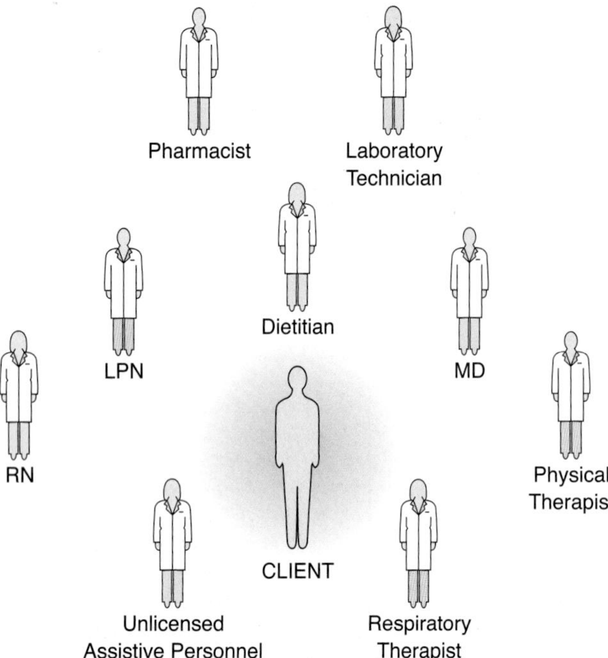

FIGURE 2-5 Members of the health care team.

to participate, either directly or indirectly, in carrying out one client's plan of care (Fig. 2-5).

The medical record is legal evidence that the plan of care has been more than just a paper trail. The information in the chart shows a correlation between the plan and the care that has been provided. In other words, the nurse's charting (see Chap. 9) reflects the written plan. Nurses are just as accountable for carrying out nursing orders as they are for physician's orders.

In addition to identifying the nursing interventions that have been provided, the record also describes the quantity and quality of the client's response. Quoting the client helps identify his or her point of view and safeguards against incorrect assumptions. In short, appropriate documentation maintains open lines of communication among members of the health care team, ensures the client's continuing progress, complies with accreditation standards, and helps ensure reimbursement from government or private insurance companies.

Evaluation

Evaluation, the fifth and final step in the nursing process, is the way by which nurses determine whether a client has reached a goal. Although this is considered the last step, the entire process is ongoing. By analyzing the client's response, evaluation helps determine the effectiveness of nursing care (Table 2-5).

Before revising a plan of care, it is important to discuss any lack of progress with the client. In this way, both the nurse and the client can speculate on what activities need to be discontinued, added, or changed. Other health team members who are familiar with a particular client or problems similar to those of the client may offer their expertise as well. The evaluation of a client's progress may be the subject of a nursing team conference. Some units even invite the client and family to participate.

USE OF THE NURSING PROCESS

Use of the nursing process is the standard for clinical nursing practice. Nurse practice acts hold nurses accountable for demonstrating all the steps in the nursing process when caring for clients. To do less implies negligence. More detailed discussions of the nursing process can be found in specialty texts and in some of the suggested readings at the end of this book. Nursing Guidelines 2-1 reiterate the sequence of the nursing process.

CONCEPT MAPPING

Concept mapping (also known as care mapping) is a method of organizing information in graphic or pictorial form. This strategy promotes learning by having the student gather data from the client and medical record or a written case study, select significant information, and organize related concepts on a one- or two-page working document. Various formats used include a spider diagram with a central theme such as the client's medical diagnosis, a hierarchy moving from general

TABLE 2-5 Outcomes from Evaluation

ANALYSIS	REASON	ACTION
The client has reached the goals	Plan was effective and implemented consistently	Discontinue the nursing orders
The client has made some progress	Care has been inconsistent	Check that nursing orders are clear and specific
	Target date was too ambitious	Continue care as planned; readjust target date
	Client's response has been less than expected	Revise the plan by adding nursing interventions or more frequent implementation
The client has made no progress	The initial diagnosis was inaccurate	Revise problem list; write new goals and nursing orders
	New problems have occurred	Add new problems, goals, and nursing orders
	The target date was unrealistic	Revise expected date for achievement
	Nursing interventions were ineffective	Add new nursing orders; discontinue ineffective measures; readjust target date

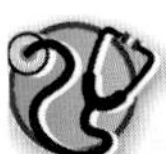

NURSING GUIDELINES 2-1

Using the Nursing Process

- Collect information about the client. Data collection is the basis for identifying problems.
- Organize the data. Organizing related data simplifies the process of analysis.
- Analyze the data for what is normal and abnormal. Abnormalities provide clues to the client's problems.
- Identify actual, risk, possible, syndrome, and wellness nursing diagnoses and collaborative problems. Problem identification directs the nurse to select methods for maintaining or restoring the client's health.
- Prioritize the problem list. Setting priorities targets problems that require the most immediate attention.
- Set goals with specific criteria for evaluating whether the problems have been prevented, reduced, or resolved. Goals predict the expected outcomes from nursing care.
- Select a limited number of appropriate nursing interventions. The nurse uses evidence-based knowledge to determine which measures will be most effective in accomplishing the goals of care.
- Give specific directions for nursing care. Specific directions promote consistency and continuity among caregivers.
- Document the plan for care using whatever written format is acceptable. A written plan provides a means of communication and reference for the nursing team to follow.
- Discuss the plan with nursing team members, the client, and the family. Verbally sharing the plan ensures that everyone is informed and goal directed.
- Put the plan into action. Work produces results.
- Observe the client's responses. Evaluating outcomes is the basis for determining the effectiveness of the plan of care.
- Chart all nursing activities and the client's responses. Documentation demonstrates that planned care has been implemented and provides information about the client's progress.
- Compare the client's responses with the goal criteria. If the planned care is appropriate, there should be some measure of progress toward accomplishing goals.
- Discuss the progress, or lack of it, with the client, family, and other nursing team members. Pooling resources may provide better alternatives when revising the plan of care.
- Change the plan in areas that are no longer appropriate. The nursing care plan changes according to the needs of the client.
- Continue to implement and evaluate the revised plan of care. The nursing process is a continuous sequence of actions that is repeated until the goals have been met.

to specific, or a flow chart (Fig. 2-6). With additional knowledge, students draw lines or arrows to link or correlate relationships within the map. Organizing the data then facilitates identifying nursing diagnoses, setting goals and expected outcomes, and evaluating the results of the care provided.

Those who use concept mapping report that the technique:

- Allows students to integrate previous knowledge with newly acquired information.

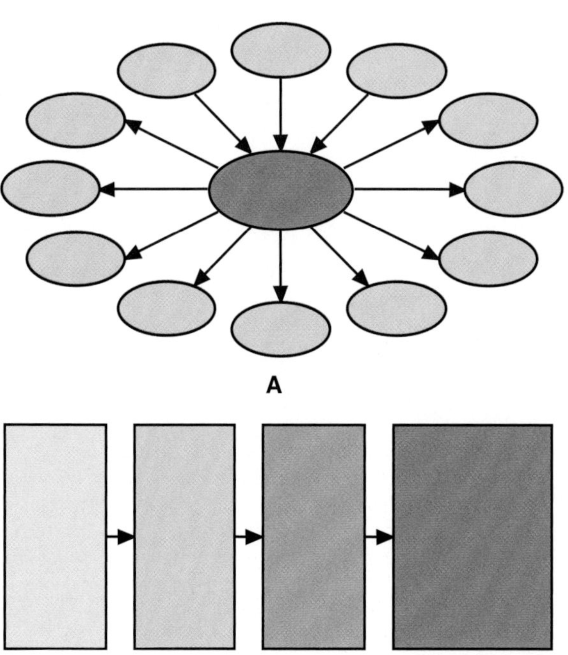

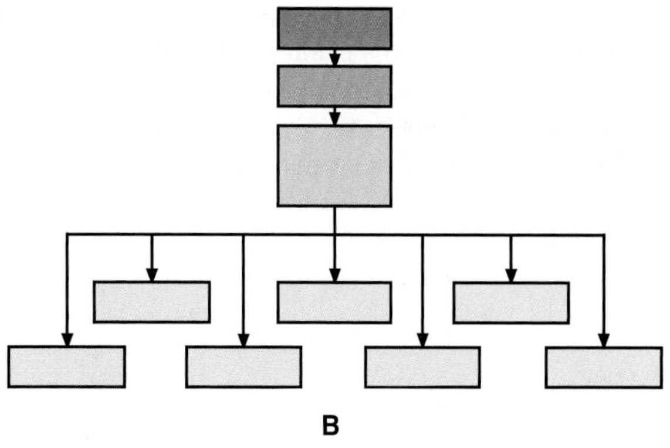

FIGURE 2-6 Three formats used in concept mapping. **A.** Spider diagram. **B.** Hierarchical arrangement. **C.** Linear flow chart.

- Enables students to organize and visualize relationships between their current academic learning and new, unique client assignments.
- Increases critical thinking and clinical reasoning skills.
- Enhances retention of knowledge.
- Correlates theoretical knowledge with nursing practice.
- Helps students recognize information that they must review or learn to promote safe, appropriate client care.
- Promotes better time management for beginning students otherwise focused on the composition requirements of nursing care plans rather than use of the nursing process itself.

CRITICAL THINKING EXERCISES

1. If an unconscious client is brought to the nursing unit, how can a nurse gather data?

2. Three nursing diagnoses are on a client's plan of care: ineffective breathing pattern, social isolation, and anxiety. Which has the highest priority, and why?

3. While reviewing a client's plan of care, a nurse notices that the client has made no progress in accomplishing the goal by its projected target date. What actions are appropriate at this time?

4. A nurse plans an 1,800 calorie diet to manage an obese client with the nursing diagnosis of Imbalanced Nutrition: More than Body Requirements, but the client rejects that intervention in lieu of exercising 30 minutes each day. What nursing action is appropriate in this situation?

NCLEX-STYLE REVIEW QUESTIONS

1. When managing the care of a client, which of the following nursing actions is most appropriate to perform first?
1. Develop a plan of care.
2. Determine the client's needs.
3. Assess the client physically.
4. Collaborate on goals for care.

2. According to most nurse practice acts, if a charge nurse assigns a licensed practical nurse to admit a new client, what is the practical nurse's primary role?
1. Create an initial nursing care plan.
2. Gather basic information from the client.
3. Develop a list of the client's nursing diagnoses.
4. Report assessment data to the client's physician.

3. At a team conference, staff members discuss a client's nursing diagnoses. Which one of the following nursing diagnoses is of highest priority?
1. Ineffective Airway Clearance
2. Ineffective Coping
3. Deficient Diversional Activity
4. Interrupted Family Processes

4. The licensed practical nurse notes that an expected outcome of bathing independently has not been reached by the target date. What action is most appropriate to take at this time?
1. Urge the client to try harder to bathe independently.
2. Limit bathing until the client can bathe independently.
3. Suggest that the staff reduce their assistance with bathing.
4. Revise the interventions or target date for achieving the goal.

5. When gathering nursing data on a newly admitted client, which of the following is an appropriate source to consult for additional information?
1. The client's visitors
2. The client's family
3. The client's clergy
4. The client's employer

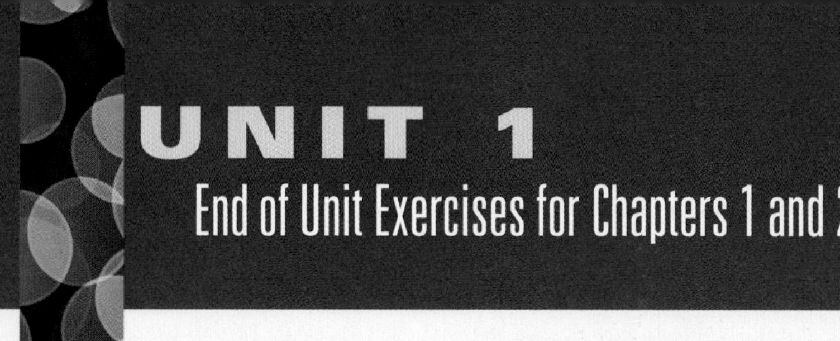

UNIT 1
End of Unit Exercises for Chapters 1 and 2

Section I: Reviewing What You've Learned

Activity A: *Fill in the blanks by choosing the correct word from the options given in parentheses.*

1. A ____________________ develops from observing and studying the relationship of one phenomenon to another. (science, skill, theory)
2. A nursing ____________________ is a health issue that can be prevented, reduced, resolved, or enhanced through independent nursing measures. (assessment, diagnosis, evaluation)
3. ____________________ defined nursing as "putting individuals in the best possible condition for nature to restore and preserve health." (Henderson, Herbert, Nightingale)
4. ____________________ data are observable and measurable facts and are referred to as signs of a disorder. (Historical, Objective, Subjective)

Activity B: *Mark each statement as either T (True) or F (False). Correct any false statements.*

1. T____F____ Concept mapping is a method of organizing information in a graphic or pictorial form.
2. T____F____ Nurses with master's degrees conduct research and advise, manage, and instruct nurses pursuing degrees.
3. T____F____ The primary health care provider refers to the plan of care, reviews it for appropriateness, and revises it according to changes in the client's condition.
4. T____F____ Nurses frequently use Maslow's Hierarchy of Human Needs to determine priorities when caring for clients.

Activity C: *Write the correct term for each description that follows.*

1. Process of identifying and evaluating outcomes __________________
2. An expected or desired outcome that helps the nursing team know whether nursing care has been appropriate for managing the client's nursing diagnoses and collaborative problems __________________
3. The standard for clinical nursing practice __________________
4. Care provided by the first health care worker assessing the person with a health need __________________

Activity D: *Match the nursing skills in Column A with their descriptions in Column B.*

Column A	Column B
1. ____________ Assessment skills	A. Assisting with activities of daily living
2. ____________ Caring skills	B. Offering pertinent health teaching
3. ____________ Counseling skills	C. Providing interventions that allow for stability and security during a health-related crisis
4. ____________ Comforting skills	D. Interviewing, observing, and examining the client

Activity E: *Differentiate between a database assessment and a focus assessment based on the criteria given.*

	Database Assessment	Focus Assessment
Definition		
Purpose		
Example		

Activity F: *The nursing process is an organized sequence of problem-solving steps used to identify and manage the health concerns of clients. When nursing practice follows the nursing process, clients receive quality care in minimal time with maximum efficiency. Write in the boxes provided the correct sequence in which the actions of the nursing process should be performed.*

1. Implementation
2. Diagnosis
3. Assessment
4. Evaluation
5. Planning

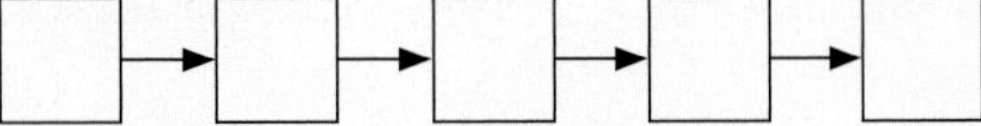

Activity G: *Answer the following questions.*

1. How did Florence Nightingale improve the image of nursing?

2. How did Virginia Henderson define nursing?

3. What are the different types of nursing diagnoses?

4. What is a collaborative problem?

Section II: Applying Your Knowledge

Activity H: *Give rationales for the following questions.*

1. Why is the use of empathy so important when nurses care for clients?

2. Why are short-term goals most appropriate for clients receiving care in acute care settings?

3. Why should the nurse document and sign a nursing order?

Activity I: *Answer the following questions focusing on nursing roles and responsibilities.*

1. A family member brings an elderly client with severe back pain following a fall to the health care facility.
   a. What should the nurse do before determining the nursing care that the client requires?

   b. What skills must the nurse possess to perform the previous intervention?

2. A nurse is providing care to a client with respiratory distress.
   a. What are the requirements for preparing a nursing diagnosis?

   b. What are the different parts of a nursing diagnosis?

3. A nurse is identifying short-term and long-term goals for a client who has been admitted to the health care facility with a fractured right leg.
   a. What should the nurse keep in mind when setting short-term goals?

   b. What are long-term goals?

   c. Identify one possible short-term goal and one possible long-term goal for this client.

Activity J: *Consider the following questions. Discuss them with your instructor or peers.*

1. A client with lung cancer is undergoing chemotherapy. Recently, he has been losing hair, looks pale and tired, and has significantly reduced his activities. His family members are worried about the drastic changes in his appearance and health. In the beginning, the client was eager to comply with the treatment, but now he tells the nurse that he would rather suffer the consequences of the disease than the side effects of the treatment. How might the nurse approach this situation using assessment, caring, counseling, and comforting skills?

2. A 50-year-old client is in a long-term care facility following a stroke. His left arm is paralyzed. The client is having problems with urinary incontinence; recently, he has also developed constipation and is not eating well. Full or partial return of the left limb's function is one of the long-term goals for this client, who eventually will undergo occupational therapy.
   a. How should the nurse prioritize care given to this client?
   b. What client needs require immediate attention?
   c. Identify some other short-term and long-term goals for this client.

Section III: Getting Ready for NCLEX

Activity K: *Answer the following questions.*

1. A nurse is assessing a client. Which of the following should the nurse record as subjective data?
   a. Temperature
   b. Abdominal pain
   c. Pulse rate
   d. Blood pressure

2. Which of the following was the primary factor that contributed to the demise of nursing in England before Florence Nightingale?
   a. Use of untrained workers, some of whom lacked good character, as nurses
   b. Recruitment of lay people by monasteries to assist in physical care
   c. Engagement of religious groups in many of the roles of nursing
   d. Lack of resources during periods of plague and pestilence

3. Which of the following programs qualify students to take the National Council Licensure Examination-Registered Nurse (NCLEX-RN)? Select all that apply.
   a. A practical nurse program
   b. A hospital-based diploma program
   c. A licensed practical nursing (LPN) program
   d. An associate degree in nursing
   e. A baccalaureate nursing program

4. Nursing diagnoses for a client with a fractured hip include "impaired skin integrity related to inactivity." To which of the following categories does this nursing diagnosis belong?
   a. Actual
   b. Possible
   c. Syndrome
   d. Wellness

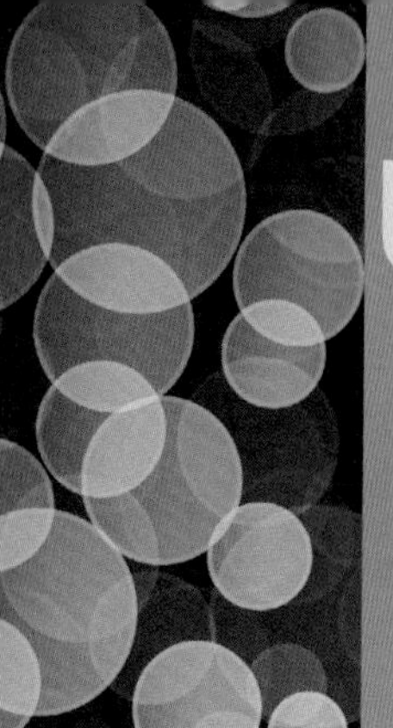

UNIT 2
Integrating Basic Concepts

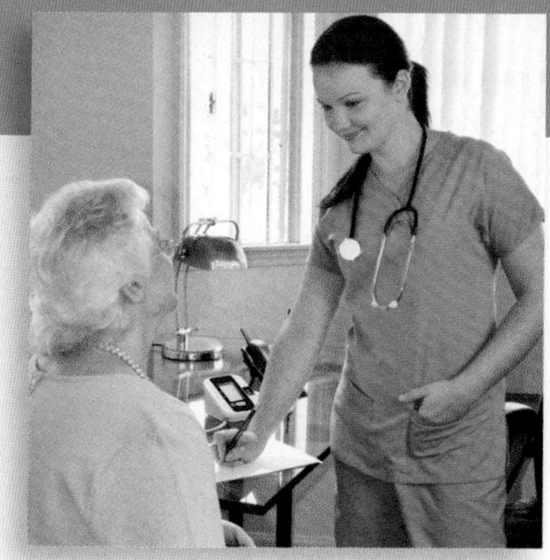

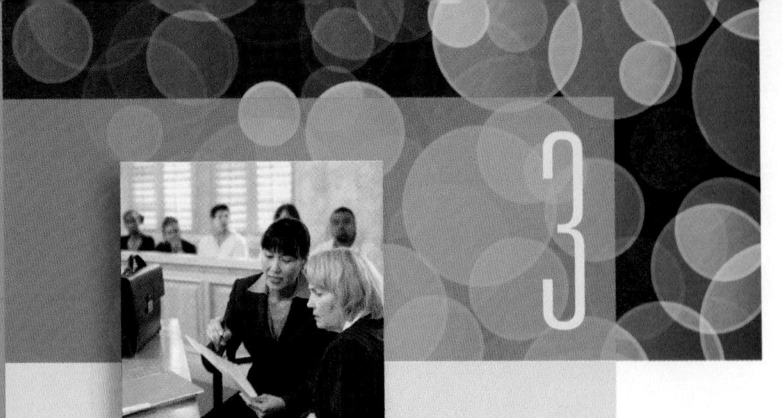

3 Laws and Ethics

Words To Know

administrative laws
advance directive
allocation of scarce resources
anecdotal record
assault
autonomy
battery
beneficence
board of nursing
civil laws
code of ethics
code status
common law
confidentiality
criminal laws
defamation
defendant
deontology
durable power of attorney for health care
duty
ethical dilemma
ethics
false imprisonment
felony
fidelity
Good Samaritan laws
incident report
intentional tort
invasion of privacy
justice
laws
liability insurance
libel
living will
malpractice
misdemeanor
negligence
nonmaleficence
nurse licensure compacts
nurse practice act
plaintiff
reciprocity
restraints
risk management
slander
statute of limitations
statutory laws

Learning Objectives

On completion of this chapter, the reader should be able to:

1. Name six types of laws.
2. Discuss the purpose of nurse practice acts and the role of the state board of nursing.
3. Explain the difference between intentional and unintentional torts.
4. Describe the difference between negligence and malpractice.
5. Identify three reasons as to why a nurse should obtain professional liability insurance.
6. List five ways that a nurse's professional liability can be mitigated in the case of a lawsuit.
7. Define the term ethics.
8. Explain the purpose of a code of ethics.
9. Describe two types of ethical theories.
10. Name and explain six ethical principles that apply to health care.
11. List five ethical issues common in nursing practice.

Laws, ethics, client rights, and nursing duties affect nurses throughout their careers. This chapter introduces basic legal and ethical concepts and issues that affect the practice of nursing.

LAWS

Laws (rules of conduct established and enforced by government) are intended to protect both the general public and each person. The six categories of laws are constitutional, statutory, administrative, common, criminal, and civil (Table 3-1).

Constitutional Law

The founders of the United States wrote the country's first formal laws within the Constitution. This document, which has endured with few amendments, divides power among three branches of government and establishes checks and balances that protect the entire nation. It also identifies the rights and privileges to which all US citizens are entitled. Two examples of rights protected by constitutional law are free speech and privacy.

Statutory Laws

Statutory laws (laws enacted by federal, state, or local legislatures) sometimes are identified as public acts, codes, or ordinances. For

Words To Know (continued)
telehealth services
telenursing
teleology
tort
truth telling
unintentional tort
values
veracity
whistle-blowing

example, state legislatures are responsible for enacting statutes that ensure the competence of health care providers. A **nurse practice act** (statute that legally defines the unique role of the nurse and differentiates it from that of other health care practitioners, such as physicians) is one example of a statutory law (Box 3-1). Although each state's nurse practice act is unique, all generally contain common elements:

- They define the scope of nursing practice.
- They establish the limits to that practice.
- They identify the titles that nurses may use, such as licensed practical nurse (LPN), licensed vocational nurse (LVN), or registered nurse (RN).
- They authorize a board of nursing to oversee nursing practice.
- They determine what constitutes grounds for disciplinary action.

Administrative Laws

Administrative laws (legal provisions through which federal, state, and local agencies maintain self-regulation) affect the power to manage governmental agencies. Some administrative laws authorize federal and state governments to ensure citizen health and safety.

State Boards of Nursing

The state board of nursing is an example of an administrative agency that enforces administrative law. Each state's **board of nursing** (regulatory agency for managing the provisions of a state's nurse practice act) has a primary responsibility to protect the public receiving nursing care within the state. Some activities of the state's board of nursing include (1) reviewing and approving nursing education programs in the state, (2) establishing criteria for licensing nurses, (3) overseeing procedures for nurse licensing examinations, (4) issuing and transferring nursing licenses, (5) investigating allegations against nurses licensed in that state, and (6) disciplining nurses who violate legal and ethical standards. The state's board of nursing is responsible for suspending and revoking licenses and reviewing applications asking for **reciprocity** (licensure based on evidence of having met licensing criteria in another state). A license in one state does not give a person a right to automatic licensure in another.

TABLE 3-1 Types of Laws

CATEGORY	PURPOSE	EXAMPLES
Constitutional law	Protects fundamental rights and freedoms of US citizens Defines the duties and limitations of the executive, legislative, and judicial branches of government	Bill of Rights, freedom of speech
Statutory law	Identifies local, state, or federal rules necessary for the public's welfare	Public health ordinances, tax laws, nurse practice acts
Administrative law	Develops regulations by which to carry out the mission of a public agency	State boards of nursing, which enact and enforce rules as they relate to nurse practice acts
Common law	Interprets legal issues based on previous court decisions in similar cases (legal precedents)	*Tarasoff v. Board of Regents of University of California* [1976], which justifies breaching a client's confidentiality if he or she reveals the identity of a potential victim of crime
Criminal law	Determines the nature of criminal acts that endanger all of society	Identifies the differences in first-degree and second-degree murder, manslaughter, etc.
Civil law	Determines the circumstances and manner in which a person may be compensated for being the victim of another person's action or omission of an action	Dereliction of duty, negligence

BOX 3-1 Scope of Nursing Practice as Defined in Sample Nurse Practice Act

The practice of nursing means the performance of services provided for purposes of nursing diagnosis and treatment of human responses to actual or potential health problems consistent with educational preparation. Knowledge and skill are the basis for assessment, analysis, planning, intervention, and evaluation used in the promotion and maintenance of health and nursing management of illness, injury, infirmity, restoration of optional function, or death with dignity. Practice is based on understanding the human condition across the human life span and understanding the relationship of the individual within the environment. This practice includes execution of the medical regime including the administration of medications and treatments prescribed by any person authorized by state law to so prescribe.

From Oklahoma Nurse Practice Act, 2003. Oklahoma Statutes, Title 59, Chapter 12, Section 567.1 et seq. Retrieved September 2009 from http://www.ok.gov/nursing/actwp.pdf.

Nurse Licensure Compacts

Several states are considering **nurse licensure compacts**, agreements between states in which a nurse licensed in one state can practice in another without obtaining an additional license (Fig. 3-1). Under this agreement, the nurse acknowledges that he or she is subject to each state's nurse practice act and discipline. Advantages include the following:

- Simplifies the licensing process and removes barriers, thus increasing employability and access to nursing care.
- Is more cost-effective than multiple licensing fees.
- Decreases barriers for nurses who live in one state and want to work in another nearby.
- Reduces the need for duplicate listings of nurses working in more than one state for disaster planning and preparedness or other times of need for qualified nursing services.
- Facilitates a cost-effective alternative when a nurse is employed to provide **telenursing**, health triage, or information from his or her state through electronic or telephonic access to residents in another state.
- Responds to the health care delivery trend in which nurses are employed in small hospitals or satellite agencies that have merged with multistate health care systems.

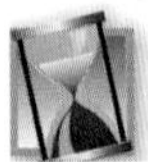

Gerontologic Considerations

■ **Telehealth services**, technology that facilitates the transmission of health assessment and monitoring data with audio, video, and Internet-based devices, contribute to the welfare of homebound elderly or those who live in rural, remote, or underserved areas for health care.

■ Telehealth, which is reimbursed by Medicare, provides quick access of home health nurses with clients, decreases client anxiety, and results in substantial cost-reduction without compromising quality of care (Miller, 2008).

The traditional method of separate licenses for each state of practice provides a legal loophole when one state revokes a nurse's license as a disciplinary measure. Some nurses move to the state where their license is still active and continue to work. Legislation has been enacted, however, to track incompetent practitioners. Since 1989, the names of licensed health care workers who have been disciplined by hospitals, courts, licensing boards, professional associations, insurers, and peer review committees are submitted to a computerized National Practitioner Data Bank. The information is made available nationwide to licensing boards and health care facilities that hire nurses, should they choose to check it. Under the nurse licensure compact, the state of licensure and the state where the client was located during an incident may take disciplinary action against a nurse working under

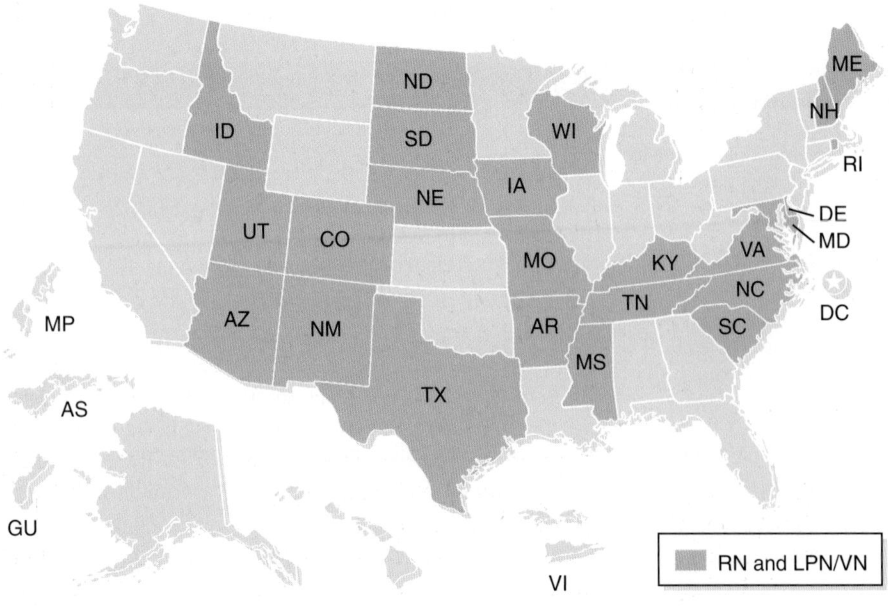

FIGURE 3-1 States participating in the Nurse Licensure Compact (NLC) as of June 2011. (From National Council of State Boards of Nursing. [2011]. Nurse Licensure Compact Administrators. Map of NLC States. Retrieved June 15, 2011 from https://www.ncsbn.org/2537.htm.)

a multistate agreement. Some employers also are requiring that potential and current employees undergo a state or federal background check and drug screen.

Common Law

Common law (decisions based on prior similar cases) is also known as *judicial law*. It is based on the principle of *stare decisis* ("let the decision stand"), in which prior outcomes guide decisions in other jurisdictions dealing with comparable circumstances. Common law refers to litigation that falls outside the realm of constitutional, statutory, and administrative laws.

Criminal Laws

Criminal laws (penal codes that protect all citizens from people who pose a threat to the public good) are used to prosecute those who commit crimes. The state represents "the people" when prosecuting those accused of crimes. Crimes are either misdemeanors or felonies. A **misdemeanor** is a minor criminal offense (eg, shoplifting). If a person is convicted of a misdemeanor, a small fine, a short period of incarceration, or both may be levied. The fine is paid to the state. A **felony** is a serious criminal offense, such as murder, falsifying medical records, insurance fraud, and stealing narcotics. Conviction is punishable by a lengthy prison term or even execution. The state generally prohibits felons from obtaining an occupational license, and the state will revoke such a license if its holder is convicted of a felony.

Civil Laws

Civil laws (statutes that protect personal freedoms and rights) apply to disputes between individual citizens. Some examples include laws that protect the right to be left alone, freedom from threats of injury, freedom from offensive contact, and freedom from character attacks. In civil cases, the **plaintiff** (person claiming injury) brings charges against the **defendant** (person charged with violating the law). The case is referred to as a **tort** (litigation in which one person asserts that a physical, emotional, or financial injury was a consequence of another person's actions or failure to act). A tort implies that a person breached his or her duty to another person. A **duty** is an expected action based on moral or legal obligations.

It does not take the same quality or quantity of evidence to be convicted in a civil lawsuit as in a criminal case. If a defendant is found guilty of a tort, he or she is required to pay the plaintiff restitution for damages. Torts are classified as intentional or unintentional.

Intentional Torts

Intentional torts are lawsuits in which a plaintiff charges that a defendant committed a deliberately aggressive act. Examples include assault, battery, false imprisonment, invasion of privacy, and defamation.

Assault

Assault is an act in which bodily harm is threatened or attempted. Such harm may be physical intimidation, remarks, or gestures. The plaintiff interprets the threat to mean that force may be forthcoming. A nurse may be accused of assault if he or she verbally threatens to restrain a client unnecessarily (eg, to curtail the use of the signal light).

Battery

Battery (unauthorized physical contact) can include touching a person's body, clothing, chair, or bed. A plaintiff can claim battery even if contact causes no actual physical harm. The criterion is that contact happened without the plaintiff's consent.

Sometimes, nonconsensual physical contact can be justified. For example, health professionals can use physical force to subdue clients with mental illness or under the influence of alcohol or drugs if their actions endanger their own safety or that of others. Documentation must show, however, that the situation required the degree of restraint used. Excessive force is never appropriate when less would have been effective. When recording information about such situations, nurses must describe the behavior and the client's response when lesser forms of restraint were used first.

To protect health care workers from being charged with battery, adult clients are asked to sign a general permission for care and treatment during admission (Fig. 3-2) and additional written consent forms for tests, procedures, or surgery. When seeking a client's consent for specific treatments, the physician must describe the proposed intervention, potential benefits, risks involved, expected outcome, available alternatives, and consequences if the intervention is not performed.

Health care personnel obtain consent from a parent or guardian if the client is a minor, is developmentally disabled, or is mentally incompetent. In an emergency, consent can be implied. In other words, it is assumed that in life-threatening circumstances, a client would give consent for treatment if he or she were able to understand the risks. In most cases, another physician must concur that the emergency procedure is essential.

False Imprisonment

A plaintiff can allege **false imprisonment** (interference with a person's freedom to move about at will without legal authority to do so) if a nurse detains a competent client from leaving the hospital or other health care agency. If a client wants to leave without being medically discharged, it is customary for him or her to sign a form indicating personal responsibility for leaving against medical advice (AMA) (Fig. 3-3). If the client refuses to sign the paper, however, health care personnel cannot bar him or her from leaving.

Forced confinement is legal under two conditions: if there is a judicial restraining order (eg, a prisoner admitted for medical care) or if there is a court-ordered commitment (eg, a client with mental illness who is dangerous to self or others).

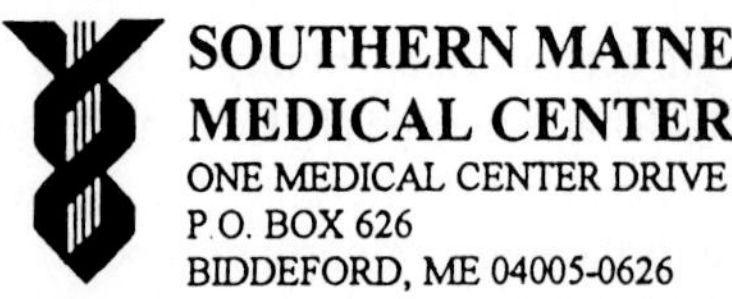

SOUTHERN MAINE MEDICAL CENTER
ONE MEDICAL CENTER DRIVE
P.O. BOX 626
BIDDEFORD, ME 04005-0626

NOTICE
You are being admitted to SMMC as an inpatient.

CONSENT TO TREAT AND/OR ADMIT
When I sign this form, I agree to let SMMC treat me in the emergency department, or as an outpatient, or to admit and treat me as an inpatient at this hospital.

1. SMMC may examine me and perform tests and treatments to help learn about, and care for, my injury or illness.
2. This could mean emergency care or outpatient services with more visits.
3. It could also mean hospital care with a need for inpatient hospital services.

I know that inpatient hospital treatment may mean medications, tests, and nursing care. I agree to this.

I know I can stop all or part of my treatment at any time.

I know my consent is needed to have me take part in any experiments or research.

I know that medicine and surgery have risks. Some tests and treatments could cause harm even death. In some cases I may be asked to sign a separate consent form. SMMC has not told me that any test or treatment will guarantee a certain result.

I know that many staff doctors are not employed by SMMC, but may use the hospital as a place to care for their patients. Other doctors at SMMC may be in post-graduate training programs. Some other health care workers at SMMC may also not be employees of SMMC.

MEDICAL RECORDS RELEASE
I know that, under Maine law, SMMC may give parts of my medical record to those who pay for health care services, check for insurance claims or do medical reviews. SMMC may also release my medical record to other people who may be responsible for my further care. Only parts of my record that relate to these purposes may be released. Maine law also allows SMMC to share health care information about me with my family and household members, unless I instruct SMMC not to do so.

I know that Maine Worker's Compensation law gives my employer(s) and their agents the right to review my record if I may have an injury or illness covered by that law. I know also, that state and federal laws may provide additional protection against giving out information regarding HIV status, mental health services, or services received from an alcohol or drug abuse treatment program.

I know that Maine law gives me the right to decide whether certain health care information may be disclosed to others. I may tell SMMC if I wish to exercise this right. If I do, one of my choices is to have my name left out of the directory that lists people being cared for at SMMC. Leaving my name out of this directory may prevent SMMC from directing visitors and telephone calls to me.

ASSIGNMENT OF INTEREST AND FINANCIAL AGREEMENT
I know I must pay any charges not covered by insurance. I agree to have the payments of insurance and plan benefits (including Medicare) go directly to SMMC. If the payment is in keeping with the provisions of the insurance policy or plan, this will end the claim on the payor to the extent of the payment. If charges are denied, or are not covered by my insurance or plan, I must pay SMMC for these charges. If my account is referred for collection, I may be responsible for all fees required to collect it (including attorney's fees).

ADVANCE APPROVAL FOR MEDICAL SERVICES
If my insurance or health plan says I need an OK for a test or treatment before it is provided, SMMC will try to help me. SMMC cannot, however, promise to get this OK for me. If some services are denied later by my payor, I must pay the balance of my bill.

MEDICARE

_____ I have received a copy of the *Important Message from Medicare.*
(Initial)

_______________ Patient   _______________ Date

_______________ Legal Representative   _______________ Relationship to Patient   _______________ Date

INPATIENT

_______________ Witness

FIGURE 3-2 Example of consent for treatment form. (From Timby, B. K., & Smith, N. E. [2010]. *Introductory medical-surgical nursing* [10th ed., p. 37]. Philadelphia: Lippincott Williams & Wilkins.)

THREE RIVERS HOSPITAL
THREE RIVERS, MICHIGAN 49093

Release from Responsibility for Discharge

Date: ______________________ Time: ____________ A.M. P.M.

CLIENT: ______________________

This is to certify that I ______________________, a client in the ______________________ Hospital, am being discharged against the advice of the attending physician and the hospital administration. I acknowledge that I have been informed of the risk involved and hereby release the attending physician and the hospital from all responsibility for any ill effects that may result from such discharge.

Witnesses:

____

(Signature of Client)

____

(To be signed by the legal representative in case of a minor or of a client who is not mentally competent, otherwise by the client.)

FIGURE 3-3 Example of a release form for discharging oneself against medical advice.

Restraints are devices or chemicals that restrict movement. They are used with the intention to subdue a client's activity. Types include cloth limb restraints, bedrails, chairs with locking lap trays, and sedative drugs. Unnecessary or unprescribed restraints can lead to charges of false imprisonment, battery, or both.

The Nursing Home Reform Act of the Omnibus Budget Reconciliation Act (OBRA) states that residents in nursing homes have "the right to be free of, and the facility must ensure freedom from, any restraints imposed or psychoactive drug administered for purposes of discipline or convenience, and not required to treat the residents' medical symptoms." This is not to say that restraints cannot be used; rather, they should be used as a last resort. Use must be justified and accompanied by informed consent from the client or a responsible relative.

Before using restraints, the best legal advice is to try alternative measures for protecting wandering clients, reducing the potential for falls (see Chap. 19), and ensuring that clients do not jeopardize medical treatment by pulling out feeding tubes or other therapeutic devices. If less restrictive alternatives are unsuccessful, nurses must obtain a medical order before each and every instance in which they use restraints. In acute care hospitals, medical orders for restraints are renewed every 24 hours. When restraints are applied, charting must indicate regular client assessment; provisions for fluids, nourishment, and bowel and bladder elimination; and attempts to release the client from the restraints for a trial period. When the client is no longer a danger to self or others, nurses must remove the restraints.

Invasion of Privacy

Civil law protects citizens from **invasion of privacy** (failure to leave people and their property alone). Nonmedical examples include trespassing, illegal search and seizure, wiretapping, and revealing personal information about someone, even if true. Examples of privacy violations in health care include photographing a client without consent, revealing a client's name in a public report, and allowing an unauthorized person to observe the client's care. To ensure and protect clients' rights to privacy, medical records and information are kept confidential. Personal names and identities are concealed or obliterated in case studies or research. Privacy curtains are used during care; permission is obtained if a nursing or medical student will observe a procedure.

Defamation

Defamation (an act in which untrue information harms a person's reputation) is unlawful. Examples include **slander** (character attack uttered orally in the presence of others) and **libel** (damaging statements written and read by others). Injury is considered to occur because the derogatory remarks attack a person's character and good name.

If a client accuses a nurse of defamation of character, the client must prove that there was malice, misuse of privileged information, and spoken or written untruths. Nurses are at risk for defamation of character suits if they make negative comments in public areas (eg, elevators), or assert opinions regarding a client's character in the medical record. To avoid accusations of defamation, nurses must avoid making or writing negative comments about clients, physicians, or other coworkers.

Unintentional Torts

Unintentional torts result in an injury, although the person responsible did not mean to cause harm. The two types of unintentional torts involve allegations of negligence and malpractice.

Negligence

Negligence (harm that results because a person did not act *reasonably*) implies that a person acted carelessly. In cases of negligence, a jury decides whether any other prudent person would have acted differently than the defendant, given the same circumstances. For example, a car breaks down on the highway. The driver moves to the side of the road, raises the hood, and activates the emergency flashing lights. If another vehicle strikes the disabled car and the driver of the second car sues, the guilt or innocence of the driver of the disabled car depends on whether the jury believes his or her action was reasonable. *Reasonableness is based on the jury's opinion of what constitutes good common sense.*

Malpractice

Malpractice is professional negligence, which differs from simple negligence. It holds professionals to a higher standard of accountability. Rather than being held accountable for acting as an ordinary, reasonable lay person, in a malpractice case the court determines whether a health care worker acted in a manner comparable to that of his or her peers. The plaintiff must prove four elements to win a malpractice lawsuit: duty, breach of duty, causation, and injury (Box 3-2).

Because the jury may be unfamiliar with the scope of nursing practice, the plaintiff may present other resources in court to prove breach of duty. Some examples include the employing agency's standards for care, written policies and procedures, care plans or clinical pathways, and the testimony of expert witnesses (Fig. 3-4).

The best protection against malpractice lawsuits is competent nursing. Nurses demonstrate competency by participating in continuing education programs, taking nursing courses at colleges or universities, and becoming certified. Defensive nursing practice also involves thorough and objective documentation (see Chap. 9).

BOX 3-2 Elements in a Malpractice Case

Duty—An obligation existed to provide care for the person who claims to have been injured or harmed
Breach of Duty—The caregiver failed to provide appropriate care, or the care provided was given negligently, that is, in a way that conflicts with how others with similar education would have acted given the same set of circumstances
Causation—The caregiver's action, or lack of it, caused the plaintiff harm
Injury—Physical, psychological, or financial harm occurred

One of the best methods for avoiding lawsuits is to administer compassionate care. The "golden rule" of doing unto others as you would have them do unto you is a good principle to follow. Clients who perceive the nurse as caring and concerned tend to be satisfied with their care. The following techniques communicate a caring and compassionate attitude:

- Smiling
- Introducing yourself
- Calling the client by the name he or she prefers
- Touching the client appropriately to demonstrate concern
- Responding quickly to the call light
- Telling the client how long you will be gone if you need to leave the unit; informing the client who will provide care in your absence; alerting the client when you return
- Spending time with the client other than while performing required care
- Being a good listener
- Explaining everything so that the client can understand it
- Being a good host or hostess—offering visitors extra chairs, letting them know where they can obtain snacks and beverages, and directing them to the restrooms and parking areas
- Accepting justifiable criticism without becoming defensive
- Saying "I'm sorry"

Clients can sense when a nurse wants to do a good job, rather than just get a job done. The relationship that develops is apt to reduce the potential for a lawsuit, even if harm occurs.

Stop, Think, and Respond Box 3-1

A nurse warns a weak and debilitated older adult that if she continues to get out of bed during the night without calling for assistance, it will be necessary to apply wrist restraints. Can the nurse legally restrain the client who may be harmed if the behavior does not change?

PROFESSIONAL LIABILITY

All professionals, including nurses, are held responsible and accountable for providing safe and appropriate care. Because nurses have specialized knowledge and proximity to clients, they have a primary role in protecting clients from preventable or reversible complications.

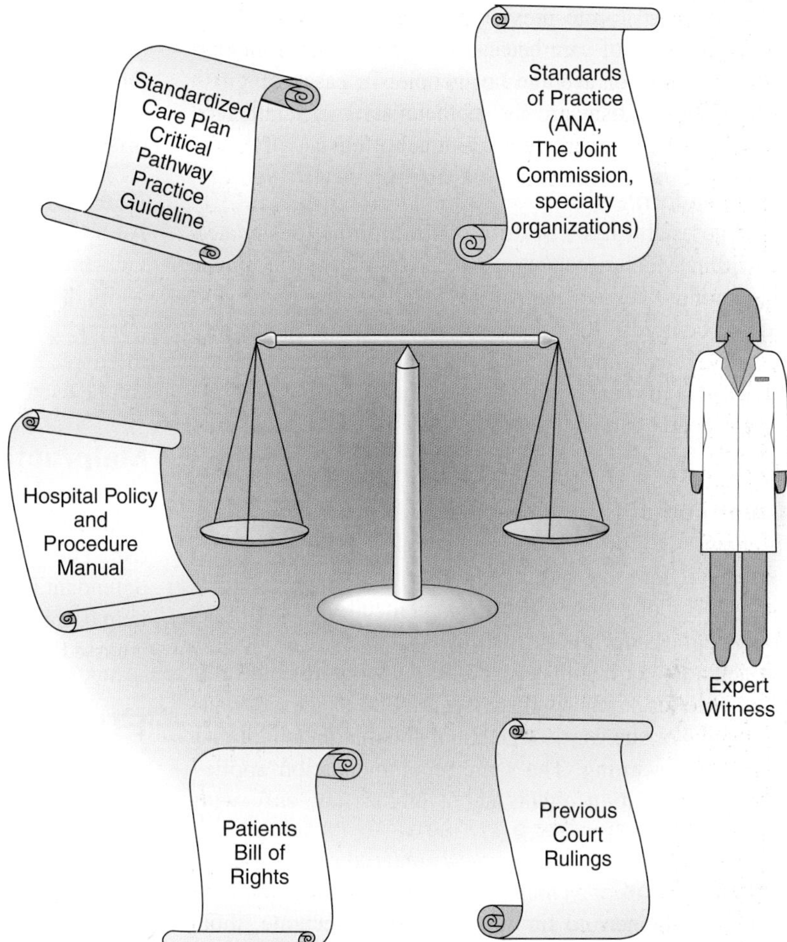

FIGURE 3-4 Data that establish standards of care. (From Timby, B. K., & Smith, N. E. [2010]. *Introductory medical-surgical nursing* [10th ed., p. 41]. Philadelphia: Lippincott Williams & Wilkins.)

The number of lawsuits involving nurses is increasing. It is to every nurse's advantage to obtain liability insurance and to become familiar with legal mechanisms, such as Good Samaritan laws and statutes of limitations, that may prevent or relieve culpability, as well as with strategies for providing a sound legal defense, such as written incident reports and anecdotal records.

Liability Insurance

Liability insurance (a contract between a person or corporation and a company willing to provide legal services and financial assistance when the policyholder is involved in a malpractice lawsuit) is necessary for all nurses. Although many agencies have liability insurance with an umbrella clause that includes its employees, nurses should obtain their own personal liability insurance. The advantage is that a nurse involved in a lawsuit will have a separate attorney working on his or her sole behalf. Because the damages sought in malpractice lawsuits are so costly, attorneys hired by health care facilities sometimes are more committed to defending the facility against liability and negative publicity, rather than defending an employed nurse whom they also are being paid to represent.

Student nurses are held accountable for their actions during clinical practice and should also carry liability insurance. Liability insurance is available through the National Federation for Licensed Practical Nurses, the National Student Nurses' Association, the American Nurses Association (ANA), and other private insurance companies.

Reducing Liability

It is unrealistic to think that lawsuits can be avoided completely. Some avenues protect nurses and other health care workers from being sued or provide a foundation for a sound legal defense. Examples include Good Samaritan laws, statutes of limitations, principles regarding assumption of risk, appropriate documentation, risk management, incident reports, and anecdotal records.

Good Samaritan Laws

Most states have enacted **Good Samaritan laws**, which provide legal immunity to passersby who provide emergency first aid to victims of accidents. The legislation is based on the biblical story of the person who gave aid to a beaten stranger along a roadside. The law defines an emergency as one occurring outside of a hospital, not in an emergency department.

Although these laws are helpful, no Good Samaritan law provides absolute exemption from prosecution in the event of injury. Paramedics, ambulance personnel, physicians, and nurses who stop to provide assistance are still held to a higher standard of care because they have training above and beyond that of average lay people. In cases of gross negligence (total disregard for another's safety), health care workers may be charged with a criminal offense.

Statute of Limitations

Each state establishes a **statute of limitations** (designated time within which a person can file a lawsuit). The length varies among states and generally is calculated from when the incident occurred. When the injured party is a minor, however, the statute of limitations sometimes does not commence until the victim reaches adulthood. When the time expires, an injured party can no longer sue, even if his or her claim is legitimate.

Assumption of Risk

If a client is forewarned of a potential safety hazard and chooses to ignore the warning, the court may hold the client responsible. For example, if a hospitalized client objects to having the side rails up or lowers the rails independently, the nurse or health care facility may not be held fully accountable for an injury. It is essential that the nurse document that he or she warned the client and that the client disregarded the warning. The same recommendation applies when nurses caution clients about ambulating only with assistance.

Documentation

A major component to limiting liability is accurate, thorough documentation. Nurses are held responsible or liable for information that they either include or exclude in reports and charting. Each health care setting requires accurate and complete documentation. The medical record is a legal document and is used as evidence in court. Records must be timely, objective, accurate, complete, and legible (see Chap. 9). The quality of the documentation, including neatness and spelling, can influence a jury's decision.

Risk Management

Risk management (the process of identifying and reducing the costs of anticipated losses) is a concept originally developed by insurance companies. Health care institutions now employ risk managers to review all the problems in the workplace, identify common elements, and then develop methods to reduce their risk. A primary tool of risk management is the incident report.

Incident Reports

An **incident report** is a written account of an unusual, potentially injurious event involving a client, employee, or visitor (Fig. 3-5). It is kept separate from the medical record. Incident reports determine how to prevent hazardous situations and serve as a reference in case of future litigation. They must include five important components: (1) when the incident occurred; (2) where it happened; (3) who was involved; (4) what happened; and (5) what actions were taken.

All witnesses are identified by name. Any pertinent statements made by the injured person, before or after the incident, are quoted. Accurate and detailed documentation often helps to prove that the nurse acted reasonably or appropriately in the circumstances.

Anecdotal Records

An **anecdotal record** (personal, handwritten account of an incident) is not recorded on any official form, nor is it filed with administrative records. The nurse retains the information, which is safeguarded and may be used later to refresh the nurse's memory if a lawsuit develops. Anecdotal notes can be used in court on advice of an attorney.

Malpractice Litigation

A successful outcome in a malpractice lawsuit depends on many variables, such as physical evidence and attorney expertise. The appearance, demeanor, and conduct of the nurse defendant inside and outside of the courtroom, however, can help or damage the case. Suggestions in Box 3-3 may help if a nurse becomes involved in malpractice litigation.

ETHICS

The word "ethics" comes from the Greek word *ethos*, meaning customs or modes of conduct. **Ethics** (moral or philosophical principles) direct actions as being either right or wrong. Various organizations, such as those representing nurses, have identified standards for ethical practice, known as a code of ethics, for members within their discipline.

Codes of Ethics

A **code of ethics** (a list of written statements describing ideal behavior) serves as a model for personal conduct. The National Association for Practical Nurse Education and Services, the National Federation for Licensed Practical Nurses, and the International Council of Nurses all have composed codes of ethics. Box 3-4 shows the ANA's current code of ethics. Because of rapidly changing technology, no code is ever specific enough to provide guidelines for every dilemma that nurses may face.

Ethical Dilemmas

An **ethical dilemma** (choice between two undesirable alternatives) occurs when individual values and laws conflict. This is especially true in relation to health care. Occasionally, nurses find themselves in situations that are legal but are personally unethical, or are ethical but illegal. For instance, abortion is legal, but some believe it is unethical. Assisted suicide is illegal (except in Oregon and Washington state), but some believe it is ethical.

Ethical Theories

Nurses generally use one of two ethical problem-solving theories to guide them in solving ethical dilemmas. These are teleology and deontology.

THREE RIVERS AREA HOSPITAL INCIDENT REPORT
CONFIDENTIAL—DO NOT DUPLICATE
Forward to Risk Managment within 48 hours

Addressograph

Indentification	Sex	Age	Incident Date	Time	Shift	Department
_ Inpatient	_ M	__	__/__/__	__:__	_ 1st	________
_ Outpatient	_ F				_ 2nd	________
_ Visitor					_ 3rd	________

Reason for hospitalization/presence on premises: ________________

I. Location of Incident:
- _ Patient room # ____
- _ Patient bathroom
- _ Corridor
- _ Other ____________

II. Type of Incident:
- _ Fall
- _ Medication
- _ Infusion
- _ Lost/found
- _ Burn
- _ Treatment/procdure
- _ Equipment
- _ Needle/sponge count
- _ Other ________

III. Description of Incident: ________________

IV. Nature of Incident:

A. FALLS:

Activity Order:	Pt. Condition Prior to:	Fall Involved:	Patient/Visitor was:
_ Restraints	_ Weak, unsteady	_ Chair, W/C	_ Lying
_ Bedrest only	_ Alert, oriented	_ Stretcher	_ Standing
_ BRP	_ Disoriented/confused	_ Tub/shower	_ Getting on/off
_ Up w/asst.	_ Senile	_ Toilet	_ Sitting
_ Up AD LIB	_ Unconscious	_ Floor condition (below)	_ Ambulating
	_ Medicated/sedated	_ Bed	_ Other ________
	Med. name ______	_ Side rails up	________
	Last dose ______	_ Side fails down	________

B. MEDICATIONS:

Incident Involved:		Factors:	
_ Wrong Med, Tx, procedure	_ Adverse reaction	_ Patient I.D not checked	_ Charting
_ Wrong patient	_ Infiltration	_ Transcription	_ Wrong med from pharmacy
_ Wrong time	_ Other ________	_ Labeling	_ Defective equipment
_ Omission	________	_ Physician orders not clear	_ Communications
_ Incorrect dose	________	_ Physician orders not checked	_ Other ________
_ Incorrect method of administration	________	_ Misread label/dose	

C. OTHER:
- _ Loss of property
- _ Struck by object, equipment
- _ Equipment malfuction
- _ Anesthesia
- _ Patient I.D.
- _ Other ________

V. Nature of Injury (Injury sustained as a result of incident):
- _ Asphyxia, strangulation, inhalation
- _ Head injury
- _ Contagious or infectious disease exposure
- _ Fracture or dislocation
- _ Viscera injury
- _ Sprain or strain
- _ Contusion, cut, laceration
- _ Burn or scald
- _ Chemical burn
- _ No injury
- _ No apparent injury
- _ Other ________

VI. Actions Taken:

Physician notified:	Pt./visitor seen by MD/T&EC:	MD Name	Time
_ Yes _ No	_ Yes _ No	____________	__:__

Physician's findings: ________________

Other follow up: _ No _ Yes–Specify ________________

____________	__/__/__	____________	__/__/__
Name of Person Reporting	*Date*	*Department Director*	*Date*
____________	__/__/__	____________	__/__/__
Supervisor	*Date*	*Risk Management*	*Date*

FIGURE 3-5 Example of an incident report form.

BOX 3-3 Legal Advice

1. Notify the claims agent of your professional liability insurance company.
2. Contact the National Nurses Claims Database through the ANA. This confidential service provides information that supports nurses involved in litigation.
3. Discuss the particulars of the case only with your attorney.
4. Tell your attorney everything.
5. Avoid giving public statements.
6. Reread the client's record, incident sheet, and your anecdotal notes before testifying.
7. Ask to reread information in court if it will help to refresh your memory.
8. Dress conservatively, in a businesslike manner. Avoid excesses in makeup, hairstyle, or jewelry.
9. Look directly at whomever asks a question.
10. Speak in a modulated but audible voice that the jury and others in the court can hear easily.
11. Tell the truth.
12. Use language with which you are comfortable. Do not try to impress the court with legal or medical terms.
13. Say as little as possible in court under cross-examination.
14. Answer the prosecuting lawyer's questions with "Yes" or "No"; limit answers to only the questions asked.
15. If you do not know or cannot remember information, say so.
16. Wait to expand on information if asked by your defense attorney.
17. Remain calm, objective, and cooperative.

BOX 3-4 Code of Ethics for Nurses

1. The nurse, in all professional relationships, practices with compassion and respect for the inherent dignity, worth, and uniqueness of every individual, unrestricted by considerations of social or economic status, personal attributes, or the nature of health problems.
2. The nurse's primary commitment is to the patient, whether an individual, family, group, or community.
3. The nurse promotes, advocates for, and strives to protect the health, safety, and rights of the patient.
4. The nurse is responsible and accountable for individual nursing practice and determines the appropriate delegation of tasks consistent with the nurse's obligation to provide optimum patient care.
5. The nurse owes the same duties to self as to others, including the responsibility to preserve integrity and safety, to maintain competence, and to continue personal and professional growth.
6. The nurse participates in establishing, maintaining, and improving health care environments and conditions of employment conducive to the provision of quality health care and consistent with the values of the profession through individual and collective action.
7. The nurse participates in the advancement of the profession through contributions to practice, education, administration, and knowledge development.
8. The nurse collaborates with other health professionals and the public in promoting community, national, and international efforts to meet health needs.
9. The profession of nursing, as represented by associations and their members, is responsible for articulating nursing values, for maintaining the integrity of the profession and its practice, and for shaping social policy.

Adapted from Fowler, M. D. M., American Nurses Association. (2010). *Guide to the Code of Ethics for Nurses: Interpretation and Application.* Silver Spring, MD, American Nurses Association.

Teleologic Theory

Teleology is ethical decision making based on final outcomes. It is also known as utilitarianism because the ultimate ethical test for any decision is based on what is best for the most people. Stated from a different perspective, teleologists believe "the end justifies the means." Thus, the choice that benefits many people justifies harm that may come to a few. A teleologist would argue that selective abortion (destroying some embryos in a multiple pregnancy) is ethical because it is done to ensure the full-term birth of those that remain. In other words, termination can be justified in some situations but may not be justified in all cases.

Teleologists analyze ethical dilemmas on a case-by-case basis. They propose that an action is not good or bad in and of itself. Instead, the consequences determine whether the action is good or bad. The primary consideration is a desirable outcome for those most affected.

Deontologic Theory

Deontology is ethical decision making based on duty or moral obligations. It proposes that the outcome is not the primary issue; rather, decisions must be based on the morality of the act itself. In other words, certain actions are always right or wrong regardless of circumstances. Deontologists would argue that destroying any fetus is wrong, whether done to save others or not, because killing is immoral. Deontology proposes that health care providers have a moral duty to maintain and preserve life. Thus, deontologists would consider it immoral for a nurse to assist with abortion, suicide for the terminally ill, or execution of a convicted prisoner.

Deontology also proposes that moral duty to others is equally as important as consequences. A duty is an obligation to perform or to avoid an action to which others are entitled. For example, deontologists believe that lying is never acceptable because it violates the duty to tell the truth to those entitled to honest information. Nurses ultimately have a professional duty to their clients, and clients have rights to which they are entitled (Box 3-5).

Stop, Think, and Respond Box 3-2

How might a teleologist and a deontologist approach an ethical dilemma such as managing the care of an infant with microcephaly (small brain and severe cognitive impairment) who develops a very high fever as a result of an infection?

BOX 3-5 A Patient's Bill of Rights

1. The patient has the right to considerate and respectful care.
2. The patient has the right to and is encouraged to obtain from physicians and other direct caregivers relevant, current, and understandable information concerning diagnosis, treatment, and prognosis.
3. The patient has the right to make decisions about the plan of care prior to and during the course of treatment and to refuse a recommended treatment or plan of care to the extent permitted by law and hospital policy and to be informed of the medical consequences of this action.
4. The patient has the right to have an advance directive (such as a living will, health care proxy, or durable power of attorney for health care) concerning treatment or designating a surrogate decision maker with the expectation that the hospital will honor the intent of that directive to the extent permitted by law and hospital policy.
5. The patient has the right to every consideration of privacy. Case discussion, consultation, examination, and treatment should be conducted so as to protect each patient's privacy.
6. The patient has the right to expect that all communications and records pertaining to his or her care will be treated as confidential by the hospital, except in cases such as suspected abuse and public health hazards when reporting is permitted or required by law.
7. The patient has the right to review the records pertaining to his or her medical care and to have the information explained or interpreted as necessary, except when restricted by law.
8. The patient has the right to expect that, within its capacity and policies, a hospital will make a reasonable response to the request of a patient for appropriate and medically indicated care and services. The hospital must provide an evaluation, a service, and/or a referral as indicated by the urgency of the case.
9. The patient has the right to ask and be informed of the existence of business relationships among the hospital, educational institutions, other health care providers, or payers that may influence the patient's treatment and care.
10. The patient has the right to consent to or decline to participate in proposed research studies or human experimentation affecting care and treatment or requiring direct patient involvement, and to have those studies fully explained prior to consent.
11. The patient has the right to expect reasonable continuity of care when appropriate and to be informed by physicians and other caregivers of available and realistic patient care options when hospital care is no longer appropriate.
12. The patient has the right to be informed of hospital policies and practices that relate to patient care, treatment, and responsibilities. The patient has the right to be informed of available resources for resolving disputes, grievances, and conflicts. The patient has the right to be informed of the hospital's charges for services and available payment methods.

Ethical Principles

It is sometimes impossible or impractical to analyze ethical issues from a teleologic or deontologic point of view. Most nurses do not exclusively use one theory's principles. They also can base ethical decisions on six principles that form a foundation for ethical practice: beneficence, nonmaleficence, autonomy, veracity, fidelity, and justice. These principles sometimes conflict with each other.

Beneficence and Nonmaleficence

Beneficence means "doing good" or acting for another's benefit. To do good, an ethical person prevents or removes any potentially harmful factor. For example, if a client has cancer, the beneficent act is to eliminate the cancer with surgery, drugs, or radiation. The difficulty, however, is that a health care worker's approach to "doing good" may not be what the client feels is best. The client may prefer no treatment of the cancer.

Nonmaleficence means "doing no harm" or avoiding an action that deliberately harms a person. Sometimes, however, "harm" is necessary to promote "good." In the previous example of cancer, available treatments can cause pain, nausea, vomiting, hair loss, and susceptibility to infection. Yet, the ultimate benefit is eradicating the cancer. This is an example of the *principle of double effect.* The following criteria can help to resolve cases involving double effect:

- The action itself must not be intrinsically wrong; it must be good or neutral.
- Only the good effect must be intended, even though the harmful effect is foreseen.
- The harmful effect must not be the means of the good effect.
- The good effect must outweigh the harmful effect (Gracyk, 2008).

Autonomy

Autonomy refers to a competent person's right to make his or her own choices without intimidation or influence. For a person to make a decision, he or she must have all relevant information, including treatment options in language he or she understands. The client always has the option of obtaining a second opinion from another practitioner. One outcome may be that the client declines all possible options for treatment, a decision that must be respected.

Conflict can arise if the client's choice poses more risk than potential benefit; is illegal (eg, requesting assistance with suicide), morally objectionable, or medically inappropriate; or interferes with the needs of another person whose case merits higher priority. An example is a young woman who seeks the removal of both breasts because she fears breast cancer. In such a case, the duty to respect the client's wishes can be nullified. One option may be to refer the client to another practitioner.

Veracity

Veracity means the duty to be honest and avoid deceiving or misleading a client. This principle causes conflict when the truth may harm the client by interfering with recovery or worsening the present condition. Avoiding the truth, however, is never justified when it is used to shield the caregiver's discomfort with sharing "bad news" (Aiken, 2004).

Fidelity

Fidelity means being faithful to work-related commitments and obligations. Its application relates to the caregiver's obligation to clients. For example, nurses are obligated to be competent in performing skills and services required for safe and appropriate care. This implies that nurses pursue continuing education and maintain current certification for cardiopulmonary resuscitation (CPR). It also requires that nurses respect clients, provide compassionate care, protect confidentiality, honor promises, and follow their employer's policies.

Justice

Justice mandates that clients be treated impartially without discrimination according to age, gender, race, religion, socioeconomic status, weight, marital status, or sexual orientation. In other words, everyone should have equal distribution of goods and services.

In reality, circumstances may force nurses to devote more attention to an unstable client. For example, a person arrives in the emergency department with fever and vomiting. Shortly thereafter, another person presents with chest pain. The nurse decides to attend to the client with chest pain first. Another example of inequity is when more than one client needs a scarce resource, such as an organ for transplantation. Although several clients have the right to the organ, only one can receive it.

When goods and services cannot be allocated equally, decisions are based on need, merit, or potential for contribution. In the example of the transplant organ, based on need, the most critically ill person would receive it. Based on merit, the organ would be given to the person who worked hardest or made the greatest effort at this point in his or her life. Based on contribution, the person with the greatest potential for positively influencing society in the future would receive the organ (Petechuk, 2006; Principle of Distributive Justice, 2007).

Values and Ethical Decision Making

When a nurse has not taken a course in ethics, his or her ethical decisions are often the result of values. **Values** are a person's most meaningful beliefs and the basis on which he or she makes most decisions about right or wrong. Values commonly are (1) acquired from parental models, life experiences, and religious tenets; (2) reinforced by a person's world view; (3) modeled in personal behavior; (4) consistent over time; and (5) defended when challenged.

The following serve as guidelines to ethical decision making:

- Make sure that whatever is done is in the client's best interest.
- Preserve and support *A Patient's Bill of Rights* (see Box 3-5).
- Work cooperatively with the client and other health practitioners.
- Follow written policies, codes of ethics, and laws.
- Follow your conscience.

Ethics Committees

Ethical decisions are complex, especially when they affect the lives of clients. Because making a judgment for another is a weighty responsibility, many health care agencies have established ethics committees. These committees consist of a broad cross section of professionals and nonprofessionals within the community with varying viewpoints. Their diversity encourages healthy debate about ethics issues. Ethics committees are best used in a policy-making capacity before any specific dilemma. They are also called on to offer advice, however, to protect clients' best interests and to avoid legal battles.

Common Ethical Issues

Several ethical issues recur in nursing practice. Examples include telling the truth, maintaining confidentiality, withholding or withdrawing treatment, advocating for ethical allocation of scarce resources, and protecting vulnerable people from unsafe practices or practitioners.

Truth Telling

Truth telling proposes that all clients have the right to complete and accurate information. It implies that physicians and nurses have a duty to tell clients the truth about matters concerning their health. Personnel demonstrate respect for this right by explaining to the client the status of his or her health problem, the benefits and risks of treatment, alternative forms of treatment, and consequences if the treatment is not administered.

It is the physician's duty to inform clients. Conflict occurs when the client has not been given full information, when facts have been misrepresented, or when a client misunderstands information. In some cases, physicians are reluctant to talk honestly with clients or present the proposed treatment in a biased manner. Often, the nurse is forced to choose between remaining silent in allegiance to the physician and providing the client with the truth. Either action may have frustrating consequences.

Confidentiality

Confidentiality, or safeguarding a person's health information from public disclosure, is the foundation for trust. Nurses must not divulge health information to unauthorized people without the client's written permission. Even giving medical information to a client's health insurance company requires a signed release. Consequently, nurses must use discretion when sharing verbal information so that others do

equality   policies mental health rights to live

LIVING WILL

TO: My family, physicians and all those concerned with my care

I, ________________________, the undersigned "principal", presently residing at ____________________, ____________, and being an adult of sound mind, make this declaration as a directive to be followed if for any reason I become unable to make or communicate decisions regarding my medical care.

I do not want medical treatment that will keep me alive if I am unconscious and there is no reasonable prospect that I will ever be conscious again (even if I am not going to die soon in my medical condition) or if I am near death from an illness or injury with no reasonable prospect of recovery. The procedures and treatment to be withheld and withdrawn include, without limitation, surgery, antibiotics, cardiac and pulmonary resuscitation, respiratory support, and artificially administered feeding and fluids. I direct that treatment be limited to measures to keep me comfortable and to relieve pain, even if such measures shorten my life.

[OPTIONAL] I wish to live out my last days at home rather than in a hospital, if it does not jeopardize the chance of my recovery to a meaningful and conscious life and does not impose an undue burden on my family.

[OPTIONAL] If, upon my death, any of my tissue or organs would be of value for transplantation, therapy, advancement of medical or dental science, research, or other medical, educational or scientific purpose, I freely give my permission to the donation of such tissue or organs.

These directions are the exercise of my legal right to refuse treatment. Therefore, I expect my family, physicians, health care facilities and all concerned with my care to regard themselves as legally and morally bound to act in accordance with my wishes, and in so doing to be free from any liability for having followed my directions.

IN WITNESS WHEREOF, I have executed this declaration, as my free and voluntary act and deed, this _______ day of ________, 2003.

________________________ ________________________

Principal's name: WITNESS:

FIGURE 3-6 A living will.

not hear it indiscriminately. Now that vast information about clients is stored on computers, the duty to protect confidentiality extends to safeguarding written and electronic data.

Withholding and Withdrawing Treatment

Technology often is used to prolong life at all costs, beyond justifying its benefits. Decisions involving life and death may sometimes continue to circumvent clients, a clear violation of ethical principles. Completing advance directives and determining a client's code status ensure that a person's health care is in accordance with his or her wishes.

Advance Directives

Legislation now mandates the discussion of terminal care with clients. Since Congress approved the Patient Self-Determination Act in 1990, health care agencies reimbursed through Medicare must ask clients whether they have executed an **advance directive** (written statement identifying a competent person's wishes concerning terminal care). The two types of advance directives are a living will and a durable power of attorney for health care.

A **living will** is an instructive form of an advance directive; that is, it is a written document that identifies a person's preferences regarding medical interventions to use—or not use—in a terminal condition, irreversible coma, or persistent vegetative state with no hope of recovery (Fig. 3-6). Clients must share advance directives with health care providers to ensure that they are implemented (see Client and Family Teaching 3-1).

A **durable power of attorney for health care** designates a proxy for making medical decisions when the client becomes so incompetent or incapacitated that he or she cannot make decisions independently. The designee can give or withhold permission for treatments on the client's behalf in end-of-life circumstances or when the client is temporarily unconscious.

Living wills and durable powers of attorney for health care are not measures reserved for older adults; any competent adult can initiate them. They are best composed before a health crisis develops to assist care providers and significant others to comply with the client's wishes. A living will and health care proxy can avoid legal expenses, delays in obtaining guardianship, or unwanted decisions made by an ethics committee or court. Thus, nurses should inform all clients about their right to self-determination, encourage them to compose advance directives, and support their decisions.

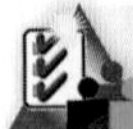

Client and Family Teaching 3-1 Advance Directives

The nurse teaches the following points:

- An advance directive is not required, but it is encouraged.
- A lawyer is not needed to create an advance directive; printed forms are available from health care agencies, organizations such as the American Association of Retired Persons, and various Internet sites such as http://www.ama-assn.org/publicbooklets/livgwill.htm.
- When filling out the form, indicate specific wishes for the initiation or withdrawal of life-sustaining medical treatments such as CPR, kidney dialysis, mechanical ventilation, use of a tube for administering food and water, obtaining comfort measures such as pain medication, and donation of organs.
- Write additional instructions if something is not addressed in the form; for example, your instructions may be different if you are pregnant.
- Obtain the signatures of two witnesses, other than your physician or spouse.
- Give a copy to your physician for your medical file.
- Tell family members or your lawyer that you have an advance directive and its location.
- Keep the original advance directive in a place where it can be found easily.
- Bring a copy of your advance directive whenever you are hospitalized or admitted to a health care facility (eg, nursing home, extended care facility).
- Change your advance directive by revoking or adding instructions at any time; share the revised copy with those who will carry out your instructions.
- A separate or different advance directive is not needed for each state; they are generally recognized universally within the United States.

Code Status

A **code status** refers to how health care personnel are required to manage care in the case of cardiac or respiratory arrest. Without a written order from the physician to the contrary, the client is designated as a full code. A full code means that all measures to resuscitate the client are used.

After a discussion with the physician, some clients indicate that they want no resuscitative efforts, that is, "no code" or "do not resuscitate (DNR)." Or they may select a combination of interventions that constitute less than a full code. Some clients specify using drugs, but refuse cardiac defibrillation or endotracheal intubation for mechanical ventilation. For anything less than a full code, the physician must write an order to that effect in the client's medical record.

Allocation of Scarce Resources

Allocation of scarce resources is the process of deciding how to distribute limited life-saving equipment or procedures among several who could benefit. Such decisions are difficult. In effect, those who receive the resources have a greater chance to live, whereas those who do not may die prematurely. One strategy is "first come, first served." Another is to project what would produce the most good for the most people, although predicting the future is impossible.

Whistle-Blowing

Whistle-blowing (reporting incompetent or unethical practices), as the name implies, calls attention to unsafe or potentially harmful situations. Usually, it occurs in the institution where the reporting person is employed. For instance, a nurse may report another nurse or physician who cares for clients while under the influence of alcohol or a controlled substance.

Whenever a problem is identified, the first step is to report the situation to an immediate supervisor. If the supervisor takes no action, the nurse faces an ethical dilemma about any further steps. Going beyond the administrative hierarchy and making public revelations may be necessary.

The decision to "blow the whistle" involves personal risks and may result in grave consequences such as character assassination, retribution in the form of crimes against one's person or property, negative evaluations, demotions, or shunning. Nevertheless, the ethical priority is protecting clients in general and the community at large.

CRITICAL THINKING EXERCISES

1. What actions might protect a nurse from being sued when a client assigned to his or her care falls out of bed?
2. A client who fell while ambulating to the bathroom sues the assigned nurse. Based on the elements necessary in a malpractice lawsuit, what must the client's lawyer prove? What defense may the nurse's lawyer offer?
3. What criteria justify assisted suicide?
4. Two people need a liver transplant; only one liver is available. What information might a teleologist and a deontologist use to determine who should receive the organ?

NCLEX-STYLE REVIEW QUESTIONS

1. If a nurse suspects that a colleague is stealing narcotics and recording their administration to assigned clients, what is the first action the nurse should take?
   1. Refer the nurse to the ethics committee
   2. Notify the local police department
   3. Share concerns with nursing peers
   4. Report suspicions to a supervisor
2. In a preoperative assessment, what information is most important for the nurse to obtain?
   1. Birth certificate
   2. Social security number
   3. Advance directive
   4. Proof of insurance

3. After checking the condition of a client who has fallen out of bed, what should be the next nursing action?
   1. Institute fall precautions
   2. Complete an incident report
   3. Call the nursing supervisor
   4. Notify the client's family
4. An unresponsive client with terminal cancer stops breathing and has no pulse. There is no advance directive or "do not resuscitate" order on the chart. What action should the nurse take next?
   1. Note the time of death
   2. Notify the physician
   3. Perform postmortem care
   4. Begin resuscitative efforts
5. An agitated and abusive client demands to leave the hospital. Which of the following nursing actions places the nurse at highest risk for being charged with false imprisonment?
   1. The nurse administers a sedative drug to the client.
   2. The nurse threatens to restrain the unruly client.
   3. The nurse calls for security to escort the client.
   4. The nurse publicly talks about the client's behavior.

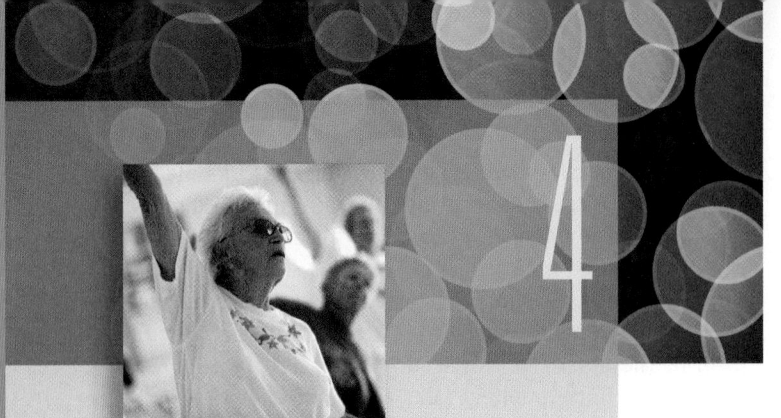

Health and Illness

Words To Know

acute illness
beliefs
capitation
case method
chronic illness
congenital disorder
continuity of care
diagnostic-related group
exacerbation
extended care
functional nursing
health
health care system
health maintenance organizations
hereditary condition
holism
human needs
idiopathic illness
illness
integrated delivery system
managed care organizations
Medicaid
Medicare
morbidity
mortality
nurse-managed care
nursing team
preferred provider organizations
primary care
primary illness
primary nursing
remission
secondary care
secondary illness
sequelae
team nursing
terminal illness
tertiary care
values
wellness

Learning Objectives

On completion of this chapter, the reader should be able to:

1. Describe how the World Health Organization (WHO) defines health.
2. Discuss the difference between values and beliefs, and list health beliefs common among Americans.
3. Explain the concept of holism.
4. Identify five levels of human needs.
5. Define illness and terms used to describe illness.
6. Differentiate primary, secondary, tertiary, and extended care.
7. Name two programs that help finance health care for the aged, disabled, and poor.
8. List four methods to control escalating health care costs.
9. Identify two national health goals targeted for the year 2020.
10. Discuss five patterns that nurses use to administer client care.

Neither health nor illness is an absolute state; rather, there are fluctuations along a continuum throughout life (Fig. 4-1). Because it is impossible to be (or get) well and stay well forever, nurses are committed to helping people prevent illness and restore or improve their health. Nurses accomplish these goals by the following:

- Helping people live healthy lives
- Encouraging early diagnosis of disease
- Implementing measures to prevent complications of disorders

HEALTH

The World Health Organization (WHO) is globally committed to "Health for All." In the preamble to its constitution, WHO defines **health** as "a state of complete physical, mental, and social well-being, not merely the absence of disease or infirmity." Each person perceives and defines health differently. Nurses must recognize the importance of respecting such differences rather than imposing standards that may be unrealistic for the person.

A person's behaviors are the outcomes of his or her values and belief systems. **Values** are ideals that a person feels are important (eg, knowledge, wealth, financial security, marital fidelity, health). **Beliefs** are concepts that a person holds to be true. Beliefs and values guide a person's actions. Both health values and beliefs demonstrate or affirm what is personally significant. When a person values health, he or she takes actions to preserve it.

Most Americans believe one or all of the following: health is a resource, a right, and a personal responsibility.

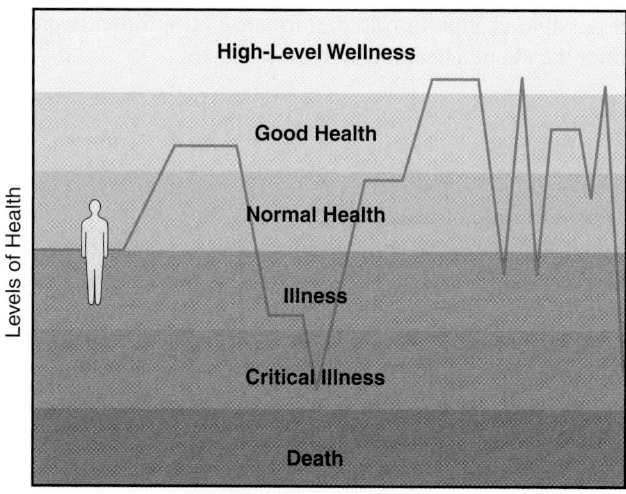

FIGURE 4-1 The health–illness continuum shows the different levels of health a person experiences over a lifetime.

Health: A Limited Resource

A resource is a possession that is valuable because its supply is limited and there is no substitute. Given that definition, health is considered quite precious. People often say, "as long as you have your health, you have everything," and "health is wealth."

Health: A Right

The United States was founded on the principle that everyone is equal and entitled to life, liberty, and the pursuit of happiness. Based on this premise, everyone, regardless of age, gender, level of education, religion, sexual orientation, ethnic origin, social position, or wealth, is entitled to equal services for sustaining health. Unfortunately, as will be discussed later, health disparities exist among various groups within the United States. These groups include the poor, racial and ethnic minorities, those affected by gender differences, older adults, and people with disabilities. Efforts are under way, however, to eliminate health barriers and to promote equal access to health care (see discussion of Healthy People 2020 later in this chapter). If all are equally deserving of health, it follows that the nation in general and nurses in particular have a duty to protect and preserve the health of those who may be unable to assert this right for themselves.

Health: A Personal Responsibility

Health requires continuous personal effort. There is as much potential for illness as there is for health. Each person is instrumental in the outcome. Pilch (1981) said, "No one can do wellness to or for another; you alone do it, but you don't do it alone." Nurses stand ready to provide assistance and to advocate on behalf of others.

WELLNESS

Wellness means a full and balanced integration of all aspects of health. It involves physical, emotional, social, and spiritual health. Physical health exists when body organs function normally. Emotional health results when one feels safe and copes effectively with the stressors of life. Social health is an outcome of feeling accepted and useful. Spiritual health is characterized as believing that one's life has purpose. The four components are collectively referred to as the concept of holism (Fig. 4-2).

Holism

Holism (the sum of physical, emotional, social, and spiritual health) determines how "whole" or well a person feels. Any change in one component, positive or negative, automatically creates repercussions in the others. Take, for example, the person who has a heart attack. Obviously, his or her physical health is immediately impaired. In addition, the heart attack affects the emotional, social, and spiritual aspects of health. For example, the client may experience psychological anxiety over this health change. His or her social roles may temporarily or permanently change. The client may explore philosophical and spiritual issues as he or she considers the potential for death.

Nurses profess to be "holistic practitioners" because they are committed to restoring balance in each of the four spheres that affect health. They base their strategies for doing so on a hierarchy of human needs.

Hierarchy of Human Needs

In the 1960s, Abraham Maslow, a psychologist, identified five levels of **human needs** (factors that motivate behavior). He grouped the needs in tiers, or a sequential hierarchy (Fig. 4-3), according to their significance: physiologic (first level), safety and security (second level), love and belonging

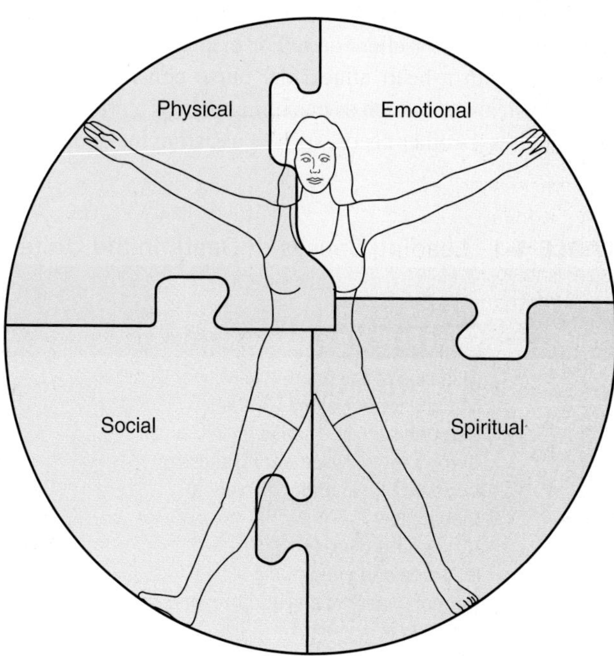

FIGURE 4-2 Holism is a concept that considers all aspects of a person.

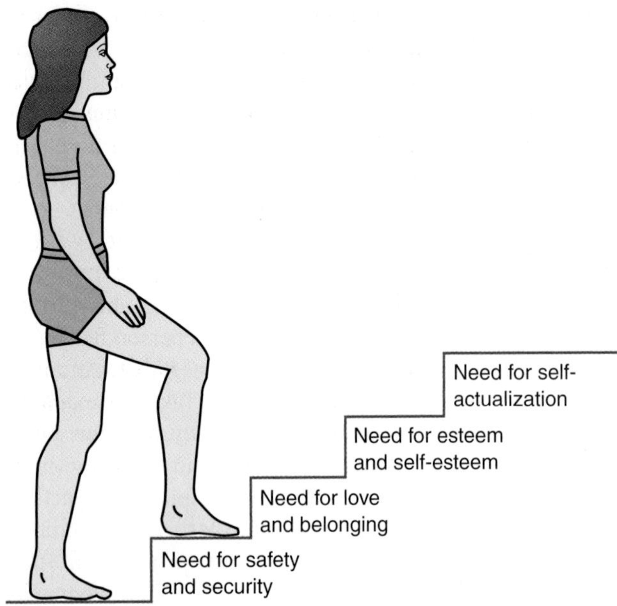

FIGURE 4-3 Maslow's hierarchy of human needs.

(third level), esteem and self-esteem (fourth level), and self-actualization (fifth level).

The first-level physiologic needs are the most important. They are the activities, such as breathing and eating, necessary to sustain life. Each higher level is less important to survival than the previous levels. Maslow believed that until a human satisfies his or her physiologic needs, he or she cannot or will not seek to fulfill other needs. By progressively satisfying needs at each level, however, people will realize their maximum potential for health and well-being.

Nurses have adopted Maslow's hierarchy as a tool for setting priorities for client care. For example, in the case of the client with a heart attack, the nurse considers the client's physical needs such as managing pain as a priority. The nurse addresses other needs, such as assisting the client with a possible change in role performance or spiritual distress, after the client's health condition stabilizes.

ILLNESS

Illness (a state of discomfort) results when disease, deterioration, or injury impairs a person's health. Several terms are used commonly when referring to illnesses: morbidity and mortality; acute, chronic, and terminal; primary and secondary; remission and exacerbation; and hereditary, congenital, and idiopathic.

Morbidity and Mortality

Morbidity (incidence of a specific disease, disorder, or injury) refers to the rate or the numbers of people affected. Federal statistics are compiled on the basis of age, gender, or per 1,000 people within the population. **Mortality** (incidence of deaths) denotes the number of people who died from a particular disease or condition. Table 4-1 lists the 10 leading causes of death among all Americans of all ages in 2006.

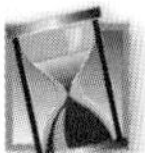

Gerontologic Considerations

- Death rates from heart disease and strokes have continued to decrease over the last three decades, whereas deaths from chronic lung disease, cancer, and diabetes increased from what some attribute to an aging population that is obese and continues to smoke (Reuters, 2005).

Acute, Chronic, and Terminal Illnesses

An **acute illness** (one that comes on suddenly and lasts a short time) is one method for classifying a change in health. Influenza is an example of an acute illness. Many acute illnesses are cured. Some lead to long-term problems

TABLE 4-1 Leading Causes of Death in the United States in 2006

			PERCENTAGE OF TOTAL DEATHS	
RANK	CAUSE OF DEATH	NUMBER	2006	2004
1	Diseases of the heart	631,636	26.03	27.2
2	Malignant neoplasms (cancer)	559,888	23.07	22.9
3	Cerebrovascular disease	137,119	5.65	6.2
4	Chronic lower respiratory diseases	124,583	5.13	5.1
5	Accidents (unintentional injuries)	121,599	5.01	4.5
6	Diabetes	72,448	2.99	3.0
7	Alzheimer's disease	72,432	2.98	2.7
8	Influenza and pneumonia	56,326	2.32	2.5
9	Nephritis, nephritic syndrome, and nephrosis	45,344	1.86	1.7
10	Septicemia	34,234	1.41	1.3

From Heron, M., Hoyert, D.L., Murphy, S.L., et al. (2009). Deaths: Final data for 2006. Accessed September 2009, from http://www.cdc.gov/nchs/data/nvsr57/nvsr57_14.pdf.

because of their **sequelae** (singular: sequela; ill effects that result from permanent or progressive organ damage caused by a disease or its treatment).

Chronic illness (one that comes on slowly and lasts a long time) increases as people age. Arthritis, a joint disease, is an example of a chronic illness.

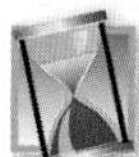

Gerontologic Considerations

- Many older adults live with persistent health problems and disabilities because they survived acute illnesses that killed others years ago.
- Four and a half million Americans now have Alzheimer's disease, which costs $100 billion to care for them. By the year 2050, the figure is expected to quadruple as more people live into their 80s and 90s (Mayo Clinic, 2009).

A **terminal illness** (one in which there is no potential for cure) is one that eventually is fatal. The terminal stage of an illness is one in which a person is approaching death.

Primary and Secondary Illnesses

A **primary illness** (one that develops independently of any other disease) differs from a **secondary illness** (disorder that develops from a preexisting condition). For example, pulmonary disease acquired from smoking is a primary illness. If pneumonia or heart failure occurs as a consequence of smoke-damaged lung tissue, it is considered a secondary problem. In essence, the primary condition predisposed the smoker, in this case, to the secondary condition.

Remission and Exacerbation

A **remission** means the disappearance of signs and symptoms associated with a particular disease. Although a remission resembles a cured state, the relief may be only temporary. The duration of a remission is unpredictable. An **exacerbation** (reactivation of a disorder, or one that reverts from a chronic to an acute state) can occur periodically in clients with long-standing diseases. Often, remissions and exacerbations are related to how well or how poorly the immune system is functioning, the stressors the client is facing, and the client's overall health status (eg, nutrition, sleep, hydration).

Hereditary, Congenital, and Idiopathic Illnesses

A **hereditary condition** (disorder acquired from the genetic codes of one or both parents) may or may not produce symptoms immediately after birth. Cystic fibrosis, a lung disease, and Huntington's chorea, a neurologic disorder, are examples of inherited illnesses. The first is diagnosed soon after birth; the second is not manifested until adulthood.

Congenital disorders (those present at birth but which are the result of faulty embryonic development) cannot be genetically predicted. Maternal illness, such as rubella (German measles) or exposure to toxic chemicals or drugs, especially during the first 3 months of pregnancy, often predisposes the fetus to congenital disorders. Several decades ago, many pregnant women took the drug thalidomide and subsequently gave birth to infants with missing arms and legs. There is a great deal of concern about the role of alcohol in producing fetal alcohol syndrome, a permanent but preventable form of cognitive impairment, and the effects of exposure to other environmental toxins. Although the etiologies for some congenital disorders are well established, they can occur randomly.

An **idiopathic illness** is an illness of unknown cause. Treatment focuses on relieving the signs and symptoms because the etiology is unknown. Examples of idiopathic conditions include hypertension for which there is no known cause or a fever of undetermined origin.

HEALTH CARE SYSTEM

The **health care system** (the network of available health services) involves agencies and institutions where people seek treatment for health problems or assistance with maintaining or promoting their health. The health care system, clients, and their diseases have drastically changed during the past 25 years (Box 4-1). Advances in technology and discoveries in science have created more elaborate methods of diagnosing and treating diseases, creating a need for more specialized care. What was once a system in which people sought medical advice and treatment from one physician, clinic, or hospital has now developed into a complex system involving primary, secondary, tertiary, and extended care.

Primary, Secondary, and Tertiary Care

Primary care (health services provided by the first health care professional or agency a person contacts) usually is given by a family practice physician, nurse practitioner, or physician's assistant in an office or clinic. Cost-conscious health care reforms advocate the provision of primary care by advanced practice nurses.

An example of **secondary care** (health services to which primary caregivers refer clients for consultation and additional testing) is the referral of a client to a cardiac catheterization laboratory. **Tertiary care** (health services provided at hospitals or medical centers where complex technology and specialists are available) may require that a client travels some distance from home. The growing trend is to provide as many secondary and tertiary care services as possible on an outpatient basis or to require no more than 24 hours of inpatient care.

Stop, Think, and Respond Box 4-1

A friend complains of having frequent bouts of indigestion. Explain how primary, secondary, and tertiary care might be involved in this client's care.

BOX 4-1 Trends in Health and Health Care

- Increased older adult population
- Greater ethnic diversity
- More chronic, but preventable illnesses
- More older adults with cognitive disorders (eg, Alzheimer's disease)
- Increased incidence of drug-resistant infections
- Decreased incidence of and death rates from HIV with increased life expectancy associated with expensive drug therapy
- Expanded application of genetic engineering (treating diseases by altering genetic codes)
- Greater success in organ transplantation
- Major efforts at cost containment
- Continued rising costs of health care despite cost-containment measures
- Fewer insured and more underinsured citizens
- More outpatient or ambulatory (1-day stay) care
- Shorter hospital stays
- Less invasive forms of treatment
- Shift to more home care
- Greater focus on disease prevention, health promotion, and health maintenance
- Movement toward more self-care and self-testing
- Approval of more prescription drugs for nonprescription use
- Greater interest in herbal supplements and other "complementary" or alternative treatments
- Nationally linked computer information systems
- Computerized medical record systems
- Shift to criterion-based treatment (clients must meet established criteria to justify treatment measures)
- Increased litigation against health professionals

Extended Care

Extended care (services that meet the health needs of clients who no longer require acute hospital care) includes rehabilitation, skilled nursing care in a person's home or a nursing home, and hospice care for dying clients. Extended care is an important component of the health care system because it allows earlier discharge from secondary and tertiary care agencies and reduces the overall expense of health care.

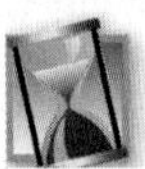

Gerontologic Considerations

- With growing numbers of older dependent persons, society is becoming burdened with providing care for aging adults (Eliopoulos, 2010).
- Older adults who require extended care are those who have generally exhausted home care and various levels of assisted living (Andrews & Boyle, 2007).

Health Care Services

As a whole, health care services include those that offer health prevention, diagnosis, treatment, or rehabilitation. As the types of health services expand, the health care delivery system becomes more complex, costly, and in many cases inaccessible.

Access to Care

According to the U.S. Census Bureau, an estimated 46.3 million citizens do not have access to health care because of the economic burden it poses. This number reflects a rate of 15.8%, a figure that is projected to rise one- or two-tenths of a percent each year. As the number of people covered by an employer's group health insurance has declined, reliance on government plans such as Medicare, Medicaid, and military health care have increased (DeNavas-Walt et al., 2009). Children, older adults, minorities, and the poor are likely to be underserved. Many of these people delay seeking early treatment for their health problems because they cannot afford to pay for services. When an illness becomes so severe that the only choice is to seek medical attention, many turn to their local hospital emergency departments for care. Inappropriate use of emergency departments is expensive and involves long waits and often no follow-up care.

Financing Health Care

Historically, private insurance, self-insurance systems, and Medicare paid for health care. Hospitals and approved providers received payment for what they charged; more charges increased income and profits. These plans offered no incentives to control costs. Disparities in access to health care and the high costs prompted evaluation of the entire health care system. Subsequently, this led to innovative cost-cutting approaches in government payment systems and those financed by private insurers and corporate health plans.

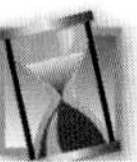

Gerontologic Considerations

- The challenge that the majority of older adults face is the high cost of paying for levels of care in skilled nursing facilities (Andrews & Boyle, 2007).
- For the majority of older American adults, the long-held value to be independent is so strong that many would rather live alone even in poor health than be a burden to his or her family (Andrews & Boyle, 2007).

Government-Funded Health Care: Medicare and Medicaid

Medicare (a federal program that finances health care costs of persons aged 65 years and older, permanently disabled workers of any age and their dependents, and those with end-stage renal disease) is funded primarily through withholdings from an employed person's income. Medicare has two parts:

- Part A covers acute hospital care, rehabilitative care, hospice, and home care services.
- Part B is purchased for an additional fee and covers physician services, outpatient hospital care, laboratory tests, durable medical equipment, and other selected services. Although Medicare is primarily used by older Americans, it does not cover long-term care and limits coverage for health promotion and illness prevention.

TABLE 4-2 Medicare Part D Prescription Drug Benefits

ANNUAL PRESCRIPTION COST TO PARTICIPANT	MEDICARE CONTRIBUTION
Monthly premium of $30, subject to increase based on date of enrolling	
$275 deductible of initial drug expenses	
25% of prescription drugs $275–$2,510	75% of prescription drug costs between $275 and $2,510
100% of drug costs $2,510–$4,050	0% of drug costs = coverage gap (also referred to as the "donut hole")
5% drug costs > $4,050	95% of drug costs > $4,050

Data from Department of Health and Human Services, Centers for Medicare & Medicaid Services (2009), and Medicare Prescription Drug Plans: Medicare Part D. Accessed September 2009, from http://www.webmd.com/medicare/medicare-part-d-prescription-plans.

In 2006, the Medicare drug benefit (Medicare Part D) became available. This and similar plans are being promoted as a means of relieving the financial burden on older Americans and those with low incomes and disabilities who require prescription drugs. Everyone eligible for Medicare can receive prescription drug coverage regardless of income, resources, health status, or current prescription expenses. Part D includes additional cost-sharing assistance for persons with incomes lower than $16,245 and assets less than $12,510 (Kaiser Family Foundation, 2009). Nevertheless, gaps in the system remain (Table 4-2). People are being advised to compare Medicare benefits with standalone prescription drug plans offered by private companies. Some may choose to purchase an additional "Medigap" insurance plan to assist with the cost of deductible and copayments.

Medicaid (a state-administered program designed to meet the needs of low-income residents) is supported by funds from federal, state, and local sources. Each state determines how the funds will be spent. In general, Medicaid programs cover hospitalization, diagnostic tests, physician visits, rehabilitation, and outpatient care. They may also cover long-term care when a person exhausts his or her private funds.

Prospective Payment Systems

In response to escalating health care costs, the federal government implemented a system of prospective payment in 1983 for people enrolled in Medicare. A prospective payment system uses financial incentives to decrease total health care charges by reimbursing hospitals on a fixed rate basis. Reimbursement is based on the **diagnostic-related group** (DRG) (a classification system used to group clients with similar diagnoses). For example, all clients receiving a hip, knee, or shoulder replacement fall into DRG 209, total joint replacement, and the surgeries are reimbursed at basically the same rate. If actual costs are less than the reimbursed amount, the hospital keeps the difference. If costs exceed the reimbursed amount, the hospital is left with the deficit. Hospitals that are inefficient in managing clients' recoveries and early discharges can potentially lose vast revenue, possibly leading to closure of the facility.

Since its inception, the DRG system has been largely responsible for marked decreases in hospital lengths of stay. Subsequently, three major criticisms have surfaced: (1) some older clients are discharged prematurely so as not to exceed the fixed reimbursement, (2) families have had to assume responsibility for the care of clients who cannot function independently after discharge, and (3) increased hospital care costs have been charged to clients with private insurance to make up for the lost Medicare revenues. In response to cost-shifting and other economic forces, private insurance companies have countered by aggressively challenging hospital charges, refusing payment for unjustified billings, and developing their own cost-containment reimbursement system known as managed care.

Managed Care

Managed care organizations (MCOs) (private insurers who carefully plan and closely supervise the distribution of their clients' health care services) control costs of health care and focus on prevention as the best way to manage costs using the following techniques:

- Using health care resources efficiently
- Bargaining with providers for quality care at reasonable costs
- Monitoring and managing fiscal and client outcomes
- Preventing illness through screening and health promotion activities
- Providing client education to decrease the risk for disease
- Minimizing the number of hospitalizations of clients with chronic illness

The two most common types of managed care systems are health maintenance organizations (HMOs) and preferred provider organizations (PPOs). Capitation is a third emerging MCO financial strategy.

Health Maintenance Organizations

Health maintenance organizations (HMOs) are corporations that charge preset, fixed, or yearly fees in exchange for providing health care for their members. The fee remains the same regardless of the type of health service required or the frequency of care. These organizations are able to remain fiscally sound because they offer preventive services, periodic screenings, and health education to keep their members healthy and out of the hospital.

HMOs provide ambulatory, hospitalization, and home care services. Some HMOs have their own health care facilities; others use facilities within the community. A member of an HMO must receive permission for seeking additional care such as second opinions from specialists or unauthorized diagnostic tests. Those members who fail to do so are responsible for the entire bill. In this way, HMOs serve as gatekeepers for health care services.

Preferred Provider Organizations

Preferred provider organizations (PPOs) are agents for health insurance companies that control health care costs on the basis of competition. PPOs create a network of a community's physicians who are willing to discount their fees for service in exchange for a steady supply of referred clients. The subscriber's clients can lower their health care costs by receiving care from any of the preferred providers. If they select providers outside the network, they pay a higher percentage of the costs.

Capitation

An approach that is fundamentally different from HMOs and PPOs is **capitation**, a payment system in which a preset fee per member is paid to a health care provider (usually a hospital or hospital system) regardless of whether the member requires services. Capitation provides an incentive to providers to control tests and services as a means of making a profit. If members do not receive costly care, the provider makes money.

Outcomes of Structured Reimbursement

In many cases, the changes in reimbursements have shifted economic and decision-making power from hospitals and physicians to insurance companies. One criticism is that it is difficult to obtain and provide health care without the economic pressure of insurers. Many claim that the profits of insurance companies come at the expense of quality care. For example, hospitals are using unlicensed assistive personnel to perform some duties that practical/vocational and registered nurses once provided. Current evidence shows that deaths in health care agencies increase as the numbers of licensed nurses decrease (Agency for Healthcare Research and Quality of Care, 2004; Aiken et al., 2008).

On the other hand, cost-driven changes have had positive effects as well. As concern for cost meets concern for quality, health care institutions, nursing personnel, and other providers search for ways to ensure that all care, teaching, and preparation before the discharge date occur without overusing expensive resources.

In an attempt to reduce duplication of health care services and to increase revenue, hospitals and other health care facilities are forming networks known as integrated delivery systems. **Integrated delivery systems** (networks that provide a full range of health care services in a highly coordinated, cost-effective manner) offer diverse options to clients (Box 4-2) and result in shorter hospital stays, fewer complications such as hospital-acquired infections, and quicker return to self-care.

BOX 4-2 Integrated Delivery Systems' Services

Integrated delivery systems provide:

- Wellness programs
- Preventive care
- Ambulatory care
- Outpatient diagnostic and laboratory services
- Emergency care
- Secondary and tertiary services
- Rehabilitation
- Long-term care
- Assisted living facilities
- Psychiatric care
- Home health care services
- Hospice care
- Outpatient pharmacies

NATIONAL HEALTH GOALS

A national ongoing health-promotion effort referred to as *Healthy People 2020* is a continuation of the 1979 Surgeon General's Report, *Healthy People*, and later, *Healthy People 2000: National Health Promotion and Disease Prevention*, and *Healthy People 2010.* The mission of Healthy People 2020 and its four main goals for promoting the nation's health in the 21st century are aimed at improving the quality of life, not just increasing life expectancy, identifying major factors that affect health and wellness, setting public health priorities, and achieving health equity among the nation's citizens (Box 4-3).

Healthy People 2020's four main goals are subdivided into multiple topic areas, each of which has identified *interventions* that consist of programs, policies, and information; *determinants* that identify social, economic, environmental factors, and individual traits; and *outcomes,* such as behaviors, specific risk factors, diseases, mental disorders, disabilities, injuries, and qualities of life (Fig. 4-4). Examples of targeted health goals for achievement are as follows:

- Increase the proportion of people with health insurance
- In the health professions, allied and associated health professions, and nursing increase the proportion of all degrees awarded to members of underrepresented racial and ethnic groups
- Increase the proportion of health and wellness, and treatment programs and facilities that provide full access for people with disabilities
- Reduce the number of new cases of cancer as well as the illness, disability, and death caused by cancer
- Reduce infections caused by key food-borne pathogens
- Improve the visual and hearing health nationally through prevention, early detection, treatment, and rehabilitation (Healthy People 2020)

BOX 4-3 Healthy People 2020 Mission and Goals

Mission

- Identify nationwide health improvement priorities
- Increase public awareness and understanding of the determinants of health, disease, and disability and the opportunities for progress
- Provide measureable objectives and goals that are applicable at the national, state, and local levels
- Engage multiple sectors to take actions to strengthen policies and improve practices that are driven by the best available evidence and knowledge
- Identify critical research, evaluation, and data collection needs

Goals

- Eliminate preventable disease, disability, injury, and premature death
- Achieve health equity, eliminate disparities, and improve the health of all groups
- Create social and physical environments that promote good health for all
- Promote healthy development and healthy behaviors across every stage of life

Fielding, J. E. (2009). Healthy People 2020: Improving our health futures. Retrieved January 11, 2010 from http:www.dialogue4health.org/webforum/PDFs_10_30_09/FIELDING02Oct2009.pdf.

The Healthy People 2020 campaign is being carried out with the combined expertise of the Public Health Service, each state's health department, national health organizations, the Institute of Medicine of the National Academy of Sciences, and selected individuals from the public at large. To meet the targeted goals, health care workers are challenged to implement strategies to improve the overall health of people living in the United States.

NURSING TEAM

The goal of the **nursing team** (personnel who care for clients directly) is to help clients attain, maintain, or regain health (Fig. 4-5). The team may include several types of professionals as well as allied health care workers with special training such as respiratory therapists, physical therapists, and technicians.

Nurses use their unique skills in the hospital as well as other employment areas. Because they have skills that assist the healthy, the dying, and all in between, nurses work in various settings such as HMOs, physical fitness centers, weight-loss clinics, public health departments, home health agencies, and hospices. Wherever nursing personnel work together, they use one of several patterns for managing client care. The five common management patterns are functional

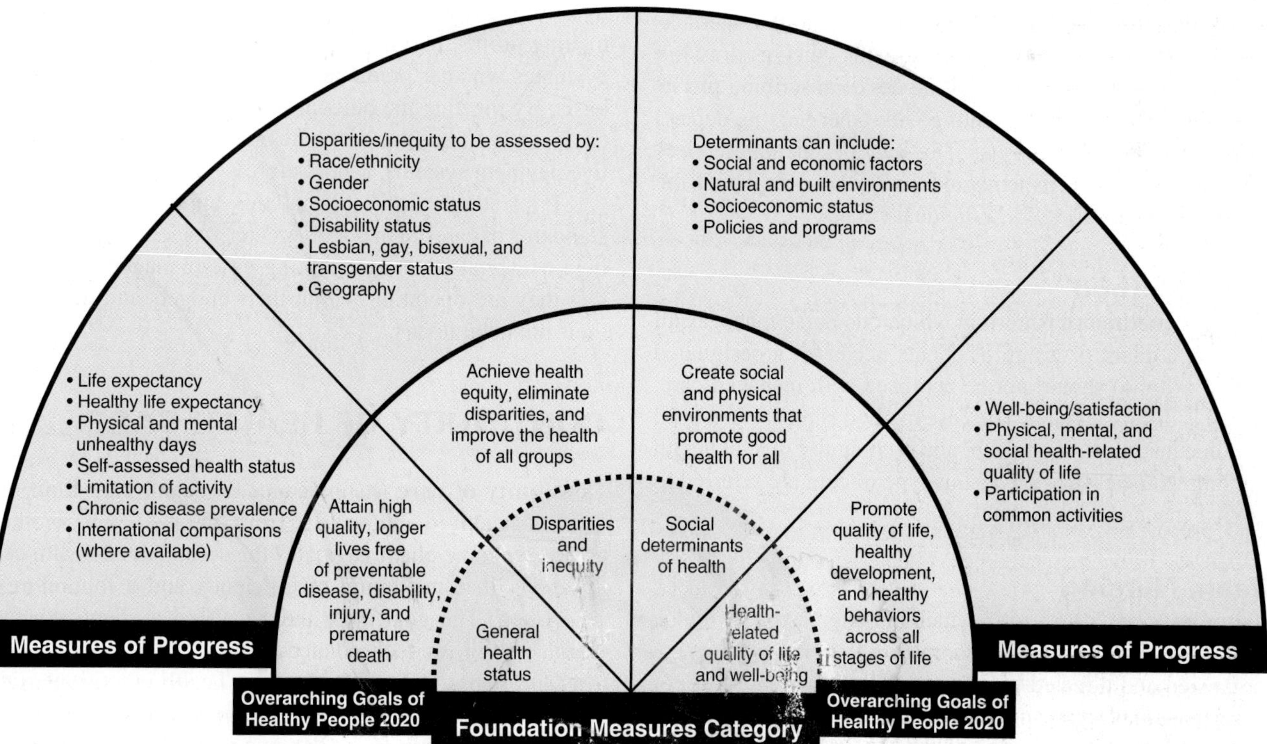

FIGURE 4-4 Components of Healthy People 2020.

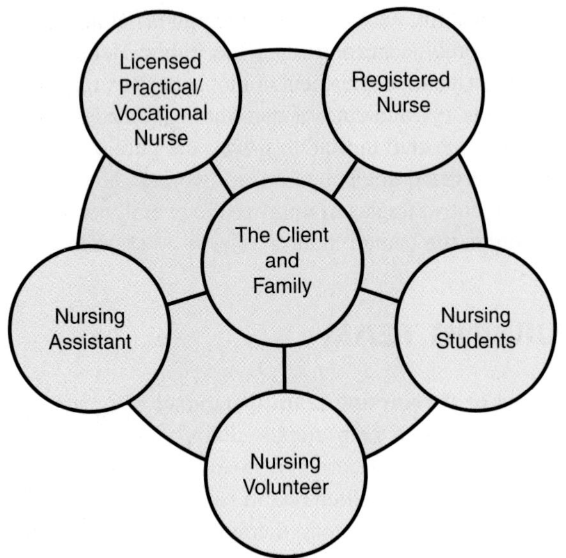

FIGURE 4-5 The nursing team.

nursing, case method, team nursing, primary nursing, and nurse-managed care. Each has advantages and disadvantages. Students are likely to encounter one or all of these methods in their clinical experience.

Functional Nursing

One method used when providing client care is **functional nursing** (a pattern in which each nurse is assigned specific tasks). For example, one is assigned to give all the medications, another performs all the treatments (such as dressing changes), and another works at the desk transcribing physicians' orders and communicating with other nursing departments about client care issues. This pattern is being used less often because its focus tends to be more on completing the task rather than caring for individual clients.

Case Method

The **case method** (a pattern in which one nurse manages all the care a client or group of clients needs for a designated period of time) should not be confused with managed care, which is discussed later. The case method is most often used in home health, public health, and community mental health nursing. Nurses who deliver this type of care are referred to as case managers.

Team Nursing

Team nursing (a pattern in which nursing personnel divide the clients into groups and complete their care together) is organized and directed by a nurse called "the team leader." The leader may assist with but usually assigns and supervises the care that other team members provide. All team members report the outcomes of their care to the team leader. The team leader is responsible for evaluating whether the goals of client care are met.

Conferences are an important part of team nursing. They may cover a variety of subjects but are planned with certain goals in mind such as determining the best approaches to each client's health problems, increasing the team members' knowledge, and promoting a cooperative spirit among nursing personnel.

Primary Nursing

In **primary nursing** (a pattern in which the admitting nurse assumes responsibility for planning client care and evaluating the client's progress), the primary nurse may delegate the client's care to someone else in his or her absence but is consulted when new problems develop or the plan of care requires modifications. The primary nurse remains responsible and accountable for specific clients until they are discharged.

Nurse-Managed Care

Another type of nursing care delivery system is **nurse-managed care** (a pattern in which a nurse manager plans the nursing care of clients based on their type of case or medical diagnosis). A clinical pathway typically is used in a managed care approach (see Chap. 1 for more information on managed care and an example of a clinical pathway).

Nurse-managed care was developed in response to several problems affecting health care delivery today such as the nursing shortage and the need to balance the costs of medical care with limited reimbursement systems. Nurse-managed care is similar to the principles used by successful businesses. In the business world, corporations pay executives to forecast trends and determine the best strategies for making profits. In nurse-managed care, a professional nurse evaluates whether predictable outcomes are met on a daily basis. By meeting the outcomes in a timely manner, the client is ready for discharge by the time designated by prospective payment systems, if not before.

Pilot studies indicate that this approach ensures that standards of care are met with greater efficiency and cost savings. Hospitals that are adopting case-managed care report that they are operating within their budgets and decreasing their financial losses.

CONTINUITY OF HEALTH CARE

Continuity of care (maintenance of health care from one level of health to another and from one agency to another) ensures that the client navigates the complicated health care system with a maximum of efficiency and a minimum of frustration. The goal is to avoid causing a client, whether healthy or ill, to feel isolated, fragmented, or abandoned. All too often, this occurs when one health practitioner fails to consult or communicate with others involved in the client's care. Chapters 9 and 10 give examples of how nurses communicate among themselves and with personnel in other institutions to ensure that the client's care is both continuous and goal directed.

CRITICAL THINKING EXERCISES

1. If you were asked to participate in planning the goals and strategies for Healthy People 2020, what suggestions would you make to promote health and to reduce chronic illness?
2. Which pattern for managing client care seems most advantageous for nurses? Which pattern might clients prefer? Give reasons for your selections.
3. What arguments would you offer to persuade others that health care reform would be beneficial for promoting wellness among citizens of the United States?
4. Why might people who manage their diabetes effectively profess that they are "healthy"?

NCLEX-STYLE REVIEW QUESTIONS

1. If all the following client problems exist, which is of highest priority for nursing management?
   1. Low self-esteem
   2. Labored breathing
   3. Feeling powerless
   4. Lack of family support
2. What is the most appropriate initial nursing referral for a person who is experiencing frequent headaches?
   1. Refer to a drug company seeking clinical trial volunteers for a headache medication
   2. Refer to a neurologic institute conducting investigational research on headaches
   3. Refer to a hospital's emergency department for immediate medical treatment
   4. Refer to a family practice physician for a baseline physical examination
3. A hospital nurse's referral to which type of organization is best for promoting continuity of care for a client with terminal cancer?
   1. Preferred provider organization
   2. Home health nursing organization
   3. Health maintenance organization
   4. Managed care organization
4. All of the following are components of Maslow's hierarchy of human needs. Place the categories in progressive sequence beginning with that which is most basic. Use all the options.
   1. Need for love and belonging
   2. Physiologic needs
   3. Need for self-actualization
   4. Need for esteem and self-esteem
   5. Need for safety and security
5. Which one of the following client problems is a nurse correct in identifying as one that compromises the human need for safety and security?
   1. Chronic anxiety
   2. Labored breathing
   3. Severe loneliness
   4. Sleep deprivation

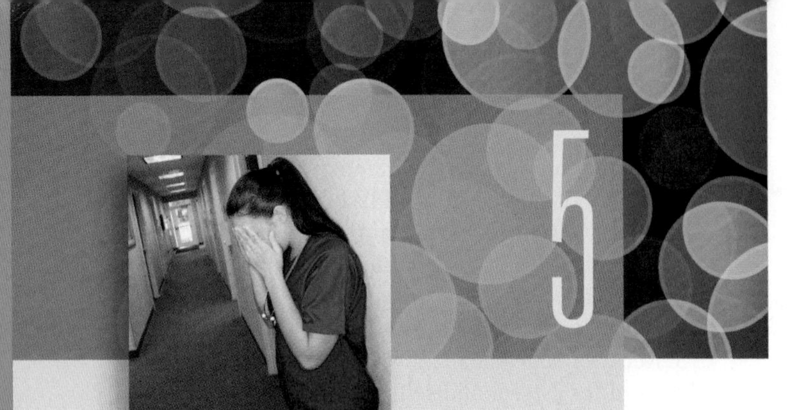

5 Homeostasis, Adaptation, and Stress

Words To Know

adaptation
alarm stage
catastrophize
coping mechanisms
coping strategies
endorphins
feedback loop
fight or flight response
general adaptation syndrome
homeostasis
hypothalamus-pituitary-adrenal (HPA) axis
neurotransmitters
primary prevention
secondary prevention
sensory manipulation
stage of exhaustion
stage of resistance
stress
stress-management techniques
stressors
stress-reduction techniques
stress-related disorders
tertiary prevention

Learning Objectives

On completion of this chapter, the reader should be able to:

1. Explain homeostasis and list categories of stressors that affect homeostasis.
2. Identify two beliefs about the body and mind based on the concept of holism.
3. Identify the purpose of adaptation and two possible outcomes of unsuccessful adaptation.
4. Trace the structures through which adaptive responses take place.
5. Differentiate between sympathetic and parasympathetic adaptive responses.
6. Define stress and list factors that affect the stress response.
7. Discuss the three stages and consequences of the general adaptation syndrome.
8. Name three levels of prevention that apply to reducing or managing stress-related disorders.
9. Explain psychological adaptation and two possible outcomes.
10. Describe the nursing activities helpful to the care of clients prone to stress and approaches for preventing, reducing, or eliminating a stress response.

Health is a tenuous state. To sustain it, the body continuously adapts to **stressors** (changes with the potential to disturb equilibrium). As long as stressors are minor, the body's responses are negligible and generally unnoticed. When stressors are intense or numerous, efforts to restore balance may cause uncomfortable signs and symptoms. With prolonged stress, related disorders and even death may occur.

HOMEOSTASIS

Homeostasis is a relatively stable state of physiologic equilibrium; it literally means "staying the same." Although it sounds contradictory, staying the same requires constant physiologic activity. The body maintains constancy by adjusting and readjusting in response to changes in the internal and external environment that foster disequilibrium.

Holism

Although homeostasis is associated primarily with a person's physical status, emotional, social, and spiritual components also affect it. As discussed in Chapter 4, holism implies that entities in all these areas contribute to the whole of a person. Based on the principles of holism, stressors may be physiologic, psychological, social, or spiritual (Box 5-1).

BOX 5-1 Common Stressors

PHYSIOLOGIC	PSYCHOLOGICAL	SOCIAL	SPIRITUAL
Prematurity	Fear	Gender, racial, age discrimination	Guilt
Aging	Powerlessness	Isolation	Doubt
Injury	Jealousy	Abandonment	Hopelessness
Infection	Rivalry	Poverty	Conflict in values
Malnutrition	Bitterness	Conflict in relationships	Pressure to join, abandon, or change religions
Obesity	Hatred	Political instability	Religious discrimination
Surgery	Insecurity	Denial of human rights	
Pain		Threats to safety	
Fever		Illiteracy	
Fatigue		Infertility	
Pollution			

Holism is the foundation of two commonly held beliefs: (1) both the mind and the body directly influence humans, and (2) the relationship between the mind and the body can potentially sustain health as well as cause illness. Consequently, it is helpful to understand how the mind perceives information and makes adaptive responses. Both physical and psychological mechanisms of perception and adaptation are discussed later in this chapter.

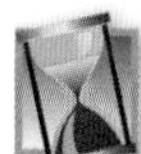

Gerontologic Considerations

■ What may be a stressor to a younger person is sometimes less so for older adults because their life experiences help them to put stressful events in a different perspective. Consequently, older adults may perceive stressors as having less priority or sense of urgency than younger age groups.

Stop, Think, and Respond Box 5-1

List physiologic, psychological, social, and spiritual stressors that can affect homeostasis among nursing students.

Adaptation

Adaptation (the response of an organism to change) requires the use of self-protective properties and mechanisms for regulating homeostasis. Neurotransmitters mediate homeostatic adaptive responses by coordinating functions of the central nervous system, autonomic nervous system, and endocrine system.

Neurotransmitters

Neurotransmitters (chemical messengers synthesized in the neurons) allow communication across the synaptic cleft between neurons, subsequently affecting thinking, behavior, and bodily functions. When released, neurotransmitters temporarily bind to receptor sites on the postsynaptic neuron and transmit their information. After this is accomplished, the neurotransmitter is broken down, recaptured for later use, or weakened (Fig. 5-1).

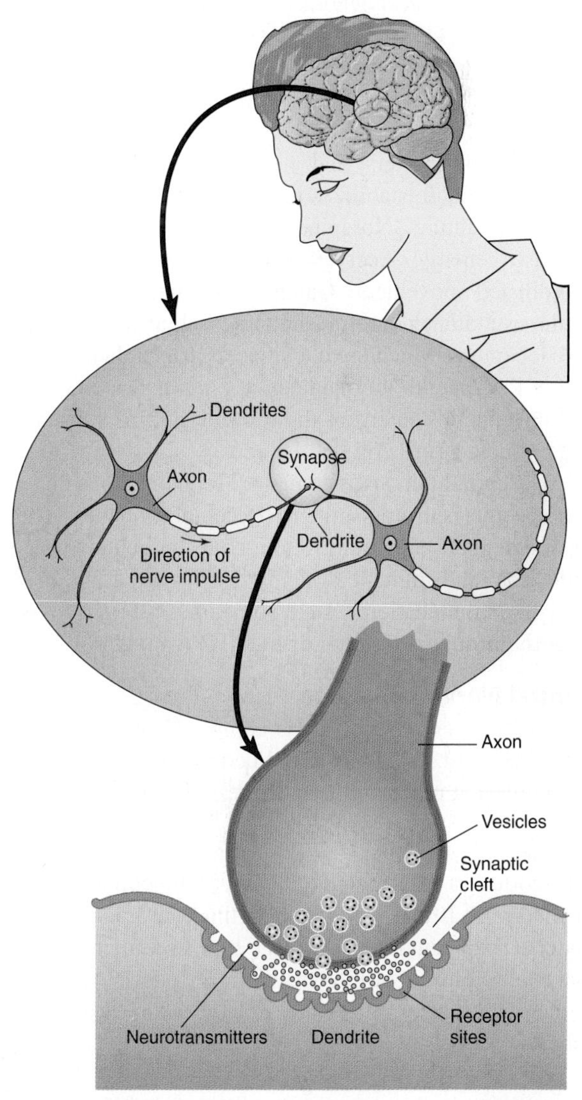

FIGURE 5-1 Neurotransmitter activity. (From Timby, B. K., & Smith, N. E. [2010]. *Introductory medical-surgical nursing* [10th ed.]. Philadelphia, PA: Lippincott Williams & Wilkins.)

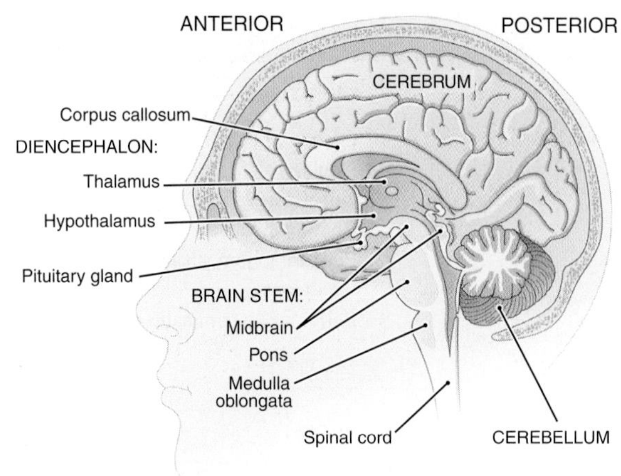

FIGURE 5-2 Central nervous system structures.

Common neurotransmitters include serotonin, dopamine, norepinephrine, acetylcholine, gamma-aminobutyric acid, and glutamate. Other chemical messengers, called "neuropeptides," are actually a separate type of neurotransmitter. Neuropeptides include substance P, endorphins, enkephalins, and neurohormones.

Neurotransmitters and neuropeptides exert different effects. Serotonin stabilizes mood, induces sleep, and regulates temperature. Norepinephrine heightens arousal and increases energy. Acetylcholine and dopamine promote coordinated movement. Gamma-aminobutyric acid inhibits the excitatory neurotransmitters, such as norepinephrine and dopamine, which are classified as catecholamines. Substance P transmits the pain sensation, whereas endorphins and enkephalins interrupt the transmission of substance P and promote a sense of well-being.

Different brain areas contain different neurons that contain specific neurotransmitters. Receptors for these chemical messengers are found throughout the central nervous, endocrine, and immune systems, suggesting a highly integrated communication system sometimes referred to as the **hypothalamus-pituitary-adrenal (HPA) axis**.

Central Nervous System

The central nervous system is composed of the brain and the spinal cord. The brain is divided into the cortex and the structures that make up the subcortex (Fig. 5-2).

Cortex

The cortex is considered the higher functioning portion of the brain. It enables people to think abstractly, use and understand language, accumulate and store memories, and make decisions about information received. The cortex also influences other primitive areas of the brain located in the subcortex.

Subcortex

The subcortex consists of the structures in the midbrain and brainstem. The midbrain, which lies between the cortex and the brainstem, includes the basal ganglia, thalamus, and hypothalamus. The brainstem, so named because it resembles a stalk, contains the cerebellum, medulla, and pons. The subcortical structures are primarily responsible for regulating and maintaining physiologic activities that promote survival. Examples include regulation of breathing, heart contraction, blood pressure, body temperature, sleep, appetite, and stimulation and inhibition of hormone production.

Reticular Activating System

The reticular activating system (RAS), an area of the brain through which a network of nerves pass, is the communication link between the body and the mind. Information about a person's internal and external environment is funneled through the RAS to the cortex on both a conscious and an unconscious level (Fig. 5-3). The cortex processes the information and generates behavioral and physiologic responses through activation by the hypothalamus. The hypothalamus, in turn, influences the autonomic nervous system and endocrine functions (Fig. 5-4).

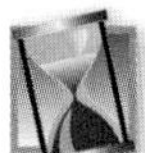

Gerontologic Considerations

- Activity in the RAS is affected by inhibitory neurotransmitters, such as gamma-aminobutyric acid (GABA), and excitatory neurotransmitters such as norepinephrine. Drugs, like alcohol, narcotic analgesics, and tranquilizers, decrease brain activity and induce sleep by simulating or increasing GABA. Drugs, like caffeine, medications for attention deficit disorder, and illegal substances like methamphetamine, increase RAS activity, alertness, and the "thinking activity" of the cortex by stimulating receptors for norepinephrine.
- Self-medication with alcohol and other sedative drugs of abuse, such as narcotic analgesics and tranquilizers, may decrease arousal and produce relaxation temporarily. However, excessive or chronic substance abuse can lead to physical impairment, drug dependence, and legal problems creating more stressors than those for which they were originally intended to relieve.
- Because an unrelieved stress response is generally accompanied by anxiety and depression, short-term prescription drug therapy with anti-anxiety medication such as alprazolam (Xanax) or antidepressant drugs like fluoxetine (Prozac) may help individuals to more realistically assess and address stressors.

Autonomic Nervous System

The autonomic nervous system is composed of peripheral nerves affecting physiologic functions that are largely automatic and beyond voluntary control. It is subdivided into the sympathetic and the parasympathetic nervous systems.

Both the sympathetic and the parasympathetic divisions supply organs throughout the body with nerve pathways. Each division takes a turn being functionally dominant, depending on the appropriate physiologic response. For example, when increased heart rate is needed, the sympathetic division

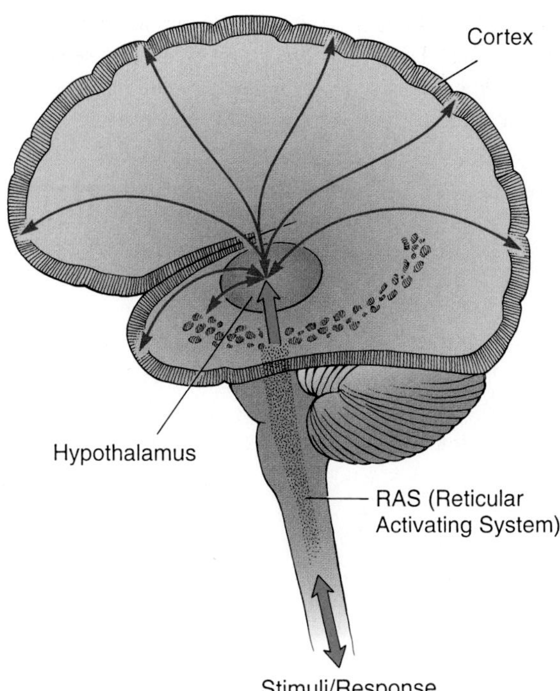

FIGURE 5-3 The reticular activating system is the link in the mind–body connection.

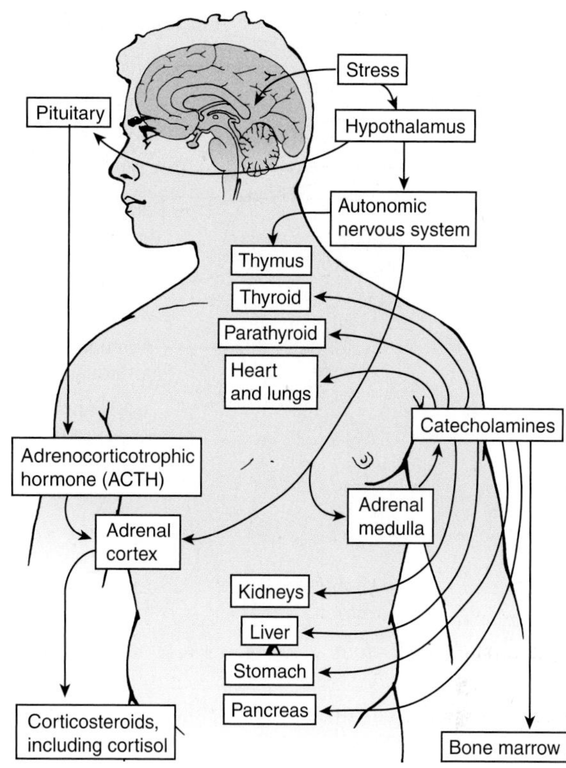

FIGURE 5-4 Homeostatic adaptive pathways.

dominates; when heart rate needs to be slowed, the parasympathetic division takes over.

Sympathetic Nervous System

When a situation occurs that the mind perceives as dangerous, the sympathetic nervous system prepares the body for a **fight or flight response**. It accelerates the physiologic functions that ensure survival through enhanced strength or rapid escape. The person becomes active, aroused, and emotionally charged.

Parasympathetic Nervous System

The parasympathetic nervous system restores equilibrium after danger is no longer apparent. It does so by inhibiting the physiologic stimulation created by its counterpart, the sympathetic nervous system. The parasympathetic nervous system, however, does not produce an opposite reaction for every sympathetic effect (Table 5-1). For this reason, some believe that the parasympathetic nervous system offers an alternate but equally effective mechanism for responding to threats from the internal or external environment. For example, physiologic deceleration, produced by the parasympathetic nervous system, has been likened to the manner in which opossums and other animals "play dead" when they sense that predators are stalking them. Simulating the appearance of death often causes the predator to leave the animal alone, thus saving its life. Therefore, it has been

TABLE 5-1 Sympathetic and Parasympathetic Effects

TARGET STRUCTURE	SYMPATHETIC EFFECT	PARASYMPATHETIC EFFECT
Iris of the eye	Dilates pupils	Constricts pupils
Sweat glands	Increases perspiration	None
Salivary glands	Inhibits salivation	Increases salivation
Digestive glands	Inhibits secretions	Stimulates secretions
Heart	Increases rate and force of contraction	Decreases rate and force of contraction
Blood vessels in the skin	Constrict, causing pale appearance	Dilate causing blush or flushed appearance
Skeletal muscles	Increased tone	Decreased tone
Bronchial muscles	Relaxed (bronchodilation)	Contracted (bronchoconstriction)
Digestive motility (peristalsis)	Decreased	Increased
Kidney	Decreased filtration	None
Bladder muscle (detrusor)	Inhibited (suppressed urination)	Stimulated (urge to urinate)
Liver	Release of glucose	None
Adrenal medulla	Stimulated	None

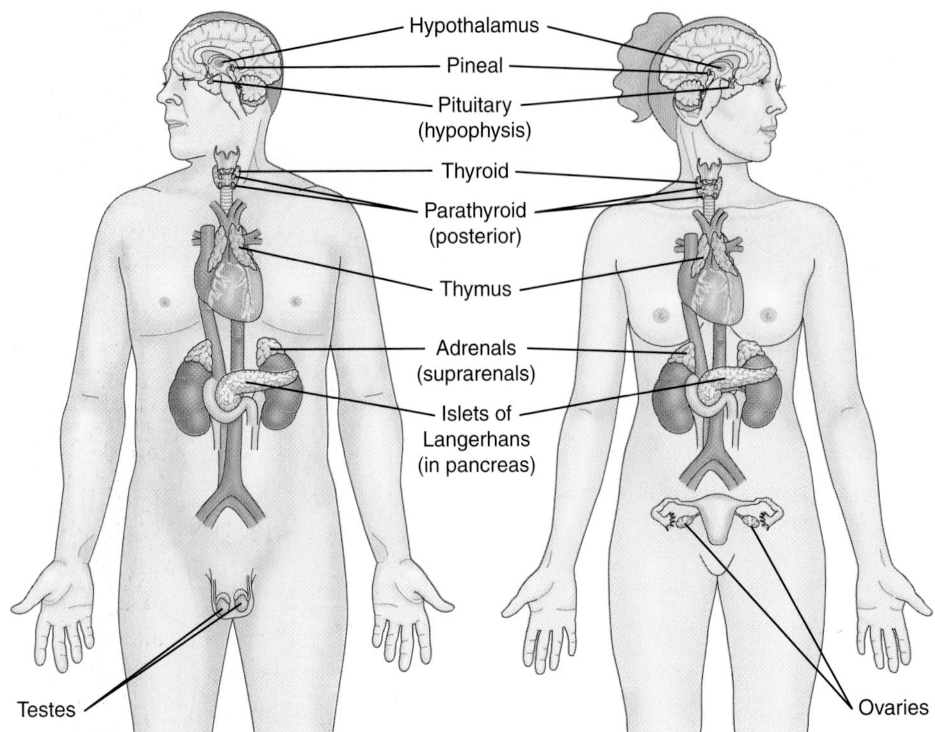

FIGURE 5-5 Endocrine glands.

proposed that humans, too, may respond to stimuli not only by speeding physiologic responses, but also by slowing them down (Nuernberger, 1981).

Endocrine System

The autonomic nervous system provides the initial and immediate response to a perceived threat through either sympathetic or parasympathetic pathways. The endocrine system, a group of glands found throughout the body that produce hormones, sustains the response (Fig. 5-5). Hormones are chemicals produced in one part of the body, the actions of which have physiologic effects on target cells elsewhere.

Neuroendocrine Control

The pituitary gland, located in the brain, is considered the master gland, producing hormones that influence other endocrine glands. The pituitary gland is connected to the hypothalamus, a subcortical structure, through both vascular connections and nerve endings. For pituitary function to occur, the cortex first stimulates the hypothalamus, which then activates the pituitary gland.

Feedback Loop

A **feedback loop** is the mechanism for controlling hormone production (Fig. 5-6). Feedback can be negative or positive. Most hormones are secreted in response to negative feedback; when a hormone level decreases, the releasing gland is stimulated. In positive feedback, the opposite occurs, keeping concentrations of hormones within a stable range at all times. Homeostasis is maintained when hormones are released as needed or inhibited when adequate.

STRESS

As long as demands on the central nervous, autonomic nervous, and endocrine systems are within adaptive capacity, the body maintains homeostasis. When internal or external changes overwhelm homeostatic adaptation, stress results. **Stress** is the physiologic and behavioral responses to disequilibrium. It has physical, emotional, and cognitive effects (Box 5-2).

Although all humans have the capacity to adapt to stress, not everyone responds to similar stressors exactly the same. Differences vary according to (1) the intensity of the stressor, (2) the number of stressors, (3) the duration of

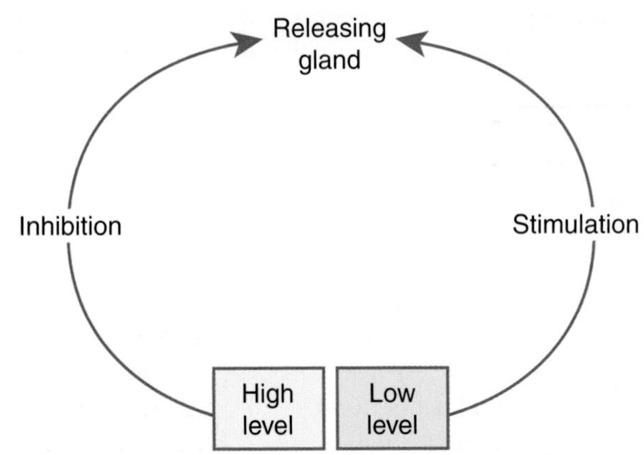

FIGURE 5-6 A feedback loop regulates hormone levels.

BOX 5-2 Common Signs and Symptoms of Stress

Physical
Rapid heart rate
Rapid breathing
Increased blood pressure
Difficulty falling asleep or excessive sleep
Loss of appetite or excessive eating
Stiff muscles
Hyperactivity or inactivity
Dry mouth
Constipation or diarrhea
Lack of interest in sex

Emotional
Irritability
Angry outbursts
Hypercritical
Verbal abuse
Withdrawal
Depression

Cognitive
Impaired attention and concentration
Forgetfulness
Preoccupation
Poor judgment

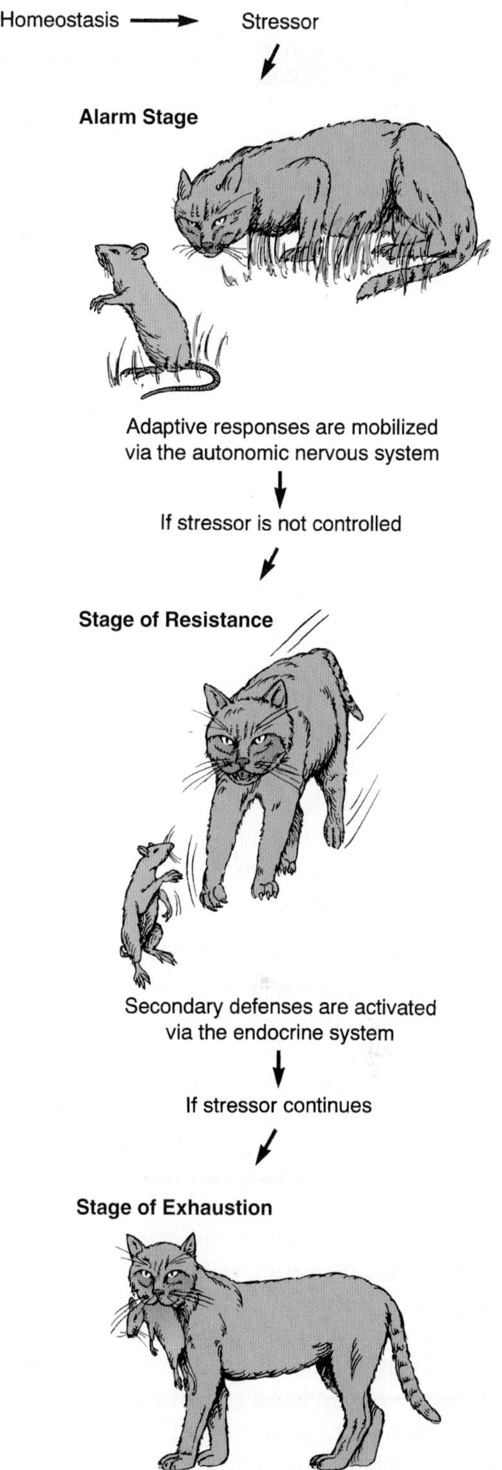

FIGURE 5-7 Stages of the general adaptation syndrome.

the stressor, (4) physical health status, (5) life experiences, (6) coping strategies, (7) social support, (8) personal beliefs, (9) attitudes, and (10) values. Because of unique differences, outcomes may be adaptive or maladaptive, depending on each person's response. Some stress-prone individuals have a tendency to **catastrophize**, choosing to focus on all the potentially negative outcomes that may result from stressors, thus perpetuating and intensifying their response to stress. In other words, they see their cup as half empty rather than half full.

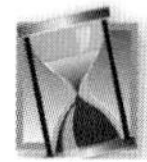

Gerontologic Considerations

■ With advanced age, networks of social support tend to dwindle or disintegrate, diminishing older adults' ability to cope. Social losses may provoke the onset of physical or emotional disorders.

Physiologic Stress Response

Hans Selye, a Canadian physician who lived in the early 1900s, devoted much of his life to researching the collective physiologic processes of the stress response, which he called the **general adaptation syndrome**. Selye observed that this syndrome occurs repeatedly and consistently regardless of the nature of the stressor. He maintained that (1) the body's physical response is always the same, and (2) it follows a one-, two-, or three-stage pattern: alarm stage, stage of resistance, and in some cases, stage of exhaustion (Fig. 5-7). The first two stages parallel the adaptation processes of maintaining homeostasis (discussed earlier). Therefore, brief stress responses generally have adaptive

TABLE 5-2 Actions of Cortisol

MAJOR INFLUENCE	EFFECT ON BODY
Glucose metabolism	Stimulates gluconeogenesis (synthesis of glucose from amino acids and sources other than carbohydrates)
	Decreases glucose use by the tissues
Protein metabolism	Increases breakdown of proteins
	Increases plasma protein levels
Fat metabolism	Increases mobilization and use of fatty acids
Anti-inflammatory action	Stabilizes membranes of inflamed cells, preventing release of proinflammatory mediators
	Decreases capillary permeability to prevent swelling of tissues
	Depresses phagocytosis by white blood cells
	Suppresses the immune response
	Causes atrophy of lymphoid tissue
	Reduces eosinophils (white blood cells active during infectious and allergic reactions)
	Decreases cell-mediated immunity
	Reduces fever
	Inhibits fibroblasts (connective tissue cells that promote wound healing)
Psychic effect	May contribute to emotional instability
Adaptive effect	Facilitates the response of tissues to physiologic changes, such as increased norepinephrine, during trauma and extreme stress

From Porth, C. M., Matfin, G. (2010). *Essentials of pathophysiology: Concepts of altered health states* (3rd ed.). Philadelphia, PA: Lippincott Williams & Wilkins.

outcomes, with restoration of equilibrium. If the stage of resistance is prolonged, however, the process can become maladaptive and pathologic. It can lead to stress-related disorders and, in some cases, death.

Alarm Stage

The **alarm stage** is the immediate physiologic response to a stressor. At its onset, storage vesicles within sympathetic nervous system neurons rapidly release norepinephrine. Shortly thereafter, the adrenal glands secrete additional norepinephrine and epinephrine. These stimulating neurotransmitters and neurohormones prepare the person for a "fight or flight" response; that is, to attack the stressor in an effort to overcome the danger it represents, or flee from the stressor to escape its threat. Almost simultaneously, the hypothalamus releases corticotropin-releasing factor (CRF), which triggers the pituitary gland to secrete adrenocorticotropic hormone (ACTH). The result is the release of cortisol, a stress hormone, from the adrenal cortex.

Cortisol plays various important roles in responding to a stressor such as raising blood glucose as a reserve for meeting increased energy requirements (Table 5-2). Prolonged elevation of norepinephrine, epinephrine, and cortisol levels, however, can predispose clients to stress-related disorders (discussed later in this chapter).

Stage of Resistance

The **stage of resistance**, the second phase in the general adaptation syndrome, is characterized by physiologic changes designed to restore homeostasis. Neuroendocrine hormones, although temporarily excessive, endeavor to compensate for the physiologic changes of the alarm stage. If stress is protracted, however, resistance efforts remain activated. Consequently, one or more organs or physiologic processes may eventually lead to increased vulnerability for stress-related disorders or progression to the stage of exhaustion.

Stage of Exhaustion

The **stage of exhaustion** is the last phase in the general adaptation syndrome. It occurs when one or more adaptive or resistive mechanisms are no longer able to protect the person experiencing a stressor. Once beneficial mechanisms now become destructive. For example, the effects of stress-related neurohormones suppress the immune system. As a result, there are reduced natural killer cells, which attack viruses and cancer cells, and decreased secretory immunoglobulin A, an antibody involved in immune defense. These changes put the person at risk for frequent or severe infections or cancer. Additional disruptions to other organs include reduced beneficial bowel microorganisms and increased bowel pathogens (Kelly, 1999). As resistance dwindles, there is physical and mental deterioration, illness, and death.

Stop, Think, and Respond Box 5-2

List the following stress-related responses in sequential order:

1. *The adrenal cortex releases cortisol.*
2. *The pituitary gland secretes ACTH.*
3. *The body prepares for fight or flight.*
4. *The blood glucose level rises.*
5. *The adrenal glands release norepinephrine and epinephrine.*
6. *The hypothalamus secretes CRF.*
7. *The immune system becomes suppressed.*
8. *Sympathetic neurons release norepinephrine.*

TABLE 5-3 Coping Mechanisms

MECHANISM	EXPLANATION	EXAMPLE
Repression	Forgetting about the stressor	Removing the experience of being sexually abused from conscious memory
Suppression	Purposely avoiding thinking about a stressor	Resolving to "sleep on a problem" or turn the problem over to a higher power, such as God
Denial	Rejecting information	Refusing to believe something like a life-threatening diagnosis
Rationalization	Relieving oneself of personal accountability by attributing responsibility to someone or something else	Blaming failure on a test to the manner in which the test was constructed
Displacement	Taking anger out on something or someone else who is less likely to retaliate	Kicking the wastebasket after being reprimanded by the boss
Regression	Behaving in a manner that is characteristic of a much younger age	Wanting to be bottle-fed like a newborn sibling
Projection	Attributing that which is unacceptable in oneself onto another	Accusing a person of another race of being prejudiced
Somatization	Manifesting emotional stress through a physical disorder	Developing diarrhea that conveniently excuses one from going to work
Compensation	Excelling at something to make up for a weakness of another kind	Becoming a motivational speaker although physically handicapped
Sublimation	Channeling one's energies into an acceptable alternative	Turning to sportscasting when an athletic career is not realistic
Reaction formation	Acting just the opposite of one's feelings	Being extremely nice to someone who is intensely disliked
Identification	Taking on the characteristics of another	Imitating the style of dress, speech, or behavior of another person

Psychological Stress Responses

Just as stress requires adaptation from the body, stress also affects the psyche (mind). The mind, in turn, mounts additional defenses.

Coping Mechanisms

Sigmund Freud posited that humans use **coping mechanisms** (unconscious tactics to defend the psyche) to prevent their ego, or reality base, from feeling inadequate (Table 5-3). These manipulations of reality act as psychological first aid, allowing people to temporarily avoid the emotional effects of stress. When appropriate and moderate, coping mechanisms enable people to maintain their mental equilibrium. Coping mechanisms that are overused or overextended may have maladaptive effects, distorting reality to such an extent that the person fails to recognize and correct his or her weaknesses. Consequently, the person may avoid taking responsibility for solving personal problems.

Coping Strategies

Coping strategies (stress-reduction activities selected consciously) help people to deal with stress-provoking events or situations. They can be therapeutic and nontherapeutic. Therapeutic coping strategies usually help the person to acquire insight, gain confidence to confront reality, and develop emotional maturity. Examples include seeking professional assistance in a crisis, using problem-solving techniques, demonstrating assertive behavior, practicing progressive relaxation, and turning to a comforting person or higher power.

Maladaptation results when people use nontherapeutic coping strategies such as mind- and mood-altering substances, hostility and aggression, excessive sleep, avoidance of conflict, and abandonment of social activities. Negative coping strategies may provide immediate temporary relief from a stressor, but they eventually cause problems.

Stress-Related Disorders

Stress-related disorders are diseases that result from prolonged stimulation of the autonomic nervous and endocrine systems (Box 5-3). Many stress-related diseases involve allergic, inflammatory, or altered immune responses. They are characterized by physical conditions that cycle through asymptomatic periods (absence of the disorder) to episodes that usually develop when the person is under stress. The brain–immune connection suggests that changes in body chemistry during periods of stress may trigger the following: (1) an autoimmune (self-attacking) response like those associated with rheumatoid arthritis and other connective tissue disorders; (2) failure to respond, as in immunosuppression;

BOX 5-3 Stress-Related Disorders

- Hypertension
- Headaches
- Gastritis
- Asthma
- Rheumatoid arthritis
- Skin disorders
- Hyper/hypoinsulinism
- Hyper/hypothyroidism
- Bruxism (teeth grinding)
- Depressive disorders
- Cancer
- Low back pain
- Irritable bowel syndrome
- Allergies
- Anxiety disorders
- Infertility
- Erectile dysfunction

or (3) a weakened immune response, which may contribute to infections and cancer. Even psychological variables such as prolonged anger, feelings of helplessness, and worry can potentially influence the onset and progression of immune system-mediated diseases (Cohen & Herbert, 1996; Godbout & Glaser, 2006).

NURSING IMPLICATIONS

Nurses must be aware of potential stressors affecting clients because they add to the cumulative effect of other stressful life events. When a person is experiencing a stressor, nurses do one or several of the following:

- Identify the stressors
- Assess the client's response to stress
- Eliminate or reduce the stressors
- Prevent additional stressors
- Promote the client's physiologic adaptive responses
- Support the client's psychological coping strategies
- Assist in maintaining a network of social support
- Implement stress reduction and stress management techniques

Assessment of Stressors

Holmes and Rahe (1967) developed, the Social Readjustment Rating Scale, a tool used to predict a person's potential for developing a stress-related disorder. The rating scale is based on the number and significance of social stressors a person has experienced within the previous 6 months (Table 5-4). The risk for a stress-related disorder increases as the person's score rises. Although the dollar amount in the mortgage-related item of the scale is outdated, being in debt is still a major stressor. Therefore, with minor modifications, the assessment tool continues to have diagnostic value.

One research study ranked hospital stressors clients experience in a list modeled after the Social Readjustment Rating Scale (Box 5-4). By being aware of how an illness or interactions with health care personnel and facilities can affect clients, nurses can be instrumental in supporting those who are especially vulnerable.

TABLE 5-4 The Social Readjustment Rating Scale

RANK	LIFE EVENT	LCU VALUE
1	Death of spouse	100
2	Divorce	73
3	Marital separation	65
4	Jail term	63
5	Death of close family member	63
6	Personal injury or illness	53
7	Marriage	50
8	Fired at work	47
9	Marital reconciliation	45
10	Retirement	45
11	Change in health of family member	44
12	Pregnancy	40
13	Sex difficulties	39
14	Gain of new family member	39
15	Business readjustment	39
16	Change in financial state	38
17	Death of close friend	37
18	Change to different line of work	36
19	Change in number of arguments with spouse	35
20	Mortgage over $10,000	31
21	Foreclosure of mortgage or loan	30
22	Change in responsibilities at work	29
23	Son or daughter leaving home	29
24	Trouble with in-laws	29
25	Outstanding personal achievement	28
26	Wife begins or stops work	26
27	Begin or end school	26
28	Change in living conditions	25
29	Revision of personal habits	24
30	Trouble with boss	23
31	Change in work hours or conditions	20
32	Change in residence	20
33	Change in schools	20
34	Change in recreation	19
35	Change in church activities	19
36	Change in social activities	18
37	Mortgage or loan less than $10,000	17
38	Change in sleeping habits	16
39	Change in number of family get-togethers	15
40	Change in eating habits	15
41	Vacation	13
42	Christmas	12
43	Minor violations of the law	11

Social events are ranked from most stressful to least stressful. Each event is assigned a life change unit (LCU) that correlates with the severity of the stressor. The sum of LCUs over the past 6 months is calculated. A score of less than 150 LCUs is considered low risk, a score between 150 and 199 is an indication of mild risk, moderate risk is associated with a score between 200 and 299, and a score over 300 places the person at major risk.

From Holmes, T. H., & Rahe, R. H. (1967). The Social Readjustment Rating Scale. *Journal of Psychosomatic Research, 11*, 216. (Copyright © 1967, Pergamon Press, Ltd.)

Prevention of Stressors

By offering appropriate interventions to people with severe or accumulated stressors, nurses can help prevent or minimize stress-related illness. Prevention takes place at three levels:

- **Primary prevention** involves eliminating the potential for illness before it occurs. An example is teaching principles of nutrition and methods to maintain normal weight and blood pressure to adolescents.
- **Secondary prevention** includes screening for risk factors and providing a means for early diagnosis of disease. An example is regularly measuring the blood pressure of a client with a family history of hypertension.
- **Tertiary prevention** minimizes the consequences of a disorder through aggressive rehabilitation or appropriate management of the disease. An example is frequently turning, positioning, and exercising a client who has had a stroke to help restore functional ability.

BOX 5-4 Client-Related Stressors

Thinking you might lose your sight
Thinking you might have cancer
Thinking you might lose a kidney or some other organ
Knowing you have a serious illness
Thinking you might lose your hearing
Not being told what your diagnosis is
Not knowing for sure what illness you have
Not getting pain medication when you need it
Not knowing the results or reasons for your treatments
Not getting relief from pain medications
Being fed through tubes
Missing your spouse
Not having your questions answered by the staff
Not having enough insurance to pay for your hospitalization
Not having your call light answered
Having a sudden hospitalization you were not planning to have
Being hospitalized far from home
Knowing you have to have an operation
Not having family visit you
Feeling you are getting dependent on medications
Having nurses or doctors talk too fast or use words you cannot understand
Having medications that cause you discomfort
Thinking about losing income because of your illness
Having the staff be in too much of a hurry
Not knowing when to expect things will be done to you
Being put in the hospital because of an accident
Being cared for by an unfamiliar doctor
Not being able to call family or friends on the phone
Having to eat cold or tasteless food
Worrying about your spouse being away from you
Thinking you might have pain because of surgery or test procedures
Being in the hospital during holidays or special family occasions
Thinking your appearance might be changed after your hospitalization
Being in a room that is too cold or too hot
Not having friends visit you
Having a roommate who is unfriendly
Having to be assisted with a bedpan
Having a roommate who is seriously ill or cannot talk with you
Being aware of unusual smells around you
Having to stay in bed or the same room all day
Having a roommate who has too many visitors
Not being able to get newspapers, radio, or TV when you want them
Having to be assisted with bathing
Being awakened in the night by the nurse
Having strange machines around
Having to wear a hospital gown
Having to sleep in a strange bed
Having to eat at different times than you usually do
Having strangers sleep in the same room with you

The events in this list are arranged in order of their perceived significance as a stressor. The first event is the most stressful, and the rest follow in descending order.

Stress-Reduction Techniques

Stress-reduction techniques are methods that promote physiologic comfort and emotional well-being. Some general interventions appropriate during the care of any client include providing adequate explanations in understandable language, keeping the client and family informed, demonstrating confidence and expertise when providing nursing care, remaining calm during crises, being available to the client, responding promptly to the client's signal for assistance, encouraging family interaction, advocating on behalf of the client, and referring the client and family to organizations or people who provide post-discharge assistance.

Stress-Management Techniques

People susceptible to intense stressors or those likely to experience stressors over a long period may benefit from additional stress management approaches. **Stress-management techniques** are therapeutic activities used to reestablish balance between the sympathetic and the parasympathetic nervous systems (Table 5-5). Techniques that counter sympathetic stimulation have a calming effect; stimulating tactics counterbalance parasympathetic dominance. Interventions that cause the release of endorphins, manipulation of sensory stimuli, and adaptive activities also mediate physical and emotional responses to stress. Nurses help clients manage stress, for example, by teaching principles of time management and assertiveness techniques.

Endorphins

Endorphins are natural body chemicals that produce effects similar to those of opiate drugs such as morphine. In addition to decreasing pain, these chemicals promote a sense of pleasantness, tranquility, and well-being.

Endorphins are produced in the pituitary gland but are present in the blood and other tissues (Porth & Matfin, 2008). Some believe that certain activities, such as massage, sustained aerobic exercise, and laughter, trigger the release of endorphins. Once released, endorphins attach themselves to receptor sites in the brain—perhaps in the limbic system, the center where emotions are experienced.

Sensory Manipulation

Sensory manipulation involves altering moods, feelings, and physiologic responses by stimulating pleasure centers in the brain using sensory stimuli. Research is being conducted on the stress-reducing effects of certain colors, full-spectrum lighting in the home and workplace, music, and specific aromas that conjure pleasant associations such as the smell of baking bread.

Adaptive Activities

To enhance adaptation, people experiencing stress may adopt techniques from the following categories: alternative thinking, alternative behaviors, and alternative lifestyles.

TABLE 5-5 Interventions for Stress Management

INTERVENTION	EXPLANATION
Modeling	Promotes the ability to learn an adaptive response by exposing a person to someone who demonstrates a positive attitude or behavior
Progressive relaxation	Eases tense muscles by clearing the mind of stressful thoughts and focusing on consciously relaxing specific muscle groups
Imagery	Uses the mind to visualize calming, pleasurable, and positive experiences
Biofeedback	Alters autonomic nervous system functions by responding to electronically displayed physiologic data
Yoga	Reduces physical and emotional tension through postural changes, muscular stretching, and focused concentration
Meditation and prayer	Reduces physiologic activation by placing one's trust in a higher power
Placebo effect	Alters a negative physiologic response through the power of suggestion

Alternative Thinking

Alternative thinking techniques are those that facilitate a change in a person's perceptions from negative to positive. *Reframing* helps a person to analyze a stressful situation from various perspectives and to ultimately conclude that the situation is not as bad as it once seemed. For instance, instead of dwelling on the negative consequences of a minor car accident, such as the expense and inconvenience of repairs, the person can choose to focus on the positive aspect of being physically unharmed in the accident.

Alternative Behaviors

A behavioral technique for modifying stress is to take control rather than become immobilized. Making choices and pursuing actions promote self-confidence over feeling victimized. Procrastination only prolongs and intensifies the original stressor.

In addition, sharing frustrations with others who are both objective and supportive is more therapeutic than brooding in isolation. Other behavioral approaches to reduce stress include prioritizing what needs to be accomplished and initially attending to that which is most important or difficult. Less important activities may be postponed or delegated to others. And although other positive behaviors can be cultivated, it is also important sometimes to say "no" to avoid becoming overwhelmed and more stressed.

Alternative Lifestyle

People prone to stress can make a conscious effort to improve their diet, become more physically active, cultivate humor, and take scheduled breaks throughout the day for leisure, power naps, or listening to uplifting music. Although pet ownership is not possible for everyone, those who do have pets find it soothing and relaxing to stroke and touch an animal that responds affectionately regardless of a person's age, physical characteristics, or accomplishments. Pets seem to improve a person's feelings of self-worth in a way that extends to human relationships as well.

CRITICAL THINKING EXERCISES

1. Identify at least five interventions that are both realistic and helpful in reducing the stressors associated with being a student.

2. What stressors are more unique to older adults than other age groups?

3. When faced with comments that a person is an alcoholic, explain how the coping mechanism of *denial* can initially protect the drinker's self-image, but can eventually cause harm.

4. How can the coping mechanism of *identification* or any other example in Table 5-3 be positive or negative?

NCLEX-STYLE REVIEW QUESTIONS

1. If a client experiences all of the following, which are the indications of a stress response? Select all that apply.
   1. Rapid heart rate
   2. Double vision
   3. Indigestion
   4. Fatigue
   5. Thirst

2. Which nursing intervention is considered primary in preventing hypertension in a client with a family history of this disorder?
   1. Assess the client's blood pressure monthly
   2. Provide information about antihypertensive medications
   3. Explain stress-management techniques
   4. Teach the client the health hazards of hypertension

3. When caring for an older adult with all the following stressors, which has the highest priority for therapeutic interventions?
   1. Death of a spouse
   2. Change in living conditions
   3. Retirement
   4. Change in financial state

4. Which coping mechanism is being demonstrated when a client refuses treatment because she believes her breast biopsy indicating cancer is incorrect?
   1. Somatization
   2. Regression
   3. Displacement
   4. Denial

5. Which one of the following nursing activities would have the most benefit toward promoting health and wellness?
   1. Encouraging teenagers to never smoke cigarettes
   2. Offering suggestions for smoking cessation
   3. Explaining how to apply nicotine patches to the skin
   4. Advocating that smokers with a chronic cough consult a physician

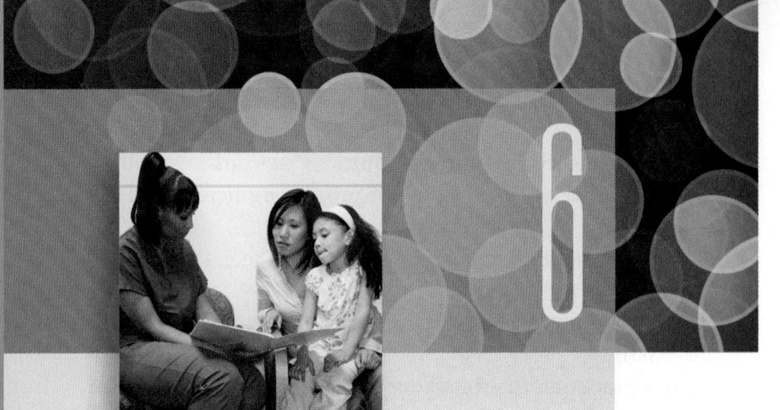

6 Culture and Ethnicity

Words To Know
acultural nursing care
African Americans
ageism
Anglo-Americans
Asian Americans
bilingual
certified interpreter
cultural shock
culturally sensitive nursing care
culture
diversity
ethnicity
ethnocentrism
folk medicine
generalization
Latinos
limited English proficiency (LEP)
minority
Native Americans
race
stereotypes
subcultures
telephonic interpreting
transcultural nursing

Learning Objectives

On completion of this chapter, the reader should be able to:

1. Differentiate culture, race, and ethnicity.
2. Discuss factors that interfere with perceiving others as individuals.
3. Explain why US culture is described as being anglicized.
4. List at least five characteristics of Anglo-American culture.
5. Define the term "subculture" and list four major subcultures in the United States.
6. List five ways in which people from subcultural groups differ from Anglo-Americans.
7. Describe four characteristics of culturally sensitive care.
8. List at least five ways to demonstrate cultural sensitivity.

Clients vary according to age, gender, race, health status, education, religion, occupation, and economic level. Culture, the focus of this chapter, is yet another characteristic that contributes to client **diversity** (differences among groups of people).

Nurses have always cared for clients with differences of some sort. Despite cultural differences, the traditional tendency has been to treat clients as though none exist. Although equal treatment may be politically correct, many nurses now believe that ignoring differences contradicts the best interests of clients. Consequently, there is a movement toward eliminating **acultural nursing care** (care that avoids concern for cultural differences) and promoting **culturally sensitive nursing care** (care that respects and is compatible with each client's culture).

This chapter provides information about cultural concepts, cultural variations among different ethnic and racial groups, and intercultural communication. Although components of culture are specific to a particular group of people, individual clients within each cultural group may deviate from the collective norm. Therefore, nurses are advised to always consider cultural needs from an individual's perspective. Every human being is in some way "like all others, like some others, and like no other" (Andrews, 2005).

CONCEPTS RELATED TO CULTURE

Culture

Culture (the values, beliefs, and practices of a particular group; Giger & Davidhizar, 2008) incorporates the attitudes and customs learned through socialization with others. It includes, but is not limited to, language, communication style, traditions, religion, art, music, dress, health beliefs, and health practices.

A group's culture is passed from one generation to the next. According to Smeltzer and Bare (2010), culture is (1) learned from birth; (2) shared by members of a group; (3) influenced by environment, technology, and the availability of resources; and (4) dynamic and ever changing.

Although the United States has been described as a "melting pot" in which culturally diverse groups have become assimilated, that is not the case. People from various cultural groups have settled, lived, and worked in the United States while continuing to sustain their unique identities (Table 6-1).

Race

Cultural groups tend to share biologic and physiologic similarities. **Race** (biologic variations) is a term used to categorize people with genetically shared physical characteristics. Some examples include skin color, eye shape, and hair texture. Despite wide ranges in physical variations, skin color has traditionally been the chief, albeit imprecise, method for dividing races into Mongoloid, Negroid, and Caucasian. Skin color is just one of a variety of inherited traits.

More importantly, nurses should not equate race with any particular cultural group. To do so leads to two erroneous assumptions: (1) all people with common physical features share the same culture and (2) all people with physical similarities have cultural values, beliefs, and practices that differ from those of **Anglo-Americans** (US whites who trace their ancestry to the United Kingdom and Western Europe).

Minority

The term **minority** is used when referring to those collective people who differ from the dominant group in terms of cultural characteristics such as language, physical characteristics such as skin color, or both. Minority does not necessarily imply that there are fewer group members in comparison with others in the society. Rather, it refers to the group's status with regard to power and control. For example, men of European ancestry are the current "majority" in the United States. Slightly more women than men make up the population of the United States, yet women are considered a minority. By the year 2050, the number of Latinos and Asian Americans living in the United States is expected to triple, and the number of African Americans will nearly double (U.S. Census Bureau, 2008). Until these groups acquire more political and economic power in society, they will continue to be classified as minorities despite the fact that the white population will decrease to only 46% of the total population in 2050.

TABLE 6-1 Culturally Diverse Groups Within the United States

CITY OR REGION	PREDOMINANT CULTURAL GROUP
New England	Irish
Detroit, Buffalo, Chicago	Polish
Upper Midwest (Minnesota, North Dakota)	Scandinavians
Ohio and Pennsylvania	Amish
Washington State and Oregon	Southeast Asians (Laotian, Vietnamese)
New York (Spanish Harlem)	Puerto Rican
Miami (Little Cuba)	Cuban
San Francisco (Chinatown)	Chinese
Manhattan (Little Italy)	Italian
Louisiana	Cajun (French/Indian)
Southwest	Latin American/Native American
Hawaiian Islands	Pacific Islanders/Japanese/Chinese

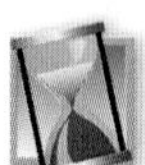

Gerontologic Considerations

- Ethnic populations of color are expected to represent 25% of the elderly by 2030 (Andrews & Boyle, 2008).

Ethnicity

Ethnicity (a bond or kinship a person feels with his or her country of birth or place of ancestral origin) may exist regardless of whether or not a person has ever lived outside of the United States. Pride in one's ethnicity is demonstrated by valuing certain physical characteristics, giving children ethnic names, wearing unique items of clothing, appreciating folk music and dance, and eating native dishes.

Because cultural characteristics and ethnic pride represent the norm in a homogeneous group, they tend to go unnoticed. When two or more cultural groups mix, however, as often happens at the borders of various countries or through the process of immigration, unique differences become more obvious. One or both groups may experience **cultural shock** (bewilderment over behavior that is culturally atypical). Consequently, many ethnic groups have been victimized as a result of bigotry based on stereotypical assumptions and ethnocentrism.

FACTORS THAT IMPACT PERCEPTION OF INDIVIDUALS

Stereotyping

Stereotypes (fixed attitudes about all people who share a common characteristic) develop with regard to age, gender, race, sexual preference, or ethnicity. Because stereotypes are preconceived ideas usually unsupported by facts, they tend to be neither real nor accurate. In fact, they can be dangerous because they interfere with accepting others as unique individuals.

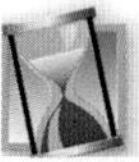

Gerontologic Considerations

- **Ageism**, a form of negative stereotypical thinking about older adults, is the basis for beliefs that the elderly are asexual, cognitively defective, physically incapacitated, and a burden to families and society.

Generalization

Generalization (supposition that a person shares cultural characteristics with others of a similar background) is different than stereotyping. Stereotyping prevents seeing and treating another person as unique, whereas generalizing suggests possible commonalities that may or may not be individually valid. Assuming that all people who affiliate themselves with a particular group behave alike or hold the same beliefs is always incorrect. Diversity exists even within cultural groups.

A generalization provides a springboard from which to explore a person's individuality. For example, when a nurse is assigned to care for a terminally ill client whose last name is Vasquez, the nurse may assume that the client is Roman Catholic because Catholicism is the religion of most Latinos. Before contacting a priest to assist with the client's spiritual needs, however, the nurse understands that the generalization concerning religion may not be accurate. A culturally sensitive nurse strives to obtain information that confirms or contradicts the original generalization.

Ethnocentrism

Ethnocentrism (belief that one's own ethnicity is superior to all others) also interferes with intercultural relationships. Ethnocentrism is manifested by treating anyone "different" as deviant and undesirable. This form of cultural intolerance was the basis for the Holocaust during which the Nazis attempted to carry out genocide, the planned extinction of an entire ethnic group (in this case, European Jews). Ethnocentrism continues to play a role in the ethnic rivalries between Shiites, Sunnis, and Kurds in Iraq; Arabs and Jews in the Middle East; Tutsis and Hutus in Rwanda; Islamic Arabs in Sudan; indigenous African tribes in Darfur, and other regions where culturally diverse groups live in close proximity. Similar conflicts also occur among US ethnic groups.

CULTURE AND SUBCULTURES IN THE UNITED STATES

US culture can be described as anglicized, or English-based, because it evolved primarily from its early English settlers. Box 6-1 provides an overview of some common characteristics of US culture. To suggest that everyone who lives in the United States embraces the totality of its culture, however, would be foolhardy.

Although it is a gross oversimplification, four major **subcultures** (unique cultural groups that coexist within the dominant culture) exist in the United States. In addition to Anglo-Americans, there are also African Americans, Latinos, Asian Americans, and Native Americans (Table 6-2). The 2010 Census allowed individuals to self-select from six race and ethnicity categories (Table 6-3).

The term **African Americans** is used to identify those whose ancestral origin is Africa. It is sometimes used interchangeably with black Americans. **Latinos**, a shortened term

BOX 6-1 Examples of US Cultural Characteristics

- English is the language of communication.
- The pronunciation or meaning of some words varies according to regions within the United States.
- The customary greeting is a handshake.
- A distance of 4 to 12 feet is customary when interacting with strangers or doing business (Giger & Davidhizar, 2008).
- In casual situations, it is acceptable for women as well as men to wear pants; blue jeans are a common mode of dress.
- Most Americans are Christians.
- Sunday is recognized as the Sabbath.
- Government is expected to remain separate from religion.
- Guilt or innocence for alleged crimes is decided by a jury of one's peers.
- Selection of a marriage partner is an individual's choice.
- Legally, men and women are equals.
- Marriage is monogamous (only one spouse); fidelity is expected.
- Divorce and subsequent remarriages are common.
- Parents are responsible for their minor children.
- Aging adults live separately from their children.
- Status is related to occupation, wealth, and education.
- Common beliefs are that everyone has the potential for success and that hard work leads to prosperity.
- Daily bathing and use of a deodorant are standard hygiene practices.
- Anglo-American women shave the hair from their legs and underarms; most men shave their faces daily.
- Licensed practitioners provide health care.
- Drugs and surgery are the traditional forms of medical treatment.
- Americans tend to value technology and equate it with quality.
- As a whole, Americans are time oriented and, therefore, rigidly schedule their activities according to clock hours.
- Forks, knives, and spoons are used, except when eating "fast foods," for which the fingers are appropriate.

TABLE 6-2 Subcultural Groups in the United States[a]

GROUP	REPRESENTATIVE COUNTRIES	US POPULATION ESTIMATE 2008
Total		304,059,724
African American	Africa, Haiti, Jamaica, West Indies, Dominican Republic	2.8%
Latino	Mexico, Puerto Rico, Cuba, South and Central America	15.4%
Asian American	China, Japan, Korea, Philippines, Thailand, Cambodia, Laos, Vietnam, Pacific Islands	4.5%
Native American	Indian and Alaskan tribes	1%

[a]As reported by the U.S. Census Bureau, 2009.

TABLE 6-3 Categories of Race and Ethnicity for Federal Statistics

CATEGORY	DESCRIPTION
White	Persons having origins in Europe, the Middle East, or North Africa
Hispanic or Latino	Persons with origins in Cuba, Mexico, Puerto Rico, South or Central America, or other Spanish culture, regardless of race
Asian	Persons with origins in East Asia, Southeast Asia, or the Indian subcontinent such as Cambodia, China, Japan, Korea, Malaysia, Pakistan, Philippine Islands, Thailand, and Vietnam
Black or African American	Persons having origins in any racial groups of Africa including Haiti
American Indian or Alaska Native	Persons with origins in any of the peoples of North and South America who maintain tribal affiliation or community attachment
Native Hawaiian or Other Pacific Islander	Persons having origins in any of the original peoples of Hawaii, Guam, Samoa, or other Pacific islands

From Revisions to the Standards for Classification of Federal Data on Race and Ethnicity, Office of Management and Budget, 1997.

for *latinoamericano* refers to those who trace their ethnic origin to Mexico, Puerto Rico, Cuba, Central and South America, or other Spanish-speaking countries, such as the Dominican Republic. However, Latinos are sometimes referred to as *Hispanics*, a term coined by the U.S. Census Bureau when referring to those residing in the eastern portion of the United States such as Florida and Texas. The term *Chicanos* is used when referring to people from Mexico, but it may have negative connotations to some. Consequently, it may be more politically correct to use the term *Mexican Americans*. **Asian Americans** (those who come from China, Japan, Korea, the Philippines, Thailand, Cambodia, Laos, and Vietnam) make up the third subculture. **Native Americans** include persons who have their origins in North, Central, and South America, as well as Eskimos and Aleuts, all of whom belong to 564 federally recognized tribes in the United States (Department of Interior, Bureau of Indian Affairs, 2009).

Although Anglo-American culture predominates in the United States, those of African, Asian, Latino/Hispanic, Native Indian, and Hawaiian/Pacific Islander descent will soon outnumber those who trace their ancestry to the United Kingdom and Western Europe. As the population of non–Anglo-Americans rises and becomes more diverse, the need for transcultural nursing is increasingly urgent.

TRANSCULTURAL NURSING

Madeline Leininger coined the term **transcultural nursing** (providing nursing care within the context of another's culture) in the 1970s. Aspects of transcultural nursing include the following:

- Assessments of a cultural nature
- Acceptance of each client as an individual
- Knowledge of health problems that affect particular cultural groups
- Planning of care within the client's health belief system to achieve the best health outcomes

To provide culturally sensitive care, nurses must become skilled at managing language differences, understanding biologic and physiologic variations, promoting health education that will reduce prevalent diseases, and respecting alternative health beliefs or practices.

Cultural Assessment

To provide culturally sensitive care, the nurse strives to gather data about the unique characteristics of clients. Pertinent data include the following:

- Language and communication style
- Hygiene practices, including feelings about modesty and accepting help from others
- Special clothing or ornamentation
- Religion and religious practices
- Rituals surrounding birth, passage from adolescence to adulthood, illness, and death
- Family and gender roles, including child-rearing practices and kinship with older adults
- Proper forms of greeting and showing respect
- Food habits and dietary restrictions
- Methods for making decisions
- Health beliefs and medical practices

Assessment of these areas is likely to reveal many differences. Examples of variations include language and communication, eye contact, space and distance, touch, emotional expressions, dietary customs and restrictions, time, and beliefs about the cause of illness.

Language and Communication

Because language is the primary way to share and gather information, the inability to communicate is one of the biggest deterrents to providing culturally sensitive care. Foreign travelers and many residents in the United States do not speak English, or they have learned it as their second language and do not speak it well. Estimates are that 47 million or 18% of those who live in the United States speak a language other than English at home; Spanish is the most often spoken language other than English in the United States (Fig. 6-1) (Shin & Bruno, 2003). Those who can communicate in English may still prefer to use their primary language, especially under stress.

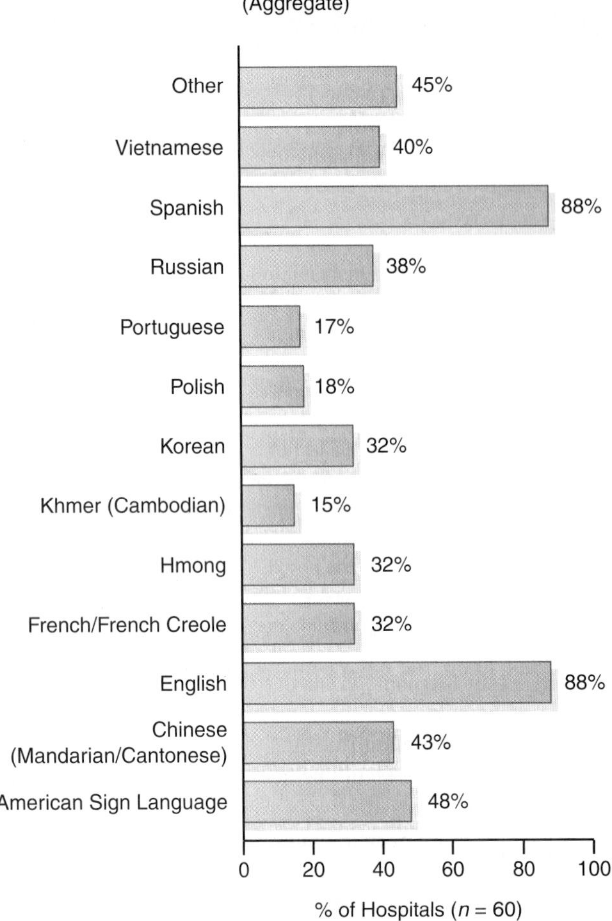

FIGURE 6-1 Spoken languages other than English in the US. A survey of hospitals in 32 states identified Spanish and American Sign Language as the two most commonly spoken languages other than English. (From Wilson-Stronks, A. & Galvez, E. Hospitals, Language, and Culture: A snapshot of the nation. The Joint Commission and The California Endowment. Retrieved November 11, 2011 from http://www.jointcommission.org/NR/rdonlyres/E64E5E89-5734-4D1D-BB4D-C4ACD4BF8BD3/0/hlc_paper.pdf.)

Equal Access. Federal law, specifically Title IV of the Civil Rights Act of 1994, states that people with limited English proficiency (LEP)—an inability to speak, read, write, or understand English at a level that permits interacting effectively—are entitled to the same health care and social services as those who speak English fluently. In other words, all clients have a right to unencumbered communication with a health provider. Using children as interpreters or requiring clients to provide their own interpreters is a civil rights violation. The Joint Commission requires that hospitals provide effective communication for each client.

The use of untrained interpreters, volunteers, or family is considered inappropriate because it undermines confidentiality and privacy. It also violates family roles and boundaries. It increases the potential for modifying, condensing, omitting, adding information, or projecting the interpreter's own values during communication between the client and the health care provider.

BOX 6-2 Characteristics of a Skilled Interpreter

- Learns the goals of the interaction
- Demonstrates courtesy and respect for the client
- Explains his or her role to the client
- Positions himself or herself to avoid disrupting direct communication between the health care worker and the client
- Has a good memory for what is said
- Converts the information in one language accurately into the other without commenting on the content
- Possesses knowledge of medical terminology and vocabulary
- Attempts to preserve the emphasis and emotions that both people express
- Asks for clarification if verbalizations from either party are unclear
- Indicates instances in which a cultural difference has the potential to impair communication
- Maintains confidentiality

The best form of communication with an LEP client is with a **certified interpreter**. A certified interpreter is a translator who is certified by a professional organization through rigorous testing based on appropriate and consistent criteria. Unfortunately, individuals who meet these qualifications are few and far between. To comply with the laws and accreditation requirements, health care agencies are strongly encouraged to train professional interpreters. A competently trained interpreter demonstrates the skills listed in Box 6-2.

When a trained or certified interpreter is not available in person or by webcam, there are a variety of other options. In descending order of preference, the following may be used: agency-employed interpreters, bilingual staff, volunteers, and least desirable, family or friends. The Joint Commission has not yet specified the type of training and competencies of individuals who are used as interpreters, but standards may be forthcoming.

When an on-site interpreter is not available, **telephonic interpreting** (over-the-phone translation) can be used as an alternative. AT&T USADirect In-Language Service provides translators in 140 languages whenever and wherever it is needed. This service costs approximately $2.50 per minute compared to $40 per hour for an on-site interpreter (Roat, 2005). In addition, although it does not meet all the needs of an LEP client, a picture or dual-language communication board may be useful for immediate bedside interactions between the client and the nursing staff (Fig. 6-2).

Culturally Sensitive Nurse–Client Communication. If the nurse is not **bilingual** (able to speak a second language) and a trained interpreter is not available, he or she must use an alternative method for communicating (see Nursing Guidelines 6-1 for more information).

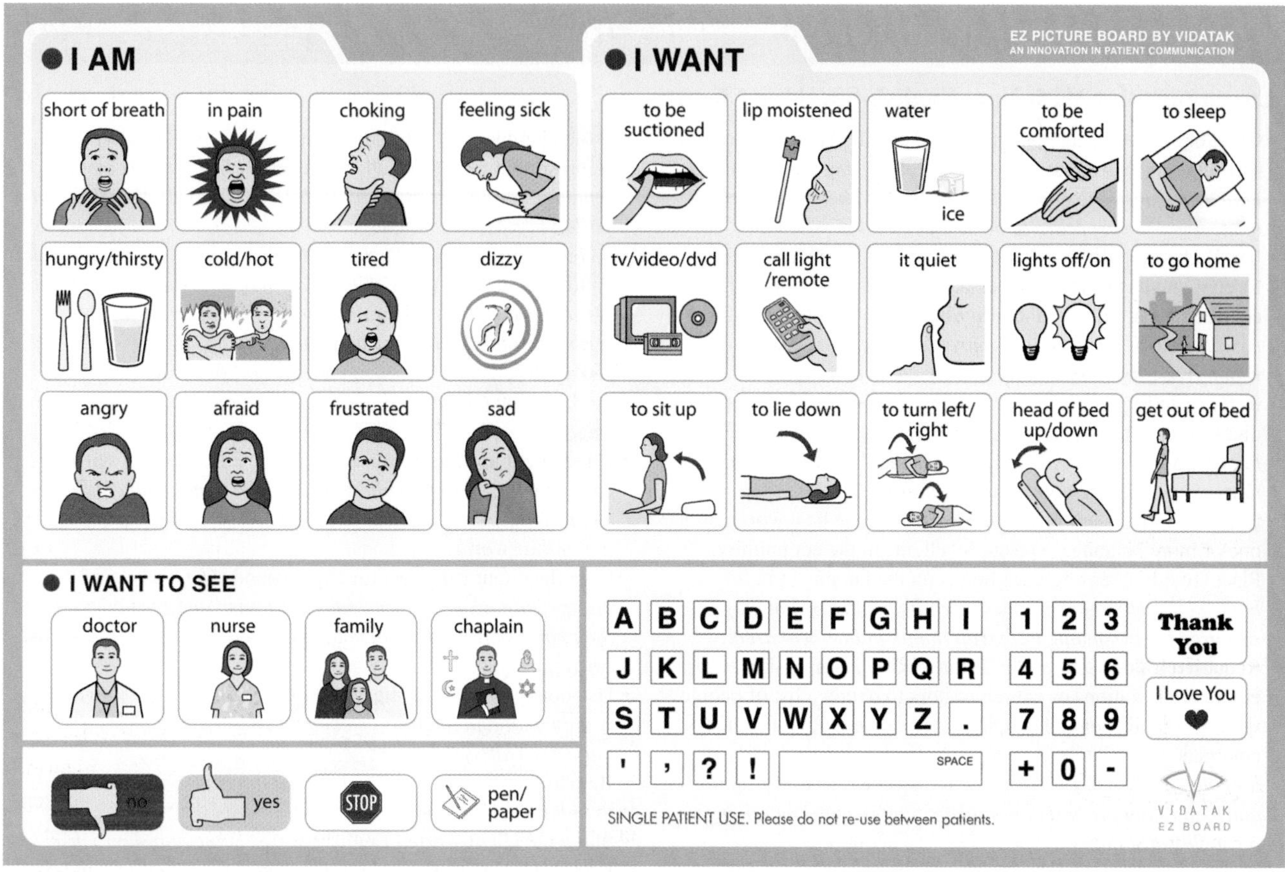

FIGURE 6-2 A picture communication board allows clients to point at appropriate images or use a wet-erase marker. (Courtesy of Vidatak, LLC. Los Angeles, CA 90069.)

Understanding some unique cultural characteristics involving aspects of communication may ease the transition toward culturally sensitive care. It is helpful to be aware of general communication patterns among the major US subcultures.

Native Americans. Native Americans tend to be private and may hesitate to share personal information with strangers. They may interpret questioning as prying or meddling. The nurse should be patient when awaiting an answer and listen carefully because people of this culture may consider impatience disrespectful (Lipson & Dibble, 2005). Navajos, currently the largest tribe of Native Americans, believe that no person has the right to speak for another and may refuse to comment on a family member's health problems.

Because Native Americans traditionally preserved their heritage through oral rather than written history, they may be skeptical of nurses who write down what they say. If possible, the nurse should write notes after, rather than during, the interview.

African Americans. African Americans may be mistrustful of the medical establishment, possibly because of unethical practices employed in past research projects such as the Tuskegee syphilis experiment (Centers for Disease Control and Prevention, 2009). They also have sometimes been treated as second-class citizens when seeking health care. The nurse must demonstrate professionalism by addressing clients by their last names and introducing himself or herself. He or she should follow-up thoroughly with requests, respect the client's privacy, and ask open-ended rather than direct questions until trust has been established. Because of their experiences as victims of discrimination, African Americans may hesitate to give any more information than what is asked.

Latinos. Latinos are characteristically comfortable sitting close to interviewers and letting interactions unfold slowly. Many Latinos speak English but still have difficulty with medical terminology. They may be embarrassed to ask the interviewer to speak slowly, so the nurse must provide information and ask questions carefully. Latino men generally are protective and authoritarian regarding women and children. They expect to be consulted in decisions concerning family members.

Asian Americans. Asian Americans tend to respond with brief or more factual answers and little elaboration, perhaps because traditionally they value simplicity, meditation, and introspection. Asian Americans may not openly disagree with

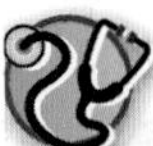

NURSING GUIDELINES 6-1

Communicating With Non–English-Speaking Clients

- Greet or say words and phrases in the client's language, even if carrying on a conversation is impossible. *Using familiar words indicates a desire to communicate with the client even if the nurse lacks the expertise to do so extensively.*
- Use Web sites with the client that translate English to several foreign languages and vice versa. Examples are found at http://ets.freetranslation.com and http://babel.altavista.com/tr. *A computer with Internet access provides sites with easy-to-use, rapid, free translations of up to 150 words at a time.*
- Refer to an English/foreign language dictionary or use appendices in references such as *Taber's Cyclopedic Medical Dictionary. Some dictionaries provide medical words and phrases that may provide pertinent information.*
- Compile a loose-leaf folder or file cards of medical words in one or more languages spoken by clients in the community. Place it with other reference books on the nursing unit. *A homemade reference provides a readily available language resource for communicating with others in the local area.*
- Request a trained interpreter. If that option is impossible, call ethnic organizations or church pastors to obtain a list of people who speak the client's language and may be willing to act as emergency translators. *Someone proficient at speaking the language is more effective at obtaining necessary information and explaining proposed treatments than is someone relying on a rough translation.*
- Contact an international telephone operator in a crisis if there is no other option for communicating with a client. *International telephone operators are generally available 24 hours a day; however, their main responsibility is the job for which they were hired.*
- When several interpreters are available, select one who is of the same gender and approximately the same age as the client. *Some clients are embarrassed relating personal information to people with whom they have little in common.*
- Look at the client, not the interpreter, when asking questions and listening for responses. *Eye contact indicates that the client is the primary focus of the interaction and helps the nurse to interpret nonverbal clues.*
- If the client speaks some English, speak slowly, not loudly, using simple words and short sentences. *Lengthy or complex sentences are barriers when communicating with someone not skilled in a second language.*
- Avoid using technical terms, slang, or phrases with a double or colloquial meaning. *The client may not understand the spoken vernacular, especially if he or she learned English from a textbook rather than conversationally.*
- Ask questions that can be answered by a yes or no. *Direct questions avoid the need to provide elaborate responses in English.*
- If the client appears confused by a question, repeat it without changing the words. *Rephrasing tends to compound confusion because it forces the client to translate yet another group of unfamiliar words.*
- Give the client sufficient time to respond. *The process of interpreting what has been said in English and then converting the response from the native language back to English requires extra time.*
- Use nonverbal communication or pantomime. *Body language is universal and tends to be communicated and interpreted quite accurately.*
- Be patient. *Anxiety is communicated interpersonally and tends to heighten frustration.*
- Show the client written English words. *Some non–English-speaking people can read English better than they can understand spoken English.*
- Work with the health agency's records committee to obtain consent forms, authorization for health insurance benefits, and copies of client's rights written in languages other than English. *Legally, clients must understand what they are consenting to.*
- Develop or obtain foreign translations describing common procedures, routine care, and health promotion. One resource is the Patient Education Resource Center in San Francisco, which provides publications in many languages on numerous health topics. *All clients are entitled to explanations and educational services.*

authority figures, such as physicians and nurses, because of their respect for harmony. Such reticence can conceal disagreement or potential noncompliance with a particular therapeutic regimen that is unacceptable from their perspective.

Eye Contact

Anglo-Americans generally make and maintain eye contact throughout communication. Although it may be natural for Anglo-Americans to look directly at a person while speaking, that is not always true of people from other cultures. It may offend Asian Americans or Native Americans who are likely to believe that lingering eye contact is an invasion of privacy or a sign of disrespect. Arabs may misinterpret direct eye contact as sexually suggestive.

Space and Distance

Providing personal care and performing nursing procedures often intrudes upon personal space, which causes discomfort for some cultural groups. For example, Asian Americans may feel more comfortable with the nurse at more than an arm's length away. The physical closeness of a nurse in an effort to provide comfort and support may threaten clients from other cultures. It is best, therefore, to provide explanations when close contact during procedures and personal care is necessary.

Touch

Some Native Americans may interpret the Anglo-American custom of a strong handshake as offensive. They may be more comfortable with just a light passing of the hands. People from Southeast Asia consider the head to be a sacred body part that only close relatives can touch. Nurses and other health care workers should ask permission before touching this area. Southeast Asians also believe that the area between a female's waist and knees is particularly private and should not be touched by any male other than the woman's husband. Before doing so, a male nurse can relieve the client's anxiety by offering an explanation, requesting permission, and allowing the client's husband to stay in the room.

Emotional Expression

Anglo-Americans and African Americans, in general, freely express positive and negative feelings. Asian and Native Americans, however, tend to control their emotions and expressions of physical discomfort (Zborowski, 1952, 1969), especially among unfamiliar people. Stoicism should not be interpreted as a lack of feeling or caring (Eliopoulos, 2010). Similarly, Latino men may not demonstrate their feelings or readily discuss their symptoms because they may interpret doing so as less than manly (Andrews & Boyle, 2008). The Latino cultural response can be attributed to *machismo*, a belief that virile men are physically strong and must deal with emotions privately. Because this behavior is atypical from an Anglo-American perspective, nurses may overlook the emotional and physical needs of people from these cultural groups.

Dietary Customs and Restrictions

Basically, food is a means of survival: it relieves hunger, promotes health, and prevents disease. Eating also has social meanings that relate to communal togetherness, celebration, reward and punishment, and relief of stress. Culture dictates the types of food and how frequently a person eats, the types of utensils used, and the status of individuals, such as who eats first and who gets larger servings.

Religious practices within some cultures impose certain rules and restrictions such as times for fasting and foods that can and cannot be consumed (Table 6-4). Nurses can jeopardize the compliance of clients with a therapeutic diet for medical disorders if dietary teaching disregards cultural and religious food preferences.

Nutrition Notes

- Dietary acculturation occurs when people change their eating behaviors after moving to a new area. Some traditional foods are rejected and new foods are added or used as substitutes for traditional foods. Availability and cost influence dietary acculturation.
- Acculturation can have a positive or negative effect on eating habits. Generally, as immigrants adopt the "typical American diet" their intake of fat, sugar, and calories increases and their intake of fruit, vegetables, fiber, and protein decreases. New Americans should be encouraged to retain healthy eating practices from their native culture.
- Hispanics and those from Central America drink *atole*, a heated mixture of masa harina (corn meal), *piloncillo* (Mexican brown sugar), cinnamon, vanilla, and sometimes chocolate or fruit, as a traditional celebration and comfort food. *Atole* is also consumed during *la cuarentena*, a 40-day period following the delivery of an infant, in the belief that it will help in recovery and increase the volume of breast milk.
- The diet of some African Americans may include greens, grits, corn bread, and beans cooked with a generous amount of fat or fatty meats, which reflects their Southern American roots.
- Some common foods in Asian American diets include rice and rice noodles; mixtures containing beef, chicken, fish, and soybean products; bok choy cabbage; and bean sprouts. Flavors are enhanced with monosodium glutamate (MSG); soy; oyster, bean, and fish sauce; and peppers resulting in food that is both spicy and salty.
- Native Americans typically consume what is grown locally like fry bread made from corn, meat that is hunted on land or fished from nearby rivers, and chicken, pigs, and cattle that are raised within the community. They may also rely on products available from commercial markets (Schlenker & Long, 2007).

Time

Throughout the world, people view clock time and social time differently (Giger & Davidhizar, 2008). Calendars and clocks define clock time, dividing it into years, months, weeks, days, hours, minutes, and seconds. Social time reflects attitudes concerning punctuality that vary among cultures. Punctuality is often less important to people from other cultures than it is to Anglo-Americans. Tolerating and accommodating cultural differences related to time facilitates culturally sensitive care.

Beliefs Concerning Illness

Generally, people embrace one of three cultural views to explain illness or disease. The *biomedical* or *scientific perspective* is shared by those from developed countries who base their beliefs about health and disease on research findings. An example of a scientific perspective is that microorganisms cause infectious diseases, and frequent handwashing reduces the potential for infection.

The *naturalistic* or *holistic perspective* espouses that humans and nature must be in balance or harmony to remain healthy; illness is an outcome of disharmony. Native Americans believe that positive outcomes result from living in congruence with Mother Earth. Another example includes Asian Americans who uphold the *Yin/Yang theory*, which refers to the belief that balanced forces promote health. Latinos embrace a similar concept referred to as the *hot/cold theory*. It implies that illness is an imbalance between components ascribed as having hot or cold attributes. Adding or subtracting heat or cold to restore balance also can restore health.

Finally, there is the *magico-religious perspective* in which there is a cultural belief that supernatural forces contribute to disease or health. Some examples of the magico-religious

TABLE 6-4 Examples of Religious Beliefs and Practices that Affect Health Care

RELIGION	EXAMPLES	NURSING IMPLICATIONS
Orthodox Judaism	Circumcision is a sacred ritual performed on the 8th day of life.	Provide information on care following circumcision before discharge.
	Kosher dietary laws allow consumption of animals that chew their cud and have cloven hoofs. Animals are slaughtered according to defined procedures; dairy products and meat are not eaten together. Seafood with fins and scales are permitted.	Notify dietary department of the client's food preferences. Packaged food labeled *kosher* indicates it was "properly preserved." *Pareve* means "made without meat or milk."
	Sabbath begins on Friday at sundown and ends on Saturday at sundown.	Avoid scheduling nonemergency tests or procedures during this time.
	Autopsies is are not allowed unless required by law.	All organs that are removed and examined during an autopsy must be returned to the body.
	Burial is preferred within 24 hours of death; Judaic law requires that the body not be left alone.	Contact the family to stay with the dying client. Expect a son or relative to close the mouth and eyes of the deceased.
Catholicism	Statues and medals of religious figures provide spiritual comfort.	Leave such items on or near the client; keep items safe and return promptly if removed.
	Artificial birth control and abortion are forbidden.	Explain how to avoid pregnancy through methods such as checking basal body temperature and characteristics of cervical mucus.
	Baptism is necessary for salvation.	In an emergency, any baptized Christian should perform baptism by pouring water over the head three times and saying, "I baptize you in the name of the Father, and of the Son, and of the Holy Spirit."
Jehovah's Witnesses	Blood transfusions are refused even in life-threatening situations because they believe that blood is the source of the soul.	Refer to physicians who practice blood conservation strategies such as autotransfusions and IV volume expanders (e.g., Dextran).
Seventh Day Adventist	Strict dietary laws are followed based on the Old Testament.	Request a consult with the dietitian to facilitate a vegetarian diet without caffeine.
	Saturday is the Sabbath.	Avoid scheduling medical appointments or procedures at this time.
Christian Scientist	Prayer is the antidote for any illness.	Expect that these clients will contact lay practitioners to assist with healing. Legal procedures may be used as an option when the well-being of minor children are threatened by parental refusal for medical care.
Church of Jesus Christ of Latter-Day Saints (Mormonism)	Coffee, tea, alcohol, tobacco, illegal drugs, and overuse of prescription drugs are prohibited.	Notify the dietary department to provide noncaffeinated beverages.
	Male members may anoint the sick with consecrated olive oil.	Facilitate anointing rituals before surgery or at the client's request.
Amish	Clients may be reluctant to spend money on health care unnecessarily.	Assess home remedies and folk healing being used. Home deliveries are preferred; expect brief overnight stays following hospital births.
	A central belief is that illness must be endured with faith and patience.	Offer comfort measures and analgesic medications rather than waiting for clients to request them.
	Clients are formally educated up to 8th grade.	Select written health educational materials at the client's level of understanding.
	Photographs are not permitted.	Avoid photographing newborns.
Hinduism	Clients highly value modesty and hygiene.	Provide a daily bath but not following a meal; add hot water to cold but not the reverse.
	The application of a *pundra*, a distinctive mark on the forehead, is religiously symbolic.	Avoid removing or replace it as soon as possible.
	Hindus value self-control.	Offer comfort measures and analgesic medications rather than waiting for Hindu clients to request them.
	Men do not participate during labor and delivery.	Keep men informed of the birthing progress
	Cleansing of the body after death symbolizes cleansing of the soul.	Inquire if the family wishes to wash a deceased client's body.
	Most clients are vegetarians: beef is forbidden, and some do not consume eggs.	Request a consult with the dietitian. Clients may refuse medication in gelatin capsules because gelatin is made from animal by-products.

RELIGION	EXAMPLES	NURSING IMPLICATIONS
Islam (Muslim)	Prayer and washing are required five times a day.	Plan care around prayer and washing rituals, which occur at sunrise, mid-morning, noon, afternoon, and sunset. Help clients face Mecca for prayer.
	Pork and alcohol are forbidden.	Clients may refuse medication in capsules and pork insulin. Request that the pharmacist omit alcohol in liquid medications, which usually contain this ingredient.
	Clients prefer to die at home.	Expect that life support will be unacceptable if there is no hope for a reasonable recovery.
	Only relatives may touch or wash the body of a deceased Muslim.	Consult the family before performing postmortem care.

Adapted from Andrews, J. D. (2005). *Cultural, ethnic and religious reference manual,* 3rd ed. Winston-Salem, NC: JAMARDA Resources.

perspective include cultural groups such as Haitians who accept faith healing or practice forms of witchcraft or voodoo. Native Americans have a strong reverence for the Great Creator's influence on health and illness. They use herbs and spiritual rituals performed by tribal leaders or medicine men known as *shamans* to relieve illness (Eliopoulos, 2010). Although nurses may disagree with a client's beliefs concerning the cause of health or illness, respect for the person helps to achieve health care goals. As long as a culturally held health belief or practice is not harmful, the nurse should incorporate it into the client's care.

Stop, Think, and Respond Box 6-1

How might a culturally sensitive nurse respond to a Vietnamese client who practices coining, which involves rubbing the skin in a symptomatic area with a heated or oiled coin to draw an illness out of the body? Coining is not painful, but it produces redness of the skin and superficial ecchymosis (bruising).

Biologic and Physiologic Variations

The biologic characteristics of primary importance to nurses are those that involve the skin, hair, and certain physiologic enzymes.

Skin Characteristics

Skin assessment techniques that are commonly taught are biased toward white clients. To provide culturally sensitive care, nurses must modify their techniques to obtain accurate data on nonwhite clients.

The best technique for observing baseline skin color in a dark-skinned person is to use natural or bright artificial light. Because the palms of the hands, the feet, and the abdomen contain the least pigmentation and are less likely to have been tanned, they are often the best structures to inspect.

According to Giger and Davidhizar (2008), all skin, regardless of a person's ethnic origin, contains an underlying red tone. Its absence or a lighter appearance indicates pallor, a characteristic of anemia or inadequate oxygenation. The color of the lips and nail beds, common sites for assessing cyanosis in whites, may be highly pigmented in other groups, and nurses may misinterpret normal findings. The conjunctiva and oral mucous membranes are likely to provide more accurate data. The sclera or the hard palate, rather than the skin, is a better location for assessing jaundice. In some nonwhites, however, the sclera may have a yellow cast from carotene and fatty deposits; nurses should not misconstrue this finding as jaundice (Andrews & Boyle, 2008).

Rashes, bruising, and inflammation may be less obvious among people with dark skin. Palpating for variations in texture, warmth, and tenderness is a better assessment technique than inspection. Keloids (irregular, elevated thick scars) are common among dark-skinned clients (Fig. 6-3). They are thought to form from a genetic tendency to produce excessive transforming-growth factor-beta (TGF-β), a substance that promotes fibroblast proliferation during tissue repair.

Some nurses, when bathing a dark-skinned person, misinterpret the brown discoloration on a washcloth as a sign of poor hygiene. In reality, this is due to the normal shedding of dead skin cells, which retain their pigmentation.

Hypopigmentation and hyperpigmentation are conditions in which the skin is not a uniform color. Hypopigmentation may result when the skin becomes damaged. Regardless of ethnic origin, damaged skin characteristically manifests

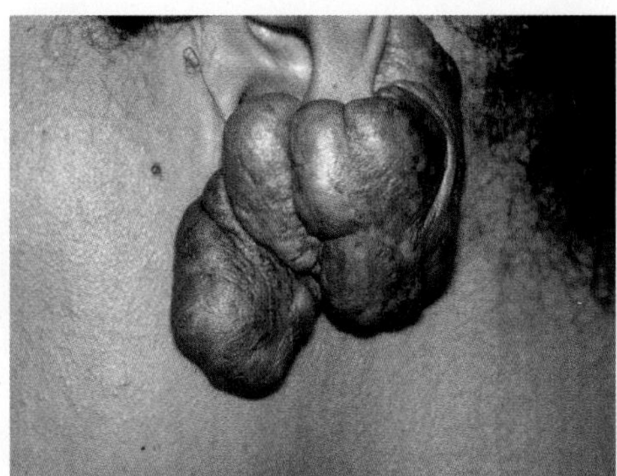

FIGURE 6-3 Keloids are raised, thick scars as is seen in this client's earlobe originally punctured to accommodate pierced earrings. (Photo by B. Proud.)

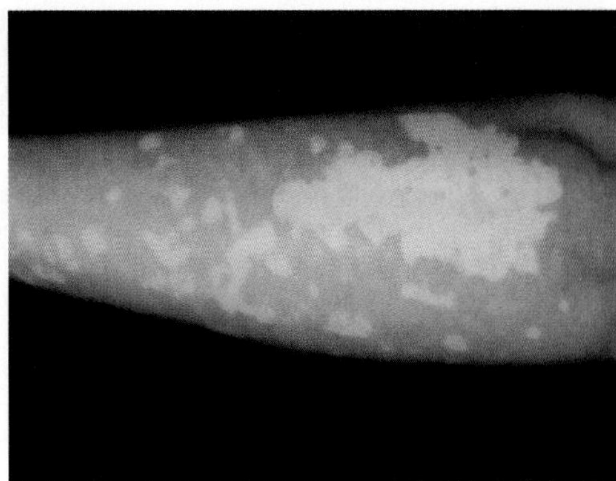

FIGURE 6-4 Vitiligo of the forearm in an African American. (Courtesy of Neutrogena Care Institute.)

temporary redness, which then fades to a lighter hue; in dark-skinned clients, the effect is much more obvious. Vitiligo, a disease that affects whites as well as those with darker skin, produces irregular white patches on the skin as a result of an absence of melanin (Fig. 6-4). Other than hypopigmentation, there are no physical symptoms, but the cosmetic effects may create emotional distress. Clients concerned about the irregularity of their skin color may use a pigmented cream to disguise noticeable areas.

Mongolian spots, an example of hyperpigmentation, are dark-blue areas on the lower back and sometimes on the abdomen, thighs, shoulders, or arms of darkly pigmented infants and children (Fig. 6-5). Mongolian spots are due to the migration of melanocytes into fetal epidermis. They are rare among whites and tend to fade by the time a child is 5 years old. Nurses unfamiliar with ethnic differences can mistake Mongolian spots as a sign of physical abuse or injury. They can differentiate between the two by pressing the pigmented area: Mongolian spots will not produce pain when pressure is applied.

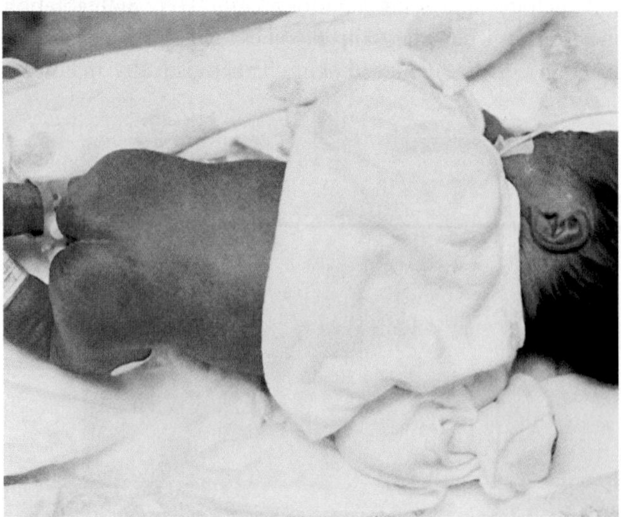

FIGURE 6-5 Mongolian spots. These bluish pigmented areas are common in dark-skinned infants. (Photo by K. Timby.)

Hair Characteristics

Hair color and texture are also biologic variants. Dark-skinned people usually have dark brown or black hair. Hair texture, also an inherited characteristic, results from the amount of protein molecules within the hair. Variations range from straight to very curly. The curlier the hair, the more difficult it is to comb. In general, using a wide-toothed comb or pick, wetting the hair with water before combing, or applying a moisturizing cream makes grooming more manageable. Some clients with very curly hair prefer to arrange it in small, tightly braided sections.

Enzymatic Variations

Three inherited enzymatic variations are prevalent among members of various US subcultures. They involve an absence or insufficiency of the enzymes lactase, glucose-6-phosphate dehydrogenase (G-6-PD), and alcohol dehydrogenase (ADH).

Lactase Deficiency. Lactase is a digestive enzyme that converts lactose, the sugar in milk, into the simpler sugars glucose and galactose. A lactase deficiency, common among African Americans, Hispanics, and Chinese, causes intolerance to dairy products. Without lactase, people have cramps, intestinal gas, and diarrhea approximately 30 minutes after ingesting milk or foods that contain it. Symptoms may continue for 2 hours (Dudek, 2009). Eliminating or reducing sources of lactose in the diet may prevent the discomfort. Liquid tube-feeding formulas and those used for bottle-fed infants can be prepared using milk substitutes. Because milk is a good source of calcium, which is necessary for health, nurses should teach affected clients to obtain calcium from other sources, such as green leafy vegetables, dates, prunes, canned sardines and salmon with bones, egg yolks, whole grains, dried peas and beans, and calcium supplements. Client and Family Teaching 6-1 provides additional points for education.

Client and Family Teaching 6-1
Reducing or Eliminating Lactose

The nurse teaches the client or the family to do the following:

- Avoid milk, dairy products, and packaged foods that list dry milk solids or whey among their ingredients (eg, some breads, cereals, puddings, gravy mixes, caramels, chocolate).
- Use nondairy creamers, which are lactose-free, instead of cream.
- Consume only small amounts of milk or dairy products at a time.
- Substitute milk that has been cultured with the *Acidophilus* organism, which converts lactose into lactic acid.
- Drink Lactaid, a commercial product in which the lactose has been preconverted into other absorbable sugars.
- Use kosher foods, which are prepared without milk; they can be identified by the word *pareve* on the label.

TABLE 6-5 Examples of Drugs that Precipitate Glucose 6-Phosphate Dehydrogenase Anemia

DRUG CATEGORY	EXAMPLE	USE
Quinine compounds	Primaquine phosphate	Prevention and treatment of malaria
Uricosurics	Probenecid (Benemid)	Treatment of gout
Sulfonamides	Sulfasalazine (Azulfidine)	Treatment of urinary infections

G-6-PD Deficiency. G-6-PD is an enzyme that helps red blood cells metabolize glucose. African Americans and people from Mediterranean countries commonly lack this enzyme. The disorder is manifested in males because the gene is sex linked, but females can carry and transmit the faulty gene.

A G-6-PD deficiency makes red blood cells vulnerable during stress, which increases metabolic needs. When this happens, red blood cells are destroyed at a much greater rate than in unaffected people. If the production of new red blood cells cannot match the rate of destruction, anemia develops.

Because several drugs can precipitate the anemic process (Table 6-5), it is important for the nurse to intervene if these drugs or those that depress red cell production are prescribed for ethnic clients who are at greatest risk. At the very least, the nurse must monitor susceptible clients and advocate for laboratory tests, such as red blood cell count and hemoglobin levels, which will indicate any adverse effects.

Alcohol Dehydrogenase (ADH) Deficiency. When a person consumes alcohol, a process of chemical reactions involving enzymes, one of which is ADH (not to be confused with antidiuretic hormone), eventually breaks down the alcohol into acetic acid and carbon dioxide. Asian Americans and Native Americans often metabolize alcohol at a different rate than other groups because of physiologic variations in their enzyme system. The result is that affected clients experience dramatic vascular effects, such as flushing and rapid heart rate, soon after consuming alcohol. In addition, middle metabolites of alcohol (those formed before acetic acid) remain unchanged for a prolonged period. Many scientists believe that the middle metabolites, such as acetaldehyde, are extremely toxic and subsequently play a primary role in causing organ damage. The rate of death from alcoholism among Native Americans is five times higher than that of whites and three times the rate in the general population (Substance Abuse and Mental Health Services Administration, 2007; Centers for Disease Control and Prevention, 2008).

Disease Prevalence

Several diseases, including sickle cell anemia, hypertension, diabetes, and stroke, occur with much greater frequency among ethnic subcultures than in the general population. The incidence of chronic illness affects morbidity differently as well (Table 6-6).

The incidence of some chronic diseases and their complications may be related partly to variations in social factors, such as poverty. Minority cultural groups tend to be less affluent; consequently, their access to expensive health care often is limited. Without preventive health care, early detection,

TABLE 6-6 Leading Causes of Death Among US Cultural Groups[a]

RANK	ALL AMERICANS	BLACK OR AFRICAN AMERICAN	HISPANIC OR LATINO	AMERICAN INDIAN OR ALASKA NATIVE	ASIAN OR PACIFIC ISLANDER
1	Heart disease	Heart disease	Heart disease	Heart disease	Heart disease
2	Cancer	Cancer	Cancer	Cancer	Cancer
3	Cerebrovascular diseases	Cerebrovascular diseases	Chronic lower respiratory diseases	Unintentional injuries	Cerebrovascular diseases
4	Chronic lower respiratory disease	Diabetes	Unintentional injuries	Diabetes	Unintentional injuries
5	Unintentional injuries	Unintentional injuries	Cerebrovascular diseases	Cerebrovascular diseases	Diabetes
6	Diabetes	Chronic lower respiratory diseases	Diabetes	Chronic lower respiratory diseases	Influenza and pneumonia
7	Influenza and pneumonia	Homicide	Influenza and pneumonia	Chronic liver disease and cirrhosis	Chronic lower respiratory diseases
8	Suicide	Influenza and pneumonia	Suicide	Influenza and pneumonia	Chronic liver disease and cirrhosis
9	Chronic liver disease and cirrhosis	Chronic liver disease and cirrhosis	Chronic liver disease and cirrhosis	Suicide	Suicide
10	Homicide	Suicide	Homicide	Homicide	Homicide

[a]Deaths, percentage of total deaths, and rank order for causes of death, by race per 100,000 population, United States, 2006. Retrieved November 2009, from http://www.cdc.gov/data/hus/hus08.pdf.

TABLE 6-7 Common Health Beliefs and Practices

CULTURAL GROUP	HEALTH BELIEF	HEALTH PRACTICES
Anglo-Americans	Illness results from infectious microorganisms, organ degeneration, and unhealthy lifestyles	Physicians are consulted for diagnosis and treatment; nurses provide physical care
African Americans	Supernatural forces can cause disease and influence recovery	Individual and group prayer is used to speed recovery
Asian Americans	Health results from a balance between *yin* and *yang* energy; illness results when equilibrium is disturbed	Acupuncture, acupressure, food, and herbs are used to restore balance
Latinos	Illness and misfortune are punishment from God (referred to as *castigo de Dios*) or results from an imbalance of "hot" or "cold" forces within the body	Prayer and penance are performed to receive forgiveness; the services of lay practitioners who are believed to possess spiritual healing power are used; foods that are "hot" or "cold" are consumed to restore balance
Native Americans	Illness occurs when the harmony of nature (Mother Earth) is disturbed	A *shaman*, or medicine man, who has both spiritual and healing power, is consulted to restore harmony

and treatment, higher death rates are bound to occur. The United States has, therefore, committed itself to reducing the disparity in health care among all Americans (see Chap. 4).

With the knowledge that special populations are at increased risk for chronic diseases, culturally sensitive nurses focus heavily on health education, participate in community health screenings, and campaign for more equitable health services.

Health Beliefs and Practices

Many differences in health beliefs exist among US subcultures. They persist as a result of strong ethnic influences. Health beliefs, in turn, affect health practices (Table 6-7).

Folk medicine (health practices unique to a particular group of people) has come to mean the methods of disease prevention or treatment outside mainstream conventional practice. Generally, lay providers rather than formally educated and licensed individuals give such treatments. In addition to culturally specific health practices, such as those sought from a *curandero* (Latino practitioner who is thought to have spiritual and medicinal powers), a *shaman*, or an herbalist, many people in the United States also turn to alternative quasi-medical therapy (Box 6-3).

Alternative medicine attracts people for various reasons: the expense of mainstream medical care, dissatisfaction with prior treatment or progress, or intimidation from the health care establishment.

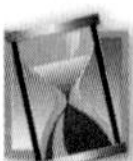

Gerontologic Considerations

■ Older adults may prefer their own culture's traditional healing practices with which they have been familiar since childhood. They may implement these practices before, during, and in spite of prescribed care by the scientific health care community.

Just because a health belief or practice is different does not make it wrong. Culturally sensitive nurses respect the client's belief system and integrate scientifically based treatment along with folk and quasi-medical practices. Refer to Table 6-7 for additional health beliefs and practices as they relate to various religions.

CULTURALLY SENSITIVE NURSING

Accepting that the United States is multicultural is the first step toward transcultural nursing. The following recommendations are ways to demonstrate culturally sensitive nursing care:

- Learn to speak a second language.
- Use culturally sensitive techniques to improve interactions such as sitting in the client's comfort zone and making appropriate eye contact.
- Become familiar with physical differences among ethnic groups.

BOX 6-3 Examples of Alternative Medical Therapy

- Homeopathy is based on the principle of similars; it uses diluted herbal and medicinal substances that cause similar symptoms of a particular illness in healthy people. For example, quinine is used to treat malaria because it causes chills, fever, and weakness (symptoms of malaria) when administered to healthy people.
- Naturopathy uses botanicals, nutrition, homeopathy, acupuncture, hydrotherapy, and manipulation to treat illness and restore a person to optimum balance.
- Chiropractic is based on the belief that illnesses and pain result from spinal misalignment; it uses manipulation and readjustments of joint articulations, massage, and physiotherapy to correct dysfunction.
- Environmental medicine proposes that allergies to environmental substances in the home and workplace affect health, particularly for supersensitive people. It advocates reduced exposure to chemicals to control conditions that mainstream physicians have failed to diagnose or underdiagnosed.

- Perform physical assessments, especially of the skin, using techniques that provide accurate data.
- Learn or ask clients about cultural beliefs concerning health, illness, and techniques for healing.
- Consult the client on ways to solve health problems.
- Never verbally or nonverbally ridicule a cultural belief or practice.
- Integrate helpful or harmless cultural practices within the plan of care.
- Modify or gradually change culturally unsafe health practices.
- Avoid removing religious medals or clothes that hold symbolic meaning for the client. If they must be removed, keep them safe and replace them as soon as possible.
- Provide culturally preferred food.
- Advocate routine screening for diseases to which clients are genetically or culturally prone.
- Facilitate rituals by the person the client identifies as a healer within his or her belief system.
- Apologize if cultural traditions or beliefs are violated.

CRITICAL THINKING EXERCISES

1. A nurse working for a home health agency is assigned to care for a non–English-speaking client from Pakistan. How would a culturally sensitive nurse prepare for this client's care?

2. A pregnant Haitian woman explains to a nurse that she is wearing a chicken bone around her neck to protect her unborn child from birth defects. Discuss how it would be best to respond to this woman from a culturally sensitive perspective.

3. Identify characteristics of a cultural group located within your community; include family patterns, dietary preferences or restrictions, health beliefs, and practices.

4. Explore approaches used to meet the health needs of a non–Anglo-American cultural group within the community in which you live; include methods for communicating and provide of non-English printed materials.

NCLEX-STYLE REVIEW QUESTIONS

1. What is the first step a nurse should take when preparing to teach a Latino client about dietary measures to control diabetes mellitus?
   1. Monitor the client's blood glucose level each day
   2. Review prescribed drug therapy
   3. Obtain a copy of a calorie-controlled exchange list
   4. Determine the client's food likes and dislikes

2. When interviewing an Asian American during admission to a health agency, what is the best technique for a culturally sensitive nurse to use when asking questions?
   1. Position himself or herself directly next to the client
   2. Position himself or herself just beyond an arm's length away
   3. Position himself or herself within the doorway to the room
   4. Position himself or herself to facilitate occasional touching

3. While assessing an African American infant during a home visit, the nurse observes a bluish area on the baby's buttocks. What is the action that is best for the nurse to take?
   1. Document the information; it is a normal assessment finding
   2. Report suspicion of physical abuse to Child Protective Services
   3. Notify the physician in charge of the infant's care about the finding
   4. Examine any and all children in the home for additional signs of abuse

4. A Native American client reports that a tribal elder used "smudging," a ritual in which a substance like sweet grass is burned and the smoke is fanned about the body with an eagle feather, to cleanse him of negative energies during his recent illness. Which response by the nurse is most appropriate?
   1. Explain that smudging will not help restore the client's health
   2. Suggest that the client include the physician's treatment regimen
   3. Report the tribal elder for practicing medicine without a license
   4. Advise the client to avoid treatment prescribed by the tribal elder

5. Which of the following hospital menu suggestions would be appropriate for a person who practices Orthodox Judaism? Select all that apply.
   1. Breaded pork chop
   2. Crab salad
   3. Tuna filet
   4. Baked chicken
   5. Bacon, lettuce, tomato sandwich

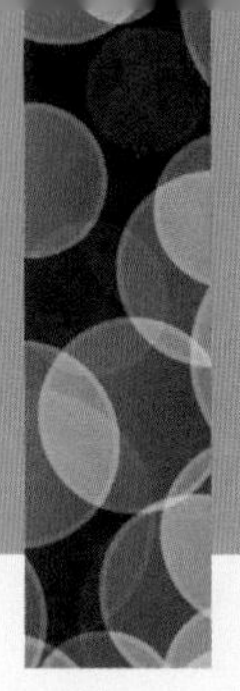

UNIT 2
End of Unit Exercises for Chapters 3, 4, 5, and 6

Section I: Reviewing What You've Learned

Activity A: *Fill in the blanks by choosing the correct word from the options given in parentheses.*

1. ________________ means damaging statements written and read by others. (Libel, Misdemeanors, Slander)
2. ________________ is the ethical principle that emphasizes the duty to be honest and to avoid deceiving or misleading clients. (Autonomy, Justice, Veracity)
3. A(n) ________________ disorder is acquired from the genetic codes of one or both parents. (congenital, hereditary, idiopathic)
4. Health services to which health care providers refer clients for consultation and additional testing, such as cardiac catheterization, are an example of ________________ care. (primary, secondary, tertiary)
5. ________________ means physiologic and behavioral responses to disequilibrium. (Adaptation, Holism, Stress)
6. ________________ stabilizes mood, induces sleep, and regulates temperature. (Dopamine, Norepinephrine, Serotonin)
7. ________________ is a bond or kinship that a person feels with his or her country of birth or place of ancestral origin. (Culture, Ethnicity, Race)
8. A fixed attitude about all people who share a common characteristic related to age, sex, race, sexual orientation, or ethnicity is called a ________________. (belief, generalization, stereotype)

Activity B: *Mark each statement as either T (True) or F (False). Correct any false statements.*

1. T____F____ An anecdotal note cannot be used as evidence in court.
2. T____F____ Malpractice is harm that results from acting carelessly in a given circumstance.
3. T____F____ Capitation is a payment system that provides incentives to control the number of tests and services rendered as a means of making a profit.
4. T____F____ In the case method of nursing, one nurse manages all the care needs of a client or group of clients for a designated period.
5. T____F____ Coping mechanisms are stress-reduction activities people select consciously to help them deal with challenging events or situations.
6. T____F____ Receptors for neurotransmitters are found throughout the central nervous, endocrine, and immune systems.
7. T____F____ Ethnocentrism refers to the belief that one's own ethnicity is superior to all others.
8. T____F____ Florence Nightingale coined the term "transcultural nursing."

Activity C: *Write the correct term for each description below.*

1. Unlawful act in which untrue information harms a person's reputation ________________
2. Person who claims injury and brings charges against another person ________________
3. Sum of physical, emotional, social, and spiritual health, which determines how "whole" or well a person feels ________________
4. Ill effect that results from permanent or progressive organ damage caused by a disease or its treatment ________________

5. A relatively stable state of physiologic equilibrium __________________

6. Natural body chemicals that produce effects similar to those of opiate drugs __________________

7. Period during which signs and symptoms of a particular disease temporarily disappear __________________

8. Digestive enzyme that converts lactose into glucose and galactose __________________

Activity D: *1. Match the terms in Column A with their definitions in Column B.*

Column A		Column B
1. __________________	Morbidity	A. The number of people who died from a particular disease or condition
2. __________________	Mortality	B. A change in health that develops slowly and lasts a long time, increasing with age
3. __________________	Acute illness	C. The number of people affected by a specific disease, disorder, or injury
4. __________________	Chronic illness	D. A change in health that happens suddenly and lasts a short time

2. Match the skin disorders in Column A with their descriptions in Column B.

Column A		Column B
1. __________________	Keloids	A. Dark-blue areas on the lower backs of darkly pigmented infants and children
2. __________________	Hypopigmentation	B. Irregular, elevated thick scars
3. __________________	Vitiligo	C. Damaged skin with temporary redness that fades to a lighter hue
4. __________________	Mongolian spots	D. Irregular white patches on the skin from a lack of melanin

Activity E: *1. Differentiate between teleologic theory and deontologic theory.*

	Teleologic Theory	*Deontologic Theory*
Definition		
Ideology		
Example		

2. Differentiate between the sympathetic and parasympathetic nervous systems.

	Sympathetic Nervous System	*Parasympathetic Nervous System*
Function		
Effect on physiologic functions		
Example		

Activity F: *Consider the following figure.*

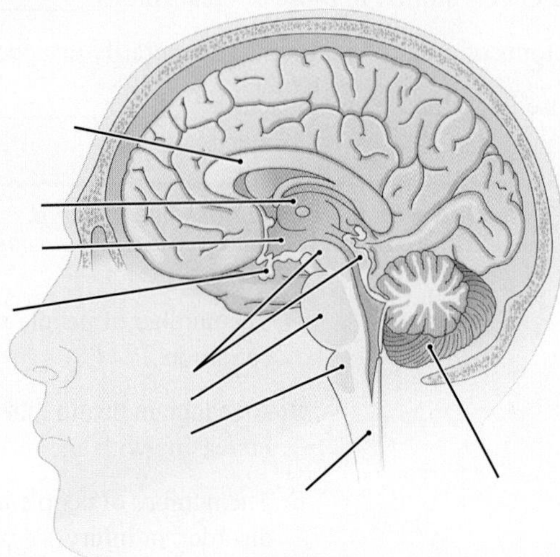

1. Label the structures in the figure.

Activity G: *In the 1960s, Abraham Maslow identified and grouped five levels of human needs in a sequential hierarchy according to their significance. In the boxes below, sequence the five levels of human needs as defined by Maslow, moving from those that are most important to those that are least important for survival.*

1. Need for esteem and self-esteem
2. Need for self-actualization
3. Need for love and belonging
4. Need for physiologic requirements
5. Need for safety and security

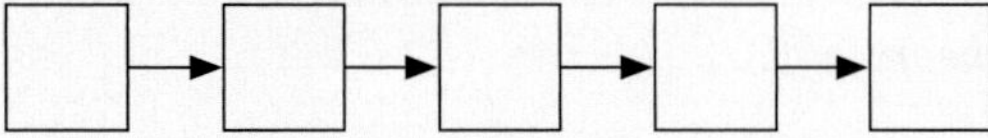

Activity H: *Answer the following questions.*

1. What are laws? What are the different types of laws?
2. What is the purpose of a nurse practice act?
3. How does the World Health Organization (WHO) define health?
4. What are the five common management patterns that nurses use to administer client care?
5. What is homeostasis? What are the four categories of stressors that affect homeostasis?
6. What factors affect the stress response?
7. What is transcultural nursing care?

Section II: Applying Your Knowledge

Activity I: *Answer the following questions.*

1. Why is it important for nurses to obtain their own personal liability insurance?

2. Why does the treatment of idiopathic illness focus on relieving signs and symptoms?

3. Why can a nurse be charged with a criminal offense in the case of gross negligence?

4. Why should the nurse refuse the assistance of untrained interpreters, volunteers, or family when caring for a client with whom the nurse does not share a common language?

5. Why is it important for the nurse to inspect the skin of the palm, foot, and abdomen during a skin assessment of a person of color?

6. Why must the nurse avoid making or writing negative comments about clients, physicians, or other coworkers?

Activity J: *Answer the following questions focusing on nursing roles and responsibilities.*

1. An unconscious client has been admitted to the health care facility after a motor vehicle crash. When the client regains consciousness, he wants to leave the facility without being medically discharged.
   a. Can the nurse prevent the client from leaving?

   b. What procedure should the nurse follow if the client refuses to stay at the facility?

2. Personnel at a health care facility follow a team nursing pattern of care, with one member as the team leader.
   a. What is team nursing?

   b. What are the roles and responsibilities of the team leader?

3. A nurse is caring for a client scheduled for minor surgery who is unusually quiet. The nurse believes that the client is under stress.
   a. What can the nurse do if the client is experiencing stress?

   b. What stress-reduction techniques can the nurse employ for this client?

4. A nurse is assessing a client who immigrated to the United States years ago and understands English well but does not speak the language fluently. The client does not want an interpreter.
   a. How should the nurse communicate with the client during the assessment?

   b. Why is it important for the nurse to be patient when communicating with this client?

5. A nurse who works in a large urban clinic assesses clients from various subcultures.
   a. What data should the nurse obtain during an assessment to provide culturally sensitive care?

   b. What variations is a nurse likely to observe when assessing these clients?

Activity K: *Consider the following questions. Discuss them with your instructor or peers.*

1. A client with a fractured left leg is learning how to use crutches. The nurse has asked the client not to leave the room without assistance. The client ignores this suggestion and falls. How should the nurse handle this situation?
2. A client is unhappy with the lunch served to him at the health care facility. When the nurse arrives to check if the client has eaten, the client pushes away the tray, spilling its contents on the floor. What should the nurse do in this case?
3. A client who is to undergo chemotherapy expresses concern about the side effects of the drug treatment and the effects that the cancer is causing on his family roles. The client mentions to the nurse that he tries to combat stress by sleeping most of the time. What interventions can the nurse suggest to help reduce the client's stress?
4. A nurse is working at a health care facility where most clients do not speak English. How should the nurse prepare to meet the challenges of this job?

Section III: Getting Ready for NCLEX

Activity L: *Answer the following questions.*

1. A nurse at a health care facility has been stealing narcotics for personal use and has been attempting to conceal the theft by altering records of narcotic drug administration. Which of the following would the nurse most likely be charged with in the case of legal proceedings?
   a. Misdemeanor
   b. Felony
   c. Malpractice
   d. Negligence
2. The nurse has asked a client who is likely to experience orthostatic hypotension to use the nurse's call light if he needs to use the bathroom. The client refuses to do so. Which of the following actions would be appropriate for the nurse to take to ensure the client's safety?
   a. Raise the side rails of the bed
   b. Obtain a medical order to use a restraint
   c. Threaten to use a restraint
   d. Use a wanderer alarm
3. A nurse has admitted a client to the health care facility. This same nurse is also responsible for planning the client's care and evaluating the client's progress until discharge. What pattern of nursing is being followed?
   a. Primary nursing
   b. Functional nursing
   c. Nurse-managed care
   d. Case method
4. A client who has been diagnosed with cancer refuses to believe this news and wants all the diagnostic tests repeated. What kind of coping mechanism is the client exhibiting?
   a. Displacement
   b. Projection
   c. Sublimation
   d. Denial
5. A nurse is caring for a client whose right hand had to be amputated following an accident. The client, whose employment involves using a computer keyboard to enter data, may have to look for another job. Which of the following is the highest contributor to stress in this client's situation?
   a. Moving to a different job
   b. Adjusting to a change in financial status
   c. Dealing with a personal injury
   d. Changing living conditions
6. The nurse is assigned to care for an Asian American woman. Which of the following is appropriate for the nurse to do when caring for this client?
   a. Touch the client's head gently
   b. Avoid touching the client's hand
   c. Provide personal care in the presence of family members
   d. Avoid lingering eye contact with the client

7. When assessing a client who does not speak the same language as the nurse, the nurse seeks the assistance of an interpreter. Which of the following is a characteristic of a skilled interpreter?
   a. Explains the role of an interpreter to the client
   b. Expresses personal views on the client's statement
   c. Informs the client's family about the client's condition
   d. Translates the client's statements without conveying the client's emotions

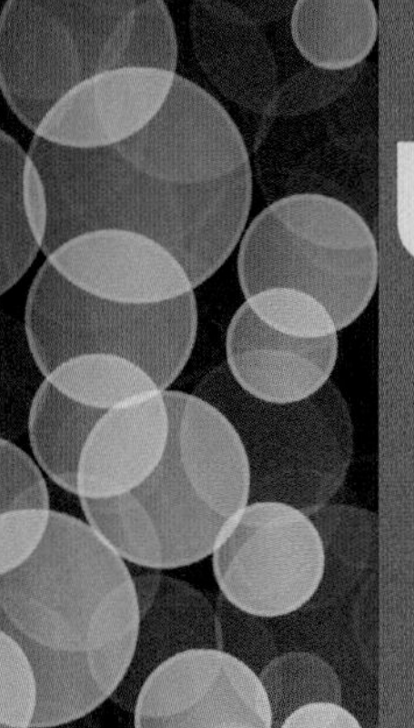

UNIT 3
Fostering Communication

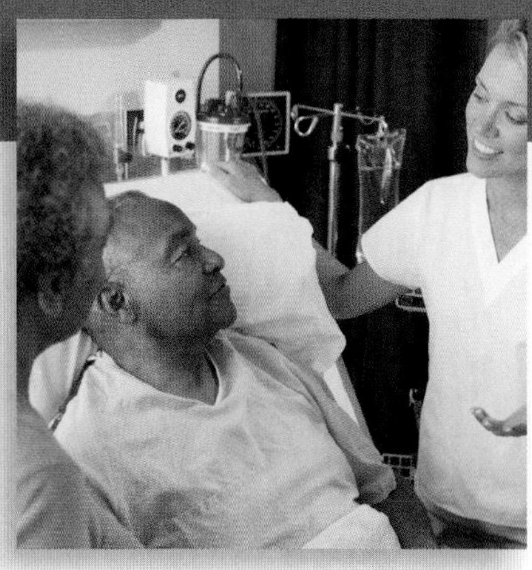

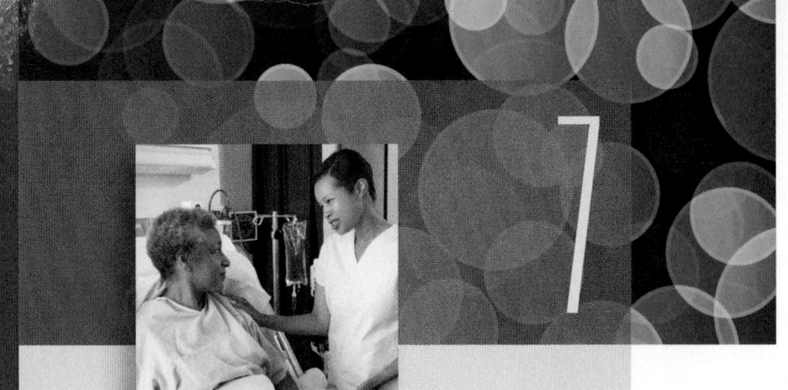

7 The Nurse–Client Relationship

Words To Know

active listening
affective touch
caregiver
collaborator
communication
delegator
educator
empathy
intimate space
introductory phase
kinesics
nonverbal communication
paralanguage
personal space
proxemics
public space
relationship
silence
social space
task-oriented touch
terminating phase
therapeutic relationship
therapeutic verbal communication
touch
verbal communication
working phase

Learning Objectives

On completion of this chapter, the reader should be able to:

1. Name four roles that nurses perform in nurse–client relationships.
2. Describe the current role expectations for clients.
3. List at least five principles that form the basis of the nurse–client relationship.
4. Identify the three phases of the nurse–client relationship.
5. Differentiate between social communication and therapeutic verbal communication.
6. Give at least five examples of therapeutic and nontherapeutic communication techniques.
7. List at least five factors that affect oral communication.
8. Describe the four forms of nonverbal communication.
9. Differentiate task-related touch from affective touch.
10. List at least five situations in which affective touch may be appropriate.

An intangible factor that helps a client hold a nurse in high regard is the relationship that develops between them. One of the primary keys to establishing and maintaining positive nurse–client relationships is the manner and style of the nurse's communication. This chapter offers information about techniques for communicating therapeutically, listening empathetically, sharing information, and providing client education, all of which are among the most basic processes within the context of nurse–client relationships.

NURSING ROLES WITHIN THE NURSE–CLIENT RELATIONSHIP

A **relationship** (an association between two or more people that develops over time) is established between the nurse and the client when nursing services are provided. Nurses provide services or skills that assist individuals (called clients or patients), promote or restore health, cope with disorders that will not improve, and die with dignity.

The nurse–client relationship requires the nurse to respond to the client's needs. The National Council of State Boards of Nursing, which develops the National Council Examination-Practical Nurse (NCLEX-PN), designates four categories of client needs as the structure for the test plan: (1) safe and effective care environment, (2) health promotion and maintenance, (3) psychosocial integrity, and (4) physiologic integrity. These four categories apply to all areas of nursing practice regardless of the stage in the client's life or the setting for health care delivery. To meet these client needs, nurses perform four basic roles: caregiver, educator, collaborator, and delegator.

The Nurse as Caregiver

A **caregiver** is one who performs health-related activities that a sick person cannot perform independently. Caregivers provide physical and emotional services to restore or maintain functional independence. Box 7-1 highlights the many differences between the services that nurses provide and those that other caring people provide.

Although the traditional nursing role is associated with physical care, it also involves developing close emotional relationships. The contemporary caregiving role incorporates an understanding that illness and injury cause feelings of insecurity that may threaten a person's ability to cope. Nurses use **empathy** (an intuitive awareness of what a client is experiencing) to perceive the client's emotional state and need for support. Empathy helps nurses become effective at providing for the client's needs while remaining compassionately detached.

The Nurse as Educator

Being an **educator** (one who provides information) is a necessity in today's complex health care arena. Nurses provide health teaching pertinent to each client's needs and knowledge base (see Chap. 8). Some examples include explanations about diagnostic test procedures, self-administration of medications after discharge, techniques for managing wound care, and restorative exercises like those performed after a mastectomy.

When it comes to treatment decisions, the nurse avoids giving advice—reserving the right of each person to make his or her own choices on matters affecting health and illness care. The nurse shares information on potential alternatives, promotes the client's freedom to choose, and supports the client's ultimate decision.

Nursing is considered a practice "without walls" because it extends beyond the original treatment facility. Consequently, nurses are resources for information about health services available in the community. This type of information empowers clients to become involved with self-help groups or those that offer rehabilitation, financial assistance, or emotional support.

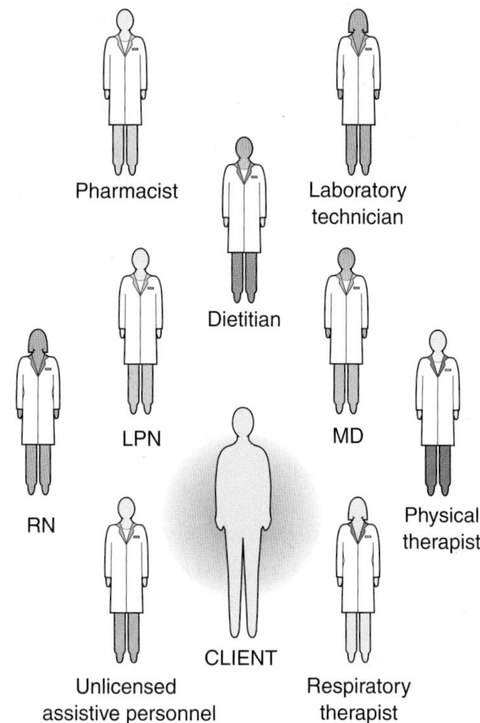

FIGURE 7-1 Collaboration may involve many members of the health care team.

The Nurse as Collaborator

The nurse also acts as a **collaborator** (one who works with others to achieve a common goal) (Fig. 7-1). The most obvious example of collaboration occurs between the nurse responsible for managing care and those to whom he or she delegates care. Collaboration also occurs when the nurse and the physician share information and exchange findings with other health care workers.

Stop, Think, and Respond Exercise 7-1

With whom would the nurse collaborate when caring for an older adult with a fractured hip?

BOX 7-1 Differentiating Caring Acts from Nursing Acts

CARING ACTS	NURSING ACTS
Prompted by observing a person in distress	Prompted by a concern for the well-being of everyone
Motivated by sympathy	Motivated by altruism
Spontaneous	Planned
Goal is to relieve crisis	Goal is to promote self-reliance
Outcomes are short term	Outcomes are long term
Assume major responsibility for resolving the person's problem	Expect mutual cooperation in resolving health problems
Experience based	Knowledge based
Modeled on a personal moral code	Modeled on a formal code of ethics
Guided by common sense	Legally defined
Accountability based on acting reasonably prudent	Accountability based on meeting professional standards

The Nurse as Delegator

Before the nurse performs the role of **delegator** (one who assigns a task to someone), he or she must know what tasks are legal and appropriate for particular health care workers to perform. It is potentially litigious to delegate a task to someone who does not have the knowledge or expertise to perform it correctly. Once a task is assigned, it is still the delegator's responsibility to check that the task has been completed and determine the resulting outcome. For example, if a nurse asks a nursing assistant to change a client's position, the nurse verifies that the assistant complied with the nurse's request and obtains additional pertinent information such as the condition of the client's skin. If the delegated task is not performed or is performed incorrectly, the nurse is accountable for the inadequate care.

Stop, Think, and Respond Exercise 7-2

Before delegating the task of taking a client's vital signs (temperature, pulse, respiratory rate, and blood pressure) to a student nurse, how might the nurse determine whether the task is appropriate for the student, and if appropriate, that it has been performed?

BOX 7-2 Responsibilities Within the Nurse–Client Relationship

Nursing Responsibilities
- Possess current knowledge
- Be aware of unique age-related differences
- Perform technical skills safely
- Be committed to client care
- Be available and courteous
- Facilitate participation of client and family in decisions
- Remain objective
- Advocate on the client's behalf
- Provide explanations in easily understood language
- Promote the client's independence

Client Responsibilities
- Identify current problem
- Describe desired outcomes
- Answer questions honestly
- Provide accurate historical and subjective data
- Participate to the fullest extent possible
- Be open and flexible to alternatives
- Comply with the plan for care
- Keep appointments for follow-up care

THE THERAPEUTIC NURSE–CLIENT RELATIONSHIP

The nurse–client relationship also can be called a **therapeutic relationship** because the desired outcome of the association is almost always moving toward improving health. A therapeutic relationship differs from a social relationship. A therapeutic relationship is client-centered with a focus on goal achievement. It is also time limited: the relationship ends when goals are achieved.

The relationship between nurses and clients has changed. In the past, the role of a sick person was passive; this allowed others to make decisions and to submit to treatments without question or protest. Nurses now encourage and expect people for whom they care to become actively involved, communicate, question, assist in planning their care, and retain as much independence as possible (Box 7-2).

Underlying Principles

A therapeutic nurse–client relationship is more likely to develop when the nurse treats each client as a unique person and respects the client's feelings. The nurse strives to promote the client's physical, emotional, social, and spiritual well-being, and encourages the client to participate in problem solving and decision making. The nurse believes that a client has the potential for growth and change and communicates using terms and language the client understands. The nurse uses the nursing process to individualize the client's care; involves people to whom the client turns for support, such as family and friends when providing care; and implements health care techniques compatible with the client's value system and cultural heritage.

Phases of the Nurse–Client Relationship

Nurse–client relationships ordinarily are brief. They begin when people seek services that will maintain or restore health or prevent disease. They end when clients can achieve their health-related goals independently. This type of relationship generally is described as having three phases: introductory, working, and terminating.

Introductory Phase

The relationship between client and nurse begins with the **introductory phase** (the period of getting acquainted). Each person usually brings preconceived ideas about the other to the initial interaction. These assumptions eventually are confirmed or dismissed.

Many experts agree that most people form their initial opinions within just a few seconds of meeting. Some techniques for facilitating a positive first impression include:

- Dressing appropriately
- Being well-groomed
- Smiling
- Making eye contact
- Greeting with a handshake
- Projecting confidence
- Avoiding offensive personal odors, such as the smell of cigarette smoke or strong scents of perfume or cologne

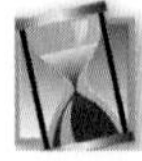

Gerontologic Considerations

■ Initially, greet the client by giving your name and title. Address the older person using formal titles of respect such as "Mr." or "Mrs." Find an appropriate time to ask the client how he or she prefers to be addressed. Avoid using familiar or endearing terms such as "dear," "sweetie," or "honey."

After the initial formalities, the client initiates the relationship by identifying one or more health problems for which he or she is seeking help. It is important for the nurse to demonstrate courtesy, active listening, empathy, competency, and appropriate communication skills to ensure that the relationship begins on a positive note.

Working Phase

The **working phase** (period during which tasks are performed) involves mutually planning the client's care and implementing the plan. Both the nurse and the client participate. Each shares in performing those tasks that lead to the desired outcomes mutually identified by the client and the nurse. During the working phase, the nurse tries not to retard the client's independence; doing too much is as harmful as doing too little.

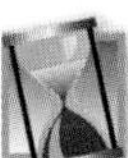

Gerontologic Considerations

- Promote an older adult's control over decisions as much as possible. Dependence is often difficult to accept; participation helps maintain self-esteem and dignity.

Terminating Phase

The nurse–client relationship is self-limiting. The **terminating phase** (the period when the relationship comes to an end) occurs when the nurse and client agree that the client's immediate health problems have improved. A caring attitude and compassion help facilitate the client's transition of care to other health care services or to independent living.

Barriers to a Therapeutic Relationship

It is impossible for a nurse to develop a positive relationship with every client. Box 7-3 lists examples of behaviors that are likely to interfere. The best approach is to treat clients in the manner one would like to be treated.

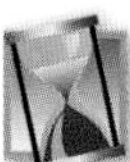

Gerontologic Considerations

- Avoid the "invisible client syndrome." Talking with someone else in the room as if the client is not there demonstrates disrespect.
- Never treat older adults as if they are children or are uneducated. Avoid using terms that are demeaning or that connote childlike or infantile behavior (eg, referring to incontinence products as "diapers").

BOX 7-3 Barriers to a Nurse–Client Relationship

- Appearing unkempt: long hair that dangles on or over the client during care, offensive body or breath odor, wrinkled or soiled uniform, dirty shoes
- Failing to identify oneself verbally and with a name tag
- Mispronouncing or avoiding the client's name
- Using the client's first name without permission
- Showing disinterest in the client's personal history and life experiences
- Sharing personal or work-related problems with the client or with staff in the client's presence
- Using crude or distasteful language
- Revealing confidential information or gossip about other clients, staff, or people commonly known
- Focusing on nursing tasks rather than the client's responses
- Being inattentive to the client's requests (eg, food, pain relief, assistance with toileting, bathing)
- Abandoning the client at stressful or emotional times
- Failing to keep promises such as consulting with the physician about a current need or request
- Going on a break or to lunch without keeping the client informed and identifying who has been delegated for the client's care during the temporary absence

COMMUNICATION

Communication (an exchange of information) involves both sending and receiving messages between two or more people followed by feedback indicating that the information was understood or requires further clarification (Fig. 7-2). Communication takes place simultaneously on a verbal and nonverbal level with the nonverbal level representing the stronger component in any interaction. Because no relationship can exist without verbal and nonverbal communication, nurses develop skills that enhance their therapeutic interactions with clients.

Verbal Communication

Verbal communication (communication that uses words) includes speaking, reading, and writing. Both the nurse and the client use verbal communication to gather facts. They also use it to instruct, clarify, and exchange ideas.

Many factors affect the ability to communicate by speech or in writing. Examples include (1) attention and concentration; (2) language compatibility; (3) verbal skills;

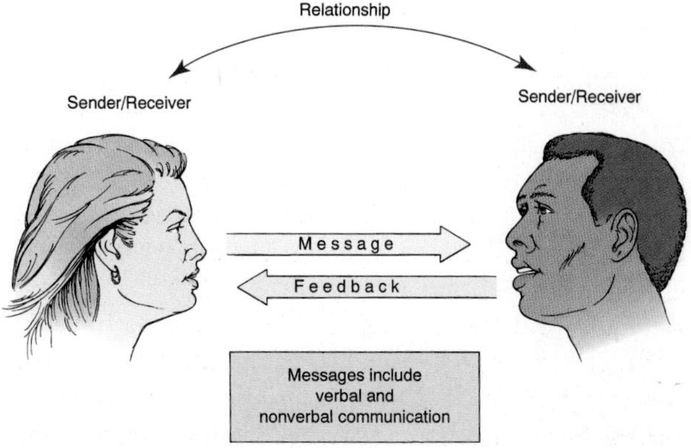

FIGURE 7-2 Communication is a two-way process between a sender and a receiver.

(4) hearing and visual acuity; (5) motor functions involving the throat, tongue, and teeth; (6) sensory distractions; (7) interpersonal attitudes; (8) literacy; and (9) cultural similarities. The nurse promotes the factors that enhance the communication of verbal content and controls or eliminates those that interfere with the accurate perception of expressed ideas.

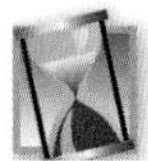

Gerontologic Considerations

■ In the event that it is difficult for older adults to read the name tag or recall the nurse's name from a previous introduction, clients may appreciate if the nurse identifies himself or herself by name and title before each interaction or posts them on a dry erase board in the room. For older clients with diminished hearing, it may be helpful to reduce noise in the immediate environment. Identify which ear has the best hearing, and take a position on that side. Speak at a normal volume with distinct pronunciation of beginning and ending consonants for each word, yet without distorting normal patterns of speaking. Because older adults with diminished hearing may rely on visual cues, avoid covering your mouth or turning away from the client when interacting verbally.

■ Encourage reminiscing. Ask about past events and relationships associated with positive experiences and feelings. Giving older adults an opportunity to talk about earlier times in their lives reinforces their value and unique identity and promotes recall of situations in which they have demonstrated coping or adaptation.

Therapeutic Verbal Communication

Communication can take place on a social or therapeutic level. Social communication is superficial; it includes common courtesies and exchanges about general topics. **Therapeutic verbal communication** (using words and gestures to accomplish a particular objective) is extremely important, especially when the nurse is exploring problems with the client or encouraging expression of feelings. Techniques that the nurse may find helpful are described in Table 7-1.

The nurse must never assume that a quiet, uncommunicative client is problem-free or understands everything. It is never appropriate to probe and pry; rather, it may be advantageous to wait and be patient. It is not unusual for reticent clients to share their feelings and concerns after they conclude that the nurse is sincere and trustworthy.

Nurses must approach vocal and/or emotional clients delicately. For instance, when clients are angry or crying, the best nursing response is to remain nonjudgmental, allow them to express their emotions, and return later with a follow-up regarding their legitimate complaints. Allowing clients to display their feelings without fear of retaliation or censure contributes to a therapeutic relationship.

TABLE 7-1 Therapeutic Verbal Communication Techniques

TECHNIQUE	USE	EXAMPLE
Broad opening	Relieves tension before getting to the real purpose of the interaction	"Wonderful weather we're having."
Giving information	Provides facts	"Your surgery is scheduled at noon."
Direct questioning	Acquires specific information	"Do you have any allergies?"
Open-ended questioning	Encourages the client to elaborate	"How are you feeling?"
Reflecting	Confirms that the nurse is following the conversation	Client: "I haven't been sleeping well." Nurse: "You haven't been sleeping well."
Paraphrasing	Restates what the client has said to demonstrate listening	Client: "After every meal, I feel like I will throw up." Nurse: "Eating makes you nauseous, but you don't actually vomit."
Verbalizing what has been implied	Shares how the nurse has interpreted a statement	Client: "All the nurses are so busy." Nurse: "You're feeling that you shouldn't ask for help."
Structuring	Defines a purpose and sets limits	"I have 15 minutes. If your pain is relieved, we could discuss how your test will be done."
Giving general leads	Encourages the client to continue	"Uh, huh," or "Go on."
Sharing perceptions	Shows empathy for the client's feelings	"You seem depressed."
Clarifying	Avoids misinterpretation	"I don't quite understand what you're asking."
Confronting	Calls attention to manipulation, inconsistencies, or lack of responsibility	"You're concerned about your weight loss, but you didn't eat any breakfast."
Summarizing	Reviews information that has been discussed	"You've asked me to check on increasing your pain medication and getting your diet changed."
Silence	Allows time for considering how to proceed or arouses the client's anxiety to the point that it stimulates more verbalization	

Although nurses often have the best intentions of interacting therapeutically with clients, some fall into traps that block or hinder verbal communication. Table 7-2 lists common examples of nontherapeutic communication.

Listening

Listening is as important during communication as speaking. In contrast to hearing, which involves perceiving sounds, **active listening** is an activity that includes attending to and becoming fully involved in what the client says. To facilitate active listening, other issues in one's personal agenda must be temporarily blocked in order to focus on the content of the present interaction.

Giving attention to what clients say provides a stimulus for meaningful interaction. It is important to avoid giving signals that indicate boredom, impatience, or the pretense of listening. For example, looking out a window or interrupting is a sign of disinterest. When communicating with most

TABLE 7-2 Nontherapeutic Verbal Communication Techniques

TECHNIQUE AND CONSEQUENCE	EXAMPLE	IMPROVEMENT
Giving False Reassurance		
Trivializes the client's unique feelings and discourages further discussion	"You've got nothing to worry about. Everything will work out just fine."	"Tell me your specific concerns."
Using Clichés		
Provides worthless advice and curtails exploring alternatives	"Keep a stiff upper lip."	"It must be difficult for you right now."
Giving Approval or Disapproval		
Holds the client to a rigid standard; implies that future deviation may lead to subsequent rejection or disfavor	"I'm glad you're exercising so regularly." "You should be testing your blood glucose each morning."	"Are you having any difficulty fitting regular exercise into your schedule?" "Let's explore some ways that will help you remember to test your blood glucose each morning."
Agreeing		
Does not allow the client flexibility to change his or her mind	"You're right about needing surgery immediately."	"Having surgery immediately is one possibility. What others have you considered?"
Disagreeing		
Intimidates the client; makes him or her feel foolish or inadequate	"That's not true! Where did you get that idea?"	"Maybe I can help clarify that for you."
Demanding an Explanation		
Puts the client on the defensive; he or she may be tempted to make up an excuse rather than risk disapproval for an honest answer	"Why didn't you keep your appointment last week?"	"I see you couldn't keep your appointment last week."
Giving Advice		
Discourages independent problem solving and decision making; provides a biased view that may prejudice the client's choice	"If I were you, I'd try drug therapy before having surgery."	"Share with me the advantages and disadvantages of your options as you see them."
Defending		
Indicates such a strong allegiance that any disagreement is unacceptable	"Ms. Johnson is my best nursing assistant. She wouldn't have let your light go unanswered that long."	"I'm sorry you had to wait so long."
Belittling		
Disregards how the client is responding as an individual	"Lots of people learn to give themselves insulin."	"You're finding it especially difficult to inject yourself with a needle."
Patronizing		
Treats the client condescendingly (less than capable of making an independent decision)	"Are *we* ready for *our* bath yet?"	"Would you like your bath now or should I check with you later?"
Changing the Subject		
Alters the direction of the discussion to a safer or more comfortable topic	Client: "I'm so scared that a mammogram will show I have cancer." Nurse: "Tell me more about your family."	Client: "I'm so scared that a mammogram will show I have cancer." Nurse: "It is a serious disease. What concerns you the most?"

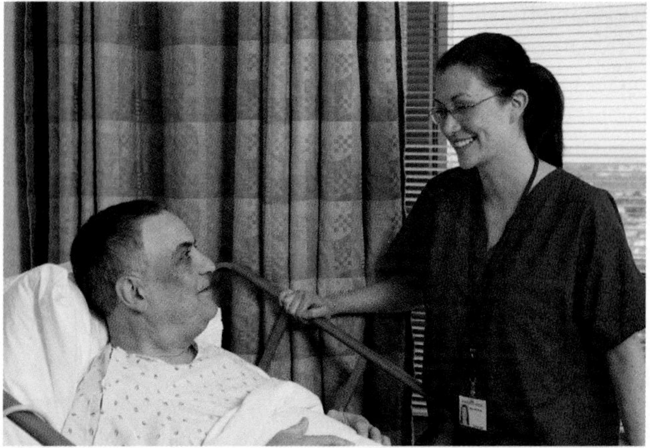

FIGURE 7-3 Appropriate positioning, space, eye contact, and attention promote therapeutic communication. (Photo by B. Proud.)

people in the United States, it is best to position oneself at the person's level and make frequent eye contact (Fig. 7-3). Refer to Chapter 6 for cultural exceptions. Nodding and making comments such as, "Yes, I see" encourages clients to continue and shows full involvement in what is being said.

Silence

Silence (intentionally withholding verbal commentary) plays an important role in communication. It may seem contradictory to include silence as a form of verbal communication. Nevertheless, one of its uses is to encourage the client to participate in verbal discussions. Other therapeutic uses for silence include relieving a client's anxiety just by providing a personal presence and offering a brief period during which clients can process information or respond to questions.

Clients may use silence to camouflage fears or to express contentment. They also use silence for introspection when they need to explore feelings or pray. Interrupting someone deep in concentration disturbs his or her thought process. A common obstacle to effective communication is ignoring the importance of silence and talking excessively.

Nonverbal Communication

Nonverbal communication (an exchange of information without using spoken or written words) involves what is not said. The manner in which a person conveys verbal information affects its meaning. It is believed that nonverbal communication has about five times the impact of verbal communication (Bennett, 2008b).

A person has less control over nonverbal than verbal communication. Words can be chosen with care, but a facial expression and other forms of body language are harder to control. As a result, people often communicate messages more accurately through nonverbal communication.

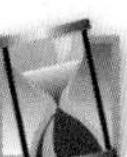

Gerontologic Considerations

- Older adults may have difficulty perceiving nonverbal forms of communication due to visual impairments.
- It is important to avoid standing in front of a sunny window when communicating with older adults because the glare may interfere with looking directly at the nurse, causing them to miss the nuances of nonverbal communication.

People communicate nonverbally through the following techniques: kinesics, paralanguage, proxemics, and touch.

Kinesics

Kinesics (body language) includes nonverbal techniques such as facial expressions, posture, gestures, and body movements. Some add that clothing style and accessories such as jewelry also affect the context of communication. Box 7-4 describes various examples of nonverbal behavior and their meaning.

Knowledge of kinesics is important for the nurse being evaluated by his or her clients and vice versa. To create a positive impression during a client interaction, the nurse should:

- Assume a position at eye level with the client; stand or sit tall
- Relax arms, legs, and feet; do not cross any body part

BOX 7-4 Examples of Body Language

POSITIVE	INTERPRETATION	NEGATIVE	INTERPRETATION
Tilt of head	Interested	Arms crossed	Blocking; oppositional
Open hands	Sincere	Clenched jaw	Angry; antagonistic
Brisk, erect walk	Confident	Downcast eyes	Remorseful; bored
Hand to cheek	Contemplative	Rubbing nose	Doubtful; deceitful
Rubbing hands	Anticipatory	Drumming fingers	Impatient
Steepled fingers	Authoritative	Fondling hair	Insecure
Nod	Agreement	Frown	Disagreement
		Stroking chin	Stalling for time
		Shifting from foot to foot	Desire to get away
		Looking at watch	Bored

Adapted from Examples of body language in use. Available at: http://www.bodylanguage training.com/examples.html; Body language, sending signals without words. Available at: http://www.uwm.edu/~ceil/career/jobs/body.htm; and Examples of body language. Available at: http://www.deltabravo.net/custody/body.php.

- Maintain eye contact approximately 60% to 70% of the time or whatever is appropriate for the culture (see Chap. 6); in a group, focus on the last person who spoke
- Keep the head level, both horizontally and vertically
- Lean forward to demonstrate interest and attention
- Keep the arms where they can be seen
- Strike a balance in arm movements—neither too demonstrative nor reserved
- Keep the legs as still as possible

Paralanguage

Paralanguage (vocal sounds that are not actually words) also communicates a message. Some examples include drawing in a deep breath to indicate surprise, clucking the tongue to indicate disappointment, and whistling to get someone's attention. Vocal inflections, volume, pitch, and rate of speech add another dimension to communication. Crying, laughing, and moaning are additional forms of paralanguage.

Proxemics

Proxemics (the use and relationship of space to communication) varies among people from different cultural backgrounds. Generally, four zones are observed in interactions between Americans (Hall, 1959, 1963, 1966): **intimate space** (within 6 in.), **personal space** (6 in. to 4 ft), **social space** (4 to 12 ft), and **public space** (more than 12 ft; Table 7-3).

Most people in the United States comfortably tolerate strangers in a 2- to 3-ft area. Venturing closer may cause some to feel anxious. Understanding the client's comfort zone helps the nurse to know how spatial relations affect nonverbal communication.

Closeness is common in nursing because, most often, nurses and clients are in direct physical contact. Therefore, some clients can misinterpret physical nearness and touching within intimate and personal spaces as having sexual connotations. Approaches that may prevent such misunderstanding include explaining beforehand how a nursing procedure will be performed, ensuring that a client is properly draped or covered, and asking that another staff person of the client's gender be present during a potentially sensitive examination or procedure.

TABLE 7-3 Communication Zones

ZONE	DISTANCE	PURPOSE
Intimate space	Within 6 in.	• Lovemaking • Confiding secrets • Sharing confidential information
Personal space	6 in. to 4 ft	• Interviewing • Physical assessment • Therapeutic interventions involving touch • Private conversations • Teaching one-on-one
Social space	4–12 ft	• Group interactions • Lecturing • Conversations that are not intended to be private
Public space	12 ft or more	• Giving speeches • Gatherings of strangers

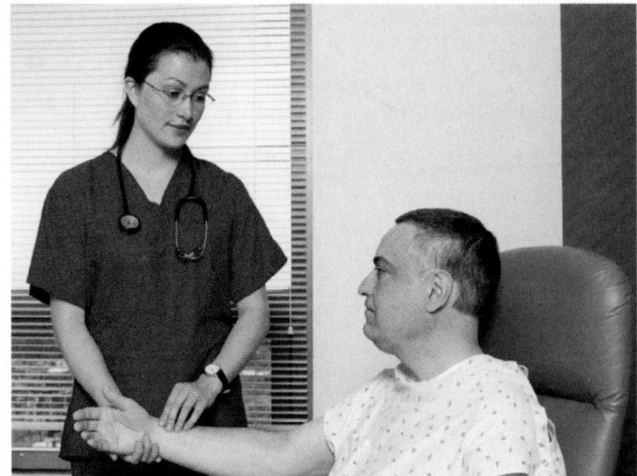

FIGURE 7-4 Examining a client involves task-oriented touch. (Photo by B. Proud.)

Touch

Touch (a tactile stimulus produced by making personal contact with another person or object) occurs frequently in nurse–client relationships. While caring for clients, touch can be task-oriented, affective, or both. **Task-oriented touch** involves the personal contact required when performing nursing procedures (Fig. 7-4). **Affective touch** is used to demonstrate concern or affection (Fig. 7-5).

Affective touch has different meanings to different people depending on how they were raised and their cultural background. Because nursing care involves a high degree of touching, the nurse is sensitive to how clients may perceive it. Most people respond positively to touch, but there are variations among individuals. Therefore, nurses use

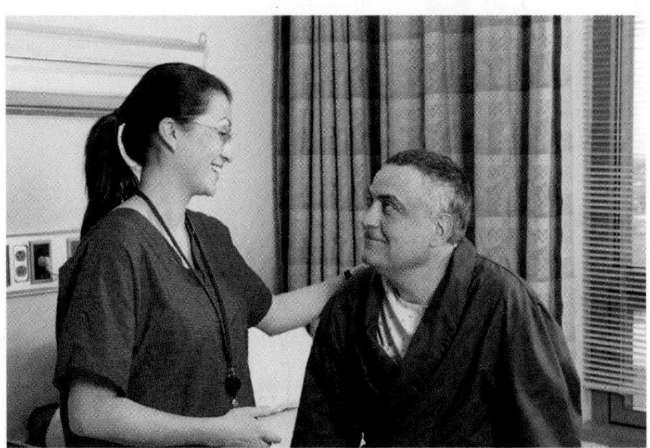

FIGURE 7-5 This nurse uses affective touch as she talks with her client. (Photo by B. Proud.)

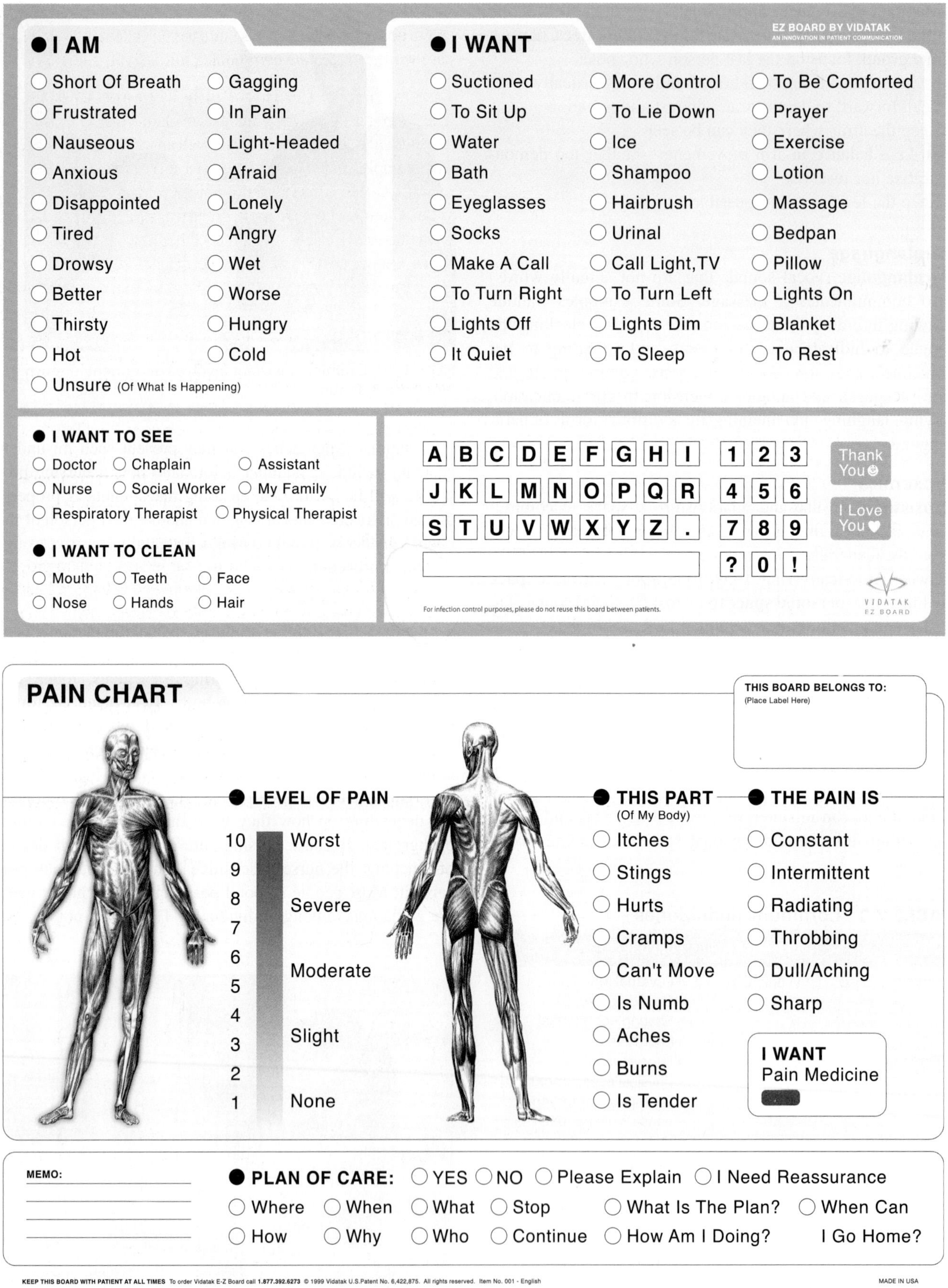

EZ BOARD BY VIDATAK
AN INNOVATION IN PATIENT COMMUNICATION

● I AM

○ Short Of Breath ○ Gagging
○ Frustrated ○ In Pain
○ Nauseous ○ Light-Headed
○ Anxious ○ Afraid
○ Disappointed ○ Lonely
○ Tired ○ Angry
○ Drowsy ○ Wet
○ Better ○ Worse
○ Thirsty ○ Hungry
○ Hot ○ Cold
○ Unsure (Of What Is Happening)

● I WANT

○ Suctioned ○ More Control ○ To Be Comforted
○ To Sit Up ○ To Lie Down ○ Prayer
○ Water ○ Ice ○ Exercise
○ Bath ○ Shampoo ○ Lotion
○ Eyeglasses ○ Hairbrush ○ Massage
○ Socks ○ Urinal ○ Bedpan
○ Make A Call ○ Call Light, TV ○ Pillow
○ To Turn Right ○ To Turn Left ○ Lights On
○ Lights Off ○ Lights Dim ○ Blanket
○ It Quiet ○ To Sleep ○ To Rest

● I WANT TO SEE

○ Doctor ○ Chaplain ○ Assistant
○ Nurse ○ Social Worker ○ My Family
○ Respiratory Therapist ○ Physical Therapist

● I WANT TO CLEAN

○ Mouth ○ Teeth ○ Face
○ Nose ○ Hands ○ Hair

A B C D E F G H I 1 2 3 Thank You
J K L M N O P Q R 4 5 6 I Love You
S T U V W X Y Z . 7 8 9
? 0 !

For infection control purposes, please do not reuse this board between patients.

VIDATAK EZ BOARD

PAIN CHART

THIS BOARD BELONGS TO:
(Place Label Here)

● LEVEL OF PAIN

10 Worst
9
8 Severe
7
6
5 Moderate
4
3 Slight
2
1 None

● THIS PART (Of My Body)

○ Itches
○ Stings
○ Hurts
○ Cramps
○ Can't Move
○ Is Numb
○ Aches
○ Burns
○ Is Tender

● THE PAIN IS

○ Constant
○ Intermittent
○ Radiating
○ Throbbing
○ Dull/Aching
○ Sharp

I WANT Pain Medicine

MEMO:

● PLAN OF CARE: ○ YES ○ NO ○ Please Explain ○ I Need Reassurance
○ Where ○ When ○ What ○ Stop ○ What Is The Plan? ○ When Can I Go Home?
○ How ○ Why ○ Who ○ Continue ○ How Am I Doing?

KEEP THIS BOARD WITH PATIENT AT ALL TIMES To order Vidatak E-Z Board call 1.877.392.6273 Item No. 001 - English MADE IN USA

FIGURE 7-6 A client who is verbally impaired due to a stroke or intubation can communicate his or her needs to the nurse using a communication board. (Courtesy of Vidatak, LLC. Los Angeles, CA 90069.)

affective touch cautiously even though its intention is to communicate caring and support. In general, affective touch is therapeutic when a client is

- Lonely
- Uncomfortable
- Near death
- Anxious, insecure, or frightened
- Disoriented
- Disfigured
- Semiconscious or comatose
- Visually impaired
- Sensory deprived

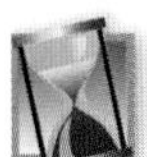

Gerontologic Considerations

- Although physical touch is an important form of nonverbal communication, use it purposefully as the primary method to reinforce verbal messages. Recognize that touch as a form of communication is usually more important to older adults than to those who are younger.
- Gender and age differences between client and care provider may determine the acceptability of touch. Appropriate use of touch, as with eye contact, requires cultural awareness.

Communicating With Special Populations

Some clients (eg, those who are verbally impaired, deaf, or have cognitive deficits such as Alzheimer's disease) pose unique challenges for communication. Nurses and other health care providers must find ways to help these clients effectively communicate their health problems and needs, give informed consent, and understand health practices that will impact their recovery or health maintenance. Regardless of the obstacles, The Joint Commission is adamant that health care workers facilitate communication with all clients.

Communicating with Verbally Impaired Clients

There are instances when nurses and clients cannot communicate verbally despite the fact that both are proficient in English. For example, clients who have had a stroke sometimes experience expressive aphasia, an inability to use verbal language skills. Clients who have artificial airways (eg, an endotracheal or tracheostomy tube) or who have their jaws wired following facial trauma cannot speak. Nevertheless, communication is still a nursing priority as mandated by the Joint Commission's National Patient Safety Goals (see Chap. 19). The nurse may provide the verbally impaired client with a paper tablet and pencil or "magic slate," although this approach is time-consuming. In some cases, the client may not have the use of the hands or the fine motor skills to use a writing device. Other communication tools such as those discussed in Chapter 6 or the example in Figure 7-6 may be used to communicate with verbally impaired clients who may point to common phrases, spell with the alphabet, and identify relevant numbers.

Communicating with Deaf Clients

A person who is deaf is unable to hear well enough to process spoken information, whereas a person who is hard of hearing has impaired hearing but is still able to perceive what is being said verbally when spoken at a louder level. If a deaf client can read and write, writing can facilitate communication. However, written communication may not be useful for all clients. Many deaf clients, especially those who were born deaf or lost their hearing at a very early age, have learned to lip read and use American Sign Language (ASL). ASL uses signs made by hand movements and finger spelling, an alphabetical substitute for words that have no sign (Fig. 7-7). However,

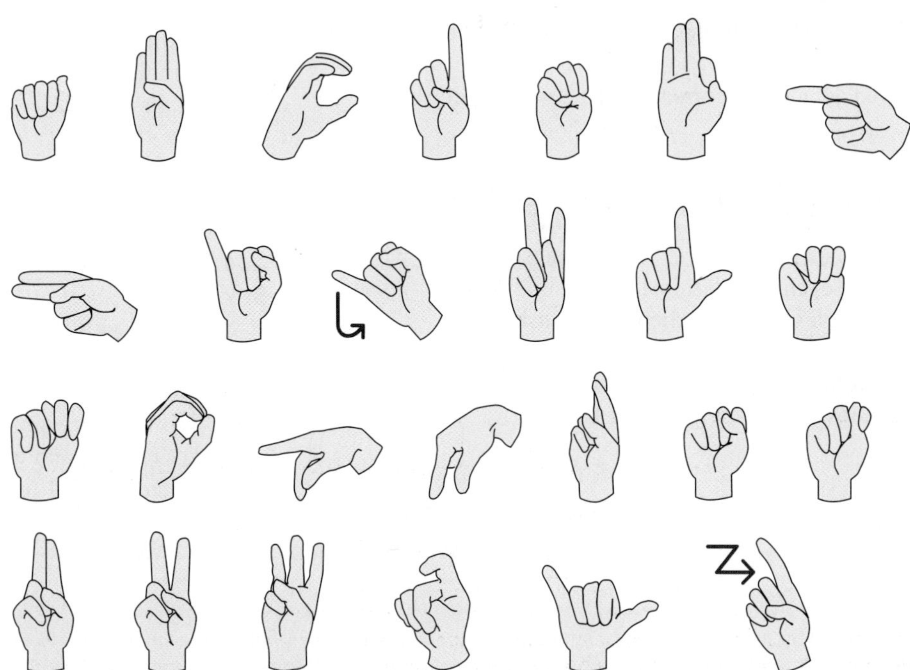

FIGURE 7-7 The alphabet in sign language.

not all health care agencies will have someone available who is proficient at ASL. To overcome this barrier, some hospitals use a webcam—a video camera that allows two-way viewing via a computerized connection. The webcam facilitates video interpreting, in which a person skilled in ASL communicates with the deaf client in the presence of the nurse.

Communicating with Clients with Alzheimer's Disease

Alzheimer's disease is a progressive, deteriorating brain disorder. Its onset is insidious, with symptoms that may develop slowly over years. Memory loss is the classic symptom, as well as disturbances in behavior and a loss in the ability to care for oneself. Problems with speaking, reading, and writing affect communication. Clients with this disease have difficulty expressing themselves verbally, such as finding correct words, organizing words into logical sentences, finishing sentences, and understanding words. Eventually, they may become mute.

Techniques that may facilitate communicating with a client who has Alzheimer's include the following:

- Gain the client's attention by approaching from the front and using the client's name
- Smile to convey friendliness
- Maintain eye contact to evaluate the client's attention and comprehension
- Assume a relaxed posture to avoid agitating the client
- Speak naturally at a normal rate and volume; avoid long sentences and difficult words
- Wait for a response while the client processes the information
- Rephrase information if the client does not seem to understand what has been said
- Show patience when the client tries to put thoughts into words
- Use visual cues like pantomimes that may clarify verbal meanings
- Avoid attempts to correct or argue with the client

CRITICAL THINKING EXERCISES

1. What specific services might a person expect within a nurse–client relationship which differ from those within a physician–client relationship?

2. Studies have shown that older adults are not touched with the same frequency as clients in other age groups. Discuss reasons for this.

3. What are the possible explanations when a client does not respond as expected during nurse–client interactions?

4. How might a nurse relieve anxiety experienced by a client who requires health care in an emergency situation?

NCLEX-STYLE REVIEW QUESTIONS

1. A discouraged client says, "I'm sure this surgery won't help any more than the others." What is the best initial nursing response?

1. "You're saying that you doubt you will improve."
2. "Do you want to talk to the surgeon again?"
3. "I'd recommend a more positive attitude."
4. "Of course it will; you'll be up and around in no time."

2. When a terminally ill client does not respond to medical treatment, which nursing action is most helpful in assisting the client to deal with his or her impending death?

1. Providing literature on death and dying
2. Allowing the client privacy to think alone
3. Listening to the client talk about his or her feelings
4. Encouraging the client to get a second opinion

3. An alarm caused by a loose cardiac monitor lead startles a client with chest pain. What nursing intervention is best to perform next?

1. Identify the client's current heart rhythm
2. Explain the reason the alarm sounded
3. Give the client a prescribed tranquilizer
4. Provide the client with a magazine to read

4. A 2-year-old child is admitted to the emergency department with a high fever of unknown origin. Which of following is the nurse correct to delegate to a nursing assistant?

1. Administer an aspirin suppository to reduce the child's fever
2. Give the toddler a popsicle or other fluid every 30 minutes
3. Call the laboratory for the results of diagnostic tests
4. Listen to the child's lungs for sounds of congestion.

5. What is the best nursing response when an 82-year-old client with Alzheimer's disease says he is looking forward to a visit from mother later today?

1. "Your mother has been deceased for years."
2. "Tell me more about your mother."
3. "Let me call and check on your mother."
4. "When did you last see your mother?"

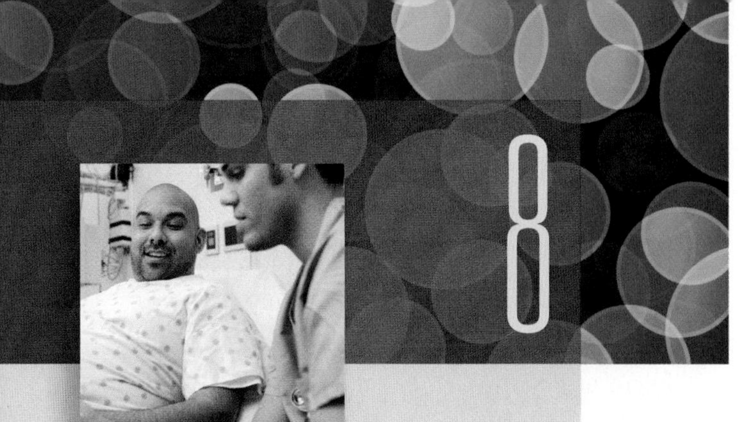

8 Client Teaching

Words To Know

affective domain
androgogy
cognitive domain
functionally illiterate
gerogogy
health literacy
illiterate
literacy
pedagogy
psychomotor domain
telehome care

Learning Objectives

On completion of this chapter, the reader should be able to:

1. Identify the authoritative bases that mandate client teaching.
2. List examples of client teaching provided by nurses.
3. List five benefits that result from client teaching.
4. Describe the three domains of learning.
5. Discuss three age-related categories of learners.
6. Discuss at least five characteristics unique to older adult learners.
7. Identify at least four factors that nurses assess before teaching clients.

Teaching is one of the most important uses of communication for nurses. Health teaching promotes the client's independent ability to meet his or her health needs. An old proverb that reinforces how education promotes self-care says, "Give a man a fish and he will eat for a day; teach a man to fish and he will eat for a lifetime."

Teaching is an essential nursing responsibility when caring for clients in a health care agency, at home, or in community settings. This chapter offers information on principles of learning and teaching.

IMPORTANCE OF CLIENT TEACHING

Health teaching is a mandated nursing activity. State nurse practice acts require health teaching, and The Joint Commission (2010) has made it a criterion for accreditation. Likewise, the American Nurses Association's Social Policy Statement addresses it (Box 8-1). Limited hospitalization time demands that nurses begin teaching as soon as possible after admission rather than waiting until discharge. Early attention to the client's learning needs is essential because learning takes place in four progressive stages:

1. Recognition of what has been taught
2. Recollection or description of information to others
3. Explanation or application of information
4. Independent use of new learning (London, 2009)

BOX 8-1 Social Policy Statement Regarding Teaching

Nursing practice includes, but is not limited to, initiating and maintaining comfort measures, promoting and supporting human functions and responses, establishing an environment conducive to well-being, providing health counseling and teaching, and collaborating on certain aspects of the health regimen.

Excerpted and reprinted with permission from American Nurses Association. (2003). *Social Policy Statement* (2nd ed., p. 8). Washington, DC: Author.

SCOPE AND CONSEQUENCES OF CLIENT TEACHING

Client teaching generally focuses on combinations of the following subject areas:

- The plan of care, treatment, and services
- Safe self-administration of medications
- The pain assessment process and methods for pain management
- Directions and practice in using equipment for self-care
- Dietary instructions
- Rehabilitation programs
- Available community resources
- Plan for medical follow-ups
- Signs of complications and actions to take

Some of the benefits of client teaching include (1) reduced length of stay, (2) cost-effectiveness of health care, (3) better allocation of resources, (4) increased client satisfaction, and (5) decreased readmission rates.

A delay in teaching retards optimum learning outcomes. If teaching standards are not met and discharged clients are readmitted or harmed because they were uninformed or failed to understand information that was taught, nurses are at risk for being sued.

The best proof of compliance with teaching standards is to document in the client's medical record who was taught, what was taught, the teaching method, and the evidence of learning.

ASSESSING THE LEARNER

To implement effective teaching, the nurse must determine the client's

- Preferred learning style
- Age and developmental level
- Capacity to learn
- Motivation
- Learning readiness
- Learning needs

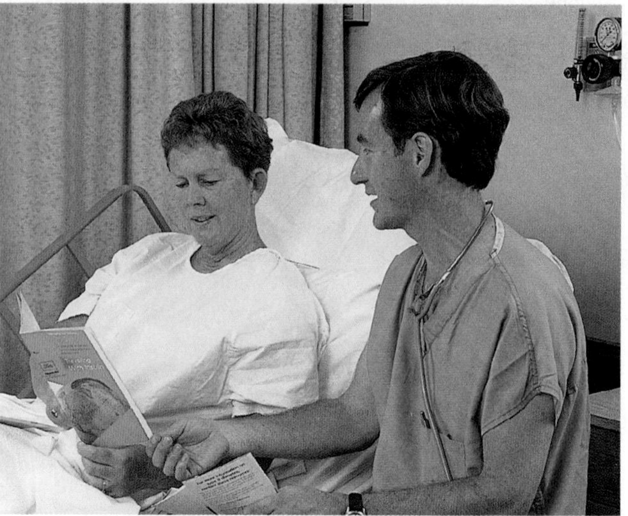

FIGURE 8-1 A nurse uses pamphlets and a book, which appeal to this client who prefers the cognitive domain of learning. (Photo by B. Proud.)

Learning Styles

Style of learning means how a person prefers to acquire knowledge. Learning styles fall within three general domains: cognitive, affective, and psychomotor. The **cognitive domain** is a style of processing information by listening or reading facts and descriptions. It is illustrated in Figure 8-1. The **affective domain** is a style of processing information that appeals to a person's feelings, beliefs, or values. The **psychomotor domain** is a style of processing information that focuses on learning by doing. Box 8-2 lists some activities associated with each learning domain.

One way to determine the client's preferred learning style is to ask a question such as, "When you learned to add fractions, what helped you most: hearing the teacher's explanation or reading about it in a mathematics book (cognitive domain), recognizing the value of the exercise (affective domain), or actually working sample problems (psychomotor domain)?" Although most clients favor one domain, nurses can optimize learning by presenting information through a combination of teaching approaches. Although the following figures (which originated in the National Training Center's Institute for Applied Behavioral Sciences in Alexandria, Virginia, in the 1960s) have been challenged, it is proposed that "learners

BOX 8-2 Activities that Promote Learning

COGNITIVE	PSYCHOMOTOR	AFFECTIVE
Listing	Assembling	Advocating
Identifying	Changing	Supporting
Locating	Emptying	Accepting
Labeling	Filling	Promoting
Summarizing	Adding	Refusing
Selecting	Removing	Defending

retain 10% of what they read, 20% of what they hear, 30% of what they see, 50% of what they see and hear, 70% of what they teach/talk, and 90% of what they talk/do" (Smaldino et al., 2007; Thalheimer, 2006). The bottom line is that learning improves when there is more active involvement.

Stop, Think, and Respond Box 8-1

Identify the learning domain that relates to each of the following teaching methods:

1. *The nurse watches as a client with diabetes practices administering an injection.*
2. *The nurse asks a client who had a mastectomy to speak to women attending a health seminar about the importance of monthly breast self-examinations.*
3. *The nurse explains the technique for performing leg exercises to a client scheduled for surgery.*
4. *The nurse helps a client self-administer nutritional formula through a gastrostomy tube.*
5. *The nurse gives a client with back strain a pamphlet on using good posture and body mechanics.*

Age and Developmental Level

Educators emphasize that learning takes place differently depending on a person's age and developmental level. Experts agree that teaching tends to be more effective when it is designed to accommodate unique age-related differences.

Nurses and all those who provide instruction must be aware of the learning characteristics of children, adult, and older adult learners (Table 8-1). Recently, a distinction has been made between learners at the early and later ends of the adult spectrum. Currently, there are three major categories:

- **Pedagogy** is the science of teaching children or those with cognitive ability comparable to children.
- **Androgogy** is the principles of teaching adult learners.
- **Gerogogy** is the unique techniques that enhance learning among older adults.

Although most clients with health problems are in their later years, nurse educators are advised to prepare themselves to teach young adults who belong to Generation X, Generation Y, and the Net Generation, as they age. Generation X refers to those born between 1961 and 1981; Generation Y refers to people who were born after 1981 through the latter part of the 20th century; and Generation Z, the Net Generation or "cyberkids," refers to those born at the beginning of the 21st century (Skiba & Barton, 2006). In general, those who represent Generations X, Y, and Z may share many learning characteristics:

- Are or will be technologically literate, having used or grown up with computers, smart phones, and tablet devices
- Crave stimulation and quick responses
- Expect immediate answers and feedback
- Become bored with memorizing information and doing repetitious tasks
- Prefer a variety of instructional methods from which they can choose
- Respond best when information is relevant
- Appreciate visualizations, simulations, and other methods of participatory learning

TABLE 8-1 Age-Related Differences among Learners[a]

PEDAGOGIC LEARNERS	ANDROGOGIC LEARNERS	GEROGOGIC LEARNERS
Physically immature	Physically mature	Undergoing degenerative changes
Lack experience	Building experience	Vast experience
Compulsory learners	Voluntary learners	Crisis learners
Passive	Active	Passive/active
Need direction and supervision	Self-directed and independent	Need structure and encouragement
Motivated to learn by potential rewards or punishment	Seek knowledge for its own sake or for personal interest	Motivated by a personal need or goal
Learning is subject centered	Learning is problem centered	Learning is self-centered
Short attention span	Longer attention span	Attention affected by low energy level, fatigue, and anxiety
Convergent thinkers (unidirectional; eg, see one application for new information)	Divergent thinkers (process multiple applications for new information)	Practical thinkers (process new information as it applies to a unique personal problem)
Need immediate feedback	Can postpone feedback	Respond to frequent feedback
Rote learning	Analytical learning	Experiential learning
Short-term retention	Long-term retention	Short-term unless reinforced by immediate use
Task oriented	Goal oriented	Outcome oriented
Think concretely	Think abstractly	Concrete/abstract
Respond to competition	Respond to collaboration	Respond to family encouragement

[a]Each learner is unique and may demonstrate characteristics associated with other age groups.

Stop, Think, and Respond Box 8-2

Identify the age-related learner for whom the following teaching techniques are most appropriate. Explain the basis for your analysis.

1. *The nurse's goal is to limit the teaching session to no more than 20 minutes.*
2. *The nurse emphasizes knowledge or techniques that the client is interested in learning.*
3. *The nurse reinforces that the client's discharge from the health agency correlates with becoming competent in self-administering insulin injections.*
4. *The nurse indicates that the client can use a computerized game for 30 minutes when he or she can name the number of recommended servings in each category within the food pyramid.*
5. *The nurse challenges the client to devise a plan for managing her colostomy when she returns to work following discharge.*

Capacity to Learn

For the person to receive, remember, analyze, and apply new information, he or she must have a certain amount of intellectual ability. Illiteracy, sensory deficits, cultural differences, shortened attention span, and lack of motivation and readiness require special adaptations when implementing health teaching.

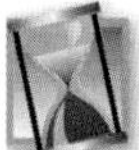

Gerontologic Considerations

■ During an initial assessment, older clients may interact in a socially appropriate manner and may indicate that they understand the material being taught. Asking a client to recall what has been discussed after approximately 15 minutes have passed may help determine what information has actually been retained. A mental status examination may be indicated (see Chap. 13). If there is cognitive impairment, a support person or caregiver should be present for the teaching sessions.

Literacy

It is essential to determine a client's level of **literacy** (ability to read and write) before developing a teaching plan. Approximately 42 million Americans cannot read at all (American Institutes for Research, 2009; Education-Portal.com, 2007). One could infer that these same adults are therefore **illiterate** (cannot read or write). Twenty percent of Americans are considered **functionally illiterate** (possess minimal literacy skills), which means they can sign their name and perform simple mathematical tasks (eg, make change) but read at or below a fifth-grade level. Functional illiteracy may be the consequence of a learning disability, not a below-average intellectual capacity.

Health literacy (the degree to which individuals have the capacity to obtain, process, and understand basic health information and services needed to make appropriate health decisions) is obviously a factor in client teaching (Kutner, Greenberg, Jin, et al., 2006). The latter affects a client's ability to evaluate information for credibility, analyze risks and benefits, calculate dosages, interpret test results, and locate health information (Glassman, 2008).

Because many illiterate or functionally illiterate people are not apt to volunteer information about their reading problems, literacy may be difficult to assess. Those who are illiterate and functionally illiterate usually develop elaborate mechanisms to disguise or compensate for their learning deficits. To protect the client's self-esteem, the nurse can ask, "How do you learn best?" and plan accordingly. Some useful approaches when teaching clients who are illiterate or functionally illiterate include the following:

- Use verbal and visual modes for instruction.
- Repeat directions several times in the same sequence so that the client can memorize the information.
- Provide pictures, diagrams, audio recordings, and videos for future review.

Sensory Deficits

The abilities to see and hear are essential for almost every learning situation. Older adults tend to have visual and auditory deficits, although such deficits are not exclusive to this population. Nursing Guidelines 8-1 presents some techniques for teaching clients with sensory impairment. Figure 8-2 shows samples of printing that can be used as an aid.

Cultural Differences

Because teaching and learning involve language, the nurse must modify approaches if the client cannot speak English or if English is a second language (see Chap. 6, Nursing Guidelines 6-1). Language barriers do not justify omitting health teaching. In most cases, if neither the nurse nor the client speaks a compatible language, a translator or acceptable alternative is needed.

Attention and Concentration

The client's attention and concentration affect the duration, delivery, and teaching methods employed. Some helpful approaches include the following:

- Observe the client and implement health teaching when he or she is most alert and comfortable.
- Keep the teaching session short.
- Use the client's name frequently throughout the instructional period; this refocuses his or her attention.
- Show enthusiasm, which you are likely to communicate to the client.
- Use colorful materials, gestures, and variety to stimulate the client.
- Involve the client in an active way.
- Vary the tone and pitch of your voice to stimulate the client aurally.

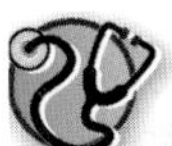

NURSING GUIDELINES 8-1

Teaching Clients with Sensory Impairments

Ensure that the client with a visual impairment is wearing prescription eyeglasses or that the client with a hearing impairment is wearing a hearing aid, if available. *Visual and auditory aids maximize the ability to perceive sensory stimuli.*

For clients with visual impairment:

- Speak in a normal tone of voice. *Clients with visual impairment do not necessarily also have hearing impairment. Increased volume does not compensate for reduced vision.*
- Use at least a 75- to 100-watt light source, preferably in a lamp that shines over the client's shoulder. *Ceiling lights tend to diffuse light rather than concentrate it on a small area where the client needs to focus.*
- Avoid standing in front of a window through which bright sunlight is shining. *It is difficult to look into bright light.*
- Provide a magnifying glass for reading. *Magnification enlarges standard or small print to a comfortable size.*
- Obtain pamphlets in large (12- to 16-point) print and serif lettering, which has horizontal lines at the bottom and top of each letter (see Fig. 8-2). *Letters and words are usually more distinct when set in large print with a style that promotes visual discrimination.*
- Avoid using materials printed on glossy paper. *Glossy paper reflects light, causing a glare that makes reading uncomfortable.*
- Select black print on white paper. *This combination provides maximum contrast and makes letters more legible.*

For clients with hearing impairment:

- Use a magic slate, chalkboard, flash cards, or writing pads to communicate. *Writing can substitute for verbal instructions.*
- Lower the voice pitch. *Hearing loss is generally in the higher pitch ranges.*
- Try to select words that do not begin with "f," "s," "k," and "sh." *These letters are formed with high-pitched sounds and are therefore difficult for clients with hearing impairment to discriminate.*
- Rephrase rather than repeat when the client does not understand. *Rephrasing may provide additional visual or auditory clues to facilitate the client's understanding.*
- Insert a stethoscope into the client's ears and speak into the bell with a low voice. *The stethoscope acts as a primitive hearing aid. It projects sounds directly to the ears and reduces background noise.*

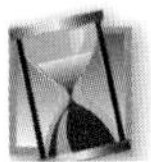

Gerontologic Considerations

■ A calm demeanor and a quiet environment can decrease anxiety or distractions that prevent new learning. Peer teaching or reinforcement in support group settings may be helpful.

12 pt. Times

Aa Bb Cc Dd Ee Ff Gg Hh Ii Jj Kk Ll
Oo Pp Qq Rr Ss Tt Uu Vv Ww Xx Yy

14 pt. Times

Aa Bb Cc Dd Ee Ff Gg Hh Ii Jj Kk
Oo Pp Qq Rr Ss Tt Uu Vv Ww Xx

16 pt. Times

Aa Bb Cc Dd Ee Ff
Oo Pp Qq Rr Ss Tt

FIGURE 8-2 Selecting printed materials with 12- to 16-point size type, black print on white paper, and serif lettering help improve visual clarity.

Motivation

Learning is optimal when a person has a purpose for acquiring new information. Relevance of learning depends on individual variables. The desire for learning may be to satisfy intellectual curiosity, restore independence, prevent complications, or facilitate discharge and return to the comfort of home. Less desirable reasons are to please others and to avoid criticism.

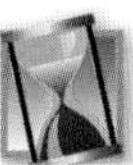

Gerontologic Considerations

■ Most people are "creatures of habit" and are reluctant to make changes without understanding the benefit. Older adults may be creative in methods for incorporating needed changes in health behavior if the purposes or anticipated benefits are made clear at the beginning of the teaching session.

■ Stating a belief that the older adult can actually make the recommended health behavioral changes and providing encouragement may increase the client's self-confidence and result in increased learning.

Learning Readiness

When a capacity and motivation for learning exist, the nurse can determine the final component—learning readiness. Readiness refers to the client's physical and psychological well-being. For example, a person who is in pain, is too warm or cold, is having difficulty breathing, or is depressed or fearful is not in the best condition to learn. In these situations, it is best to restore comfort and then attend to teaching.

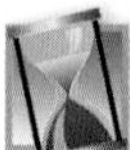

Gerontologic Considerations

- Beginning the teaching session with a reference to the older person's actual experience will help provide a link to which the new learning can connect.

Learning Needs

The best teaching and learning take place when both are individualized. To be most efficient and personalized, the nurse must gather pertinent information from the client. Second-guessing what the client wants and needs to know often leads to wasted time and effort.

The following are questions a nurse can ask to assess the client's learning needs:

- What does being healthy mean to you?
- What things in your life interfere with being healthy?
- What don't you understand as fully as you would like?
- What activities do you need help with?
- What do you hope to accomplish before being discharged?
- How can I help you at this time?

INFORMAL AND FORMAL TEACHING

Informal teaching is unplanned and occurs spontaneously at the bedside. Formal teaching requires a plan. Without a plan, teaching becomes haphazard. Furthermore, without some organization of time and content, the potential for reaching goals, providing adequate information, and ensuring comprehension is jeopardized. Potential teaching needs are generally identified at the client's admission, but they may be amended as care and treatment progress. If ongoing teaching is necessary, furnishing clients with technology for **telehome care** (visiting clients electronically in their home for the purpose of seeing and communicating in real time) may be beneficial, especially for clients located in rural areas. A student nurse may work with a staff nurse or instructor in developing a teaching plan. Usually, one or more nurses carry out certain specific parts of a teaching plan (Fig. 8-3). This approach is the most desirable so that a client is not overwhelmed with processing volumes of new information or learning skills that are difficult for novices to perform. Skill 8-1 serves as a model when an adult client needs teaching.

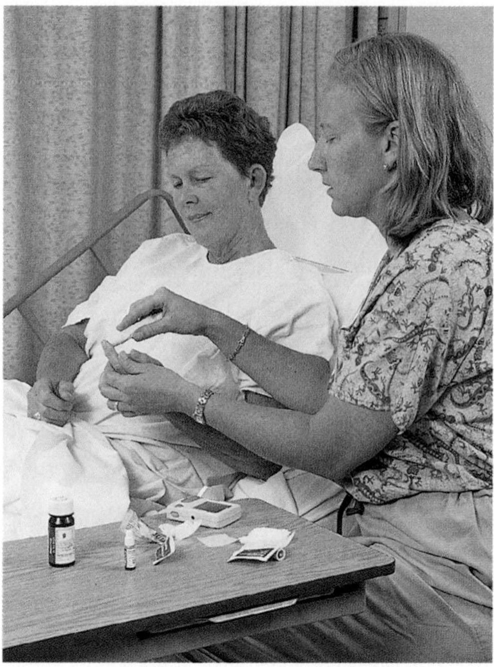

FIGURE 8-3 The nurse teaches about diabetes at the bedside. Multisensory stimulation is promoted by giving the client explanations and encouraging her to watch the technique for testing blood sugar as it is being performed. (Photo by B. Proud.)

CRITICAL THINKING EXERCISES

1. Identify reasons why health literacy is especially important in the 21st century.
2. How would a nurse teach techniques for toothbrushing differently to a child; to a person from the Y, X, or Net generations; to a young adult; to a middle-aged adult; and to an older adult?
3. What teaching strategies could the nurse use to teach toothbrushing within the cognitive, affective, and psychomotor domains of learning?
4. Give two examples of how you could determine whether a client actually learned information you taught such as toothbrushing.

NCLEX-STYLE REVIEW QUESTIONS

1. Which of the following are examples of activities that are best performed by a client whose learning style is primarily in the cognitive domain? Select all that apply.
   1. Assembling equipment
   2. Listing needed equipment
   3. Identifying pieces of equipment
   4. Defending the choice of equipment
   5. Summarizing the use of equipment

2. Arrange the following steps in the order in which they should occur when teaching a client. Use all the options:
   1. Encourage feedback from the client
   2. Divide information into manageable amounts
   3. Find out what the client wants to know
   4. Document the client's evidence of learning
   5. Determine the client's recall of information
3. Which of the following is most essential before teaching the mother of a 6-year-old child about nutrition?
   1. Assess the child's height and weight
   2. Obtain a nutrition guidelines pamphlet
   3. Develop a plan for 1 week of menus
   4. Collect various nutritional recipes
4. After teaching a client how to perform breathing exercises, what is the best method for evaluating the effectiveness of the teaching?
   1. Request that the client explain the importance of breathing exercises
   2. Ask the client to perform the breathing exercises as they were taught
   3. Ask the client if he is performing the breathing exercises as required
   4. Monitor the client's respiratory rate several times a day
5. Which of the following teaching aids is developmentally appropriate when preparing a preschool child for a diagnostic test such as a bone marrow puncture?
   1. Dolls or puppets
   2. Pamphlets or booklets
   3. Colored diagrams
   4. Commercial videotapes

SKILL 8-1 Teaching Adult Clients

Suggested Action	Reason for Action
ASSESSMENT	
Find out what the client wants to know.	Personal interest facilitates learning.
Establish what the client should know to remain healthy.	Clients are not always aware of what information is vital to maintain their health and safety.
Determine the client's learning style.	Teaching is more effective when techniques support the client's preferred learning method.
PLANNING	
Collaborate with the client on content, goals, and realistic time frames.	Adult learners tend to prefer collaboration and active involvement in the learning process.
Develop a written plan that builds from simple to complex, familiar to unfamiliar, and normal to abnormal.	Adult learners learn best by applying information from present knowledge or past experiences.
Divide information into manageable amounts.	Too much information at once tends to overwhelm learners.
Select teaching strategies and resources that are compatible with the client's preferred style for learning.	Adult learners generally prefer one learning style, but multiple approaches enhance learning.
Use a variety of instructional methods from the cognitive, affective, and psychomotor domains.	Adults tend to retain more knowledge when a variety of instructional techniques are used.
Review the content that will be used during teaching.	Preparation and knowledge evoke self-confidence.
IMPLEMENTATION	
Teach when the client appears interested and physically and emotionally ready to learn, if possible.	Learning takes place more easily when the client can focus on the task at hand.
Provide an environment that promotes learning.	Learning occurs best in a well-lit room with a comfortable temperature. Distractions and interruptions interfere with concentration.
Identify how long the teaching session will last.	Clarifying the length of time prepares the client for the demands on his or her time and attention.
Begin with basic concepts.	Learning that builds from simple to complex is best.
Review previously taught information.	Repetition increases retention of information.
Use vocabulary within the client's personal level of understanding.	Teaching at the learner's level preserves dignity. The nurse is accountable for ensuring the client's comprehension.
Explain any and all new terms.	Clients are sometimes embarrassed to admit they do not understand.
Involve the client actively by encouraging feedback and handling of equipment.	Adult learners prefer active rather than passive learning situations.
Stimulate as many senses as possible.	Involvement of more than one sense enhances learning.
Invent songs, rhymes, or a series of key terms that correspond with the teaching content.	Creativity stimulates the right hemisphere of the brain where information is retrieved more easily.
Use equipment as similar as possible to what the client will use at home.	Becoming familiar with equipment is the best preparation for self-care at home.
Allow time for questions and answers.	Providing this opportunity helps the client clarify information and prevents misunderstandings.
Summarize the key points covered during the current teaching.	Reviewing reinforces important concepts.
Determine the client's level of learning.	The ability to recall or apply information and to demonstrate skills is proof of short-term learning.
Identify the time, place, and content for the next teaching session.	Planning the next meeting provides a time frame during which the client may review and practice what has been taught.
Arrange an opportunity for the client to use or apply the new information as soon as possible after it was taught.	Immediate application reinforces learning and promotes long-term retention.
Document the information taught and evidence demonstrating the client's understanding.	Documentation provides a written record of the client's progress and avoids omissions or duplications during future teaching sessions.
Review with the client the progress made toward goals.	Collaboration keeps the client focused on expected outcomes.
Evaluate the need for further teaching.	Evaluation is the basis for revising the teaching plan.

(continues)

Teaching Adult Clients (continued)

Evaluation

- The planned teaching content was covered.
- The client participated in the teaching process.
- The client recalled at least 50% of the concepts with accuracy.

Document

- Date and time
- Content taught
- Evidence of the client's learning

SAMPLE DOCUMENTATION

Date and Time Explained the times for taking two drugs that require self-administration after discharge. States, "I take the yellow pill once in the morning before breakfast and I take one blue pill three times a day when I eat breakfast, lunch, and supper." ——— SIGNATURE/TITLE

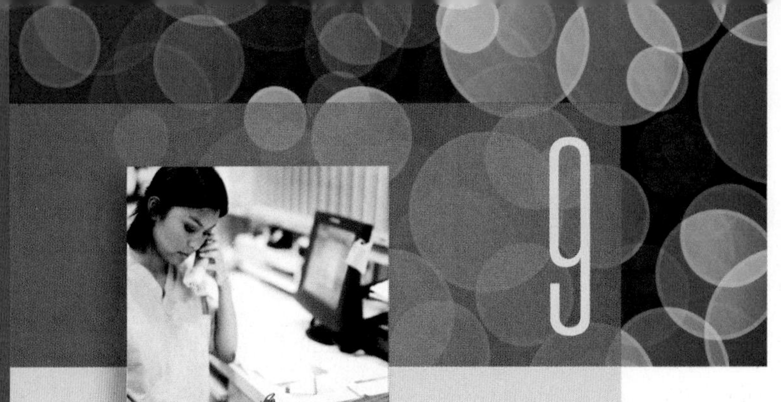

9 Recording and Reporting

Words To Know

auditors
beneficial disclosure
change-of-shift report
chart
charting
charting by exception
checklist
computerized charting
continuous quality improvement
documenting
double charting
flow sheet
focus charting
Kardex
medical records
military time
minimum disclosure
narrative charting
nursing care plan
PIE charting
problem-oriented record
quality assurance
recording
rounds
SOAP charting
source-oriented record
total quality improvement
traditional time

Learning Objectives

On completion of this chapter, the reader should be able to:

1. Identify seven uses for medical records.
2. List six components generally found in any client's medical record.
3. Differentiate between source-oriented and problem-oriented records.
4. Identify six methods of charting.
5. Explain the purpose and applications associated with the Health Insurance Portability and Accountability Act (HIPAA).
6. List four aspects of documentation required in the medical records of all clients cared for in acute settings.
7. Discuss why it is important to use only approved abbreviations when charting.
8. Explain how to convert traditional time to military time.
9. List at least 10 guidelines that apply to charting.
10. Identify four written forms used to communicate information about clients.
11. List five ways that health care workers exchange client information other than by reading the medical record.

Nurses must communicate information clearly, concisely, and accurately, both when writing and when speaking. This chapter describes various written and spoken forms of communication and nursing responsibilities for record keeping and reporting.

MEDICAL RECORDS

Medical records are collections of information about a person's health, the care provided by health practitioners, and the client's progress. They are also referred to as *health records* or *client records*. The medical record may consist of various agency-approved paper forms (Table 9-1), or the forms may be stored on the hard drive of a computerized electronic medical record. Physicians who provide care to Medicare and Medicaid clients have an incentive to use electronic information technology to maintain computerized health records as early as 2011 and no later than 2015 if they wish to qualify for government funds under the American Recovery and Reinvestment Act (Amatayakul, 2009).

Hard copy paper forms are placed in a **chart** (a binder or folder that promotes the orderly collection, storage, and safekeeping of a person's medical records). The paper forms in the chart are color-coded or separated by tabbed sheets. A computerized medical record is

TABLE 9-1 Common Agency Chart Forms

NAME OF FORM	CONTENT
Fact sheet	Provides information such as the client's name, date of birth, address, phone number, religion, insurer, admitting physician, admitting diagnosis, person to contact in case of emergency, and emergency phone number
Advance directive	Provides instructions about the client's choices for care should he or she be unable to make decisions later
History and physical examination	Contains the physician's review of the client's current and past health problems, results of a body system examination, medical diagnosis, and tentative plan for treatment
Physician's orders	Identifies laboratory and diagnostic tests, diet, activity, medications, intravenous fluids, and clinical procedures (instructions for changing a dressing, inserting tubes, and so forth) on a day-by-day basis
Physician's or multidisciplinary progress notes	Describes the client's ongoing status and response to the current plan of care, and potential modifications in the plan
Nursing admission database	Documents information concerning the client's health patterns and initial physical assessment findings
Nursing or multidisciplinary plan of care	Identifies client problems, goals, and directions for care based on an analysis of collected data
Graphic sheet	Displays trends in the client's vital signs, weight, and daily summary of fluid intake and output
Daily nursing assessment and flow sheet	Indicates focused physical assessment findings by individual nurses during each 24-hour period and the routine care that was provided
Nursing notes	Provides narrative details of subjective and objective data, nursing actions, response of the client, outcomes of communication with other health care personnel, or the client's family
Medication administration record	Identifies the drug name, date, time, route, and frequency of drug administration as well as the name of the nurse who administered each medication
Laboratory and diagnostic reports	Contains the results of tests in a sequential order
Discharge plan	Indicates the information, skills, and referral services that the client may need before being released from the agency's care
Teaching summary	Identifies content that was taught, evidence of the client's learning, and need for repetition or reinforcement

accessed by using a password and selecting the desired form from a menu. Computerized records can be printed if a hard copy is desired. All personnel involved in a client's health care contribute to the medical record by **charting**, **recording**, or **documenting** (the process of entering information).

Uses

Besides serving as a permanent health record, the collective information about a client provides a means to share information among health care workers, thus ensuring client safety and continuity of care. Occasionally, medical records also are used to investigate quality of care in a health agency, demonstrate compliance with national accreditation standards, promote reimbursement from insurance companies, facilitate health education and research, and provide evidence during malpractice lawsuits.

Permanent Account

The medical record is a written, chronologic account of a person's illness or injury and the health care provided from the onset of the problem through discharge or death. The record is filed and maintained for future reference. Previous health records often are requested during subsequent admissions so that the client's health history can be reviewed.

Sharing Information

Because it is impossible for all health care workers to meet and exchange information on a personal basis at the same time, the written record becomes central to communication (ie, sharing information among personnel). The documentation serves as a way to inform others about the client's status and plan for care.

Sharing information prevents duplication of care and helps reduce the chance of error or omission. For example, if a client requests medication for pain, the nurse checks the client's record to determine when the last pain-relieving drug was administered. Accurate and timely documentation prevents medication from being administered too frequently or withheld unnecessarily. Maintaining immunization records is an example of how documentation promotes continuity—the record ensures the administration of subsequent immunizations according to an appropriate schedule.

Quality Assurance

To maintain a high level of care, hospitals and other health care agencies use medical records to promote **quality assurance**, **continuous quality improvement**, or **total quality improvement** (an agency's internal process for self-improvement to ensure that the level of care reflects or exceeds established standards). One quality assurance method involves investigating the documentation in a sample of medical records. If the analyzed data indicate less-than-acceptable compliance with standards of care, the committee recommends corrective measures and reevaluates the outcomes later.

Accreditation

The Joint Commission is a private association that has established criteria reflecting high standards for client safety and institutional health care. Representatives of The Joint Commission periodically inspect health care agencies to determine whether they demonstrate evidence of quality care.

The documentation in randomly selected medical records is just one component examined during an accreditation visit. To support a health care agency's accreditation, nursing documentation should include the following:

- Initial assessment and reassessments of physical, psychological, social, environmental, and self-care status; education; and discharge planning
- Identification of nursing diagnoses or client needs
- Planned nursing interventions or nursing standards of care for meeting the client's nursing care needs
- Nursing care provided
- Client's response to interventions and outcomes of care, including pain management, discharge planning activities, and the client's or significant other's ability to manage continuing care needs

If documentation is substandard, accreditation may be withheld or withdrawn.

Reimbursement

The costs of most clients' hospital and home care are billed to third-party payers such as Medicare, Medicaid, and private insurance companies. **Auditors** (inspectors who examine client records) survey medical records to determine whether the care provided meets the established criteria for reimbursement. Undocumented, incomplete, or inconsistent documentation of care may result in a denial of payment.

Education and Research

Published references are primary resources for health education. Examining the medical records of clients with specific disorders, however, provides a valuable supplement that enhances learning and future problem solving. Client records also facilitate research. For example, some types of clinical investigations are difficult to conduct because few participants are in a particular locale or test facilities are limited. Consequently, stored, microfilmed, or computerized medical records serve as an alternative resource for scientific data.

Nevertheless, to protect confidentiality, only authorized persons are allowed access to client records (see later discussion on protecting health information). Formal permission must be obtained from the client, the health agency's administrator, or other authority whenever a client's record is used for a purpose other than treatment and record keeping.

BOX 9-1 Criteria for Legally Defensible Charting

When making an entry in a client's medical record, the nurse should:

- Ensure that the client's name appears on each page.
- Never chart for someone else.
- Use the specified color of ink and ballpoint pen, or enter data on a computer.
- Date and time each entry as it is made.
- Chart promptly after providing care.
- Make entries in chronologic order.
- Identify documentation that is out of chronologic sequence with the words "late entry."
- Write or print legibly.
- Use correct grammar and spelling.
- Reflect the plan of care.
- Describe the outcomes of care.
- Record relevant details.
- Use only approved abbreviations.
- Never scribble over entries or use correction fluid to obliterate what has been written.
- Draw a single line through erroneous information so that it remains readable, add the date, initial, and then document the correct information.
- Record facts, not subjective interpretations.
- Quote the client's verbal comments.
- Write "duplicate" or "recopied" on documentation that is not original; include the date, time, initials, and reason for the duplication.
- Never imply criticism of another's care.
- Document the circumstances for notifying a physician, the specific data reported, and the physician's recommendations.
- Identify specific information provided when teaching a client and the evidence that indicates the client has understood the instructions.
- Leave no empty spaces between entries and signature.
- Sign each entry by name and title.

Legal Evidence

The medical record is considered a legal document. Therefore, entries in medical records must follow legally defensible criteria (Box 9-1). Portions of the medical record can be subpoenaed as evidence by the defense or prosecuting attorney to prove or disprove allegations of malpractice. It is especially important to document safety precautions taken to protect the client, individuals who were notified about concerns and issues, and outcomes of the communication.

Each person who makes entries in the client's medical record is responsible for the information he or she records and can be summoned as a witness to testify concerning

TABLE 9-2 Common Components of a Problem-Oriented Record

COMPONENT	DESCRIPTION
Data base	Contains initial health information
Problem list	Consists of a numeric list of the client's health problems
Plan of care	Identifies methods for solving each identified health problem
Progress notes	Describes the client's responses to what has been done and revisions to the initial plan

what has been documented. Any written documentation that cannot be clearly read or that is vague, scribbled through, whited out, written over, or erased makes for a poor legal defense.

Stop, Think, and Respond Box 9-1

Discuss how the nurse could improve each of the following documentation samples:
1. 01/11 0800 Ate well.
2. 1400 Hygiene provided and ambulated.
3. 1500 Depressed all day. S. Rogers.

Client Access to Records

Historically, clients were not allowed to see their medical records. Since the passing of federal legislation in 1996 known as the HIPAA, with further revisions in 2001 and 2002, clients now have the right to see their own medical and billing records, request changes to anything they feel is inaccurate, and be informed about who has seen their medical records (US Department of Health and Human Services, 2005). Consequently, many institutions have written policies that describe the guidelines by which clients can access their own medical records. Policies range from complete, unrestricted access within 30 days of the client's written request to arranging access in the presence of the client's physician or hospital administrator. Nurses must follow the established agency policy.

Types of Client Records

Health records in most agencies contain similar information. They generally are organized in one of two ways: either a source-oriented or a problem-oriented format.

Source-Oriented Records

The traditional type of client record is a **source-oriented record** (records organized according to the source of documented information). This type of record contains separate forms on which physicians, nurses, dietitians, physical therapists, and other health care providers make entries about their own specific activities in relation to the client's care.

One of the criticisms of source-oriented records is that it is difficult to demonstrate a unified, cooperative approach for resolving the client's problems among caregivers. Frequently, the fragmented documentation gives the impression that each professional is working independently of the others.

Problem-Oriented Records

A second type of client record is the **problem-oriented record** (records organized according to the client's health problems). In contrast to source-oriented records that contain numerous locations for information, problem-oriented records contain four major components: the database, the problem list, the plan of care, and the progress notes (Table 9-2). The information is compiled and arranged to emphasize goal-directed care to promote the recording of pertinent information and to facilitate communication among health care professionals.

METHODS OF CHARTING

Nurses use various styles to record information within the client's record. Examples include narrative notes, SOAP charting, focus charting, PIE charting, charting by exception, and computerized charting.

Narrative Charting

Narrative charting (the style of documentation generally used in source-oriented records) involves writing information about the client and client care in chronologic order. There is no established format for narrative notations; the content resembles a log or journal (Fig. 9-1).

Narrative charting is time-consuming to write and read. The caregiver must sort through the lengthy notation for specific information about care and progress that correlates with the client's problems. Depending on the skill of the person writing a narrative entry, he or she may omit pertinent documentation or include insignificant information.

SOAP Charting

SOAP charting (the documentation style more likely to be used in a problem-oriented record) acquired its name from the four essential components included in a progress note:

- S = subjective data
- O = objective data
- A = analysis of the data
- P = plan for care

Some agencies have expanded the SOAP format to SOAPIE or SOAPIER (I = interventions, E = evaluation, R = revision to the plan of care; Table 9-3).

Any variations in the SOAP format tend to focus the documentation on pertinent information that is required by The Joint Commission. SOAP charting also helps demonstrate

Three Rivers Area Hospital
214 SPRING STREET
THREE RIVERS, MICHIGAN 49093

NURSING NOTES

ROOM NO. ______
NAME ______
DOCTOR ______

Date Time	NURSES REMARKS	Signature
1330	States "I'm having chest pain. It's like an elephant is sitting on me."	B. Zook, RN
1340	BP $^{150}/_{90}$, P-122 and irregular. Skin is pale and moist. O_2 started at 5L/min. Nitroglycerin ī tab. administered sublingually.	B. Zook, RN.
1350	Dr. Johnson notified of the change in condition. EKG ordered. 1000 cc 5% D/W started IV c̄ #20 gauge angiocath in (L) arm. IV running at 20 gtts/minute.	B. Zook, RN
1410	EKG obtained. BP $^{140}/_{84}$ P-110 and still irregular, skin pink but moist. No relief from Nitroglycerin. States "It's still pretty bad."	B. Zook, RN.
1420	Morphine 10 mg. administered sub-q for chest pain and anxiety.	B. Zook, RN
1430	Transferred to CCU per bed. Clothing, dentures, and eyeglasses accompanied transfer.	B. Zook RN
1440	Family notified of transfer.	B. Zook, RN

FIGURE 9-1 Sample of narrative charting. (Courtesy of Three Rivers Area Hospital, Three Rivers, MI.)

TABLE 9-3 SOAPIER Charting Format

LETTER	EXPLANATION	EXAMPLE OF RECORDING
S = Subjective information	Information reported by the client	S—"I don't feel well."
O = Objective information	Observations made by the nurse	O—Temperature 102.4°F
A = Analysis	Problem identification	A—Fever
P = Plan	Proposed treatment	P—Offer extra fluids and monitor body temperature
I = Intervention	Care provided	I—750 mL of fluid intake in 8 hours; temperature assessed every 4 hours
E = Evaluation	Outcome of treatment	E—Temperature reduced to 101°F
R = Revision	Changes in treatment	R—Increase fluid intake to 1,000 mL per shift until temperature is ≤100°F

6/30/2007	D(ata) –	Bladder distended 2 fingers above pubis.
1015		Has not urinated in 8 hrs. since
		catheter was removed. ————
	A(ction) –	Assisted to toilet. Water turned on at
		faucet. Instructed to press over bladder
		with hands. ————
	R(esponse) –	Voided 525 mL of clear urine. L. Cass, SN

FIGURE 9-2 Example of DAR charting.

interdisciplinary cooperation because everyone involved in the care of a client makes entries in the same location in the chart.

Focus Charting

Focus charting (a modified form of SOAP charting) uses the word *focus* rather than problem because some believe that the word *problem* carries negative connotations. A focus can be the client's current or changed behavior, significant events in the client's care, or even a North American Nursing Diagnosis Association (NANDA) nursing diagnosis. Instead of using the SOAP format to make entries, focus charting follows a DAR model (D = data, A = action, R = response; Fig. 9-2). DAR notations tend to reflect the steps in the nursing process.

PIE Charting

PIE charting (a method of recording the client's progress under the headings of problem, intervention, and evaluation) is similar to the SOAPIE format. The PIE style prompts the nurse to address specific content in a charted progress note.

When nurses use the PIE method, they document assessments on a separate form and give the client's problems a corresponding number. They use the numbers subsequently in the progress notes when referring to interventions and the client's responses (Fig. 9-3).

Charting by Exception

Charting by exception is a documentation method in which nurses chart only abnormal assessment findings or care that deviates from the standard. Proponents of this efficient method say that charting by exception provides quick access to abnormal findings because it does not describe normal and routine information.

NURSING NOTES

Date Time	NURSES REMARKS	Signature
6/19	P#1 Crackles heard on inspiration in	
0750	the bases of R and L lungs. ——	
	I#1 Incision splinted with pillow.	
	Instructed to breathe deeply,	
	open mouth, and cough at the	
	end of expiration ————	
	E#1 Lungs clear with coughing.	
	———— A. Walker, LPN	

FIGURE 9-3 Sample of PIE charting.

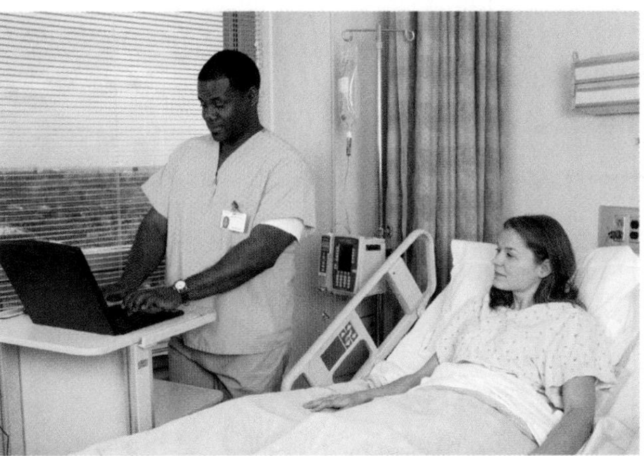

FIGURE 9-4 Portable computers allow for point of care documentation. (From Craven, R.F., Hirnle, C.J. *Fundamentals of Nursing* [6th ed.]. Philadelphia: Lippincott Williams & Wilkins.)

Computerized Charting

Computerized charting (documenting client information electronically) is most efficient for nurses when documentation is done at the point of care or bedside (Fig. 9-4). Having a terminal at the nursing station is a less desirable option because this removes the nurse from the source of the data; however, this may be the only alternative when there are limited computers for charting available. Centralized terminals generally are connected to large information systems that link departments in the institution (eg, pharmacy, laboratory, admissions office, accounting); therefore, they are less specific for nursing use.

Although each computer system varies, computerized charting generally is done by using a portable laptop and keyboard, or touching the monitor screen with a finger or electronic device such as a light pen to select from a list of menu options. Some systems allow a combination of keyboarding and touch-screen technology. Data entry by voice activation is on the horizon. A single keystroke saves the information displayed on the monitor to the client's record (Fig. 9-5).

Computerized charting has many advantages:

- The information is always legible.
- It automatically records the date and time of the documentation.
- The abbreviations and terms are consistent with agency-approved lists.
- It eliminates trivia.
- Omissions are fewer because the computer prompts the nurse to enter specific information.
- It saves time because it eliminates delays in obtaining the chart.
- It reduces overtime costs for uncompleted end-of-shift charting.

Washington Hospital Center

Requested by Page – 1

RoutneNurseCare

DATE (2012)	1/18	1/19		1/20	1/21		
TIME	2200	0400	1300	2200	0200	2000	2310
Bath Care	Complt	None	Partl	Complt	Partl	Complt	None
Oral Care	q4h	q8h	q4h	q2h	q4h	q4h	q4h
Skin Care	Yes	Yes	Yes	Yes	Yes	Yes	Yes
Freq. Turned	q2h	q2h	q2h	q2h	q2h	q2h	q2h
ROMq4	Ys-Act	No	Ys-Act	Ys-Pas	Ys-Pas	Ys-Pas	
Decubitus care	None	None	None			None	None
Foly/Texs Care	Yes	Yes	Yes	Yes	Yes	Yes	Yes
Line Dressing	Ok	Ok	Ok	None	None	Ok	Ok
IV tubing	Ok	Ok	Chnged	Ok	Chnged	Chnged	Chnged
HeprinLk Flush	None	None		Yes	None		None
OOB	Assist	Bedrst	Assist			Assist	Bedrst
OOB-hrs	>1hr		>2hr			>1hr	
Slept-hrs	1–4hr	>4hr	1–4hr			<1hr	>4hr
Nares Care	q8h	q8h		q8h	q8h	q8h	q8h
ET/Trach Care	q8h	q8h	q8h	q8h	q8h	q4h	q8h
Chest PT	q6h	q6h		q6h	q6h	q6h	q6h
Restr.check q2		Yes	None				
Pulse check q8	Palp	Palp	Palp	Palp	Palp	Palp	Palp
NG/Dobpatentq4	Yes	Yes	Yes	Yes	Yes	Yes	Yes
BowelSounds q8	Normal	Normal	Normal	Normal	Normal	Normal	Normal
Wound Dressing						Ok	
Daily Wght (kg)			66.1	65.5			
Alrmlmitchk q4	Yes	Yes	Yes	Yes	Yes	Yes	Yes
Stop cock chk					No	Yes	
CXR done			No	No	No		Yes
12 Lead EKG			No	No	No		
Pt.Clasificati	B	B	B	B	B	B	B

Critical Care Data RoutneNurseCare	Date: 1/22/12	Patient : Hosp. No.: Location : 4G08

FIGURE 9-5 Sample of computerized charting.

Computerized documentation and electronic medical records have additional advantages for institutions, but there are also disadvantages (Table 9-4).

Besides charting, there are other nursing benefits from computer applications. Computers are being used to generate nursing care plans, develop staffing patterns that meet the current unit census and client acuity levels, analyze assessment data from monitoring equipment, and reduce medication errors by calling attention to drugs that have been newly ordered or not administered and by alerting the nurse to incompatibilities or contraindications to prescribed drugs.

TABLE 9-4 Advantages and Disadvantages of Electronic Medical Records

ADVANTAGES	DISADVANTAGES
• Increased capacity to store information for longer periods of time • Eliminates loss of entire record or portions thereof due to misplacement or misfiling • Instant access to the record from remote locations when needed by a particular health care worker • Multiple health care workers can use the medical record simultaneously from many different workstations • Legibility and spelling are no longer issues • Reduces medication errors because the system alerts and prompts the physician regarding miscalculations of drug doses, medication interactions, or the client's allergies • Firewalls and passwords prevent breaches in confidentiality by protecting unauthorized access to confidential information • Electronic records are periodically backed up on systems elsewhere than in the agency of origin and are therefore protected from destruction should there be a fire or other type of disaster	• Competency in using the system requires significant learning time • Passwords must be changed regularly • Power or electronic failures can interrupt and delay documentation and access to the full record • Fewer narrative entries due to structured options that are limited to multiple lists • Information is scattered among various files • Promotes **double charting** (repetitious entry of same information)

PROTECTING HEALTH INFORMATION

Congress enacted the first HIPAA legislation to protect the rights of US citizens to retain their health insurance when changing employment. To do so required transmitting health records from one insurance company to another. Transmission of the information resulted in the disclosure of personal health information to nonclinical individuals, a process that, in essence, jeopardized the individual's right to privacy. Subsequently, the original HIPAA legislation was expanded in 2001 and 2002 to enact further measures to protect the privacy of health records and the security of that data. All health care agencies have been mandated to comply with the newest HIPAA regulations since 2003.

Privacy Standards

HIPAA regulations require health care agencies to safeguard written, spoken, and electronic health information in the following ways:

1. Submit a written notice to all clients identifying the uses and disclosures of their health information such as to third parties for use in treatment or for payment for services.
2. Obtain the client's signature indicating that he or she has been informed of the disclosure of information and his or her right to learn who has seen the records. The law also indicates that agencies must limit released information from a health record to **minimum disclosure**, or information necessary for the immediate purpose only. In other words, it is inappropriate to release the entire health record when only portions or isolated pieces of information are needed.

Health care agencies must obtain specific authorization from the client to release information to family or friends, attorneys, and to other parties for uses such as research, fundraising, and marketing. The client retains the right to withhold health information for any of these. There are some exceptions when health information can be revealed without the client's prior approval. Box 9-2 identifies examples of **beneficial disclosures** (exemptions when agencies can release private health information without the client's prior authorization).

Workplace Applications

In an effort to limit casual access to the identity of clients and health information, HIPAA legislation has created several changes that affect the workplace. Some examples of these regulations include the following:

- The names of clients on charts can no longer be visible to the public.
- Clipboards must obscure identifiable names of clients and private information about them.
- Whiteboards must be free of information linking a client with a diagnosis, procedure, or treatment.
- Computer screens must be oriented away from public view; flat screen monitors are recommended because they are more difficult to read at obtuse angles.
- Conversations regarding clients must take place in private places where they cannot be overheard. This has led to a trend of providing private rooms for all hospitalized clients so that personal health information cannot be overheard by someone else sharing the room.

BOX 9-2 Exemptions for Beneficial Disclosures

- Reporting vital statistics (births and deaths)
- Informing the US Food and Drug Administration of adverse reactions to drugs or medical devices
- Disclosing information for organ or tissue donation
- Notifying the public health department about communicable diseases

- Facsimile (fax) machines, filing cabinets, and medical records must be located in areas off-limits to the public.
- A cover sheet and a statement indicating that faxed data contain confidential information must accompany electronically transmitted information.
- Light boxes for examining X-rays or other diagnostic scans on which the client's name appears must be in private areas.
- Documentation must be kept of people who have accessed a client's record.

Data Security

Maintaining confidentiality is more difficult with computerized data keeping. Because multiple people who enter and retrieve information from computer files can access electronically stored data, it has been difficult to monitor use or to limit access to only authorized people within and outside a health care institution.

As a result of HIPAA legislation, health agencies are adopting the following methods to ensure the protection of electronic data:

- Assigning an access number and password to authorized personnel who use a computer for health records. These are kept secret and changed regularly.
- Using automatic save, use of a screen saver, or return to a menu if data have been displayed for a specific period.
- Issuing a plastic card or key that authorized personnel use to retrieve information.
- Locking out client information except to those who have been authorized through a fingerprint or voice-activation device.
- Blocking the type of information that personnel in various departments can retrieve. For example, laboratory employees can obtain information from the medical orders, but they cannot view information in the client's personal history.
- Storing the time and location from which the client's record is accessed in case there is an allegation concerning a breach in confidentiality.
- Encrypting any client information transmitted through the Internet.

DOCUMENTING INFORMATION

Each agency sets its own documentation policies. In addition to identifying the method for charting, such policies generally indicate the type of information recorded on each chart form, the people responsible for charting, and the frequency for making entries on the record. Box 9-3 lists the general content of nursing documentation. Current standards of The Joint Commission require that the medical records of clients cared for in acute care agencies (eg, hospitals) must identify the steps of the nursing process (assessment, diagnosis, planning, implementation, and evaluation of outcomes).

BOX 9-3 Content of Nursing Documentation

Nurses or those to whom they delegate client care are responsible for documenting:

- Assessment data[a]
- Client care needs
- Routine care such as hygiene measures
- Safety precautions that have been used
- Nursing interventions described in the care plan
- Medical treatments prescribed by the physician
- Outcomes of treatment and nursing interventions
- Client activity
- Medication administration
- Percentage of food consumed at each meal
- Visits or consults by physicians or other health professionals
- Reasons for contacting the physician and the outcome of the communication
- Transportation to other departments, like the radiography department, for specialized care or diagnostic tests, and time of return
- Client teaching and discharge instructions
- Referrals to other health care agencies

[a]In acute care settings, The Joint Commission requires a registered nurse to document the admission nursing assessment findings and develop the initial plan of care. The registered nurse may delegate some aspects of the initial data collection to the practical or vocational nurse.

Because consistency in charting is important for legal purposes, nurses must follow the agency's documentation policy. Deviating from the charting policy reduces a nurse's protection if the record is subpoenaed (see Chap. 3).

Using Abbreviations

Abbreviations shorten the length of documentation and the time required for this task. Brevity, however, must never take priority over completeness and accuracy. It is better to write at length than to omit information or make vague entries.

Many abbreviations have common meanings; however, nurses cannot assume that all abbreviations are interpreted the same universally. Some may have one meaning in one locale or agency but may mean something different or be unfamiliar in another. To avoid confusion among caregivers and misinterpretation if the chart is subpoenaed as legal evidence, each agency provides a written or computerized list of approved abbreviations and their meanings. When documenting, nurses must use only those abbreviations on the agency's approved list. The Joint Commission has identified specific abbreviations that should not be used in order to protect the safety of clients (available via The Joint Commission's Web site; see Web Resources on the Point). There may be future deletions as The Joint Commission monitors and evaluates compliance. Some common abbreviations are listed in Table 9-5; more can be found in Appendix B.

TABLE 9-5 Commonly Used Abbreviations

ABBREVIATION	MEANING	ABBREVIATION	MEANING
abd.	abdomen	NSS	normal saline solution
a.c.	before meals	O_2	oxygen
ad lib	as desired	OB	obstetrics
AMA	against medical advice	OOB	out of bed
amt.	amount	OR	operating room
approx.	approximately	per	by or through
b.i.d.	twice a day	P	pulse
BM	bowel movement	p.c.	after meals
BP	blood pressure	p.o.	by mouth
bpm	beats per minute	postop.	postoperative
BRP	bathroom privileges	preop.	preoperative
c̄	with	pt.	patient
C	Centigrade	PT	physical therapy
CCU	coronary care unit	q	every
c/o	complains of	q.i.d.	four times a day
dc	discontinue	q.s.	quantity sufficient
ED	emergency department	R, Rt, or R	right
et	and	R	respirations
H_2O	water	s̄	without
I & O	intake and output	SS	soap suds
IM	intramuscular	stat	immediately
IV	intravenous	t.i.d.	three times a day
kg	kilogram	TPR	temperature, pulse, respirations
L, Lt, or L	left	UA	urinalysis
L	liter	via	by way of
lb	Pound	WC	wheelchair
NKA	no known allergies	WNL	within normal limits
NPO	nothing by mouth	Wt.	weight

Indicating Documentation Time

The nurse dates and times each entry in the record. Some hospitals use **traditional time** (time based on two 12-hour revolutions on a clock), which is identified with the hour and minute, followed by AM or PM. Other agencies prefer **military time** (time based on a 24-hour clock), which uses a different four-digit number for each hour and minute of the day (Fig. 9-6 and Table 9-6). The first two digits indicate the hour within the 24-hour period and the last two digits indicate the minutes.

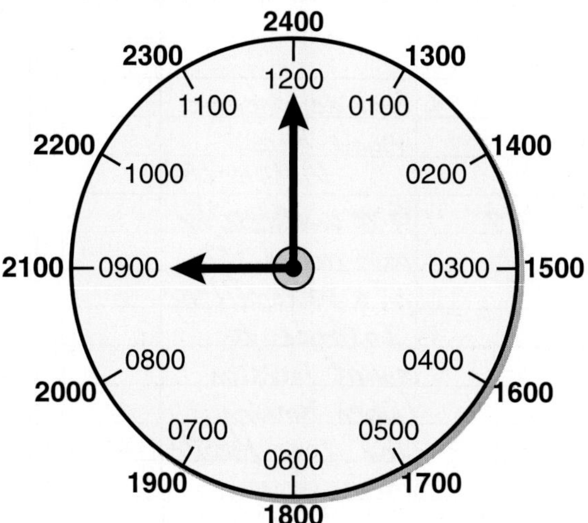

FIGURE 9-6 The military clock uses one 24-hour time cycle instead of two 12-hour cycles (eg, 9:00 AM is 0900 and 9:00 PM is 2100).

The use of military time avoids confusion because no number is ever duplicated, and the labels AM, PM, midnight, and noon are not needed. Military time begins at midnight (2400 or 0000). One minute after midnight is 0001. A zero is placed before the hours of one through nine in the morning; for example, 0700 refers to 7 AM and is stated as "oh seven hundred." After noon, 12 is added to each hour; therefore, 1 PM is 1300. Minutes are given as 1 to 59. See Skill 9-1.

TABLE 9-6 Examples of Military Time Conversions

TRADITIONAL TIME	MILITARY TIME
Midnight	0000 or 2400
12:01 AM	0001
1:30 AM	0130
Noon	1200
1:00 PM	1300
3:15 PM	1515
7:59 PM	1959
10:47 PM	2247

Stop, Think, and Respond Box 9-2

Convert the following from traditional time to military time:

1. *6:30 PM*
2. *Midnight*
3. *8:45 AM*
4. *9:05 PM*
5. *4:15 AM*

COMMUNICATION FOR CONTINUITY AND COLLABORATION

Although the record serves as an ongoing source of information about the client's status, nurses use other methods of communication to promote continuity of care and collaboration among the health personnel involved in the client's care. These methods are in written or verbal form.

Written Forms of Communication

Examples of written forms of communication include the nursing care plan, the nursing Kardex, checklists, and flow sheets.

Nursing Care Plans

A **nursing care plan** is a written list of the client's problems, goals, and nursing orders for client care. It promotes the prevention, reduction, or resolution of health problems. The principles and style for writing a diagnostic statement, goals, and nursing orders are described in Chapter 2.

Presently, The Joint Commission's standards require that the record show evidence of a plan of care. Many agencies require a separate nursing care plan as a means of demonstrating compliance. Nurses revise the plan of care as the client's condition changes.

Most nursing care plans are handwritten on a form that the agency develops (Fig. 9-7). Some agencies use preprinted care plans, computer-generated care plans, standards

DISCHARGE GOALS:

Client will be discharged home with approximated incision, pain within tolerable level, normal vital signs, voiding well, able to eat sufficient food, clear lungs, and active bowel sounds

DIRECTIONS: Each entry must be signed with nurse's name and title.

DATE	PATIENT PROBLEM/NURSING DIAGNOSIS	GOAL/EXPECTED OUTCOMES	GOAL REVIEWED WITH PT./S.O.	NURSING ORDER/ACTIONS	DATE RESOLVED
1/7	Risk for infection related to impaired skin integrity 2° to surgical incision	Client will remain free of infection as evidenced by absence of redness, swelling, drainage from wound and afebrile for length of stay	1/7	1. Observe appropriate handwashing before and after client care. 2. Keep dressing dry and intact. 3. Provide aseptic wound care. D. Miller, LPN	
1/7	Risk for ineffective breathing pattern related to abdominal incisional pain	Client's respiratory rate will remain within normal limits (16-20/min) for length of stay.	1/7	1. Give analgesic for pain rated >5 on a scale of 1-10 2. Instruct to splint incision when turning and deep breathing. D. Miller, LPN	

FIGURE 9-7 Sample nursing care plan.

of care, clinical pathways, or cite the plan of care within progress notes.

Because the nursing care plan is part of the permanent record and thus is a legal document, it is compiled and maintained following documentation principles. All entries and revisions are dated. The written components are clear, concise, and legible. The information is never obliterated; only approved abbreviations are used. Each addition or revision to the plan is signed.

Nursing Kardex

The nursing **Kardex** is a quick reference for current information about the client and his or her care (Fig. 9-8). The Kardex forms for all clients are centrally located in a folder at the nursing station to allow caregivers to flip from one client's data to another. The Kardex has the following uses:

- Locate clients by name and room number
- Identify each client's physician and medical diagnosis
- Serve as a reference for a change of shift report
- Serve as a guide for making nursing assignments
- Provide a rapid resource for current medical orders on each client
- Specify the client's code or DNR (do not resuscitate) status
- Check quickly on a client's diet
- Alert nursing personnel to a client's scheduled tests or test preparations
- Inform staff of a client's current level of activity
- Identify comfort or assistive measures a client may require
- Provide a tool for estimating the personnel-to-client ratio for a nursing unit

The information in the Kardex changes frequently, sometimes several times in a day. The Kardex is not a part of the permanent record. Therefore, nurses can write information in pencil and erase.

Checklists

A **checklist** is a form of documentation in which the nurse indicates with a check mark or initials the performance of routine care. It is an alternative to writing a narrative note. Nurses use paper checklists or a designated file on a computer primarily to avoid documenting types of care that are regularly repeated such as bathing and mouth care. This charting technique is especially helpful when the care is similar each day and the client's condition does not differ much for extended periods.

Flow Sheets

A **flow sheet** is a form of documentation with sections for recording frequently repeated assessment data. It enables nurses to evaluate trends because similar information is located on one form. Some flow sheets provide room for recording numbers or brief descriptions.

3/10/11 539 Page 001

Stevens, James M 65
MR #: 00310593 Acct #: 9400037290
DR: J. Carrio 2/W 204-01
DX: Unstable angina Date: 3/10/11

SUMMARY : 3/10 0701 to 1501

PATIENT INFORMATION
3/10 ADVANCE DIRECTIVE: No.
Advance directive does not exist
3/10 ORGAN DONOR: Yes
3/10 ADMIT DX: Unstable angina
3/10 MED ALLERGY: None known
3/10 ISOLATION: Standard precautions

MISC. PATIENT DATA

NURSING CARE PLAN PROBLEMS
3/10 Acute pain R/T: anginal pain

ALL CURRENT MEDICAL ORDERS

NURSING ORDERS:
3/10 Activity, OOB, up as tol.
3/10 Routine V/S q & h
3/10 Telemetry
3/10 If 1800 PTT < 50, increase heparin drip to 1200 units/hr. If 50 to 100, maintain 1000 units/hr. If > 100, reduce to 900 units/hr.

DIET:
3/10 Diabetic: 1600 cal., start with lunch today

I.V.s.:
3/10 Peripheral line #1. . . . Start D2W 250 ml with heprin 25,000 units: rate, 1000 units/hr.

(continued)

3/10/11 539 Page 002

Stevens, James M 65
MR #: 00310593 Acct #: 9400037290
DR: J. Carrio 2/W 204-01
DX: Unstable angina Date: 3/10/11

SUMMARY: 3/10 0701 to 1501

SCHEDULED MEDICATIONS:
3/10 Nitroglycerin oint 2%, 1-1/2 inches, apply to chest wall q 8 h, starting on 3/10, 1800 hrs.
3/10 Diltiazem tab 90 mg, #1, P.O., q 6 h 0800, 1400, 2000, 0200
3/10 Furosemide tab 40 mg, #1, P.O., daily 0900
3/10 Potassium chloride tab 10 mEq, #1, P.O. daily 0900
3/10 Labetalol tab 100mg, #1/2, P.O. bid 0900, 1800

STAT/NOW MEDICATIONS:
3/10 Furosemide tab 40 mg, #1, P.O. now
3/10 Potassium chloride tab 10 mEq, #1, P.O., now

PRN MEDICATIONS:
3/10 Procardia nifedipine cap 10 mg, #1, subling. q 6 n, prn SBP > 170 or DSBP > 105
3/10 Acetaminophen tab 325 mg, #2, P.O., q 4 h, prn for pain
3/10 Temazepan cap 15 mg, #1, P.O. q HS, prn
3/10 Alprazolam tab 0.25 mg, #1/2, P.O., q 8 h, prn

LABORATORY:
3/10 CK & MB 1800 today
3/10 CK & MB 0200 tomorrow
3/10 Urinalysis floor to collect
3/10 PTT 1800 today

LABORATORY:
3/10 Stress test persantine, perp H1, Patient handling: Wheelchair, Schedule: tomorrow

Last page

FIGURE 9-8 A computer-generated Kardex. (Used with permission. Holmes, H. N. [Ed.]. [2006]. *Documentation in Action* [pp. 231–232]. Philadelphia: Lippincott Williams & Wilkins.)

Interpersonal Communication

In addition to using written resources (eg, the medical record) to exchange information, communication also takes place during personal interactions among health professionals. Some examples are as follows:

- Change of shift reports
- Client assignments
- Team conferences
- Rounds
- Telephone calls

Change of Shift Report

A **change of shift report** is a discussion between a nursing spokesperson from the shift that is ending and the arriving personnel (Fig. 9-9). It includes a summary of each client's condition and current status of care (Box 9-4).

To maximize the efficiency of change of shift reports, nurses should do the following:

- Be prompt so that the report can start and end on time.
- Come prepared with a pen and paper or clipboard.
- Avoid socializing during reporting sessions.
- Take notes.
- Clarify unclear information.
- Ask questions about pertinent information that may have been omitted.

Some agencies tape-record the report, which saves time because there are no interruptions or digressions. In addition, nurses can replay portions of the tape if information needs to be repeated. A taped report, however, does not allow direct questions, elaboration, or clarification with the person who recorded the report.

BOX 9-4 Change of Shift Report

A change of shift report usually includes:

- Name of client, age, and room number
- Name of physician
- Medical diagnosis or surgical procedure and date
- Range in vital signs
- Abnormal assessment data
- Characteristics of pain, medication, amount, time last administered, and outcome achieved
- Type of diet and percentage consumed at each meal
- Special body position and level of activity, if applicable
- Scheduled diagnostic tests
- Test results, including those performed by the nurse, such as blood glucose levels
- Changes in medical orders, including newly prescribed drugs
- Intake and output totals
- Type and rate of infusing intravenous fluid
- Amount of intravenous fluid that remains
- Settings on electronic equipment such as amount of suction
- Condition of incision and dressing, if applicable
- Color and amount of wound or suction drainage

Client Care Assignments

Client care assignments are made at the beginning of each shift. Assignments are posted, discussed with team members, or written on a worksheet (Fig. 9-10). Each assignment identifies the clients for whom the staff person is responsible and describes their care. Meals and break times also may be scheduled, as well as special tasks such as checking and restocking supplies.

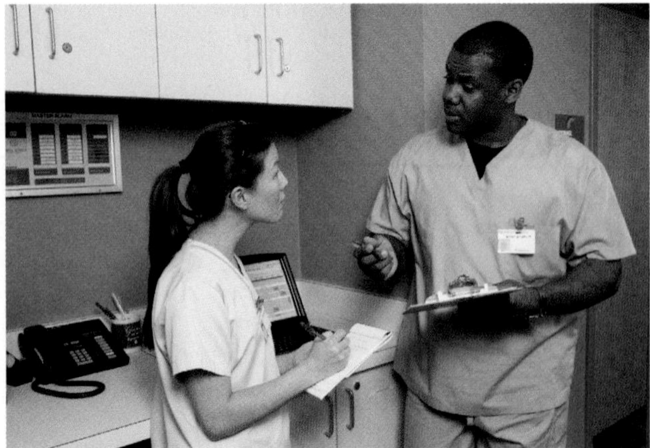

FIGURE 9-9 Nurses begin their shift by receiving a report on their clients. (From Craven, R. F., Hirnle, C. J. *Fundamentals of Nursing* [6th ed.]. Philadelphia: Lippincott Williams & Wilkins.)

Team Conferences

Conferences are commonly used to exchange information. Topics generally include client care problems, personnel conflicts, new equipment or treatment methods, and changes in policies or procedures. Team conferences often include the nursing staff, staff from other departments involved in client care, physicians, social workers, personnel from community agencies, and, in some cases, clients and their significant others. Usually, one person organizes and directs the conference. Responsibilities for certain outcomes that result from the team conference may be delegated to various staff members who attend the meeting.

Client Rounds

Rounds (visits to clients on an individual basis or as a group) are used as a means of learning firsthand about clients. The client is a witness to and often an active participant in the interaction (Fig. 9-11).

Some nurses use walking rounds as a method of giving a change of shift report. Giving the report in the client's presence provides oncoming staff with an opportunity to survey the client's condition and to determine the status of equipment used in his or her care. It also tends to boost the client's confidence and security in the transition of care. Since the passage of HIPAA regulations, however, agencies

NURSING ASSIGNMENT SHEET									
TEAM MEMBER Jane Doe L.P.N.				BREAK 9:15 AM. CONFERENCE 10:30 AM. LUNCH 12:00 N. DATE:					
TEAM LEADER Mary Black RN				ASSIGNMENT Filling and distributing water carafes on the Northwing					
ROOM	PATIENT	BATH	ACTIVITY	DIET	FLUIDS	TO BE CHECKED	TREATMENTS	SPECIMEN	COMMENTS
296[1]	Flora Brown Duodenal Ulcer	BED SELF * SHOWER TUB SITZ	BED DANGLE B R P B R P . HELP AMB AMB . HELP WALKER CRUTCHES W C	REGULAR SOFT SURG LIQ FULL LIQ SPECIAL Bland III FASTING TUBE FEEDING	FORCE N P O LIMIT SIPS WATER ICE CHIPS I V DIST WATER	BLOOD PRESSURE 8A T P R 8A TEST URINE A C & HS SLIDING SCALE I & O LEVIN TUBE CHEST TUBE FOLEY OXYGEN	ENEMA DOUCHE PERI CARE . LIGHT WEIGH ORAL HYGIENE SPECIAL BACK CARE PREPARE FOR SURG PREPARE FOR X-RAY O T . P T . E C T	STOOL OB. URINE SPUTUM BLOOD CULTURE TISSUE	
296[2]	Mary Green Coronary	BED SELF * SHOWER TUB SITZ	BED DANGLE B R P B R P HELP AMB AMB . HELP WALKER CRUTCHES W C	REGULAR SOFT SURG LIQ FULL LIQ SPECIAL 2Gm Na FASTING TUBE FEEDING	FORCE N P O LIMIT SIPS WATER ICE CHIPS I V DIST WATER	BLOOD PRESSURE 8-12 T P R 8-12 TEST URINE A C & HS SLIDING SCALE I & O LEVIN TUBE CHEST TUBE FOLEY OXYGEN 4L/M - 1hr pc + HS	ENEMA DOUCHE PERI CARE . LIGHT WEIGH . 8A ORAL HYGIENE SPECIAL BACK CARE PREPARE FOR SURG PREPARE FOR X-RAY O T . P T . E C T	STOOL URINE SPUTUM BLOOD CULTURE TISSUE	
298[1]	John Snapp C.O.P.D.	BED SELF * SHOWER TUB SITZ	BED DANGLE B R P B R P . HELP AMB c̄ O₂ AMB . HELP WALKER CRUTCHES W C	REGULAR SOFT SURG LIQ FULL LIQ SPECIAL FASTING TUBE FEEDING	FORCE N P O LIMIT SIPS WATER ICE CHIPS I V DIST WATER	BLOOD PRESSURE T P R TEST URINE A C & HS SLIDING SCALE I & O LEVIN TUBE CHEST TUBE FOLEY OXYGEN 1L/M CONT.	ENEMA FLEETS DOUCHE PERI CARE . LIGHT WEIGH ORAL HYGIENE SPECIAL BACK CARE PREPARE FOR SURG PREPARE FOR X-RAY O T . P T . E C T	STOOL URINE SPUTUM BLOOD CULTURE TISSUE	1000 mL 5% D/W c̄ 500mg Aminophylline @ 100mL/hr CONT.
298[2]	Tom Henry C.H.F.	BED SELF * SHOWER TUB SITZ	BED DANGLE B R P B R P HELP AMB AMB HELP WALKER CRUTCHES W C	REGULAR SOFT SURG LIQ FULL LIQ SPECIAL 1/2Gm Na FASTING TUBE FEEDING	FORCE N P O LIMIT - 300/8h SIPS WATER ICE CHIPS I V DIST WATER	BLOOD PRESSURE q2h T P R q2h TEST URINE A C & HS SLIDING SCALE I & O LEVIN TUBE CHEST TUBE FOLEY OXYGEN 4L/M CONT.	ENEMA DOUCHE PERI CARE . LIGHT WEIGH 8 ORAL HYGIENE 8-12 SPECIAL BACK CARE PREPARE FOR SURG PREPARE FOR X-RAY O T . P T . E C T	STOOL URINE SPUTUM BLOOD CULTURE TISSUE	Change position q 2hr.
299	Jim Smith Diabetes Mellitus	BED SELF * SHOWER TUB SITZ	BED DANGLE B R P B R P . HELP AMB AMB . HELP WALKER CRUTCHES W C	REGULAR SOFT SURG LIQ FULL LIQ SPECIAL 1300Cal Diabetic FASTING TUBE FEEDING	FORCE N P O LIMIT SIPS WATER ICE CHIPS I V DIST WATER	BLOOD PRESSURE T P R 8 TEST URINE A C & HS SLIDING SCALE I & O LEVIN TUBE CHEST TUBE FOLEY OXYGEN	ENEMA DOUCHE PERI CARE . LIGHT WEIGH ORAL HYGIENE SPECIAL BACK CARE PREPARE FOR SURG PREPARE FOR X-RAY O T . P T . E C T	STOOL URINE SPUTUM BLOOD CULTURE TISSUE	
		BED SELF * SHOWER TUB SITZ	BED DANGLE B R P B R P HELP AMB AMB HELP WALKER CRUTCHES W C	REGULAR SOFT SURG LIQ FULL LIQ SPECIAL FASTING TUBE FEEDING	FORCE N P O LIMIT SIPS WATER ICE CHIPS I V DIST WATER	BLOOD PRESSURE T P R TEST URINE A.C. & HS SLIDING SCALE I & O LEVIN TUBE CHEST TUBE FOLEY OXYGEN	ENEMA DOUCHE PERI CARE . LIGHT WEIGH ORAL HYGIENE SPECIAL BACK CARE PREPARE FOR SURG PREPARE FOR X-RAY O T . P T . E C T	STOOL URINE SPUTUM BLOOD CULTURE TISSUE	
		BED SELF * SHOWER TUB SITZ	BED DANGLE B R P B R P HELP AMB AMB . HELP WALKER CRUTCHES W C	REGULAR SOFT SURG LIQ FULL LIQ SPECIAL FASTING TUBE FEEDING	FORCE N P O LIMIT SIPS WATER ICE CHIPS I V DIST WATER	BLOOD PRESSURE T P R TEST URINE A C & HS SLIDING SCALE I & O LEVIN TUBE CHEST TUBE FOLEY OXYGEN	ENEMA DOUCHE PERI CARE . LIGHT WEIGH ORAL HYGIENE SPECIAL BACK CARE PREPARE FOR SURG PREPARE FOR X-RAY O T . P T . E C T	STOOL URINE SPUTUM BLOOD CULTURE TISSUE	
		BED SELF * SHOWER TUB SITZ	BED DANGLE B R P B R P HELP AMB AMB HELP WALKER CRUTCHES W C	REGULAR SOFT SURG LIQ FULL LIQ SPECIAL FASTING TUBE FEEDING	FORCE N P O LIMIT SIPS WATER ICE CHIPS I V DIST WATER	BLOOD PRESSURE T P R TEST URINE A C & HS SLIDING SCALE I & O LEVIN TUBE CHEST TUBE FOLEY OXYGEN	ENEMA DOUCHE PERI CARE . LIGHT WEIGH ORAL HYGIENE SPECIAL BACK CARE PREPARE FOR SURG PREPARE FOR X-RAY O T . P T . E C T	STOOL URINE SPUTUM BLOOD CULTURE TISSUE	

CODE

*	You wash back and legs	W C	Wheelchair	E C T	Electrical Convulsive Therapy
B R P	Bathroom privileges	B P	Blood pressure	O T	Occupational Therapy
AMB	Ambulatory	N P O	Nothing by mouth	P T	Physical Therapy
I & O	Intake and output	DIST	Distilled water		

FIGURE 9-10 Sample of a nursing assignment sheet.

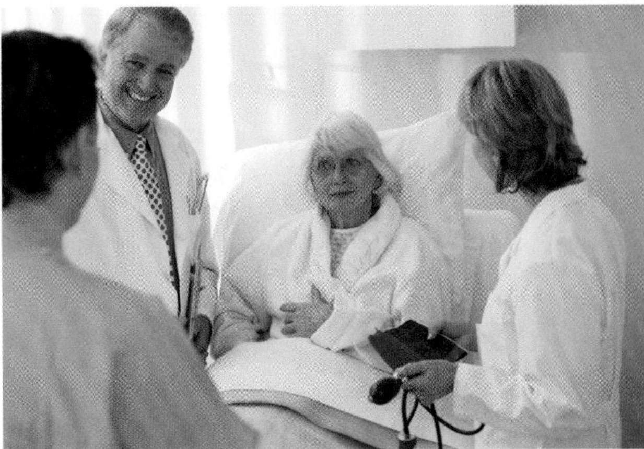

FIGURE 9-11 Rounds help acquaint oncoming staff with the client.

avoid this type of communication if another client shares the room or if the client has not authorized family members or friends who may be visiting to have access to his or her health information.

Telephone

Nurses use the telephone to exchange information when it is difficult for people to get together or when they must communicate information quickly. When using the telephone, the nurse does the following:

- Answers as promptly as possible
- Speaks in a normal tone of voice
- Identifies himself or herself by name, title, and nursing unit
- Obtains or states the reason for the call
- Discretely identifies the client being discussed to avoid being publicly overheard
- Spells the client's name if there is any chance of confusion
- Converses in a courteous and business-like manner
- Repeats information to ensure it has been heard accurately

When notifying a physician about a change in a client's condition, the nurse documents in the client's record the information reported and the instructions received. If the nurse believes that the physician has not responded in a safe manner to the information given, he or she notifies the nursing supervisor or the head of the medical department.

CRITICAL THINKING EXERCISE

1. What are some reasons for protecting the information within a client's health record?
2. In your opinion, what is the most important reason for compiling and maintaining a client's health record?
3. When initially employed, how can the nurse ensure that he or she is documenting information appropriately?
4. Explain the possible consequences if a nurse's documentation contains illegible writing, unapproved abbreviations, and misspelled words. How would you help the nurse improve his or her documentation?

NCLEX-STYLE REVIEW QUESTIONS

1. If a charge nurse does all of the following, which practice could jeopardize the health agency's accreditation?
   1. The nurse assigns five clients to each person on the team.
   2. The nurse writes the names of clients on a dry erase board in a public area.
   3. The nurse posts the names of the current staff at the nursing station.
   4. The nurse reviews the Kardex of each client on the nursing unit.
2. All of the following are poor examples of documentation practices. Which one places the writer in the most legal jeopardy?
   1. The writer squeezes information into a line written hours earlier.
   2. The writer misspells several words while completing documentation.
   3. The writer uses blue rather than black ink as the agency specifies.
   4. The writer signs the documentation but omits his or her title.
3. Which method of documentation is used when the nurse charts only abnormal assessment findings or care that deviates from the agency's standard?
   1. PIE (problem, intervention, evaluation) charting
   2. Narrative charting
   3. Charting by exception
   4. Focus charting
4. For which of the following situations is breaching confidentiality appropriate?
   1. The client is treated for an attempted suicide.
   2. The client has a substance abuse problem.
   3. The client wishes to terminate further treatment.
   4. The client has a highly contagious disease.
5. When using the SOAP method of documentation, what does the "A" represent?
   1. Assessment
   2. Analysis
   3. Abnormality
   4. Action

SKILL 9-1 Making Entries in a Client's Record

Suggested Action	Reason for Action
ASSESSMENT	
Review the agency's policy for the charting format it uses.	Some agencies require personnel to use a specific style (eg, SOAP charting, narrative charting, PIE charting) for documentation.
Locate the agency's list of approved abbreviations.	Abbreviations must be compatible with those that have been approved for legally defensible reasons.
Determine the paper form that is appropriate to use for documenting the information or locate the file within an electronic record used for nursing documentation via a computer.	Data obtained initially from the client are entered on the admission form; periodic additions about the client's condition and care are entered on a form commonly called "nurses' notes" or on a progress sheet. A graphic sheet or flow sheet is used to document numbers or trends in assessment data.
Check that the client's name is identified on the chart form or computer file.	If a sheet of paper becomes separated from the chart, proper identification ensures that it is reinserted into the appropriate record. Electronic records are opened and stored using the client's name.
PLANNING	
Resolve to document information as soon as it is obtained or at least every 1–2 hours.	The potential for inaccuracies or omissions increases when documentation is delayed.
Use a pen or keyboard to make entries; use the color of ink indicated by the agency's policy.	Ink is permanent. Black ink photocopies better than other colors.
IMPLEMENTATION	
Record the date and time.	Information is recorded in chronologic order. The time of documentation is when the notation is written. Legal issues often involve the timing of events.
Write, print, or type information so that it can be read easily. Take care that keyboarding is accurate when a computer is used.	The entry loses its value for exchanging information if it is unreadable. Illegible entries become questionable in a court of law.
Use accurate spelling and grammar.	Literacy skills reflect a person's knowledge and education.
Be brief but complete; delete articles (a, an, the).	Extra words add length to the entry.
Do not state the client's name; do not use *pt.* as an abbreviation for "patient."	It is understood that all the entries refer to the person identified on the chart form.
Use only agency-approved abbreviations and symbols.	Using approved abbreviations promotes consistent interpretation.
Document information clearly and accurately without any subjective interpretation. Quote the client if a statement is pertinent.	The chart is a record of facts, not opinions.
Avoid phrases such as "appears to be" or "seems to be."	Phrases implying uncertainty suggest that the nurse lacks reasonable knowledge.
Never use ditto marks.	Even if information is repetitious, it must be documented separately.
Identify actual or approximate sizes when describing assessment data rather than using relative descriptions such as large, moderate, or small.	Nonspecific measurements are subject to wide interpretation and are therefore less accurate and informative.
Record adverse reactions; include the measures used to manage them.	Documentation may be necessary to demonstrate that the nurse acted reasonably and that the care was not substandard.
Identify the specific information that is taught and the evidence of the client's learning.	Ensures continuity in preparing the client for discharge.
Fill all the space on each line of the form; draw a line through any blank space on an unfilled line.	Filling space reduces the possibility that someone else will add information to the current documentation.
Never chart nursing activities before they have been performed.	Making early entries can cause legal problems, especially if the client's condition suddenly changes.
Follow agency policy for the interval between entries.	Frequent charting indicates that the client has been observed and attended to at reasonable periods.
Indicate the current time when charting a late entry (documentation of information that occurred earlier but was unintentionally omitted); write "late entry for ...," identifying the date and time to which the documentation refers.	Correlating time with actual events promotes logic and order when evaluating the client's progress.
Draw a line through a mistake rather than scribbling through or in any other way obscuring the original words.	Corrections are done in such a way that all words are readable. Obliterated words can cast suspicion that the record was tampered with to conceal damaging information.

(continued)

Making Entries in a Client's Record (continued)

IMPLEMENTATION (CONTINUED)	
Put the word error followed by a date and initials next to the entry and immediately enter the corrected information. Some agencies specify that the nurse must indicate the nature of the error (eg, "wrong medical record").	A jury seeing the word *error* without any explanation might assume that the nurse made an error in care rather than in documentation.
Sign each entry with a first initial, last name, and title.	The signature demonstrates accountability for what has been written.
Log off the computer after documenting in an electronic client record.	Logging off returns the computer to a home or menu page, which prevents anyone else from entering information under the name of the person who originally logged in. Exiting to a home or menu page prevents those who are unauthorized from viewing anything confidential on the computer screen.

Evaluation

The writer's entries are:

- Dated and timed
- Accurate, comprehensive, and up-to-date
- Legibly written according to the agency's format
- Spelled correctly without grammatical errors
- Objectively written
- Free of unapproved abbreviations
- Identified with the writer's name and title

SAMPLE DOCUMENTATION

Date and Time Dressing changed. Abdominal incision and sutures are intact. No evidence of redness, swelling, or drainage. ——— SIGNATURE/TITLE

UNIT 3

End of Unit Exercises for Chapters 7, 8, and 9

Section I: Reviewing What You've Learned

Activity A: *Fill in the blanks by choosing the correct word from the options given in parentheses.*

1. The ________________ domain is a learning style through which information is presented in such a way as to appeal to a person's feelings, beliefs, or values. (affective, cognitive, psychomotor)
2. Charting by exception is a documentation method in which nurses chart only ________________ assessment findings. (abnormal, physical, psychological)
3. ________________ includes nonverbal components such as facial expressions, posture, gestures, and body movements. (Kinesics, Paralanguage, Proxemics)
4. ________________ is the technique of restating what the client has said to demonstrate listening. (Paraphrasing, Reflecting, Structuring)
5. The nursing ________________ is a quick reference for current information about the client and his or her care. (checklist, Kardex, care plan)
6. ________________ charting follows a data, action, response (DAR) model to reflect the steps in the nursing process. (Exception, Flow, Focus)

Activity B: *Mark each statement as either T (True) or F (False). Correct any false statements.*

1. T____F____ Health teaching promotes the client's ability to meet his or her health needs independently.
2. T____F____ People belonging to Generation X are technologically literate, having grown up with computers.
3. T____F____ Therapeutic verbal communication involves the use of words alone to accomplish a particular objective.
4. T____F____ Silence is a form of therapeutic communication that encourages the client to participate in verbal discussions.
5. T____F____ PIE charting is a method of recording the client's progress under the headings of patient, implementation, and education.
6. T____F____ A change-of-shift report is a discussion between a nurse from a shift that is ending and the personnel coming on duty.

Activity C: *Write the correct term for each description below.*

1. Learning style in which a person processes information by listening or reading facts and descriptions ________________
2. Science of teaching children or those with cognitive ability comparable to that of children ________________
3. Nursing role that involves assigning a task, checking on completion of that task, and evaluating the resulting outcome ________________
4. Person who performs health-related activities that a sick person cannot perform independently ________________
5. Written collections of information about a person's health, the care provided by health practitioners, and the client's progress ________________
6. Method of documentation that involves writing information about the client and his or her care in chronologic order ________________

Activity D: *1. Match the terms in Column A with their descriptions in Column B.*

Column A	Column B
1. ___________ Psychomotor domain	A. The principle of teaching adult learners
2. ___________ Androgogy	B. A style of processing information that focuses on learning by doing
3. ___________ Gerogogy	C. A term given to a person who possesses minimal literacy skills
4. ___________ Functionally illiterate	D. A technique that enhances learning in older adults

2. Match the phases of the nurse–client relationship in Column A with the descriptions of what happens during those phases in Column B.

Column A	Column B
1. ___________ Introductory phase	A. The nurse and client plan and implement the client's care
2. ___________ Working phase	B. The nurse and client mutually agree that the client's immediate health problems have improved
3. ___________ Terminating phase	C. The client identifies one or more health problems for which he or she is seeking help

Activity E: *1. Differentiate between informal and formal teaching based on the components listed below.*

	Informal Teaching	Formal Teaching
Definition		
Requirements		
Disadvantages		

2. Differentiate between source-oriented records and problem-oriented records based on the items listed below.

	Source-Oriented Records	Problem-Oriented Records
Definition		
Components		

Activity F: *Consider the following figures.*

1. 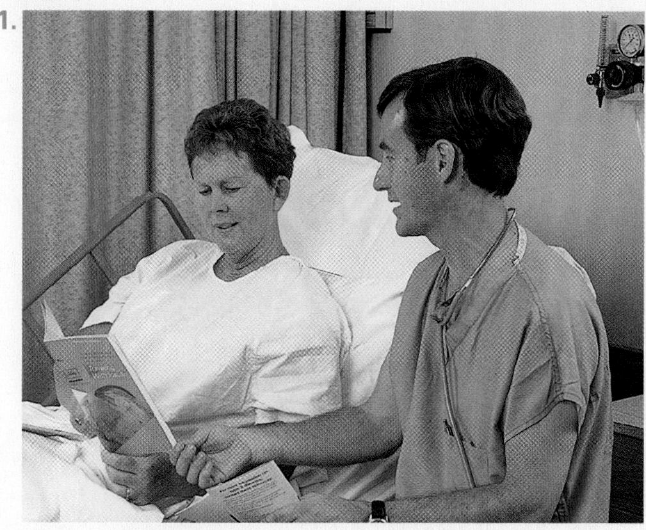

a. Identify what is happening in the figure shown above.
b. What learning style might this client prefer?

2. 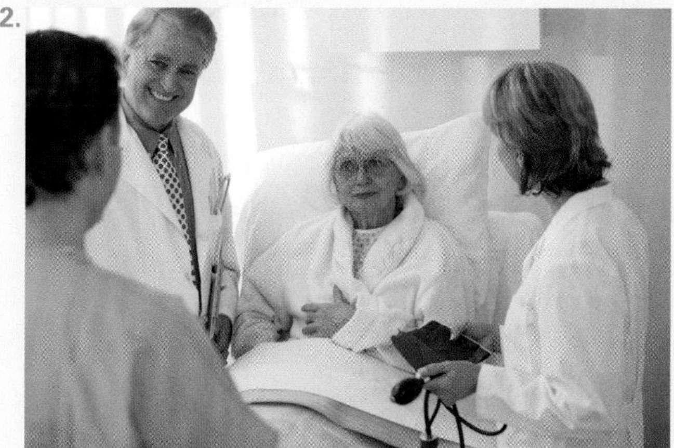

a. Identify what is happening in the figure shown above.
b. What are its benefits?

Activity G: *Limited hospitalization time demands that nurses begin teaching as soon as possible after admission rather than waiting until discharge. Early attention to the client's educational needs is essential because learning takes place in four progressive stages. Write down the correct sequence of the progressive stages of learning in the boxes below:*

1. Using new learning independently
2. Recalling or describing information to others
3. Recognizing what has been taught
4. Explaining or applying information

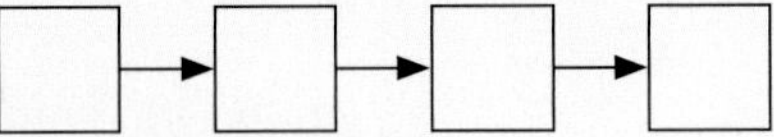

Activity H: *Answer the following questions.*

1. What subject areas should the nurse focus on when teaching a client?

2. How can the nurse implement effective teaching?

3. How does task-related touch differ from affective touch?

4. What factors affect the ability to communicate by speech or in writing?

5. What are the seven uses of medical records?

6. What are the steps for converting traditional time into military time?

Section II: Applying Your Knowledge

Activity I: *Give rationales for the following questions.*

1. Why should the nurse select black print on white paper when providing instructions to a visually impaired client?

2. Why should the nurse document information he or she has taught and evidence demonstrating the client's understanding?

3. Why is the nurse–client relationship called a therapeutic relationship?

4. Why is it important for nurses to follow their agency's documentation policy?

5. Why do some health care agencies use military time instead of traditional time?

Activity J: *Answer the following questions focusing on nursing roles and responsibilities.*

1. A nurse at an extended-care facility is caring for a client with impaired hearing who has undergone knee surgery. How might the nurse approach teaching this client?

2. A nurse at a dermatology clinic is caring for a 12-year-old boy who has just had a cyst removed from the soft tissue on his forearm.
   a. What important first step should the nurse follow after the surgical procedure?

   b. Describe skin care techniques that the nurse should explain to this client.

3. A young male client is bedridden with limited use of his arms following a motorcycle accident. A female nurse needs to assist this client with activities of daily living, such as bathing and shaving.
   a. What actions can the nurse take to prevent the client from misinterpreting physical nearness and hands-on nursing procedures as sexual advances?

   b. Why should nurses use affective touch cautiously?

4. A nurse caring for multiple clients in a health care facility has completed shift duties and is preparing to leave for the day.
   a. How should the nurse proceed when completing a shift and preparing to leave the facility?

   b. What actions should the nurse receiving the shift report take to ensure maximum efficiency during this process?

5. A physician returns a nurse's call about a change in a client's health condition.
   a. What actions should the nurse take when answering the telephone and reporting information about the client's condition?

   b. What information should the nurse document following communication with the physician?

Activity K: *Think over the following questions. Discuss them with your instructor or peers.*

1. A nurse is caring for three clients in a health care facility:
   - A functionally illiterate elderly man who has undergone cataract surgery.
   - A 58-year-old woman with diabetes who has undergone hand amputation.
   - An 18-year-old Asian American girl who cannot speak English and has to learn how to use a hearing aid.

   a. How can the nurse determine each client's preferred learning style and developmental level?
   b. How should the nurse provide teaching to these clients?
   c. What kind of processes or techniques should the nurse follow?

2. A nurse is caring for a middle-aged client who has been diagnosed with cancer. The client is worried about the expenses involved in treatment, his future, and his dependent family members.
   a. How can the nurse begin to build a therapeutic relationship with this client?
   b. What communication techniques should the nurse use with this client?

3. A nurse is working at a health care facility that has a computer terminal at every client's bedside. The nurse is required to use computerized charting for each client.
   a. What actions should the nurse take when completing computerized charting?
   b. What are the advantages and disadvantages of this documentation system?

Section III: Getting Ready for NCLEX

Activity L: *Answer the following questions.*

1. Which one of the following methods should a nurse use when teaching a client who uses prescription eyeglasses?
   a. Provide pamphlets in 12- to 16-point type and serif lettering.
   b. Provide teaching material printed on glossy paper.
   c. Ensure that the room is well lit by a ceiling light.
   d. Stand in front of a window letting in bright sunlight.
2. Which of the following are characteristics of pedagogic learners? Select all that apply.
   a. Need direction and supervision
   b. Need immediate feedback
   c. Think abstractly
   d. Learn analytically
   e. Respond to competition
3. A nurse is caring for an elderly client who lives alone and is recovering from a fall. The client is in severe pain and angry that the fall could have been avoided if somebody else has been in the home. Which of the following responses by the nurse is most appropriate when caring for this client?
   a. Ask why the client is living alone.
   b. Allow the client to express emotions.
   c. Ask the client to stop complaining.
   d. Tell the client to stay calm and take pain medication.
4. A nurse is teaching an American-born client about a medication regimen. What is the appropriate distance that the nurse should maintain from the client during teaching?
   a. 12 or more feet
   b. 4 to 12 feet
   c. 6 inches to 4 feet
   d. 6 inches or less
5. A nurse is caring for a client undergoing treatment following a stroke. The nurse needs to document routine care, such as bathing and oral hygiene. Which of the following forms should the nurse use to document this routine nursing care?
   a. Kardex
   b. Flow sheet
   c. Care plan
   d. Checklist
6. A nurse is caring for a client who cannot have any food or oral fluids for 4 hours before the scheduled surgery. Which of the following abbreviations should the nurse note on the client's chart?
   a. AMA
   b. NKA
   c. NPO
   d. NSS

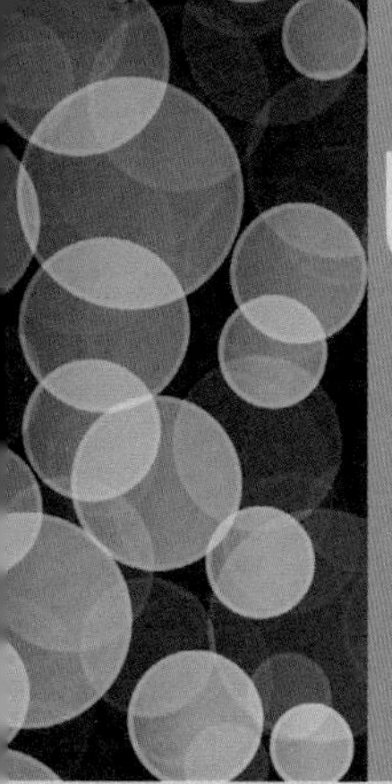

UNIT 4
Performing Basic Client Care

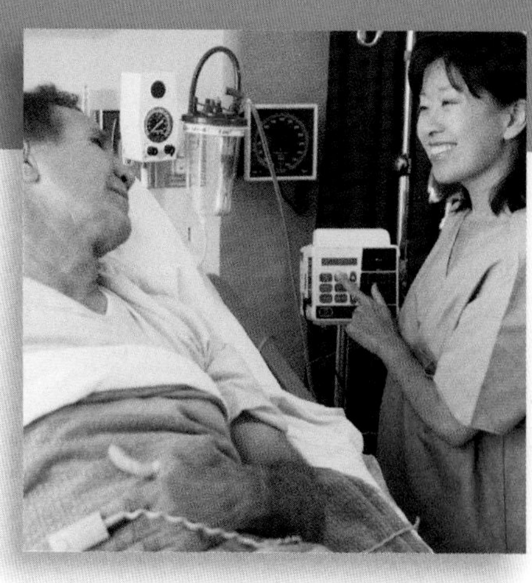

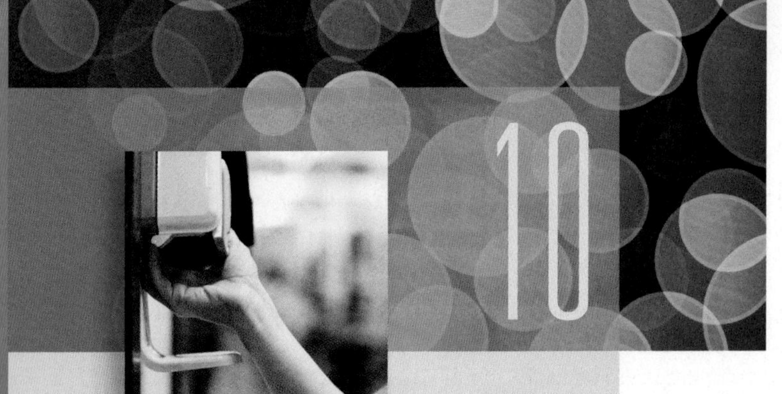

10 Asepsis

Words To Know

aerobic bacteria
anaerobic bacteria
antimicrobial agents
antiseptics
asepsis
aseptic techniques
biologic defense mechanisms
carriers
chain of infection
communicable diseases
community-acquired infections
concurrent disinfection
contagious diseases
disinfectants
exit route
fomites
hand antisepsis
hand hygiene
hand washing
means of transmission
medical asepsis
microorganisms
nonpathogens
normal flora
nosocomial infections
opportunistic infections
pathogens
portal of entry
reservoir
resident microorganisms
spore
sterile field
sterile technique
sterilization
surgical asepsis
surgical hand antisepsis
susceptible host
terminal disinfection
transient microorganisms
viral load
virulence

Learning Objectives

On completion of this chapter, the reader should be able to:

1. Describe microorganisms.
2. Name eight specific types of microorganisms.
3. Differentiate between nonpathogens and pathogens, resident and transient microorganisms, and aerobic and anaerobic microorganisms.
4. Give two examples of the ways some microorganisms have adapted for their survival.
5. Name the six components in the chain of infection.
6. Cite examples of biologic defense mechanisms.
7. Define nosocomial infection.
8. Discuss the concept of asepsis.
9. Differentiate between medical and surgical asepsis.
10. Identify at least three principles of medical asepsis.
11. List five examples of medical aseptic practices.
12. Name at least three techniques for sterilizing equipment.
13. Identify at least three principles of surgical asepsis.
14. List at least three nursing activities that require application of the principles of surgical asepsis.

Preventing infections is one of the most important priorities in nursing. The most effective method is hand hygiene, an essential nursing activity that must be performed repeatedly when caring for clients. This chapter discusses how microorganisms survive and how to use **aseptic techniques**, measures that reduce or eliminate microorganisms.

MICROORGANISMS

Microorganisms, living animals or plants visible only through a microscope, are commonly called "microbes" or "germs." What they lack in size, they make up for in numbers. Microorganisms are present everywhere: in the air, soil, and water, and on and within virtually everything and everyone.

Once microorganisms invade, one of three events occurs: the body's immune defense mechanisms eliminate them, they reside within the body without causing disease, or they cause an infection or an infectious disease. Factors that influence whether an infection develops include the type and number of microorganisms, the characteristics of the microorganism (such as its virulence), and the person's state of health.

Types of Microorganisms

Microorganisms are divided into two main groups: **nonpathogens**, or **normal flora** (harmless, beneficial microorganisms), and **pathogens** (microorganisms that cause illness).

Nonpathogens live abundantly and perpetually on and within the human body, which is their host. They are found in areas of the body exposed to the external environment, such as the skin, nose, mouth, throat, lower urethra, and intestines. They have adapted to human defense mechanisms like acidic sweat and oil secretions on the skin. Most exist in the large intestine, having been introduced from food or substances on fingers, pencils, tableware, and other items placed in the mouth. Nonpathogens assume one of two relationships with their human host: mutually beneficial, or neither harming nor helping the host. They inhibit pathogenic growth and reproduction by competing for nutrients, vying for space, or producing substances that interfere with the pathogens. They thus ensure a hospitable habitat for themselves.

Pathogens have a high potential for causing infectious **communicable diseases** (diseases that can be transmitted to other people), also called **contagious diseases** and **community-acquired infections**. Some examples of communicable diseases are measles, streptococcal sore throat, sexually transmitted infections, and tuberculosis (TB). Although pathogenic infections can result in death, most of them lead only to temporary illness. They may cause illness in various ways. They may become established, grow, and proliferate when numbers of nonpathogens are reduced when broad-spectrum antibiotics are prescribed. Pathogens may also cause infections when the host is immunosuppressed from acquired immunodeficiency syndrome (AIDS), cancer chemotherapy, or steroid drug therapy.

In addition, their structures and functions may promote **virulence** (the extent of dangerousness) of pathogens. Some have *fimbriae,* tiny hairs used to attach themselves to the host's tissue to avoid expulsion. Fimbriae prevent pathogens that reach the bladder from being eliminated during urination. Some pathogens use *flagella,* long tails that promote motility to reach a site less hostile to survival. Others release *toxins* (harmful chemicals). Many enter the host's cells and use their content to support their life cycle.

Nonpathogens and pathogens include bacteria, viruses, fungi, rickettsiae, protozoans, mycoplasmas, helminths, and prions.

Bacteria

Bacteria are single-celled microorganisms. They appear in various shapes: round (cocci), rod-shaped (bacilli), and spiral (spirochetes) (Fig. 10-1). **Aerobic bacteria** require oxygen to live, whereas **anaerobic bacteria** exist without oxygen; this difference demonstrates how varied these life-forms have become.

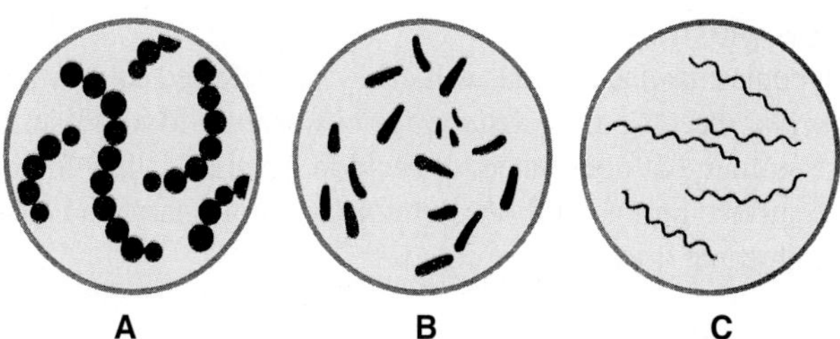

FIGURE 10-1 Classification of bacteria according to shape: cocci **(A)**, bacilli **(B)**, and spirochetes **(C)**.

Viruses

Viruses, the smallest microorganisms known to cause infectious diseases, are visible only through an electron microscope. They are filterable, which means that they can pass through very small barriers. Viruses are unique because they do not possess all the genetic information necessary to reproduce; they require metabolic and reproductive materials from other living species. Some can remain dormant in a human and reactivate sporadically, causing recurrence of an infectious disorder. An example is the herpes simplex virus, which can cause cold sores (fever blisters) to repeatedly flare up years after an initial infection.

Some viral infections, such as the common cold, are minor and self-limiting, that is, they terminate with or without medical treatment. Others, such as rabies, poliomyelitis, hepatitis, and AIDS, are more serious or fatal.

Fungi

Fungi include yeasts and molds. Only a few types of fungi produce infectious diseases in humans. The three types of fungal (mycotic) infections are superficial, intermediate, and systemic. Superficial fungal infections affect the skin, mucous membranes, hair, and nails. Examples include tinea corporis (ringworm), tinea pedis (athlete's foot), and candidiasis (a yeast infection that infects mucous membranes in the mouth and the vagina). Intermediate fungal infections affect subcutaneous tissues such as fungal granuloma (an inflammatory lesion under the skin). Systemic fungi infect deep tissues and organs, such as histoplasmosis in the lungs.

Rickettsiae

Rickettsiae resemble bacteria; like viruses, however, they cannot survive outside another living species. Consequently, an intermediate life-form, such as fleas, ticks, lice, or mites, transmits rickettsial diseases to humans. For example, tiny deer ticks transmit Lyme disease, a problem found where people live, work, or enjoy activities in wooded areas.

Protozoans

Protozoans are single-celled animals classified according to their ability to move. Some use ameboid motion, by which they extend their cell walls and their intracellular contents flow forward. Others move by cilia (hairlike projections) or flagella (whiplike appendages). Some cannot move independently at all.

Mycoplasmas

Mycoplasmas lack a cell wall. They are referred to as *pleomorphic* because they assume various shapes. Mycoplasmas are similar, but not related, to bacteria. Primarily, they infect the surface linings of the respiratory, genitourinary, and gastrointestinal tracts.

Helminths

Helminths are infectious worms, some of which are microscopic. They are classified into three major groups: nematodes (roundworms), cestodes (tapeworms), and trematodes (flukes). Some helminths enter the body in the egg stage, whereas others spend the larval stage in an intermediate life-form before finding their way into humans. Helminths mate and reproduce after they invade a species; they are then excreted, and the cycle begins again.

Prions

Until recently, it was believed that all infectious agents contain nucleic acid—either deoxyribonucleic acid (DNA) or ribonucleic acid (RNA). The idea of an atypical infectious agent (initially referred to as rogue proteins) was proposed in 1967. Dr. Stanley Prusiner won a Nobel Prize in 1997 for his discovery of such proteins called prions.

A prion is a protein containing no nucleic acid. Research suggests that a normal prion, which is present in brain cells, protects against dementia (diminished mental function). When a prion mutates, however, it can become an infectious agent that alters other normal prion proteins into similar mutant copies. The mutants, which can result from either genetic predisposition or transmission between same or similar infected animal species, cause transmissible spongiform encephalopathies. These are so named because they cause the brain to become spongy (ie, full of holes). As a result, brain tissue withers, leading to uncoordinated movements. Examples of transmissible spongiform encephalopathies include bovine spongiform encephalopathy (mad cow disease), scrapie in sheep, and Creutzfeldt–Jakob disease in humans. Researchers are currently trying to determine whether prions are the cause of neurologic disorders such as Alzheimer's disease, Parkinson's disease, and Huntington's disease; whether people with these disorders lack prions; and whether prions in people with these disorders are ineffective.

Survival of Microorganisms

Each species of microorganism is unique, but all microorganisms share one characteristic; that is, although infinitesimally small, they are powerful enough to cause disease. All they need is a favorable environment to survive. Conditions that promote survival include warmth, darkness, oxygen, water, and nourishment. Humans offer all these and so are optimal hosts for supporting the growth and reproduction of microorganisms.

Many pathogens have mutated to adapt to hostile environments and unfavorable living conditions. Such adaptability has ensured that they continue to pose a threat to humans. One example of biologic adaptation is the ability of some microorganisms to form spores. A **spore** is a temporarily inactive microbial life-form that can resist heat and destructive chemicals and can survive without moisture. Consequently, spores are more difficult to destroy than their more biologically active counterparts. When conditions are favorable, spores can reactivate and reproduce.

Another example of adaptation is the development of antibiotic-resistant bacterial strains of *Staphylococcus aureus, Enterococcus faecalis* and *E. faecium,* and *Streptococcus pneumoniae.* Such strains no longer respond to drugs that once were effective against them (Box 10-1). Researchers speculate that resistant species can transmit their resistant genes to totally different microbial species (National Institute of Allergy and Infectious Diseases, 2009).

BOX 10-1 Causes of Antibiotic Drug Resistance

- Prescribing antibiotics for minor or self-limiting bacterial infections
- Administering antibiotics prophylactically (for prevention) in the absence of an infection
- Failing to take the full course of antibiotic therapy
- Taking someone else's prescribed antibiotic without knowing whether it is effective for one's illness or symptoms
- Prescribing antibiotics for viral infections (antibiotics are ineffective for treating infections caused by viruses)
- Dispersing antibiotic solutions into the environment:
  - Depositing partially empty IV bags containing antibiotic drugs in waste containers
  - Releasing droplets while purging IV tubing attached to secondary bags of antibiotic solution
  - Expelling air from syringes before injecting antibiotics
- Administering antibiotics to livestock, leaving traces of drug residue that humans consume after their slaughter
- Spreading nosocomial pathogens via unwashed or poorly washed hands

CHAIN OF INFECTION

By interfering with the conditions that perpetuate the transmission of microorganisms, humans can avoid acquiring infectious diseases. The six essential components in the **chain of infection** (the sequence that enables the spread of disease-producing microorganisms) must be in place if pathogens are to be transmitted from one location or person to another:

1. An infectious agent
2. A reservoir for growth and reproduction
3. An exit route from the reservoir
4. A means of transmission
5. A portal of entry
6. A susceptible host (Fig. 10-2)

Infectious Agents

Some microorganisms are less dangerous than others. Just as some animal species coexist *symbiotically* (for mutual

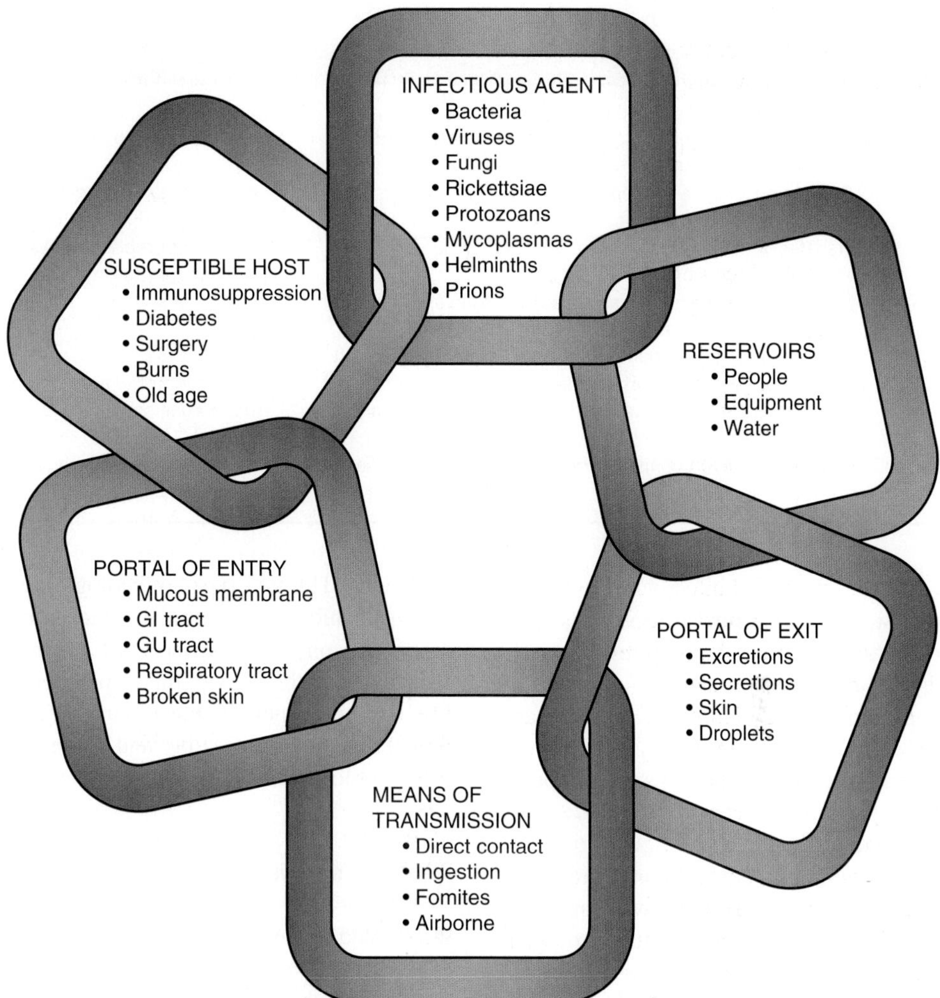

FIGURE 10-2 The chain of infection. GI, gastrointestinal; GU, gastrourinary.

benefit), some normal flora help maintain healthy functioning. For example, intestinal bacteria help produce vitamin K, which, in turn, helps control bleeding. Vaginal bacteria create an acid environment hostile to the growth of pathogens.

Unless the supporting host becomes weakened, normal flora remain controlled. If the host's defenses are weakened, however, even benign microorganisms can cause **opportunistic infections** (infectious disorders among people with compromised health). More commonly, however, infections result from pathogens that, by their very nature, produce illness after invading body tissues and organs.

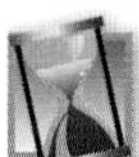

Gerontologic Considerations

■ Pneumonia, influenza, urinary tract and skin infections, and TB are common in older adults. Most cases of TB occur in people aged 65 years or older living in long-term care facilities (Toughy & Jett, 2010). The incidence of TB in community-living older adults is twice that of the general population (Miller, 2008).

Reservoir

A **reservoir** is a place where microbes grow and reproduce, providing a haven for their survival. Microorganisms thrive in reservoirs such as tissues within the superficial crevices of the skin, on shafts of hair, in open wounds, in the blood, inside the lower digestive tract, and in nasal passages. Some grow abundantly in stagnant water, in uncooked and unrefrigerated food, and on used utensils or equipment. They are present in intestinal excreta and the earth's organic material.

Asymptomatic clients or animals that harbor pathogens but do not show evidence of an infectious disease are known as **carriers**. Nonliving reservoirs are **fomites**.

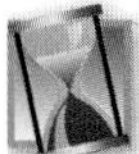

Gerontologic Considerations

■ Many long-term care residents, older hospitalized clients, and health care personnel are colonized with antibiotic-resistant bacteria, possibly with few or no symptoms.

TABLE 10-1 Methods of Transmission

ROUTE	DESCRIPTION	EXAMPLE
Contact transmission		
Direct contact	Actual physical transfer from one infected person to another (body surface to body surface contact)	Sexual intercourse with an infected person
Indirect contact	Contact between a susceptible person and a contaminated object	Use of a contaminated surgical instrument
Droplet transmission	Transfer of moist particles from an infected person who is within a radius of 3 ft	Inhalation of droplets released during sneezing, coughing, or talking
Airborne transmission	Movement of microorganisms attached to evaporated water droplets or dust particles that have been suspended and carried over distances greater than 3 ft	Inhalation of spores
Vehicle transmission	Transfer of microorganisms present on or in contaminated items such as food, water, medications, devices, and equipment	Consumption of water contaminated with microorganisms
Vector transmission	Transfer of microorganisms from an infected animal carrier	Diseases spread by mosquitoes, fleas, ticks, or rats

Exit Route

The **exit route** is how microorganisms escape from their original reservoir and move about. When present within or on humans, they are displaced by handling or touching objects or whenever blood, body fluids, secretions, and excretions are released. In the environment, factors such as flooding and soil erosion provide mechanisms for escape.

Means of Transmission

The **means of transmission** is how infectious microorganisms move to another location. This component is important to the microorganism's survival because most microorganisms cannot travel independently. Microorganisms are transmitted by one of five routes: contact, droplet, airborne, vehicle, and vector (Table 10-1).

Portal of Entry

The **portal of entry** is where microorganisms find their way onto or into a new host, thus facilitating their relocation. One of the most common ports of entry is an opening in the skin or mucous membranes. Microorganisms also can be inhaled, swallowed, introduced into the blood, or transferred into body tissues or cavities through unclean hands or contaminated medical equipment.

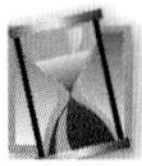

Gerontologic Considerations

- Pathogens may find a portal of entry into vulnerable older adults through devices such as indwelling urinary catheters, humidifiers, oxygen administration devices, and tissues compromised by equipment used for administering intravenous fluids, parenteral nutrition, or tube feedings.

Although microorganisms exist in reservoirs everywhere, **biologic defense mechanisms** (anatomic or physiologic methods that stop microorganisms from causing an infectious disorder) often prevent them from producing infections. The two types of biologic defense mechanisms are mechanical and chemical. Mechanical defense mechanisms are physical barriers that prevent microorganisms from entering the body or that expel them before they multiply. Examples include intact skin and mucous membranes, reflexes such as sneezing and coughing, and infection-fighting blood cells called "phagocytes" or "macrophages."

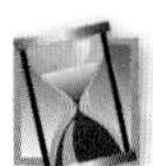

Gerontologic Considerations

- Thinning, drying, and decreased vascular supply to the skin predispose the older person to infections.

Chemical defense mechanisms destroy or incapacitate microorganisms through natural biologic substances. For example, lysozyme, an enzyme found in tears and other secretions, can dissolve the cell wall of some microorganisms. Gastric acid creates an inhospitable microbial environment. Antibodies, complex proteins also called "immunoglobulins," form when macrophages consume microorganisms and display their distinct cellular markers.

Susceptible Host

Humans become susceptible to infections when their defense mechanisms are diminished or impaired. A **susceptible host**, the last link in the chain of infection, is one whose biologic defense mechanisms are weakened in some way (Box 10-2). Ill clients are prime targets for infectious microorganisms because their health is already compromised. Health care workers who are ill should stay at home rather than exposing clients, who are already ill, to infectious microorganisms.

Particularly susceptible clients include those who:

- Are burn victims
- Have suffered major trauma
- Require invasive procedures such as endoscopy (see Chap. 14)
- Need indwelling equipment such as a urinary catheter

BOX 10-2 Factors Affecting Susceptibility to Infections

- Inadequate nutrition
- Poor hygiene practices
- Suppressed immune system
- Chronic illness
- Insufficient white blood cells
- Prematurity
- Advanced age
- Compromised skin integrity
- Weakened cough reflex
- Diminished blood circulation

- Receive implantable devices such as intravenous catheters
- Are given antibiotics inappropriately, which promote microbial resistance
- Are receiving anticancer drugs and anti-inflammatory drugs such as corticosteroids that suppress the immune system
- Are infected with HIV

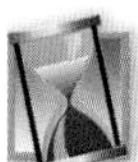

Gerontologic Considerations

■ Older adults are more susceptible to infections because of diminished functioning of the immune system.

Stop, Think, and Respond Box 10-1

Use the chain of infection to trace the transmission of the common cold from one person to another.

ASEPSIS

Health care institutions are teeming reservoirs of microorganisms because of the sheer numbers of confined sick people. Add to this the number of caretakers, equipment, and treatment devices in constant use, and it is easy to understand why infection control is so important. Nurses must understand and practice methods to prevent **nosocomial infections** (infections acquired while a person is receiving care in a health care agency).

Asepsis refers to those practices that decrease or eliminate infectious agents, their reservoirs, and vehicles for transmission. It is the major method for controlling infection. Health care professionals use medical and surgical asepsis to accomplish this goal.

Medical Asepsis

Medical asepsis means those practices that confine or reduce the numbers of microorganisms. Also called *clean technique,* it involves measures that interfere with the chain of infection in various ways. The following principles underlie medical asepsis:

- Microorganisms exist everywhere except on sterilized equipment.
- Frequent hand hygiene and maintaining intact skin are the best methods for reducing the transmission of microorganisms.
- Blood, body fluids, cells, and tissues are considered major reservoirs of microorganisms.
- Personal protective equipment such as gloves, gowns, masks, goggles, and hair and shoe covers serve as a barrier to microbial transmission.
- A clean environment reduces microorganisms.
- Certain areas—the floor, toilets, and the insides of sinks—are more contaminated than others.
- Cleaning should be done from cleaner to dirtier areas.

Examples of medical aseptic practices include using antimicrobial agents, performing hand hygiene, wearing hospital garments, confining and containing soiled materials appropriately, and keeping the environment as clean as possible. Measures used to control the transmission of infectious microorganisms are discussed in more detail in Chapter 22.

Using Antimicrobial Agents

Antimicrobial agents are chemicals that destroy or suppress the growth of infectious microorganisms (Table 10-2). Some antimicrobial agents are used to clean equipment, surfaces, and inanimate objects. Others are applied directly to the skin or administered internally. Examples are antiseptics, disinfectants, and anti-infective drugs.

Antiseptics

Antiseptics, also known as *bacteriostatic agents*, inhibit the growth of, but do not kill, microorganisms. An example is alcohol. Antiseptics generally are applied to the skin or mucous membranes. Some are also used as cleansing agents.

Disinfectants

Disinfectants, also called *germicides* and *bactericides*, destroy active microorganisms but not spores. Phenol, household bleach, and formaldehyde are examples. Disinfectants are rarely applied to the skin because they are very strong; rather, they are used to kill and remove microorganisms from equipment, walls, and floors.

Anti-infective Drugs

The two groups of drugs used most often to combat infections are antibacterials and antivirals.

The chemical actions of antibacterials, which consist of antibiotics and sulfonamides, alter the metabolic processes of bacteria but not viruses. They damage or destroy bacterial cell walls or the mechanisms that bacteria need to reproduce. When used, the intent is to kill or control pathogens; however, these drugs have the capacity to similarly affect normal nonpathogenic bacteria. Before the advent of antibacterial therapy, wound infections, dysentery, and many contagious diseases cut short life expectancy. Some believe that humans will return to the days of epidemics, plagues,

TABLE 10-2 Antimicrobial Agents

TYPE	MECHANISM	EXAMPLE	USE
Soap	Lowers the surface tension of oil on the skin, which holds microorganisms; facilitates removal during rinsing	Dial, Safeguard	Hygiene
Detergent	Acts as soap, except detergents do not form a precipitate when mixed with water	Dreft, Tide	Sanitizing eating utensils, laundry
Alcohol	Injures the protein and lipid structures in the cellular membrane of some microorganisms (70% concentration)	Isopropyl ethanol	Cleansing skin, instruments
Iodine	Damages the cell membrane of microorganisms and disrupts their enzyme functions; not effective against *Pseudomonas*, a common wound pathogen	Betadine	Cleansing skin
Chlorine	Interferes with microbial enzyme systems	Bleach, Clorox	Disinfecting water, utensils, blood spills
Chlorhexidine	Damages the cell membrane of microorganisms, but is ineffective against spores and most viruses	Hibiclens	Cleansing skin and equipment
Mercury	Alters microbial cellular proteins	Merthiolate, Mercurochrome	Disinfecting skin
Glutaraldehyde	Inactivates cellular proteins of bacteria, viruses, and microbes that form spores	Cidex	Sterilizing equipment

and pestilence if antibacterial agents can no longer control microorganisms.

Antiviral agents were developed more recently, most likely in response to the rising incidence of influenza and blood-borne viral diseases such as AIDS. Antivirals do not destroy the infecting viruses; rather, they control viral replication (copying) or their release from the infected cells. The virus remains alive and can potentially cause reactivation of the illness. The goal of antiviral therapy is to limit the **viral load** (the number of viral copies).

Hand Hygiene

Hand hygiene refers to removing surface contaminants on the skin by either hand washing or hand antisepsis. **Hand washing** is a medical aseptic practice that involves cleaning the hands with soap, water, and friction to mechanically remove dirt and organic substances. It is the preferred method of hand hygiene when the hands are visibly dirty, when the hands are soiled with blood or other body fluids, after using the toilet, or when exposure to potential spore-forming pathogens is strongly suspected or proven (Barclay & Murata, 2009). Hand washing removes **resident microorganisms** (generally, nonpathogens constantly present on the skin) and **transient microorganisms** (pathogens picked up during brief contact with contaminated reservoirs).

Although transient microorganisms are more pathogenic, hand washing more easily removes them. They tend to cling to grooves and gems in rings, the margins of chipped nail polish and broken or separated artificial nails, and long fingernails. Thus, these items are contraindicated when caring for clients. Without conscientious hand washing, transient microorganisms become residents, thereby increasing the potential for transmission of infection. One possible explanation for the increase of antimicrobial-resistant pathogens is that nosocomial pathogens are replacing the normal flora of clients when health care workers fail to wash their hands at appropriate times for a minimum of 15 seconds (Goldmann, 2006). Considering how often health care personnel use their hands when touching or using equipment in their care, it is no surprise that *hand hygiene is the single most effective way to prevent infections.* Skill 10-1 describes the steps of hand washing.

Certain situations require hand washing; in others, nurses may substitute hand antisepsis (Box 10-3).

Performing Hand Antisepsis

Research has shown that approximately 36% to 59% of health care workers comply with the minimum requirements for hand washing (Boyce & Pittet, 2002) as recommended by the Centers for Disease Control and Prevention (CDC). To improve compliance with hand hygiene, guidelines for hand antisepsis with alcohol-based hand rubs have been developed. **Hand antisepsis** means the removal and destruction of transient microorganisms without soap and water (Skill 10-2). It involves products such as alcohol-based liquids, thick gels, and foams. Alcohol-based hand rubs are not substitutes for hand washing in all situations (see Box 10-3). Alcohol does not remove soil or dirt with organic material; however, it does produce antisepsis when the hands are visibly clean. Alcohol-based hand rubs remove microorganisms on the hands, including gram-positive and gram-negative bacteria, fungi, multidrug-resistant pathogens, and viruses (Kovach, 2003; Paul-Cheadle, 2003). Because alcohol formulations have a brief rather than sustained antiseptic effect, however, nurses must reuse them over the course of a day (Kovach, 2003).

Advantages of alcohol-based hand rubs over hand washing are that they (1) take less time considering drying does not require the use of paper towels, (2) are more accessible because they do not require sinks or water, (3) increase compliance because they are easier to perform, (4) provide convenience based on their location at the client's point of care, (5) provide the fastest and greatest reduction in microbial counts on the skin, (6) reduce costs

BOX 10-3 Hand Washing and Hand Antisepsis Guidelines

Hand washing with either a nonantimicrobial or an antimicrobial soap and water is performed:

- When hands are visibly dirty
- When hands are contaminated with proteinaceous material
- When hands are visibly soiled with blood or other body fluids
- Before eating and after using the restroom
- If exposure to spore-forming pathogens is suspected or proven

Hand antisepsis with an alcohol-based hand rub can be substituted for hand washing:

- Before having direct contact with clients
- After contact with a client's intact skin (eg, when taking a pulse or blood pressure and lifting a client)
- Before donning sterile gloves to insert invasive devices such as urinary catheters, peripheral vascular catheters, central intravascular catheters, or other devices that do not require a surgical procedure
- After contact with body fluids or excretions, mucous membranes, nonintact skin, and wound dressings if hands are not visibly soiled
- If moving from a contaminated body site to a clean body site during client care
- After contact with inanimate objects (including medical equipment) in the immediate vicinity of the client
- After taking off gloves because gloves are not an impervious barrier

Boyce, J. M., & Pittet, D. (2002). Guideline for hand hygiene in health-care settings: Recommendations of the Healthcare Control Practice Advisory Committee and the HICPAC/SHEA/APIC/IDSA Hand Hygiene Task Force. *Morbidity & Mortality Weekly Report, 51* (RR16), 1–44. Retrieved January 2010, from http://www.cdc.gov/mmwr/preview/mmwrhtml/rr5116a1.htm

by eliminating paper towels and waste management, and (7) are less irritating and drying than soap because they contain emollients (Hand Hygiene Resource Center, 2009; Paul-Cheadle, 2003). The CDC believes that with higher compliance, there is a greater potential for reducing the rate of nosocomial infections.

Stop, Think, and Respond Box 10-2

Discuss actions for ensuring appropriate hand washing before and after caring for a client in his or her home. Use a scenario in which the client has bar soap that rests on the bathroom sink and terrycloth hand towels shared among an entire family.

Performing Surgical Hand Antisepsis

Surgical hand antisepsis, previously referred to as a surgical scrub, is a medically aseptic hand-hygiene procedure that is performed before donning sterile gloves and garments when the nurse is actively involved in an operative or obstetric procedure. The purpose is to more extensively remove transient microorganisms from the nails, hands, and forearms. In fact, the cleanser should reduce microbial growth for increasingly longer periods when repeatedly performed. Table 10-3 lists several differences between surgical hand antisepsis and routine hand washing.

To maximally reduce the number of microorganisms, the fingernails must be short—no more than ¼ in. long, a length that does not extend beyond the tip of the fingers (Arbique, 2006; Gile, 2009). Artificial nails are prohibited. Nail polish is discouraged, especially if it is chipped, worn, or on for more than 4 days because it is conducive to harboring an increased number of microorganisms. All rings, watches, and jewelry are removed and safeguarded before surgical hand antisepsis (Skill 10-3).

TABLE 10-3 Differences Between Hand Washing and Surgical Hand Antisepsis

HAND WASHING	SURGICAL HAND ANTISEPSIS
Plain wedding band may be worn	All hand jewelry, including watches, are removed
Faucets with hand controls are used; elbow, knee, or foot controls are preferred	Faucets are regulated with elbow, knee, or foot controls
Liquid, bar, leaflet, or powdered soap or detergent is used	Liquid antibacterial soap is used; devices such as sponges may be incorporated with antibacterial soap
Washing lasts a minimum of 15 seconds	Antisepsis lasts 2–6 min, depending on the antibacterial agent and time interval between subsequent repetitions
Hands are held lower than the elbows during washing, rinsing, and drying	Hands are held higher than the elbows during washing, rinsing, and drying
Areas beneath fingernails are washed	Areas beneath fingernails are cleaned with an orange stick or similar nail cleaner
Friction is produced by rubbing the hands together	Friction is produced by scrubbing with a brush and/or sponge
Hands are dried with paper towels; the paper is used to turn off hand-regulated faucet controls	Hands are dried with sterile towels
Clean gloves are donned if the nurse has open skin or if there is a potential for contact with blood or body fluids	Sterile gloves are donned immediately after the hands are dried

Wearing Personal Protective Equipment

To reduce the transfer of microorganisms between themselves and clients, health care personnel wear various garments: uniforms, scrub suits or gowns, masks, gloves, hair and shoe covers, and protective eyewear. They wear some of these items when caring for any client regardless of diagnosis or presumed infectious status (see Chap. 22).

Uniforms

Health care professionals should wear their uniforms only while working with clients. Some nurses wear a clean laboratory coat over their uniform to reduce the spread of microorganisms onto or from the surface of clothing worn from home. When caring for clients, they wear a plastic apron or cover gown over the uniform if there is a potential for soiling it with blood or body fluids. When not wearing a cover, nurses take care to avoid touching the uniform with any soiled items such as bed linens. After work, they should change the uniform as soon as possible to avoid exposing their family and the public to the microorganisms present on work clothing.

Scrub Suits and Gowns

Scrub suits and gowns are hospital garments worn instead of a uniform. Their use is mandatory in some areas of a hospital, such as the nursery, the operating room, and the delivery room. These garments prevent personnel from bringing microorganisms on their clothes into the working environment. Employees in other departments sometimes wear their own scrub suits or gowns because they are comfortable and practical. Personnel who work in mandatory-wear areas don scrub suits and gowns when they arrive for work. They wear cover gowns over the scrubs when taking coffee or lunch breaks. Nurses discard mandatory-wear scrub suits and gowns in a laundry receptacle and change into street clothes before leaving the place of employment.

Masks

Masks are disposable, loose-fitting covers for the nose and mouth (Fig. 10-3). They help prevent droplet and airborne transmission of microorganisms, but not necessarily viruses, by keeping splashes or sprays from reaching the wearer's nose and mouth. They are worn once and then disposed.

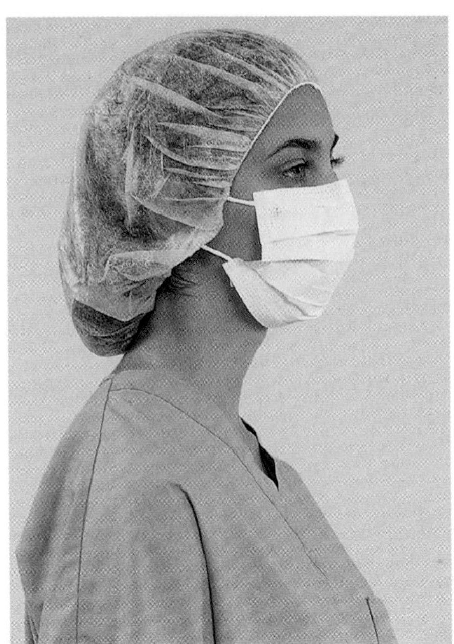

FIGURE 10-3 Face mask and hair cover. (Photo by B. Proud.)

Respirators

To prevent the transmission of TB, the National Institute for Occupational Safety and Health (NIOSH, 2008) recommends the use of a disposable or replaceable particulate air filter respirator that fits snugly to the face (Fig. 10-4). The minimum specification for a particulate air filter respirator is N-95; N refers to "not resistant to oil" (ie, it is effective at blocking particulate aerosols that are free of oil). An N-95 air filter respirator can filter very small particles that may contain viruses with a minimum efficiency of 95% (CDC, 2009).

Particulate respirators are custom sized and fitted for each health care worker to ensure that there is less than 10% leakage between the seal of the mask and the wearer's face. Once fitted, the health care worker can reuse his or her own N-95 respirator as long as it remains intact and clean, and the wearer does not grow facial hair, gain or lose 10 lb, or incur other facial changes that interfere with a tight facial seal (Nursing Guidelines 10-1).

In certain high-risk situations, such as when a bronchoscopy or autopsy is performed on a client with TB, a respirator that exceeds the minimum standard is used. In those

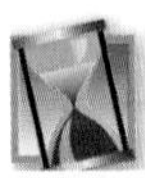

Gerontologic Considerations

- Visitors with respiratory infections need to wear a mask or avoid contact with older adults in their home or long-term care settings until their symptoms have subsided. In addition to the mask, frequent and thorough hand washing can help prevent the transfer of organisms.
- Older adults, family members in close contact with older people, and all personnel in health care settings should obtain annual immunizations against influenza, a virus spread via respiratory secretions. Those 65 years and older should receive an initial dose of the pneumococcal vaccine.

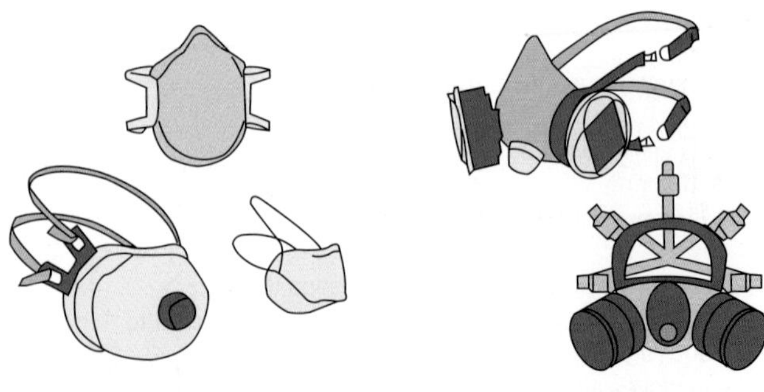

FIGURE 10-4 Replaceable filters and disposable respirators.

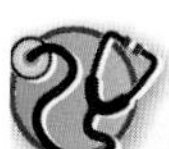

NURSING GUIDELINES 10-1

Using a Mask or Particulate Filter Respiratory

- Wear a mask if there is a risk for coughing or sneezing within a radius of 3 ft. *The mask blocks the route of exit.*
- Wear a mask or particulate filter respirator if there is a potential for acquiring diseases caused by droplet or airborne transmission. *The mask blocks the port of entry.*
- Position the mask or respirator so that it covers the nose and mouth. *The mask provides a barrier to nasal and oral ports of entry.*
- Tie the upper strings of a mask snugly at the back of the head and the lower strings at the back of the neck. *Proper placement reduces the exit and entry routes for microorganisms.*
- Avoid touching the mask or respirator once it is in place. *Touching the mask transfers microorganisms to the hands.*
- Change the mask or respirator every 20 to 30 minutes or when it becomes damp; particulate filter respirators can be worn multiple times, but they must be rechecked for leakage and fit. *Changing the mask preserves its effectiveness.*
- Touch only the strings of the mask or the respirator strap during removal. *Touching the mask transfers microorganisms to the hands.*
- Discard used masks into a lined or waterproof waste container. *Proper disposal reduces the transmission of microorganisms to others.*
- Perform hand washing or hand antisepsis after removing a mask or respirator. *Hand washing and hand antisepsis remove microorganisms from the hands.*

cases, a powered air-purifying respirator or positive-pressure airline respirator equipped with a half- or full-face mask is required (CDC, 2005). This type of respirator removes air contaminants by blowing them through a high efficiency particulate air (HEPA) filter, thus providing purified air to enter a facepiece, hood, or helmet.

Gloves

Nurses wear clean gloves, sometimes called "examination gloves," in the following circumstances:

- As a barrier to prevent direct hand contact with blood, body fluids, secretions, excretions, mucous membranes, and nonintact skin
- As a barrier to protect clients from microorganisms transmitted from nursing personnel when performing procedures or care involving contact with the client's mucous membranes or nonintact skin
- When there is a potential transfer of microorganisms from one client or object to another during subsequent nursing care

Examination gloves are generally made of latex or vinyl, although other types are available (see Chap. 19). Latex and vinyl gloves are equally protective with nonvigorous use, but latex gloves have some advantages. They stretch and mold to fit the wearer almost like a second layer of skin, permitting greater flexibility with movement. Perhaps most importantly, they can reseal tiny punctures.

Unfortunately, some nurses and clients are allergic to latex. Reactions vary and range from annoying symptoms such as skin rash, flushing, itching and watery eyes, and nasal stuffiness to life-threatening swelling of the airway and low blood pressure. Nurses who are sensitive to latex can wear alternative types of gloves, or they can wear a double pair of vinyl gloves when the risk for contact with blood or body fluids is high.

Nurses should change gloves if they become perforated, after a period of use, and between the care of clients. Vinyl gloves are not as protective as latex gloves after 5 minutes of wear. By using aseptic techniques, nurses should remove gloves without directly touching their more contaminated outer surface (see Nursing Guidelines 10-2).

Hair and Shoe Covers

Hair and shoe covers reduce the transmission of pathogens present on the hair or shoes. Health care personnel generally wear these garments during surgical or obstetric procedures. Shoe covers are fastened so that they cover the open ends of pant legs. Hair covers should envelop the entire head. Men with beards or long sideburns wear specially designed head covers that resemble a cloth or paper helmet. Even though hair covers are not required during general nursing care, health care workers should keep their hair short or contained with a clip, band, or by some other means.

Protective Eyewear

Protective eyewear is essential when there is a possibility that body fluids will splash into the eyes. Goggles are worn along with a mask, or a multipurpose face shield is used (Fig. 10-6).

Confining Soiled Articles

Health care agencies use several medically aseptic practices to contain reservoirs of microorganisms, especially those on soiled equipment and supplies. They include using designated clean and dirty utility rooms and various waste receptacles.

Utility Rooms

Health care agencies have at least two utility rooms: one designated clean and the other considered dirty. Personnel must not place soiled articles in the clean utility room.

The dirty or soiled utility room contains covered waste receptacles, at least one large laundry hamper, and a flushable hopper. This room also houses equipment for testing stool or urine. A sink is located in the soiled utility room for hand washing and for rinsing grossly contaminated equipment.

Waste Receptacles

Agencies rely on various methods to contain soiled articles until they can be discarded. Most clients have a paper bag at the

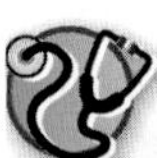

NURSING GUIDELINES 10-2

Removing Gloves

- Grasp one of the gloves at the upper, outer edge at the wrist (Fig. 10-5). *This position maintains a barrier between contaminated surfaces.*
- Stretch and pull the upper edge of the glove downward while inverting the glove as it is removed. *This action encloses the soiled surface, blocking a potential exit route for microorganisms.*
- Insert the fingers of the ungloved hand within the inside edge of the other glove. *The inside edge is the cleaner surface of the glove.*
- Pull the second glove inside out while enclosing the first glove within the palm. *This action contains the reservoir of microorganisms.*
- Place the gloves within a lined waste container. *Proper disposal confines the reservoir of microorganisms.*
- Wash hands or perform hand antisepsis with an alcohol-based rub immediately after removing gloves. *Hand washing and hand antisepsis remove transient and resident microorganisms that have proliferated within the warm, dark, and moist environment inside the gloves.*

bedside for tissues or other small, burnable items. Wastebaskets generally are lined with plastic. Suction and drainage containers are kept covered and emptied at least once during each shift. Most client rooms have a wall-mounted puncture-resistant container for needles or other sharp objects (Fig. 10-7).

Keeping the Environment Clean

Health agencies employ laundry staff and housekeeping personnel to assist with cleaning. In general, if soiled linen is bagged appropriately or handled with gloves, the detergents and heat from the water and the dryer are sufficient to rid linens of pathogenic organisms.

Housekeeping personnel are responsible for collecting and disposing of accumulated refuse and for performing concurrent and terminal disinfection. Housekeepers who follow the principles of medical asepsis carry out **concurrent disinfection** or measures that keep the client environment clean on a daily basis, which include:

- They clean less soiled areas before grossly dirty ones.
- They wet-mop floors and damp-dust furniture to avoid dispersing microorganisms on dust particles and air currents.
- They frequently discard solutions used for mopping in a flushable hopper.
- They never place clean items on the floor.

Terminal disinfection is more thorough than concurrent disinfection and consists of measures used to clean a client's environment after discharge. It includes scrubbing the mattress surface and the insides of drawers and bedside stands.

Nurses who work in home health care can teach the client and the family simple aseptic practices for cleaning contaminated articles (see Client and Family Teaching 10-1).

Stop, Think, and Respond Box 10-3

Describe the methods of medical asepsis that are helpful in controlling the chain of infection of the common cold.

Surgical Asepsis

Surgical asepsis refers to those measures that render supplies and equipment totally free of microorganisms. **Sterile techniques** include practices that avoid contaminating microbe-free items. Both begin with the process of sterilization.

Sterilization

Sterilization consists of physical and chemical techniques that destroy all microorganisms, including spores. Sterilization of equipment is done within the health agency or by

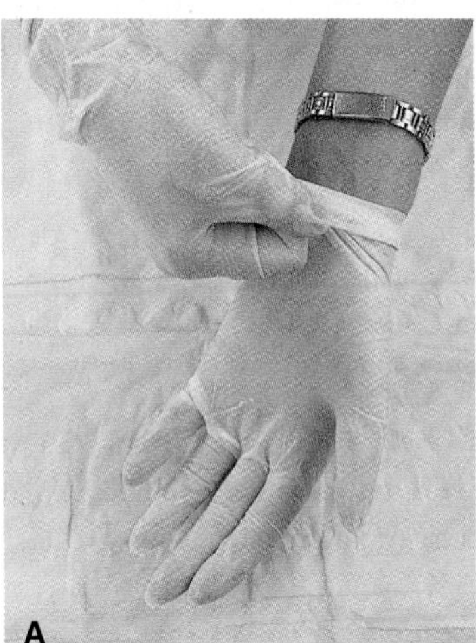

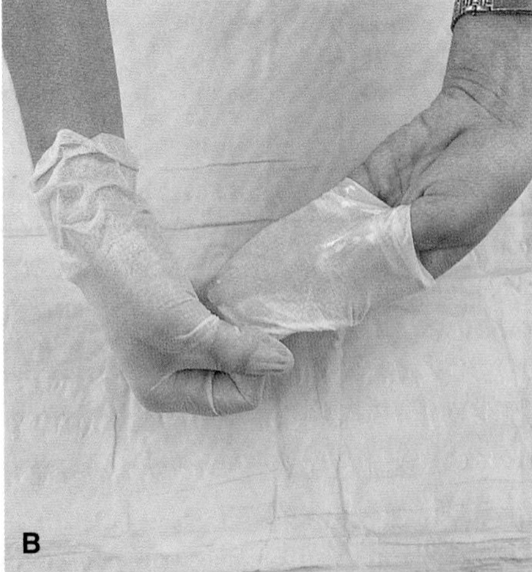

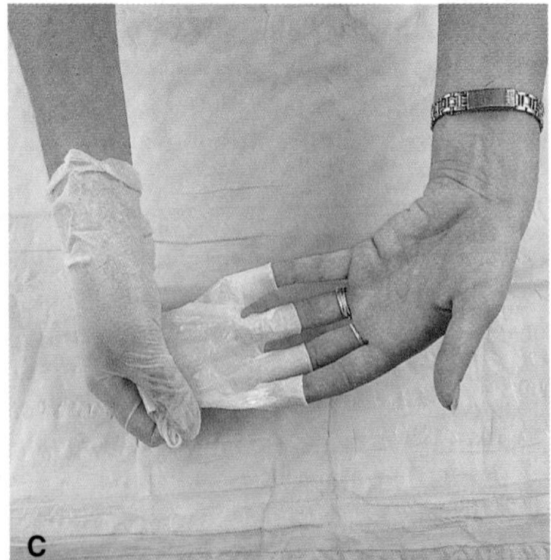

FIGURE 10-5 A. Pulling at the cuff. **B.** Inverting the glove. **C.** Enclosing contaminated surfaces. (Photo by B. Proud.)

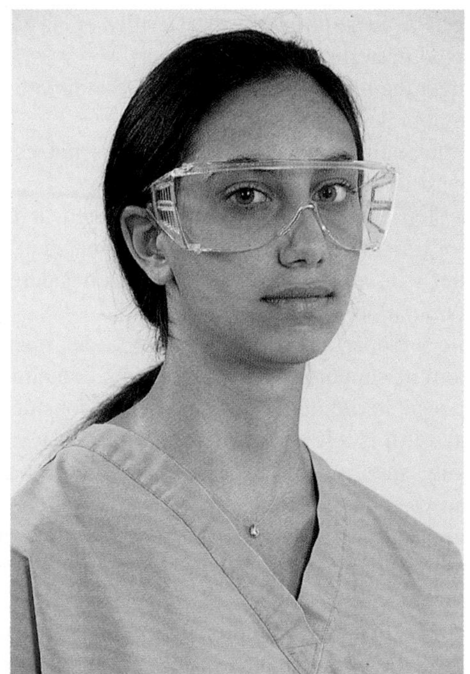

FIGURE 10-6 Protective goggles. (Photo by B. Proud.)

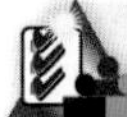

Client and Family Teaching 10-1
Cleaning Potentially Infectious Equipment

The nurse teaches the client and the family to do the following:

- Wear waterproof gloves when handling heavily contaminated items or if there are open skin areas on the hands.
- Designate one container for the sole purpose of cleaning contaminated articles.
- Disassemble and rinse reusable equipment as soon as possible after use.
- Rinse grossly contaminated items first under cool, running water; hot water causes protein substances in body fluids to thicken or congeal.
- Soak reusable items in a solution of water and detergent or disinfectant if a thorough cleaning is not immediately possible.
- Use a sponge, scrub brush, or cloth to create friction and loosen dirt, body fluids, and microorganisms from the surface of contaminated articles.
- Force sudsy water through the hollow channels of items to remove debris.
- Rinse washed items well under running water.
- Drain rinsed equipment and air dry.
- Wash hands for at least 15 seconds after cleaning equipment if the hands are visibly dirty, soiled with blood or other body fluids, or contaminated with proteinaceous material; substitute an alcohol-based hand rub in other circumstances.
- Store clean, dry items in a covered container or in a clean, folded towel.

manufacturers of hospital supplies. Labels on commercially sterilized equipment identify a safe use date.

Physical Sterilization

Microorganisms and spores are destroyed physically through radiation or heat, boiling water, free-flowing steam, dry heat, and steam under pressure.

Radiation. Ultraviolet radiation can kill bacteria, especially the organism that transmits TB. This process is generally combined with other aseptic methods, however, its efficacy depends on circulating organisms by air currents from lower areas of a room to wall- or ceiling-mounted units (CDC, 2008). Exposure to sunlight was used in the past to eliminate microorganisms.

Boiling Water. Boiling water is a convenient way to sterilize items used in the home. To be effective, contaminated equipment needs to be boiled for 15 minutes at 212°F (100°C)—longer in places at higher altitudes.

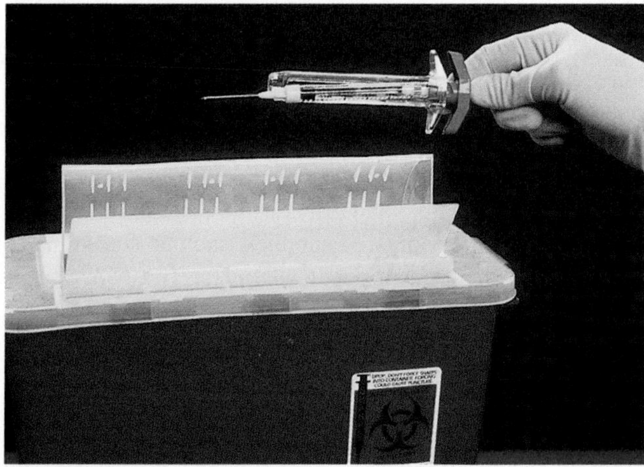

FIGURE 10-7 A sharps container.

Free-Flowing Steam. Free-flowing steam is a method in which items are exposed to the heated vapor that escapes from boiling water. It requires the same time and temperature as the boiling method. Free-flowing steam is less reliable than boiling because exposing all the surfaces of some contaminated items to the steam is difficult.

Dry Heat. Dry heat, or hot air sterilization, is similar to baking items in an oven. To destroy microorganisms with dry heat, temperatures of 330° to 340°F (165° to 170°C) are maintained for at least 3 hours. Dry heat is a good technique for sterilizing sharp instruments and reusable syringes because moist heat damages cutting edges and the ground surfaces of glass. Dry heat prevents the rusting of objects that are not made of stainless steel.

Steam Under Pressure. Steam under pressure is the most dependable method for destroying all forms of organisms and spores. The *autoclave* is a type of pressure steam sterilizer that most health care agencies use (Fig. 10-8). Pressure makes it possible to achieve much hotter temperatures than the boiling point of water or free-flowing steam. Heat-sensitive tape that changes color or displays a pattern when exposed to high temperatures is used on sterilized packages as a visual indicator that the wrapped item is sterile.

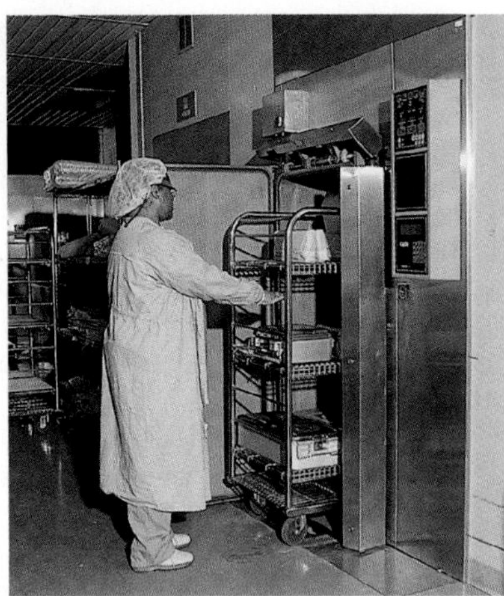

FIGURE 10-8 An autoclave. (Photo by B. Proud.)

Chemical Sterilization

Both gas and liquid chemicals are used to sterilize invasive equipment. Until peracetic acid was perfected as a sterilizing agent, sterilization using liquid chemicals was difficult and some questioned its reliability. The use of peracetic acid, however, and performic acid, a second liquid sterilizing agent, is considered a reliable method for sterilizing heat-sensitive instruments such as endoscopes (Rutola & Weber, 2001). Gas sterilization, using ethylene oxide gas, is a traditional method for destroying microorganisms if heat or moisture is likely to damage items or if no better method is available.

Peracetic Acid. Peracetic acid is a liquid sterilizing agent, which is a combination of acetic acid and hydrogen peroxide. When compared with other liquid sterilizing agents, peracetic acid is the most effective agent against bacteria, viruses, yeasts, and molds. It sterilizes equipment quickly, is effective in the presence of organic material such as blood and stool, and decomposes into environmentally safe byproducts (Steris Corporation, 2006).

Ethylene Oxide Gas. Ethylene oxide gas destroys a broad spectrum of microorganisms, including spores and viruses, when contaminated items are exposed for 3 hours at 86ºF (30ºC). Gassed items, however, must be aired for 5 days at room temperature or 8 hours at 248ºF (120ºC) to remove traces of the gas, which can cause chemical burns.

Principles of Surgical Asepsis

Surgical asepsis is based on the premise that once equipment and areas are free of microorganisms, they can remain in that state if contamination is prevented. Consequently, health care professionals observe the following principles:

- They preserve sterility by touching one sterile item with another that is sterile.
- Once a sterile item touches something that is not sterile, it is considered contaminated.
- Any partially unwrapped sterile package is considered contaminated.
- If there is a question about the sterility of an item, it is considered unsterile.
- The longer the time since sterilization, the more likely it is that the item is no longer sterile.
- A commercially packaged sterile item is not considered sterile past its recommended expiration date.
- Once a sterile item is opened or uncovered, it is only a matter of time before it becomes contaminated.
- The outer 1-in. margin of a sterile area is considered a zone of contamination.
- A sterile wrapper, if it becomes wet, wicks microorganisms from its supporting surface, causing contamination.
- Any opened sterile item or sterile area is considered contaminated if it is left unattended.
- Coughing, sneezing, or excessive talking over a sterile field causes contamination.
- Reaching across an area that contains sterile equipment has a high potential for causing contamination and is therefore avoided.
- Sterile items that are located or lowered below waist level are considered contaminated because they are not within critical view.

Health care professionals observe the principles of surgical asepsis during surgery, when performing invasive procedures such as inserting urinary catheters, and when caring for open wounds. Practices that involve surgical asepsis include creating a sterile field, adding sterile items to the sterile field, and donning sterile gloves.

Creating a Sterile Field

A **sterile field** means a work area free of microorganisms. It is formed using the inner surface of a cloth or paper wrapper that holds sterile items, much like a table cloth. The field enlarges the area where sterile equipment or supplies are placed. When opening the sterile package, the nurse must be careful to keep the inside of the wrapper and its contents sterile. Refer to Skill 10-4.

Adding Items to a Sterile Field

Sometimes it is necessary to add sterile items or sterile solutions to the sterile field (see Skill 10-4).

Sterile Items. Agency-sterilized items or those that have been commercially prepared may be added to the sterile field. The former are generally wrapped in cloth. The nurse unwraps the cloth by supporting the wrapped item in one hand rather than placing it on a solid surface. He or she holds each of the four corners to prevent the edges of the wrap from hanging loosely. The nurse places the unwrapped item on the sterile field and discards the cloth cover.

Commercially prepared supplies, such as sterile gauze squares, are enclosed in paper wrappers. The paper cover usually has two loose flaps that extend above the sealed edges. After separating the flaps, the nurse drops the sterile contents onto the sterile field.

Sterile Solutions. Sterile solutions, such as normal saline, come in various volumes. Some containers are sealed with

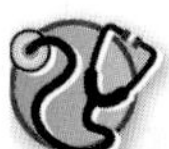

NURSING GUIDELINES 10-3

Donning a Sterile Gown

- Apply a mask and hair cover. *This sequence prevents contamination of the hands after they are washed.*
- Perform surgical hand antisepsis (see Skill 10-3). *This removes resident and transient microorganisms.*
- Pick up the sterile gown at the inner neckline. *This action preserves the sterility of the outer gown surface.*
- Hold the gown away from the body and other unsterile objects (see Fig. 10-9A). *This prevents contamination.*
- Allow the gown to unfold while holding it high enough to avoid contact with the floor. *This prevents contamination.*
- Insert an arm within each sleeve without touching the outer surface of the gown. *This action maintains sterility.*
- Have an assistant pull at the inside of the gown to adjust the fit, expose the hands, and then tie it closed (see Fig. 10-9B). *This action preserves the sterility of the front of the gown.*
- Don sterile gloves. *Wearing sterile gloves ensures the sterile condition of the hands and cuff of the gown.*

a rubber cap or screw top. Either is replaced if the inside surface is contaminated. To avoid contamination, the nurse places the cap upside down on a flat surface or holds it during pouring.

Before each use of a sterile solution, the nurse pours and discards a small amount to wash away airborne contaminants from the mouth of the container. This is called *lipping* the container. While pouring, the nurse holds the container in front of himself or herself. The nurse avoids touching any sterile areas within the field. He or she controls the height of the container to avoid splashing the sterile field, causing a wet area of contamination. Agencies replace sterile solutions daily even if the entire volume is not used.

Donning Sterile Gloves

When applied correctly, nurses can use sterile gloves to handle sterile equipment and supplies without contaminating them. Sterile gloves also provide a barrier against transmitting microbes to clients. Some packages of supplies include sterile gloves; they are also packaged separately in glove wrappers (Skill 10-5).

Stop, Think, and Respond Box 10-4

What is the best action to take if while donning sterile gloves, a nurse touches the thumb of an already gloved finger to his or her ungloved wrist?

Donning a Sterile Gown

A sterile gown protects the client and the sterile equipment from microorganisms that collect on the surface of uniforms, scrub suits, or scrub gowns. Sterile gowns are required during surgery and childbirth. They are used during other sterile procedures as well.

Sterile gowns usually are made of cloth and are laundered and sterilized after each use. Before wrapping a gown for sterilization, it is folded so that the inside surface can be touched while putting it on. To avoid contamination, the nurse should follow the steps outlined in Nursing Guidelines 10-3.

NURSING IMPLICATIONS

Everyone is susceptible to infections, especially if sources of microorganisms among personnel, clients, equipment, and

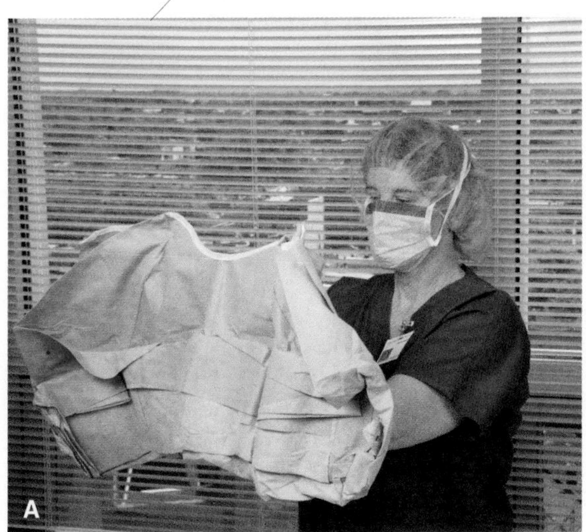

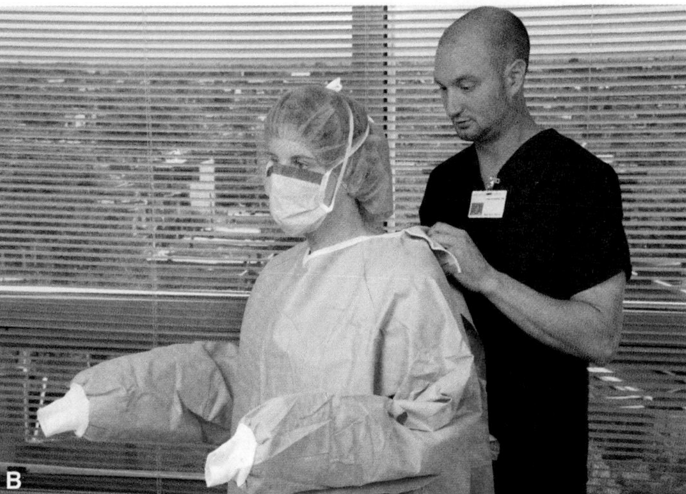

FIGURE 10-9 A. Unfolding a sterile gown. **B.** Assisting with donning a sterile gown. (Photo by B. Proud.)

the agency are not controlled. Nurses generally identify pertinent nursing diagnoses like those that follow when caring for particularly susceptible clients:

- Risk for Infection
- Risk for Infection Transmission
- Ineffective Protection
- Delayed Surgical Recovery
- Deficient Knowledge

Nursing Care Plan 10-1 illustrates how nurses incorporate aseptic principles into a teaching plan for the nursing diagnosis of Deficient Knowledge. The NANDA taxonomy (2012) defines Deficient Knowledge as an absence or deficiency of cognitive information related to a specific topic. Carpenito-Moyet (2008) uses the definition, "the state in which an individual or group experiences a deficiency in cognitive knowledge or psychomotor skills concerning the condition or treatment plan." Some have argued that this

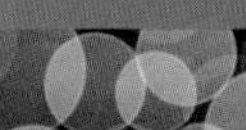

NURSING CARE PLAN 10-1 Deficient Knowledge

Assessment

- Explore the client's level of knowledge in a particular area of health care.
- Provide opportunities during which a client can request health-related information.
- Listen for statements that reflect inaccurate health information.
- Observe if a client performs health-related self-care incorrectly.
- Watch for signs of emotional distress that reflect inaccurate information.

Nursing Diagnosis. **Deficient Knowledge** related to unfamiliarity with infectious disease (hepatitis A) transmission as evidenced by the statements, "The school nurse sent this note home saying there's been a case of hepatitis in my daughter's fifth-grade class. Isn't that what drug users get? Should I keep my daughter home from school? What will prevent her from catching it?"

Expected Outcome. The client will (1) state the difference in transmission of hepatitis A and hepatitis B, (2) list at least three signs and symptoms of hepatitis A, (3) verbalize how to avoid infection with hepatitis A, and (4) demonstrate how to wash hands appropriately by the end of the office visit.

Interventions	Rationales
Explain that hepatitis A is primarily transmitted from the stool of an infected person to the oral route of the susceptible person and that hepatitis B is spread by blood and body fluids.	This discussion provides accurate information concerning the mode of disease transmission.
Provide health-related information about hepatitis A, which includes: • The incubation period for hepatitis A is 25–30 days. • Signs and symptoms that may develop are low-grade fever, reduced activity, loss of appetite, nausea, abdominal pain, dark urine, light-colored stool, and yellowing of the skin and sclera of the eyes. • Hand washing is an excellent preventive measure especially when performed before eating and after using the toilet. • An injection of immune serum globulin is a method of providing temporary passive immunity when exposed to hepatitis A.	Specific information increases the client's knowledge, clarifies misinformation, and helps relieve anxiety.
Demonstrate hand washing and observe a return demonstration emphasizing the following: • Turn handles of the faucet on and let the water run. • Wet hands and lather with soap. • Rub lathered hands for at least 15 seconds. • Rinse, letting the water flow from wrists to fingers. • Dry hands with a paper towel. • Use the paper towel to turn the faucet off.	A demonstration provides health teaching by visual learning; returning a demonstration reinforces learning via a psychomotor activity.

Evaluation of Expected Outcomes

- The client identifies the mode of transmitting hepatitis A as the fecal/oral route.
- The client lists low fever, loss of appetite, and yellow sclera as indications of hepatitis A infection.
- The client states that frequent and thorough hand washing is a method for preventing the acquisition of hepatitis A.
- The client demonstrates appropriate hand washing and is prepared to teach her daughter the same skill.
- The client makes an appointment for her daughter to receive an injection of immune serum globulin.

nursing diagnosis is used erroneously because it is more often an etiology than a nursing diagnosis (Carpenito-Moyet, 2008).

CRITICAL THINKING EXERCISES

1. If the rate of infections increased on your nursing unit, what would you investigate to determine the contributing factors?
2. If the cause of nosocomial infections is related to inadequate hand washing among health care personnel, what suggestions would you give for correcting the problem?
3. What methods could be used to evaluate if health care workers are performing hand hygiene appropriately?
4. What recommendations might you suggest to prevent transferring microorganisms from health care workers' homes to clients for whom they care?

NCLEX-STYLE REVIEW QUESTIONS

1. What is the minimum amount of time required for performing an alcohol-based hand rub?
   1. 5 seconds
   2. 10 seconds
   3. 15 seconds
   4. 20 seconds
2. Which of the following are appropriate aseptic practices in relation to hand hygiene? Select all that apply.
   1. The health care worker has freshly applied artificial nails.
   2. The fingernails are less than 1/4 in.
   3. The nurse removed all remnants of fingernail polish.
   4. The nurse rubs the tips of the fingers against the opposite palm containing an alcohol-based product.
   5. The nurse rubs the hands up to, but not including, the wrists.
3. What is the most important health teaching the nurse can provide to a client with an eye infection?
   1. Eat a well-balanced, nutritious diet.
   2. Wear sunglasses in bright light.
   3. Cease sharing towels and washcloths.
   4. Avoid products containing aspirin.
4. If the nurse provides the following information to a person who has just had his or her earlobes pierced, which is most important for reducing the potential for infection?
   1. Use earrings made of 14-carat gold.
   2. Leave the earrings in place for 2 weeks.
   3. Turn the earrings frequently.
   4. Swab the earlobes daily with alcohol.
5. When donning sterile gloves, which actions are correct? Select all that apply.
   1. The nurse performs hand hygiene.
   2. The finger ends of the opened glove wrapper are positioned nearest the nurse.
   3. The nurse picks up the first glove cuff at the folded edge with the fingers and thumb.
   4. The nurse pulls the glove on without touching the glove's outer surface.
   5. The second glove is donned by holding the cuff with the finger and thumb of the first glove.

SKILL 10-1 Hand Washing

Suggested Action	Reason for Action
ASSESSMENT	
Review the medical record to determine whether it is appropriate to perform hand washing for longer than 15 seconds.	Demonstrates concern for immunosuppressed clients, newborns, or other susceptible hosts.
Check that there are soap and paper towels near the sink and a waste receptacle nearby.	Promotes effective hand washing and disposal of paper towels; bar soap is supplied in small cakes, which are changed frequently and placed on a drainable holder to avoid colonization with microorganisms; liquid soap is stored in closed containers that are replaced, or cleaned, dried, and refilled on a regular schedule.
PLANNING	
Trim long fingernails so that they are less than ¼ in. long, a length at which the nails cannot be seen when the palms are held in front of the nose.	Reduces the reservoir where the majority of hand flora reside; prevents tearing gloves.
Remove all jewelry; a plain, *smooth* wedding band can be worn; roll up long sleeves.	Facilitates removing transient and resident microorganisms; bacterial counts are higher when rings are worn during client care.
Explain the purpose for hand washing to the client.	Reinforces and demonstrates concern for client safety.
IMPLEMENTATION	
Turn on the water using faucet handles; an automated faucet; or elbow, knee, or foot controls (Fig. A).	Serves as a wetting agent and facilitates lathering; using automated faucets, elbow, knee, or foot controls prevents recontamination of hands after they are washed.

Turning on faucet.

Suggested Action	Reason for Action
If a lever-operated paper towel dispenser is available, activate it to dispense the paper towel.	Electronic sensors decrease hand contamination before and after hand washing, but they are not generally available in most health care agencies.
Wet your hands with comfortably warm water from the wrists toward the fingers (Fig. B).	Allows water to flow from the least contaminated area to the most contaminated area.

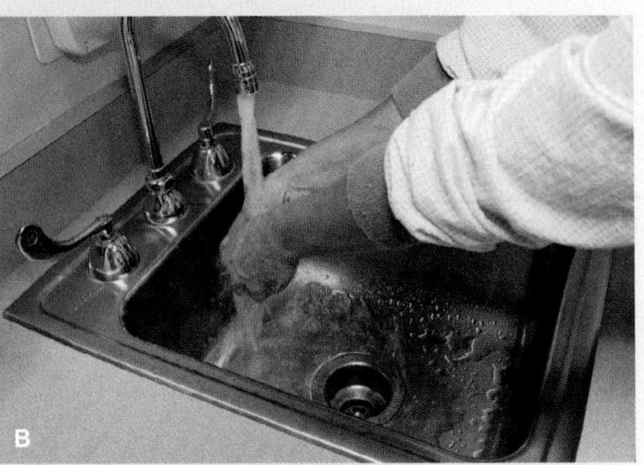

Wetting hands.

Suggested Action	Reason for Action
Avoid splashing water from the sink onto your uniform.	Prevents transferring microorganisms to clothing via a wicking action.

(continued)

Hand Washing (continued)

IMPLEMENTATION (CONTINUED)

Dispense about 3–5 mL (1 tsp) of liquid soap into your hands, or wet a cake of bar soap.
Provides an agent for emulsifying body oils and releasing microorganisms.

Work the soap into a lather and generate friction.
Expands the volume and distribution of the soap; begins to soften the keratin layer of the skin; loosens debris and directs soap into crevices of skin.

Rinse the bar soap, if used, and replace it within a drainable soap dish.
Flushes microorganisms from the surface of the soap; drained bar soap is less likely to support the growth of microorganisms.

Rub the lather vigorously over all surfaces of the hands including thumbs and backs of fingers and hands and under the fingernails for a minimum of 15 seconds–the time it takes to sing two rounds of the song, "Happy Birthday" (Fig. C).
Frees microorganisms that are lodged in skin creases and crevices.

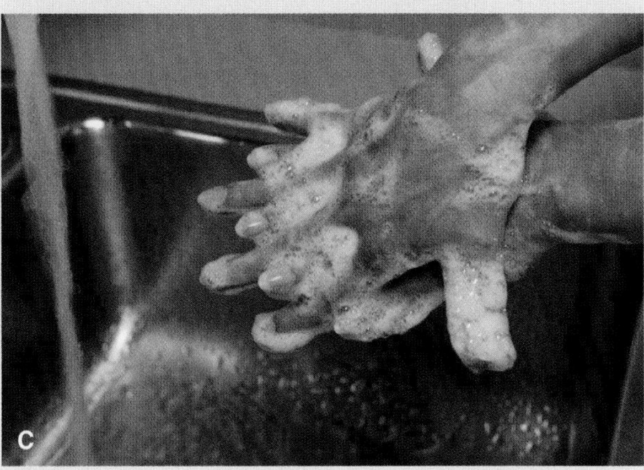

Cleaning backs of fingers.

Rinse the soap from your hands by letting the water run from the wrists toward the fingers (Fig. D).
Avoids transferring microorganisms to cleaner areas.

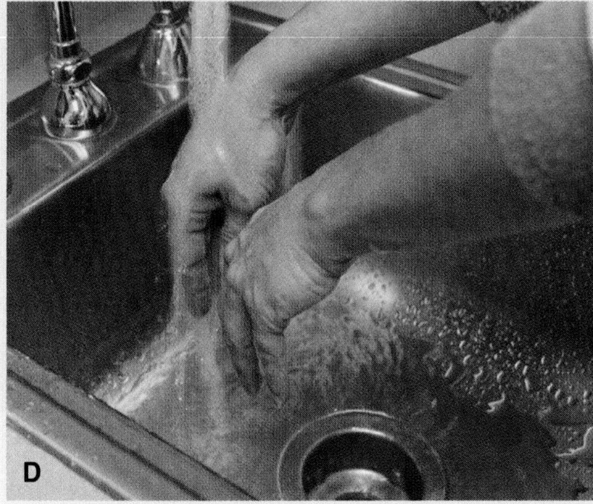

Rinsing hands.

Stop the flow of water if it is controlled by an elbow or knee lever, or a foot pedal.
Terminates the flow of water without recontaminating the hands.

Hold your draining hands lower than your wrists.
Promotes drainage by gravity flow toward the fingers.

(continued)

Hand Washing (continued)

Suggested Action	Reason for Action
IMPLEMENTATION (CONTINUED)	
Dry your hands thoroughly with paper towels or similar items (Fig. E).	Prevents chapping. Cloth towels are the least desirable method of drying because they are prone to contamination. A warm air dryer (rarely available in client environments) is the best. Paper towels dispensed from a holder mounted high enough to avoid splash contamination are acceptable and effective.
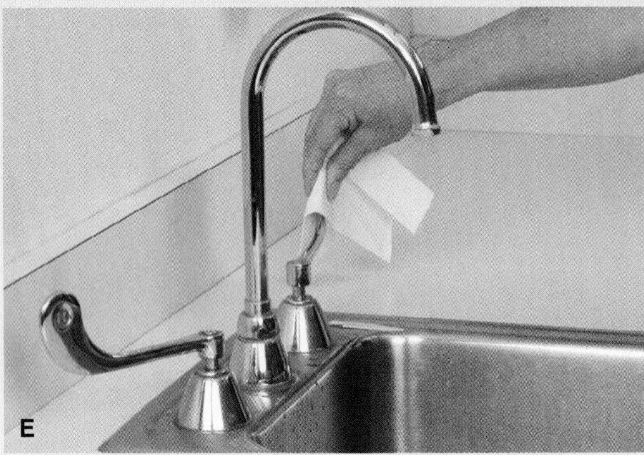	Drying hands.
Turn the hand controls of the faucet off using a paper towel.	Prevents recontamination of washed hands.
Apply hand lotion from time to time.	Maintains the integrity of the skin because skin that becomes irritated and abraded from frequent hand washing increases the risk of acquiring pathogens by direct skin contact.

Evaluation

- Hand washing has met time requirements.
- Hands are clean.
- Skin is intact.

Document

Because hand washing is performed so frequently, it is not documented, but it is expected as a standard for care among all health care personnel.

SKILL 10-2 Hand Antisepsis with an Alcohol-Based Rub

Suggested Action	Reason for Action
ASSESSMENT	
Determine that the hands are *not* visibly dirty or contaminated with proteinaceous material, blood, or other body fluids.	Hand washing is required when the hands are visibly soiled.
Identify the location of the alcohol-based dispenser.	Compliance increases when the dispenser is close to the point of client care such as at the entrance to the client's room or at the bedside.
PLANNING	
Prepare to perform routine hand antisepsis with an alcohol-based product when the hands are not visibly soiled such as before and after touching a client, before and after performing a procedure, after touching within the immediate vicinity of the client, and after removing gloves.	Hands acquire 100–1,000 colony-forming units, a measure of microbial load, during "clean activities." Products containing alcohol have better antimicrobial activity than soap (Boyce & Pittet, 2002).

(continued)

Hand Antisepsis with an Alcohol-Based Rub (continued)

IMPLEMENTATION	
Dispense approximately 3 mL of the alcohol-based product into a cupped palm (Fig. A).	Achieving effective antisepsis is related to a sufficient volume necessary to cover all hand and wrist surfaces.

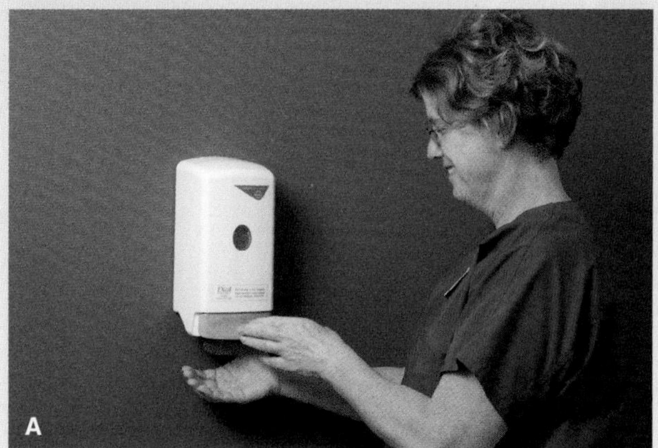

Accessing an alcohol-based product.

Distribute and rub the alcohol-based product over all surfaces of the hands and fingers.	Effective antisepsis requires contact between the alcohol-based product and the skin surfaces where microorganisms reside.
Rub the back of each hand with the opposite palm.	Rubbing spreads the alcohol-based product over the dorsum of the hands and creates friction that loosens surface debris.
Spread the fingers and rub the webbed areas of exposed skin on each hand.	Microorganisms tend to collect and accumulate in the folds of skin.
Rub down the length of each thumb using a rotating motion.	A rotational movement ensures that the entire thumb is included.
Rub the tips of the fingers against the opposite palm on each hand in a circular fashion.	The areas that are cleaned less effectively during hand hygiene include the thumbs, fingertips, and webs between the fingers.
Rub the wrists of both hands in a rotating manner.	Cleaning the wrists is the final step in reducing surfaces in close proximity of clients.
Proceed with nursing activities after rubbing the hands for at least 15 seconds and the hands are dry.	After sufficient rubbing and evaporation, bacterial counts on the hands are significantly reduced.

Evaluation

Hand antisepsis is completed when the product containing alcohol has totally evaporated.

Documentation

Hand hygiene is not documented, but it is expected to be performed conscientiously as a standard of care for all health care personnel.

SKILL 10-3 Performing Surgical Hand Antisepsis

Suggested Action	Reason for Action
ASSESSMENT	
Locate the area designated for performing surgical hand antisepsis. Verify that the sink is deep and has a faucet with either a knee or a foot control. Ensure that there is a sufficient supply of liquid cleanser that can be dispensed with a foot pump; also check to see whether a hand sponge and nail cleaner are available.	This action reduces the potential for recontamination or repeating surgical hand antisepsis because of a lack of necessary supplies.
PLANNING	
Change from uniform or street clothes into a scrub gown or suit.	Changing attire decreases the number of microorganisms transferred from other areas of the health care agency.
Place uniform and valuables, which may include rings and a wristwatch, in a locker.	Storage ensures the safekeeping of items that contain abundant microorganisms.
Don a mask and hair and shoe covers.	These items prevent recontaminating the skin after the hands have been cleaned.
Verify that a sterile towel, gloves, and long-sleeved cover gown are in the operative or obstetric room adjacent to the cleansing area.	Checking ensures that clean hands can be dried and covered quickly to avoid transferring additional microbes to the cleansed areas.

(continued)

Performing Surgical Hand Antisepsis (continued)

IMPLEMENTATION

Turn on the water to a comfortably warm temperature; wet the hands to the forearms and lather the liquid cleanser to all the wet areas, using friction for approximately 15 seconds.
This measure removes surface debris, oil, and some microorganisms before beginning surgical hand antisepsis.

Use a brush, if one is provided, to scrub under the nails, around the cuticles, and the creases in the palms.
A brush may be used initially to remove superficial debris from the hands.

Clean beneath each fingernail with a nail file or orange stick (Fig. A); dispose of this item in a foot-operated waste container before rinsing.
This device removes deeper debris and microorganisms from beneath the nails.

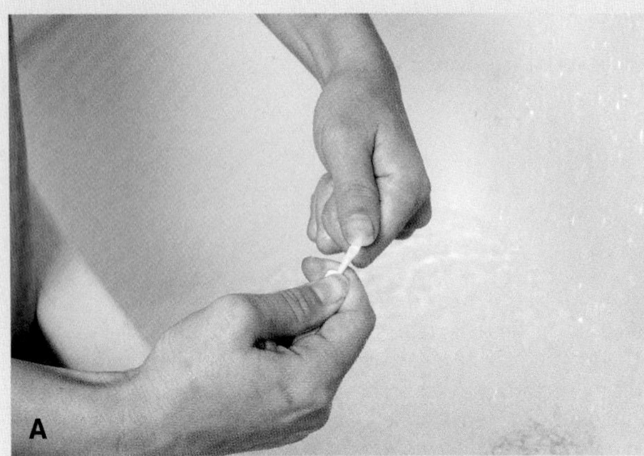

A Cleaning the fingernails.

Rinse the lather while keeping the hands above the elbows.
Gravity prevents soiled lather from adhering to the hands.

Dispense the antimicrobial cleanser into the palm of a hand or use a wetted sponge that has been presaturated with the cleanser.
Doing so decreases microorganisms.

Using friction, wash the nails and all surfaces of each finger; proceed to the thumb, palm, and back of the hand (Fig. B).
These steps follow the principle of cleaning from most to least contaminated areas.

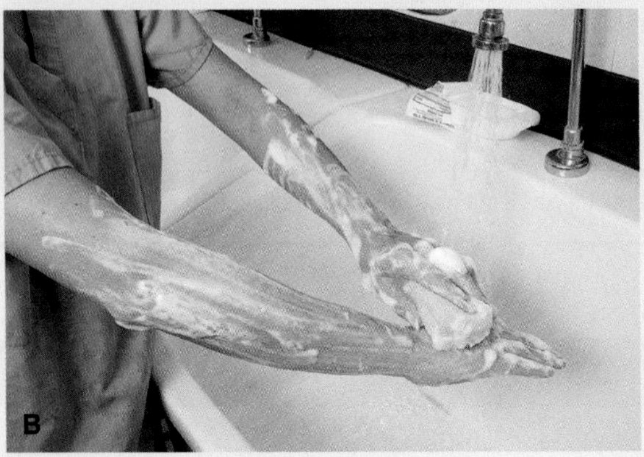

B Washing all surfaces of the hands using friction.

Go over all areas with at least 10 strokes each; repeat on the other side.
This amount ensures adequate cleansing.

Avoid splashing water or lather onto the surface of the scrub gown or suit.
Doing so wicks microorganisms beneath the surface of the cover gown or suit to the surface.

Proceed to wash the forearms with circular strokes from lower to middle to upper areas.
Cleanse in the direction of cleaner areas of the body.

Ensure that washing continues for the time identified by the manufacturer of the cleansing agent (generally a total of 2–6 minutes; Boyce & Pittet, 2002).
Adequate time is necessary to reduce microorganisms. Current studies are being conducted to determine whether surgical hand antisepsis using hand rubbing products that contain alcohol or chlorhexidine may be used in lieu of using traditional hand antiseptics such as povidone iodine or whether the duration of surgical hand antisepsis could be shortened with their use (Al Naami & Afzal, 2006; Tanner, 2008).

(continued)

Performing Surgical Hand Antisepsis (continued)

IMPLEMENTATION (CONTINUED)

Drop the soapy sponge in the sink or discard it within a foot-operated waste container. Rinse lather by allowing the water to run from fingers to elbows (Fig. C).	These steps prevent touching unclean surfaces, as well as debris and loosened microorganisms from dripping over previously cleaned hands.

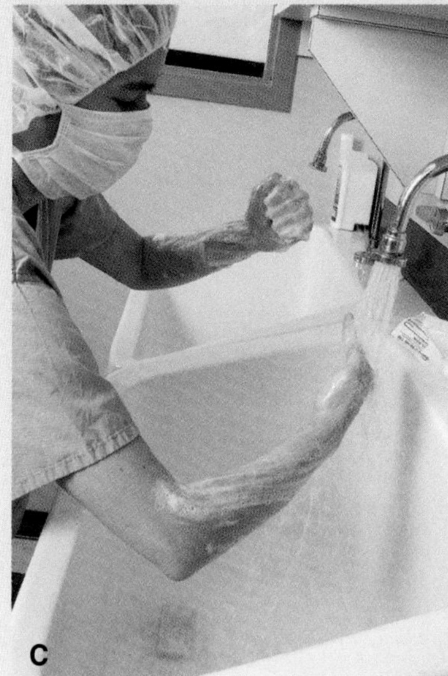

Rinse water flowing toward the elbows.

Keep the hands elevated above the waist, well in front of the scrub gown or suit with the elbows flexed; enter the room where the sterile towel, gloves, and gown are located (Fig. D).	Proceeding this way maintains cleanliness during relocation to the operating room or obstetric suite.

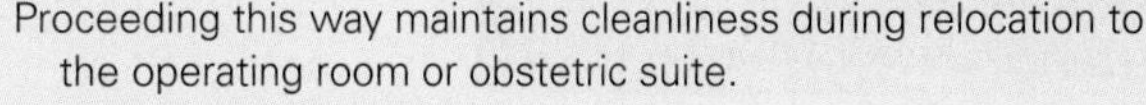

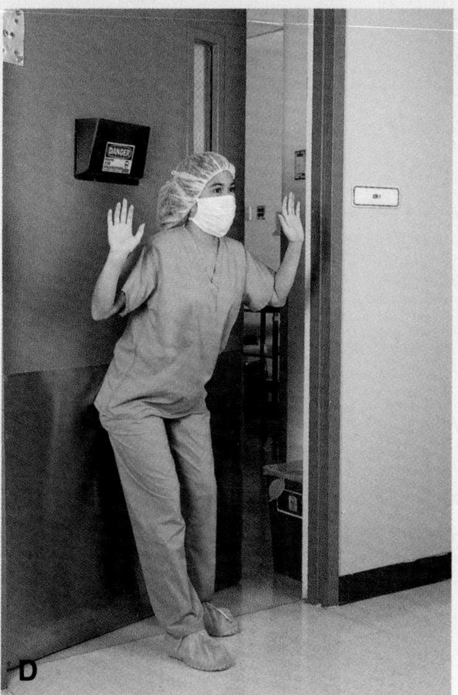

Holding the hands and arms upward and away from the body.

(continued)

Performing Surgical Hand Antisepsis (continued)

IMPLEMENTATION (CONTINUED)

Suggested Action	Reason for Action
Walk to the table containing an unwrapped sterile towel while keeping a slight distance from it.	This step prevents transferring organisms from the scrub gown or suit to a sterile area.
Pick up the sterile towel by its folded edge. After allowing it to unfold without touching anything, use one end to dry the hands and forearm in that order. Use the other end to dry the opposite hand and forearm (Fig. E).	This process avoids transferring organisms from an unclean to a clean area.

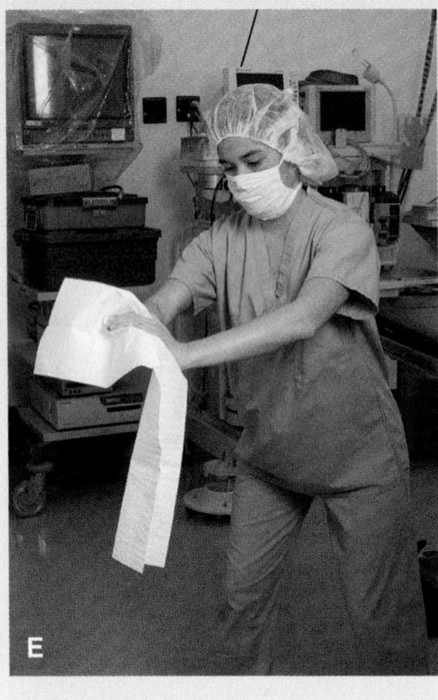

Drying the hands with a sterile towel.

Suggested Action	Reason for Action
Discard the towel within a linen hamper.	Such disposal confines soiled items.
Pick up and don a sterile gown with assistance from another person (see Nursing Guidelines 10-3) and don sterile gloves.	This step keeps the front surface of the gown sterile and covers the clean hands.

Evaluation

- Nails, hands, and forearms have been washed for the designated time.
- The sequence of cleansing supports principles of asepsis.
- The procedure and the use of equipment have followed principles to avoid recontamination.

Document

Surgical hand antisepsis is not documented, but it is expected to be performed conscientiously following agency policies and procedures that are standards of care for all health care personnel.

SKILL 10-4 Creating a Sterile Field and Adding Sterile Items

Suggested Action	Reason for Action
ASSESSMENT	
Inspect the work area to determine the cleanliness and orderliness of the surface on which you will work.	Working in a clean area is a principle of medical asepsis.
Obtain the prepared package that contains items needed for performing the clinical procedure.	Contents within a prepared package contain sterile items.
Check that the package is sealed and that its use date has not expired.	Items are not used if there is a question as to their sterility.
Determine whether additional sterile items are needed but not contained in the sterile package.	Gathering all necessary items facilitates organization and time management.

(continued)

Creating a Sterile Field and Adding Sterile Items (continued)

PLANNING

Explain what is about to take place to the client.
Promotes understanding and cooperation.

Plan to perform the procedure that requires a sterile field when the client is comfortable and there are no potential interruptions.
Once a sterile field is created, it has a potential for contamination when items are uncovered and the field is exposed for a any length of time.

Remove objects from the area where the field will be created.
Removing unsterile items provides room for working and reduces the potential for accidental contamination.

IMPLEMENTATION

Perform hand washing or hand antisepsis with an alcohol-based rub.
Removes transient microorganisms and reduces the potential for transmitting infection.

Place the wrapped package on a surface at or above waist level.
Placement above the waist keeps the sterile field and its contents within sight and reduces the potential for contamination.

Position the package so that the outermost triangular edge of the wrapper can be moved away from the front of the body (Fig. A).
This placement prevents reaching over the sterile area while the package is opened and reduces the potential for contamination.

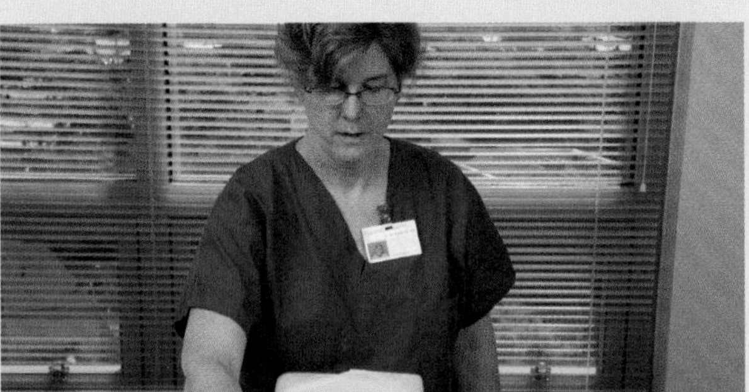
A

Unfolding away from the body.

Unfold each side of the wrapper by touching the area that will be in direct contact with the table or stand, or touch no more than the outer 1 in. of the edge of the wrapper (Fig. B).
This action maintains a sterile area.

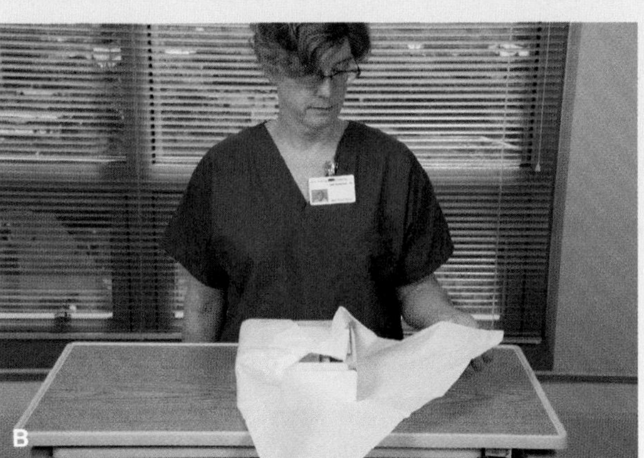
B

Unfolding the sides.

(continued)

Creating a Sterile Field and Adding Sterile Items (continued)

IMPLEMENTATION (CONTINUED)

Unfold the final corner of the wrapper by pulling it toward the body (Fig. C).

This action avoids reaching over an uncovered sterile area, which has the potential for contaminating the sterile field and the items that rest upon it.

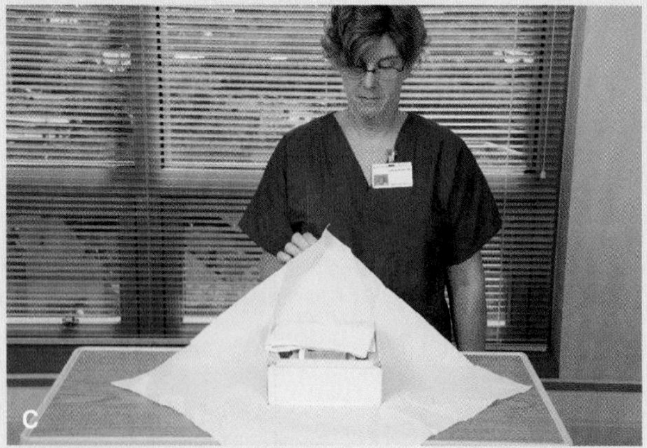

Unfolding toward the body.

Add additional wrapped sterile items by unwrapping them, securing the edges of the wrapper in one hand, and placing them on the sterile field (Fig. D).

Placing sterile items on a sterile field without touching anything that is unsterile preserves a sterile condition.

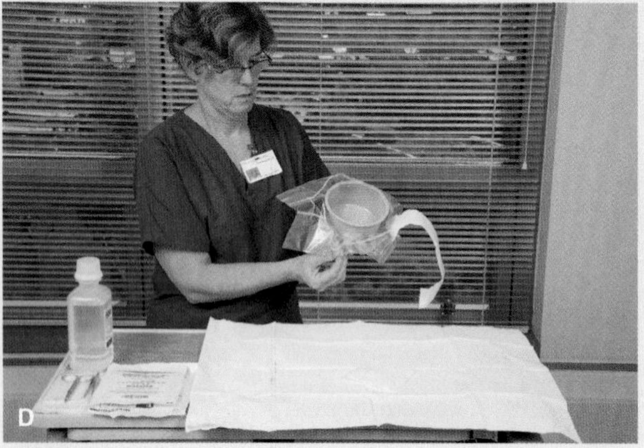

Adding an agency-sterilized item.

Add additional paper-wrapped sterile items by separating the sealed flaps and dropping the contents onto the sterile field (Fig. E).

Placing sterile items on a sterile field without touching anything that is unsterile preserves a sterile condition.

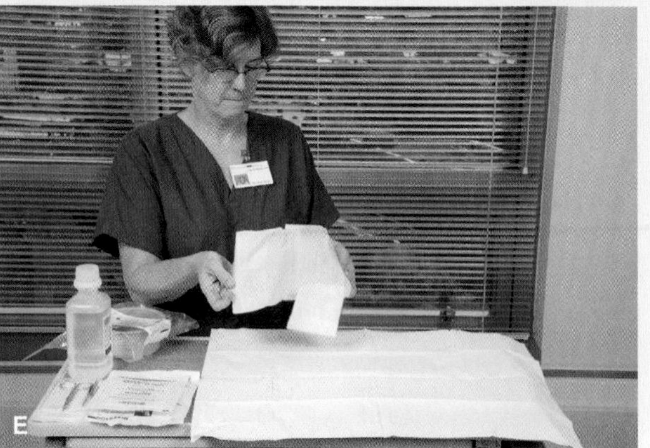

Adding sterile gauze.

(continued)

Creating a Sterile Field and Adding Sterile Items (continued)

IMPLEMENTATION (CONTINUED)

Suggested Action	Reason for Action
Add a sterile solution to a sterile container, if it is needed, by: • Opening the cap on the solution without touching the inner surface with anything that is unsterile • Pouring and discarding a small amount into a waste container • Pouring the amount desired into the container on the sterile field without splashing the surface of the field (Fig. F)	Placing sterile items on a sterile field without touching anything that is unsterile preserves a sterile condition.

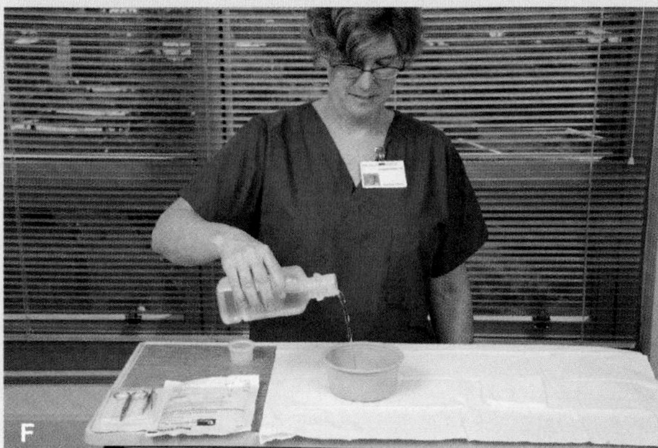

Adding sterile solution.

Evaluation

- The exposed area of the field is sterile; nothing unsterile has touched the surface inside the 1-in. outer margin.
- Additional items have been added to the sterile field in such a way as to preserve the sterility of the items and the surface of the sterile field.

Document

Preparation of a sterile field and the addition of sterile items is not documented, but it is expected as a standard for care among all health professionals. The procedure that required the sterile field and the outcome of the procedure are documented (refer to the sample documentation that accompanies Skill 10-5).

SKILL 10-5 Donning Sterile Gloves

Suggested Action	Reason for Action
ASSESSMENT	
Determine whether the procedure requires surgical asepsis.	Complies with infection control measures.
Read the contents of prepackaged sterile equipment to determine whether sterile gloves are enclosed.	Indicates whether extra supplies are needed.
Discover how much the client understands about the subsequent procedure.	Provides a basis for teaching.
PLANNING	
Explain what is about to take place to the client.	Promotes understanding and cooperation.
Select a package of sterile gloves of the appropriate size.	Ensures ease when donning and using gloves.
Remove unnecessary items from the overbed table or bedside stand.	Ensures an adequate, clean work space.

(continued)

Donning Sterile Gloves (continued)

IMPLEMENTATION

Perform hand washing or alcohol-rub hand antisepsis. — Reduces the potential for transmitting microorganisms.

Open the outer wrapper of the gloves (Fig. A). — Provides access to inner wrapper.

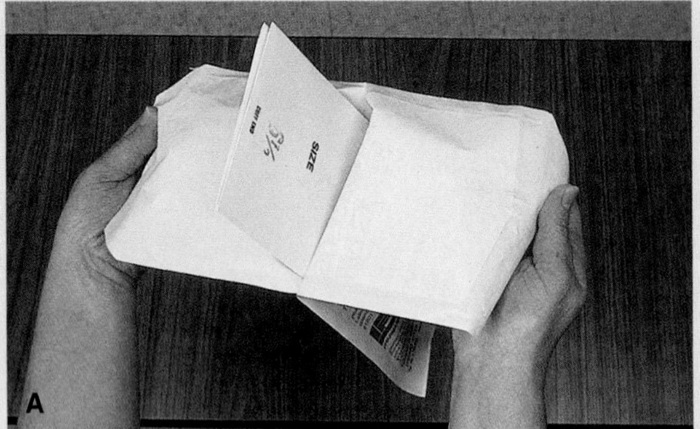

Opening the outer package.

Carefully open the inner package and expose the sterile gloves with the cuff ends closest to you (Fig. B). — Facilitates donning gloves.

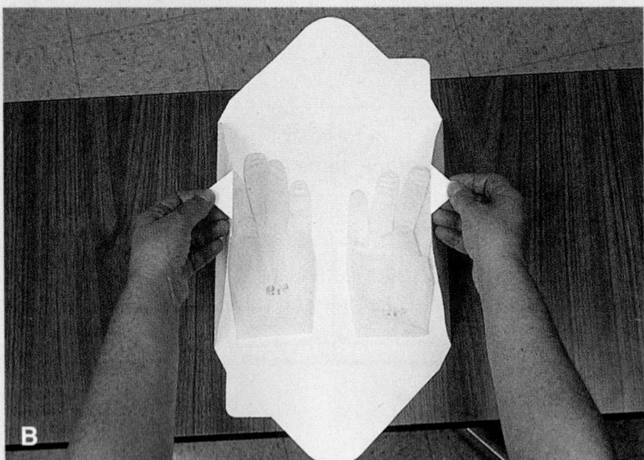

Positioning the inner wrapper.

Pick up one glove at the folded edge of the cuff using your thumb and fingers (Fig. C). — Avoids contaminating the outer surface of the glove.

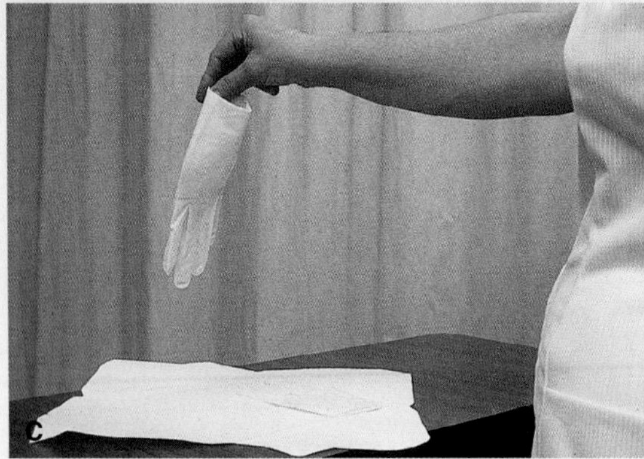

Picking up the first glove.

Insert your fingers while pulling and stretching the glove over your hand, taking care not to touch the outside of the glove to anything that is unsterile. — Avoids contaminating the outer surface of the glove.

Unfold the cuff so that the glove extends above the wrist, but touch only the surface that will be in direct contact with the skin. — Extends the sterile area.

(continued)

Donning Sterile Gloves (continued)

IMPLEMENTATION (CONTINUED)

Insert the gloved hand beneath the sterile folded edge of the remaining glove (Fig. D).	Maintains the sterility of each glove.

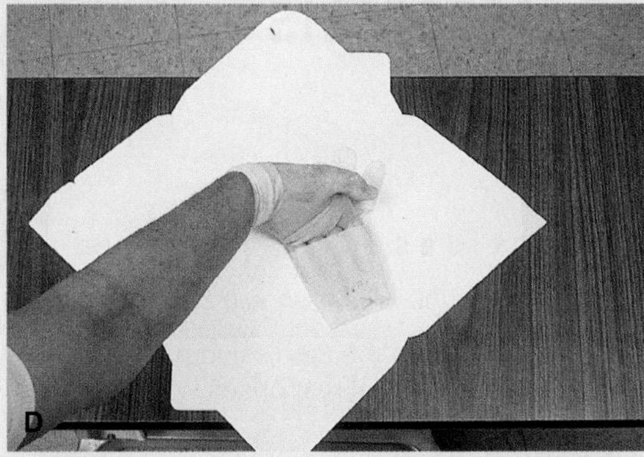

Picking up the second glove.

Insert the fingers within the second glove while pulling and stretching it over the hand (Fig. E).	Facilitates donning the glove.

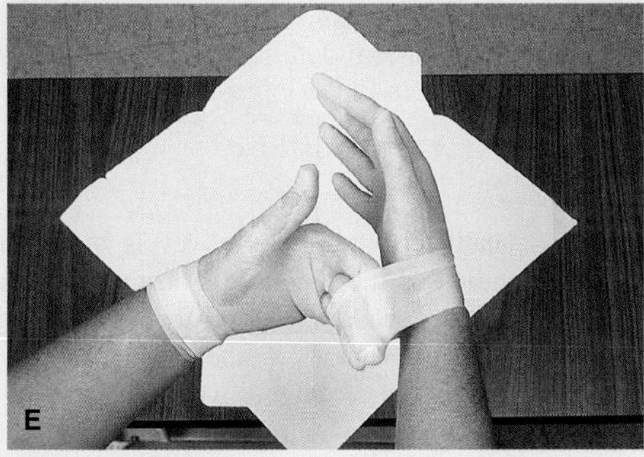

Pulling on the second glove.

Take care to avoid touching anything that is unsterile.	Maintains sterility.
Maintain your gloved hands at or above waist level.	Prevents the potential for contamination.
Repeat the procedure if contamination occurs.	Protects the client from acquiring an infection.

Evaluation

- Gloves are donned.
- Sterility is maintained.

Document

- The procedure that was performed.
- The outcome of the procedure.

SAMPLE DOCUMENTATION

Date and Time Sterile dressing changed over abdominal incision. Wound edges are approximated, with no evidence of redness or drainage. ———— SIGNATURE/TITLE

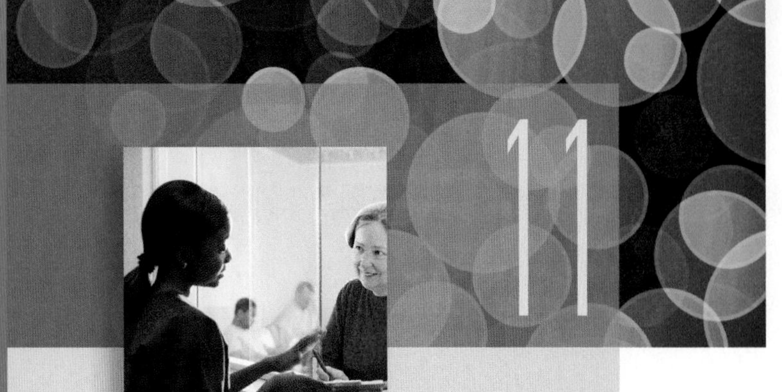

11 Admission, Discharge, Transfer, and Referrals

Words To Know

admission
basic care facility
clinical résumé
continuity of care
discharge
discharge planning
extended care facility
home health care
intermediate care facility
orientation
progressive care units
referral
skilled nursing facility
stepdown units
transfer
transfer summary
transitional care units

Learning Objectives

On completion of this chapter, the reader should be able to:

1. List four major steps involved in the admission process.
2. Identify four common psychosocial responses when clients are admitted to a health agency.
3. List the steps involved in the discharge process.
4. Give three examples of the use of transfers in client care.
5. Explain the difference between transferring clients and referring clients.
6. Describe three levels of care that nursing homes provide.
7. Discuss the purpose of a minimum data set (MDS).
8. Identify two contributing factors to the increased demand for home health care.

EVERYONE experiences health changes. Several levels of health care are available, depending on the seriousness of the condition (see Chap. 4). Some people recover with self-treatment or by following health instructions from nurses or other health care team members.

This chapter describes skills used in caring for clients who become seriously ill, are injured, or have chronic health problems that require admission and temporary care in a facility such as a hospital. This chapter also addresses nursing skills involved in the subsequent discharge, transfer, or referral of clients to community agencies that provide health care.

THE ADMISSION PROCESS

Admission means entering a health care agency for nursing care and medical or surgical treatment. It involves the following:

- Authorization from a physician that the person requires specialized care and treatment
- Collection of billing information by the admitting department of the health care agency
- Completion of the agency's admission database by nursing personnel
- Documentation of the client's medical history and findings from physical examination
- Development of an initial nursing care plan
- Initial medical orders for treatment

The various types of admissions are listed in Table 11-1.

TABLE 11-1 Types of Admissions

TYPE	EXPLANATION	EXAMPLE
Inpatient	Length of stay generally more than 24 hours	Acute pneumonia
Planned (nonurgent)	Scheduled in advance	Elective or required major surgery
Emergency admission	Unplanned; stabilized in emergency department and transferred to nursing care unit	Unrelieved chest pain, major trauma
Direct admission	Unplanned; emergency department bypassed	Acute condition such as prolonged vomiting or diarrhea
Outpatient	Length of stay less than 24 hours; possible return on a regular basis for continued care or treatment	Minor surgery, cancer therapy, physical therapy
Observational	Monitoring required; need for inpatient admission determined within 23 hours	Head injury, unstable vital signs, premature or early labor

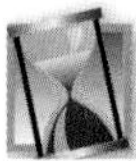

Gerontologic Considerations

- Many older adults fear that admission to a hospital or long-term care facility will eventually prevent their return to independent living. They may, therefore, minimize symptoms to protect their independent-living status.
- Aging directly correlates with increased incidence of acute disease and exacerbations of chronic conditions.
- Adults 65 years and older accounted for one third of the hospital admissions in 2007 (Stranges & Friedman, 2009).
- Pets are an integral social support system and contribute to the general well-being of older adults. Those who live alone may be concerned about the welfare of pets. This should be considered during admission, with arrangements made for the care of the pet.

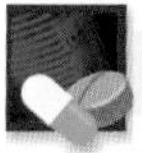

Pharmacologic Considerations

- Nonadherence to medication regimens accounts for more than 10% of older adult hospital admissions, nearly one fourth of nursing home admissions, and 20% of preventable adverse drug events among older persons in the ambulatory setting (American Society on Aging and American Society of Consultant Pharmacists Foundation, 2006).

Medical Authorization

Before admission, a physician determines whether a client's condition requires special tests, technical care, or treatment unavailable anywhere other than in a hospital or other health care agency. Some clients are scheduled for nonurgent care, such as some types of surgery, on a mutually agreeable date and time. Most clients, however, see a primary care or emergency department physician just before admission. The physician advises both the client and the nursing staff to proceed with the admission process.

The Admitting Department

In the admitting department, clerical personnel begin to gather information from the prospective client or his or her family. They initiate the medical record with data obtained at this time. They prepare a form with the client's address, place of employment (if the client works), insurance carrier and policy numbers, Medicare information, and other personal data. The hospital's business office uses this information for record keeping and billing.

Clients who are extremely unstable or in severe discomfort may bypass the admitting department and go directly to the nursing unit. Personnel eventually will direct someone from the family to the admitting department on the client's behalf or go to the client's bedside to obtain the needed information.

Generally, the admissions clerk prepares an identification bracelet for the client, which contains the client's name, an identification number, and, in some cases, a bar code for computerized scanning purposes. Someone in the admitting department or the admitting nurse applies the bracelet. For the client's safety, he or she must wear the bracelet throughout the stay. Other than asking a client's name, the bracelet is the single most important method for identifying the client. If the identification bracelet is missing or has been removed, the nurse is responsible for replacing it as soon as possible.

Once personnel have collected preliminary data, they notify the nursing unit and escort the client to the site where he or she will receive care. They deliver the form initiated in the admitting department to the nursing unit along with a plastic card called an addressograph plate. The card identifies the pages within the client's medical record. Nurses use it to stamp laboratory test request forms, forms that accompany a laboratory specimen, and charge slips for special items such as dressing supplies used in the client's care.

Nursing Admission Activities

Preparing the Client's Room

When the admissions department informs the nursing unit that the client is about to arrive, nurses check the room to ensure it is clean and stocked with basic equipment for initial care (Box 11-1). They later provide personal care items such as soap, skin lotion, a toothbrush, toothpaste, razors, paper tissues, and denture containers for clients who do not have them. They also place oxygen administration equipment, a stand for supporting intravenous fluids, and anything else required at the time of initial treatment.

BOX 11-1 Basic Room Supplies

Each bedside stand is generally stocked with the following:

- A wash basin
- A soap dish
- An emesis basin
- A water carafe
- A bedpan and a urinal

Welcoming the Client

One of the most important steps in admission is to make the client feel welcome. On arrival, the admitting nurse greets the client warmly with a smile and a handshake. He or she wears a name tag, introduces himself or herself, and also introduces other clients sharing the room. Being treated courteously helps relax the client. A client who feels unexpected or unwanted is likely to have a poor, and lasting, first impression of the unit.

Orienting the Client

Orientation (helping a person become familiar with a new environment) facilitates comfort and adaptation. When orienting a client, the nurse describes the following:

- The location of the nursing station, toilet, shower or bathing area, and lounge available to the client and visitors
- Where to store clothing and personal items
- How to call for nursing assistance from the bed and bathroom
- How to adjust the hospital bed
- How to regulate the room lights
- How to use the telephone and any policy about diverting incoming calls to the nursing station during the night
- How to operate the television
- The daily routine such as meal times
- When the doctor usually visits
- When surgery is scheduled
- When laboratory or diagnostic tests are performed

Some hospitals provide booklets with information about the agency, such as gift shop hours, newspaper deliveries, and the location of the chapel or name of the chaplain. Such booklets, however, should never replace a nurse's individualized explanations.

Safeguarding Valuables and Clothing

Nurses give certain items, such as prescription and nonprescription medications, valuable jewelry, and large sums of money, to family members to take home. If this is not possible, *the nurse must carefully observe the agency's policies.* Some institutions provide clients who are not expected to stay longer than 24 hours with a locker to store personal effects. The nurse may place the clients' valuables in the hospital's safe temporarily. He or she notes in the medical record the type of valuables and how they have been safeguarded. It is best to be as descriptive as possible. For example, rather than indicating that the nurse placed a ring in the safe, it is better to describe the type of metal and stones in the ring.

CLOTHING LIST:
(Please check articles of clothing with client and describe.)

Dress	1-BLUE & WHITE	Pants	
Slip	1-WHITE (½ SLIP)	Shirt	
Bra	1-WHITE	Undershirt	
Panties	1-WHITE	Undershorts	
Hose		Socks	
Girdle		Tie	
Slippers	1-PINK	Shoes	1-WHITE
Nightgown	1-BLUE, 1-PINK	Pajamas	
Suit		Robe	
Sweater		Coat	
Slacks		Truss	
Blouse		Backsupport	
Shorts		Belt	
Skirt		Hat	

Other items not listed:

Check valuables below and describe if necessary:

Watch ____ Earrings ____
Medals ____ Rings-Type & Number 1-YELLOW METAL, PLAIN BAND
Other Jewelry ____

Dentures-Yes ✓ No ____ Prosthesis-Yes ____ No ✓
Contact Lenses-Yes ____ No ✓ Glasses-Yes ✓ No ____
Removed-Yes ____ No ____ Hearing Aid-Yes ____ No ✓

Wallet ✓ Color RED With Pt. ✓ In Safe ____ To Family or Friend ____
Purse ✓ Color WHITE With Pt. ✓ In Safe ____ To Family or Friend ____
Cash $25.00 With Pt. ____ In Safe ✓ To Family or Friend ____
Checks/Check Book ____ With Pt. ____ In Safe ____ To Family or Friend ____

The above list is correct:

Client's signature Helen Jones Witness Nancy Smith, L.P.N.

Clothing taken home by ____

Relationship ____

Witness ____

Received by on Nursing Unit ____

FIGURE 11-1 An inventory of a client's personal belongings.

Losing a client's personal items can have serious legal implications for both the nurse and the health care agency. The client may sue, claiming the belongings were lost or stolen because of careless handling. Therefore, it is best to have a second nurse's, supervisor's, or security person's signature on the envelope containing the secured valuables.

One method for avoiding discrepancies between the items entrusted to the nurse and those eventually returned is to make an inventory (Fig. 11-1), which both the nurse and the client sign. The nurse gives one copy to the client and attaches another copy to the chart. When adding items or returning them to the client, the nurse revises the list and the client signs the new inventory. Problems with theft or loss may occur without subsequent documentation.

The nurse identifies client-owned equipment, such as a walker or wheelchair, with a large, easily read label. Labeling prevents confusing such equipment with that belonging to the facility. Most agencies have places in the client's room for storing street clothing.

Because clients occasionally remove eyeglasses and dentures, such items may be lost or broken. Generally, the health care agency is responsible for replacing these items if negligence of the staff causes accidental damage or loss.

Helping the Client Undress

To facilitate a physical examination, the client must undress. If the client cannot undress without the nurse's help, the nurse does the following:

- Provides privacy.
- Has the client sit on the edge of the bed, which has already been lowered.
- Removes the client's shoes.
- Gathers each stocking, sliding it down the leg and over the foot.
- Helps the client lie down if weak or tired.
- Releases fasteners such as zippers and buttons and removes the item of clothing in whatever way is most comfortable and least disturbing. For example, the nurse folds or gathers a garment and works it up and over the body. He or she has the client lift the hips to slide clothes up or down.
- Lifts the client's head to guide garments over it.
- Rolls the client from side to side to remove clothes that fasten up the front or back.
- Covers the client with a bath blanket after removing the outer clothing, or puts a hospital gown on the client, explaining that hospital gowns fasten in the back.

Compiling the Nursing Database

On admission, the nurse begins assessing the client and collecting information for the database (Fig. 11-2). Although the registered nurse is responsible for the admission assessment, he or she may delegate some aspects to the practical nurse, nursing student, or other ancillary staff. Physical assessment skills, which include taking vital signs, are discussed in more depth in Chapters 12 and 13.

Skill 11-1 describes the basic steps in admitting a client. Additions or modifications to the procedure depend largely on the client's condition and agency policies.

Stop, Think, and Respond Box 11-1

What aspects of admission could the registered nurse delegate to a practical nurse, a nursing student, or a nursing assistant? What are the responsibilities of the nurse who has delegated admission tasks?

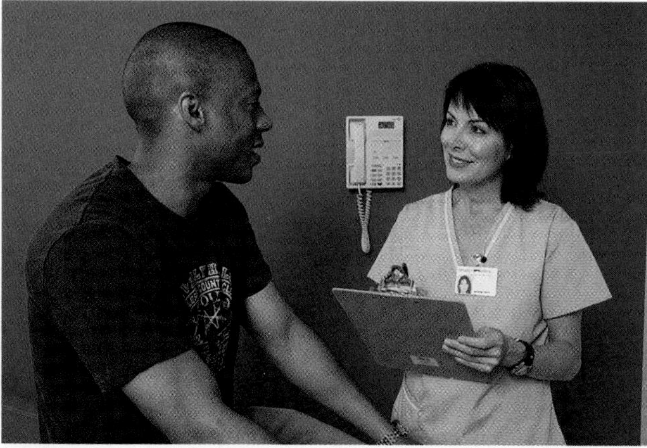

FIGURE 11-2 Beginning to compile the nursing database.

Initial Nursing Plan for Care

Once all admission data are collected, the nurse develops an initial plan for the client's care as soon as possible but no later than 24 hours following admission (see Chap. 2). The initial plan generally identifies priority problems and includes the client's projected needs for teaching and discharge planning. The nurse revises the care plan as more data accumulate or if the client's condition changes.

Medical Admission Responsibilities

The nurse notifies the physician once the admission procedure is completed. The physician provides medical orders for medications and other treatments, laboratory and diagnostic tests, activity, and diet. He or she also obtains a medical history and performs a physical examination within 24 hours of admission. The physician may delegate this task to another member of the medical team such as a medical student, an intern, or a resident.

The medical history and physical examination generally include identifying data, reason for seeking care, history of present illness, personal history, past health history, family history, review of body systems, and conclusions (Box 11-2). If the physician is unsure of the actual medical diagnosis, he or she uses the term *rule out* or the abbreviation *R/O* to indicate that the condition is suspected, but additional diagnostic data must be obtained before confirmation.

Common Responses to Admission

Nurses and physicians must remember that no matter how often they have admitted clients, it is a unique and emotionally traumatic experience for each client. Leaving the security of the home and entering an unfamiliar environment compound the stress of physical illness and contribute to emotional and social distress.

Although specific responses to admission are unique, common reactions include anxiety, loneliness, decreased privacy, and loss of identity. In addition, the nurse may identify one or more of the following nursing diagnoses as a consequence of admission:

- Anxiety
- Fear
- Decisional conflict
- Situational low self-esteem
- Powerlessness
- Social isolation
- Ineffective self-health managment

Anxiety

Anxiety is an uncomfortable feeling caused by insecurity. The NANDA International (NANDA-I, 2012, p. 344) has defined it as "a vague uneasy feeling of discomfort or dread accompanied by an autonomic response (the source is often nonspecific or unknown to the individual); a feeling of apprehension caused by anticipation of danger. It is an alerting signal that warns of impending danger and enables the individual to take measures to deal with threat."

BOX 11-2 Components of a Medical History and Physical Examination

Identifying Data
- Age, gender, marital status
- General appearance
- Circumstances surrounding physician involvement
- Reliability of client as historian
- Others providing information about the client's history

Chief Complaint
- Reason for seeking care (from client's perspective)

Present Illness
- Chronologic description of onset, frequency, and duration of current signs and symptoms
- Outcomes of earlier attempts at self-treatment and medical treatment

Personal History
- Occupation
- Highest level of education
- Religious affiliation
- Residence
- Country of origin
- Primary language
- Military service
- Foreign travel or residence (date, location, length)

Past Health History
- Childhood disease summary
- Physical injuries
- Major illnesses and surgeries
- Previous hospitalizations (medical or psychiatric)
- Drug history
- Alcohol and tobacco use
- Allergy history

Family History
- Health problems in immediate family members (living and deceased)
- Longevity and cause of death among deceased blood relatives (especially parents and grandparents)

Review of Body Systems
- Results of physical examination

Conclusions
- Primary diagnosis (from chief complaint and physical examination)
- Secondary diagnoses reflecting stable or preexisting conditions possibly affecting client's treatment

Many adults do not manifest their anxiety in obvious ways. Observant nurses may note that adults appear sad or worried, are restless, have a reduced appetite, and have trouble sleeping (see Chap. 5). Because adults have a greater capacity to process information than children, it is helpful to acknowledge their uneasiness and to provide explanations and instructions before any new experience. Nursing Care Plan 11-1 provides an example of how to use the nursing process when planning the care of a client with anxiety.

Loneliness

Loneliness occurs when a client cannot interact with family and friends. Although nurses can never replace significant others, they act as temporary surrogates and should make frequent contact with the client. To help combat loneliness, many hospitals and nursing homes have adopted liberal visiting hours. They also are lifting age restrictions to allow more contact between children and their sick relatives.

Decreased Privacy

Privacy is at a premium in most health care agencies. Providing private rooms for all hospitalized clients is becoming a trend because of *Health Insurance Portability and Accountability Act* (HIPAA) legislation (see Chap. 9). Although most prefer a private room, not all clients have one; in fact, clients may have little more than a few feet that they can consider their personal space. For most, it is stressful to share a room with a stranger. To ensure privacy, the nurse closes room doors unless safety issues require observation. Doors may be open at the client's request, but this results in being observed by many people who pass by at all hours.

Nurses demonstrate respect for and protect each client's right to privacy. They always shield clients from the view of others when giving personal care. If a client's door is closed or the curtains are pulled, the nurse knocks and asks permission to enter. If the health care agency has a place where clients can find solitude, such as a chapel or reading room, the nurse includes this information in the admission orientation.

Stop, Think, and Respond Box 11-2

What actions are appropriate if a family member or significant other chooses to remain with the client after he or she has been escorted to a room on the nursing unit at admission?

Loss of Identity

Admission to a health care facility may temporarily deprive a person of his or her identity. For example, clients required to wear hospital gowns tend to look somewhat alike. As a result, personnel may treat clients impersonally—simply as a face or a warm body with no name. This attitude makes clients feel like they are receiving care but without caring.

Nurses learn and use the client's name. They use first names only at the client's request. They encourage clients to display pictures or other small personal objects that reaffirm their unique life and personality. Many long-term care facilities urge clients to dress in their own clothing and invite them to furnish their rooms with personal items from home.

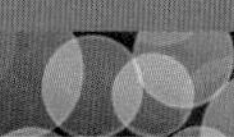

NURSING CARE PLAN 11-1 Anxiety

Assessment

- Observe evidence of anxiety such as rapid heart rate, elevated blood pressure, sleep disturbance, restlessness, worry, irritability, facial tension, impaired attention, difficulty concentrating, talking excessively, crying, or being withdrawn.
- Encourage the client to validate observations by asking open-ended questions such as "How are you feeling now?" If anxiety exists, ask the client to rate the level of anxiety by using a scale from 0 to 10, in which 0 represents no anxiety and 10 represents the most anxiety the client has ever experienced.
- Also ask the client to indicate the level at which he or she can tolerate or cope with anxiety.
- Inquire as to methods the client uses to control anxiety when it exists and the effectiveness of the identified methods.

Nursing Diagnosis. **Anxiety** related to the perception of danger as evidenced by a heart rate of 92 beats/minute at rest, elevated blood pressure of 156/92, awareness of feelings of apprehension in the statement, "I feel like a rubber band that's stretched and ready to snap," and rate of 7 as level of emotional discomfort.

Expected Outcome. The client's anxiety will be reduced to a self-rated level of tolerance of "5."

Interventions	Rationales
Encourage the client to use methods that have successfully relieved anxiety in the past.	Interventions that the client has relied upon and that have had beneficial outcomes can increase the potential for effectiveness in current and future episodes of anxiety.
Reduce external stimuli such as bright lights, noise, sudden movement, and unnecessary activity.	Numerous stimuli escalate anxiety because they interfere with attention and concentration. Dealing simultaneously with multiple stimuli can tax the client's energy and compromise the ability to cope.
Maintain a calm manner when interacting with the client.	People communicate anxiety to one another; an anxious nurse can increase anxiety in a client. Modeling a controlled state promotes a similar response in the client.
Take a position at least an arm's length away from the client.	Invading an anxious client's personal space may increase his or her discomfort.
Avoid touching the client without first asking permission.	An anxious client may misinterpret unexpected touching as threatening.
Establish trust by being available to the client and keeping promises.	Insecurity can be relieved if the client knows he or she can depend on assistance from the nurse.
Advise the client to seek out the nurse or another supportive person when feeling heightened anxiety.	The earlier the anxiety is de-escalated, the sooner the client will experience relief of symptoms.
Stay with the client during periods of severe anxiety.	The nurse's presence can help the client stay in control or restore control to a more comfortable level.
Follow a consistent schedule for routine activities.	Unpredictability heightens anxiety; consistency helps a client manage time and cope with personal demands.
Encourage the client to identify what he or she perceives to be a threat to emotional equilibrium.	Processing situations verbally may give the client perspective on perceived threats so that they are more realistic and less exaggerated.
Use a soft voice, short sentences, and clear messages when exchanging information.	Anxious clients have a short attention span and reduced ability to concentrate; they may be unable to follow lengthy or complicated information.
Provide specific, succinct directions for tasks the client should complete or assist the client who becomes agitated.	Anxious clients have difficulty following instructions and performing tasks in correct sequence. Assistance relieves unnecessary distress.
Instruct and help the client with moderate or severe anxiety to perform one or more of the following until anxiety is within a tolerable level:	
• Count slowly backward from 100.	Distraction redirects the client's attention from distressing physiologic symptoms to a simple task.
• Breathe slowly and deeply in through the nose and out through the mouth.	Slowing respirations aborts hyperventilation and subsequent potential for fainting, peripheral tingling, and numbness from respiratory alkalosis.
• Offer a warm bath or back rub.	Sitting in warm running water promotes relaxation; massage relaxes tense muscles and possibly releases endorphins (natural chemicals that create a feeling of well-being).

(continued)

NURSING CARE PLAN 11-1 Anxiety (continued)

Interventions	Rationales
Help the client to progressively relax groups of muscles from the toes to the head.	Consciously relaxing skeletal muscles relieves tension and fatigue.
Suggest that the client repeat positive statements such as, "I am relaxed," "I am in control," "I am safe."	Positive self-talk can be transformed into reality.
Encourage the client to visualize a pleasant, relaxing place.	Imagery can transform a person's aroused state to one that is more relaxed.
Have the client listen to a relaxation tape or soothing music.	Distraction helps to refocus attention to less anxiety-provoking stimuli.
Advise the client to reduce dietary intake of substances that contain caffeine such as colas and coffee.	Caffeine is a central nervous system stimulant that contributes to the symptoms the client experiences with anxiety.

Evaluation of Expected Outcomes

- The client deals with anxiety-provoking stimuli realistically and implements interventions that reduce anxiety.
- The client has extended periods during which his or her anxiety is at a tolerable level.
- The client has a reduced perception of being apprehensive.

THE DISCHARGE PROCESS

Regardless of where or why clients are admitted, the goal is to keep the admission brief and to discharge clients to the home or to another health care facility of their choice as soon as possible. **Discharge** (the termination of care from a health care agency) generally consists of discharge planning, obtaining a written medical order, completing discharge instructions, notifying the business office, helping the client leave the agency, writing a summary of the client's condition at discharge, and requesting that the room be cleaned.

Discharge Planning

Discharge planning is a process that improves client outcomes by (1) predetermining his or her postdischarge needs in a timely manner and (2) coordinating the use of appropriate community resources to provide a continuum of care. If effective, discharge planning shortens the hospital stay, decreases the cost of in-hospital care, reduces the necessity for readmission, and eases the transition between the hospital and the next level of care.

Activities involved in discharge planning, which are incorporated within the plan of care, ideally begin at admission or shortly thereafter (Fig. 11-3). Although the discharge planner may be a nurse consultant or social worker, the planning often involves a multidisciplinary team of personnel from a skilled intermediate or basic care nursing facility, home health agency, and hospice provider; a physical, occupational, or speech therapist; a medical equipment supplier; and others.

Gerontologic Considerations

■ Early discharge planning and the appropriate use of community resources may return many older adults to their own homes. Discharge planning for older adults should consider the needs of caregivers, which may include family, friends, or paid helpers. Delaying discharge planning or teaching until immediately before the discharge may not meet the educational needs of older clients and family members, which can result in readmissions.

■ Resources available to discharged older adults include senior centers, adult day care centers, churches, and care management services. In addition, support and education may come from advocacy groups such as the Alzheimer's Association, Area Councils on Aging, Parkinson's support groups, and the American Cancer Society.

■ Barriers to the use of community-based services by older adults include the following:

- Lack of financial assets to pay for services
- Reluctance to spend assets for services
- Unwillingness to acknowledge or accept the need for services
- Mistrust of service providers
- Lack of time, energy, or problem-solving ability to select appropriate services

Discharge planning usually is simple and routine. Clients with one or more of the following characteristics may have special considerations related to discharge planning:

- Age older than 75 years
- Multiple, chronic, or terminal health problems
- Cognitive impairment, motivational problems, or confusion
- Inability to perform self-care
- Impaired mobility
- Safety risks associated with independent living or that pose a burden to potential caregivers
- A treatment regimen involving multiple medications, dietary management, or complicated medical equipment
- History of multiple treatments in the emergency department

Discharge Care Plan

Date & Sign.	Plan and Outcome *(check those that apply)*	Target Date:	Nursing Interventions *(check those that apply)*	Date Achieved:
	☐ The client/family's discharge planning will begin on day of admission including preparation for education and/or equipment. ☐ On the day of discharge, the client/family will receive verbal and written instructions concerning: - Medications - Diet - Activity - Treatment - Follow-up appointments - Signs and symptoms to observe for (when to contact the doctor) - Care of incisions, wounds, etc. ☐ Other:		☐ Assess needs of client/family beginning on the day of admission and continue assessment during hospitalization. ☐ Anticipated needs/services: - Respiratory equipment - Hospital bed - Wheelchair - Walker - Home health nurse - Home PT/OT/ST ☐ Involve client/family in the discharge process. ☐ Discuss with physician the discharge plan and obtain orders if needed. ☐ Contact appropriate personnel with orders. ☐ Provide written and verbal instructions at the client/family's level of understanding. ☐ Verbally explain instructions to client/family prior to discharge and provide client/family with a written copy. ☐ Ascertain that client has follow-up care arranged at discharge. ☐ Provide verbal and written information on what signs and symptoms to observe and when to contact the physician. ☐ Assess if any community resources should be used (i.e., Home Health Nurse), and contact appropriate personnel. ☐ Document all discharge teaching on Discharge Instruction Sheet and Nursing notes. ☐ Other: ____________	

Client/Significant other signature ____________

RN signature ____________

FIGURE 11-3 A discharge care plan. (Used with permission of RN Central. Available at: http://www.rncentral.com/careplans/plans/dc. Accessed January 21, 2010.)

Obtaining Authorization for Medical Discharge

The physician determines when the client is well enough for discharge. Generally, he or she waits to write the medical order until after examining the client. Before leaving the nursing unit, the physician writes the discharge order, provides written prescriptions for the client, and indicates when and where a follow-up appointment should occur.

Leaving against medical advice (AMA) is a term that applies to situations in which the client leaves before the physician authorizes the discharge. Many times, it happens because the client is unhappy with an aspect of care. In some cases, the nurse may negotiate a compromise or persuade the client to delay such action. In the meantime, the nurse informs the physician and nursing supervisor of the client's wish to leave.

If the client is determined to leave, the nurse asks him or her to sign a special form (see Chap. 3). This signed form may release the physician and agency from future responsibility for any complications. If the client refuses to sign, personnel cannot prevent him or her from leaving. They note in the client's medical record, however, that they presented the form and that the client subsequently refused it.

Providing Discharge Instructions

When the nurse anticipates that a client will be discharged home, he or she establishes the anticipated knowledge, skills, and community resources that the client will need to maintain a safe level of self-care. One discharge planning technique uses the acronym METHOD (Table 11-2). The nurse provides the

TABLE 11-2 The METHOD Discharge Planning Guide

TOPIC	NURSING ACTIVITY	EXAMPLE
M—Medications	Instruct the client about drugs that will be self-administered	Insulin
E—Environment	Explore how the home environment can be modified to ensure the client's safety	Remove scatter rugs
T—Treatments	Demonstrate how to perform skills involved in self-care and provide opportunities for returning the demonstration	Dressing changes
H—Health teaching	Identify information that is necessary for maintaining or improving health	Signs and symptoms of complications
O—Outpatient referral	Explain what community services are available that may ease the client's transition to independent living	Physical therapy
D—Diet	Arrange for the dietitian to provide verbal and written instructions on modifying or restricting certain foods or suggestions for altering their methods of preparation	Low-fat diet

teaching identified in the discharge plan periodically during the client's stay and documents it in the record (see Chap. 8).

Before the client leaves, the nurse reviews teaching that has been provided, gives the client prescriptions to have filled, and advises the client to make an office appointment for the date specified by the physician. He or she provides a written summary of discharge instructions. The client signs and keeps the original; the nurse attaches a copy to the client's medical record.

Notifying the Business Office

Before the client leaves the agency, the nurse notifies the business office. At that time, clerical personnel verify that all insurance information is complete and that the client has signed a consent form authorizing the release of medical information to the insurance carrier. If records are incomplete or the client has no health insurance, the client may be asked to make arrangements for future financial payments before discharge.

Discharging a Client

When all the preliminary business is complete, the nurse helps the client gather his or her belongings, plan for transportation, and actually leave the agency.

Gathering Belongings

If necessary, the nurse helps the client to repack personal items. The nurse uses the inventory of valuables to ensure that nothing has been lost or forgotten. Because most hospitals dispose of the plastic supplies (eg, basin, bedpan, urinal), the nurse can offer them to the client; otherwise, he or she discards them in the soiled utility room. A wheeled cart is helpful to transport the client's belongings.

Arranging Transportation

The nurse informs clients about the agency's "check-out time"—the time before which they can avoid being charged for another full day. In most cases, the client contacts a family member or friend for assistance with transportation. If no transportation is available, the client may use public transportation, a taxicab, or an ambulance to get home. Van transportation may be available for older adults through the local Commission on Aging, but 24-hour advance notification is usually required.

Escorting the Client

When the client is ready, the nurse takes him or her to the door in a wheelchair or allows the client to walk there with assistance. The client may choose to have discharge prescriptions filled at the hospital's pharmacy before leaving. Generally, the nurse remains with the client until he or she is safely inside a vehicle or waiting in the lobby for a ride. Skill 11-2 provides a step-by-step description of the discharge process.

Stop, Think, and Respond Box 11-3

What information is helpful to obtain to ensure a safe transition from a health agency to self-management before discharge?

Writing a Discharge Summary

After the client has left the health care agency, the nurse documents the discharge activities and client's condition (see Skill 11-2).

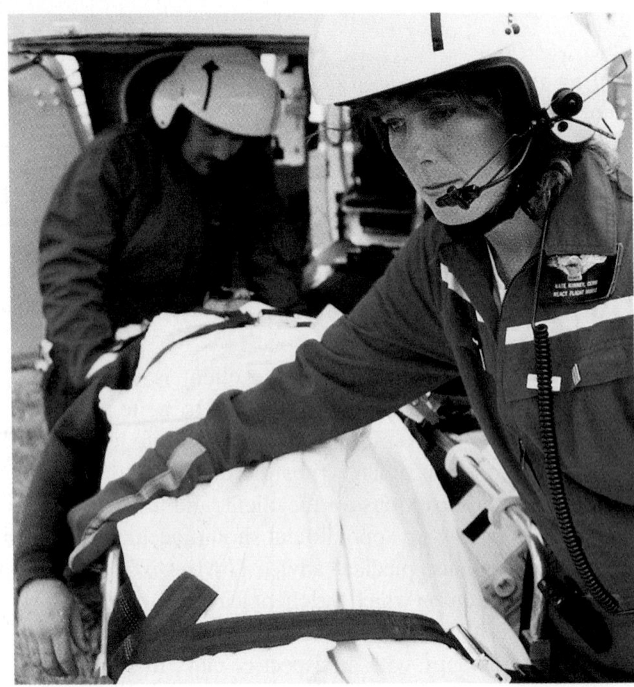

FIGURE 11-4 Transferring a client rapidly may be a life-saving measure.

Terminal Cleaning

Except in unusual circumstances, housekeeping personnel prepare the client's room for the next admission. They strip the bed of linen and clean it with disinfectant, and they restock the bedside cabinet with basic equipment. They then notify the admitting department that the unit is ready. These measures prevent assigning a client to a room that still requires cleaning.

THE TRANSFER PROCESS

A **transfer** (discharging a client from one unit or agency and admitting him or her to another without going home in the interim) may occur when a client's condition improves or worsens. Generally, a transfer has some advantage for the client. It may facilitate more specialized care in a life-threatening situation (Fig. 11-4), or it may reduce health care costs. Many hospitals are creating **stepdown units, progressive care units,** or **transitional care units.** These units are for clients who were once in a critical or unstable condition but have recovered sufficiently to require less intensive nursing care.

Transfer Activities

Transferring a client to a different nursing unit is less complex than to another agency. In a transfer within the same agency, the nurse does the following:

- Informs the client and family about the transfer
- Completes a **transfer summary** (a written review of the client's current status) briefly describing the client's current condition and reason for transfer (Fig. 11-5)

PATIENT TRANSFER FORM
(INTER-AGENCY REFERRAL)

1. PATIENT'S LAST NAME: Carver | FIRST NAME: Anna | MIDDLE: B | 2. SEX: ☐ M ☒ F | 3. HEALTH INSURANCE CLAIM NUMBER: 66585-83-2G

4. PATIENT'S ADDRESS (Street number, City, State, Zip Code): 358 W. York Three Rivers, MI 49093 | 5. DATE OF BIRTH: 9/03/17 | RELIGION: Protestant

7. DATE OF THIS TRANSFER: 12/5/07 | 8. FACILITY NAME AND ADDRESS TRANSFERRING TO: Twin Oaks Nursing Home 215 Riverside, Sturgis, MI

11. Dates of qualifying stay FROM: 11 07 11 | 12-A. FACILITY NAME AND ADDRESS TRANSFERRING FROM: Three Rivers Area Hospital 1111 Broadway, Three Rivers, MI

THRU: 11 18 11 | 12-B. QUALIFYING AND OTHER PRIOR STAY INFORMATION (Including Medical Record Numbers): 11

EMPLOYMENT RELATED: ☐ YES ☒ NO | MEDICAID ELIGIBLE: ☐ YES ☒ NO

13. INSURING ORGANIZATION OR STATE AGENCY NAME AND ADDRESS: Medicare (Blue Cross of Michigan) | 14. POLICY OR MEDICAL ASSISTANCE NO.: 311425609

CLINIC APPOINTMENT DATE: 1/08/12 | TIME: 10 AM | ATTACH CLINIC APPOINTMENT CARD | DATE OF LAST PHYSICAL EXAMINATION: 11/18/11 | WEIGHT: 167

ATTENDING PHYSICIAN INFORMATION

1. NAME AND ADDRESS OF PHYSICIAN AT NEW FACILITY: Chester Sweder MD (Sturgis)

2. FINAL DIAGNOSIS(ES), OR PHOTOCOPY ATTACHED ☐
PRIMARY: Fractured Ⓡ hip
ALL OTHER CONDITIONS: CHF

3. SURGICAL PROCEDURE(S) AND DATE(S) OR, CHECK NONE ☐
Open reduction c̄ Ⓡ hip pin 11/07/11

4. PHYSICIAN ORDERS ON TRANSFER:
Low Na (0.5Gm) Soft diet
Lanoxin 0.25mg daily
Diupres 250 mg B.I.D.

5. ESTIMATED MEDICALLY NECESSARY STAY: 30 DAYS ____ WEEKS OR ____ MONTHS

6. DRUG SENSITIVITIES OR, CHECK NONE ☐
Allergic to Penicillin

7. DIETARY REGIMEN: see above #4

8. PHYSICIAN'S SIGNATURE: Chester Sweder MD | DATE: 11/18/11

NURSING EVALUATION

9. SPEECH	NORMAL ☒	Impaired ☐	Unable To Speak ☐	
10. HEARING	NORMAL ☒	Impaired ☐	Deaf ☐	
11. SIGHT	NORMAL ☐	Impaired ☒	Blind ☐	
12. MENTAL STATUS	ALWAYS ALERT ☒	Occasionally Confused ☐	Always Confused ☐	
13. FEEDING	INDEPENDENT ☒	Help With Feeding ☐	Cannot Feed Self ☐	
14. DRESSING	INDEPENDENT ☐	Help With Dressing ☒	Cannot Dress Self ☐	
15. ELIMINATION	INDEPENDENT ☐	Help To Bathroom ☒	Bedpan or Urinal Required ☐	Incontinent ☐
16. BATHING	INDEPENDENT ☐	Bathing With Help ☒	Bed Bath With Help ☐	Bed Bath ☐
17. AMBULATORY STATUS	INDEPENDENT ☐	Walks With Assistance ☒	Help From Bed To Chair ☐	Bed Bound ☐

18. DRESSINGS AND BANDAGES: OR, CHECK NONE ☒

19. APPLIANCES OR SUPPORTS: OR, CHECK NONE ☐
Uses walker; only partial weight bearing on Ⓡ leg

20. NURSING ASSESSMENT AND RECOMMENDATIONS:
Incision healed
Wears glasses and dentures
Help with shoes
Likes to take pills with apple juice rather than water
Needs reassurance and encouragement with ambulation

SUMMARY ATTACHED ☐ Yes ☒ No

21. SIGNATURE: Laurie Highfield | TITLE: LPN | DATE: 11/18/11

SOCIAL EVALUATION

22. NAME AND ADDRESS OF PERSON TO CONTACT: Thomas Carver, 110 Armitage, Three Rivers, MI | RELATIONSHIP TO PATIENT: Son | TELEPHONE NUMBER: 279-6013

23. PATIENT LIVES: ALONE ☒ WITH FAMILY ☐ WITH SPOUSE ☐ OTHER ☐ EXPLAIN:

24. PATIENT ATTITUDE: Motivated and Cooperative | 25. SUMMARY ATTACHED SOCIAL/EMOTIONAL FACTORS ☐ YES ☒ NO

26. POST STAY PLANS: Family + neighbors will check daily

27. SIGNATURE: Susan Adams | DATE: 11/18/11 | TITLE: Discharge Planner / Coordinator

0880-5 FEB. 75

TRANSFERRING HOSPITAL

FIGURE 11-5 A transfer summary provides information that promotes continuity of care.

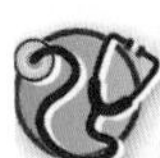

NURSING GUIDELINES 11-1

Transferring a Client

- Be sure to inform the client and the family of the need for a transfer as early as possible. *Communication promotes cooperation.*
- If time permits and the client and family have some choice, encourage them to investigate various facilities and collaborate on the one they prefer. *The people most affected should make the decisions.*
- Communicate with the agency or unit where the client will be transferred. *Other personnel need time to prepare for the client's arrival.*
- Make a photocopy of the medical record. *A copy aids in continuity of care and avoids duplicating services.*
- Provide a written **clinical résumé**, which is a summary of previous care (see Fig. 11-5). It should include (1) the reason for the hospitalization, (2) significant findings, (3) the treatment rendered, (4) the current condition of the client, and (5) instructions, if any, to the client and family (JCAHO, 1998). Check that the client has been notified and given consent for the release of his or her personal health information. *To comply with privacy rules and data security standards set by HIPAA in 1996 and further modified in 2001 and 2002 (see Chap. 9), the client must be informed and approve the release of health information among third parties for routine use in treatment.*
- Place the written information in a large manila envelope or send it via facsimile (fax) machine with a cover sheet. Call the transfer agency to inform them to momentarily expect the fax. *Under the revisions to the HIPAA privacy rules (2002), agencies must systematically protect the client's personal health information within and outside of the institution.*
- Collect all the client's belongings. *Carelessness can lead to the loss of the client's clothing or valuables and can cause inconvenience in returning them.*
- Accompany emergency medical staff or paramedics to the client's room. *Seeing a familiar face may reduce the client's anxiety.*
- Help transfer the client onto the stretcher. *Assistance reduces the physical demands on the client.*
- Give the transfer personnel a copy of the medical record in a folder or envelope. *Enclosing the record protects confidentiality and prevents loss.*
- Complete the original medical record by adding a summary of the client's discharge. *Each medical record includes a discharge summary.*
- Send the completed chart within a file folder to the medical records department. *All charts are filed for future reference.*
- Notify the business office, admitting office, and housekeeping department of the client's transfer. *Each department has its own responsibilities when a client leaves.*

- Speaks with a nurse on the transfer unit to coordinate the transfer (the change of shift report in Chap. 9 can be used as a model)
- Transports the client and his or her belongings, medications, nursing supplies, and chart to the other unit

When transferring the client to a nursing home or other facility, the nurse conducts the process similarly to a discharge: the client is discharged from the hospital and admitted to the transfer facility. See Nursing Guidelines 11-1.

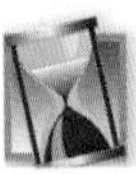

Gerontologic Considerations

■ When admitting, discharging, or transferring older adults, nurses should allow additional time because of possible functional impairments.

Extended Care Facilities

Older adults, in particular, may be transferred directly from an acute care hospital to a facility that provides extended care (Fig. 11-6). An **extended care facility** (a health care agency that provides long-term care) is designed for people who do not meet the criteria for hospitalization. Although group homes for assisted living, adult day care centers, senior residential communities, home health care agencies, and hospice organizations (see Chap. 38) all fit this description, extended care is generally associated with nursing homes.

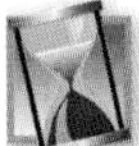

Gerontologic Considerations

■ Approximately 5% of US adults 65 years or older reside in long-term care facilities. The range of housing options for older adults is increasing (Table 11-3).

Nursing homes are classified as skilled nursing facilities or those that provide intermediate or basic care.

Skilled Nursing Facilities

A nursing home licensed as a **skilled nursing facility** provides 24-hour nursing care under the direction of a registered nurse. The facility is reimbursed for the care of clients who require specific technical nursing skills. To qualify for skilled care, the client must be referred by a physician and must require daily skilled nursing care. The following are examples of common procedures that qualify:

- Care for a pressure ulcer
- Enteral feedings or intravenous fluids
- Bowel or bladder retraining
- Injectable medications
- Sterile dressing changes
- Tracheostomy care

Skilled care is provided from a multidisciplinary perspective. In addition to a 24-hour team of nurses, a skilled nursing facility must provide rehabilitation services such as

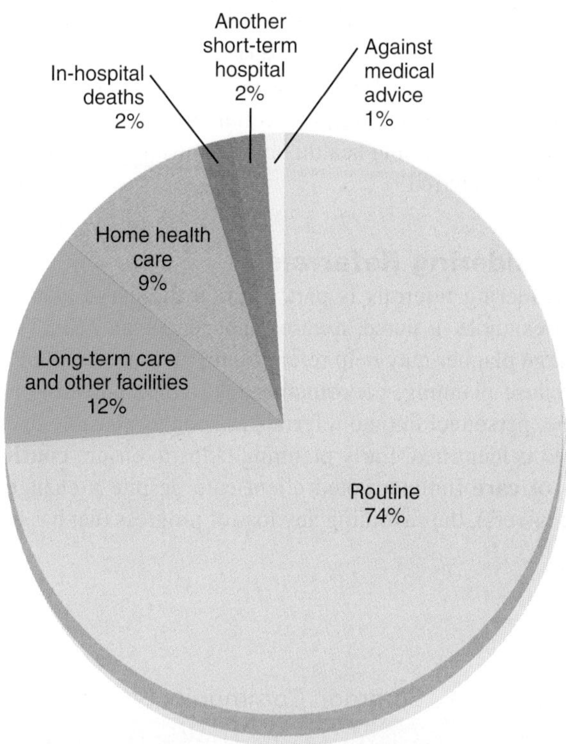

FIGURE 11-6 More than 21% of all clients admitted to hospitals require additional health care services after discharge. (From Agency for Healthcare Research and Quality. [2009]. *HCUP Facts and Figures: Statistics on Hospital-based Care in the United States, 2007.* Available at: http://www.hcup-us.ahrq.gov/reports/factsandfigures/2007/hcup_partnersV2.jsp. Accessed November 20, 2011.)

TABLE 11-3 Housing Options for Older Adults

TYPE	DESCRIPTION
Shared housing	The older person shares a house or apartment and living expenses with one or more unrelated people.
Foster care or board-and-care home	The older person lives in a residence where an unrelated person provides a room, meals, housekeeping, and supervision or assistance with activities of daily living
Congregate housing	Older adults occupy individual apartments and receive supportive services within a multiunit dwelling
Retirement community	Self-sufficient older people live in owned or rented units within a residential development exclusively for retired people
Life care or continuing care community	Older adults live in a residential complex that provides services and accommodations as each resident's needs change
Assisted living facility	Older adults live in their own small apartments and share common areas for meals and social activities. These facilities provide some support and 24-hour emergency services

(Adapted from Miller, C. A. [2008]. *Nursing for wellness in older adults* [5th ed.]. Philadelphia: Lippincott Williams & Wilkins.)

physical therapy and occupational therapy, pharmaceutical services, dietary services, diversional and therapeutic activities, and routine and emergency dental services. Many of the latter services are provided by qualified people on a contractual basis rather than through full-time employment.

To qualify for Medicare benefits in a nursing home, a person must have been hospitalized for three or more days within 30 days before needing skilled nursing care. Clients who meet the criteria are eligible for 100 days of assistance with the costs. There is no charge for the first 20 days; for the next 80 days, Medicare pays most, but not all of the expenses.

Some older adults have private insurance policies that assist with Medicare co-payments. If not, or if clients continue to require skilled care beyond 100 days, they must bear the cost personally until they are considered indigent. After clients have exhausted their own financial resources and those of their spouse, they may apply to the state for Medicaid or its equivalent.

Intermediate Care Facilities

A nursing home also may be licensed as an **intermediate care facility**. This type of agency provides health-related care and services to people who, because of their mental or physical condition, require institutional care but not 24-hour nursing care. Clients who require intermediate care may need supervision because they tend to wander or are confused. They need assistance with oral medications, bathing, dressing, toileting, and mobility.

Medicare does not provide reimbursement for intermediate care. Clients assume the costs. For impoverished residents, state welfare programs, such as Medicaid, will pay. Some nursing homes do not accept Medicaid clients, however, because states fix the fees for reimbursement at much lower amounts than Medicare and private insurance provide.

Basic Care Facilities

A third type of nursing home is a **basic care facility** (an agency that provides extended custodial care). The emphasis is on providing shelter, food, and laundry services in a group setting. These clients assume much responsibility for their own activities of daily living such as hygiene and dressing, preparing for sleep, and joining others for meals. Intermediate and basic care may be provided at a skilled nursing facility but usually in separate wings.

Determining the Level of Care

The level of care is determined at or prior to admission. Each client is assessed using a standard form developed by the Health Care Financing Association called a *Minimum Data Set for*

Nursing Home Resident Assessment and Care Screening. By federal law, the MDS is repeated every 3 months or whenever a client's condition changes. The MDS requires an assessment of the following:

- Cognitive patterns
- Communication and hearing patterns
- Vision patterns
- Physical functioning and structural problems
- Continence patterns in the last 14 days
- Psychosocial well-being
- Mood and behavior patterns
- Activity pursuit patterns
- Disease diagnoses
- Health conditions
- Oral and nutritional status
- Oral and dental status
- Skin condition
- Medication use
- Special treatments and procedures

Problems identified on the MDS are then reflected in the nursing care plan.

Selecting a Nursing Home

When the need arises, family members are often ill-prepared for selecting a nursing home. A discharge planner can assist with arranging nursing home care. Brochures on selection are available from the American Association of Retired Persons, the Commission on Aging, and each state's public health and welfare departments. Web sites also provide valuable information. See Client and Family Teaching 11-1.

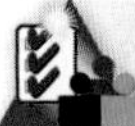

Client and Family Teaching 11-1
Selecting a Nursing Home

The nurse teaches the client or family to do the following:

- Find out the levels of care (skilled, intermediate, or basic) that the nursing home is licensed to provide.
- Review inspection reports on each home. This information is available from the state's public health department on a fee-per-page basis.
- Ask others in the community, including the family physician, for recommendations.
- Visit nursing homes with, and again without, an appointment. Go at least once during a meal.
- Note the appearance of residents and how staff members respond to their needs.
- Observe the cleanliness of the surroundings and any unpleasant odors.
- Request brochures that identify medical care, nursing services, rehabilitation therapy, social services, activities programs, religious observances, and residents' rights and privileges.
- Clarify charges and billing procedures.
- Analyze if the overall impression of the home is positive or negative.

THE REFERRAL PROCESS

A **referral** is the process of sending someone to another person or agency for special services. Referrals generally are made to private practitioners or community agencies. Table 11-4 lists some common community services to which people with declining health, physical disabilities, or special needs are referred.

Considering Referrals

Considering referrals is part of good discharge planning. For example, a nurse, a case manager, or an agency discharge planner may help refer clients for home health care. Because planning, coordinating, and communicating take time, personnel initiate referrals as soon as possible once a need is identified. Early planning helps to ensure **continuity of care** (uninterrupted client care despite a change in caregivers), thus avoiding any loss of progress that has been made.

TABLE 11-4 Common Community Services

ORGANIZATION	SERVICE
Commission on Aging	Assists older adults with transportation to medical appointments, outpatient therapy, and community meal sites
Hospice	Supports the family and terminally ill clients who choose to stay at home
Visiting Nurses' Association	Offers intermittent nursing care to homebound clients
Meals on Wheels	Provides one or two hot meals per day delivered either at home or at a community meal site
Homemaker Services	Sends adults to the home to assist in shopping, meal preparation, and light housekeeping
Home health aides	Assist with bathing, hygiene, and medications
Adult protective services	Investigates and pursues accountability of individuals who are physically, socially, emotionally, or financially victimizing vulnerable adults
Respite care	Provides short-term, temporary relief to full-time caregivers of homebound clients
Older Americans' Ombudsman	Investigates and resolves complaints made by or on behalf of nursing home residents; at least one full-time ombudsman is mandated for each state

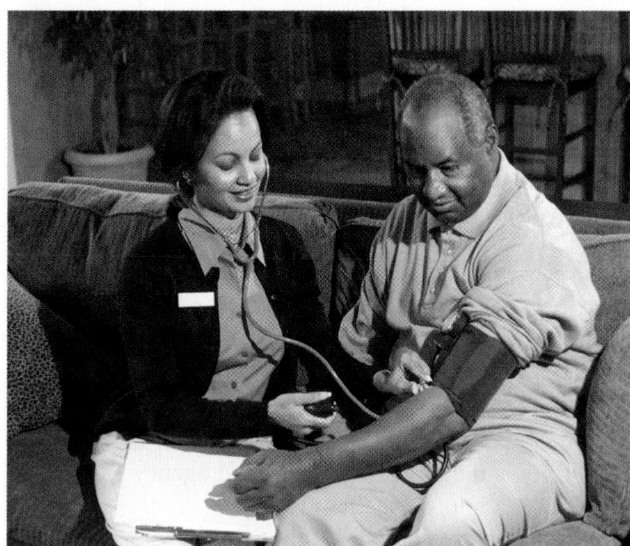

FIGURE 11-7 A home health care assessment.

Home Health Care

Home health care is health care provided in the home by an employee of a home health agency (Fig. 11-7). Public agencies (regional, state, or federal, such as the public health department) or private agencies may provide home health care.

The number of clients who receive home health care continues to rise, partly as an outcome of limitations imposed by Medicare and insurance companies on the number of hospital and nursing home days for which they reimburse care. Another factor is the growing number of chronically ill older adults in the population in need of assistance.

According to the Administration on Aging (2008), 52% of older Americans reported having some type of disability. Almost 35% of those over the age of 80 with disabilities need assistance (American Association of Retired Persons, 2005) (Fig. 11-8). Types of assistance older adults may need include basic activities of daily living (bathing, dressing, eating, and getting around the house), preparing meals, shopping, housework, managing money, using the phone, and taking medications.

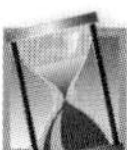

Gerontologic Considerations

- Medicare requires that a client meet all the following eligibility criteria for coverage of home care services:
1. A physician has signed or will sign a care plan.
2. The person is homebound. Homebound status is met if leaving home requires a considerable and taxing effort, such as needing personal assistance or the help of a wheelchair, crutches, etc. Occasional but infrequent "walks around the block" are allowable. Attendance at an adult day care center or religious services is *not* an automatic bar to meeting the homebound requirement.
3. The person needs skilled nursing care or physical or speech therapy intermittently. Intermittency may vary from every day to once every 60 days.
4. The care must be provided by, or under arrangements with, a Medicare-certified provider.
- Some older adults have difficulty accepting help from others even though they recognize the need for it. They may resist changes related to how they accomplish familiar tasks. Nurses should consider methods to facilitate required changes and minimize any unnecessary alterations when planning a transition to an institutional setting.

Home care nursing services help shorten the time spent recovering in the hospital, prevent admissions to extended care facilities, and reduce readmissions to acute care facilities. Box 11-3 identifies the responsibilities assumed by home health nurses who provide community-based care.

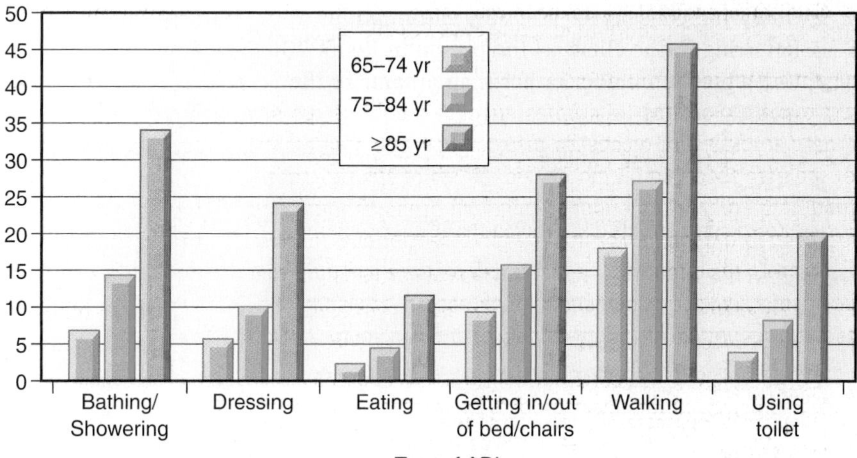

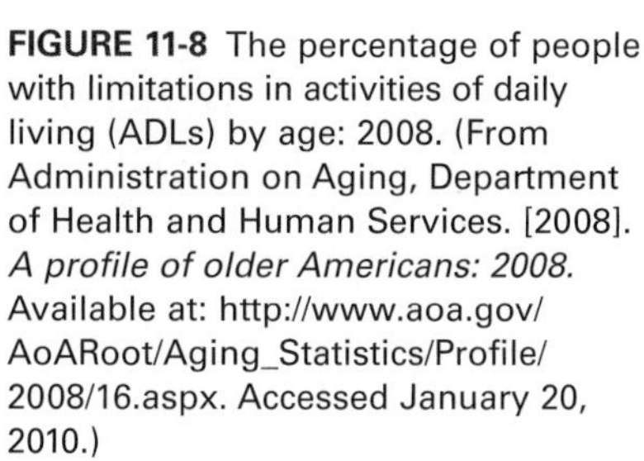

FIGURE 11-8 The percentage of people with limitations in activities of daily living (ADLs) by age: 2008. (From Administration on Aging, Department of Health and Human Services. [2008]. *A profile of older Americans: 2008.* Available at: http://www.aoa.gov/AoARoot/Aging_Statistics/Profile/2008/16.aspx. Accessed January 20, 2010.)

BOX 11-3 Responsibilities of Home Health Nurses

- Assess the readiness of the client and the home environment
- Treat each client with respect regardless of the person's standard of living
- Identify health or social problems that require nursing, allied health, or supportive care services
- Plan, coordinate, and monitor home care
- Give skilled care to clients requiring part-time nursing services
- Teach and supervise the client in self-care activities and family members who participate in the client's home care
- Assess the safety of health practices that are being used
- Observe, evaluate, and modify environmental and social factors that affect the client's progress
- Evaluate the urgency and complexity of each client's changing health needs
- Keep accurate written records and submit documentation to the agency for the purpose of reimbursement
- Arrange for referrals to other health care agencies
- Discharge clients who have reached a level of self-reliance

CRITICAL THINKING EXERCISES

1. Discuss how the admission of a child might differ from that of an adult.

2. Compare and contrast admission to a hospital and to a nursing home.

3. Describe the criteria you would use when selecting a nursing home for a relative.

4. If it becomes apparent that a relative cannot continue to live independently, what options would you pursue?

NCLEX-STYLE REVIEW QUESTIONS

1. Which of the following is essential for complying with federal regulations that ensure the client's right to privacy?
   1. Addressing clients by their first names only
   2. Obtaining consent for releasing information
   3. Referring to the client as the person in Room 201
   4. Using a code number rather than a name in the medical record

2. Which of the following information is essential for the nurse to obtain at the time of a client's admission to a health care agency?
   1. Social security number
   2. Medicare status
   3. Advance directive
   4. Health insurance policy

3. Which of the following observations is most suggestive that a newly admitted client is anxious?
   1. The client is unusually quiet and withdrawn.
   2. The client is restless and awakens frequently.
   3. The client eats very little food at each meal.
   4. The client misses his or her spouse and children.

4. If there is a suspicion that an older adult in the community is the target of abuse, what agency would be appropriate to contact?
   1. The Commission on Aging
   2. Visiting Nurses Association
   3. Older Americans' Ombudsman
   4. Adult Protective Services

5. Which type of extended care facility referral would be appropriate for an older adult who needs further rehabilitation for mobility at the time of discharge from an acute care facility?
   1. Skilled care facility
   2. Intermediate care facility
   3. Basic care facility
   4. Assisted living facility

SKILL 11-1 Admitting a Client

Suggested Action	Reason for Action
ASSESSMENT	
Obtain the name, admitting diagnosis, and condition of the client and the room to which he or she has been assigned.	Provides preliminary data from which to plan the activities that may be involved in admitting the client.
Check the appearance of the room and the presence of basic supplies.	Demonstrates concern for cleanliness, order, and client convenience.
PLANNING	
Assemble the needed equipment: admission assessment form, thermometer, blood pressure cuff (if not wall mounted), stethoscope, scale, urine specimen container.	Enhances organization and efficient time management.
Obtain special equipment, such as an intravenous pole or oxygen, that may be needed according to the client's needs.	Facilitates immediate care of the client without causing unnecessary delay or discomfort.
Arrange the height of the bed to coordinate with the expected mode of arrival.	Reduces the physical effort in moving from a wheelchair or stretcher to the bed.
Fold the top linen to the bottom of the bed if the client will be immediately confined to bed.	Reduces obstacles that may interfere with the client's comfort and ease of transfer.
IMPLEMENTATION	
Greet the client by name and demonstrate a friendly smile; extend a hand as a symbol of welcome.	Promotes feelings of friendliness and personal regard to help reduce initial anxiety.
Introduce yourself to the client and those who have accompanied the client.	Establishes the nurse–client relationship on a personal basis.
Observe the client for signs of acute distress.	Determines if the admission process requires modification.
Attend to urgent needs for comfort and breathing.	Demonstrates concern for the client's well-being.
Introduce the client to his or her roommate, if there is one, and anyone else who enters the room.	Promotes a sense of familiarity to relieve social awkwardness; demonstrates concern for the client's emotional comfort.
Offer the client a chair unless the client requires immediate bed rest.	Demonstrates concern for the client's physical comfort.
Check the client's identification bracelet.	Enhances safety by accurately identifying the client.
Orient the client to the physical environment of the room and the nursing unit.	Aids in adapting the client to unfamiliar surroundings.
Demonstrate how to use the equipment in the room such as the adjustments for the bed, how to signal for a nurse, and use of the telephone and television.	Promotes comfort and self-reliance; ensures safety.
Explain the general routines and schedules that are followed for visiting hours, meals, and care.	Reduces uncertainty about when to expect activities.
Explain the need to examine the client and ask personal health questions.	Prepares the client for what will follow next.
Ask if the client would like family members to leave or remain.	Promotes a sense of control over decisions and outcomes.
Make provisions for privacy.	Demonstrates respect for the client's dignity.
Request that the client undress and don a hospital or examination gown; assist as necessary.	Facilitates physical assessment.
Ask the client about the need to urinate at the present time, and obtain a urine specimen if ordered.	Shows concern for the client's immediate comfort; facilitates physical assessment of the abdomen.
Weigh the client before helping him or her into bed.	Avoids disturbing the client once settled in bed.
Assist the client to a comfortable position in bed.	Shows concern for the client's comfort; facilitates the examination.
Take care of the client's clothing and valuables according to agency policy.	Provides safeguards for the client's possessions.
Ask the client to identify allergies to food, drugs, or other substances and to describe the type of symptoms that accompany a typical allergic reaction.	Aids in preventing the potential for an allergic reaction during care; prepares staff for the manner in which the client reacts to the allergen.
Apply a second bracelet that is color-coded to the client's arm that identifies the client's allergies.	Calls staff's attention to the fact that the client has allergies.
Wash hands or perform hand antisepsis with an alcohol rub (see Chap. 10).	Reduces the direct transmission of microorganisms from the nurse's hands to the client.
Obtain the client's temperature, pulse, respiratory rate, and blood pressure.	Contributes to the initial database assessment.
Place the signal cord where it can be conveniently reached.	Reduces the potential for accidents by ensuring that the client can make his or her needs known.

(continued)

Admitting a Client (continued)

Suggested Action	Reason for Action
IMPLEMENTATION (CONTINUED)	
Make sure the bed is in low position, and follow agency policy about raising the side rails on the bed.	Promotes safety. Side rails are considered a form of physical restraint in a nursing home; their use may require written permission from the client.
Remove the urine specimen if obtained at this time, attach a laboratory request form, and place it in the refrigerator or take it to the laboratory.	Ensures proper identification of the specimen, specifies the test to be performed, and prevents changes that may affect test results.
Wash hands or perform hand antisepsis with an alcohol rub (see Chap. 10).	Removes microorganisms acquired from contact with the client or the urine specimen.
Report the progress of the client's admission to the registered nurse, who may perform the nursing interview and physical assessment or delegate components at this time.	Complies with The Joint Commission standards; the entire admission assessment must be completed within 24 hours; parts of the assessment may be performed at periodic intervals until it is completed.
Inform family or friends that they may resume visiting when the nursing activities are completed.	Facilitates the client's network of support.

Evaluation

- Client is comfortable and oriented to the room and to routines.
- Safety measures are implemented.
- Database assessments are initiated.
- Status and progress are communicated to nursing team.

Document

- Date and time of admission
- Age and gender of client
- Overall appearance
- Mode of arrival to unit
- Room number
- Initial vital signs and weight
- List of allergies, if any; quote the client's description of a typical reaction or indicate if the client has no allergies by using the abbreviation NKA (no known allergies) or whatever abbreviation is acceptable
- Disposition of urine specimen
- Present condition of client

SAMPLE DOCUMENTATION

Date and Time Sixty-eight-year-old female admitted to Room 258 by wheelchair from admitting dept. with moderate dyspnea. O_2 running at 2 L per nasal cannula. Weighs 173 lb on bed scale wearing only a hospital gown. T 98.4°, P 92, R 32, BP 146/68 in R arm while sitting up. Cannot void at present. Allergic to penicillin, which causes "hives and difficulty breathing." In high Fowler's position at this time with a respiratory rate of 24 at rest.

____________________ SIGNATURE/TITLE

SKILL 11-2 Discharging a Client

Suggested Action	Reason for Action
ASSESSMENT	
Determine that a medical order has been written.	Provides authorization for discharging the client.
Check for written prescriptions and other medical discharge instructions.	Enables the client to continue self-care.
Note if any new medical orders must be carried out before the client's discharge.	Ensures that the client will leave in the best possible condition.
Review the nursing discharge plan.	Determines if the client needs more health teaching or if instructions have been completed.

(continued)

Discharging a Client (continued)

PLANNING*

Action	Rationale
Discuss the client's time frame for leaving the hospital.	Helps coordinate nursing activities within the client's schedule.
Coordinate the discharge with the home health care agency, hospice organization, or company supplying oxygen or other medical equipment.	Facilitates continuity of care.
Determine the client's mode of transportation.	Clarifies if the client needs the services of a cab company or other resource.
*Notify the business office of the client's impending discharge.	Allows time for the clerical department to review the client's billing information and determine the necessity for further actions.
*Inform the housekeeping department that the client will be leaving.	Alerts cleaning staff that the unit will need terminal cleaning.
*Cancel any meals that the client will miss after discharge.	Avoids wasting food.
*Notify the pharmacy of the approximate time of discharge.	Eliminates wasted drugs.
Plan to provide hygiene and medical treatments early.	Prevents delays in the client's departure.

IMPLEMENTATION

Action	Rationale
Wash hands or perform hand antisepsis with an alcohol rub (see Chap. 10).	Reduces transmission of microorganisms.
Provide for hygiene but omit changing the bed linen.	Eliminates unnecessary work.
Complete medical treatment and nursing interventions according to the plan for care.	Promotes continuation of nursing care.
Help the client dress in street clothing or clothing appropriate for leaving the agency.	Demonstrates concern for the client's appearance and appropriateness for the weather.
Review discharge instructions and complete health teaching.	Promotes safe self-care.
Have the client sign the discharge instruction sheet, paraphrase the information it contains, and provide the client with the original form containing the discharge instructions and prescriptions that should be filled.	Validates that the client has understood instructions for maintaining health and can refer to the information at a future time.
Assist the client with packing personal items; if appropriate, have the client sign the clothing inventory or valuables list.	Reduces claims that personal items were lost or stolen; signing a clothing inventory or valuables list is more likely to apply when a client is discharged from a nursing home or rehabilitation center.
Obtain a cart for the client's belongings.	Eases the work of transporting multiple or heavy items.
Assist the client into a wheelchair when transportation is available.	Reduces the potential for a fall if the client is weak or unsteady.
Stop, if necessary, at the business office.	Complies with billing procedures.
Escort the client to the waiting vehicle.	Promotes safety while still in the hospital.
Return any forms from the business office.	Confirms that the client has left the hospital.
Replace the wheelchair in its proper location on the nursing unit.	Makes equipment available for others to use.
Wash hands or perform hand antisepsis with an alcohol rub (see Chap. 10).	Reduces the transmission of microorganisms.
Complete a discharge summary in the medical record.	Closes the medical record for this admission.

Evaluation

- Health condition is stable (if being transferred in unstable condition, is accompanied by qualified personnel who have the knowledge and skills to intervene in emergencies).
- Client can paraphrase discharge instructions accurately.
- Business office indicates that billing records are in order.
- Client experiences no injuries during transport from room to vehicle.

Document

- Date and time of discharge
- Condition at the time of discharge
- Include a copy of discharge instructions
- Mode of transportation
- Identity of person(s) who accompanied the client

(continued)

Discharging a Client (continued)

SAMPLE DOCUMENTATION

Date and Time No fever or wound tenderness at this time. Sutures removed. Abdominal incision intact. No dressing applied. Given prescription for Keflex. Can repeat how many capsules to self-administer per dose, appropriate times for administration, and possible side effects. Repeated signs and symptoms of infection and the need to report them immediately. Instructed to shower as usual and temporarily avoid lifting objects over 10 lb. Informed to make follow-up appointment in 1 week with physician as indicated on discharge instruction sheet. Given copy of written discharge instructions. Escorted to automobile in wheelchair accompanied by spouse. Assisted into private car without any unusual events. ———————— SIGNATURE/TITLE

*Activities marked with asterisk may be delegated to a clerk.

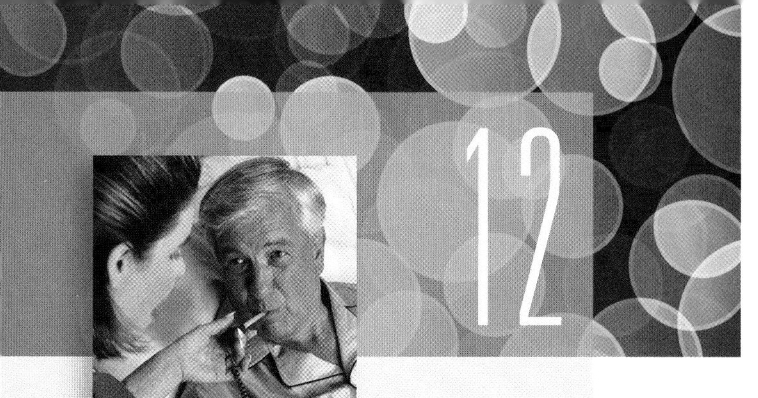

Vital Signs

Words To Know

afebrile
afterload
antipyretics
apical heart rate
apical–radial rate
apnea
arrhythmia
auscultatory gap
automated monitoring devices
blood pressure
bradycardia
bradypnea
cardiac output
centigrade scale
cerumen
clinical thermometers
core temperature
diastolic pressure
Doppler stethoscope
drawdown effect
dyspnea
dysrhythmia
Fahrenheit scale
febrile
fever
frenulum
hypertension
hyperthermia
hyperventilation
hypotension
hypothalamus
hypothermia
hypoventilation
Korotkoff sounds
metabolic rate
offsets
orthopnea
orthostatic hypotension
palpitation
piloerection
postural hypotension
preload
pulse
pulse deficit
pulse pressure
pulse rate
pulse rhythm

Learning Objectives

On completion of this chapter, the reader should be able to:

1. List four physiologic components measured during an assessment of vital signs.
2. Differentiate between shell and core body temperature.
3. Identify the two scales used to measure temperature.
4. List four temperature assessment sites and indicate the sites considered the closest to core temperature.
5. Name four types of clinical thermometers.
6. Discuss the difference between fever and hyperthermia.
7. Name the four phases of a fever.
8. List at least four signs or symptoms that accompany a fever.
9. Give two reasons for using an infrared tympanic thermometer when body temperature is subnormal.
10. List at least four signs and symptoms that accompany subnormal body temperature.
11. Identify three characteristics noted when assessing a client's pulse.
12. Name the most commonly used site for pulse assessment and three other assessment techniques that may be used.
13. Explain the difference between systolic and diastolic blood pressure.
14. Name and explain at least four terms used to describe abnormal breathing characteristics.
15. Discuss the physiologic data that can be inferred from a blood pressure assessment.
16. Name three pieces of equipment for assessing blood pressure.
17. Describe the five phases of Korotkoff sounds.
18. Identify three alternative techniques for assessing blood pressure.

Vital signs (body temperature, pulse rate, respiratory rate, and blood pressure) are four objective assessment data that indicate how well or how poorly the body is functioning. Pain assessment is considered a fifth vital sign. A subjective pain assessment is performed at least daily and whenever vital signs are taken (see Chap. 20).

Vital signs are very sensitive to alterations in physiology; therefore, nurses measure them at regular intervals (Box 12-1) or whenever they determine it is appropriate to assess a client's health status. This chapter describes how to obtain each component of the vital signs and explains what findings indicate based on established norms.

Words To Know (continued)

pulse volume
pyrexia
respiration
respiratory rate
set point
shell temperature
speculum
sphygmomanometer
stertorous breathing
stethoscope
stridor
systolic pressure
tachycardia
tachypnea
temperature translation
thermistor catheter
thermogenesis
training effect
ventilation
vital signs
white-coat hypertension

BODY TEMPERATURE

Body temperature refers to the warmth of the human body. Body heat is produced primarily from exercise and metabolism of food. Heat is lost through the skin, the lungs, and the body's waste products through the processes of radiation, conduction, convection, and evaporation (Table 12-1).

The body's **shell temperature** (warmth at the skin surface) is usually lower than its **core temperature** (warmth in deeper sites within the body like the brain and heart). Core temperature is much more significant than shell temperature because there is a narrow range within which core temperature can fluctuate without resulting in negative outcomes.

BOX 12-1 Recommendations for Measuring Vital Signs

Vital signs are taken:

- On admission, when obtaining database assessments
- According to written medical orders
- Once per day when a client is stable
- At least every 4 hours when one or more vital signs are abnormal
- Every 5 to 15 minutes when a client is unstable or at risk for rapid physiologic changes such as after surgery
- Whenever a client's condition appears to have changed
- A second time, or more frequently, when there is a significant difference from the previous measurement
- When a client is feeling unusual
- Before, during, and after a blood transfusion
- Before administering medications that affect any of the vital signs and after to monitor the drug's effect

Temperature Measurement

Physicists studying *thermokinetics*, or heat in motion, have developed various scales for measuring heat and cold. Some examples include Kelvin (K), Rankine (R), Fahrenheit (F), and centigrade (C) scales, all of which are based on increments at which water freezes and boils. The centigrade temperature scale is also known as Celsius. Health care professionals commonly use the Fahrenheit and centigrade scales.

The **Fahrenheit scale** (a scale that uses 32°F as the temperature at which water freezes and 212°F as the point at which it boils) generally is used in the United States to measure and report body temperature. The **centigrade scale** (a scale that uses 0°C as the temperature at which water freezes and 100°C as the point at which it boils) is used more often in scientific research and in countries that use the metric system. Nurses are required to use both scales occasionally and to convert between the two measurements (Box 12-2).

Normal Body Temperature

In normal, healthy adults, shell temperature generally ranges from 96.6° to 99.3°F or 35.8° to 37.4°C (Porth & Matfin, 2008). Core body temperature, according to Nicholl (2002), ranges from 97.5° to 100.4°F (36.4° to 37.3°C). If a client's temperature is above or below normal, the nurse records and reports the temperature, implements nursing and medical interventions for restoring a normal body temperature when appropriate, and reassesses the client frequently.

TABLE 12-1 Mechanisms of Heat Transfer

	RADIATION	CONVECTION	EVAPORATION	CONDUCTION
Definition	The diffusion or dissemination of heat by electromagnetic waves.	The dissemination of heat by motion between areas of unequal density.	The conversion of a liquid to a vapor.	The transfer of heat to another object during direct contact.
Example	The body gives off waves of heat from uncovered surfaces.	An oscillating fan blows currents of cool air across the surface of a warm body.	Body fluid in the form of perspiration and insensible loss is vaporized from the skin.	The body transfers heat to an ice pack, causing the ice to melt.
Illustration				

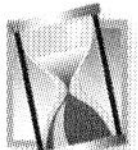

Gerontologic Considerations

■ Older adults tend to have lower "normal" or baseline temperatures; therefore, a temperature in the normal range may actually be elevated for an older adult. An older person's usual temperature should be assessed and documented to enable accurate comparison when assessing for elevations. Nevertheless, with changes in an older adult's thermoregulation system, temperature elevations may not accompany infections.

Temperature Regulation

The temperature of *poikilothermic* animals, such as reptiles, fluctuates widely depending on environmental temperature. Humans, on the other hand, are *homeothermic*; that is, various structural and physiologic adaptations keep their body temperature within a narrow stable range regardless of the environmental temperature.

In humans, the **hypothalamus** (a structure within the brain that helps control various metabolic activities) acts as the center for temperature regulation. The anterior hypothalamus promotes heat loss through vasodilation and sweating. The posterior hypothalamus promotes two functions: *heat conservation* and *heat production*. It produces heat conservation in the following ways:

1. Adjusting where blood circulates
2. Causing **piloerection** (the contraction of arrector pili muscles in skin follicles), which stiffens body hairs and gives the appearance of what commonly is described as "goose flesh"
3. Promoting a shivering response

The hypothalamus promotes heat production by increasing metabolism through secretion of thyroid hormone as well as epinephrine and norepinephrine from the adrenal medulla.

When functioning appropriately, the hypothalamus maintains the core temperature **set point** (an optimal body temperature) within 1°C by responding to slight changes in the skin surface and blood temperatures. Other physiologic responses accompany the temperature-regulating mechanisms of the hypothalamus, as shown in Figure 12-1.

Temperatures above 105.8°F (41°C) and below 93.2°F (34°C) indicate impairment of the hypothalamic regulatory center. According to Porth and Matfin (2008), the chance of survival is diminished when body temperatures exceed 110°F (43.3°C) or fall below 84°F (28.8°C).

BOX 12-2 Temperature Conversion Formulas

To convert Fahrenheit to centigrade, use the formula:

$$°C = \frac{(°F - 32)}{1.8}$$

Example: Step 1: 98.6°F − 32 = 66.6
Step 2: 66.6 ÷ 1.8 = 37°C

To convert centigrade to Fahrenheit, use the formula:

$$°F = (°C \times 1.8) + 32$$

Example: Step 1: 15°C × 1.8 = 27
Step 2: 27 + 32 = 59°F

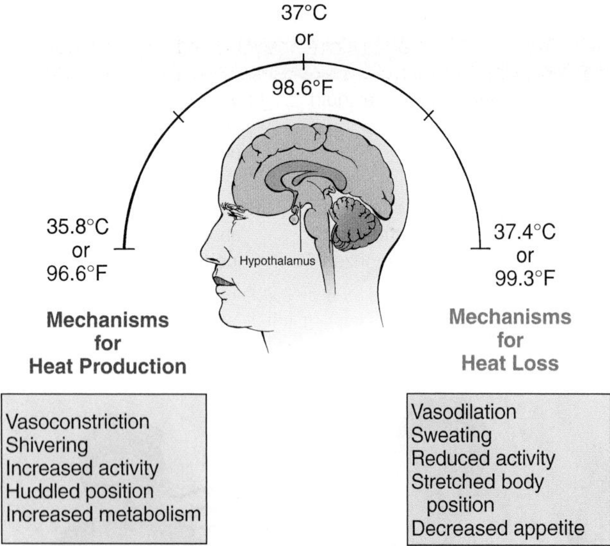

FIGURE 12-1 The hypothalamus regulates body temperature.

Factors Affecting Body Temperature

Various factors affect body temperature. Examples include food intake, age, climate, gender, exercise and activity, circadian rhythm, emotions, illness or injury, and medications.

Food Intake

Food intake, or lack of it, affects **thermogenesis** (heat production). When a person consumes food, the body requires energy to digest, absorb, transport, metabolize, and store nutrients. The process is sometimes described as the *specific dynamic action of food* or the *thermic effect of food* because it produces heat. Protein foods have the greatest thermic effect. Thus, both the amount and the type of food eaten affect body temperature. Dietary restrictions can contribute to decreased body heat as a result of reduced processing of nutrients.

Age

Infants and older adults have difficulty maintaining normal body temperature for several reasons. Both have limited subcutaneous *white adipocytes* (fat cells that provide heat insulation and cushioning of internal structures). The ability of both young and old to shiver and perspire also may be inadequate, putting them at risk for abnormally low or high body temperatures. Another problem for both populations is an inability to independently forestall or reverse heat loss or gain without the assistance of a caretaker.

Newborns and young infants tend to experience temperature fluctuations because they have a three times greater surface area from which heat is lost (Nicholl, 2002) and a **metabolic rate** (use of calories for sustaining body functions) twice that of adults. Older adults are compromised further by progressively impaired circulation, which interferes with losing or retaining heat through the dilation or constriction of blood vessels near the skin.

Climate

Climate affects mechanisms for temperature regulation. Heat and cold produce neurosensory stimulation of thermal receptors in the skin, which transmit information through the autonomic nervous system to the hypothalamus. Cool environmental temperatures result in vasoconstriction of surface blood vessels with subsequent shunting of blood to vital organs. This physiologic phenomenon helps to explain how brain cells are protected temporarily in cold-water drownings.

People who live in predominately cold climates have more *brown adipocytes* (fat cells uniquely adapted for thermogenesis) (Austgen & Bowen, 2009). Thermogenesis from brown fat occurs when norepinephrine triggers lipolysis (the breakdown of fat). Those who live in arctic regions are highly cold adaptive because they have increased brown adipocytes. They tend to have an overall 10% to 20% higher metabolic rate compared with those who live in geographic areas with less severe environmental temperatures (Lichtenbelt et al., 2009; Iatropoulos & Williams, 2004). Conversely, those who live in the tropics have a 10% to 20% lower metabolic rate than those in milder climates.

Gender

Body temperature increases slightly in women of childbearing age during ovulation. This probably results from hormonal changes affecting metabolism or tissue injury and repair after the release of an ovum (egg). The change in body temperature is so slight that most women are unaware of it unless they are monitoring their temperature daily (to plan or avoid pregnancy).

Exercise and Activity

Both exercise and activity involve muscle contraction. As muscle groups and tendons repeatedly stretch and recoil, the friction produces body heat. Shivering is another example of contractile thermogenesis.

Muscles also are the largest mass of metabolically active tissue. This means that muscle activity generates additional heat from chemical reactions during the muscle cells' combustion of nutrients for cellular functions. To provide adequate calories that will give the energy necessary for muscle activity, the body adjusts its metabolic rate through endocrine hormones released from the pituitary, thyroid, and adrenal glands. In contrast, inactivity and reduced metabolism or nutrient intake may lead to a lower body temperature.

Circadian Rhythm

Circadian rhythms are physiologic changes, such as fluctuations in body temperature and other vital signs, over 24-hour cycles. Body temperature fluctuates from 0.5° to 2.0°F (0.28° to 1.1°C) during a 24-hour period. It tends to be lowest from midnight to dawn and highest in the late afternoon to early evening. People who routinely work at night and sleep during the day have temperature fluctuations that cycle in reverse.

Emotions

Emotions affect metabolic rate by triggering hormonal changes through the sympathetic and parasympathetic pathways of the autonomic nervous system (see Chap. 5). People who tend to be consistently anxious and nervous are likely to have slightly increased body temperatures. Conversely, people who are apathetic or depressed are prone to have slightly lower body temperatures.

Illness or Injury

Diseases, disorders, or injuries that affect the function of the hypothalamus or mechanisms for heat production and loss alter body temperature, sometimes dramatically. Some examples include tissue injury, infections and inflammatory disorders, fluid loss, injury to the skin, impaired circulation, and head injury.

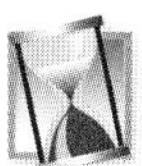

Gerontologic Considerations

- Some older adults have a delayed and diminished febrile response to illnesses. A careful assessment is essential to identify temperature elevations or disease symptoms other than increased temperature. Often, a change in cognitive function, restlessness, or anxiety are initial signs of illness.

Medications

Various medications affect body temperature by increasing or decreasing metabolic rate and energy requirements. Drugs, such as aspirin, acetaminophen, and ibuprofen, directly lower body temperature by acting on the hypothalamus itself. In the absence of fever, however, their use will not lower body temperature to subnormal levels. Stimulant drugs, like those containing dextroamphetamine (Dexedrine) or ephedrine, increase metabolic rate and body temperature.

Stop, Think, and Respond Box 12-1

Explain how infants and older adults are particularly vulnerable to alterations in temperature regulation.

Assessment Sites

Body temperature can be assessed at various locations, some of which are more practical than others. The most accurate locations for measuring core body temperature are the brain, heart, lower third of the esophagus, and the urinary bladder. Measuring the temperature in the brain is currently prohibitive because of a lack of technology. The temperature of blood circulating through the heart, esophagus, or bladder is measured using a **thermistor catheter** (heat-sensing device at the tip of an internally placed tube). The required skill for insertion and risks associated with the use of thermistor catheters, however, restricts their use to clients with highly acute illnesses.

The most practical and convenient temperature assessment sites are the ear (tympanic membrane and temporal artery on the forehead and behind the ear lobe), mouth, rectum, and axilla. These areas are anatomically close to superficial arteries containing warm blood, enclosed areas where heat loss is minimal, or both. Of the four sites, the ear is the peripheral site that most closely reflects core body temperature.

TABLE 12-2 Equivalent Thermometer Measurements According to Site

ASSESSMENT SITE	FAHRENHEIT	CENTIGRADE
Oral	98.6°	37.0°
Rectal equivalent	99.5°	37.5°
Axillary equivalent	97.5°	36.4°
Tympanic membrane	99.5°	37.5°
Temporal artery	99.4°	37.4°

Rectal and arterial temperatures are generally 1°F (0.5°C) higher than oral temperatures and 2°F (1°C) higher than axillary temperatures; axillary temperature is lower than any measured site. Report the temperature and site used.

Temperature measurements vary slightly depending on the assessment site (Table 12-2). To evaluate trends in body temperature, the nurse documents the assessment site as O for oral, R for rectal, AX for axillary, and T for tympanic membrane, and TA for temporal artery. He or she takes the temperature by the same route each time.

The Ear

Research indicates that the temperature within the ear near the tympanic membrane and behind the ear over the path of the temporal artery have the closest correlation to core temperature.

Tympanic Membrane Thermometry

The tympanic membrane is just 1.4 in. (3.8 cm) from the hypothalamus; blood from the internal and external carotid arteries, the same vessels that supply the hypothalamus, also warms the tympanic membrane. For these reasons, temperatures obtained at this site, if the thermometer is inserted correctly (Fig. 12-2), are considered more reliable than those

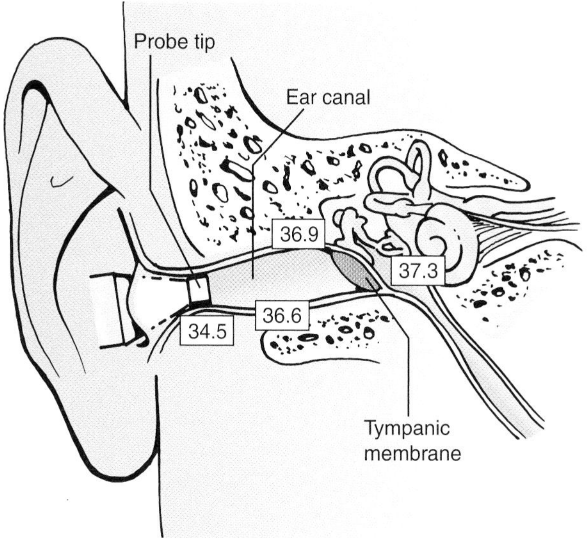

FIGURE 12-2 Obtain the most accurate tympanic temperature by aiming the probe toward the anterior inferior third of the ear canal.

obtained at the oral and axillary sites. They also correlate closely with those taken at the rectal site. Also, because the tympanic membrane is fairly deep within the head, warm or cool air temperatures affect it less.

Temporal Artery Thermometry

The superficial branch of the temporal artery, which receives blood from the aorta, lies less than 2 mm below the skin surface at the forehead. Because of this anatomic relationship, the temperature of blood flowing through the temporal artery is analogous to the temperature of blood within the heart, that is, core body temperature. In research studies, temperatures measured with an infrared temporal artery thermometer demonstrated measurements that were more accurate than the tympanic membrane thermometry; as accurate, or more so, than rectal measurements; interchangeable with esophageal probes; and similar to measurements obtained with pulmonary artery catheters (Medical News Today, 2007; Pompei & Pompei, 2004). Besides its accuracy, the temporal artery thermometer is the most noninvasive device when compared with others because it scans the artery at the skin surface, poses no risk for injury, and is suitable for nearly all ages. However, continuing research is reporting mixed reviews concerning the use of these thermometers in certain populations (Holzhauer et al., 2009; Langham et al., 2009; Marable et al., 2009). Before adopting their use universally, practitioners should investigate continuing scientific data.

Oral Site

The oral site, or mouth, is convenient. It generally measures temperatures 0.8° to 1.0°F (0.5° to 0.6°C) below the core temperature. The area under the tongue is in direct proximity to the sublingual artery. As long as the client keeps the mouth closed and breathes normally, the tissue remains at a fairly consistent temperature. Valid measurement also depends on accurate placement and maintenance of an oral thermometer in the rear sublingual pocket at the base of the tongue (Fig. 12-3). Poor placement or premature removal of the thermometer can result in inaccurate measurements, deviating by as much as 1.5°F (0.9°C) from the actual temperature.

The oral site is contraindicated for clients who are uncooperative, very young, unconscious, shivering, prone to seizures, or mouth breathers; those who have had oral surgery; and those who continue to talk during temperature assessment. To ensure accuracy, the nurse delays the oral temperature assessment for at least 30 minutes after the client has been chewing gum, smoking a cigarette, or eating hot or cold food or beverages.

Rectal Site

A rectal temperature differs only about 0.2°F (0.1°C) from the core temperature. Rapid fluctuations in temperature may not be identified for as long as 1 hour, however, because this area retains heat longer than other sites. In addition, this site can be embarrassing and emotionally traumatic for alert clients. Furthermore, stool in the rectum, improper placement of the thermometer, and premature removal affect the accuracy of rectal temperature assessment.

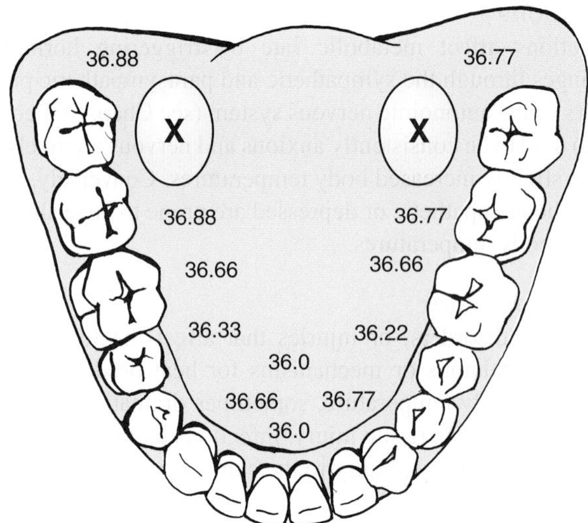

FIGURE 12-3 Temperature measurements vary with the placement of the oral thermometer. A thermometer placed at the rear sublingual pockets provides the most accurate measurement.

Axillary Site

The axilla, or underarm, is an alternative site for assessing body temperature. Temperature measurements from this site are generally 1°F (0.6°C) lower than those obtained at the oral site and reflect shell rather than core temperature (except in newborns). Because infants can be injured internally with rectal thermometers and because they lose heat through their skin at a greater rate than other age groups, the axilla and the groin, areas where there is skin-to-skin contact, have traditionally been the preferred sites for temperature assessment in this age group.

The axillary site has several advantages for all age groups. It is readily accessible in most instances. It is safe. There is less potential for spreading microorganisms than with the oral and rectal sites, and it is less disturbing psychologically than the rectal site. This route, however, requires the longest assessment time of 5 minutes or longer depending on the electronic monitoring mode being used (discussed later). Poor circulation, recent bathing, or rubbing the axillary area dry with a towel also affects the accuracy of the axillary site.

Thermometers

There are several types of **clinical thermometers** (instruments used to measure body temperature): electronic, infrared, chemical, digital, and glass (Table 12-3).

Electronic Thermometers

An electronic thermometer (Fig. 12-4) uses a temperature-sensitive probe covered with a disposable sheath attached by a coiled wire to a display unit. Electronic thermometers are portable. They are recharged when not in use.

Electronic thermometers generally have two types of probes: one for oral or axillary use and the other for rectal use. Some models offer the option of providing the measurement in Fahrenheit or centigrade.

TABLE 12-3 Types of Clinical Thermometers

TYPE	ADVANTAGES	DISADVANTAGES
Electronic	Faster than glass Accurate No sterilization or disinfection needed Easy to use	Expensive Recharging is necessary Probe needs to be held by the client or nurse Interference with simultaneously taking the client's pulse while holding the probe with one hand and unit in the other
Infrared (tympanic)	Fast Convenient Close approximation of core temperature Less invasive Accuracy unaffected by eating, drinking, or breathing Sanitary	Expensive in comparison with others Battery recharging is necessary Accuracy is affected by improper placement and probe size Actual ear and core temperature ranges are slightly different from oral, rectal, and axillary sites Tip requires cleaning with a paper tissue or alcohol swab Extreme hot or cold environmental temperatures may affect electronics No sterilization or disinfection is required
Infrared (temporal artery)	Closest approximate of core temperature Most sanitary Most convenient for clients Records within 2 seconds Initial cost is similar to other types of electronic and tympanic membrane thermometers Probe covers are not needed; decreases volume of disposal waste Can be used over the femoral artery or lateral thoracic artery if the temporal artery is inaccessible due to bandaging or trauma	User error if the thermometer is moved too quickly across the skin Hair, clothing, or bandages between the probe and the skin can result in falsely high readings Infrared probe requires cleaning between uses with an alcohol prep pad and dry swab
Chemical	Inexpensive Safe; nonbreakable Sanitary Temperature registers in approximately 45 seconds to 3 minutes Resets in 30 seconds Cleans easily in hot soapy water Easily used by untrained people	Varying measurements at different body sites depending on blood flow and room temperature
Digital	Inexpensive Safe; no glass to break or potential mercury spill Memory displays last temperature Fast; records in 1–3 minutes Audible signal during or after assessment Automatic shut-off to prolong battery Battery life of 200 hours Water resistant, which facilitates cleaning Large, lighted numerical display for ease of reading	Requires a battery (1.55 V) Accuracy of ±0.2°F compared with glass thermometer at 95–102.2°F Accuracy is ±0.4°F compared with glass thermometer at <95 or >102.2°F
Glass	Inexpensive Small Portable	Breakable Difficult to read Cleaning necessary before use by another client Cannot sterilize using heat Time-consuming Accuracy affected by eating, drinking, smoking, talking, mouth breathing, stool in rectum, vasoconstriction of skin and mucous membranes Porous; possible inaccuracy from mercury evaporation High risk for injury if broken during use Environmental pollution from mercury is possible if not properly disposed

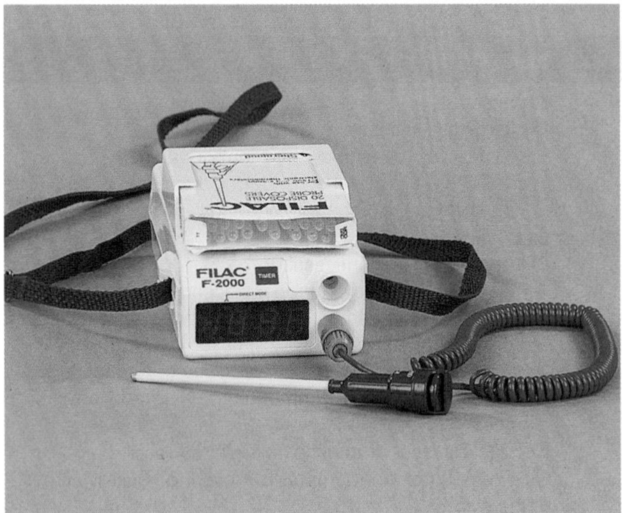

FIGURE 12-4 An electronic thermometer. (Copyright B. Proud.)

Electronic thermometers operate in either a *predictive mode* or a *monitor mode.* If used in the predictive mode, the thermometer takes multiple measurements that a computer chip processes in only a few seconds to determine what the temperature would be if the thermometer was left in place for several minutes. The monitor mode requires that the thermometer remain at the assessment site for a longer, more steady time to obtain the actual temperature. There is no significant difference in temperature measurements obtained by the predictive versus the monitor mode (Nicholl, 2002). The electronic unit senses when the temperature ceases to change and emits a beep. The audible signal alerts the nurse to remove the probe and read the displayed measurement.

Infrared (Tympanic) Thermometers

An infrared tympanic thermometer is a battery-operated device that contains an infrared sensor for detecting the warmth radiating from the tympanic membrane (eardrum) when a handheld covered probe is inserted into the ear canal (Fig. 12-5). When not in use, it rests in a base-charging unit, referred to as its cradle.

A tympanic membrane thermometer converts the heat it detects into a temperature measurement in 2 to 5 seconds. The potential for transferring microorganisms from one client to another is reduced because the probe cover is changed after each use and because the ear does not contain mucous membranes or their accompanying secretions.

Despite the advantages of tympanic thermometers, infrared thermometers can produce inaccurate measurements in the following circumstances:

- The ear canal is not straightened appropriately.
- The probe, which measures 6 to 8 mm, is too large for the ear canal (a problem with infants and small children whose ear canals are 5 mm or smaller). The size difference alters the location where infrared light must be precisely directed. Consequently, use of a tympanic thermometer is contraindicated for children younger than 2 years.
- The sensor is directed at the ear canal rather than directly at the tympanic membrane.
- There is impacted **cerumen** (ear wax), a common problem among older adults.
- There is fluid behind the tympanic membrane, a problem that occurs with middle-ear infections.
- The **drawdown effect** (cooling of the ear when it comes in contact with the probe) occurs.

The first use of a tympanic thermometer after recharging is not always as accurate as a second reading. Another criticism of the tympanic temperature measurement is that currently there is no standard for actual ear or core temperatures. At present, tympanic thermometers use internally calculated **offsets** (predictive mathematical conversions) for oral and rectal temperatures. These offsets vary among manufacturers.

Infrared Temporal Artery Thermometer

The temporal artery thermometer (Fig. 12-6) contains an infrared sensor that uses computerized algorithms to compute temperature measurements. It does so by calculating

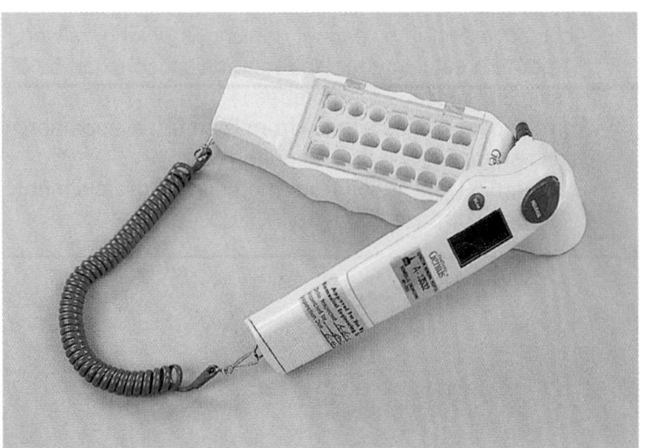

FIGURE 12-5 An infrared tympanic thermometer. (Copyright B. Proud.)

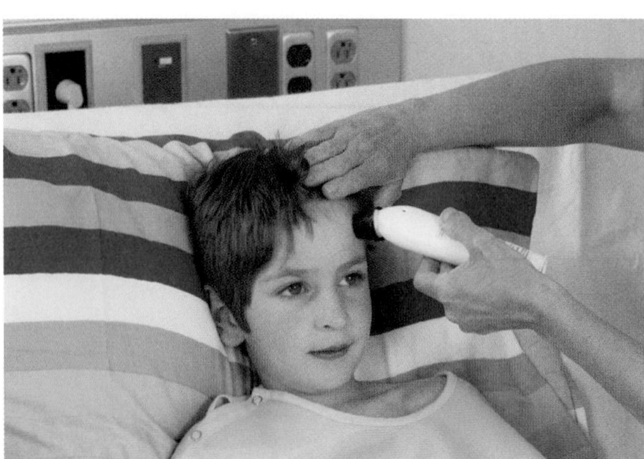

FIGURE 12-6 A temporal artery thermometer.

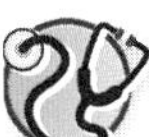

NURSING GUIDELINES 12-1

Using a Temporal Artery Thermometer

- Perform hand hygiene.
- Place the probe at the center of the forehead.
- Depress the sensing button on the thermometer throughout the procedure.
- Slide the thermometer laterally across the forehead to the hairline.
- Lift the probe while keeping the button depressed.
- Relocate the probe behind the ear.
- Slide the probe to the depression behind the ear lobe.
- Release the button.
- Read and record the displayed temperature.
- Wait 30 seconds if a sequential measurement is needed or use the opposite side.
- Clean the thermometer probe with an alcohol pad and a dry swab.
- Replace the 9 V alkaline battery when "BATT" display indicates the battery is low.

the difference between the heat radiating from the temporal artery at the center of the forehead and the heat loss at the skin. Because there may be evaporative cooling on the exposed skin on the forehead, *the thermometer is secondarily moved to scan the skin behind the ear lobe*, which tends to remain relatively dry (Nursing Guidelines 12-1). An assessment over the temporal artery alone is sufficient for infants.

Glass Thermometers

Electronic and infrared tympanic thermometers have replaced glass mercury thermometers in health care agencies. Glass thermometers contain mercury and are considered environmentally toxic and obsolete because safer alternatives are available and preferred.

The Mercury Reduction Act, passed in 2002 and amended in 2005, prohibits the sale or supply of mercury fever thermometers to consumers, except by prescription. It further requires manufacturers to provide clear instructions on handling mercury thermometers to avoid breakage and proper cleanup in the event of a breakage (United States 109th Congress, 2002, 2005). Health care institutions are making their facilities mercury free.

Nurses may be required to use a client's glass thermometer or to teach a client to use one because that is all the client has available. If a glass thermometer is the only option, the nurse teaches clients and their family members how to clean the glass thermometer (see Client and Family Teaching 12-1).

If a glass thermometer breaks, the mercury is disposed of following the actions discussed in Nursing Guidelines 12-2.

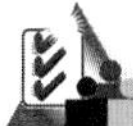

Client and Family Teaching 12-1
Cleaning Glass Thermometers

The nurse teaches the client or the family the following:

- Don gloves if there is the potential for contact with blood or stool (as with a rectal assessment).
- Hold the thermometer at the tip of the stem. Keep the bulb downward and away from your hand.
- Using a firm twisting motion and a clean, soft tissue, wipe the soiled thermometer toward the bulb.
- Wash the thermometer with soap or detergent solution, again using friction, while holding the thermometer over a towel or other soft material to reduce the potential for breaking if dropped.
- Rinse the thermometer under cold running water.
- Dry the thermometer with a soft towel.
- Soak the thermometer in 70% to 90% isopropyl alcohol or a 1:10 solution of household bleach (1 part bleach to 10 parts water).
- Rinse the thermometer after disinfecting it.
- Store the thermometer in a clean, dry container.

Chemical Thermometers

Various chemical thermometers are available. One example is a paper or plastic strip with chemically treated dots (Fig. 12-7). The temperature is determined by noting how many dots change color after the strip is held in the mouth. Chemical dot thermometers are discarded after one use. They are used to assess the temperature of clients who require isolation precautions for infectious diseases. Their use eliminates the need to clean a multiuse electronic or infrared thermometer. Some physician's offices also use chemical dot thermometers because they are disposable.

A second type of chemical thermometer is made of heat-sensitive tape or patch applied to the abdomen or forehead (Fig. 12-8). The tape or patch changes color according to body temperature. Heat-sensitive tapes and patches can be reused several times before being thrown away.

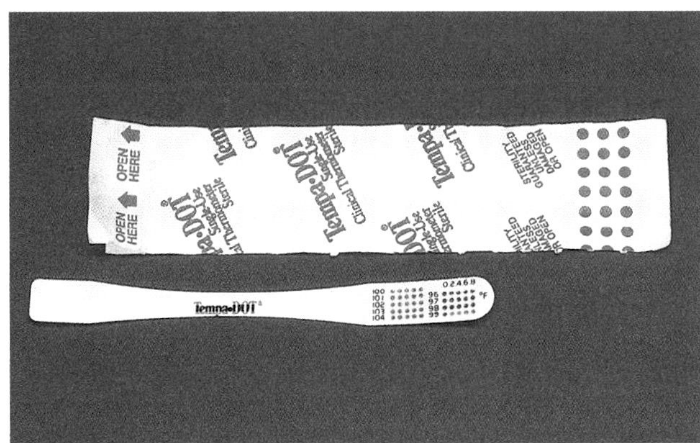

FIGURE 12-7 A chemical thermometer.

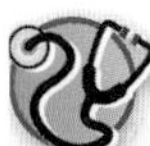

NURSING GUIDELINES 12-2

Disposing of Heavy Metals Safely

- Don gloves.
- Pick up shards of glass and place in a puncture-resistant container.
- Use an index card to pool the droplets of mercury.
- Collect the droplets with a syringe, pipette, adhesive tape, or wet paper towel.
- Seal the mercury in a glass or plastic jar or sturdy plastic bag.
- Affix a label identifying the contents as "mercury spill debris."
- Deliver the mercury spill debris to the waste manager of the health care institution or the county public health department (Princeton University Environmental Health and Safety, 2004).

Digital Thermometers

A plastic digital thermometer looks similar to a glass thermometer (Fig. 12-9) and can be used at oral, axillary, and rectal sites. It has a sensing tip at the end of the stem, an on/off button, and a display area that lights up during use. The battery used to operate the thermometer requires occasional replacement.

Digital thermometers are designed for multiple uses; for this reason, they require cleaning after use. Digital thermometers are cleaned similarly to glass thermometers except that they are wiped rather than soaked with isopropyl alcohol. Disposable plastic sheaths can be used to cover the probe with each use as an alternative sanitary measure.

Automated Monitoring Devices

Some agencies use **automated monitoring devices** (equipment that allows for the simultaneous collection of multiple data). They may measure the temperature, blood pressure, and pulse, as well as other information such as heart rhythm and pulse oximetry (Fig. 12-10). Some models can store and display the trends in vital signs. Their chief advantage is that they save time and money. Agencies favor the use of automated monitors for potentially unstable clients who require frequent assessments. To ensure reliable data, the accuracy of automated devices is compared with data measured with manual devices on a regular basis.

Continuous Monitoring Devices

Continuous temperature monitoring devices are used primarily in critical care areas. They measure body temperature using internal thermistor probes within the esophagus of anesthetized clients, inside the bladder, or attached to a pulmonary artery catheter. These measurements are generally required when caring for clients with extreme hypothermia or hyperthermia. Warming or cooling blankets are also generally used at the same time (see Chap. 28). Temperature assessments aid in evaluating the effectiveness of these treatment devices.

Skill 12-1 describes how to assess body temperature using electronic, infrared tympanic membrane, and glass thermometers. Some agencies also use automated and continuous monitoring devices.

Stop, Think, and Respond Box 12-2

When caring for an older adult who has chronic disorders but is currently stable, what type of thermometer and site is best for a temperature assessment? Explain your choice.

Elevated Body Temperature

A **fever** (a body temperature that exceeds 99.3°F [37.4°C]) is a common indication of illness. **Pyrexia** (Greek word for

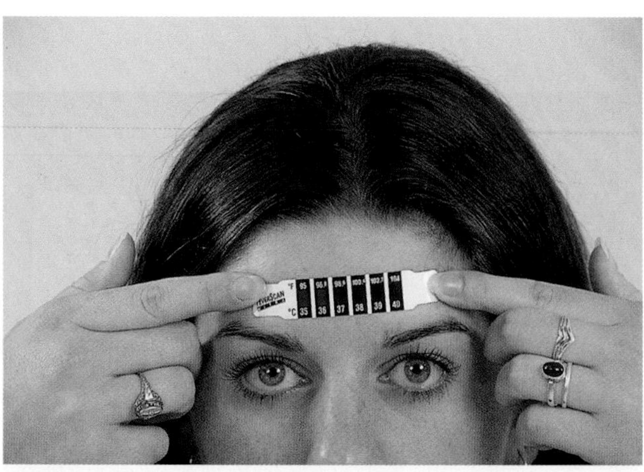

FIGURE 12-8 A disposable chemical thermometer with heat-sensitive liquid crystals. (Photo by B. Proud.)

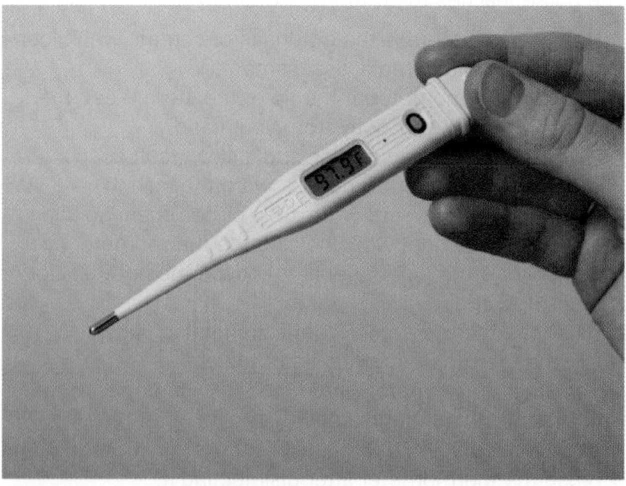

FIGURE 12-9 A digital thermometer is a nonmercury alternative considered as accurate as a glass mercury thermometer.

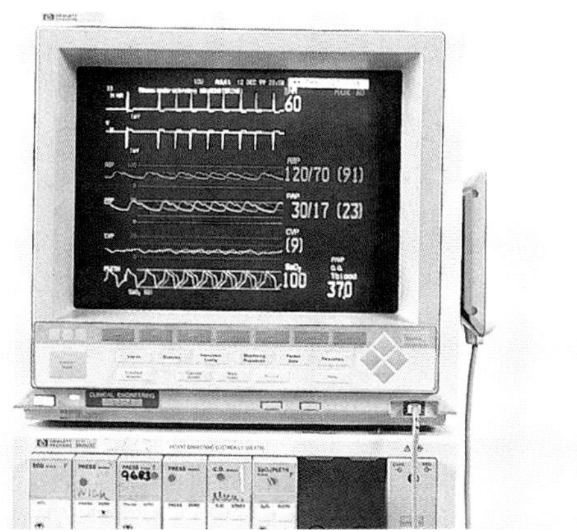

FIGURE 12-10 An automated monitoring device. (Photo by B. Proud.)

fire) is a term used to describe a warmer-than-normal set point. A person with a fever is said to be **febrile** (a condition in which the temperature is elevated) as opposed to **afebrile** (no fever).

The following are common signs and symptoms associated with a fever:

- Pinkish, red (flushed) skin that is warm to the touch
- Restlessness or, in others, excessive sleepiness
- Irritability
- Poor appetite
- Glassy eyes and a sensitivity to light
- Increased perspiration
- Headache
- Above-normal pulse and respiratory rates
- Disorientation and confusion (when the temperature is very high)
- Convulsions in infants and children (when the temperature is very high)
- Fever blisters around the nose or lips in clients who harbor the herpes simplex virus

Hyperthermia (excessively high core temperature) describes a state in which the temperature exceeds 105.8°F (40.6°C). At this level, the person is at extremely high risk for brain damage or death from complications associated with increased metabolic demands.

Phases of a Fever

A fever generally progresses through four distinct phases:

1. *Prodromal phase:* The client has nonspecific symptoms just before the temperature rises.
2. *Onset* or *invasion phase:* Obvious mechanisms for increasing body temperature, such as shivering, develop.
3. *Stationary phase:* The fever is sustained.
4. *Resolution* or *defervescence phase:* The temperature returns to normal (Fig. 12-11).

Common variations in fever patterns are described in Table 12-4. Fevers also subside in different ways. If an elevated temperature suddenly drops to normal, it is referred to as a resolution by crisis. If the descent is gradual, it is referred to as a resolution lysis.

Nursing Management

A fever is considered an important body defense for destroying infectious microorganisms. Therefore, as long as a fever remains below 102°F (38.9°C) and the person does not have a chronic medical condition, fluids or rest may be all that is necessary.

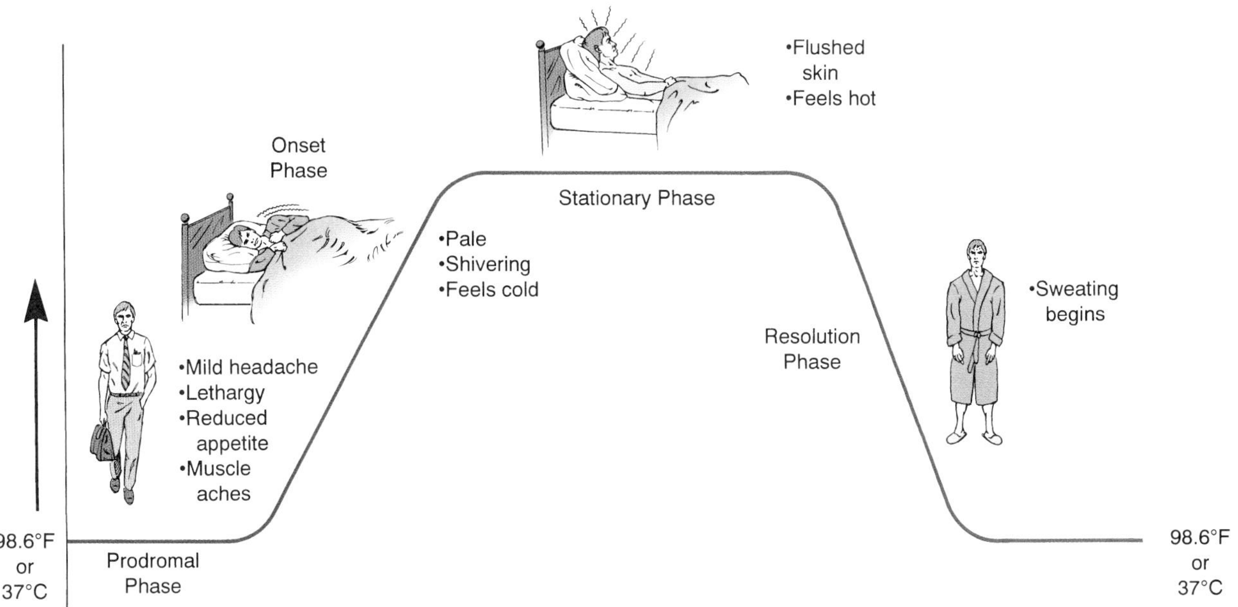

FIGURE 12-11 Phases of a fever and physiologic changes.

TABLE 12-4 Variations in Fever Patterns

TYPE OF FEVER	DESCRIPTION
Sustained fever	Remains elevated with little fluctuation
Remittent fever	Fluctuates several degrees but never reaches normal between fluctuations
Intermittent fever	Cycles frequently between periods of normal or subnormal temperatures and spikes of fever
Relapsing fever	Recurs after a brief but sustained period during which temperature has been normal

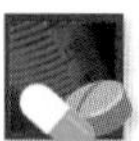

Pharmacologic Considerations

- **Antipyretics** (drugs that reduce fever), such as aspirin, acetaminophen, or ibuprofen, are helpful when a temperature is 102° to 104°F (38.9° to 40°C).

Physical cooling measures are used for temperatures between 104° and 105.8°F (40° to 40.6°C). If the temperature is higher than 105.8°F (40.6°C) or if a high temperature is unchanged after a sufficient response time with conventional interventions, more aggressive treatment is warranted.

Nursing Care Plan 12-1 describes nursing actions used for a client with a nursing diagnosis of Hyperthermia. NANDA-I (2012; p. 468) defines hyperthermia as a "body temperature elevated above normal range." If the fever is so severe that it requires medical interventions, it is a collaborative problem.

Subnormal Body Temperature

There are several ranges of **hypothermia** (a core body temperature less than 95°F [35°C]). A person is considered *mildly hypothermic* at temperatures of 95° to 93.2°F (35° to 34°C), *moderately hypothermic* at 93° to 86°F (33.8° to 30°C), and *severely hypothermic* below 86°F (30°C).

Cold body temperatures are best measured with a tympanic thermometer for two reasons. First, other clinical thermometers do not have the capacity to measure temperatures in hypothermic ranges. Second, the blood flow in the mouth, rectum, or axillae generally is so reduced that measurements taken from these sites are inaccurate.

The following are common signs and symptoms associated with hypothermia:

- Shivering until body temperature is extremely low
- Pale, cool, and puffy skin
- Impaired muscle coordination
- Listlessness
- Slow pulse and respiratory rates
- Irregular heart rhythm
- Decreased ability to think coherently and use good judgment
- Diminished ability to feel pain or other sensations

In some illnesses, such as hypothyroidism and starvation, the client typically has a subnormal temperature. Therefore, the nurse must assess clients just as closely when body temperature falls below normal ranges as when it is elevated.

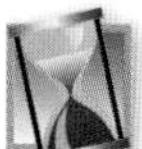

Gerontologic Considerations

- Older adults are more susceptible to hypothermia and heat-related conditions. Environmental factors, such as extreme heat and cold conditions and inadequately heated or cooled living environments, pose additional risk factors for developing hypothermia and heat-related illnesses.

Clients with severe hypothermia usually die. Nevertheless, clients have been known to live even with very low temperatures, as in near-drowning in cold water and exposure in extremely cold environments. This phenomenon has led to the saying among paramedics and emergency department personnel that "a person isn't dead until he or she is warm and dead." Various supportive measures are implemented when clients have subnormal body temperatures (see Nursing Guidelines 12-3).

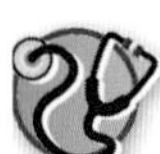

NURSING GUIDELINES 12-3

The Client With a Subnormal Temperature

- Raise the room temperature. *Doing so warms the body surface.*
- Remove wet clothing. *This measure reduces heat loss.*
- Apply layers of dry clothing and loosely woven blankets. *Layers trap body heat next to the skin.*
- Warm blankets and clothing in an oven or microwave if body temperature is quite low. *Heating raises the temperature of woven fabrics above ambient (room) temperature.*
- Position the client so that the arms are next to the chest and the legs are tucked toward the abdomen. *This position prevents heat loss.*
- Cover the head with a cap or towel. *Covering the head reduces heat loss.*
- Provide warm fluids. *Fluids conduct heat to internal organs.*
- Massage the skin unless it has been frostbitten. *Massage produces mechanical friction, which produces warmth.*
- Apply bags filled with warm water between areas of skin folds, or place an electronic warming pad beneath the back and hips (see Chap. 28) according to medical orders. *These measures transfer heat to the blood as it circulates through the skin.*

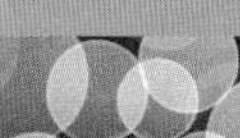

NURSING CARE PLAN 12-1 The Client With a Fever

Assessment

Determine the following:

- Current temperature
- Contributing factors such as dehydration, illness, inability to perspire, exposure to warm environment or excessive layers of clothing, prolonged physical activity, current drug history
- Trend in temperature measurements to determine whether the fever is sustained, remittent, intermittent, or relapsing
- Additional assessment data such as if the client is flushed, restless, sleepy, confused, shivering, perspiring, or sensitive to light, or has an accompanying headache or poor appetite
- Results of latest white blood cell count and thyroid hormone levels
- Exposure to others with similar symptoms

Nursing Diagnosis. Hyperthermia related to imbalance between heat production and heat loss secondary to known or unknown etiology.

Expected Outcome. The client's body temperature will be between 96.6° and 99.3°F (35.8° to 37.4°C) within 24 hours following implementation of fever-relieving interventions.

Interventions	Rationales
Cover a client who is shivering.	Covering prevents heat loss; shivering will not cease until the hypothalamus readjusts to a higher set point.
Keep the client in a warm but not hot environment.	A warm environment provides comfort while the client's body adapts to the new set point.
Remove blankets or heavy clothing once shivering subsides.	Decreasing layers of insulating fabric facilitates heat loss by radiation and convection.
Limit activity.	Restriction of activity reduces contractile thermogenesis from muscle movement.
Provide liberal oral fluids.	They replace fluid loss from perspiration and increased metabolism.
Provide light but high-calorie nourishment.	Modifying dietary intake compensates for increased metabolic rate, delayed gastric emptying, and decreased intestinal motility.
Administer antipyretics according to medical orders; aspirin is contraindicated for children with fevers because it is associated with Reye's syndrome.	Antipyretics block the set point elevation in the hypothalamus.
Apply cool cloths or an ice pack to the forehead, behind the neck, and between the axillary and the inguinal skin folds.	Cooling the skin lowers the temperature of blood by conduction as the warmer blood flows near the peripheral skin surface.
Promote room ventilation or use an electric fan if an air conditioner is not available.	Convection disperses heat via air currents.
Keep the humidity level low.	Reducing environmental moisture facilitates heat loss via evaporation.
Apply tepid water to the skin, as in a sponge bath, 30 minutes after administering an antipyretic.	Heat loss via convection and evaporation after an antipyretic helps to alter the set point in the hypothalamus.
Discontinue physical cooling measures if the client begins to shiver.	Shivering raises body heat and defeats the purpose of the sponge bath.
Apply an electronically regulated cooling pad beneath the client as directed by a physician (see Chap. 28).	A cooling pad lowers the body temperature by conduction as blood circulates through vessels in the skin.

Evaluation of Expected Outcome

The client's temperature returns to normal range.

PULSE

A **pulse**, a wavelike sensation that can be palpated in a peripheral artery, is produced by the movement of blood during the heart's contraction. In most adults, the heart contracts 60 to 100 times per minute at rest.

Pulse Rate

The **pulse rate** (the number of peripheral pulsations palpated in 1 minute) is counted by compressing a superficial artery against an underlying bone with the tips of the fingers.

Rapid Pulse Rate

The pulse rate of adults is considered rapid if it exceeds 100 beats per minute (bpm) at rest. **Tachycardia** (100 to 150 bpm) is a fast heart rate, but heart and pulse rates can exceed 150 bpm. Rapid contraction, if sustained, tends to overwork the heart and may not oxygenate cells adequately because the heart has such little time between contractions to fill with blood.

The term **palpitation** (awareness of one's own heart contraction without having to feel the pulse) can accompany tachycardia. Clients with rapid pulse rates are monitored closely, and the results are reported and recorded according to agency policy.

Slow Pulse Rate

The pulse rate of adults is considered slower than normal if it falls below 60 bpm. **Bradycardia** (less than 60 bpm) is less common than tachycardia; it merits prompt reporting and continued monitoring.

Factors Affecting Pulse and Heart Rates

Any factors that affect the rate of heart contraction also cause comparable effects in pulse rate. Because one depends on the other, the pulse rate can never be faster than the actual heart rate. Heart and pulse rates may vary depending on the following:

- *Age.* Some common rates are listed in Table 12-5.
- *Circadian rhythm.* Rates tend to be lower in the morning and increase later in the day.
- *Gender.* Men average approximately 60 to 65 bpm at rest; the average rate for women is about 7 or 8 bpm faster.
- *Body build.* Tall, slender people usually have slower heart and pulse rates than short, stout people.

TABLE 12-5 Normal Pulse Rates Per Minute at Various Ages

AGE	APPROXIMATE RANGE	APPROXIMATE AVERAGE
Newborn	120–160	140
1–12 months	80–140	120
1–2 years	80–130	110
3–6 years	75–120	100
7–12 years	75–110	95
Adolescence	60–100	80
Adulthood	60–100	80

- *Exercise and activity.* Rates increase with exercise and activity and decrease with rest. With regular aerobic exercise, however, a **training effect** occurs, in which the heart rate and, consequently, the pulse rate become consistently lower than average. This effect develops because the heart muscle becomes more efficient at supplying body cells with sufficient oxygenated blood with fewer beats. Those who are physically fit exhibit slower pulse rates even during exercise.
- *Stress and emotions.* Stimulation of the sympathetic nervous system and emotions such as anger, fear, and excitement increase heart and pulse rates. Pain, which is stressful (especially when moderate to severe), can trigger faster rates.
- *Body temperature.* For every degree of Fahrenheit elevation, the heart and pulse rates increase by 10 bpm. A 1° increase in centigrade measurement causes a 15-bpm increase (Porth, 2004). With a fall in body temperature, the opposite effect occurs.
- *Blood volume.* Excessive blood loss causes the heart and pulse rates to increase. With decreased red blood cells or inadequate hemoglobin to distribute oxygen to cells, the heart rate accelerates in an effort to keep cells adequately supplied.
- *Drugs.* Certain drugs can slow or speed the rate of heart contraction. Digitalis preparations and sedatives typically slow the heart rate. Caffeine, nicotine, cocaine, thyroid replacement hormones, and epinephrine increase heart contractions and subsequently, pulse rates.

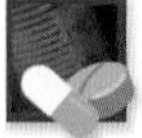

Pharmacologic Considerations

- Older adults generally have more profound responses to cardiovascular medications than younger adults. Changes such as dizziness or fainting, diminished appetite, nausea, or visual changes may indicate the need for evaluation of cardiovascular medications.

Pulse Rhythm

The **pulse rhythm** (the pattern of the pulsations and the pauses between them) is normally regular. That is, the beats and the pauses occur similarly throughout the time the pulse is palpated.

An **arrhythmia** or **dysrhythmia** (an irregular pattern of heartbeats) with a consequently irregular pulse rhythm is reported promptly. Some types indicate potentially life-threatening cardiac dysfunctions that may warrant more sophisticated monitoring and treatment. Details about dysrhythmias and their causes can be found in textbooks that discuss cardiac disorders.

Pulse Volume

Pulse volume (the quality of pulsations felt) is usually related to the amount of blood pumped with each heartbeat, or the

TABLE 12-6 Identifying Pulse Volume

NUMBER	DEFINITION	DESCRIPTION
0	Absent pulse	No pulsation is felt despite extreme pressure.
1+	Thready pulse	Pulsation is not easily felt; slight pressure causes it to disappear.
2+	Weak pulse	Pulse is stronger than thready; light pressure causes it to disappear.
3+	Normal pulse	Pulsation is felt easily; moderate pressure causes it to disappear.
4+	Bounding pulse	Pulsation is strong and does not disappear with moderate pressure.

force of the heart's contraction. When a pulse can be felt with mild pressure over the artery, it is described as being *strong*. A *feeble, weak,* or *thready pulse* refers to a pulse that is difficult to feel or, once felt, is obliterated easily with slight pressure. A rapid, thready pulse is usually a serious sign and reported promptly. A *bounding* or *full pulse* produces a pronounced pulsation that does not easily disappear with pressure.

Another way to describe the volume or quality of the pulse is with corresponding numbers (Table 12-6). When documenting pulse volume, the nurse should follow the agency policy about using descriptive terms or a numbering system.

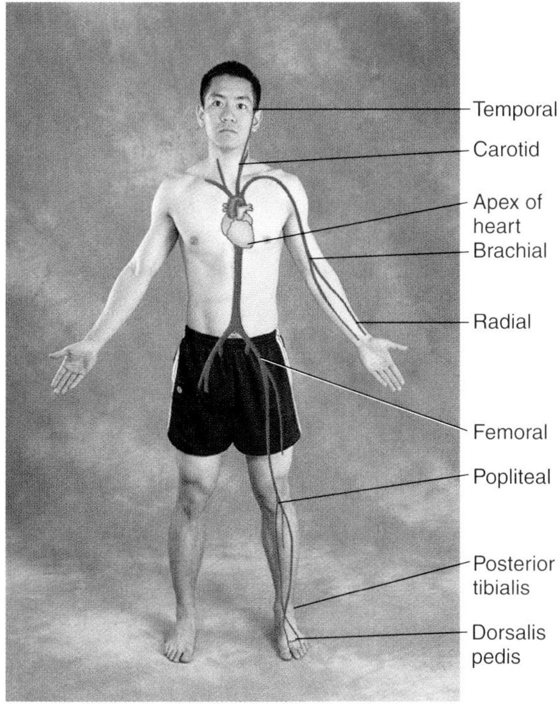

FIGURE 12-12 The peripheral pulse sites.

Assessment Sites

The arteries used for pulse assessment lie close to the skin. Most, but not all, are named for the bone over which they are located (Fig. 12-12). These pulse sites are collectively called "peripheral pulses" because they are distant from the heart. Of all the peripheral pulses, the radial artery, located on the inner (thumb) side of the wrist, is the site most often used for pulse assessment. Three alternative assessment techniques can be used instead of or in addition to the assessment of a peripheral pulse. These techniques include counting the apical heart rate, obtaining an apical–radial rate, and using a Doppler ultrasound device over a peripheral artery.

The **apical heart rate** (the number of ventricular contractions per minute) is considered more accurate than the radial pulse for two reasons. First, the sound of each heartbeat is obvious and distinct. Second, sometimes the heart contraction is not strong enough to be felt at a peripheral pulse site. Counting the apical rate, however, is less convenient than counting a radial pulse. An apical heart rate generally is assessed when the peripheral pulse is irregular or difficult to palpate because of a rapid rate or thready quality or when it is necessary to obtain an actual heart rate.

The apical heart rate is counted by listening at the chest with a stethoscope or by feeling the pulsations in the chest for 1 full minute at an area called the "point of maximum impulse". As the name suggests, the heartbeats are best heard or felt at the apex, or lower tip, of the heart. The apex in a healthy adult is slightly below the left nipple in line with the middle of the clavicle (Fig. 12-13).

When assessing the apical heart rate by listening to the chest—which is generally the more accurate technique—the nurse listens for the "lub/dub" sound. The lub sound is louder if the stethoscope has been correctly applied. These

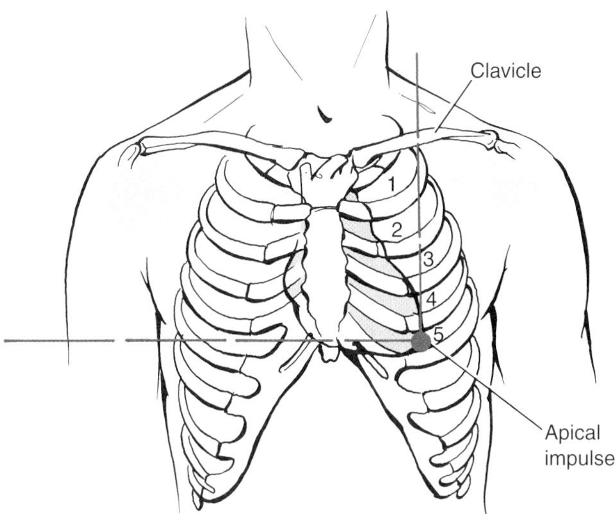

FIGURE 12-13 Assess the apical heart rate to the left of the sternum at the interspace below the fifth rib in midline with the clavicle.

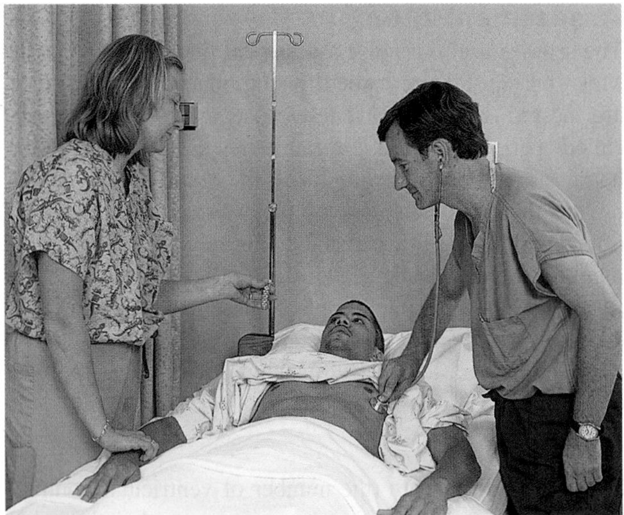

FIGURE 12-14 One nurse counts the radial pulse while the other counts the apical rate. (Photo by B. Proud.)

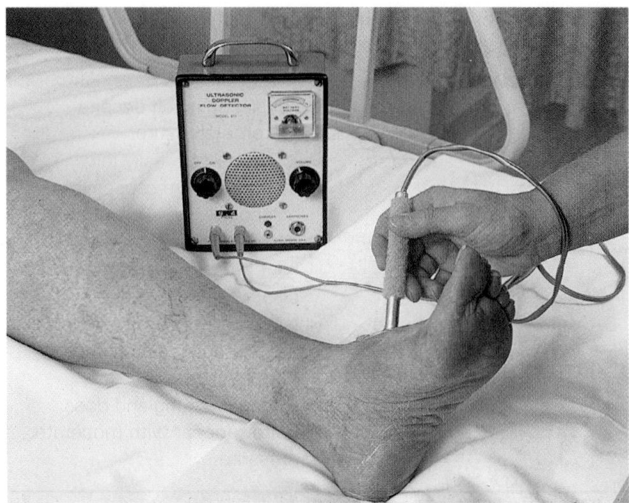

FIGURE 12-15 Using a Doppler ultrasound device. (Photo by B. Proud.)

two sounds equal one pulsation at a peripheral pulse site. The apical heart rate is counted for 1 full minute, and the rhythm is also evaluated.

Apical–Radial Rate

The **apical–radial rate** (the number of sounds heard at the heart's apex and the rate of the radial pulse during the same period) is counted by separate nurses at the same time using one watch or clock (Fig. 12-14). The apical and radial rates should be the same, but in some clients, they are not. The **pulse deficit** (the difference between the apical and the radial pulse rates) is noted. If a pulse deficit is significant—and the rates have been counted accurately—the nurse reports the findings promptly and documents them in the client's medical record.

DOPPLER ULTRASOUND DEVICE

A Doppler ultrasound device is an electronic instrument that detects the movement of blood through peripheral blood vessels and converts the movement to a sound. This instrument is most helpful when slight pressure occludes pulsations or when arterial blood flow is severely compromised.

When the device is used, conductive gel is applied over the arterial site, and the probe is moved at an angle over the skin until a pulsating sound is heard (Fig. 12-15). The pulsating sounds are counted, much like the palpated pulsations. The nurse documents the assessment site and the rate, followed by the abbreviation D to indicate the use of a Doppler device.

Skill 12-2 describes how to assess the rate, rhythm, and volume of the pulse at the radial artery.

Stop, Think, and Respond Box 12-3

If assessing the radial pulse is difficult or impossible, what alternatives could be taken?

RESPIRATION

Respiration is the exchange of oxygen and carbon dioxide. When it occurs between the alveolar and the capillary membranes, it is called "external respiration." The exchange of oxygen and carbon dioxide between the blood and the body cells is called "internal" or "tissue respiration."

Ventilation (the movement of air in and out of the chest) involves *inhalation* or *inspiration* (breathing in) and *exhalation* or *expiration* (breathing out). The medulla, which is the primary respiratory center in the brain, controls ventilation. The medulla is sensitive to the amount of carbon dioxide in the blood and adapts the rate of ventilations accordingly. Breathing can be voluntarily controlled to a certain extent.

Respiratory Rate

The **respiratory rate** (the number of ventilations per minute) varies considerably in healthy people, but normal ranges have been established (Table 12-7). Factors that influence pulse rate generally also affect respiratory rate. The faster the pulse rate, the faster the respiratory rate, and vice versa. The ratio of one respiration to approximately four or five heartbeats is fairly consistent in healthy adults.

TABLE 12-7 Normal Respiratory Rates at Various Ages

AGE	AVERAGE RANGE
Newborn	30–80
Early childhood	20–40
Late childhood	15–25
Adulthood	
Men	14–18
Women	16–20

Rapid Respiratory Rates

Resting respiratory rates that exceed the standards for a client's age are considered abnormal. **Tachypnea** (a rapid respiratory rate) often accompanies an elevated temperature or diseases that affect the cardiac and respiratory systems.

Slow Respiratory Rates

Bradypnea (a slower-than-normal respiratory rate at rest) can result from medications; for instance, morphine sulfate slows the respiratory rate. Slow respirations also may be observed in clients with neurologic disorders or who are experiencing hypothermia.

Breathing Patterns and Abnormal Characteristics

Various breathing patterns and abnormal characteristics may be identified when assessing respiratory rates. *Cheyne–Stokes respiration* refers to a breathing pattern in which the depth of respirations gradually increases, followed by a gradual decrease, and then a period when breathing stops briefly before resuming again. Cheyne–Stokes respiration is a serious sign that may occur as death approaches.

Hyperventilation (rapid or deep breathing or both) and **hypoventilation** (diminished breathing) affect the volume of air entering and leaving the lungs. Changes in ventilation may occur in clients with airway obstruction or pulmonary or neuromuscular diseases.

Dyspnea (difficult or labored breathing) is almost always accompanied by a rapid respiratory rate as clients work to improve the efficiency of their breathing. Clients with dyspnea usually appear anxious and worried. The nostrils flare (widen) as they fight to fill the lungs with air. They may use the abdominal and neck muscles to assist other muscles in breathing. When observing these clients, the nurse should note how much and what type of activity brings on dyspnea. For example, walking to the bathroom may bring on dyspnea in a client but sitting in a chair may not.

Orthopnea (breathing facilitated by sitting up or standing) occurs in clients with dyspnea who find it easier to breathe this way. The sitting or standing position causes organs in the abdominal cavity to fall away from the diaphragm with gravity. This gives more room for the lungs to expand within the chest cavity, allowing the person to take in more air with each breath.

Apnea (the absence of breathing) is life threatening if it lasts more than 4 to 6 minutes. Prolonged apnea leads to brain damage or death. Brief periods of apnea lower oxygen levels in the blood and can trigger serious abnormal cardiac rhythms (see Chap. 21 for more on sleep apnea).

Terms such as **"stertorous breathing"** (noisy ventilation) and **"stridor"** (a harsh, high-pitched sound heard on inspiration when there is laryngeal obstruction) are used to describe sounds that accompany breathing. Infants and young children with croup often have stridor when breathing. The nurse uses a stethoscope to listen to the sounds of air moving through the chest. The assessment technique and the characteristics of lung sounds are described in Chapter 13.

Skill 12-3 lists techniques to use when counting the respiratory rate.

Stop, Think, and Respond Box 12-4

What nursing actions are appropriate if a client has an abnormal respiratory rate?

BLOOD PRESSURE

Blood pressure is the force that the blood exerts within the arteries. Several physiologic variables create blood pressure:

- Circulating blood volume averages 4.5 to 5.5 L in adult women and 5.0 to 6.0 L in adult men. Lower-than-normal volumes decrease blood pressure; excess volumes increase it.
- Contractility of the heart is influenced by the stretch of cardiac muscle fibers. Based on *Starling's law of the heart,* the force of heart contraction is related to **preload** (the volume of blood that fills the heart and stretches the heart muscle fibers during its resting phase). A common analogy is to compare the effect of preload and contractility with the snap of a rubber band stretched to various lengths—the longer the rubber band is stretched, the greater it snaps when released. Tissue damage that scars the heart, such as after a heart attack, impairs stretching and reduces contractility. Regular aerobic exercise increases the tone of the heart muscle, making it an efficient muscular pump.
- **Cardiac output** (the volume of blood ejected from the left ventricle per minute) is approximately 5 to 6 L (slightly more than a gallon) in adults at rest. It is estimated by multiplying the heart rate by the stroke volume (amount of blood that leaves the heart with each contraction). The average stroke volume in adults is 70 mL. With exercise, cardiac output can increase as much as five times the resting volume. Bradycardia can severely reduce cardiac output and thus, blood pressure.
- Blood viscosity (thickness) creates a resisting force when the heart contracts. The resistance compromises stroke volume and cardiac output. Blood thickens when there are more cells and proteins than water in plasma. Circulating viscous blood also causes cardiac fatigue and weakens the heart's ability to contract.
- Peripheral resistance, referred to as **afterload** (the force against which the heart pumps when ejecting blood), increases when the valves of the heart and arterioles (small subdivisions of arteries) are narrowed or calcified. Afterload is decreased when arteries dilate.

In healthy people, the arterial walls are elastic and easily stretch and recoil to accommodate the changing volume of circulating blood. Measuring the blood pressure helps to assess the efficiency of the circulatory system. Blood pressure measurements reflect (1) the ability of the arteries to stretch, (2) the volume of circulating blood, and

(3) the amount of resistance the heart must overcome when it pumps blood.

Factors Affecting Blood Pressure

Besides the physiologic variables that create blood pressure, other factors that cause temporary or permanent alterations are as follows:

- *Age.* Blood pressure tends to become elevated with age as a result of arteriosclerosis, a process in which arteries lose their elasticity and become more rigid, and atherosclerosis, a process in which the arteries become narrowed with fat deposits. The rate of these conditions depends on heredity and lifestyle habits such as diet and exercise.
- *Circadian rhythm.* Blood pressure tends to be lowest after midnight, begins rising at approximately 4 or 5 AM, and peaks during late morning or early afternoon.
- *Gender.* Women tend to have lower blood pressure than men of the same age.
- *Exercise and activity.* Blood pressure rises during exercise and activity, when the heart pumps more blood. Regular exercise, however, helps to maintain blood pressure within normal levels.
- *Emotions and pain.* Strong emotional experiences and pain tend to increase blood pressure from sympathetic nervous system stimulation.
- *Miscellaneous factors.* As a rule, a person has lower blood pressure when lying down than when sitting or standing, although the difference in most people is insignificant. Blood pressure also seems to rise somewhat when the urinary bladder is full, when the legs are crossed, or when the person is cold. Drugs that stimulate the heart such as nicotine, caffeine, cocaine, and methamphetamine also tend to constrict the arteries and raise blood pressure.

Pressure Measurements

When assessing blood pressure, nurses obtain both systolic and diastolic measurements. **Systolic pressure** (pressure within the arterial system when the heart contracts) is higher than **diastolic pressure** (pressure within the arterial system when the heart relaxes and fills with blood). Blood pressure measurements are expressed as a fraction. The numerator is the systolic pressure, the pressure during systole, and the denominator is the diastolic pressure, the pressure during diastole (Fig. 12-16).

Currently, blood pressure measurement is expressed in millimeters of mercury (mm Hg) because the mercury sphygmomanometer, an instrument for measuring blood pressure using a graduated column of mercury, has been the standard for use. Thus, a recording of 118/78 means the systolic blood pressure measured 118 mm Hg and the diastolic blood pressure measured 78 mm Hg. Because mercury within the sphygmomanometer is a toxin that persists and accumulates within the environment and living species, mercury sphygmomanometers have been eliminated. As a result, some propose that the pressure measurements should be changed to something other than millimeters of mercury. One possible alternative is to use the kilopascal (kPa), a measurement from the European Système International (SI) in which 1 mm Hg equals 0.133 kPa. Using this system, the equivalent of a normal blood pressure such as 118/78 mm Hg would be 16/11 kPa when rounded to the nearest decimal point. Although the conversion to kPa for measuring blood pressure has been discussed by experts from the National Heart, Lung, and Blood Institute and the American Heart Association (NHLBI, 2002), it has not been adopted as yet.

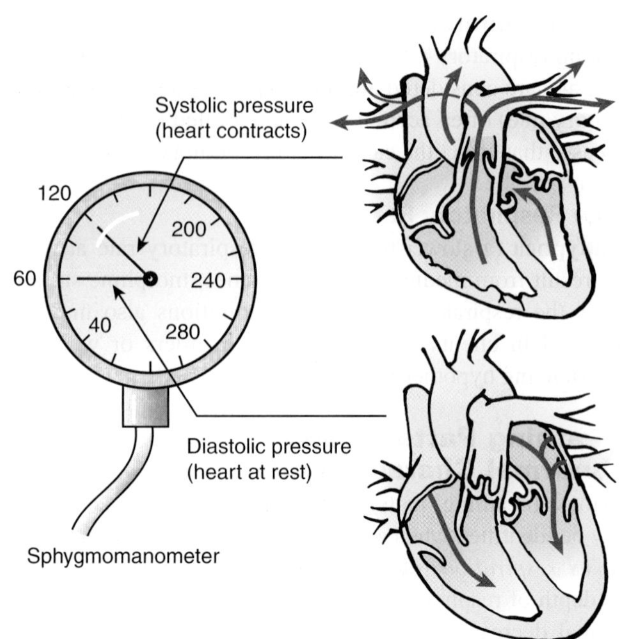

FIGURE 12-16 The pressure of blood in the arteries is higher during systole when the heart contracts and is lower during diastole when the heart muscle relaxes, hence the terms systolic and diastolic pressure.

The **pulse pressure** (the difference between systolic and diastolic blood pressure measurements) is computed by subtracting the smaller measurement from the larger. For example, when the blood pressure is 126/88 mm Hg, the pulse pressure is 38. A pulse pressure between 30 and 50 is considered normal, with 40 being a healthy average.

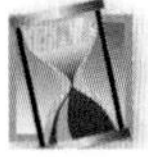

Gerontologic Considerations

■ Some older adults have a wide pulse pressure because of a rising systolic pressure exceeding the rate of diastolic elevation. Such people have a higher incidence of hypertension.

Studies of healthy people show that blood pressure can fluctuate within a wide range and still be normal. Because individual differences can be considerable, analyzing the usual ranges and patterns of blood pressure measurements for each person is important. A rise or fall of 20 to 30 mm Hg in usual pressure is significant, even if it is well within the generally accepted range for normal.

Assessment Sites

Blood pressure usually is assessed over the brachial artery at the inner aspect of the elbow. It is also possible to use the lower arm and radial artery. There are situations in which the nurse must use an alternative to brachial or radial measurement, such as in the following circumstances:

- When the client's arms are missing
- When both of a client's breasts have been removed
- When a client has had vascular surgery (such as that which permits dialysis treatments for kidney failure)
- When dressings or plaster or fiberglass casts obscure the brachial and radial sites

In these and other unusual circumstances, blood pressure is measured over the popliteal artery behind the knee (see sections "Alternative Assessment Techniques" and "Measuring Thigh Blood Pressure"). Documentation of the site is essential because measurements vary depending on the site used.

Equipment for Measuring Blood Pressure

Blood pressure most often is measured with a **sphygmomanometer** (a device for measuring blood pressure), an inflatable cuff, and a stethoscope.

Sphygmomanometer

A sphygmomanometer may be portable or wall mounted. It contains a gauge for measuring the pressure of a gas or liquid. Mercury manometers have always been considered the gold standard; however, health care agencies have eliminated devices containing mercury. Presently, two types of devices are available for measuring blood pressure noninvasively: the aneroid and electronic oscillometric manometers (Fig. 12-17).

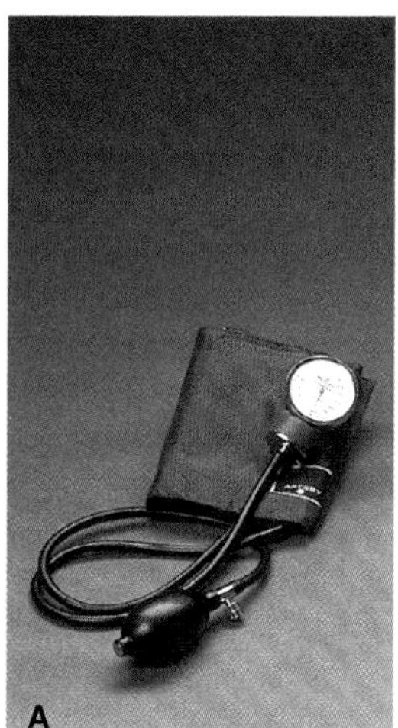

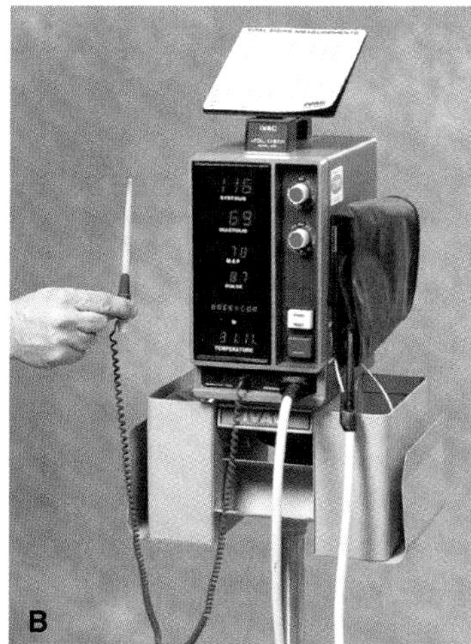

FIGURE 12-17 An aneroid (**A**) and an electronic oscillometric manometer (**B**).

Aneroid Manometer

An aneroid manometer, named from the French word *aneroide*, which means "no liquid," measures pressure using a spring mechanism. Its gauge features a needle that moves around a numbered dial. The numbers correspond to the measurements obtained with a mercury manometer. Before using an aneroid manometer, the needle on the gauge must be positioned at zero to ensure an accurate measurement.

Electronic Oscillometric Manometer

An electronic oscillometric manometer is battery operated or uses power from an electrical outlet. Unlike an aneroid manometer, an electronic oscillometric manometer does not require a stethoscope for auscultating sounds that correspond to pressure measurements. It measures blood pressure with a transducer within the cuff. The transducer is a device that receives sound waves, in this case, from the flow of blood within the artery. The device actually measures the mean arterial pressure and then electronically calculates the systolic and diastolic pressure using a preprogrammed formula. The calculated pressures are visually displayed. Models vary from those used in intensive care settings to others intended for home use.

Aneroid and electronic monitors have advantages and disadvantages (Table 12-8). Either can be used to assess blood pressure, provided they are working properly and are used correctly.

Inflatable Cuff

The cuff of a sphygmomanometer contains an inflatable bladder to which two tubes are attached. One is connected to the manometer, which registers the pressure. The other is attached to a bulb that is used to inflate the bladder with air. A screw valve on the bulb allows the nurse to fill and empty the bladder. As the air escapes, the pressure is measured.

Cuffs come in various sizes. A common guide (Fig. 12-18) is to use a cuff that has a bladder width of at least 40% and a length that is 80% to 100% of midlimb circumference (Pickering et al., 2005). *Note that it is not the width and length of the cuff itself, but rather the inflatable bladder that must be the correct size.*

If the cuff is too wide, the blood pressure reading will be falsely low. If the cuff is too narrow, the blood pressure reading will be falsely high. At the working meeting on blood pressure measurement under the auspices of the National High Blood Pressure Education Program, the National Heart, Lung, and Blood Institute, and the American Heart Association in April 2002, it was noted that the mean arm circumference of US adults is increasing because of the growing trend toward obesity. This means that the standard adult blood pressure cuff no longer corresponds to a "standard adult" because more and more adults require a "large adult" cuff when the blood pressure is measured. The nurse must select a cuff with an appropriate bladder size for the body proportions of each client.

TABLE 12-8 Comparisons of Sphygmomanometer Equipment

TYPE	ADVANTAGES	DISADVANTAGES
Aneroid	Inexpensive Easy to carry and store Ability to read the gauge from any position	Delicate Periodic equipment checking against a second sphygmomanometer necessary for accuracy Gauge possibly clumsy to attach to cuff Stethoscope and accurate hearing necessary Calibration check and readjustment recommended yearly Manufacturer repair required
Electronic	Digital display of measurement No stethoscope required Accurate for people with hearing loss Facilitation of blood pressure measurement of newborns and infants in whom auscultation (listening with a stethoscope) is difficult	Expensive depending on quality Batteries necessary Body movements and improper cuff application can influence accuracy Calibration check and readjustment recommended every 6 months Manufacturer repair needed

Adapted from Blood pressure: Buying and caring for home equipment. *American Heart Association*, 1999.

Stethoscope

A **stethoscope** (an instrument that carries sound to the ears) is composed of eartips, a brace and binaurals, and tubing leading to a chest piece that may be a bell, diaphragm, or both (Fig. 12-19). The eartips are generally rubber or plastic. When the stethoscope is used, the eartips are positioned downward and forward within the ears to produce the best sound perception. If various people are using stethoscopes in common, they must clean the eartips with alcohol pads between uses. Personal stethoscopes also need periodic cleaning to keep the eartips free of cerumen and dirt.

The brace and binaurals are generally made of metal. They connect the eartips to the tubing and chest piece. The brace prevents the tubing from kinking and distorting the sound. Stethoscope tubing is rubber or plastic. The best length for good sound conduction is about 20 in. (50 cm).

The bell, or cup-shaped chest piece, is used to detect low-pitched sounds such as those produced in blood vessels.

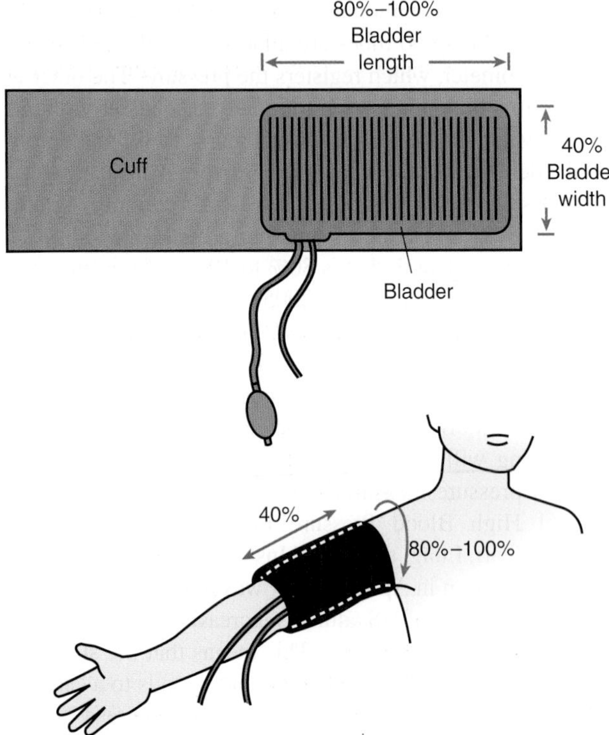

FIGURE 12-18 To determine the appropriate size of blood pressure cuff, the width of the bladder should be 40% of the midarm circumference and the length should be at least 80%.

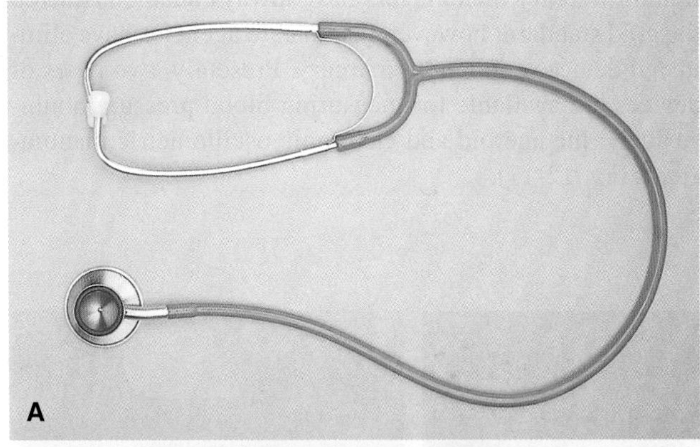

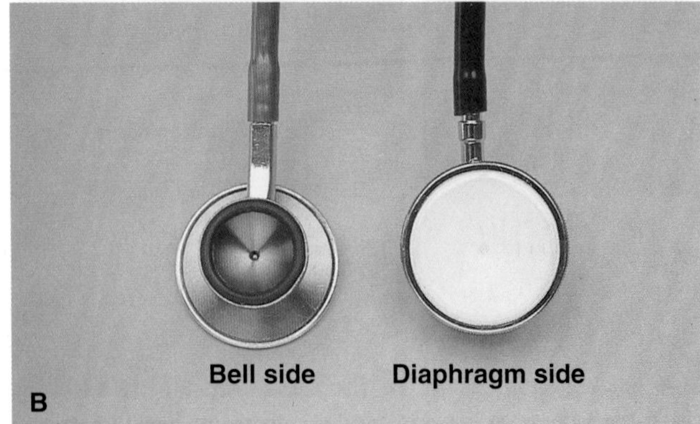

FIGURE 12-19 A stethoscope (**A**) and a chest piece (**B**).

The diaphragm, or disk-shaped chest piece, detects high-pitched sounds such as those in the lungs, heart, or abdomen. A cracked diaphragm must be replaced. When the bell is used, care is taken to position it lightly over the anatomic area because pressure flattens the skin and creates the same effect as a diaphragm.

Measuring Blood Pressure

The first time blood pressure is measured, it is assessed in each arm. The two blood pressure measurements should not vary more than 5 to 10 mm Hg unless pathology (disease) is present. Some agencies include a blood pressure assessment of the client in lying, sitting, and standing positions for the initial database. Several variables can result in inaccurate blood pressure measurements (Table 12-9).

Korotkoff Sounds

Most blood pressure recordings are obtained indirectly. That is, they are determined by applying a blood pressure cuff, briefly occluding arterial blood flow, and listening for **Korotkoff sounds** (sounds that result from the vibrations of blood within the arterial wall or changes in blood flow). Blood pressure measurements are determined by correlating the phases of Korotkoff sounds with the numbers on the sphygmomanometer. If Korotkoff sounds are difficult to hear, they can be intensified in one of two ways:

- Have the client elevate the arm before and during cuff inflation, then lower the arm after full inflation.
- Have the client open and close the fist after cuff inflation.

Korotkoff sounds have five unique phases (Fig. 12-20). *Phase I* begins with the first faint but clear tapping sound that follows a period of silence as pressure is released from the cuff. When the first sound occurs, it corresponds to the peak pressure in the arterial system during heart contraction, or the systolic pressure measurement. It is recorded as the first number in the fraction.

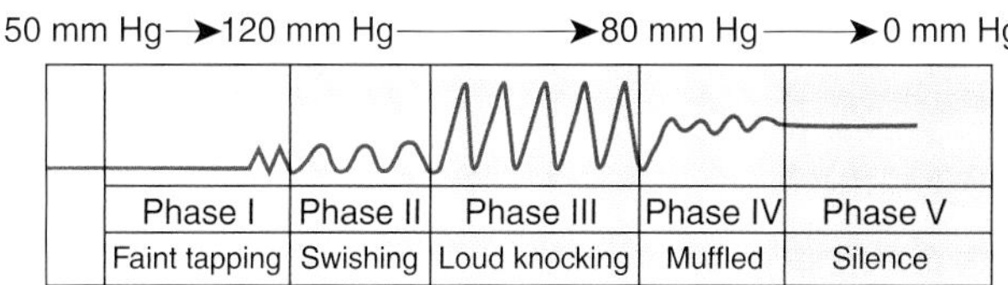

FIGURE 12-20 Characteristics of Korotkoff sounds.

The first sound, which is heard for at least two consecutive beats, may be missed if the cuff pressure is not initially pumped high enough. Palpating for the disappearance of a distal pulse when inflating the cuff helps to ensure that the cuff pressure is above arterial pressure.

Phase I sounds may disappear briefly before they become reestablished, especially in older adults and in clients with high blood pressure or peripheral arterial disease. An **auscultatory gap** (a period during which sound disappears) can range as much as 40 mm Hg. Failure to identify the first sound preceding an auscultatory gap results in an inaccurate blood pressure assessment from undermeasurement of the systolic pressure. Consequently, many clients with hypertension may be unidentified and thus, undiagnosed and untreated.

Phase II is characterized by a change from tapping sounds to swishing sounds. At this time, the diameter of the artery is widening, allowing more arterial blood flow.

Phase III is characterized by a change to loud and distinct sounds described as crisp knocking sounds. During this phase, blood flows relatively freely through the artery once more.

Phase IV sounds are muffled and have a blowing quality. The sound change results from a loss in the transmission of pressure from the deflating cuff to the artery. The point at which the sound becomes muffled is considered the first diastolic pressure measurement. It is generally preferred when documenting blood pressure measurements in children.

Phase V is the point at which the last sound is heard, or the second diastolic pressure measurement. This is considered the best reflection of adult diastolic pressure because phase IV

TABLE 12-9 Common Causes of Blood Pressure Assessment Errors

CAUSE	EFFECT	CORRECTION
Inaccurate manometer calibration	False high or low readings	Recalibrate, repair, or replace gauge
Loosely applied cuff	High reading	Wrap snugly with equal pressure about extremity
Cuff too small for extremity	High reading	Select appropriate size
Cuff too large for extremity	Low reading	Select appropriate size
Cuff applied over clothing	Creates noise or interferes with sound perception	Remove arm from sleeve or have client don a gown
Tubing that leaks	Rapid loss of pressure	Replace or repair
Improper positioning of eartips	Poor sound conduction	Reposition and retake blood pressure
Impaired hearing	Altered sound perception	Use an alternative assessment technique or equipment
Loud environmental noise	Interferes with sound perception	Reduce noise and reassess
Impaired vision	Inaccurate observation of gauge	Correct vision; reposition gauge in adequate range
Rapid cuff deflation	Inaccurate observation of gauge	Reassess and deflate at 2 to 3 mm Hg/second
Number bias	Falsely high or low measurements	Use an electronic sphygmomanometer

is often 7 to 10 mm Hg higher than direct diastolic pressure measurements. When recording adult blood pressure measurements, the pressures at phases I and V are used.

Studies have shown that some health care workers do not record auscultated measurements accurately because they have a number bias. In other words, they prefer recording auscultated measurements in even numbers or zero. Blood pressure measurements using an electronic sphygmomanometer or other nonauscultatory hybrid sphygmomanometers that are being developed could eliminate number biases and provide more accurate measurements (National Institutes of Health, Working Meeting on Blood Pressure Measurement, 2002).

Directions for standard auscultatory blood pressure measurements are given in Skill 12-4.

Alternative Assessment Techniques

When Korotkoff sounds are difficult to hear in the usual manner no matter how conscientious the effort to augment them, nurses can assess blood pressure using alternative methods. They can measure blood pressure by palpation or by using a Doppler stethoscope. When blood pressure requires frequent or prolonged assessment, an automated blood pressure machine is necessary. When the brachial or radial artery is inaccessible in both arms or assessing blood pressure at these sites is contraindicated, the thigh is an optional alternative.

Palpating the Blood Pressure

When palpating the blood pressure, the nurse applies a blood pressure cuff. Instead of using a stethoscope, however, he or she positions the fingers over the artery while releasing the cuff pressure. The point at which the nurse feels the first pulsation corresponds to the systolic pressure. The diastolic pressure cannot be measured because there is no perceptible change in the quality of pulsations like there is in the sounds. When recording a blood pressure taken this way, it is important to indicate that palpation was used.

Doppler Stethoscope

A **Doppler stethoscope** (Fig. 12-21) helps to detect sounds created by the velocity of blood moving through a blood vessel. The sounds of moving blood cells are reflected toward the ultrasound receiver, producing a tone. The nurse notes the pressure at which the sound occurs. The onset of sound represents the peak pressure of arterial blood flow. A description of how Doppler is used was given earlier in this chapter. When documenting the pressure measurement, the nurse writes a D to indicate the use of Doppler.

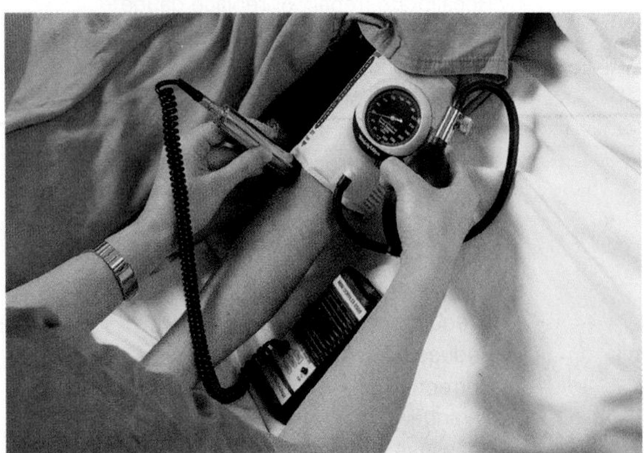

FIGURE 12-21 A Doppler stethoscope is used when Korotkoff sounds are difficult to hear.

Automatic Blood Pressure Monitoring

An automatic electronic blood pressure monitoring device consists of a blood pressure cuff attached to a microprocessing unit. Such devices diagnose unusual fluctuations in blood pressure that single or sporadic monitoring cannot identify. When used, the device records the client's blood pressure every 10 to 30 minutes or as needed over 24 hours. It stores the data in the microprocessor's memory. Measurements are printed or transferred by hand to a flow sheet for vital signs. Outpatients can wear a portable model supported either at the shoulder or waist to help diagnose conditions in which blood pressure is altered.

Measuring Thigh Blood Pressure

The thigh is a structure that corresponds anatomically to the upper arm. Nurses use this site for blood pressure assessment when they cannot obtain readings in either of the client's arms. The systolic measurement tends to be 10% to 20% higher than that obtained in the arms, but the diastolic measurement is similar (Brownfield, 2004). Skill 12-5 describes the technique for obtaining a thigh blood pressure measurement.

Stop, Think, and Respond Box 12-5

What suggestions would you offer to a nurse who has difficulty hearing Korotkoff sounds when assessing a client's blood pressure?

Abnormal Blood Pressure Measurements

Blood pressures above or below normal ranges may indicate significant health problems.

High Blood Pressure

Hypertension (high blood pressure) exists when the systolic pressure, diastolic pressure, or both are sustained above normal levels for the person's age. For adults 18 years or older, the Joint National Committee on Prevention, Detection, Evaluation, and Treatment of High Blood Pressure (2004) considers a systolic pressure of 140 mm Hg or greater and a diastolic pressure of 90 mm Hg or greater to be abnormally high (Table 12-10); these guidelines are due to be updated in Spring 2012. An occasional elevation in blood pressure does not necessarily mean a person has hypertension. It does mean that the blood pressure should be monitored at various intervals depending on the significance of the measurements (Table 12-11). Monitoring is especially important to determine whether the elevated blood pressure is sustained or is the result of **white-coat hypertension** (a condition in which the blood pressure is elevated when taken by a health care worker but normal at other times).

TABLE 12-10 Classification of Adult Blood Pressure Measurements

CATEGORY	SYSTOLIC (MM HG)		DIASTOLIC (MM HG)
Normal[a]	<120	and	<80
Prehypertension	120–139	or	80–89
Hypertension[b]			
Stage 1	140–159	or	90–99
Stage 2	160 or higher	or	100 or higher

[a]Normal blood pressure with respect to cardiovascular risk is below 120/80 mm Hg. However, unusually low readings should be evaluated for clinical significance.

[b]Based on the average or two or more readings taken at each of two or more visits after an initial screening.

Classification terms and measurements from the seventh report of the Joint National Committee on Prevention, Detection, Evaluation, and Treatment of High Blood Pressure, 2004.

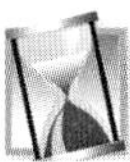

Gerontologic Considerations

■ Older adults may use self-monitoring devices or blood pressure monitors at community settings, but these monitors should be validated for accuracy.

Hypertensive blood pressure measurements often are associated with the following:

- Anxiety
- Obesity
- Vascular diseases
- Stroke
- Heart failure
- Kidney diseases

TABLE 12-11 Recommendations for Follow-up Based on Initial Set of Blood Pressure Measurements

INITIAL BLOOD PRESSURE (MM HG)[a]		RECOMMENDED FOLLOW-UP[b]
Systolic	Diastolic	
<120	<80	Recheck in 2 years
120–139	80–89	Recheck in 1 year[c]
140–159	90–99	Confirm within 2 months[d]
160–179	100–109	Evaluate or refer to source of care within 1 month
≥180	≥110	Evaluate or refer to source of care immediately or within 1 week depending on clinical situation

[a]If systolic and diastolic categories are different, follow recommendations for shorter follow-up (eg, client with 160/86 mm Hg should be evaluated or referred to source of care within 1 month).

[b]Modify the scheduling of follow-up according to reliable information about past blood pressure measurements, other cardiovascular risk factors, or target organ disease.

[c]Provide advice about lifestyle modifications.

From the seventh report of the Joint National Committee for the Detection, Evaluation, and Treatment of High Blood Pressure, National Heart, Lung, and Blood Institute, National Institutes of Health, 2004.

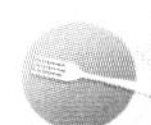

Nutrition Notes

■ Individuals who are prehypertensive or who have hypertension may lower their blood pressure by adopting the Dietary Approaches to Stop Hypertension (DASH) eating plan. It features generous amounts of fruits, vegetables, and low-fat or nonfat milk and milk products, and encourages whole grains, fish, poultry, and nuts. Red meats, sweets, and foods with added sugars are limited. Reducing sodium intake to 2,300 mg (the amount in 1 teaspoon of salt) or lower (1,500 mg/day) improves the blood pressure lowering effect of DASH (National Heart Lung and Blood Institute, 2006).

Low Blood Pressure

Hypotension (low blood pressure) is when blood pressure measurements are below the normal systolic values for the person's age. Having a consistently low pressure, 96/60 mm Hg, for example, seems to cause no harm. In fact, low blood pressure usually is associated with efficient functioning of the heart and blood vessels. People with low blood pressure, however, should continue to be monitored to evaluate its significance. Low blood pressure measurements may indicate shock, hemorrhage, or side effects from drugs.

Postural Hypotension

Postural or **orthostatic hypotension** (a sudden but temporary drop in blood pressure when rising from a reclining position) is most common in those with circulatory problems, those who are dehydrated, and those who take diuretics or other drugs that lower blood pressure. A consequence of a sudden drop in blood pressure is dizziness and fainting. Skill 12-6 describes an assessment of postural hypotension for clients in high-risk categories or who become symptomatic during care.

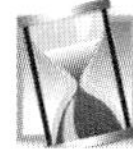

Gerontologic Considerations

■ Older adults are more susceptible to postural and postprandial hypotension (a drop in blood pressure of 20 mm Hg within 1 hour of eating a meal). If hypotension is assessed in a client, plan for limited activities during the hour following eating or for frequent, smaller food consumption throughout the day.

DOCUMENTING VITAL SIGNS

Once nurses have obtained vital sign measurements, they are documented in the medical record for analysis of patterns and trends (Fig. 12-22). They also may be entered as data, along with any other subjective or objective information, elsewhere in the client's record such as in the narrative nursing notes.

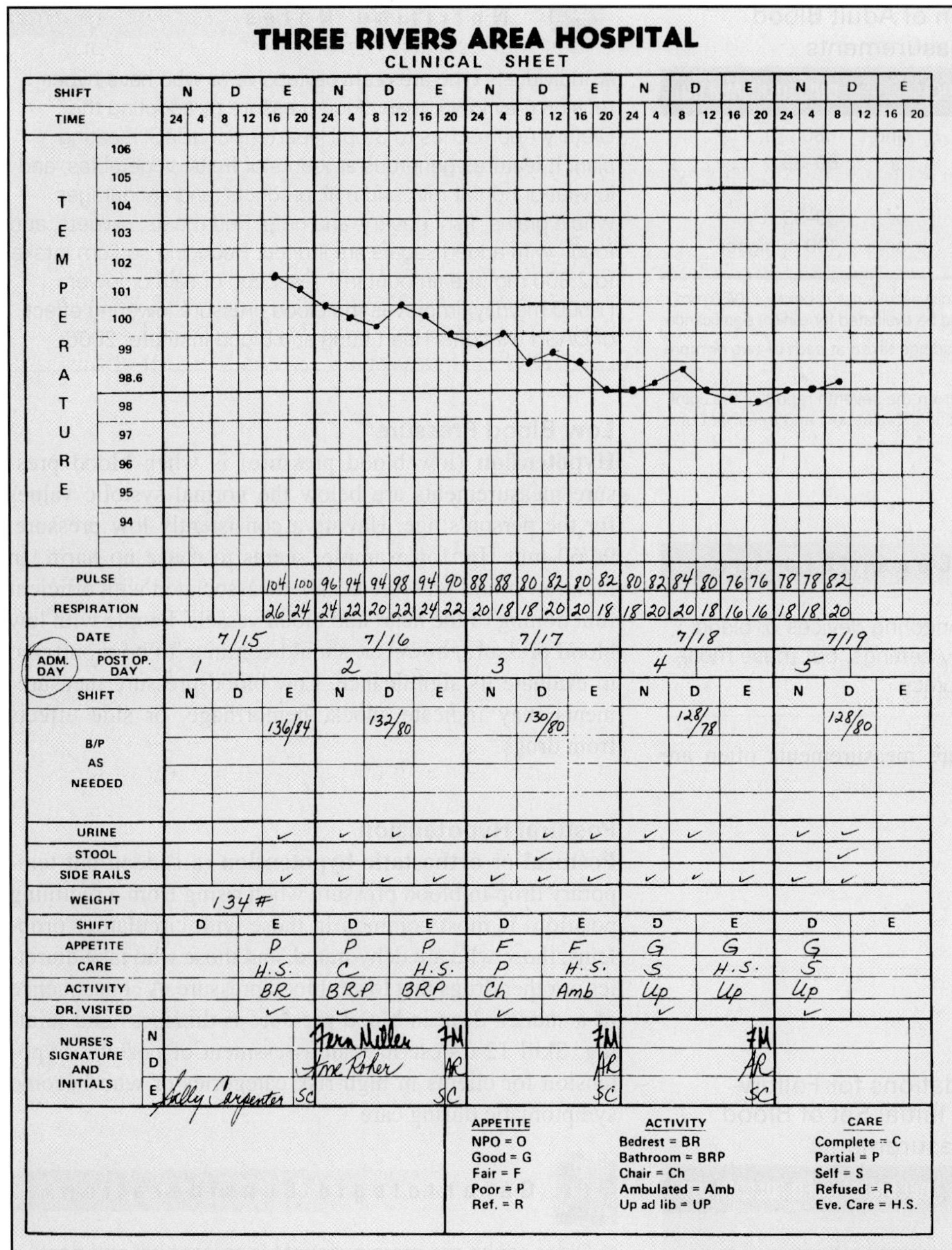

THREE RIVERS AREA HOSPITAL

CLINICAL SHEET

TEMPERATURE: 106, 105, 104, 103, 102, 101, 100, 99, 98.6, 98, 97, 96, 95, 94

SHIFT	N		D		E		N		D		E		N		D		E		N		D		E		N		D		E	
TIME	24	4	8	12	16	20	24	4	8	12	16	20	24	4	8	12	16	20	24	4	8	12	16	20	24	4	8	12	16	20
PULSE					104	100	96	94	94	98	94	90	88	88	80	82	80	82	80	82	84	80	76	76	78	78	82			
RESPIRATION					26	24	24	22	20	22	24	22	20	18	18	20	20	18	18	20	20	18	16	16	18	18	20			

DATE	7/15			7/16			7/17			7/18			7/19		
ADM. DAY / POST OP. DAY	1			2			3			4			5		
SHIFT	N	D	E	N	D	E	N	D	E	N	D	E	N	D	E
B/P AS NEEDED			136/84		132/80			130/80			128/78			128/80	
URINE			✓	✓	✓		✓	✓	✓	✓	✓		✓	✓	
STOOL								✓						✓	
SIDE RAILS			✓	✓	✓	✓	✓	✓	✓	✓	✓	✓	✓	✓	
WEIGHT	134#														

SHIFT	D	E	D	E	D	E	D	E	D	E
APPETITE		P	P	P	F	F	G	G	G	
CARE		H.S.	C	H.S.	P	H.S.	S	H.S.	S	
ACTIVITY		BR	BRP	BRP	Ch	Amb	Up	Up	Up	
DR. VISITED		✓	✓		✓		✓		✓	

NURSE'S SIGNATURE AND INITIALS
N: Fern Miller FM FM FM
D: Anne Roher AR AR AR
E: Sally Carpenter SC SC SC SC

APPETITE	ACTIVITY	CARE
NPO = O	Bedrest = BR	Complete = C
Good = G	Bathroom = BRP	Partial = P
Fair = F	Chair = Ch	Self = S
Poor = P	Ambulated = Amb	Refused = R
Ref. = R	Up ad lib = UP	Eve. Care = H.S.

FIGURE 12-22 A graphic recording of vital signs.

NURSING IMPLICATIONS

Vital sign assessment is part of every client's care and forms the basis for identifying problems. Based on the analysis of assessment data, the nurse may identify one or more of the following nursing diagnoses:

- Hyperthermia
- Hypothermia
- Ineffective thermoregulation
- Decreased cardiac output
- Risk for injury
- Ineffective breathing pattern

CRITICAL THINKING EXERCISES

1. When visiting a friend with a fever, you see that the only thermometer available is made of glass and contains mercury. What suggestions for replacement would you offer when your friend feels better?
2. A neighbor with no medical experience asks how to tell if her 4-year-old child has a fever. What advice would you give?

3. An 80-year-old client explains that, as an economy measure, she keeps her thermostat set at 65°F. What health information would be appropriate, considering this woman's age?
4. While participating in a community health assessment, you discover a person with a blood pressure that measures 190/110 mm Hg. What actions are appropriate at this time?

NCLEX-STYLE REVIEW QUESTIONS

1. Upon observing a nursing assistant taking a client's vital signs (oral temperature, pulse rate, respiratory rate, and blood pressure) immediately after breakfast, what instruction should the nurse give the nursing assistant?
   1. Obtain the client's apical-radial heart rate.
   2. Wait 15 minutes to assess the client's pulse.
   3. Assess the client's temperature in 30 minutes.
   4. Take the blood pressure with the client lying down.
2. What nursing action is best when a client with a temperature of 103.6°F is shivering?
   1. Offer the client a cup of hot soup.
   2. Cover the client with a light blanket.
   3. Direct a fan in the client's direction
   4. Darken the room to provide rest.
3. While assessing a client's radial pulse, the nurse notes that it disappears with very slight pressure. What is the best description for the nurse to use when documenting the quality of the pulse?
   1. Normal
   2. Weak
   3. Thready
   4. Diminished
4. Before assessing an adult client's blood pressure, the nurse is most correct in selecting a blood pressure cuff with a bladder width that is 40% and a bladder length that encircles at least what percent of the client's upper arm?
   1. 40%
   2. 60%
   3. 80%
   4. 100%
5. If the nurse detects that a client has symptoms associated with orthostatic hypotension, what is the best instruction the nurse can offer the client?
   1. Limit consumption of fluids during the day.
   2. Rise slowly from a lying or sitting position.
   3. Remain on bed rest throughout care in the health agency.
   4. Ambulate about the health agency at least four times a day.

SKILL 12-1 Assessing Body Temperature

Suggested Action	Reason for Action
ASSESSMENT	
Determine when and how frequently to monitor the client's temperature (see Box 12-1) and the type of thermometer previously used.	Demonstrates accountability for making timely and appropriate assessments; ensures consistency in the technique for gathering data.
Review previously recorded temperature measurements.	Aids in identifying trends and analyzing significant patterns.
If using an oral electronic or digital thermometer:	
Observe the client's ability to support a thermometer within the mouth and breathe adequately through the nose with the mouth closed.	Shows consideration for accuracy because thermal energy is transferred from the oral cavity to the thermometer probe; escape of heat invalidates the measurement.
Read the client's history for any reference to recent seizures or a seizure disorder.	Shows consideration for safety and identifies possible contraindication for oral site.
Determine whether the client consumed any hot or cold substances or smoked a cigarette within the past 30 minutes.	Shows consideration for accuracy because the temperature in the oral cavity can be temporarily altered from substances recently placed within the mouth.
PLANNING	
Arrange to take the client's temperature as near to the scheduled routine as possible.	Ensures consistency and accuracy.
Gather supplies including a thermometer, watch, and probe cover or disposable sleeve if needed. Include lubricant, paper tissues, and gloves if using the rectal site or other route if there is a potential for contact with body secretions.	Promotes efficiency, accuracy, and safety.
(Use of gloves is determined on an individual basis. The virus that causes AIDS has not been shown to be transmitted through contact with oral secretions unless they contain blood; thorough handwashing or hand antisepsis is always appropriate after any client contact.)	
IMPLEMENTATION	
Introduce yourself to the client if you have not done so during earlier contact.	Demonstrates responsibility and accountability.
Explain the procedure to the client.	Reduces apprehension and promotes cooperation.
Wash hands or perform hand antisepsis with an alcohol rub (see Chap. 10).	Reduces the spread of microorganisms.
Electronic Thermometer	
Remove the electronic unit from the charging base.	Promotes portability.
Select the oral or rectal probe depending on the intended site for assessment.	Ensures appropriate use.
Insert the probe into a disposable cover until it locks into place (Fig. A).	Protects the probe from contamination with secretions containing microorganisms.

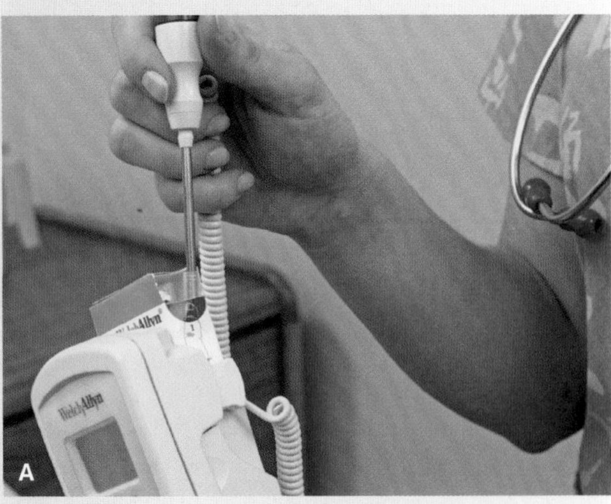

Inserting the probe into a disposable cover. (Photo by Rick Brady.)

(continued)

Assessing Body Temperature (continued)

IMPLEMENTATION (CONTINUED)

Oral Method

Place the covered probe beneath the tongue to the right or left of the **frenulum** (structure that attaches the underneath surface of the tongue to the fleshy portion of the mouth) (Fig. B).

Locates the probe near the sublingual artery to ensure correct location.

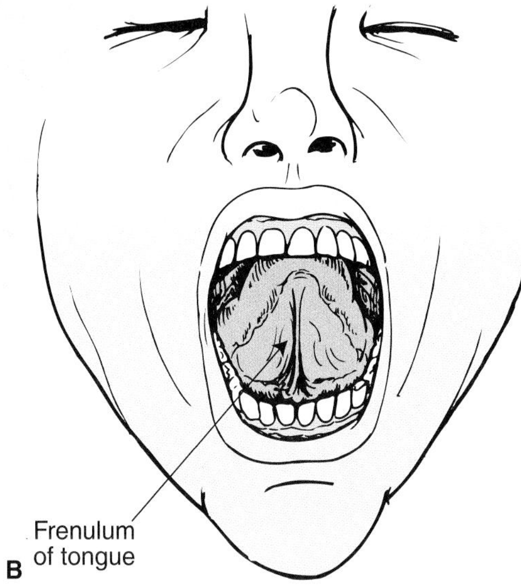

Location for oral temperature assessment.

Hold probe in place (Fig. C).

Supports the probe so that it does not drift away from its intended location; ensures valid data collection.

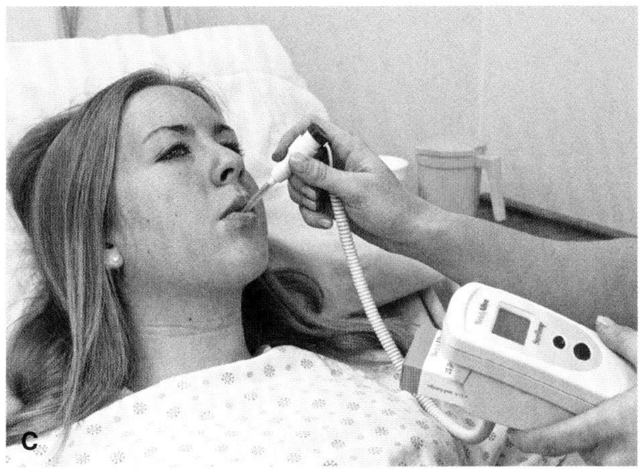

Maintaining the probe in position. (Photo by Rick Brady.)

Maintain the probe in position until an audible sound occurs.

Signals when the sensed temperature remains constant.

Observe the numbers displayed on the electronic unit.

Indicates temperature measurement.

(continued)

Assessing Body Temperature (continued)

IMPLEMENTATION (CONTINUED)

Remove the probe and eject the probe cover into a lined receptacle (Fig. D). — Confines contaminated objects to an area for proper disposal without direct contact.

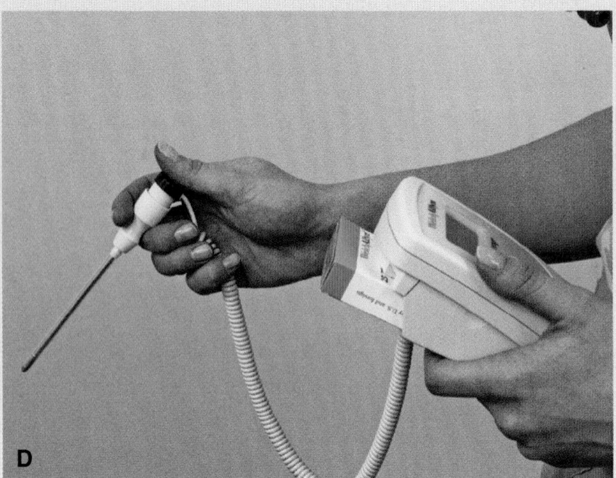

D — Releasing the probe cover. (Photo by Rick Brady.)

Replace the probe in the storage holder within the electronic unit. — Prevents damage to the probe attachment.

Rectal Method

Provide privacy. — Demonstrates respect for the client's dignity.

Lubricate approximately 1″ (2.5 cm) of the rectal probe cover. — Promotes comfort and ease of insertion.

Position the client on the side with the upper leg slightly flexed at the hip and knee (Sims' position). — Helps to locate the anus and facilitate probe insertion.

Instruct the client to breathe deeply. — Relaxes the rectal sphincter and reduces discomfort during insertion.

Insert the thermometer approximately 1.5 in. (3.8 cm) in an adult, 1 in. (2.5 cm) in a child, and 0.5 in. (1.25 cm) in an infant (Fig. E).

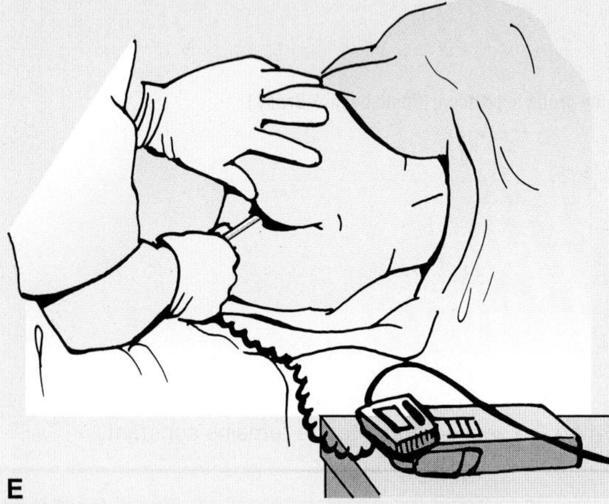

E — Rectal thermometer insertion.

Maintain the probe in position until an audible sound occurs. — Signals when the sensed temperature remains constant.

Observe the numbers displayed on the electronic unit. — Indicates temperature measurement.

Remove the probe and eject the probe cover into a lined receptacle (see Fig. D). — Confines contaminated objects to an area for proper disposal without direct contact.

Replace the probe in the storage holder within the electronic unit. — Prevents damage to the probe attachment.

Wipe lubricant and any stool from around the client's rectum. — Demonstrates concern for the client's hygiene and comfort.

Remove and discard gloves, if worn; wash hands or perform hand antisepsis with an alcohol rub (see Chap. 10). — Reduces the transmission of microorganisms.

(continued)

Assessing Body Temperature (continued)

IMPLEMENTATION (CONTINUED)

Axillary Method

Insert the thermometer into the center of the axilla and lower the client's arm to enclose the thermometer between the two folds of skin (Fig. F). — Confines the tip of the thermometer so that room air does not affect it.

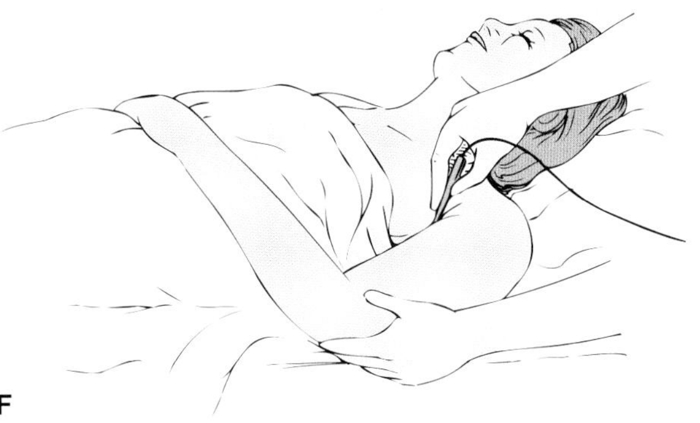

F

Placement for an auxiliary temperature assessment.

Hold the probe in place. — Supports the probe so it does not drift away from its intended location; ensures valid data collection.

Maintain the probe in position until an audible sound occurs. — Signals when the sensed temperature remains constant.

Remove the probe and eject the probe cover into a lined receptacle (see Fig. D). — Confines contaminated objects to an area for proper disposal without direct contact.

Replace the probe in the storage holder within the electronic unit. — Prevents damage to the probe attachment.

Return the electronic unit to its charging base. — Facilitates reuse.

Record the assessment measurement on the graphic sheet or flow sheet, or in the narrative nursing notes. — Provides documentation for future comparisons.

Verbally report elevated or subnormal temperatures. — Alerts others to monitor the client closely and make changes in the care plan.

Infrared Tympanic Thermometer

Remove the thermometer component from its holding cradle (Fig. G). — Facilitates insertion of the tympanic **speculum** (funnel-shaped instrument used to widen and support an opening in the body).

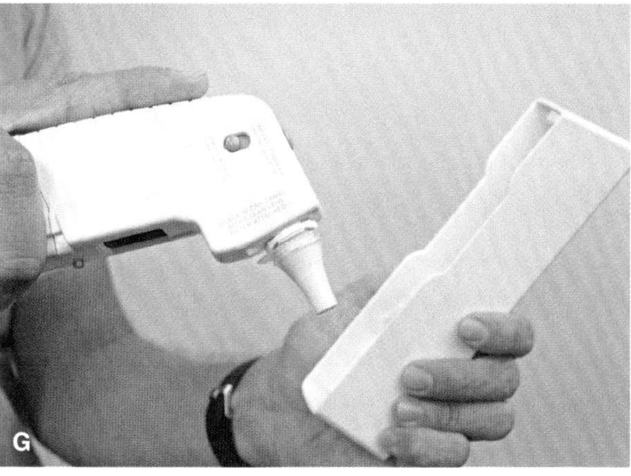

G

A tympanic thermometer and cradle. (Photo by Rick Brady.)

Inspect the tip of the thermometer for damage and the lens for cleanliness. — Promotes safety and hygiene.

Replace a cracked or broken tip; clean the lens with a dry wipe or lint-free swab moistened with a small amount of isopropyl alcohol, and then wipe to remove the alcohol film. — Ensures accurate data collection.

(continued)

Assessing Body Temperature (continued)

IMPLEMENTATION (CONTINUED)

Action	Rationale
Wait 30 min after cleaning with alcohol.	Allows the thermometer to readjust after the cooling effect created by alcohol evaporation.
Cover the speculum with a disposable cover until it locks in place.	Maintains cleanliness of the tip.
Press the mode button to select the choice of **temperature translation** (conversion of tympanic temperature into an oral, rectal, or core temperature).	Adjusts the tympanic measurement, norms for which have not been established, into more common frames of reference. The rectal equivalent is recommended for children younger than 3 years.
Depress the mode button for several seconds to select either Fahrenheit or centigrade.	Eliminates the need to calculate conversion measurements by hand.
Hold the probe in your dominant hand.	Improves motor skill and coordination.
Position the client with the head turned 90 degrees, exposing the ear with the hand holding the probe.	Promotes proper probe placement; if the right hand is holding the probe, the left ear is assessed.
Wait for display of a "Ready" message.	Indicates offset has been programmed.
Pull the external ear of adults up and back by grasping the external ear at its midpoint with your nondominant hand; for children 6 years and younger, pull the ear down and back.	Straightens the ear canal.
Insert the probe into the ear, advancing it with a gentle back-and-forth motion until it seals the ear canal.	Seals the tip of the probe within the ear canal and confines the radiated heat within the area of the probe.
Point the tip of the probe in an imaginary line between the sideburn hair and the eyebrow on the opposite side of the face (Fig. H).	Positions the probe in direct alignment with the tympanic membrane; if pointed elsewhere, the infrared sensor detects the temperature of surrounding tissue rather than membrane temperature.

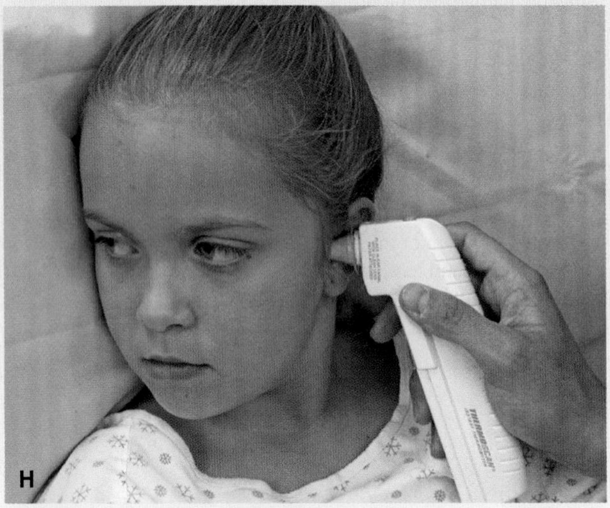

H

The placement of a probe for accurate tympanic assessment. (Photo by Rick Brady.)

Action	Rationale
Press the button that activates the thermometer as soon as the probe is in position.	Initiates electronic sensing; for some models, this action must be done within 25 seconds of having removed the thermometer from its holding cradle.
Keep the probe within the ear until the thermometer emits a sound or flashing light.	Indicates that the procedure is complete.

(continued)

Assessing Body Temperature (continued)

IMPLEMENTATION (CONTINUED)

Repeat the procedure after waiting 2 minutes if this is the first use of the tympanic thermometer since it was recharged.	Ensures accuracy with a second assessment.
Read the temperature, remove the thermometer from the ear, and release the probe cover into a lined receptacle (Fig. I).	Controls the transmission of microorganisms.

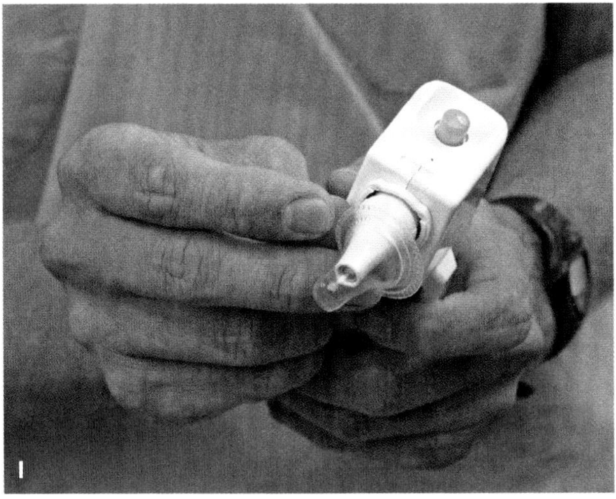

Disposing of the probe cover. (Photo by Rick Brady.)

Record the assessment measurement on the graphic sheet or flowsheet, or in the narrative nursing notes.	Provides documentation for future comparisons.
Verbally report elevated or subnormal temperatures.	Alerts others to monitor the client closely and make changes in the plan for care.

Evaluation

- Thermometer remained inserted the appropriate time.
- Level of temperature is consistent with accompanying signs and symptoms.
- Thermometer and surrounding tissue remain intact.

Document

- Date and time
- Degree of heat to the nearest tenth
- Temperature scale
- Site of assessment
- Accompanying signs and symptoms
- To whom abnormal information was reported and the outcome of the interaction

SAMPLE DOCUMENTATION

Date and Time T 102.4°F (O). States, "I feel cold and my throat hurts." Pharynx looks beefy red. Reported to Dr. Washington. New orders for throat culture. ——— SIGNATURE/TITLE

SKILL 12-2 Assessing the Radial Pulse

Suggested Action	Reason for Action
ASSESSMENT	
Determine when and how frequently to monitor the client's pulse (see Box 12-1).	Demonstrates accountability for making timely and appropriate assessments.
Review data collected in previous assessments of the pulse or abnormalities in other vital signs.	Aids in identifying trends and analyzing significant patterns.
Read the client's history for any reference to cardiac or vascular disorders.	Demonstrates an understanding of factors that may affect the pulse rate.
Review the list of prescribed drugs for any that may have cardiac effects.	Helps in analyzing the results of assessment findings.
PLANNING	
Arrange to take the client's pulse as near to the scheduled routine as possible.	Ensures consistency and accuracy.
Make sure a watch or wall clock with a second hand is available.	Ensures accurate timing when counting pulsations.
Plan to assess the client's pulse after 5 minutes of inactivity.	Reflects the characteristics of the pulse at rest rather than data that may be influenced by activity.
Plan to use the right or left radial pulse site unless it is inaccessible or difficult to palpate.	Provides consistency in evaluating data.
IMPLEMENTATION	
Introduce yourself to the client, if you have not done so earlier.	Demonstrates responsibility and accountability.
Explain the procedure to the client.	Reduces apprehension and promotes cooperation.
Raise the height of the bed.	Reduces musculoskeletal strain.
Wash hands or perform hand antisepsis with an alcohol rub (see Chap. 10).	Reduces the spread of microorganisms.
Help the client to a position of comfort.	Avoids stress or pain from influencing the pulse rate.
Rest or support the client's forearm with the wrist extended (Fig. A).	Provides access to the radial artery and relaxes the arm.

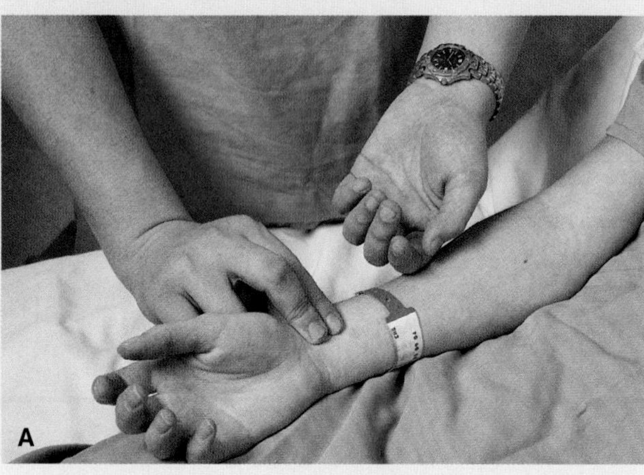

Locating the radial pulse.

Suggested Action	Reason for Action
Press the first and second fingertips toward the radius while feeling for a recurrent pulsation.	Ensures accuracy because the nurse may feel his or her own pulse if using the thumb; light palpation should not obliterate the pulse.
Palpate the rhythm and volume of the pulse once it is located.	Provides comprehensive assessment data.
Note the position of the second hand on the clock or watch.	Identifies the point at which the assessment begins.
Count the number of pulsations for 15 or 30 seconds and multiply the number by 4 or 2, respectively. If the pulse is irregular, count for a full minute.	Provides pulse rate data. A regular pulse rate should not vary whether it is counted for a full minute or some portion thereof, whereas the rate of an irregular pulse may be significantly inaccurate if assessed for less than a full minute.
Write down the pulse rate.	Ensures accurate documentation.
Restore the client to a therapeutic position or one that provides comfort, and lower the bed.	Demonstrates responsibility for client care, safety, and comfort.
Record the assessed measurement on the graphic sheet or the flow sheet, or in the narrative nursing notes.	Provides documentation for future comparisons.
Verbally report rapid or slow pulse rates.	Alerts others to monitor the client closely and to make changes in the plan for care.

(continued)

Assessing the Radial Pulse (continued)

Evaluation

- Pulse rate remained palpable throughout the assessment.
- Pulse rate is consistent with the client's condition.

Document

- Date and time
- Assessment site
- Rate of pulsations per minute, pulse volume, and rhythm
- Accompanying signs and symptoms, if appropriate
- To whom abnormal information was reported and the outcome of the interaction

SAMPLE DOCUMENTATION

Date and Time Radial pulse 88 bpm full and regular. ——— SIGNATURE/TITLE

SKILL 12-3 Assessing the Respiratory Rate

Suggested Action	Reason for Action
ASSESSMENT	
Determine when and how frequently to monitor the client's respiratory rate (see Box 12-1).	Demonstrates accountability for making timely and appropriate assessments.
Review data collected in previous assessments of the respiratory rate and other vital signs.	Aids in identifying trends and analyzing significant patterns.
Read the client's history for any reference to respiratory, cardiac, or neurologic disorders.	Demonstrates an understanding of factors that may affect the respiratory rate.
Review the list of prescribed drugs for any that may have respiratory or neurologic effects.	Helps in analyzing the results of assessment findings.
PLANNING	
Arrange to count the client's respiratory rate as close to the scheduled routine as possible.	Ensures consistency and accuracy.
Make sure a watch or wall clock with a second hand is available.	Ensures accurate timing.
Plan to assess the client's respiratory rate after a 5-minute period of inactivity.	Reflects the characteristics of respirations at rest rather than under the influence of activity.
IMPLEMENTATION	
Introduce yourself to the client, if you have not done so previously.	Demonstrates responsibility and accountability.
Explain the procedure to the client.	Reduces apprehension and promotes cooperation.
Raise the height of the bed.	Reduces musculoskeletal strain.
Wash hands or perform hand antisepsis with an alcohol rub (see Chap. 10).	Reduces the spread of microorganisms.
Help the client to a sitting or lying position.	Facilitates the ability to observe breathing.
Note the position of the second hand on the clock or watch.	Identifies the point at which assessment begins.
Choose a time when the client is unaware of being watched; it may help to count the respiratory rate while appearing to count the pulse or while the client holds a thermometer in the mouth.	Discourages conscious control of breathing or talking during the assessment of the rate of breathing.
Observe the rise and fall of the client's chest for a full minute, if breathing is unusual. If breathing appears noiseless and effortless, count ventilations for a fractional portion of 1 minute and then multiply to calculate the rate.	Determines the respiratory rate per minute.
Write down the respiratory rate.	Ensures accurate documentation.
Restore the client to a therapeutic position or one that provides comfort, and lower the bed.	Demonstrates responsibility for client care, safety, and comfort.
Record the assessed measurement on the graphic sheet or flow sheet, or in the narrative nursing notes.	Provides documentation for future comparisons.

(continued)

Assessing the Respiratory Rate (continued)

Suggested Action	Reason for Action
IMPLEMENTATION (CONTINUED)	
Verbally report rapid or slow respiratory rates or any other unusual characteristics.	Alerts others to monitor the client closely and make changes in the plan for care.

Evaluation

- Respiratory rate is counted for an appropriate time.
- Respiratory rate is consistent with the client's condition.

Document

- Date and time
- Rate per minute
- Accompanying signs and symptoms, if appropriate
- To whom abnormal information was reported and the outcome of the interaction

SAMPLE DOCUMENTATION

Date and Time Respiratory rate of 20/minute at rest. Breathing is noiseless and effortless. ———— SIGNATURE/TITLE

SKILL 12-4 Assessing Blood Pressure

Suggested Action	Reason for Action
ASSESSMENT	
Determine when and how frequently to monitor the client's blood pressure (see Box 12-1).	Demonstrates accountability for making timely and appropriate assessments.
Review the data collected in previous assessments.	Aids in identifying trends and analyzing significant patterns.
Determine in which arm and in what position previous assessments were made.	Ensures consistency when evaluating data.
Read the client's history for any reference to cardiac or vascular disorders.	Demonstrates an understanding of factors that may affect the blood pressure.
Review the list of prescribed drugs for any that may have cardiovascular effects.	Helps in analyzing the results of assessment findings.
PLANNING	
Gather the necessary supplies: blood pressure cuff, sphygmomanometer, and stethoscope.	Promotes efficient time management. A recently calibrated aneroid or a validated electronic device can be used.
Select an appropriately sized cuff for the client.	Ensures valid assessment findings.
Arrange to take the client's blood pressure as near to the scheduled routine as possible.	Ensures consistency.
Plan to assess the blood pressure after at least 5 minutes of inactivity unless it is an emergency.	Reflects the blood pressure under resting conditions.
Wait 30 minutes after the client has ingested caffeine or used tobacco.	Avoids obtaining a higher-than-usual measurement from arterial constriction.
Plan to use the right or left arm unless inaccessible.	Provides consistency in evaluating data.
IMPLEMENTATION	
Introduce yourself to the client if you have not done so earlier.	Demonstrates responsibility and accountability.
Explain the procedure to the client.	Reduces apprehension and promotes cooperation.
Raise the height of the bed.	Reduces musculoskeletal strain.
Wash hands or perform hand antisepsis with an alcohol rub (see Chap. 10).	Reduces the spread of microorganisms.
Help the client to a sitting position or one of comfort.	Relaxes the client and reduces elevations caused by stress or discomfort.
Support the client's forearm at the level of the heart with the palm of the hand upward.	Ensures collecting accurate data and facilitates locating the brachial artery.
Expose the inner aspect of the elbow by removing clothing or loosely rolling up a sleeve.	Facilitates application of the blood pressure cuff and optimum sound perception.

(continued)

Assessing Blood Pressure (continued)

IMPLEMENTATION (CONTINUED)

Center the cuff bladder so that the lower edge is about 1–2 inches (2.5–5 cm) above the inner aspect of the elbow (Fig. A).

Places the cuff in the best position for occluding the blood flow through the brachial artery.

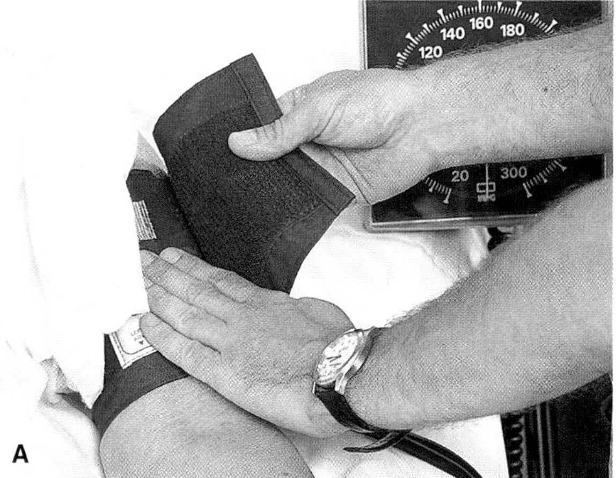

A — Applying the blood pressure cuff. (Photo by B. Proud.)

Wrap the cuff snugly and uniformly about the circumference of the arm.

Ensures the application of even pressure during inflation.

Make sure the aneroid gauge can be clearly seen.

Prevents errors when observing the gauge.

Palpate the brachial pulse (Fig. B).

Determines the most accurate location for assessing and hearing Korotkoff sounds.

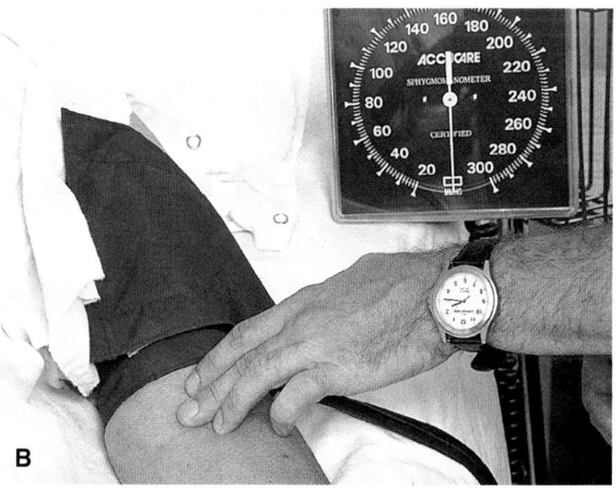

B — Palpating the brachial artery. (Photo by B. Proud.)

Tighten the screw valve on the bulb (Fig. C).

Prevents loss of pumped air.

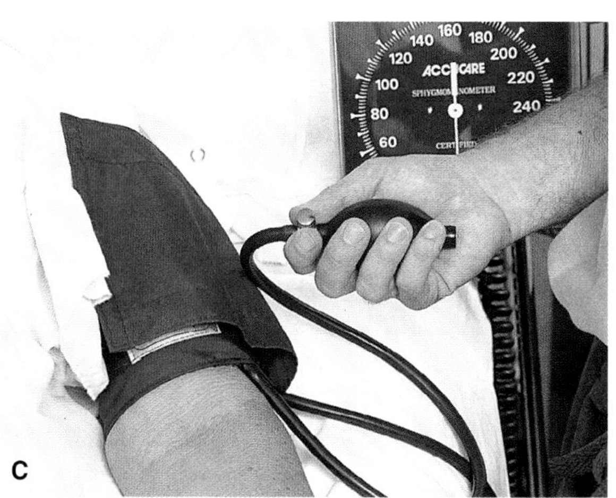

C — Tightening the screw valve. (Photo by B. Proud.)

(continued)

Assessing Blood Pressure (continued)

IMPLEMENTATION (CONTINUED)

Compress the bulb until the pulsation within the artery stops and note the measurement at that point.	Provides an estimation of systolic pressure.
Deflate the cuff and wait 15–30 seconds.	Allows the return of normal blood flow.
Place the eartips of the stethoscope within the ears and position the bell of the stethoscope lightly over the location of the brachial artery (Fig. D). The diaphragm may be used, but it is not preferred.	Ensures accurate assessment.

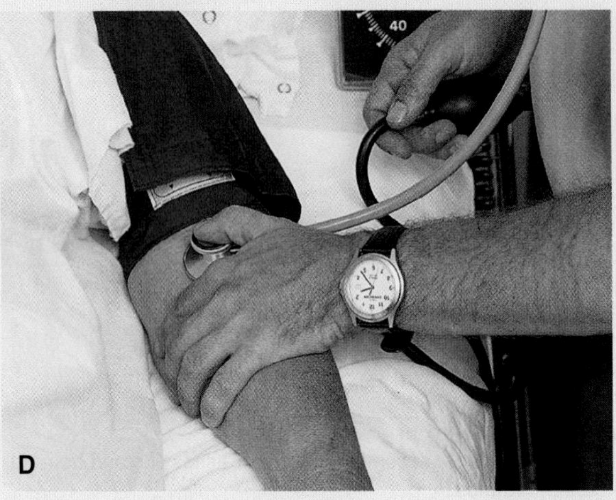

Placing the stethoscope. (Photo by B. Proud.)

Keep the tubing free from contact with clothing.	Reduces sound distortion.
Pump the cuff bladder to a pressure that is 30 mm Hg above the point where the pulse previously disappeared (Fig. E).	Facilitates identifying phase I of Korotkoff sounds.

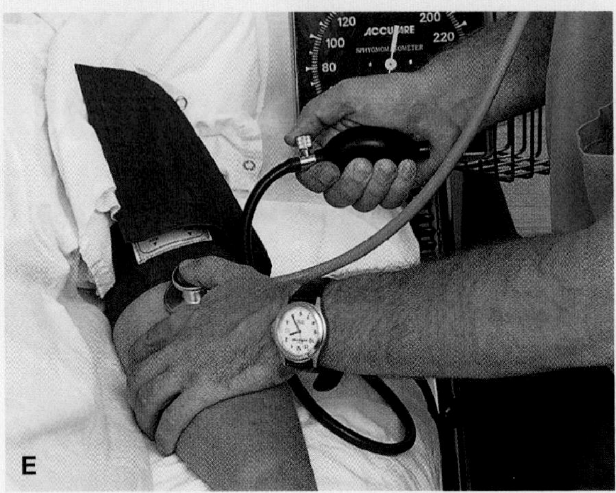

Pumping the bulb. (Photo by B. Proud.)

Loosen the screw on the valve.	Releases air from the cuff bladder.
Control the release of air at a rate of approximately 2–3 mm Hg/second.	Ensures an accurate assessment between the perception of a sound and noting the numbers on the gauge.
Listen for the onset and changes in Korotkoff sounds.	Aids in determining the systolic and diastolic pressures.
Read the manometer gauge to the closest even number when phase I, IV, or V is noted.	Follows recommended standards for children or adults.
Release the air quickly when there has been silence for at least 10 mm Hg.	Indicates phase V is complete.
Write down the blood pressure measurements.	Ensures accurate documentation.
Repeat the assessment after waiting at least 1 minute if unsure of the pressure measurements.	Allows time for the arterial pressure to return to baseline before another assessment.
Restore the client to a therapeutic position or one that provides comfort, and lower the bed.	Demonstrates responsibility for client care, safety, and comfort.
Wash hands or perform hand antisepsis with an alcohol rub (see Chap. 10).	Reduces the spread of microorganisms.

(continued)

Assessing Blood Pressure (continued)

Suggested Action	Reason for Action
IMPLEMENTATION (CONTINUED)	
Record the assessed measurement on the graphic sheet or flow sheet, or in the narrative nursing notes.	Provides documentation for future comparisons.
Verbally report elevated or low blood pressure measurements.	Alerts others to monitor the client closely and make changes in the plan for care.

Evaluation

- Korotkoff sounds are heard clearly.
- Blood pressure is consistent with the client's condition.

Document

- Date and time
- Systolic and diastolic pressure measurements
- Assessment site
- Position of the client
- Accompanying signs and symptoms, if appropriate
- To whom abnormal information was reported and the outcome of the interaction

SAMPLE DOCUMENTATION

Date and Time BP 136/72 in R arm while in sitting position. ——— SIGNATURE/TITLE

SKILL 12-5 Obtaining a Thigh Blood Pressure

Suggested Action	Reason for Action
ASSESSMENT	
Determine when and how frequently to monitor the client's blood pressure (see Box 12-1).	Demonstrates accountability for making timely and appropriate assessments.
Review the data collected in previous assessments.	Aids in identifying trends and analyzing significant patterns.
Determine on which thigh previous assessments were made.	Ensures consistency when evaluating data.
Read the client's history for any reference to cardiac or vascular disorders.	Demonstrates an understanding of factors that may affect blood pressure.
Review the list of prescribed drugs for any that may have cardiovascular effects.	Helps in analyzing the results of assessment findings.
PLANNING	
Gather the necessary supplies: thigh blood pressure cuff, sphygmomanometer, and stethoscope (Fig. A).	Promotes efficient time management and ensures an accurate measurement when a wider and longer blood pressure cuff is used.

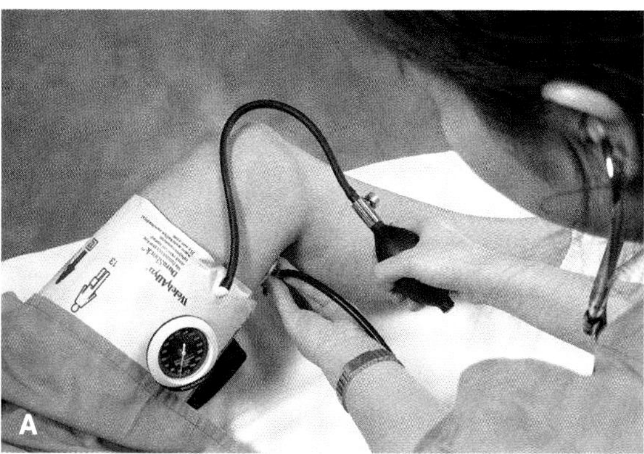

A Application of blood pressure cuff to the thigh.

(continued)

Obtaining a Thigh Blood Pressure (continued)

PLANNING (CONTINUED)

Action	Rationale
Plan to assess blood pressure after the client has been reclining for at least 10 minutes.	Promotes conditions for obtaining accurate measurements.
Wait 30 minutes from the time the client has ingested caffeine, used tobacco, consumed a heavy meal, exercised vigorously, or taken a hot shower or bath.	Eliminates factors that contribute to the constriction or dilation of blood vessels.

IMPLEMENTATION

Action	Rationale
Introduce yourself to the client if you have not done so earlier.	Demonstrates responsibility and accountability.
Explain the procedure to the client.	Reduces apprehension and promotes cooperation.
Provide privacy.	Demonstrates respect for the client's dignity.
Raise the height of the bed.	Reduces musculoskeletal strain.
Wash hands or perform hand antisepsis with an alcohol rub (see Chap. 10).	Reduces the spread of microorganisms.
Place the client in either the supine or the prone position, with the knee slightly flexed and the hip abducted.	Facilitates application of the blood pressure cuff.
Make sure the manometer can be seen clearly.	Prevents observational errors.
Palpate the popliteal pulse.	Determines the most accurate location for hearing Korotkoff sounds.
Warn the client that he or she may experience discomfort when the cuff is inflated but that remaining still will facilitate accuracy.	Prepares the client for sensation and provides an explanation for its necessity.
Tighten the screw valve on the bulb.	Prevents the loss of air from the cuff bladder.
Compress the bulb until the pulsation within the artery stops and note the pressure measurement.	Provides an estimation of systolic pressure.
Deflate the cuff and wait 15 to 30 seconds.	Allows the return of normal blood flow.
Place the eartips of the stethoscope within the ears, and position the bell of the stethoscope lightly over the location of the popliteal artery. (Note: The diaphragm of the stethoscope may be used, but it is not preferred.)	Ensures an accurate assessment.
Keep the tubing free from contact with clothing and bed linens.	Reduces sound distortion.
Pump the cuff bladder to a pressure that is 30 mm Hg above the point where the pulse previously disappeared.	Facilitates identifying phase I of Korotkoff sounds.
Loosen the screw on the valve.	Releases air from the cuff bladder.
Control the release of air at a rate of approximately 2 to 3 mm Hg/second.	Ensures accurate assessment between perception of the sound and noting the numbers on the gauge.
Listen for the onset and changes in Korotkoff sounds.	Aids in determining systolic and diastolic pressure.
Read the manometer when phase I, IV, and V are noted.	Follows recommended standards for adults or children.
Release the air quickly when there has been silence for at least 10 mm Hg.	Indicates that phase V is complete.
Write down the blood pressure measurements.	Ensures accurate documentation.
Restore the client to a therapeutic position or one that provides comfort.	Demonstrates responsibility for client care, safety, and comfort.
Wash hands or perform hand antisepsis with an alcohol rub (see Chap. 10).	Reduces the spread of microorganisms.
Record assessed measurements on the graphic sheet or the flow sheet, or in the narrative nursing notes.	Provides documentation for future comparisons.
Verbally report blood pressure measurements to the nurse in charge.	Alerts others to monitor the client closely or to modify the client's plan of care.

Evaluation

- Korotkoff sounds are heard clearly.
- Blood pressure is consistent with the client's condition.

Document

- Date and time
- Systolic and diastolic pressure measurements
- Assessment site
- Accompanying signs and symptoms, if appropriate
- To whom abnormal information was reported, and the outcome of the interaction

SAMPLE DOCUMENTATION

Date and Time BP 176/88 at popliteal artery of left thigh. States, "It hurts when the blood pressure cuff gets tight."

———————————————————— SIGNATURE/TITLE

SKILL 12-6 Assessing for Postural Hypotension

Suggested Action	Reason for Action
ASSESSMENT	
Determine when and how frequently to monitor the client's blood pressure (see Box 12-1).	Demonstrates accountability for making timely and appropriate assessments.
Review the data collected in previous assessments.	Aids in identifying trends and analyzing significant patterns.
Determine in which arm previous assessments were made.	Ensures consistency when evaluating data.
Read the client's history for any reference to cardiac or vascular disorders.	Demonstrates an understanding of factors that may affect the blood pressure.
Review the list of prescribed drugs for any that may have cardiovascular effects.	Helps in analyzing the results of assessment findings.
PLANNING	
Gather the necessary supplies: blood pressure cuff, sphygmomanometer, and stethoscope.	Promotes efficient time management.
Select a cuff that is an appropriate size for the client.	Ensures valid assessment findings.
Arrange to take the client's blood pressure as near to the scheduled routine as possible.	Ensures consistency.
Plan to assess the blood pressure after the client has been reclining for at least 5 minutes.	Promotes conditions for obtaining accurate baseline measurements for comparison.
Wait 30 minutes from the time the client has ingested caffeine, used tobacco, consumed a heavy meal, exercised vigorously, or taken a hot shower or bath.	Eliminates factors that contribute to constriction or dilation of blood vessels.
IMPLEMENTATION	
Introduce yourself to the client if you have not done so earlier.	Demonstrates responsibility and accountability.
Explain the procedure to the client.	Reduces apprehension and promotes cooperation.
Provide privacy.	Demonstrates respect for the client's dignity.
Raise the height of the bed.	Reduces musculoskeletal strain.
Wash hands or perform hand antisepsis with an alcohol rub (see Chap. 10).	Reduces the spread of microorganisms.
Assess the client's pulse.	Provides a baseline for evaluating heart rate in relation to postural changes.
Support the client's forearm at the level of the heart with the palm of the hand upward.	Ensures collecting accurate data and facilitates locating the brachial artery.
Expose the inner aspect of the elbow by removing clothing or loosely rolling up a sleeve.	Facilitates the application of the blood pressure cuff and optimum sound perception.
Center the cuff bladder so that the lower edge is about 1–2 inches (2.5–5 cm) above the inner aspect of the elbow.	Places the cuff in the best position for occluding blood flow through the brachial artery.
Wrap the cuff snugly and uniformly about the circumference of the arm.	Ensures the application of even pressure during inflation.
Make sure the manometer can be clearly seen.	Prevents observational errors.
Palpate the brachial pulse.	Determines the most accurate location for hearing Korotkoff sounds.
Tighten the screw valve on the bulb.	Prevents loss of air from the cuff bladder.
Compress the bulb until the pulsation within the artery stops and note the pressure measurement.	Provides an estimation of systolic pressure.
Deflate the cuff and wait 15–30 seconds.	Allows the return of normal blood flow.
Place the eartips of the stethoscope within the ears and position the bell of the stethoscope lightly over the brachial artery. (Note: The diaphragm of the stethoscope may be used, but it is not preferred.)	Ensures accurate assessment.
Keep the tubing free from contact with clothing.	Reduces sound distortion.
Pump the cuff bladder to a pressure that is 30 mm Hg above the measurement where the pulse previously disappeared.	Facilitates identifying phase I of Korotkoff sounds.
Loosen the screw on the valve.	Releases air from the cuff bladder.
Control the release of air at a rate of approximately 2–3 mm Hg/second.	Ensures accurate assessment between the perception of a sound and noting of numbers on the gauge.
Listen for the onset and changes in pressure.	Aids in determining systolic and diastolic Korotkoff sounds.
Read the manometer when phase I, IV, and V are noted.	Follows the recommended standards for adults or children.
Release the air quickly when there has been silence for at least 10 mm Hg.	Indicates that phase V is complete.
Write down the blood pressure measurements.	Ensures accurate documentation.
Assist the client with standing or sitting.	Stimulates reflexes for maintaining blood flow to the brain.

(continued)

Assessing for Postural Hypotension (continued)

IMPLEMENTATION (CONTINUED)

Action	Rationale
Be prepared to steady or assist the client should he or she become dizzy or faint.	Promotes safety and reduces the potential for injury.
Repeat the blood pressure and pulse measurement within 3 minutes of quiet standing (Pickering et al., 2005).	Provides data for comparison.
Use a head-up tilt at 60 degrees if the client cannot stand (Pickering et al., 2005).	Provides an alternative for unstable or mobility challenged clients.
Determine if the systolic blood pressure falls 20 mm Hg or more, the diastolic blood pressure falls 10 mm Hg or more, or the pulse rises 20 beats or more.	Hypotension accompanied by tachycardia is an abnormal response (Carlson, 1999).
Restore the client to a therapeutic position or one that provides comfort.	Demonstrates responsibility for client care, safety, and comfort.
Instruct the client to rise slowly from a sitting or lying position if the data indicate the client experiences postural hypotension.	Allows time for the physiologic adaptation in blood flow to the brain.
Wash hands or perform hand antisepsis with an alcohol rub (see Chap. 10).	Reduces the spread of microorganisms.
Record assessed measurements on the graphic or flow sheet, or in the narrative nursing notes.	Provides documentation for future comparisons.
Verbally report blood pressure measurements to the nurse in charge.	Alerts others to monitor the client closely or to modify the client's plan of care.

Evaluation

The data validate or disprove that the client experiences postural hypotension.

Document

- Date and time
- Systolic and diastolic pressure measurements and pulse rate in lying and standing or sitting positions
- Assessment site
- Accompanying signs and symptoms, if appropriate
- To whom abnormal information was reported, and the outcome of the interaction

SAMPLE DOCUMENTATION

Date and Time P-68, BP 136/72 in R arm while lying down. BP 110/60 and P-90 in standing position. States, "I feel very light-headed." Assisted to lie down in bed. Cautioned to call for assistance when there is a need to ambulate or get out of bed. Signal cord attached to bed. —— SIGNATURE/TITLE

13 Physical Assessment

Words To Know

accommodation
audiometry
auscultation
body systems approach
capillary refill time
cerumen
consensual response
drape
edema
extraocular movements
head-to-toe approach
hearing acuity
inspection
Jaeger chart
mental status assessment
palpation
percussion
physical assessment
Rinne test
smelling acuity
Snellen eye chart
turgor
visual acuity
visual field examination
Weber test

Learning Objectives

On completion of this chapter, the reader should be able to:

1. List four purposes of a physical assessment.
2. Name four assessment techniques.
3. List at least five items needed when performing a basic physical assessment.
4. Discuss at least three criteria for an appropriate assessment environment.
5. Identify at least five assessments that can be obtained during the initial survey of clients.
6. State two reasons for draping clients.
7. Differentiate a head-to-toe and a body systems approach to physical assessment.
8. List six ways in which the body may be divided for organizing data collection.
9. Identify two self-examinations that nurses should teach their adult clients.

The first step in the nursing process is assessment, or gathering of information. The **physical assessment** (a systematic examination of body structures) is one method for gathering health data. This chapter describes how to perform a physical assessment from a generalist's or beginning nurse's point of view and identifies common assessment findings. Students can learn advanced physical assessment skills through additional education and experience or by consulting specialty texts.

OVERVIEW OF THE PHYSICAL ASSESSMENT

Health care practitioners use various techniques and equipment to perform the physical assessment. Although the settings for a physical assessment vary, each environment must facilitate accurate data collection and be conducive to the client's privacy and comfort.

Purposes

The overall goal of a physical assessment is to gather objective data about a client. To achieve this goal, nurses thoroughly examine clients on admission, briefly at the start of each shift, and any time a client's condition changes. The purposes of assessment are as follows:

- To evaluate the client's current physical condition
- To detect early signs of developing health problems
- To establish a baseline for future comparisons
- To evaluate the client's responses to medical and nursing interventions

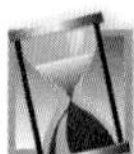

Gerontologic Considerations

■ The nurse shows consideration for alterations in hearing, vision, or movement before starting the examination. Before the physical assessment, the nurse may ask, "Is there anything you want me to know before we begin?" or "How can I make you as comfortable as possible during this examination?"

■ If limitations are identified, the nurse makes appropriate adjustments to the examination such as speaking into the ear with the best hearing or modifying positions to reduce discomfort.

■ Physical limitations from chronic diseases (eg, difficulty breathing, limited movement, weakness) may require modifying assessment techniques during the examination.

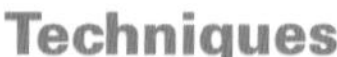

Techniques

The four basic physical assessment techniques are inspection, percussion, palpation, and auscultation.

Inspection

Inspection (purposeful observation) is the most frequently used assessment technique. It involves examining particular body parts and looking for specific normal and abnormal characteristics (Fig. 13-1A). With advanced instruction, some nurses learn to use special instruments to inspect parts of the body, such as the interior of the eyes, that are potentially inaccessible to ordinary vision and inspection techniques.

Percussion

Percussion, the least used assessment technique by nurses, is the striking or tapping a part of the client's body with the fingertips to produce vibratory sounds (see Fig. 13-1B) (Table 13-1). The quality of the sounds aids in determining the location, size, and density of underlying structures. A sound different from expected suggests a pathologic change in the area being examined. If percussion is performed correctly, the client experiences no discomfort. Pain could indicate a disease process or tissue injury.

Palpation

Palpation involves lightly touching or applying pressure to the body. *Light palpation* involves using the fingertips, the back of the hand, or the palm of the hand (Fig. 13-2A). It is best used when feeling the surface of the skin, structures that lie just beneath the skin, pulsations from peripheral arteries, and vibrations in the chest. *Deep palpation* is performed by depressing tissue approximately 1 in. (2.5 cm) with the forefingers of one or both hands (Fig. 13-2B).

Palpation provides information about the following:

- The size, shape, consistency, and mobility of normal tissue and unusual masses
- The symmetry or asymmetry of bilateral (both sides of the body) structures such as the lobes of the thyroid gland
- Skin temperature and moisture
- Any tenderness
- Unusual vibrations

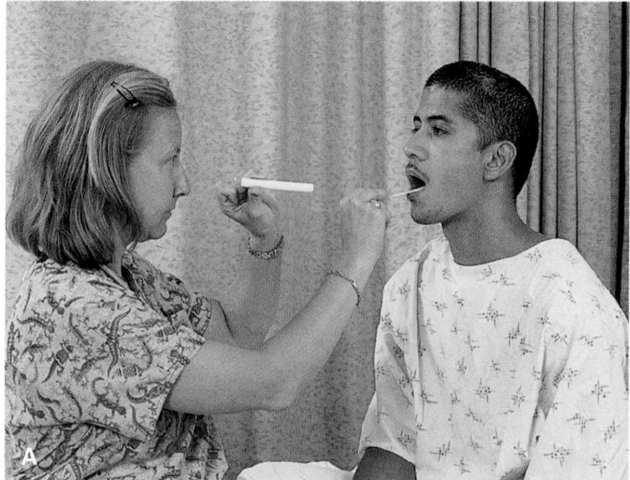

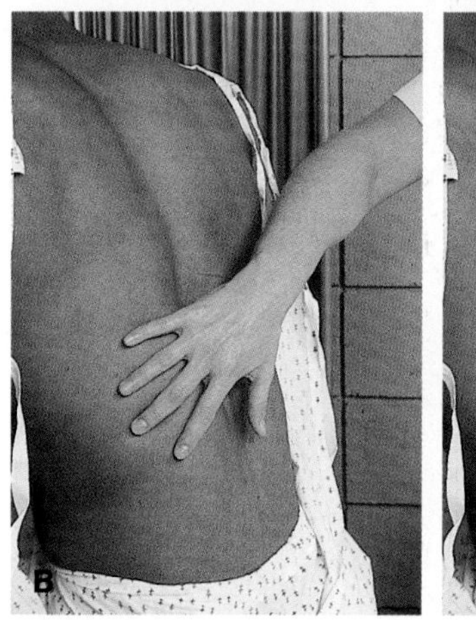

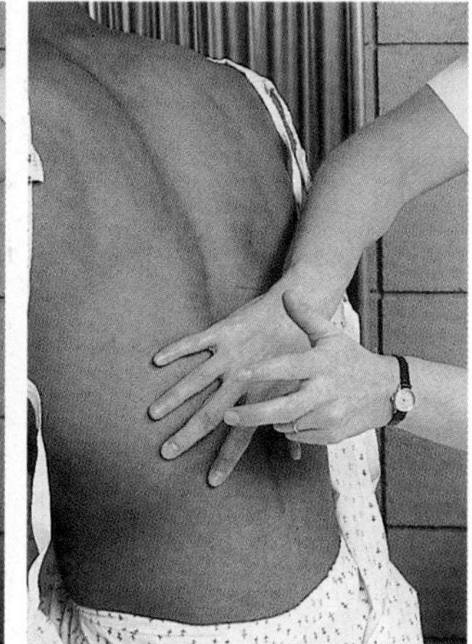

FIGURE 13-1 A. Inspection. (Copyright B. Proud.) **B.** Percussion. (Copyright Ken Kasper.)

TABLE 13-1 Percussion Sounds

SOUND	INTENSITY	DESCRIPTIVE TERM	COMMON LOCATIONS
Muted	Soft	Flat	Muscle, bone
Thud	Soft to moderate	Dull	Liver, full bladder, and tumorous mass
Empty	Moderate to loud	Resonant	Normal lung
Cavernous	Loud	Tympanic	Intestine filled with air
Booming	Very loud	Hyperresonant	Barrel-shaped chest overinflated with trapped air as a result of chronic lung disease

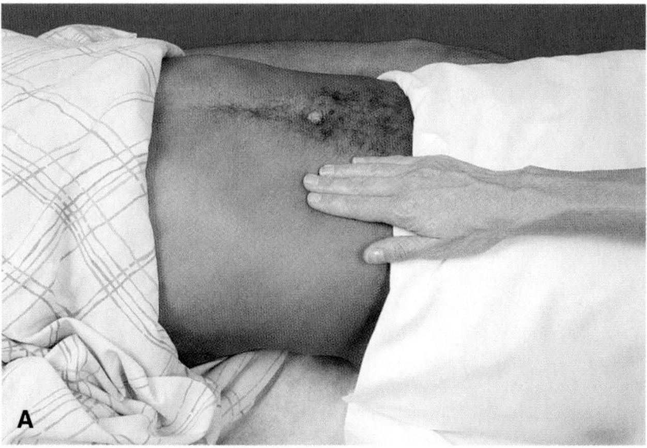

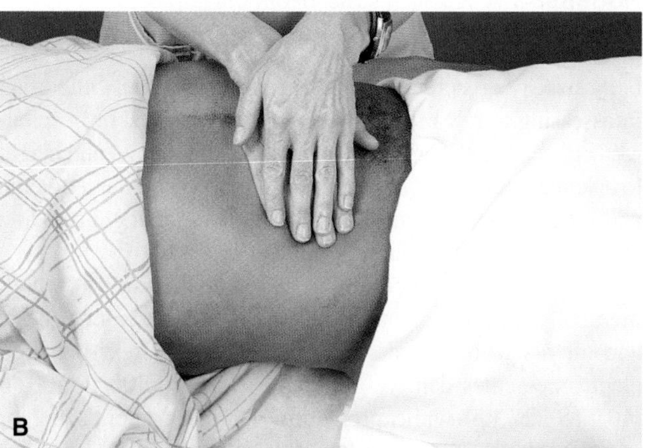

FIGURE 13-2 Palpation techniques. A. Light palpation. B. Deep palpation. (From Craven, 2009.)

Auscultation

Auscultation (listening to body sounds) is used frequently, most often to assess the heart, lungs, and abdomen. A stethoscope is required to hear most internal sounds (Fig. 13-3), but in some cases, loud sounds, such as those associated with intestinal hyperactivity, are audible with gross hearing (ie, listening without any instrumentation).

Nurses must practice auscultation repeatedly on various healthy and ill people to gain proficiency with the equipment and experience in interpreting data. To ensure the accuracy of findings, it is best to eliminate or reduce environmental noise as much as possible.

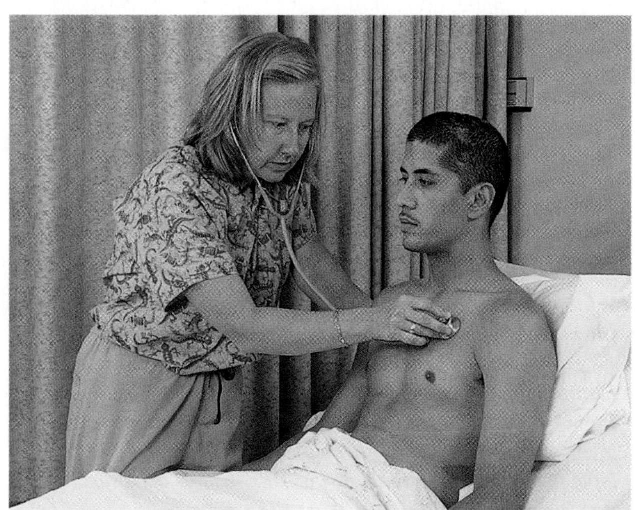

FIGURE 13-3 Auscultation. (Photo by B. Proud.)

BOX 13-1 Physical Assessment Equipment

For a basic physical assessment, the nurse needs:

- Gloves
- Examination gown
- Cloth or paper drapes
- Scale
- Stethoscope
- Sphygmomanometer
- Thermometer
- Pen light or flashlight
- Tongue blade
- Assessment form and pen

Equipment

The items generally needed for a basic physical assessment are listed in Box 13-1. More advanced practitioners use additional examination equipment.

Environment

Nurses assess clients in a special examination room or at the bedside. Regardless of the assessment location, the area should have easy access to a restroom; a door or curtain that ensures privacy; adequate warmth for client comfort; a padded, adjustable table or bed; sufficient room for moving to either side of the client; adequate lighting; facilities for hand hygiene; a clean counter or surface for placing examination equipment; and a lined receptacle for soiled articles.

PERFORMING A PHYSICAL ASSESSMENT

Basic activities involved in a physical assessment include gathering general data, draping and positioning the client, selecting a systematic approach for collecting data, and examining the client.

Gathering General Data

The nurse obtains general data during the first contact with the client. At this time, the nurse appraises the client's overall condition. By observing and interacting with the client before the actual physical examination, the nurse notes the following:

- Physical appearance with regard to clothing and hygiene
- Level of consciousness

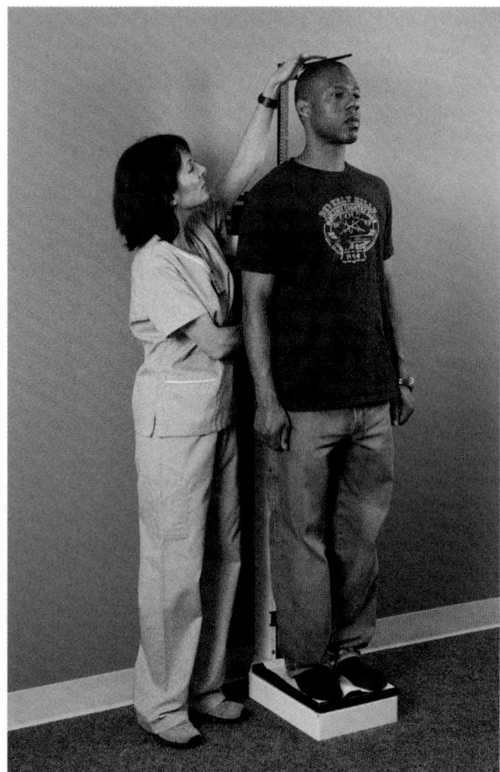

FIGURE 13-4 An assessment of height and weight. (From Taylor, 2011.)

- Body size
- Posture
- Gait and coordinated movement (or lack of it)
- Use of ambulatory aids
- Mood and emotional tone

The nurse also gathers some preliminary data, such as vital signs (see Chap. 12), weight, and height, at this time.

The nurse documents the client's weight and height because they provide more reliable data than a subjective assessment of body size. The recorded measurements are extremely important in assessing trends in future weight loss or gain. For hospitalized clients, health care practitioners also use weight and height to calculate dosages of some drugs. In most cases, nurses weigh and measure adult clients and older children using a standing scale (Fig. 13-4) (see Nursing Guidelines 13-1.)

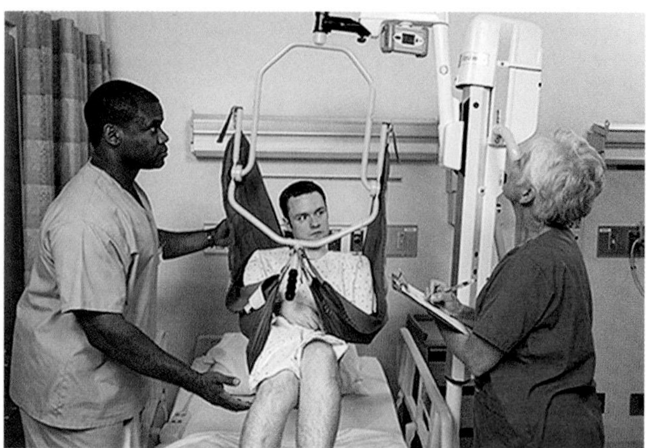

FIGURE 13-5 A bed-sling scale. (From Craven, 2009.)

Nurses use an electronic bed or chair scale to weigh medically unstable clients, clients who are extremely obese, and clients who cannot stand (Fig. 13-5). Battery-powered electronic scales can weigh people who are 400 to 500 lb (181 to 227 kg) while protecting against a client's fall or injury to the nurse. Several models store the client's weight in its memory, allowing it to be automatically recalled until another client is weighed. Electronic scales can be transported from storage to a client's room when needed.

Draping and Positioning

Because assessment takes place while clients are naked (or wearing only a loose examination gown), they generally appreciate being covered with a **drape** (a sheet of soft cloth or paper). A drape provides more modesty than warmth.

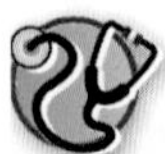

NURSING GUIDELINES 13-1

Obtaining Weight and Height

- Check to see that the scale is calibrated at zero. *Doing so ensures accuracy.*
- Ask or assist the client to remove shoes and all but a minimum of clothing. *Doing so facilitates measuring body weight.*
- Place a paper towel on the scale before the client stands on it in bare feet. *This helps to reduce contact with microorganisms on equipment that other people use.*
- Assist the client onto the scale. *Doing so helps to prevent injury should the client become dizzy or unstable.*
- Position the heavier weight in a calibrated groove of the scale arm. *Doing so provides a rough approximation of the gross body weight.*
- Move the lighter weight across the calibrations for individual pounds and ounces until the bar balances in the center of the scale. *This positioning correlates with the actual weight.*
- Read the weight and write it down. *Doing so ensures accurate documentation.*
- Raise the measuring bar well above the client's head. *This provides room for positioning the client without injury.*
- Ask the client to stand straight and look forward. *Doing so facilitates measuring height.*
- Lower the measuring bar until it lightly touches the top of the client's head. *This positioning correlates with actual height.*
- Note the height and write it down. *This ensures accurate documentation.*

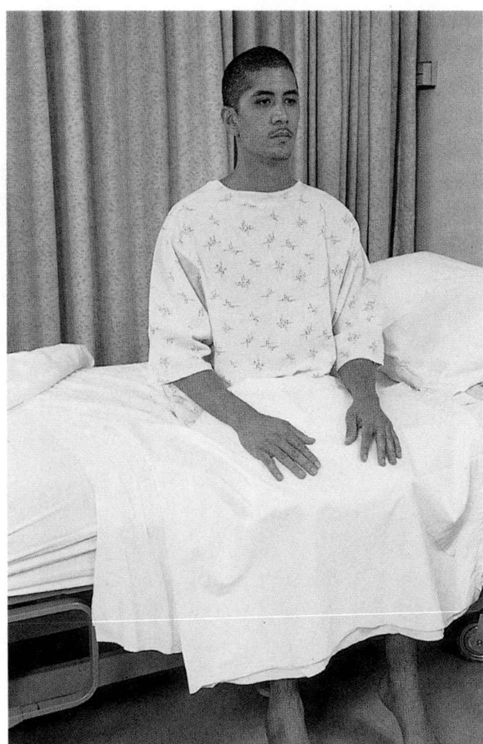

FIGURE 13-6 A client is prepared for examination. (Photo by B. Proud.)

The examination usually begins with the client standing or sitting (Fig. 13-6). Some components of the physical assessment require the client to recline and turn from side to side. Specific positions for special examinations are described and illustrated in Chapters 14 and 23.

Selecting an Approach for Data Collection

Once the client is draped and positioned, selection of a systematic, organized pattern facilitates further data collection. Two common approaches are the head-to-toe approach and the body systems approach. The objective of both methods is to obtain the same basic data. Consequently, each nurse develops his or her own order and sequence for examining clients or uses an assessment form as a guide. Nurses should conduct the assessment consistently each time to avoid omitting essential information.

Head-to-Toe Approach

A **head-to-toe approach** means assessing the client from the top of the body to the feet. This has three advantages:

1. It helps to prevent overlooking some aspect of data collection.
2. It reduces the number of position changes required of the client.
3. It generally takes less time because the nurse is not constantly moving around the client in what may appear to be a haphazard manner.

Body Systems Approach

A **body systems approach** means assessing the client according to the functional systems of the body. It involves examining the structures in each system separately. For example, the nurse assesses the skin, mucous membranes, nails, and hair because they are all parts of the integumentary system. When assessing the cardiovascular system, the nurse palpates peripheral pulses, listens to heart sounds, and so on. One advantage of this method is that findings tend to be clustered, making problems more easily identifiable. Disadvantages are that the nurse examines the same areas of the body several times before completing the assessment; also, frequent position changes during the examination may tire the client.

Examining the Client

The procedure for performing a physical assessment is described in Skill 13-1. Specific assessment techniques, their purpose, and the data they provide are described later in the chapter.

Stop, Think, and Respond Box 13-1

You have been asked to assess two new clients. One arrived by wheelchair and has been walking around the nursing unit. The other was transported by ambulance, has intravenous fluid infusing, and is receiving oxygen. Which client would you assess first? Why? What differences might you use in the physical assessment of each client?

DATA COLLECTION

When collecting data, the nurse may divide the body into six general areas: the head and neck, the chest, the extremities, the abdomen, the genitalia, and the anus and rectum. The following discussion identifies structures commonly assessed, specific techniques used, and common findings.

Head and Neck

Head

The nurse begins at the client's head by assessing his or her mental status and the symmetry and function of craniofacial structures (eyes, ears, nose, mouth). The nurse also assesses the client's skin, oral and nasal mucous membranes, hair, and scalp.

Mental Status Assessment

A **mental status assessment** (a technique for determining the level of a client's cognitive functioning) provides information about a client's attention, concentration, memory, and ability to think abstractly. For most clients, documenting that they are alert and oriented is all that is necessary. More objective assessment data are important, however, when caring for the following clients:

- Clients who were previously unconscious
- Clients who were recently resuscitated
- Clients with periods of confusion
- Clients with a head injury
- Clients who took an overdose of drugs
- Clients with a history of chronic alcoholism
- Clients with a psychiatric diagnosis

Eyes. When examining the head, one of the most obvious assessments is the appearance of the eyes, which generally are of similar size and distance from the center of the face. Each iris is the same color, the sclerae (plural of sclera) appear white, the corneas are clear, and eyelashes are present along the margins of each eye. More advanced practitioners use an instrument called an ophthalmoscope (Fig. 13-7) to examine structures within the eye. After gross inspection, the nurse assesses functions such as visual acuity, pupil size and response, and ocular movements.

Visual acuity (the ability to see both far and near) is not assessed in every client. It is always appropriate, however, to ask if a client wears glasses or contact lenses, has a prosthetic eye, or considers himself or herself blind.

To assess far vision grossly, the nurse asks the client to cover one eye at a time and, from a distance of approximately 20 ft, count the number of fingers the nurse raises. Clients can wear corrective lenses during this assessment. For close vision, the nurse asks literate clients to read newsprint from approximately 14 in. away.

A **Snellen eye chart** (a tool for assessing far vision) is a more objective technique (Fig. 13-8). Each line on the chart is printed in progressively smaller letters or symbols. The nurse asks the client to read the smallest line he or she can see comfortably from a distance of 20 ft, both with and without any corrective lenses. The nurse then compares the client's vision against norms.

Normal vision is the ability to read printed letters that most people can see at a distance of 20 ft without prescription lenses. This number is written as a fraction (eg, 20/20). If, at 20 ft from the chart, a person sees only the first line—one that people with normal vision can see from 200 ft

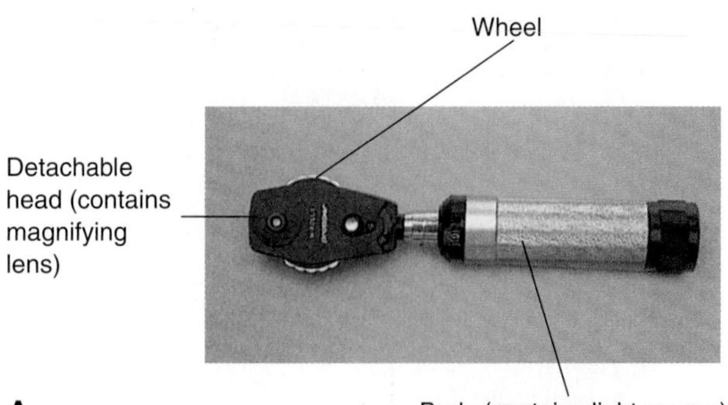

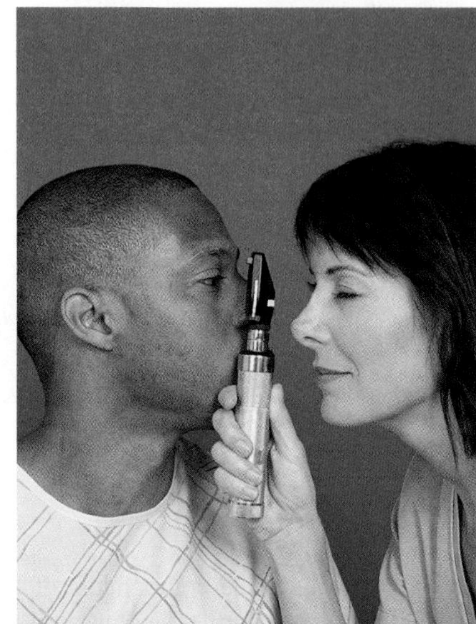

FIGURE 13-7 A. Components of an ophthalmoscope. **B.** Performing an ophthalmoscopic examination. (From Craven, R. F, Hirnle, C. J. (2008). *Fundamentals of Nursing* (6th ed.).

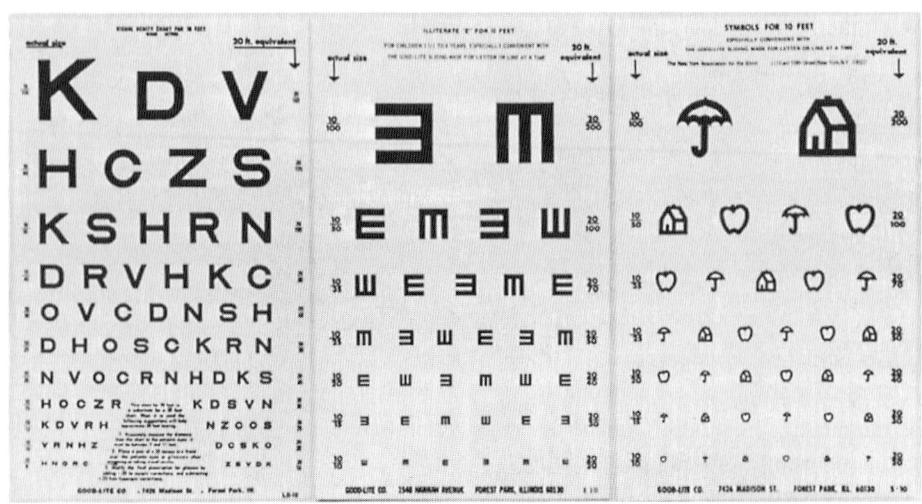

FIGURE 13-8 Three examples of Snellen eye charts. (Photo by Ken Timby.)

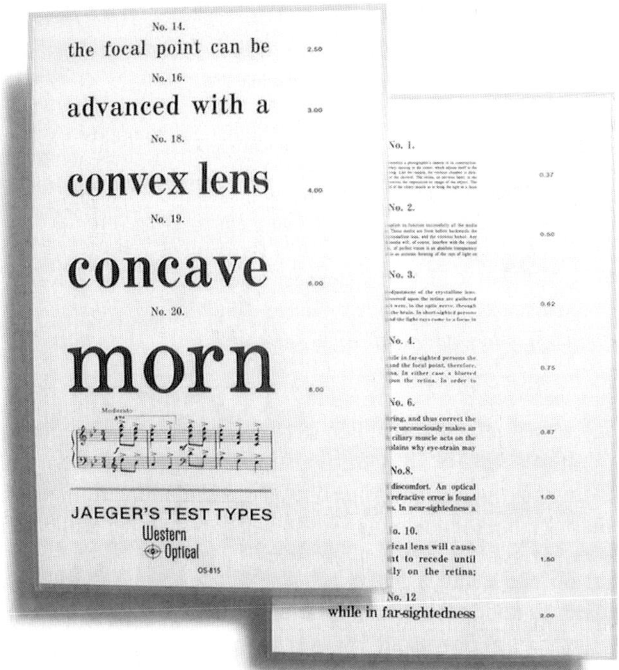

FIGURE 13-9 A Jaeger reading test card used for assessing near visual acuity. (Source: Western Ophthalmics, Lynnwood, WA http://www.west-op.com)

away—the client's visual acuity is recorded as 20/200. The nurse tests near vision using a **Jaeger chart**, a visual assessment tool with small print (Fig. 13-9).

The size of each pupil is estimated in millimeters under normal light conditions (Fig. 13-10). Normal pupils are round and equal in size. There is also a **consensual response** (a brisk, equal, and simultaneous constriction of both pupils when one eye then the other is stimulated with light) (Fig. 13-11A). In addition, the nurse assesses the pupils for **accommodation** (the ability to constrict when looking at a near object and dilate when looking at an object in the distance) (see Fig. 13-11B).

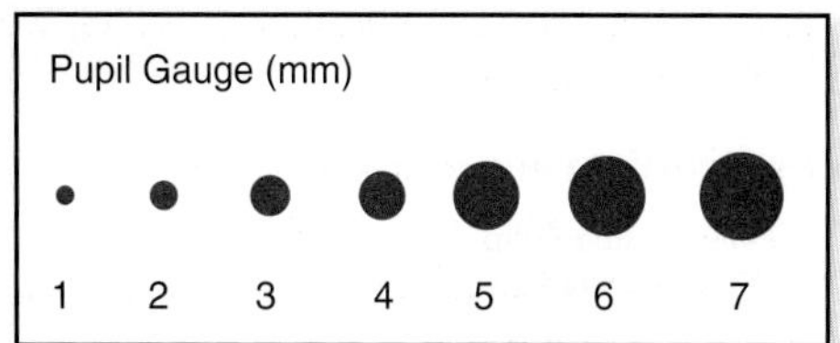

FIGURE 13-10 Pupil size assessment guide.

The nurse documents normal findings using the abbreviation PERRLA: *p*upils *e*qually *r*ound and *r*eact to *l*ight and *a*ccommodation (see Nursing Guidelines 13-2).

The nurse observes **extraocular movements**, which are eye movements controlled by several pairs of eye muscles. He or she asks the client to focus on and track the nurse's finger or some other object as it moves in each of six positions (see Fig. 13-11C). During the assessment, both eyes should move in a coordinated manner. No movement in one eye may indicate cranial nerve damage; irregular or uncoordinated movement may suggest other neurologic pathology.

A **visual field examination** is the assessment of peripheral vision and continuity in the visual field. The nurse may perform a gross assessment or test using more sophisticated ophthalmic equipment. For gross assessment, the nurse stands directly in front of the client, and each person covers his or her eye. The nurse instructs the client to look straight ahead and indicate when he or she sees a light or the nurse's finger as the nurse brings it from several sectors of the periphery toward the center. If the client's and the nurse's visual fields are normal, they see the object at the same time. Certain eye and neurologic disorders are associated with changes in the visual field.

Ears. The nurse inspects and palpates the external ears. More advanced practitioners use an *otoscope* to examine the tympanic membrane, or eardrum.

The nurse performs a gross examination of the ear by observing the appearance of the ears. Both should be similar

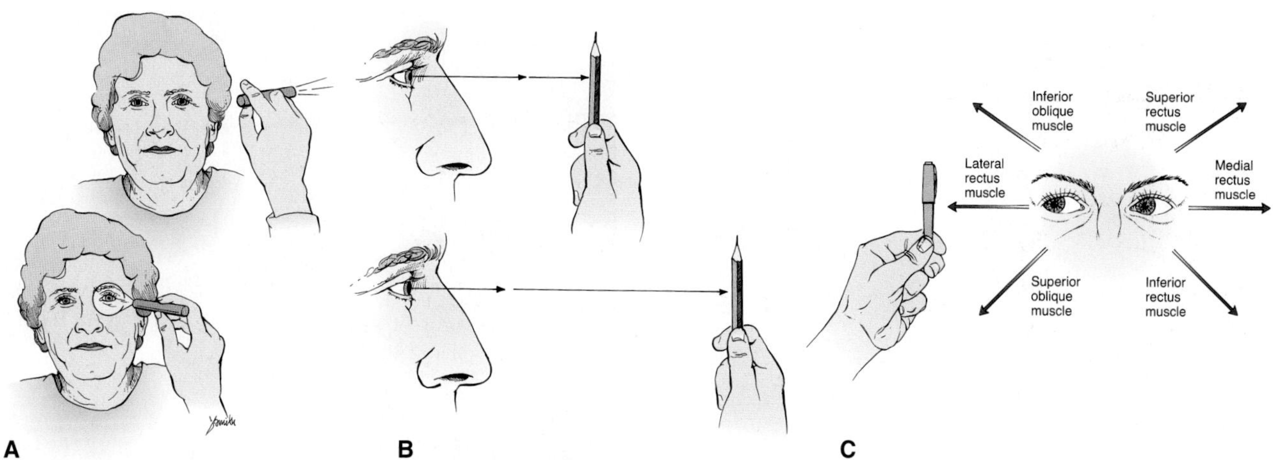

FIGURE 13-11 **A.** Testing pupil response to light. **B.** Testing accommodation. **C.** Assessing extraocular movements.

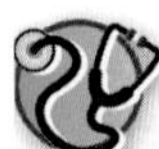

NURSING GUIDELINES 13-2

Assessing Pupillary Response

- Dim the lights in the examination area and instruct the client to stare straight ahead. *Doing so facilitates pupil dilation.*
- Bring a narrow beam of light, like that from a pen light or small flashlight, from the temple toward the eye. *This step provides a direct stimulus for pupil constriction.*
- Observe the pupil of the stimulated eye as well as the unstimulated pupil. The response should be the same. *This assessment indicates the status of brain function.*
- Repeat the assessment by directly stimulating the opposite eye. *Doing so provides comparative data.*
- Ask the client to look at a finger or object approximately 4 inches (10 cm) from his or her face. *This measure produces a situation in which the pupils should get smaller.*
- Tell the client to look from the near object to another that is more distant. *This measure produces a situation in which the pupils should get larger.*

in size, shape, and location. He or she moves the skin behind and in front of the ears as well as the underlying cartilage to determine whether there is any tenderness. The nurse shines a penlight or other light source within each ear to illuminate the ear canal. For optimal visualization, the nurse straightens the curved ear canal as much as possible. For children, this is done by pulling the ear down and back; for an adult, the ear is pulled up and back (Fig. 13-12). **Cerumen** (a yellowish-brown, waxy secretion produced by glands within the ear) is a common finding. Any other drainage is abnormal, and the nurse describes and reports its characteristics.

If the client relies on a hearing aid to amplify sound, the nurse notes that information on the assessment form. The nurse may discover changes in **hearing acuity** (the ability to hear and discriminate sound) by performing a voice test or the Weber or Rinne test (see Nursing Guidelines 13-3 and Fig. 13-13).

The Weber and Rinne tests help to determine hearing impairment resulting from sensory nerve damage or disorders that interfere with sound conduction through the ear. To perform the **Weber test** (an assessment technique for determining equality or disparity of bone-conducted sound), the nurse strikes a tuning fork on his or her palm and places the vibrating stem in the center of the client's head (Fig. 13-14). He or she then asks the client if the sound is audible equally in both ears. A positive response indicates either a normal finding or that hearing in both ears is equally diminished. Hearing the sound louder in one ear is a sign of unequal hearing (hearing loss greater in one ear).

A tuning fork is also necessary in the **Rinne test** (an assessment technique for comparing air versus bone conduction of sound). First, the nurse strikes the tuning fork and then places the stem on the client's mastoid area behind the ear (Fig. 13-15). This test is for bone conduction of sound waves in the tested ear. The client reports when the sound stops. The nurse then moves the tines of the still-vibrating tuning fork near the ear canal and asks the client if he or she perceives sound. This tests air conduction of sound in the tested ear. Both ears are assessed separately. Normally, sound is heard longer by air conduction. If the client does not continue to hear sound when the tuning fork is beside the ear, it indicates a problem with the ear structures that collect and transmit sound through the ear.

Audiometry measures hearing acuity at various sound frequencies. An *audiologist* is a professional trained to test hearing with standardized instruments. Audiometric hearing tests measure exact pitch and volume deficits. They measure hearing in decibels (intensity of sound)—the greater the

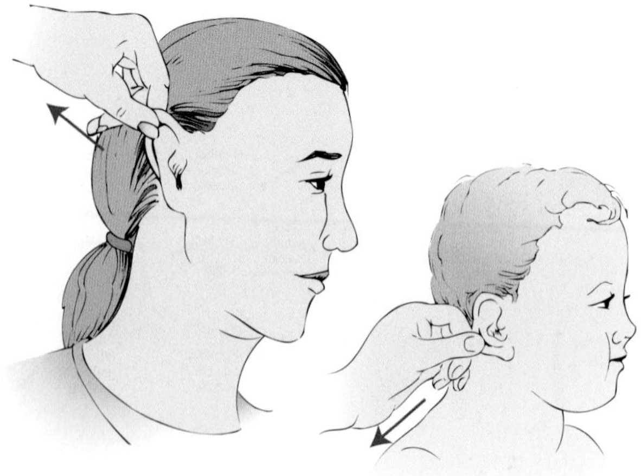

FIGURE 13-12 Technique for straightening the ear canal of an adult and child.

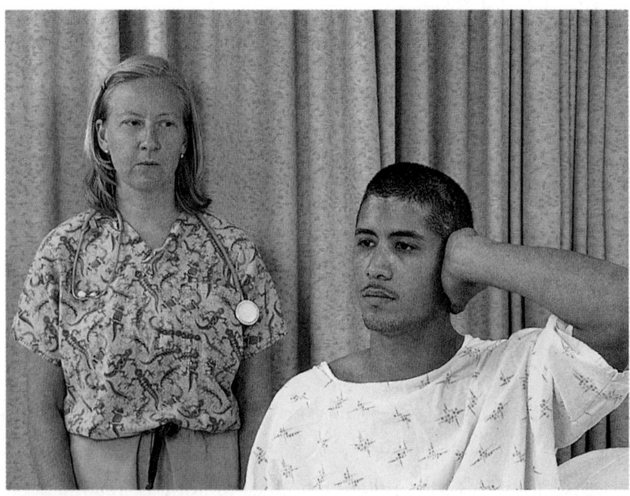

FIGURE 13-13 Voice test. (Photo by B. Proud.)

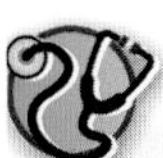

NURSING GUIDELINES 13-3

Performing a Voice Test for Hearing Acuity

- Stand approximately 2 ft behind and to the side of the client. *This placement simulates the distance between most people during social interaction and prevents the client from observing visual cues.*
- Instruct the client to cover the ear on the opposite side (see Fig. 13-13). *This step facilitates sound conduction to the tested ear only.*
- Whisper a color, number, or name toward the uncovered ear. *Doing so delivers a high-pitched sound, the most common type of hearing loss, toward the tested ear.*
- Instruct the client to repeat the whispered word. *This reveals the client's ability to discriminate sound.*
- Continue the same pattern using several more words; increase the volume from a soft to medium to loud whisper or spoken voice if the client's response is inaccurate. *Variations provide more reliable data.*
- Repeat the test on the opposite ear. *Doing so provides separate assessment findings for each ear.*

intensity of sound that can be heard by the client, the more impaired the hearing (Table 13-2).

Nose. The nurse inspects the nose and nasal passages by having the client assume a "sniffing" position. The septum (the tissue that divides the nose in half) should be in midline with equal-sized nasal passages. Pressing at the tip of the nose facilitates deeper inspection. Air should move fairly quietly through the nose during breathing. Normal nasal mucous membrane is pink, moist, and free of obvious drainage. The nurse documents a deviated septum, lesions, growths, flaring of the nostrils, or unusual drainage.

Smelling acuity (the ability to smell and identify odors) is not commonly checked unless impairment is suspected. To test smelling acuity:

1. Have the client occlude one nostril and close his or her eyes.
2. Place substances with strong odors, such as lemon, vanilla extract, coffee, peppermint, or alcohol, one at a time beneath the patent (open) nostril.
3. Ask the client to sniff and identify the substance.

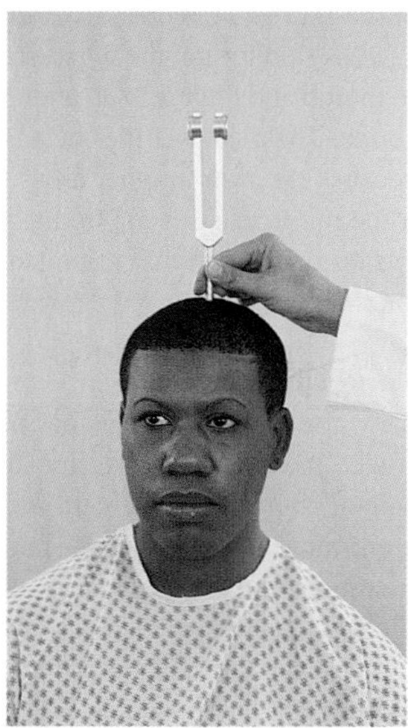

FIGURE 13-14 The Weber test assesses sound conducted through bone. (Photo by B. Proud.)

Mouth and Oral Mucous Membranes

The lips surround the mouth, which contains the tongue and teeth. The nurse inspects these structures by having the client open the mouth widely. The protruding tongue is normally in midline. The nurse documents any dentures, missing or malpositioned teeth, or a partial plate. Some unusual breath odors are diagnostic. For example, the odor of alcohol or acetone suggests additional health problems.

Normal oral mucous membranes are pink, intact, and kept moist by salivary glands located below the tongue. When the client smiles, purses the lips as though preparing to whistle, or shows the teeth, the lips should look the same.

The tongue contains many taste buds that detect particular taste characteristics. Although assessing taste is rarely

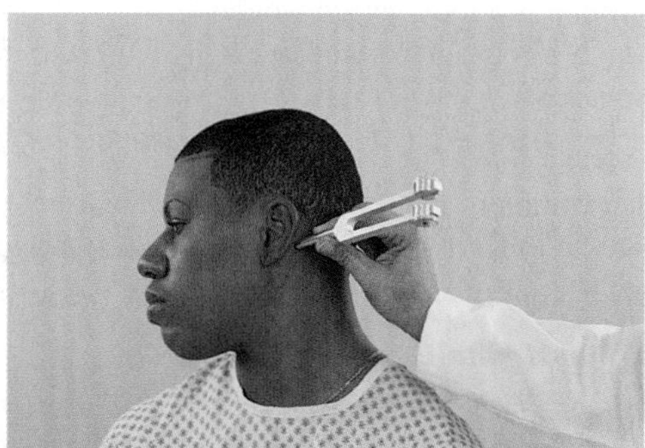

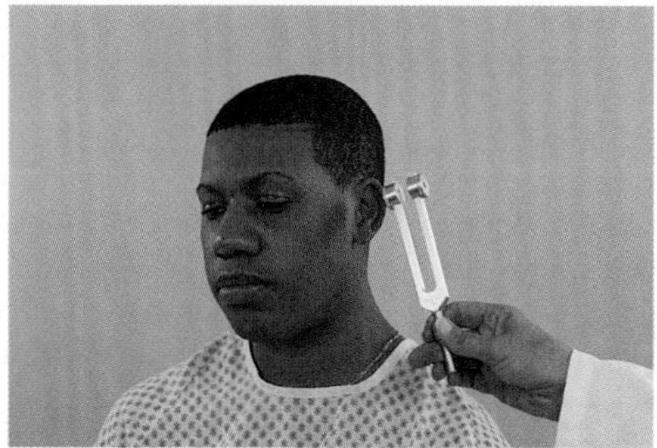

FIGURE 13-15 For the Rinne test, the tuning fork base is placed first on the mastoid process (*top*), after which the prongs are moved to the front of the external auditory canal (*bottom*). (Photo by B. Proud.)

TABLE 13-2 Hearing Acuity Levels

HEARING LEVEL	DECIBEL RANGE (dB)
Normal	0–25
Mildly impaired	26–30
Moderately impaired	31–55
Moderately to severely impaired	56–70
Severely impaired	71–90
Profoundly impaired	91 or greater

done, it is facilitated by placing substances on the tongue and asking the client to identify them with the eyes closed. To ensure valid results, the nurse instructs the client to sip water between assessments.

Facial Skin. The nurse notes characteristics of the facial skin while assessing the head. Although skin assessment begins here, it continues as the nurse examines other body areas. Regardless of location, skin should be smooth, unbroken, of uniform color consistent with the client's ethnicity or race, warm, and resilient. It should not be wet or unusually dry. Diagnostic variations in skin color are listed in Table 13-3.

While examining the skin, the nurse may detect one or more alterations in its integrity:

- A *wound* is a break in the skin.
- An *ulcer* is an open, crater-like area.
- An *abrasion* is an area that has been rubbed away by friction.
- A *laceration* is a torn, jagged wound.
- A *fissure* is a crack in the skin especially in or near mucous membranes.
- A *scar* is a mark left by the healing of a wound or lesion.

Other common skin lesions and their characteristics are described in Table 13-4. Additional skin assessments are described later as related to other body areas.

Stop, Think, and Respond Box 13-2

A nurse has documented that a client has maculopapular skin lesions over her body. Describe how these would appear.

Hair. Assessment of the hair includes scalp hair, eyebrows, and eyelashes. The nurse notes the color, texture, and distribution (presence or absence in unusual locations for gender or age). He or she also inspects the hair for debris such as blood in a client with head trauma, nits (eggs from a lice infestation), or scales from scalp lesions. As the physical assessment progresses, the nurse also observes the characteristics of body hair.

Scalp. The nurse assesses the scalp by randomly separating the hair and inspecting the skin. He or she looks for signs that the scalp is smooth, intact, and free of lesions. The nurse also palpates the skull for any unusual contour.

TABLE 13-3 Common Skin Color Variations

COLOR	TERM	POSSIBLE CAUSES
Pale, regardless of race	Pallor	Anemia, blood loss
Red	Erythema	Superficial burns, local inflammation, carbon monoxide poisoning
Pink	Flushed	Fever, hypertension
Purple	Ecchymosis	Trauma to soft tissue
Blue	Cyanosis	Low tissue oxygenation
Yellow	Jaundice	Liver or kidney disease, destruction of red blood cells
Brown	Tan	Ethnic variation, sun exposure, pregnancy, Addison's disease

Neck

The neck supports the head in midline. The client should be able to bend the head forward, backward, and to either side, as well as to rotate it 180 degrees. The trachea (windpipe) should be in the center of the neck. Pulsations in the carotid arteries (see Chap. 12) are visible and easy to palpate. There should be no unusual bulges or fullness in the neck. Some nurses lightly palpate the lymph nodes in the neck area or assess anteriorly for an enlarged thyroid gland.

Chest and Spine

The chest is a cavity surrounded by the ribs and vertebrae and houses the heart and lungs. The nurse observes the chest's shape and movement with breathing, notes the curved appearance of the spine, and assesses skin turgor, breasts, heart sounds, and lung sounds.

Turgor (the resiliency of the skin) is a combination of the elastic quality of the skin and the pressure exerted on it by the fluid within. To assess skin turgor, the nurse grasps the client's skin between the thumb and fingers in an attempt to lift it from the underlying tissue. The area over the chest is a good assessment location because the skin in other areas tends to loosen with age. When the nurse releases the tissue, it should return immediately to its original position. Prolonged "tenting" indicates dehydration.

Chest Shape and Movement

In normal adults, the lateral dimension of the chest is approximately twice the anterior–posterior dimension. Various musculoskeletal abnormalities, cardiac or respiratory diseases, or trauma can cause changes in shape (Fig. 13-16). With normal breathing, the chest expands equally on both sides. To assess chest expansion, the nurse places his or her thumbs side by side over the client's posterior vertebrae at about the level of the 10th rib (Fig. 13-17). As the client inhales, the nurse notes how far the thumbs separate; normally the distance is 1 to 2 in. (3 to 5 cm).

TABLE 13-4 Common Skin Lesions

TYPE OF LESION	DESCRIPTION	EXAMPLE	ILLUSTRATION
Macule	Flat, round, colored, nonpalpable area	Freckles	
Papule	Elevated, palpable, solid	Wart	
Vesicle	Elevated, round, filled with serum	Blister	
Wheal	Elevated, irregular border, no free fluid	Hives	
Pustule	Elevated, raised border, filled with pus	Boil	
Nodule	Elevated, solid mass, deeper and firmer than papule	Enlarged lymph node	
Cyst	Encapsulated, round, fluid-filled or solid mass beneath the skin	Tissue growth	

Spine

The spine, or vertebral column, appears in midline with gentle concave and convex curves when viewed from the side. The shoulders are at equal height. Some common deviations may be noted (Fig. 13-18). *Lordosis* is an exaggerated natural lumbar curve of the spine. *Kyphosis* is an increased thoracic curve. *Scoliosis* is a pronounced lateral curvature of the spine.

Breasts

Although breast abnormalities such as tumors can occur in men, they are more common in women. Usually, more advanced practitioners examine the breasts manually. In November 2009, the U.S. Preventive Services Task Force made several controversial recommendations: (1) that teaching breast self-examination (BSE) is unnecessary because there is no net benefit and (2) that routine mammography

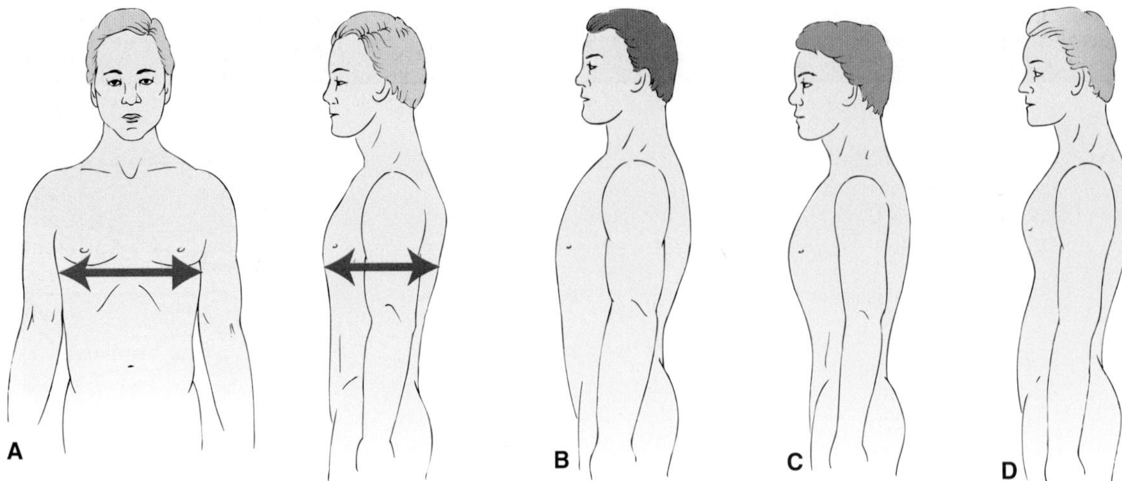

FIGURE 13-16 **A.** Normal chest size and shape; anterolateral dimension is twice the anteroposterior dimension. **B.** Barrel chest. **C.** Pigeon chest. **D.** Funnel chest.

screening should begin at age 50 and every 2 years thereafter because earlier screenings rarely saved lives and more often resulted in misdiagnoses (Agency for Health Care Research and Quality, 2009). However, the Society of Breast Imaging, the American College of Radiology, and the American Cancer Society continue to advocate that mammography screening should begin at age 40. Furthermore, the American Cancer Society recommends that although BSE plays a small role in finding breast cancer, its benefit lies in helping women assess the look and feel of their breasts to detect changes (American Cancer Society, 2009). For those women who wish to perform BSE, nurses are the ideal health practitioner to teach this self-assessment technique (Client and Family Teaching 13-1, Table 13-5, and Fig. 13-19).

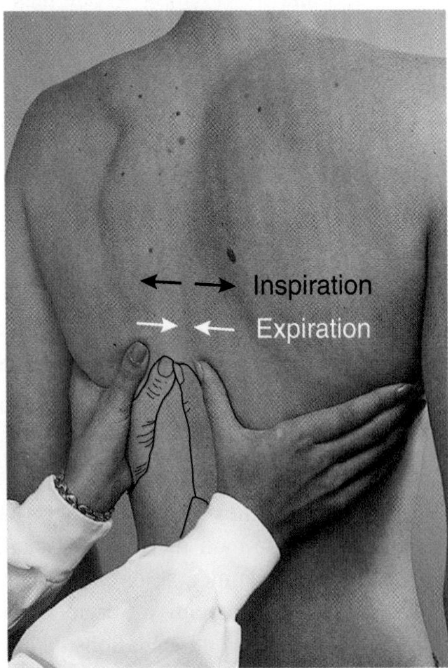

FIGURE 13-17 Palpation of thoracic excursion. In the posterior approach, the nurse places the hands at the level of the 10th rib and observes for equal movement as the client inhales.

Heart Sounds

When assessing the anterior chest, the nurse listens to the heart sounds, which presumably are caused by the closing of the atrial and ventricular valves. A beginning nurse may limit assessment to the apical area (see Chap. 12). Experienced nurses expand their skills to auscultate at the aortic, pulmonic, tricuspid, and mitral areas (Fig. 13-20).

Normal Heart Sounds

The two normal heart sounds are S1 and S2. S1, the first heart sound, correlates with the "lub" sound and is louder at the apex or mitral area when using the diaphragm of a stethoscope. Although the second heart sound, S2 or the "dub" sound, can be heard in the mitral area, it is louder over the aortic area.

Sometimes there is a slight slurring, or splitting, of one or both sounds that lasts just a fraction of a second longer. It may sound like "lubba-dub" or "lub-dubba." Split sounds generally are attributed to the fact that the valves between the atria (or ventricles) do not always close in exact unison. Splitting, if heard at all, generally is noted with the stethoscope at point P or T on the chest.

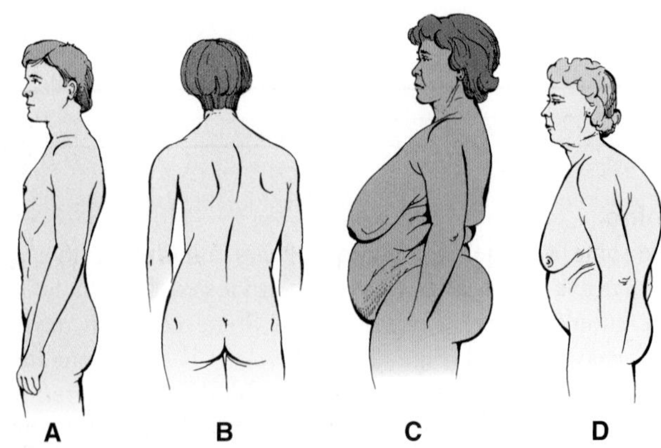

FIGURE 13-18 Variations in spinal curves: normal (**A**), scoliosis (**B**), lordosis (**C**), and kyphosis (**D**).

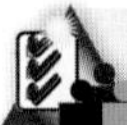

Client and Family Teaching 13-1 Breast Self-Examination

The nurse teaches the client as follows:

- Examine the breasts monthly about 1 week after the menstrual period or on a specific date postmenopause.
- Begin the examination in the shower.
- Use the right hand to examine the left breast and the left hand to examine the right breast.
- Place the hand on the side that will be examined behind the head.
- Glide the flat portion of the fingers over each breast up to the collarbone, out to the armpit, to the middle of the chest, and down to the bottom of the rib cage (see Fig. 13-19) in an up-and-down or vertical pattern.
- Determine if there are any lumps, hard knots, or thickened areas.
- Next, stand in front of a mirror.
- Look at both breasts with the arms relaxed at the side, with the hands pressing on the hips, and with the hands elevated above the head.
- Look for dimpling in the skin or retraction of either nipple.
- Lie down for the remainder of the examination.
- Put a pillow or folded towel under the shoulder on the side where the first breast will be examined; reverse the pillow before examining the second breast.
- Again, place the arm behind the head.
- Press the flat surface of the fingers in small circular motions from the outer margin of the breast toward the nipple, feeling for changes in any area of the breast (see Fig. 13-19).
- Feel upward toward the axilla of each arm.
- Complete at least three revolutions about the breast.
- Squeeze the nipple gently between the thumb and index finger to determine if there is any clear or bloody discharge.
- Repeat the examination on the opposite breast and axilla.
- Report any unusual findings or changes to a physician.
- Breast self-examination may be combined with a clinical examination and mammography to ensure early diagnosis and treatment of cancerous tumors (see Table 13-5).

TABLE 13-5 Breast Examination Guidelines

TECHNIQUE	AGE	FREQUENCY
Self-examination (optional)	≥20 years	Once per month
Clinical examination by a nurse or physician	20–39 years	Every 3 years
	≥40 years	Every year
Mammography	40 years	First examination and yearly thereafter
Clinical exam, mammography, magnetic resonance imaging (MRI)	Any age, high risk	Yearly

Source: American Cancer Society, 2009.

Abnormal Heart Sounds

The nurse may hear two additional sounds, S3 and S4, when auscultating the chest. S3, which is normal in children but abnormal in most adults, appears after S2. S3 sounds like "lub-dub-**dub**" or the cadence of sounds in "Ken-tuck-**y**." An S3 is much more pronounced than a split second sound. S4 is heard just before S1. It may sound like "**lub**-lub-dub" or the syllables in "**Ten**-nes-see."

Identifying abnormal heart sounds—S3, S4, heart murmurs, clicks, and rubs—is a skill that nurses master after they become proficient at distinguishing S1 from S2. A beginning nurse should consult with an experienced nurse or physician if there are any unusual characteristics in a client's S1 and S2 heart sounds.

Lung Sounds

Listening to the lungs is another skill that requires frequent and repeated practice because some sounds are normal and others are abnormal (see Nursing Guidelines 13-4 and Figure 13-21).

Normal Lung Sounds

Normal lung sounds are created by air moving in and out of passageways. The sounds vary in pitch and duration in

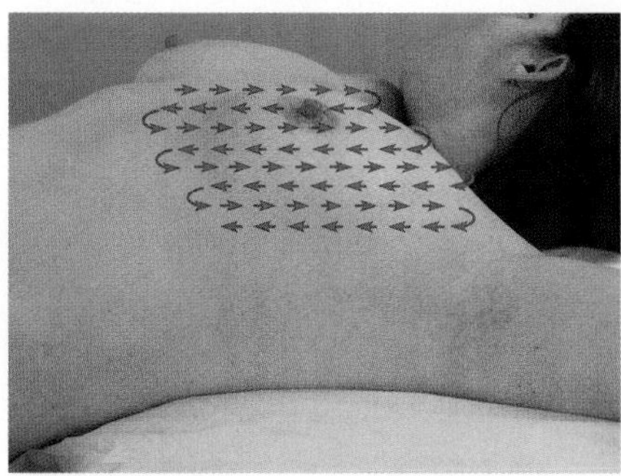
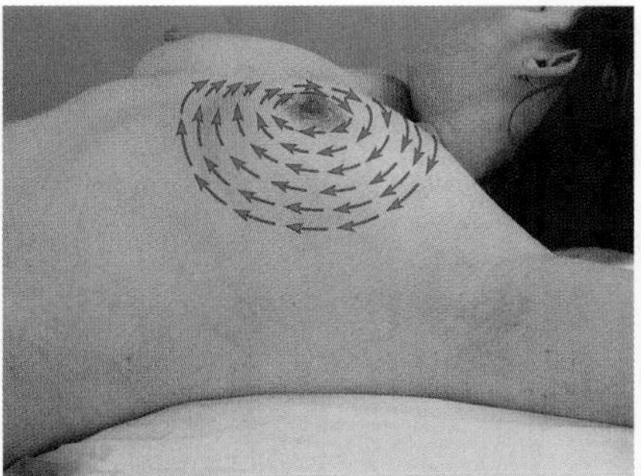
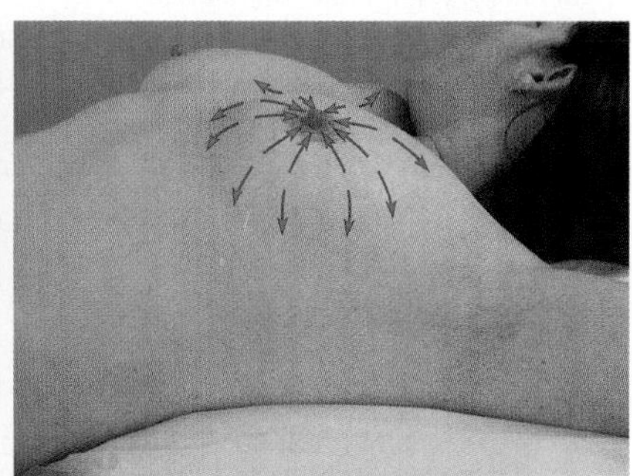

FIGURE 13-19 Patterns for assessment of breast tissue. The vertical up-and-down pattern starting at an imaginary line drawn straight down the side from the underarm and moving across the breast from the clavicle to the base of the ribs is the most effective pattern for covering the entire breast without missing any breast tissue (American Cancer Society, 2009). (From Taylor, 2011.)

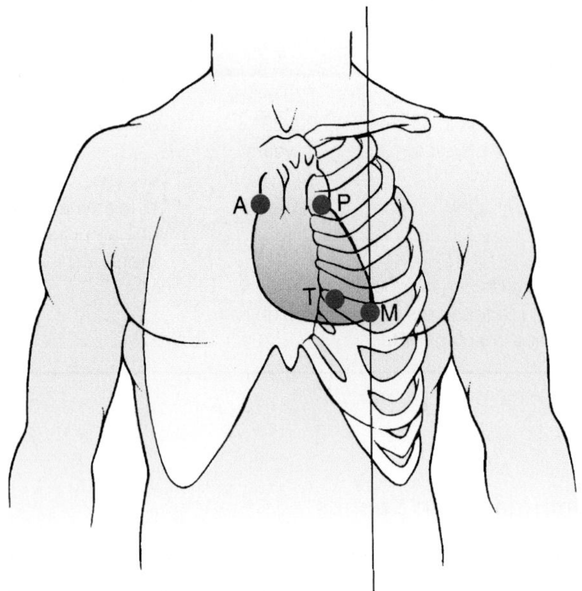

FIGURE 13-20 Locations for assessing heart sounds: M, mitral area; T, tricuspid area; P, pulmonic area; A, aortic area.

relation to the size and location of the air passages (Fig. 13-22). There are four normal lung sounds:

- *Tracheal sounds* are loud and coarse. They are equal in length during inspiration and expiration and are separated by a brief pause.
- *Bronchial sounds,* heard over the upper sternum and between the scapulae, are harsh and loud. They are shorter on inspiration than expiration with a pause between them.
- *Bronchovesicular sounds* are heard on either side of the central chest or back. These medium-range sounds of equal length during inspiration and expiration have no noticeable pause.
- *Vesicular sounds* are located in the periphery of all the lung fields. Their soft, rustling quality is longer on inspiration than expiration, with no pause between.

Abnormal Lung Sounds

Abnormal lung sounds, known as *adventitious sounds,* are those heard in addition to normal lung sounds. Most adventitious sounds are created by air moving through secretions or narrowed airways. Adventitious sounds are divided into four categories:

- *Crackles,* also called *rales,* are intermittent, high-pitched, popping, and heard in distant areas of the lungs, primarily during inspiration. They resemble the sound of crisped rice cereal when milk is added. They are attributed to the opening of partially collapsed alveoli (terminal air sacs) or the movement of air over minute amounts of fluid in the periphery of the lungs during deep inspiration.
- *Gurgles,* also called *rhonchi,* are low-pitched, continuous, bubbling, and heard in larger airways. They are more prominent during expiration. Some describe gurgles as

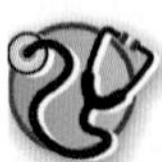

NURSING GUIDELINES 13-4

Assessing Lung Sounds

- Wash hands or perform hand antisepsis with an alcohol rub (see Chap. 10). *These measures reduce the spread of infection.*
- Provide privacy. *Doing so demonstrates concern for client modesty.*
- Raise the bed to a comfortable position for you. *Doing so reduces strain on the musculoskeletal system.*
- Assist the client to a sitting position, if possible. *This position facilitates auscultating the anterior, posterior, and lateral aspects of the chest with minimal client exertion.*
- Remove or loosen the client's upper clothing. *Doing so aids in identifying anatomic landmarks.*
- Reduce or eliminate environmental noise such as suction motors and oxygen equipment. *Quiet conditions promote the accurate identification of lung sounds.*
- Ask the client to refrain from talking. *Talking interferes with concentration and distorts lung sounds.*
- Warm the diaphragm of the stethoscope in the palm of your hand. *Warmth reduces discomfort when the diaphragm is applied to the chest.*
- Instruct the client to breathe in and out through an open mouth deeply but slowly. *This type of breathing reduces noise from air turbulence and prevents hyperventilation.*
- Apply the chest piece to the upper back, but avoid placement over the scapulae or ribs. *This method facilitates hearing sounds in the upper and lower lobes and reduces competing sounds from the heart.*
- Listen for one complete ventilation (inspiration and expiration) at each area auscultated. *This method ensures hearing characteristics during each phase of ventilation.*
- If body hair causes noise, wet it or press harder with the chest piece. *This technique reduces sound distortion.*
- Move the diaphragm from side to side from the apices (top) to the bases (bottom) of the lungs (see Fig. 13-21). *This sequence facilitates comparison of sounds.*
- Auscultate the lateral and anterior chest in a similar fashion. *Doing so ensures a comprehensive assessment.*
- Ask the client to cough or breathe deeply if crackles or gurgles are audible. *This method helps to clear the air passages and open the alveoli.*
- Reapply clothing and lower the bed. *Doing so restores comfort and safety.*
- Wash hands or perform hand antisepsis with an alcohol rub (see Chap. 10). *Doing so reduces the spread of microorganisms.*
- Record assessment findings. *Documented data can be used for future comparisons.*
- Repeat lung sound assessments according to agency policy or the client's condition. *Doing so demonstrates responsibility, accountability, and good clinical judgment.*

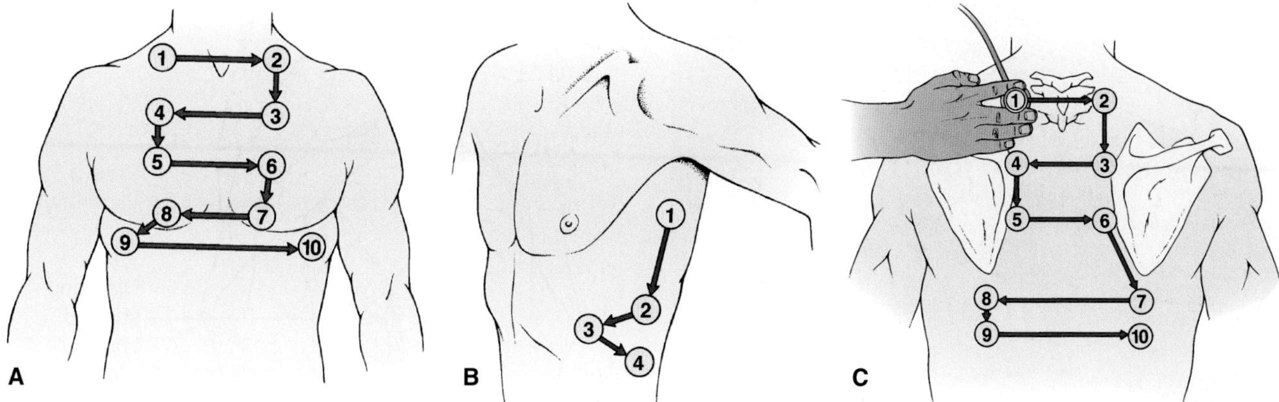

FIGURE 13-21 The auscultation sequence: anterior (A), lateral (B), and posterior (C).

sounding like wet snoring. Gurgles may clear with deep breathing or coughing.

- *Wheezes* are whistling or squeaking sounds caused by air moving through a narrowed passage. They can be heard anywhere in the chest during inspiration or expiration. Wheezes may be audible without a stethoscope. Coughing and deep breathing do not usually alter a wheeze; in fact, if wheezing suddenly stops, it may mean that the air passage is totally occluded.
- *Rubs* are grating, leathery sounds caused by two dry pleural surfaces moving over each other.

Whenever adventitious sounds are heard, the nurse also assesses the characteristics of any cough and the appearance of raised sputum.

Stop, Think, and Respond Box 13-3

What physical assessments are appropriate when a client is coughing frequently?

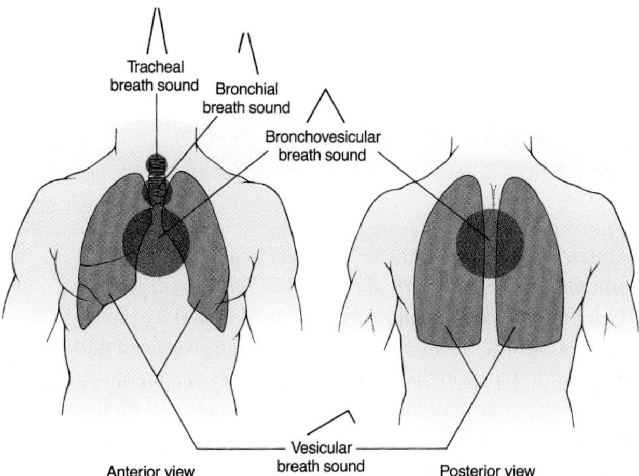

FIGURE 13-22 Locations of normal lung sounds. The symbols indicate the ratio of time they may be heard during inspiration and expiration, as well as the presence or absence of pauses between the two.

Extremities

The nurse notes the alignment, mobility, and strength of the extremities and compares their size. He or she feels the skin temperature, notes the characteristics of the nails, times the capillary refill, palpates local peripheral pulses (see Chap. 12), checks for edema, and may test the perception of skin sensations. Advanced practitioners assess deep tendon reflexes with a reflex hammer.

Muscle Strength

The nurse assesses all four extremities separately to determine muscle strength. He or she asks the client to grasp, squeeze, and release the nurse's fingers. As the nurse pulls and pushes on the forearm and upper arm, he or she instructs the client to resist. To test strength in the lower extremities, the nurse has the client push and pull against resistance (Fig. 13-23).

Fingernails and Toenails

Changes in the shape and thickness of the fingernails and toenails are often signs of chronic cardiopulmonary disease (Fig. 13-24) or fungal infections. The nurse documents any unusual characteristics of the nails or surrounding tissues.

Capillary refill time (the time it takes blood to resume flowing in the base of the nail beds) is normally less than 3 seconds after compression and release of the nail bed. To assess capillary refill time:

1. Observe the color in the nail bed.
2. Depress the nail bed, displacing capillary blood.
3. Release the pressure.
4. Note how many seconds it takes for the preassessment color to reappear. Watching a clock would interfere with an accurate assessment, so count, "one-one thousand, two-one thousand, three-one thousand" to estimate the time in seconds.

Edema

Edema is excessive fluid within tissue and signifies abnormal fluid distribution. Clients with cardiovascular, liver,

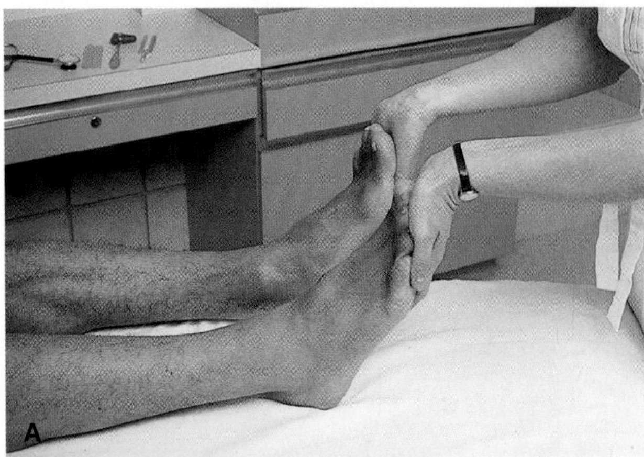

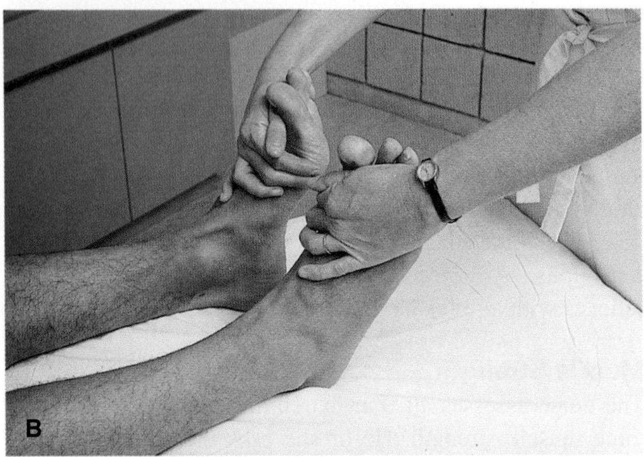

FIGURE 13-23 Assessing muscle strength of lower extremities. **A.** Resisting the push of a nurse. **B.** Resisting the pull by a nurse.

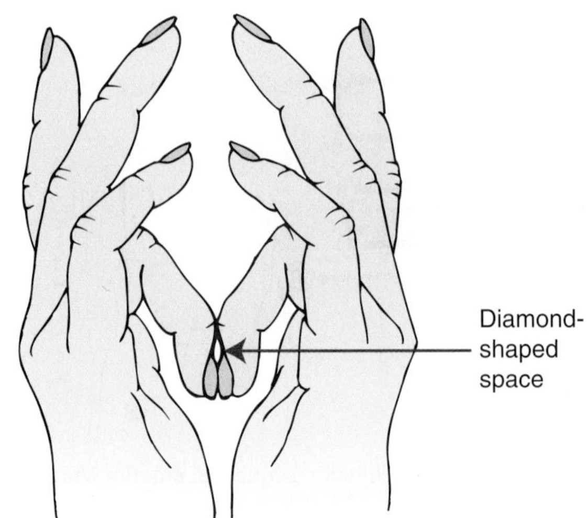

FIGURE 13-24 A technique for assessing clubbed fingernails. A diamond-shape space between the nails of the ring fingers is normal.

and kidney dysfunction are prone to edema. Subtle signs of edema include weight gain, tight rings, and patterns in the skin after removing socks or shoes. To determine the extent of any edema, the nurse presses a thumb or finger into the tissue over a bone. If an indentation remains (*pitting edema*), the nurse attempts to quantify its severity (Box 13-2).

Skin Sensation

During a comprehensive rather than a basic assessment, the nurse tests the client's ability to differentiate between light touch, warmth, cold, sharp, dull, and vibration (see Nursing Guidelines 13-5).

ABDOMEN

Most gastrointestinal and accessory digestive organs lie within the abdomen. The bladder, if distended, may rise into the abdomen.

For assessment purposes, the abdomen is divided into four quadrants (Fig. 13-25). *The abdomen is always inspected and then auscultated—in that sequence—before using palpation or percussion techniques.* Touching or manipulating the abdomen can alter bowel sounds, thus producing invalid findings.

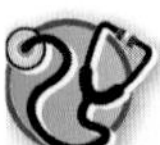

NURSING GUIDELINES 13-5

Assessing Sensory Skin Perception

- Gather a cotton ball, a safety pin, or other pointed object; a small container of warm water and one of ice water; and a tuning fork. *These materials provide for a variety of test resources.*
- Instruct the client to shut both eyes. *Doing so reduces the potential for gathering invalid data.*
- Explain that you will touch the skin with test objects at various places and on both sides of the body and that you will ask the client to identify the location and characteristics of the sensation. *This information identifies the test method and how the client is expected to respond.*
- Touch the client with the test objects in a random pattern. *A random pattern prevents the potential for correct guessing.*
- Use both the pointed and curved ends of the safety pin to determine if the client can discriminate between sharp and dull. Take care not to puncture the skin. *Doing so prevents injury.*
- Stroke the skin with the cotton ball; touch areas with the warm and cold containers. *These tests assess the client's ability to identify fine touch and differences in temperature.*
- Strike a tuning fork and place the stem against bony areas such as the wrists and along the length of the shins. *This tests the client's ability to sense vibration.*

BOX 13-2 Criteria for Estimating Pitting Edema

1+ Pitting Edema
- Slight indentation (2 mm)
- Normal contours
- Associated with interstitial fluid volume 30% above normal

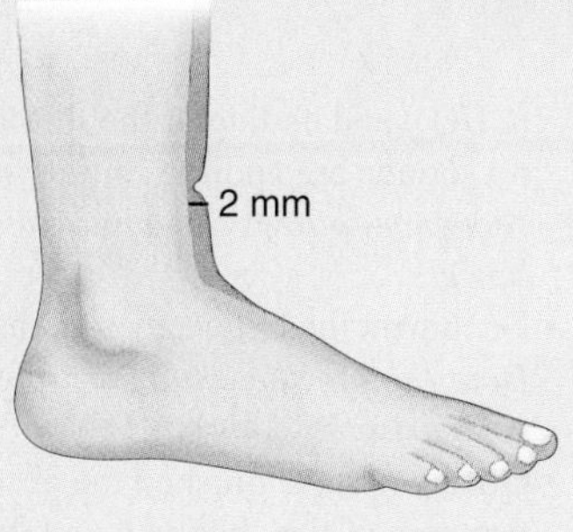

2+ Pitting Edema
- Deeper pit after pressing (4 mm)
- Lasts longer than 1+
- Fairly normal contour

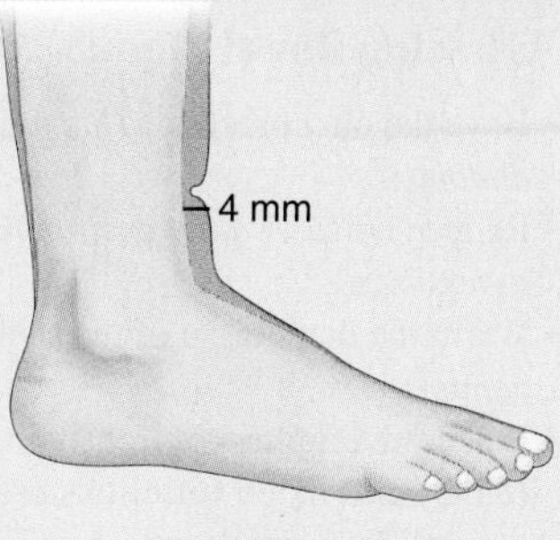

3+ Pitting Edema
- Deep pit (6 mm)
- Remains several seconds after pressing
- Skin swelling obvious by general inspection

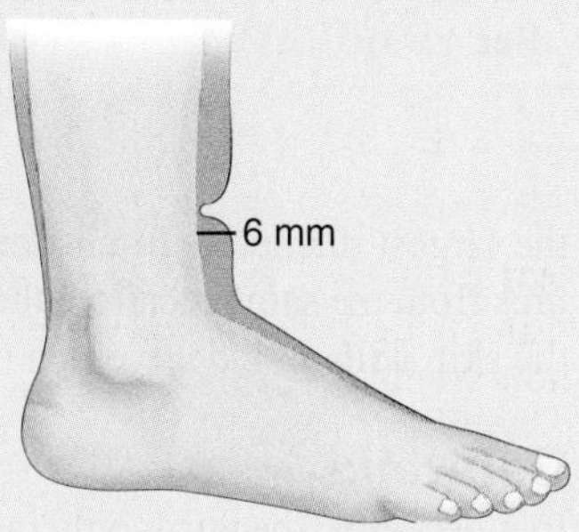

4+ Pitting Edema
- Deep pit (8 mm)
- Remains for a prolonged time after pressing, possibly minutes
- Frank swelling

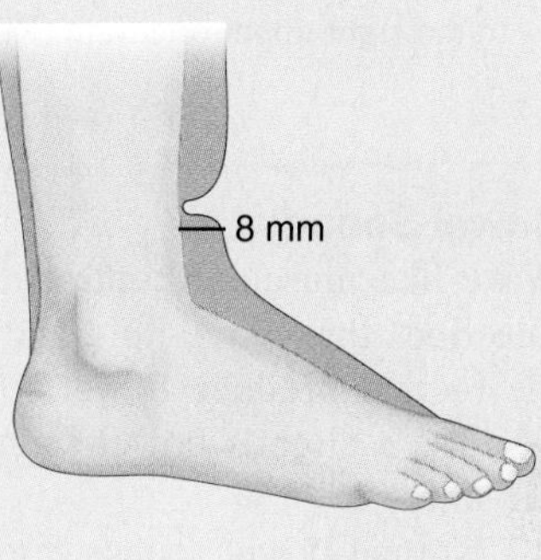

5+ Brawny Edema
- Fluid can no longer be displaced secondary to excessive interstitial fluid accumulation
- No pitting
- Tissue palpates as firm or hard
- Skin surface shiny, warm, moist

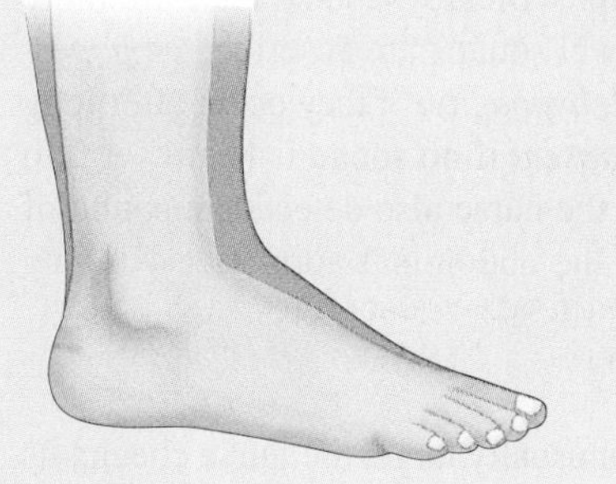

Midline

A B
RUQ LUQ
RLQ LLQ
C D

Right Upper Quadrant
- Pylorous
- Duodenum
- Liver
- Right kidney and adrenal gland
- Hepatic flexure of colon
- Head of pancreas

Left Upper Quadrant
- Stomach
- Spleen
- Left kidney and adrenal gland
- Splenic flexure of colon
- Body of pancreas

Right Lower Quadrant
- Cecum
- Appendix
- Right ovary and fallopian tube (female)
- Right ureter and lower kidney pole
- Right spermatic cord (male)

Left Lower Quadrant
- Sigmoid colon
- Left ovary and fallopian tube (female)
- Left ureter and lower kidney pole
- Left spermatic cord (male)

Midline
- Urinary bladder
- Urethra (female)

FIGURE 13-25 The four abdominal quadrants. **A.** The right upper quadrant (RUQ). **B.** The left upper quadrant (LUQ). **C.** The right upper quadrant (LUQ). **D.** The left lower quadrant (LLQ). (From Taylor, 2011.)

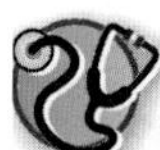

NURSING GUIDELINES 13-6

Assessing Bowel Sounds

- Have the client recline. *This position provides access to the abdomen.*
- Reduce noise. *A quiet environment facilitates an accurate assessment.*
- Warm the diaphragm of the stethoscope. *Warmth promotes comfort.*
- Place the diaphragm lightly in the right lower quadrant (RLQ) and listen for clicks or gurgles. Move the chest piece over all four quadrants in a clockwise pattern from the RLQ to the right upper quadrant (RUQ) to the left upper quadrant (LUQ), and ending at the left lower quadrant (LLQ)). If no sounds are audible initially, listen for 2 to 5 min. *This sequence follows the anatomic areas of the upper to lower bowel.*
- Document the frequency and character of the bowel sounds. *Doing so provides data for problem identification and future comparisons.*
- Once you have finished the auscultation, note the softness or firmness of the abdomen and feel for palpable masses (see Box 13-3).

Bowel Sounds

Wave-like muscular contractions of the large and small intestines that move fluid and intestinal contents toward the rectum produce bowel sounds. The nurse routinely assesses a client's bowel sounds on admission and once per shift.

Normal bowel sounds resemble clicks or gurgles and occur 5 to 34 times a minute (Bickley, 2008). They are more frequent after eating. Bowel sounds are described as *hyperactive* if they are frequent, *hypoactive* if they occur after long intervals of silence, and *absent* if no sound is heard for 2 to 5 minutes. Occasionally, the nurse also detects the sound of blood pulsating through the abdominal aorta (see Nursing Guidelines 13-6 and Box 13-3).

Abdominal Girth

If the abdomen appears unusually large, the nurse checks its girth (circumference) daily by using a tape measure around the largest diameter. To ensure that he or she always measures from the same location, the nurse makes guide marks on the skin with an indelible pen (Fig. 13-26).

BOX 13-3 Characteristics of Palpated Masses

CHARACTERISTIC	DESCRIPTION
Mobility	Fixed—does not move Mobile—can be moved with palpation
Shape	Round—resembles a ball Tubular—is elongated Ovoid—resembles an egg Irregular—has no definite shape
Consistency	Edematous—leaves indentation when palpated Nodular—feels bumpy to touch Granular—feels gritty to touch Spongy—feels soft to touch Hard—feels firm to touch
Size	Measured in centimeters (1 cm = approximately 0.4 in.)
Tenderness	Amount of discomfort when palpated—none, slight, moderate, or severe

Genitalia

In most cases, the nurse only inspects the genitalia. If contact with genital structures or secretions is required, the nurse dons gloves. To eliminate the possibility of being falsely accused of sexual impropriety, it is a good practice to ask someone of the client's gender to be present when the nurse touches the genitalia.

During inspection, the nurse notes the condition of the skin and the distribution and characteristics of pubic hair (lice may infest pubic hair). A physician or nurse with advanced skills examines females internally with an instrument called a speculum (see Chap. 14); in men, the prostate gland is palpated during a digital rectal examination.

The nurse observes if the male is circumcised and if the scrotum appears to be of normal size. Whenever possible, he or she instructs male clients how to examine their testicles (see Client and Family Teaching 13-2 and Fig. 13-27).

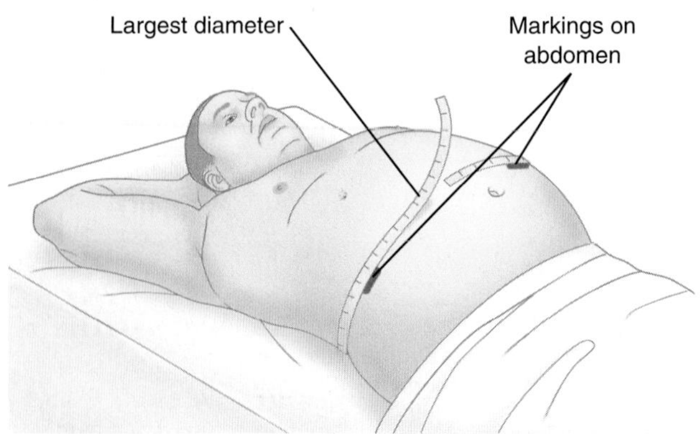

FIGURE 13-26 Measuring abdominal girth.

Client and Family Teaching 13-2 Testicular Self-Examination

The nurse teaches the client as follows:

- Examine the testes monthly at a time when the testicles are warm and positioned loosely within the scrotum (eg, during bathing or showering).
- Elevate the penis with one hand.
- Gently roll each testicle within the scrotum between the thumb and index finger.
- Feel each testicle vertically and horizontally (see Fig. 13-27).
- Check for any unusual lumps; cancerous lumps are located most often on the upper and outer sides of the testes.
- Continue palpation following the spermatic cord from the testicle to where it ascends into the abdomen.
- Report any unusual findings to a physician as soon as possible; an early diagnosis carries a better prognosis.

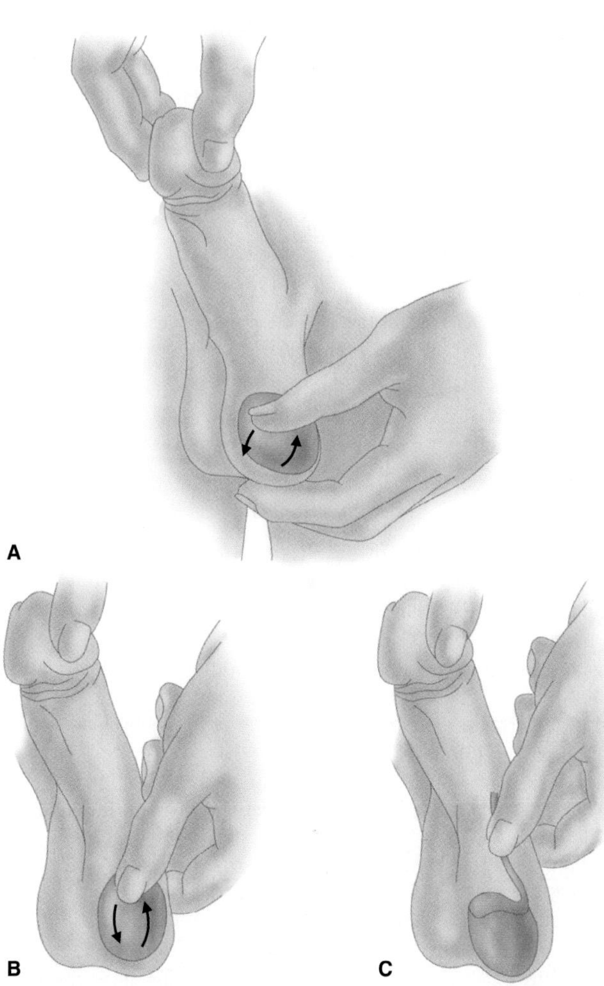

FIGURE 13-27 A testicular self-examination. **A.** Horizontal palpation. **B.** Vertical palpation. **C.** Palpation of spermatic cord. (From Taylor, 2011.)

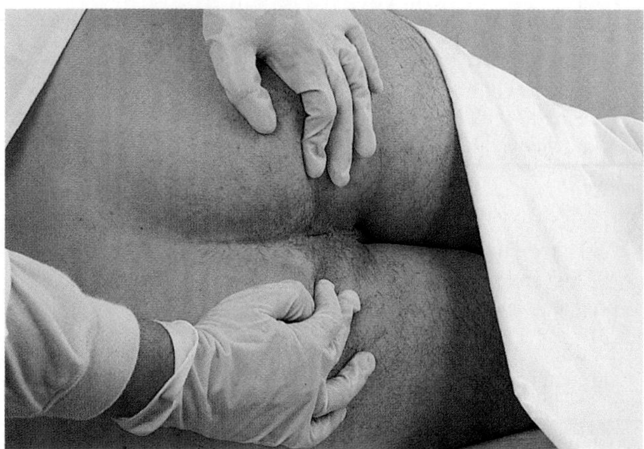

FIGURE 13-28 An inspection of the anus.

Anus and Rectum

Unless a client has specific symptoms, the nurse inspects only the anus. If touching is required, gloves are necessary. To examine the anus, the nurse positions the client on the side with the knees bent. He or she separates the client's buttocks and inspects the external orifice (Fig. 13-28). The area should appear intact but more pigmented than adjacent skin; it should be moist and hairless. External hemorrhoids (saccular protrusions filled with blood) may extend beyond the external sphincter muscle. There may be rectal fissures (cracks) if the client has a history of chronic constipation. Trauma also may be present if the client has anal intercourse.

NURSING IMPLICATIONS

Assessment findings form the basis for identifying health problems. Often during a physical assessment, clients reveal situations that caused their health to fail, or they indicate a desire for more health information. The following are some nursing diagnoses that may apply:

- Readiness for Enhanced Knowledge
- Ineffective Health Maintenance
- Ineffective Self-Health Management
- Deficient Knowledge
- Noncompliance
- Readiness for Enhanced Self-Health Management

Nursing Care Plan 13-1 is an example of how the nursing process is used when a client has the nursing diagnosis of Readiness for Enhanced Self-Health Management, defined by NANDA-I (2012, p. 164) as "a pattern of regulating and integrating into daily living a therapeutic regimen … that is sufficient for meeting health-related goals and can be strengthened."

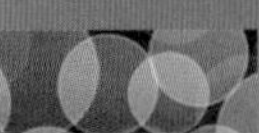

NURSING CARE PLAN 13-1 Readiness for Enhanced Self-Health Management

Assessment

- Interact with the client to determine if he or she expresses a desire to seek a higher level of wellness or manifests a lack of knowledge about health promotional activities.
- Other evidence that validates the nursing diagnosis of Readiness for Enhanced Self-Health Management is that the client voices an interest in making choices in daily living that are appropriate for meeting goals that reduce health risk factors and prevent illness.

Nursing Diagnosis. **Readiness for Enhanced Self-Health Management** related to prevention of sexually transmitted diseases (STDs) and pregnancy as evidenced by the following statements, "I've been having sex with many women. None of them has gotten pregnant, and I haven't caught any diseases as far as I know. But I don't want to take chances anymore."

Expected Outcome. The client will describe safer sexual practices within 24 hours (time of anticipated discharge), following a surgical repair of an inguinal hernia.

Interventions	Rationales
Determine the client's knowledge regarding various common STDs and how they are transmitted.	Effective health teaching builds on a foundation of knowledge that the client already has acquired.
Explore the client's views concerning nonpermanent measures that men can implement to reduce the potential for pregnancy.	The client's ability to incorporate new health behaviors depends on his acceptance of and willingness to integrate such changes.
Provide pamphlets titled "Choices" and "Understanding Safer Sex" from the Reproductive Control Clinic. These describe birth control measures and illustrate the technique for applying a condom to prevent STDs.	Information from an authoritative resource provides scientifically based information.
Give the client a supply of free condoms from the Reproductive Control Clinic.	An initial supply of condoms facilitates implementation of new health behaviors until the client acquires his own personal supply.
Review the following health information and illustrations (A and B) in the pamphlets.	

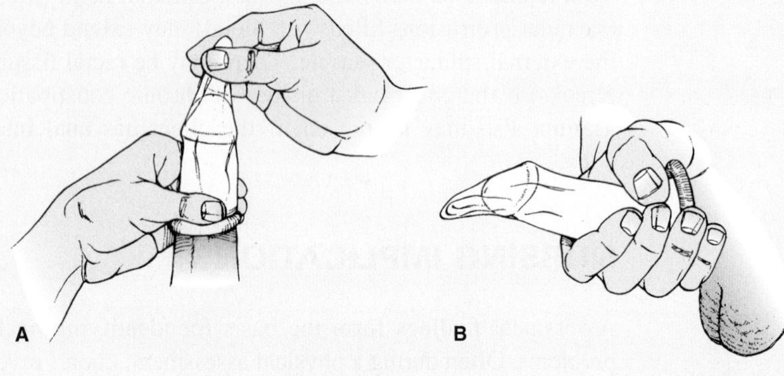

A. To apply, roll the condom completely over the erect penis while pinching the space at the condom tip. **B.** Hold the condom at the base of the penis during its removal from the vagina.

Interventions	Rationales
Reduce sexual partners to one noninfected, faithful person.	Sex with a monogamous, disease-free partner reduces the potential for acquiring an STD.
Use a latex condom and apply nonoxynol-9 either over the tip of the condom or as a vaginal application.	A condom provides a barrier for sperm and microorganisms. Nonoxynol-9 is a chemical spermicide.
Roll the condom completely over the erect penis while pinching a space at the condom tip.	Leaving a space provides an area where semen can collect without breaking the condom.
Hold the condom at the base of the penis and promptly remove the condom-covered penis from the vagina before the penis becomes limp.	Prompt removal of a condom reduces the potential for leaking sperm within the vagina, which can lead to pregnancy.
Do not have sexual contact again unless you apply another condom.	For maximum effectiveness, condoms are recommended for single use.
If a condom breaks or leaks, urinate immediately and wash the penis with soap and water.	Urination helps to eliminate microorganisms that cause STDs through the male urethra. Washing with soap and water removes microorganisms from the surface of the penis.

Evaluation of Expected Outcomes

- The client reads the pamphlets provided.
- The client states, "Condoms are inconvenient, but they're better than getting a disease. They're also cheaper than babies. I plan to use them from now on until I find the right life partner."

CRITICAL THINKING EXERCISES

1. A client reports that he has not had a bowel movement for 3 days, which is unusual for him. Discuss the physical assessments important to perform at this time.

2. Describe the characteristics of lung sounds normally heard at the midchest area below the nipple line.

3. What action is appropriate if an older adult becomes fatigued during a physical assessment?

4. What information could the nurse provide to a female client who is confused about the change in the breast examination guidelines?

NCLEX-STYLE REVIEW QUESTIONS

1. Although all the following information is appropriate to gather when assessing a client with a cough, besides documenting the characteristics of the cough, what other assessment information is essential?

1. The client's family history of respiratory disease
2. A current assessment of the client's heart rate
3. The appearance of respiratory secretions
4. Any self-treatment that the client is using

2. Which explanation is best when teaching a client how to palpate breast tissue during a breast self-examination?

1. Move up and down beginning in the axilla
2. Move in small circles from the nipple outward
3. Move laterally from the sternum across the breast
4. Move diagonally in four breast quadrants

3. A nurse caring for a client with a head injury performs all of the following assessments. Which one is most important at this time?

1. Assessing the client's lung sounds
2. Assessing the client's skin integrity
3. Assessing the client's urine characteristics
4. Assessing the client's pupillary responses

4. Where is the best location for the nurse to auscultate an S1 heart sound?

1. The fifth intercostal space in the left midclavicular line
2. The fourth intercostal space to the left of the sternum
3. The second intercostal space to the right of the sternum
4. The second intercostal space to the left of the sternum

5. What is the most accurate instruction a nurse can provide before using a Snellen chart to assess a client's vision?

1. "Read the words in a sample newsprint."
2. "Read the letters standing at a distance of 20 feet."
3. "Look at the colored picture and identify the image."
4. "Look at the screen and indicate when you see an object."

SKILL 13-1 Performing a Physical Assessment

Suggested Action	Reason for Action
ASSESSMENT	
Identify the client.	Ensures that the assessment is being performed on the correct person.
Determine the client's age, gender, and race.	Forms the basis for planning techniques for physical assessment.
Observe the client's state of alertness and ability to move.	Aids in determining the best location for the assessment and if the nurse, client, or both will require assistance.
Ask the client's opinion about his or her health status and any current or recent signs and symptoms.	Helps to focus attention during the assessment on particular structures and their functions.
PLANNING	
Give the client a specimen container, if a urine sample is needed.	Takes advantage of an opportunity when the client's bladder contains urine.
Have the client empty his or her bladder before undressing.	Facilitates the examination and reduces discomfort.
Pull the curtain or close the door and give the client a drape or examination gown to put on after undressing.	Prepares the client for an accurate assessment and ensures privacy.
Gather assessment equipment and supplies (see Box 13-1 for basic necessities).	Promotes organization and efficient time management.
Decide to examine the client using either a head-to-toe or a body systems approach.	Establishes the plan for assessment and ensures that comprehensive data will be gathered.
IMPLEMENTATION	
Explain how the assessment will be conducted.	Reduces anxiety.
Explain that all information will be kept confidential among those involved in the client's care.	Encourages the client to be honest and open in identifying health problems.
Wash hands or perform hand antisepsis with an alcohol rub (see Chap. 10), preferably in the client's presence.	Provides reassurance that the nurse is clean and conscientious about controlling the spread of microorganisms.
Warm your hands before touching the client.	Demonstrates concern for the client's comfort.
Obtain the client's height, weight, and vital signs.	Contributes to the general survey of the client.
Assist the client to sit at the bottom of the examination table.	Facilitates examination of the upper body without requiring the client to change positions.
Modify the client's position if the examination is being conducted in locations other than an examination room.	Demonstrates adaptability.
Explain each assessment technique before performing it.	Reduces anxiety.
Try to avoid tiring the client and apologize if the client experiences discomfort.	Demonstrates concern for the client's comfort.
Help the client to resume sitting after the examination.	Places the client in the best position for communicating.
Wash hands or perform hand antisepsis with an alcohol rub (see Chap. 10) once again.	Shows responsibility for controlling the spread of microorganisms.
Review pertinent findings, both normal and abnormal, without making medical interpretations.	Demonstrates compliance with the client's right to information.
Offer the client an opportunity to ask questions.	Encourages active participation in learning and decision making.
Begin organizing assessment findings outside the examination room while the client dresses or dons a bathrobe.	Ensures privacy.
Help the client leave the examination room.	Demonstrates courtesy and concern for the client's safety.
Dispose of soiled equipment, restore cleanliness and order to the examination room, and restock used supplies.	Shows consideration for the next person who uses the examination room.

Evaluation

- All aspects of the assessment have been carried out, and comprehensive data have been collected.
- The client remained safe, warm, and comfortable.
- The client's questions or concerns have been addressed.

Document

- Date and time
- Normal and abnormal findings
- Any unexpected outcomes during the procedure and the nursing actions taken
- To whom abnormal findings were verbally reported, and the outcome of the interaction

SAMPLE DOCUMENTATION

Date and Time A 67-year-old man transported from bed to examination room by wheelchair for physical assessment. Can cooperate without distress. Refer to assessment form for examination findings. ——— SIGNATURE/TITLE

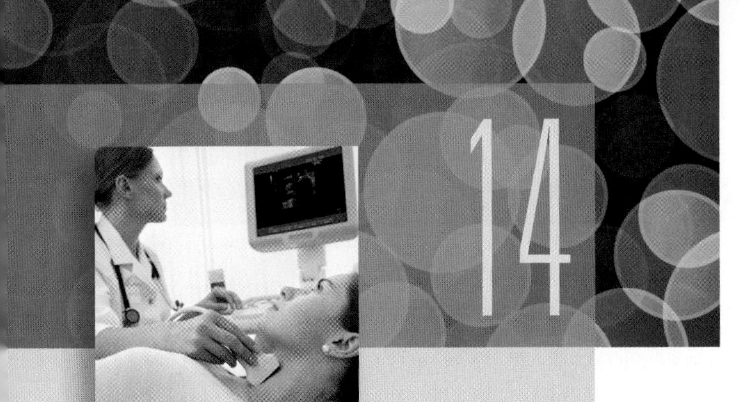

14 Special Examinations and Tests

Words To Know

cold spot
computed tomography
contrast medium
culture
diagnostic examination
dorsal recumbent position
echography
electrocardiography
electroencephalography
electromyography
endoscopy
fluoroscopy
glucometer
Gram staining
hot spot
knee–chest position
laboratory test
lithotomy position
lumbar puncture
magnetic resonance imaging
modified standing position
nuclear medicine department
Pap (Papanicolaou) test
paracentesis
pelvic examination
positron emission tomography
radiography
radionuclides
roentgenography
Sims' position
specimens
speculum
spinal tap
transducer
ultrasonography

Learning Objectives

On completion of this chapter, the reader should be able to:

1. Differentiate between an examination and a test.
2. List 10 general nursing responsibilities related to assisting with special examinations and tests.
3. Name five positions commonly used during tests or examinations.
4. Explain what is involved in a pelvic examination and a Pap test.
5. List six commonly performed categories of tests or examinations.
6. Identify four word endings and their meanings that provide clues as to how tests or examinations are performed.
7. Explain the following procedures: sigmoidoscopy, paracentesis, lumbar puncture, throat culture, and measurement of capillary blood glucose.
8. Discuss at least three factors to consider when performing examinations and tests on older adults.

In addition to obtaining a health history and performing a physical assessment, the nurse gains assessment data by evaluating the results of special examinations and tests. This chapter gives an overview of some common diagnostic examinations and tests and related nursing responsibilities. Tests involving the collection of urine and stool specimens are discussed in Chapters 30 and 31, respectively.

EXAMINATIONS AND TEST

A **diagnostic examination** is a procedure that involves the physical inspection of body structures and evidence of their functions. It is facilitated through the use of technical equipment and techniques, such as the following:

- Radiography (X-rays)
- Endoscopy (optical scopes)
- Radionuclide imaging (radioactive chemicals)
- Ultrasonography (high-frequency sound waves)
- Electrical graphic recordings

By learning root words and suffixes (word endings), which are primarily of Latin and Greek origin, it is possible to decipher many unfamiliar names of diagnostic examinations and tests (Table 14-1).

TABLE 14-1 Deciphering Diagnostic Terms

SUFFIX	MEANING	EXAMPLES	DESCRIPTION
-graphy	To record	Angiography	Test that records an image of blood vessels
-gram	An image	Angiogram	The actual image recorded during angiography
-scopy	To see	Sigmoidoscopy	Test in which the lower intestine is inspected
-scope	Examination instrument	Sigmoidoscope	A tube with a light and lens for looking within the lower intestine
-centesis	To puncture	Thoracentesis	Procedure in which a needle is used to puncture the thorax and withdraw fluid
-metry	To measure	Pelvimetry	Procedure in which the pelvis is measured
-meter	Instrument for obtaining measurements	Glucometer	Instrument for measuring glucose

A **laboratory test** is a procedure that involves the examination of body fluids or specimens. It involves comparing the components of a collected specimen with normal findings. A diagnostic examination may or may not include the collection of specimens.

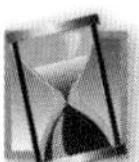

Gerontologic Considerations

■ Some laboratory values change minimally or not at all with age. Parameters are often determined by using averaged statistics. Failure to appreciate age-related differences in laboratory test results can lead to overdiagnoses or underdiagnoses and, therefore, inappropriate treatment.

■ Many prescription and over-the-counter medications, as well as herbal therapies, may affect laboratory values. Therefore, nurses must take care to review and evaluate all medications and alternative therapies before any laboratory procedures.

■ Knowing the usual range of laboratory results for older adults who have chronic conditions is important. A chronic disorder or its treatment can cause abnormal test findings that may be normal or acceptable for older adults. It is also important to know the client's previous results for the diagnostic test being done as a baseline for comparison.

General Nursing Responsibilities

When clients undergo diagnostic examinations and laboratory tests, nurses have specific responsibilities before, during, and after the procedures (Box 14-1).

Preprocedural Care

Before a client agrees to a procedure, the nurse determines whether the client understands its purpose and the activities involved. Once the client's consent for a diagnostic test is obtained, the nurse prepares the client, obtains the equipment and supplies, and readies the examination area.

Clarifying Explanations. In some cases, a signed consent form is required before performing examinations or tests. To be legally sound, consent must contain three elements: *capacity, comprehension,* and *voluntariness* (Box 14-2).

Although physicians are responsible for giving clients sufficient information to obtain their informed consent, not all clients fully understand the information. Some are too anxious to process details, others feel too insecure to ask questions, and still others express additional concerns after the physician has left. Often the nurse must repeat, simplify, clarify, or expand the original explanation.

There are no exact rules for clarifying explanations. In general, it is best to find out how much of the physician's

BOX 14-1 General Nursing Responsibilities for Examinations and Tests

- Determine the client's understanding of the procedure.
- Witness the client's signature on a consent form.
- Teach or follow test preparation requirements.
- Obtain equipment and supplies.
- Arrange the examination area.
- Position and drape the client.
- Assist the examiner.
- Provide the client with physical and emotional support.
- Care for specimens.
- Record and report appropriate information.

BOX 14-2 Elements of Informed Consent

Capacity	Indicates that the client has the ability to make a rational decision; if not, a spouse, parent, or legal guardian must do so.
Comprehension	Indicates that the client understands the physician's explanation of the risks, benefits, and alternatives that are available.[a]
Voluntariness	Indicates that the client is acting on his or her own free will without coercion or the threat of intimidation.

[a]Sedative drugs or the effects of anesthesia may temporarily affect capacity and comprehension.

explanation the client understands and use the client's questions as a guide for providing further information. Nurses should follow the suggestions for teaching and providing emotional support given in Chapter 8.

Preparing Clients. Some examinations and tests require special preparation of the client such as withholding food and fluids or modifying the diet.

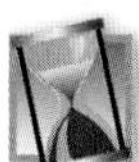

Gerontologic Considerations

- When working with an older adult who is cognitively compromised (eg, dementia), consult the person who has a medical durable power of attorney. Include the caregiver or family member in the procedure as much as possible.
- Older adults, especially those who are medically frail, may not be able to tolerate the withholding of food or fluids for long periods before tests or examinations. Assessing urinary output, blood pressure, and mental status provides data on how well an older adult is tolerating a fasting state.
- When older adults must abstain from food or fluid before a test or examination, administration of their prescribed medications with a small amount of water may be allowed based on consultation with the physician.
- Frail older adults fatigue easily; therefore, coordinate tests and examinations with diagnostic personnel to eliminate long periods of fasting or waiting in uncomfortable environments.

Because test preparation requirements vary among health care agencies, the nurse refers to written protocols in the agency's manual rather than relying on memory.

Once he or she understands the specific requirements for a test, the nurse provides directions to the client, nursing staff, and other hospital departments, such as the dietary department, involved in the test. Everyone involved must cooperate to ensure test accuracy. The nurse reports any incorrect test preparations promptly because the procedure may need to be canceled and rescheduled.

Because many tests and examinations are done on an outpatient basis, the nurse must understand the client's responsibilities and instruct him or her accordingly (see Client and Family Teaching 14-1).

Regardless of the type of examination or test, the nurse helps the client to change into an examination gown, applies an identification bracelet, takes vital signs, and suggests that the client empty his or her bladder. The nurse continues to monitor the condition of waiting clients who can experience adverse effects from fatigue, delayed food consumption, or medical symptoms.

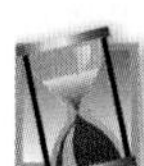

Gerontologic Considerations

- Older adults are likely to need additional clothing, slippers, and extra covers to keep them warm in waiting rooms and examination areas.

Client and Family Teaching 14-1
Preparation for Special Examinations or Tests

The nurse teaches the client who is not hospitalized to:

- Call (specify the number) if test preparation instructions are not clearly understood or cannot be followed.
- Refrain from eating or drinking anything for at least 8 hours before a test or examination that requires a fasting state.
- Follow all dietary specifications for eating or omitting certain foods exactly as directed.
- Check with the physician about taking or readjusting the time schedule for taking prescribed medications on the day of the test or examination.
- Bathe or shower as usual on the day of the test or examination.
- Dress casually and in layers so that items of clothing can be removed or added to maintain comfort in the test environment.
- Ask a friend or family member to provide transportation to and from the site if there is a potential for drowsiness, lingering pain, or weakness after the procedure.
- Arrive at least 30 minutes before the test is scheduled.
- Identify oneself at the information or appointment desk upon arrival.
- Bring information to verify insurance or Medicare coverage.

Obtaining Equipment and Supplies. If an examination or test is performed at the bedside or in an examination room on the nursing unit, the nurse obtains equipment and supplies ahead of time. Nurses are relieved of this responsibility if the examination or test is carried out in other locations or when a special technician performs the procedure.

Some items that nurses may need are in packaged kits (such as a lumbar puncture kit) kept in a clean utility room (Fig. 14-1) or may be obtained from a central supply department (also called "materials management" in some health care agencies). If using a packaged kit, the nurse checks the list of contents to determine what, if any, additional items are needed. Clean gloves, goggles, masks, and gowns are required to prevent direct contact with blood or body secretions (see section on "Standard Precautions" in Chap. 22).

Arranging the Examination Area. If the procedure is performed at the bedside, the nurse removes unnecessary articles from the area and provides privacy. Many nursing units contain an examination room that is clean, well lit, and stocked with frequently used equipment. The nurse covers the examination table with a sheet or paper dispensed from a roll. A lined receptacle is nearby for the disposal of soiled items.

The nurse arranges equipment and supplies for easy access by the examiner (Fig. 14-2). Sterile items remain wrapped or covered until just before their use. Before the examiner arrives, nurses check instruments that require

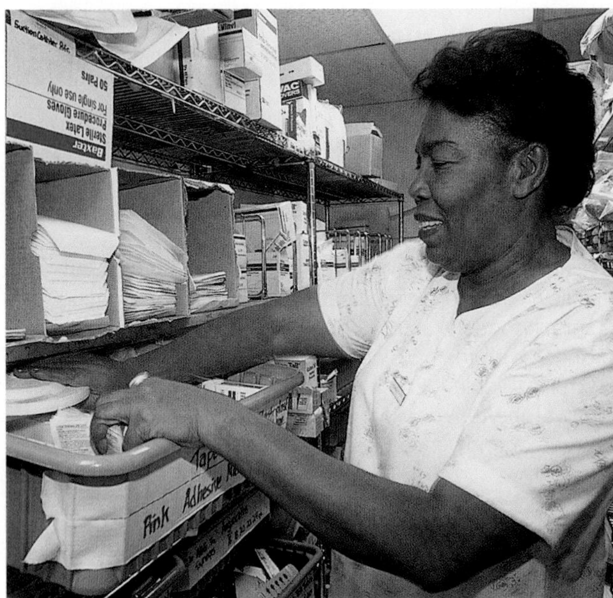

FIGURE 14-1 Obtaining equipment from the supply room. (Photo by Sharon Gynup.)

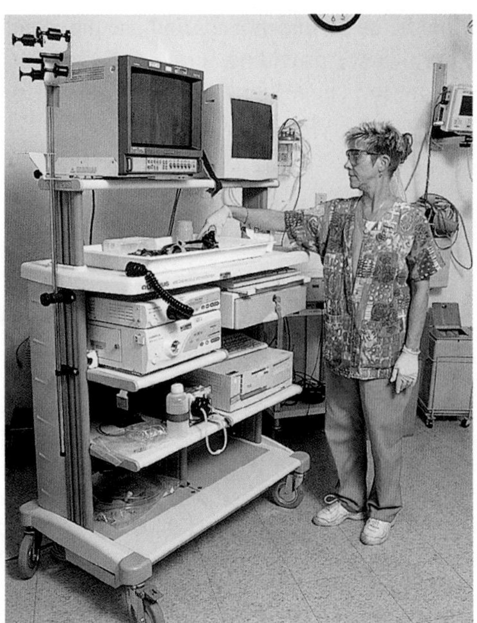

FIGURE 14-2 The nurse arranges supplies and equipment in an endoscopic examination room. (Photo by B. Proud.)

electric power, batteries, or lights so that they can replace nonfunctioning equipment.

Procedural Responsibilities

During the examination or test, the nurse positions and drapes the client, provides the examiner with technical assistance, and supports the client physically and emotionally.

Positioning and Draping. Five positions are commonly used depending on the type of examination, the condition of the client, and the preference of the examiner. They include the dorsal recumbent position, Sims' or left lateral position, lithotomy position, knee–chest or genupectoral position, and modified standing position (Table 14-2).

The **dorsal recumbent position** is a reclining position with the knees bent, hips rotated outward, and feet flat. It is commonly used for various examinations. The nurse uses a bath blanket to drape the client and places examination paper or a disposable pad under the client's buttocks to absorb drainage.

The **lithotomy position** is a reclining position with the feet in metal supports called "stirrups." It is used to facilitate gynecologic (female reproductive), urologic, and sometimes rectal examinations. The nurse uses a drape to cover the client's exposed perineum and legs.

In the **Sims' position**, the client lies on the left side with the chest leaning forward, the right knee bent toward the head, the right arm forward, and the left arm extended behind the body. Indications are similar to those for the lithotomy position. It is an alternative gynecologic or urologic position when a client cannot abduct the hips (move the legs outward from midline) because of restricted joint movement such as that caused by arthritis. This position also provides access to the anus and rectum when the client requires rectal administration of medication or the instillation of an enema solution.

In the **knee–chest position**, also called a "genupectoral position," the client rests on the knees and chest. He or she turns the head, which is supported on a small pillow, to one side. The nurse places a pillow under the client's chest for added comfort. The arms are above the head or bent at the elbows so that they rest alongside the client's head. The nurse places a drape to cover the client's back, buttocks, and thighs. This position is very difficult for most clients—especially older adults—to assume for any length of time. Therefore, the nurse waits to place the client in this position until just before the examination. Some examination tables have movable sections that facilitate maintaining this position without much client effort.

In the **modified standing position**, the client stands with the upper half of the body leaning forward. It is used primarily for examining the prostate gland in men. For comfort and safety, the draped client stands in front of the examination table and leans forward from the waist.

Assisting the Examiner. The nurse must be familiar with the examination equipment and the order of its use. He or she places instruments and equipment on the side of the examiner's dominant hand, if possible. If not, the nurse anticipates what will be needed during the procedure and hands the examiner one item at a time.

If the skin and underlying tissue require local anesthesia, the nurse holds a container of the medication as the physician withdraws some of its contents. The nurse always carefully checks the drug name and concentration on the label.

TABLE 14-2 Indications for Common Examination Positions

POSITION	USES
A. Dorsal recumbent position 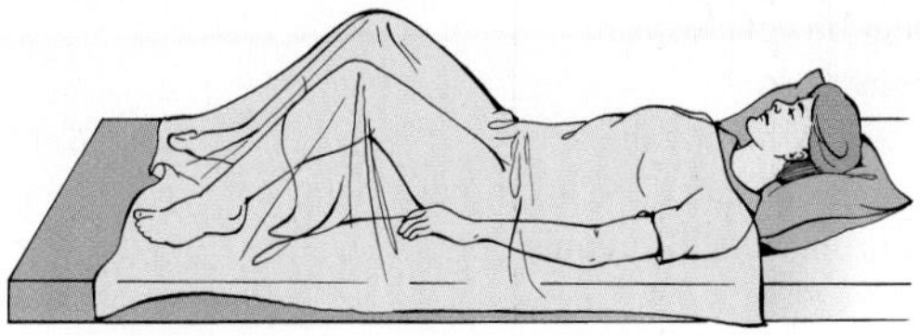	• External genitalia inspection • Vaginal examination • Rectal examination • Urinary catheter insertion
B. Lithotomy position 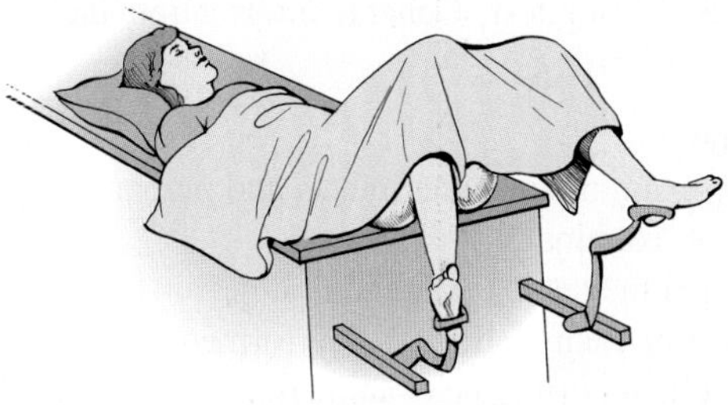	• Internal pelvic examination (female) • Obstetric delivery • Cystoscopic (bladder) examination • Rectal examination
C. Sims' position 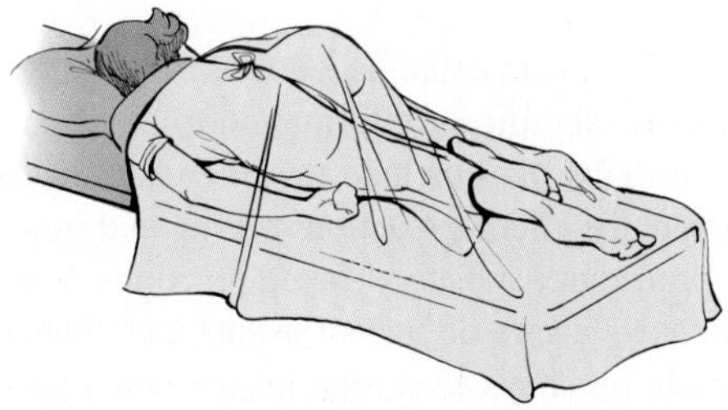	• Rectal examination • Vaginal examination • Rectal temperature assessment • Suppository insertion • Enema administration
D. Knee–chest position 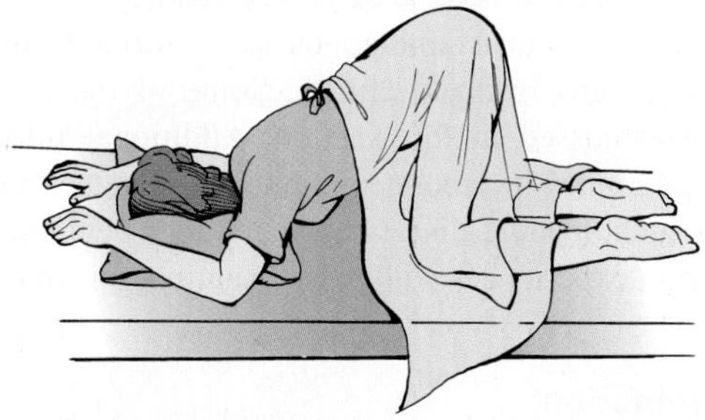	• Rectal and lower intestinal examinations • Prostate gland examination
E. Modified standing position 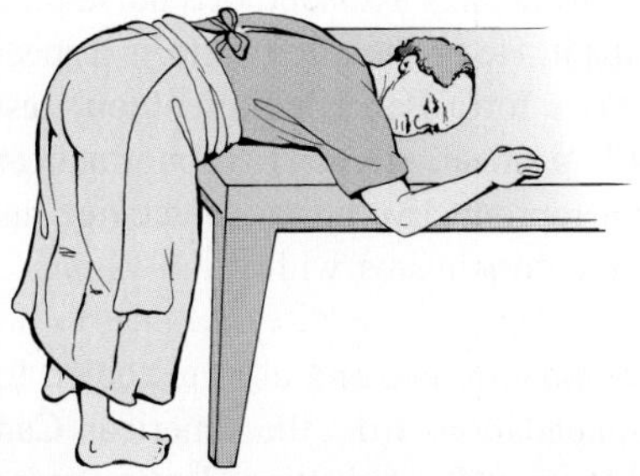	• Prostate gland examination

A second method for ensuring the use of the correct drug is to hold the container so that the examiner can read the label.

If the nurse is responsible for performing the test or examination, he or she cannot leave the client to obtain equipment and supplies. If he or she needs assistance or additional equipment, the nurse summons help with a telephone or call light in the examination room.

Providing Physical and Emotional Support. Throughout any examination or test, the nurse continuously observes the client's physical and emotional reactions and responds accordingly. For example, comfort measures are in order if the client is cold or in pain. Holding the client's hand and offering words of encouragement help the client to endure temporary discomfort. The nurse communicates assessments of the client to the examiner, who may choose to shorten or modify the examination in some manner.

Postprocedural Care

After the completion of an examination and/or test, the nurse attends to the client's comfort and safety, cares for specimens, and records and reports pertinent data.

Attending to the Client. First, the nurse helps the client to a position of comfort. He or she rechecks vital signs to verify that the client's condition is stable. The nurse cleans any substances from the client that caused soiling. He or she offers hospitalized clients a clean gown or directs outpatients to dress in their own clothing. When it is safe to do so, the nurse escorts clients to their rooms or to the discharge area and provides instructions for follow-up care.

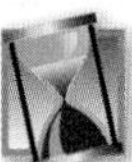

Gerontologic Considerations

- After a diagnostic examination, offer older adults food and fluid and a period of rest before they resume physically taxing activities. Encourage fluids because older adults may have a diminished thirst sensation and may not realize the need for fluid replacement.

Caring for Specimens. Sometimes **specimens** (samples of tissue or body fluids) are collected during an examination or test. To ensure their accurate analysis, the nurse does the following:

- Collects the specimen in an appropriate container
- Labels the specimen container with the correct information
- Attaches the proper laboratory request form
- Ensures that the specimen does not decompose before it can be examined
- Delivers the specimen to the laboratory as soon as possible

Box 14-3 lists factors that often interfere with accurate examinations or that invalidate test results.

Recording and Reporting Data. The nurse must document certain information whenever a client undergoes a special examination or test. General information includes the following:

- Date and time
- Pertinent pre-examination assessments and preparations
- Type of test or examination
- Who performed the test or examination
- Where the test or examination was performed
- Response of client during the examination and afterward
- Type of specimen obtained, if any
- Appearance, size, or volume of specimen
- Where the specimen was transported

In addition to the documented account of the examination, the nurse reports significant information to other nursing team members. This may include that the examination has been completed, the client's reactions during and immediately after the procedure, and any delayed reactions. When the nursing team stays aware of current events and changes in the client's condition, they can revise and keep the plan of care current.

BOX 14-3 Common Factors That Invalidate Examination or Test Results

- Incorrect diet preparation
- Failure to remain fasting
- Insufficient bowel cleansing
- Drug interactions
- Inadequate specimen volume
- Failure to deliver specimen in a timely manner
- Incorrect or missing test requisition

Common Diagnostic Examinations

Many types of diagnostic examinations are performed commonly to assess and evaluate clients. Some of the most common are discussed in this section. Additional information can be found in laboratory and test manuals and courses in which specific diseases are studied; beginning nurses also gain experiences with these examinations in the clinical setting.

Pelvic Examination

A **pelvic examination** is the physical inspection of the vagina and the cervix with palpation of the uterus and the ovaries. A physician, a physician's assistant, or a nurse practitioner usually performs it. He or she often collects a specimen of cervical secretions for a **Pap (Papanicolaou) test.** This test, also called a Pap smear, screens for abnormal cervical cells, the status of reproductive hormone activity, and normal or infectious microorganisms within the vagina or uterus (Table 14-3).

When a pelvic examination is being used to screen for cervical cancer, recommendations from the American Cancer Society, the Association of Reproductive Health Professionals, and the American Congress of Obstetricians and

TABLE 14-3 Pap Test Results

TEST COMPONENT	INTERPRETATION
Cellular Examination	
Class I	Negative; no abnormal cells
Class II	Unusual, but not cancerous
Class III	Suggestive of cancer, but not definite
Class IV	Strongly suggestive of cancer
Class V	Definitely cancerous
Hormonal Effects (on a 6-point scale)	
1	Marked estrogen effect
2	Moderate estrogen effect
3	Slight estrogen effect
4	Absent estrogen effect
5	Compatible with pregnancy
6	Too bloody, inflamed, or scanty to analyze
Identifiable Microorganisms (on a 5-point scale)	
1	Normal microorganisms
2	Scanty or absent microorganisms
3	*Trichomonas vaginalis* (protozoan organism)
4	*Candida* (yeastlike fungus)
5	Other or mixed collection of microorganisms

Adapted from Fischbach F. (2008). *A manual of laboratory and diagnostic tests* (8th ed.). Philadelphia: Lippincott, Williams & Wilkins.

Gynecologists (ACOG) have slight variations. ACOG's latest (2009) recommendations are that women:

1. Receive their first Pap test approximately 3 years after the onset of vaginal intercourse, but no later than 21 years of age.
2. Have annual Pap tests thereafter until 30 years of age.
3. Be screened every 2 to 3 years at or after 30 years of age when three prior consecutive tests were normal or negative. More frequent screenings are advocated for women who have a history of risk factors for cervical cancer, such as being HIV positive, immunosuppressed secondary to an organ transplantation, exposed to diethylstilbestrol as a fetus, or previously diagnosed with cervical cancer, or continuing to shed abnormal cells after a hysterectomy. As an alternative, physicians may opt to perform a Pap test and a second test on women 30 years and older to detect human papillomavirus DNA. If both yield negative results, the client can be retested, using the same two tests every 3 years; if one test is positive, the client is screened more frequently.
4. At or beyond age 65, women should continue to have gynecologic examinations, but the physician determines the frequency of cervical cancer screening on a case-by-case basis. When three prior Pap tests within the previous 10 years were normal or negative, screening guidelines may be relaxed because cervical cancer in women older than 70 years is almost entirely confined to women who have not been previously screened or who have deviated from screening guidelines in the previous 10 years.

Related Nursing Responsibilities. Skill 14-1 identifies the nursing responsibilities involved in assisting with a pelvic examination and collecting cervical secretions for a Pap test.

Radiography

Radiography, or **roentgenography** (a general term for procedures that use roentgen rays, or X-rays), produces images of body structures. The actual film image is technically called a "roentgenogram," but is commonly known as an X-ray. Roentgen rays produce electromagnetic energy that passes through body structures, leaving an image of dense tissue on special film. Table 14-4 lists common radiographic examinations and indications for their use.

X-rays cannot be seen or felt, but cells absorb the energy. Repeated exposure to X-rays, even at small doses, or a single exposure to a high dose causes cell damage that can lead to cancerous cell changes. Consequently, practitioners tend to be cautious about the number of X-ray studies that they request. X-rays are avoided during pregnancy if at all possible because a developing fetus is at greater risk for cellular damage from X-rays. **Magnetic resonance imaging** (MRI) is a technique for producing an image by using atoms subjected to a strong electromagnetic field. This diagnostic alternative does not involve exposure to the type of radiation produced with roentgenography (Fig. 14-3).

Some hospitals are offering open MRIs that eliminate being enclosed within a tube. Claustrophobic and anxious clients prefer the open system, which also is ideal for pediatric clients and clients weighing more than 500 lb. Some metal

TABLE 14-4 Common Radiographic Examinations

EXAMINATION	EXAMPLES OF INDICATIONS FOR USE
Chest X-ray (anterior, posterior, lateral views)	Detects pneumonia, broken ribs, lung tumors, enlarged heart
Upper gastrointestinal X-ray (upper GI or barium swallow)	Aids in diagnosis of ulcers, GI tumors, narrowing of the esophagus
Lower gastrointestinal X-ray (lower GI or barium enema)	Helps in diagnosis of polyps or tumors of the bowel, intestinal obstruction, and structural changes within the intestine
Cholecystography (X-ray of the gallbladder and ducts)	Facilitates determining the presence of gallstones and obstruction in the flow of bile
Intravenous pyelography (IVP)	Helps identify urinary malformations, tumors, stones, cysts, and obstructions in the kidneys and ureters
Retrograde pyelography	Same as for IVP, but the contrast medium is instilled through a urinary catheter
Angiography (X-ray of blood vessels)	Determines the location where and the extent to which blood vessels have narrowed, or evaluates improvement after treatment
Myelography (X-ray of spinal canal)	Detects spinal tumors, ruptured intervertebral disks, and bony changes in the vertebrae

GI, gastrointestinal.

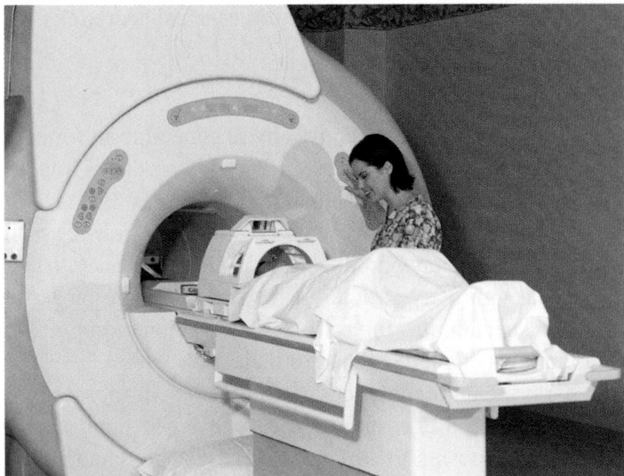

FIGURE 14-3 Magnetic resonance imaging.

devices that are within the body prohibit performing an MRI; metal objects on a client's person must be removed before an MRI (Box 14-4). MRIs can now be done on clients with metal joint implants, but it requires that the radiologist use an adjustment called metal artifact reduction sequence (MARS) to avoid radiographic distortion of the image.

Contrast Medium. A **contrast medium** is a substance, such as barium sulfate or iodine, that adds density to a body organ or cavity. It makes hollow body areas appear more distinct when imaged on X-ray film. Some people are sensitive to substances used in contrast media and have an immediate allergic reaction to them.

Contrast media are administered orally or rectally or injected intravenously. **Fluoroscopy** is a form of radiography that displays an image in real time. It is used to observe the movement of contrast media—for example, as it is being swallowed, instilled, or injected. **Computed tomography** (CT) scanning is a form of roentgenography that shows planes of tissue. This and other types of X-ray examinations use contrast media. The CT contrast medium makes it possible to identify differences in tissue density when obtaining X-ray images from various angles and levels in the body (Fig. 14-4).

BOX 14-4 Metal Devices That Prohibit an MRI

WITHIN THE BODY	ON THE BODY (MUST BE REMOVED)
Wound staples	Watch
Implanted pacemaker	Jewelry
Artificial heart valve	Hearing aid
Metallic pins, screws, plates	Hair clips or pins
Implanted drug delivery device	Pocket knives
Metal intrauterine device	Keys
Aneurysm clips	Credit cards or bank cards
Implanted cardiac defibrillator	
Implanted brain stimulator	
Tattooed eyeliner	

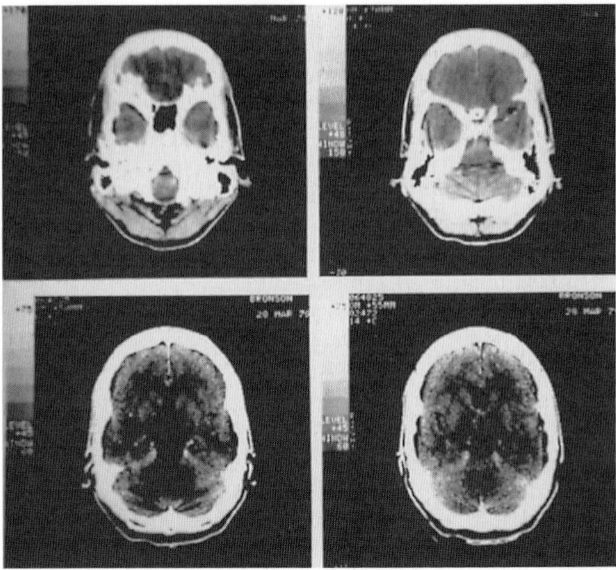

FIGURE 14-4 Cross-sections of a cranial computed tomography (CT) scan. (Photo by Ken Timby.)

Related Nursing Responsibilities. For the client undergoing a radiographic examination, nursing responsibilities include the following:

- Assess vital signs before the examination to provide a baseline and to help detect changes in the client's condition during or after the procedure.
- Remove any metal items such as a religious medal or clothing that contains metal such as the hooks and eyes on a bra. Metal produces a dense image that may be confused with a tissue abnormality.
- Request a lead apron or collar to shield a fetus or vulnerable body parts during X-rays (Fig. 14-5).

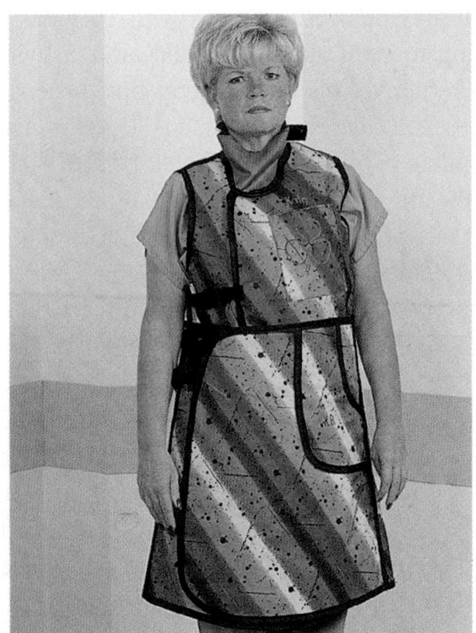

FIGURE 14-5 A lead thyroid collar, apron, and skirt. (Photo by B. Proud.)

- If the radiographic study involves administration of a contrast medium, ask the client about allergies, especially to seafood or iodine, or previous adverse reactions during a diagnostic examination. A reaction can range from mild nausea and vomiting to shock and death.
- Know the location of emergency equipment and drugs in case there is an unexpected allergic reaction to the contrast medium.
- To avoid interference with subsequent visual imaging, schedule procedures requiring iodine before those that use barium.
- To promote urinary excretion, encourage the client to drink a large amount of fluid after an examination involving iodine to promote its excretion.
- Check on bowel elimination and stool characteristics for at least 2 days after the administration of an oral barium contrast medium. Barium retention can lead to constipation and bowel obstruction. Report an absence of bowel elimination beyond 2 days. The administration of a prescribed laxative is often necessary.

Endoscopic Examinations

Endoscopy (a visual examination of internal structures) is performed using optical scopes. Endoscopes have lighted mirror-lens systems attached to a tube and are quite flexible so that they can be advanced through curved structures.

Endoscopic examinations are named primarily for the structure being examined (Box 14-5). In addition to allowing the examiner to inspect the appearance of a structure, endoscopes also have attachments that permit various forms of treatment or the collection of specimens for microscopic analysis. Endoscopic examinations that produce discomfort or anxiety are performed under a light, short-acting form of anesthesia, sometimes referred to as *conscious sedation.* When conscious sedation is used, clients may have no memory of having had the test even though they communicate and interact with staff during its performance.

Endoscopic examinations are being performed more frequently on an outpatient basis and in the physician's office. They are an economical alternative to invasive tests and procedures that previously required surgery to determine a diagnosis.

Related Nursing Responsibilities. For the client undergoing an endoscopy, nursing responsibilities include the following:

- To prevent aspiration, withhold food and fluids or advise the client to do so for at least 6 hours before any procedure in which an endoscope is inserted into the upper airway or upper gastrointestinal tract.
- If conscious sedation is used, monitor the client's vital signs, breathing, oxygen saturation (using pulse oximetry; see Chap. 21), and cardiac rhythm. Have oxygen and resuscitation equipment readily available.
- If topical anesthesia is used to facilitate the passage of an endoscope into the airway or upper gastrointestinal tract, withhold food or fluids for at least 2 hours after the procedure and until swallow, cough, and gag reflexes return.
- Relieve the client's sore throat with ice chips, fluids, or gargles when it is safe to do so.
- Confirm that a bowel preparation using laxatives and enemas has been completed before endoscopic procedures of the lower intestine.
- Report difficulty in arousing a client or any sharp pain, fever, unusual bleeding, nausea, vomiting, or difficulty with urination after any endoscopic examination.

BOX 14-5 Examples of Endoscopic Examinations

- *Bronchoscopy*—inspection of the bronchi
- *Gastroscopy*—inspection of the stomach
- *Colonoscopy*—inspection of the colon
- *Esophagogastroduodenoscopy*—inspection of the esophagus, stomach, and duodenum
- *Laparoscopy*—inspection of the abdominal cavity
- *Cystoscopy*—inspection of the urinary bladder

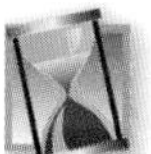

Gerontologic Considerations

■ Some older adults become exhausted by preparations for gastrointestinal examinations that require the use of laxatives and enemas. Harsh laxatives or multiple enemas may also deplete electrolyte balance, leading to weakness or dizziness. Providing a bedside commode and hands-on assistance is helpful for older adults, especially those with impaired mobility, when they are undergoing preparation for gastrointestinal examinations.

Skill 14-2 describes the nurse's role when assisting with a sigmoidoscopy.

Stop, Think, and Respond Box 14-1

Explain why it is important for clients to have a sigmoidoscopy.

Radionuclide Imaging

Radionuclides are elements whose molecular structures are altered to produce radiation. They are identified by a number followed by a chemical symbol, such as ^{131}I (radioactive iodine) and ^{99}Tc (radioactive technetium). When radionuclides are instilled in the body, usually by the intravenous route, particular tissues or organs absorb them. A scanning device that detects radiation creates an image of the size, shape, and concentration of the organ containing the radionuclide. The terms "**hot spot**" (area where the radionuclide is intensely concentrated) and "**cold spot**" (area with little if any radionuclide concentration) refer to the amount of radiation that the tissue absorbs. **Positron emission tomography** (PET) combines the technology of radionuclide scanning with the layered analysis of tomography.

Radionuclide imaging offers two advantages over standard radiography: it visualizes areas within organs and tissues that are not possible with standard X-rays, and it involves less exposure to radiation than with roentgenography. Tests using radionuclides, however, are contraindicated for women who are pregnant or breast-feeding; the energy released is harmful to the rapidly growing cells of an infant or fetus.

Related Nursing Responsibilities. For the client undergoing radionuclide imaging, nursing responsibilities include the following:

- Inquire about a woman's menstrual and obstetric history. Notify the **nuclear medicine department** (the unit responsible for radionuclide imaging) if the client is pregnant, could possibly be pregnant, or is breast-feeding.
- Ask about the allergy history because iodine commonly is used in radionuclide examinations.
- Assist the client with a gown, robe, and slippers. Make sure that the client has no internal metal devices or external metal objects because these interfere with diagnostic findings.
- Obtain an accurate weight because the dose of radionuclide is calculated according to weight.
- Inform the client that he or she will be radioactive for a brief period (usually less than 24 hours) but that body fluids, such as urine, stool, and emesis, can be safely flushed away.
- Instruct premenopausal women to abstain from intercourse or use an effective contraceptive method for the short period during which radiation continues to be present.

Ultrasonography

Ultrasonography (a soft tissue examination that uses sound waves in ranges beyond human hearing) is also known as **echography**. During ultrasonography, which is similar to the echolocation used by bats, dolphins, and sonar devices on submarines, a hand held probe called a **transducer** projects sound through the body's surface. The sound waves cause vibrations within body tissues, producing images as the waves are reflected back toward the machine. The reflected sound waves are converted into a visual image called an ultrasonogram, sonogram, or echogram, which can be viewed in real time on a monitor and recorded for future analysis. Doppler ultrasound, discussed in Chapter 12, is a variation of this type of technology.

Ultrasound examinations are used to visualize breast, abdominal, and pelvic organs; male reproductive organs; structures in the head and neck; the heart and valves; and structures within the eyes. Air-filled structures such as the lungs or the intestines and extremely dense tissue such as bones do not image well. This type of examination is used in obstetrics to determine fetal size, more than one fetus, and location of the placenta. The outline of fetal anatomy during pregnancy is sometimes visible on ultrasound, alerting the client to the gender of the fetus. Because ultrasound examinations do not involve radiation or contrast media, they are extremely safe diagnostic tools.

Related Nursing Responsibilities. For the client undergoing ultrasonography, nursing responsibilities include the following:

- Schedule abdominal and pelvic ultrasonography before any examinations that use barium for the best visualization.
- Instruct clients undergoing an abdominal ultrasonography to drink five to six full glasses of fluid approximately 1 to 2 hours before the test. To ensure a full bladder, urination should be avoided until after the test is completed.
- Explain that acoustic gel is applied over the area where the transducer is placed.

Electrical Graphic Recordings

Machines can record electrical impulses from structures such as the heart, brain, and skeletal muscles. These tests are identified by the prefix "electro-" as in **electrocardiography** (ECG or EKG; an examination of the electrical activity in the heart), **electroencephalography** (EEG; an examination of the energy emitted by the brain), and **electromyography** (EMG; an examination of the energy produced by stimulated muscles).

To detect electrical activity, wires called electrodes are attached to the skin (or muscle in the case of an EMG). They transmit electrical activity to a machine that converts it into a series of waveforms (Fig. 14-6). Except for an awareness of the electrodes, the client undergoing an ECG or EEG usually does not experience any other sensations. Occasionally, there is slight discomfort during an EMG.

Related Nursing Responsibilities. For the client undergoing an ECG, nursing responsibilities include the following:

- Clean the skin and clip hair in the area where the electrode tabs will be placed to ensure adherence and to reduce discomfort on removal.
- Attach the adhesive electrode tabs to the skin where the electrode wires will be fastened.
- Avoid attaching the adhesive tabs over bones, scars, or breast tissue.

For the client undergoing an EEG, nursing responsibilities include the following:

- Instruct the client to shampoo the hair the evening before the procedure to facilitate firm attachment of the electrodes. He or she should shampoo the hair after the test to remove adhesive from the scalp.
- Withhold coffee, tea, and cola beverages for 8 hours before the procedure. Consult with the physician about withholding scheduled medications, especially those that affect neurologic activity.

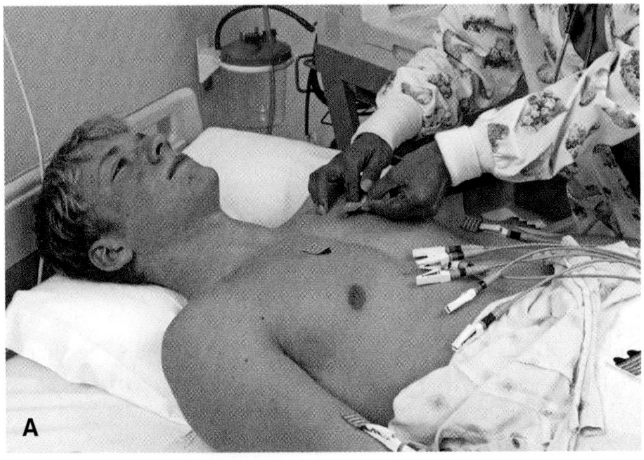

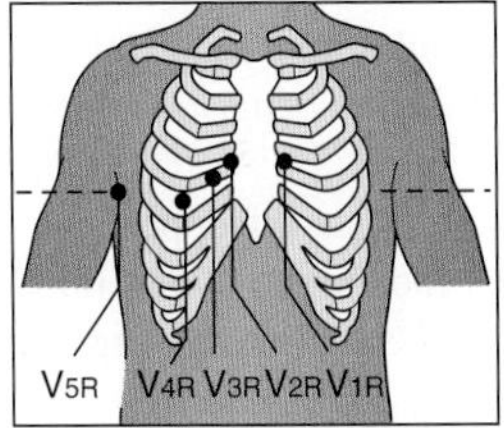

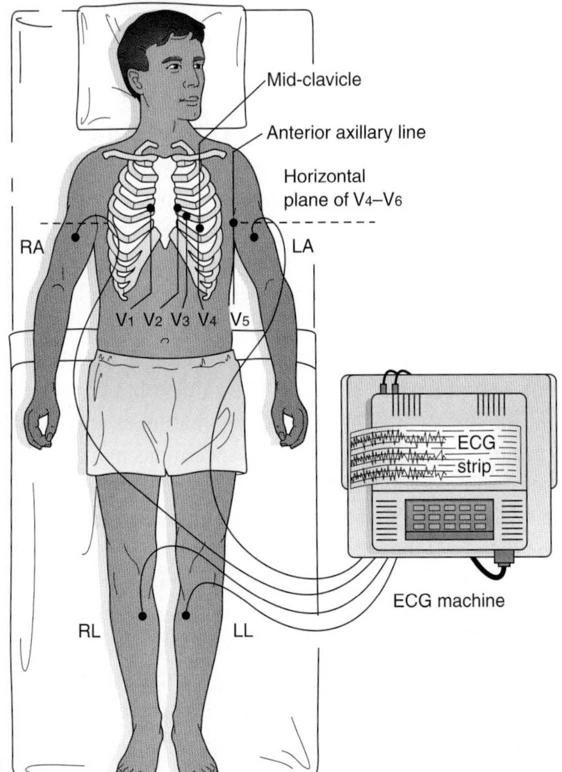

FIGURE 14-6 The nurse attaches electrodes to the patient's chest and limbs before an ECG.

- If a sleep-deprived EEG is scheduled, instruct the client that he or she must stay awake after midnight before the examination.

For the client undergoing an EMG, nursing responsibilities include the following:

- Tell the client he or she will be instructed to contract and relax certain muscles during the examination.
- Explain that electrical current is applied to muscles during an EMG but that the sensation is not usually painful. Also, a muscle electrode is inserted with a small-gauge needle in 10 or more locations, but the experience is painless unless it touches a terminal nerve in the area.

Diagnostic Laboratory Tests

Nurses, laboratory personnel, and physicians collect specimens such as blood, urine, stool, sputum, intestinal secretions, spinal fluid, and drainage from wounds or infected tissue. They repeat tests on collected specimens at intervals to monitor the progress of clients. Students can refer to laboratory manuals to learn the purpose of specific tests and the associated nursing responsibilities.

Several examples of specimen collection are discussed in future chapters where they are more pertinent. Nursing responsibilities for assisting with a paracentesis and a lumbar puncture, collecting a specimen for a throat culture, and measuring capillary blood glucose follow.

Assisting With a Paracentesis

A **paracentesis** is a procedure for withdrawing fluid from the abdominal cavity. A physician always performs it with the assistance of a nurse. A paracentesis is done most commonly to relieve abdominal pressure and to improve breathing, which generally becomes labored when fluid crowds the lungs. Sometimes, paracentesis removes 1 L (approximately 1 quart) or more of fluid. The physician may send a specimen of the fluid to the laboratory for microscopic examination (see Nursing Guidelines 14-1 and Fig. 14-7).

Assisting With a Lumbar Puncture

The physician requires nursing assistance when performing a **lumbar puncture** or **spinal tap**. This procedure involves inserting a needle between lumbar vertebrae in the spinal canal but below the spinal cord itself. The physician advances the tip of the needle until it is beneath the middle layer of the membrane surrounding the spinal cord. He or she measures the spinal fluid pressure and then withdraws a small amount of fluid.

This test is performed for various reasons. It is used to diagnose conditions that raise the pressure within the brain, such as brain or spinal cord tumors, or infections such as meningitis. Spinal fluid also is withdrawn before instilling a contrast medium for X-rays of the spinal column. Finally, the treatment of some conditions requires the instillation of drugs directly into the spinal fluid after withdrawing a similar amount (see Nursing Guidelines 14-2 and Fig. 14-8).

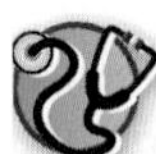

NURSING GUIDELINES 14-1

Assisting With a Paracentesis

- Explain the procedure or clarify the physician's explanation to the client. *Explanations prepare the client for an unfamiliar experience or promote a clearer understanding.*
- Ensure that the client has signed the consent form, if needed. *A consent form provides legal protection.*
- Measure and record the client's weight, blood pressure, and respiratory rate; measure abdominal girth at its widest point with a tape measure. *These data serve as a basis for postprocedural comparisons.*
- Obtain a prepackaged paracentesis kit along with a vial of local anesthetic. *Gathering supplies promotes efficient time management.*
- Make sure that extra gloves, gown, mask, and goggles are available. *These items protect against contact with microorganisms, such as HIV, that may be in the blood or other body fluids.*
- Encourage the client to empty the bladder just before the procedure. *An empty bladder prevents accidental puncture of the bladder.*
- Place the client in a sitting position. *This position pools abdominal fluid in the lower areas of the abdomen and displaces the intestines posteriorly.*
- Hold the container of local anesthetic so the physician can withdraw a sufficient amount. *Doing so prevents contaminating the physician's sterile gloves.*
- Offer the client support as an area of the abdomen is anesthetized then pierced with an instrument called a trocar and a hollow sheath called a cannula is inserted (see Fig. 14-7). *Empathetic concern helps to relieve anxiety.*
- Reassess the client periodically after the cannula insertion; expect that blood pressure and respiratory rate may decrease. *Assessment indicates the client's response.*
- Place a Band-Aid or small dressing over the puncture site after withdrawal of the cannula. *The dressing acts as a barrier to microorganisms and absorbs drainage.*
- Assist the client to a position of comfort. *Doing so demonstrates concern for the client's welfare.*
- Measure the volume of fluid withdrawn. *This measurement contributes to an accurate assessment of fluid volume.*
- Label the specimen, if ordered, and send it to the laboratory with the appropriate requisition form. *Doing so facilitates an appropriate analysis.*
- Document pertinent information such as the appearance and volume of the fluid, client assessments, and disposition of the specimen. *Such documentation adds essential data to the client's medical record.*

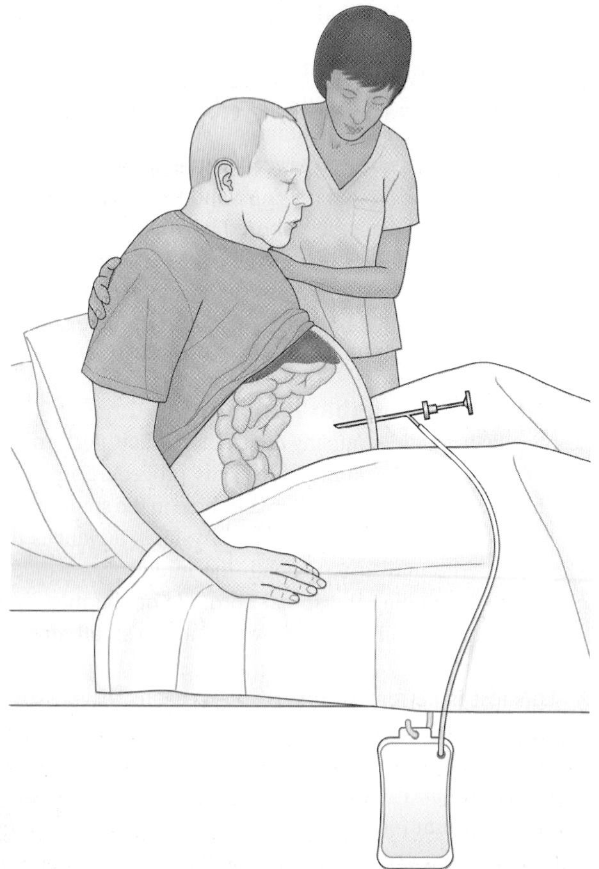

FIGURE 14-7 The nurse offers support during an abdominal paracentesis.

Collecting a Specimen for a Throat Culture

A **culture** (an incubation of microorganisms) is performed by collecting body fluid or substances suspected of containing infectious microorganisms, growing the living microorganisms in a nutritive substance, and examining their characteristics with a microscope. Cultures are performed commonly on urine, blood, stool, wound drainage, and throat secretions.

To identify and treat the cause of a throat infection (commonly streptococcal bacteria), the nurse obtains a specimen from the throat. An abbreviated test that takes approximately 10 minutes is performed on throat specimens in many doctors' offices and student health clinics. A rapid preliminary diagnosis is made so that appropriate treatment can be initiated immediately. If the quick test is not clearly negative and symptoms strongly suggest a streptococcal infection, a follow-up specimen is obtained and sent to the laboratory for culturing. Conclusive results of a bacterial culture generally require 24 to 72 hours for sufficient microbial growth to take place.

Once bacteria grow within the nutritive medium, they are identified microscopically by their shape and by the color they acquire when stained with special dyes. **Gram staining** (a process of adding a dye to a microscopic specimen) is named for the Danish physician who developed the technique. The Gram stain helps determine whether bacteria are gram-positive or gram-negative. *Gram-positive bacteria* appear violet after staining. Those that repel the violet dye but appear red, the color of a counterstain, are called gram-negative bacteria (Fischbach & Dunning, 2008). Streptococci are round, grow in chains, and are gram-positive bacteria.

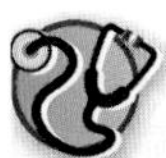

NURSING GUIDELINES 14-2

Assisting With a Lumbar Puncture

- Explain the procedure or clarify the physician's explanation to the client. *Explanations prepare the client for an unfamiliar experience or promote a clearer understanding.*
- Ensure that the client has signed the consent form, if needed. *A consent form provides legal protection.*
- Perform a basic neurologic examination including the client's pupil size and response and muscle strength and sensation in all four extremities. *This information provides a baseline for future comparisons.*
- Encourage the client to empty the bladder. *An empty bladder promotes comfort during the procedure.*
- Administer a sedative drug if ordered. *Sedatives reduce anxiety.*
- Obtain a prepackaged lumbar puncture kit along with a vial of local anesthetic. *Gathering supplies promotes efficient time management.*
- Make sure that extra gloves, gown, mask, and goggles are available. *These items offer protection from contact with microorganisms, such as HIV, that may be present in the blood or other body fluids.*
- Place the client on his or her side with the knees and neck acutely flexed (see Fig. 14-8) or in a sitting position, bent from the hips. *These positions separate the bony vertebrae.*
- Instruct the client that once the needle is inserted, he or she must avoid movement. *This measure prevents injury.*
- Hold the container of local anesthetic so the physician can withdraw a sufficient amount. *Doing so prevents contaminating the physician's sterile gloves.*
- Stabilize the client's position at the neck and knees. *This reinforces the need to remain motionless.*
- Support the client emotionally as the needle is inserted and the skin is injected with local anesthesia. *Empathetic concern helps to relieve anxiety.*
- Tell the client that it is not unusual to feel pressure or a shooting pain down the leg. *This information prepares the client for expected sensations.*
- Perform *Queckenstedt's test*, if asked, by compressing each jugular vein separately for approximately 10 seconds while pressure is being measured. *Queckenstedt's test helps demonstrate if there is an obstruction in the circulation of spinal fluid. If so, the pressure remains unchanged, rises slightly, or takes longer than 20 seconds to return to baseline.*
- Observe that the physician fills three separate numbered containers with 5 to 10 mL in their appropriate sequence if laboratory analysis is desired. *In this way, if blood is present but in the least amount in the third container, its source is most likely trauma from the procedure rather than central nervous system pathology.*
- Place a Band-Aid or small dressing over the puncture site after the needle has been withdrawn. *The dressing acts as a barrier to microorganisms and absorbs drainage.*
- Position the client flat on the back or abdomen; instruct the client to remain flat and roll from side to side for the next 6 to 12 hours. *These measures reduce the potential for severe headache.*
- Reassess the client's neurologic status. Check the puncture site for bleeding or clear drainage. *Comparative data help the nurse to evaluate changes in the client's condition.*
- Offer oral fluids frequently. *They restore the volume of spinal fluid.*
- Label the specimens, if ordered, and send them to the laboratory with the appropriate requisition form. *Doing so facilitates an appropriate analysis.*
- Document pertinent information such as the appearance of the fluid, client assessments, and disposition of the specimen. *Doing so adds essential data to the client's medical record.*

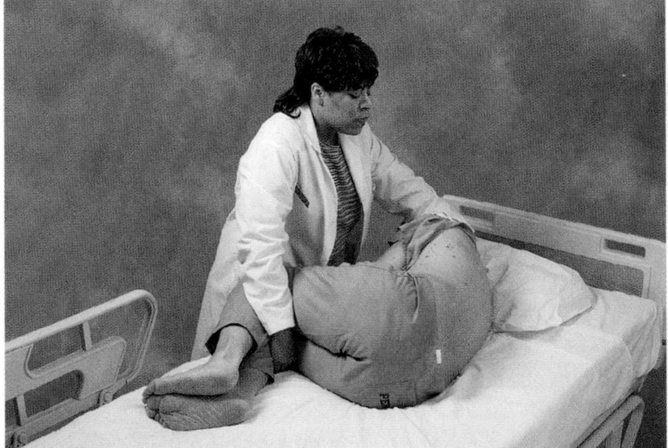

FIGURE 14-8 Positioning for lumbar puncture. (Photo by B. Proud.)

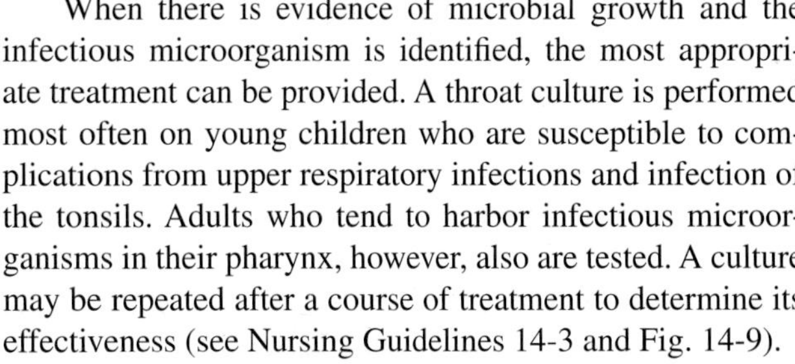

When there is evidence of microbial growth and the infectious microorganism is identified, the most appropriate treatment can be provided. A throat culture is performed most often on young children who are susceptible to complications from upper respiratory infections and infection of the tonsils. Adults who tend to harbor infectious microorganisms in their pharynx, however, also are tested. A culture may be repeated after a course of treatment to determine its effectiveness (see Nursing Guidelines 14-3 and Fig. 14-9).

Measuring Capillary Blood Glucose

Glucose is the type of sugar in blood that results from eating carbohydrates. A certain amount is always present to supply cells with a source of instant energy. The American Diabetes Association (2008, 2010) recommends that the amount of blood glucose before meals should range between 70 and 130 mg/dL (milligrams per deciliter) and less than 180 mg/dL within 1 to 2 hours after eating when using a blood sample drawn from a finger. The body produces the hormones glucagon and insulin,

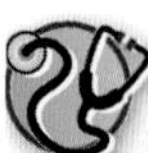

NURSING GUIDELINES 14-3

Collecting a Specimen for a Throat Culture

- Check with the physician about proceeding with the throat culture if the client is taking antibiotics. *Antibiotics affect test results.*
- Delay collecting a specimen if the client has recently used an antiseptic gargle. *Such gargles affect the test's diagnostic value.*
- Explain the purpose of and the technique for obtaining the culture. *Explanations help to reduce anxiety and promote cooperation.*
- Collect supplies: sterile culture swab, glass slide, tongue blade, gloves, mask if the client is coughing, paper tissues, and an emesis basin if the client gags. *Doing so facilitates organization and efficient time management.*
- Have the client sit where light is optimum. *Light enhances inspection of the throat anatomy.*
- Don gloves and a mask, if necessary. *Their use reduces the potential for transferring microorganisms.*
- Loosen the cap on the tube in which the swab is located. *Doing so facilitates hand dexterity.*
- Tell the client to open the mouth wide, stick out the tongue, and tilt the head back. *This position promotes access to the back of the throat.*
- Depress the middle of the tongue with a tongue blade in your nondominant hand (see Fig. 14-9). *Doing so opens the pathway for the swab.*
- Rub and twist the tip of the swab around the tonsil areas and the back of the throat without touching the lips, teeth, or tongue. *Doing so transfers microorganisms from the inflamed tissue to the swab.*
- Be prepared for the client's gagging. *Stroking the back of the throat stimulates the gag reflex.*
- Remove the swab and discard the tongue blade in a lined receptacle. *This measure controls the spread of microorganisms.*
- Spread the secretions on the swab across the glass slide. *Doing so prepares a specimen for quick staining and microscopic examination.*
- Replace the swab securely within the tube, taking care not to touch the outside of the container. *This method avoids collecting unrelated microorganisms and provides containment for the collected specimen.*
- Crush the packet in the bottom of the tube. *Crushing releases nourishing fluid to promote bacterial growth.*
- Remove gloves, discard them in a lined receptacle, and wash your hands or perform hand antisepsis with an alcohol rub (see Chap. 10). *These steps reduce the transmission of microorganisms.*
- Label the culture tube with the client's name, the date and time, and the source of the specimen. *These steps provide laboratory personnel with essential information.*
- Attend to the staining and examination of the prepared glass slide, if appropriate. *Doing so provides tentative identification of streptococcal bacteria.*
- Deliver the sealed culture tube to the laboratory or refrigerate it if there will be a delay of longer than 1 hour. *These steps ensure that the microorganisms will grow when transferred to other culture media.*

which regulate glucose metabolism and maintain normal blood glucose levels.

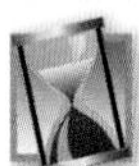

Gerontologic Considerations

■ Older adults are more susceptible to dehydration. The resulting concentration of blood can cause false elevations of laboratory blood tests.

People with diabetes have an impaired ability to produce insulin and have difficulty regulating blood glucose levels. They control their disease with diet, exercise, and in some cases, medications. People with diabetes may experience low or high blood glucose levels, both of which can have life-threatening consequences. Therefore, many clients with diabetes measure their own capillary blood glucose levels rather than having venous blood drawn for laboratory analysis.

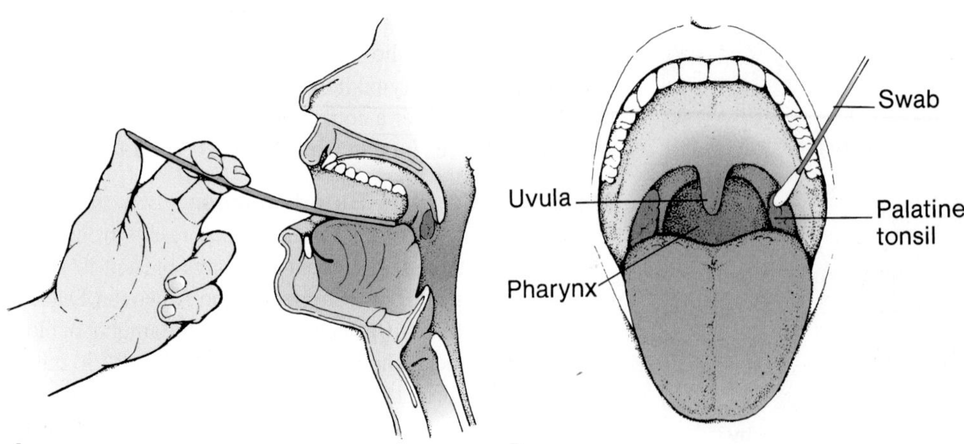

FIGURE 14-9 A throat culture. **A.** Depressing the tongue. **B.** Obtaining a specimen.

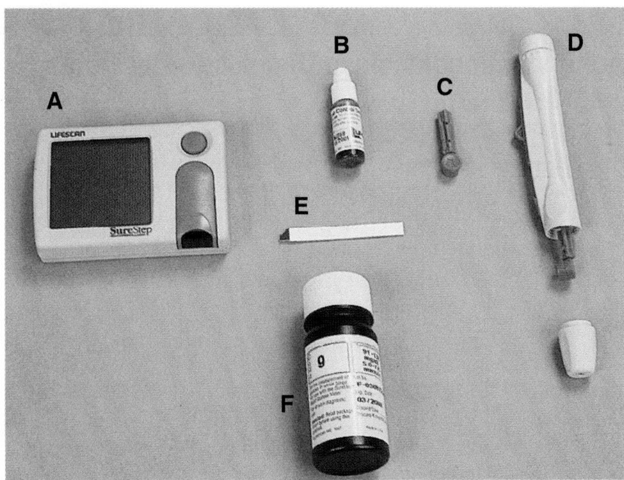

FIGURE 14-10 Equipment used to perform capillary blood glucose testing: a glucometer (**A**), control solution (**B**), a lancet (**C**), a lancet holder (**D**), a test strip (**E**), and a container of test strips (**F**). (Photo by B. Proud.)

A **glucometer** is an instrument that measures the amount of glucose in capillary blood. It operates by assessing the amount of light reflected through a chemical test strip (Fig. 14-10). Based on the amount of measured glucose in the blood, clients with diabetes adjust their intake of food or medication.

Because diabetes is so common, nurses frequently are called on to teach people who have been recently diagnosed with this problem how to test their own blood glucose levels. Nurses measure blood glucose levels for clients with diabetes who are hospitalized or being cared for in long-term care facilities.

There are several important points to remember about measuring blood glucose:

1. Several types of glucometers are available. The user must follow the manufacturer's instructions for accurate use.
2. The blood glucose level usually is measured about 30 minutes before eating and before bedtime to determine what are likely to be the lowest levels of glucose. This allows time for the client to increase or decrease food consumption or, if insulin-dependent, to administer additional prescribed insulin (see Chap. 34), referred to as coverage.
3. Measuring blood glucose involves a risk for contact with blood. Because blood may contain infectious viruses, nurses *always* wear gloves when performing this test.

Researchers are working on developing noninvasive devices that will not require piercing the skin with a lancet, but such devices are not available at present.

Skill 14-3 presents the steps involved in using a Lifescan glucometer.

NURSING IMPLICATIONS

Most clients who undergo special examinations and tests have emotional needs from the stress of a potential diagnosis or the anxiety created by undergoing something unfamiliar. The following are some nursing diagnoses that nurses may identify during preprocedural and postprocedural stages of examinations and tests:

- Anxiety
- Fear
- Decisional conflict
- Readiness for enhanced self-health management
- Powerlessness
- Spiritual distress

Nursing Care Plan 14-1 illustrates the nursing process as it relates to the nursing diagnosis of Decisional Conflict, defined in the NANDA-I taxonomy (2012, p. 396) as "uncertainty about the course of action to be taken when choice among competing actions involves risk, loss, or challenge to values and beliefs."

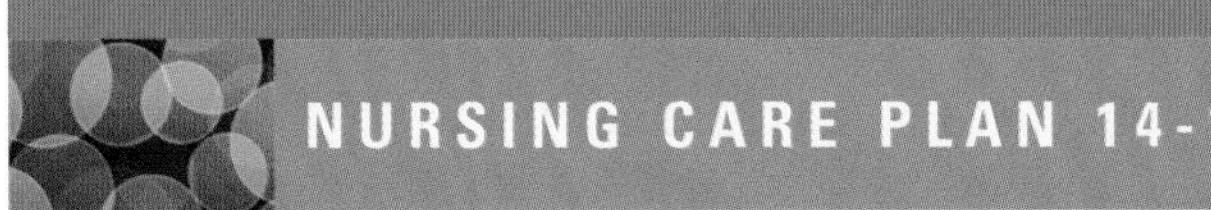

A Client Undergoing Amniocentesis to Diagnose a Possible Fetal Genetic Disorder

Assessment

Determine the following:

- Signs of distress such as restlessness, tachycardia, increased muscle tension, and rapid respirations
- Values and beliefs about terminating a pregnancy
- Remarks indicating uncertainty about subsequent choices pending the outcome of the amniocentesis
- Feelings of anguish or ambivalence regarding the decision to either carry the fetus to term or abort it

Nursing Diagnosis. **Decisional conflict** related to birthing options as evidenced by tearfulness, sleep disturbance, heart rate of 90 to 100 beats/min at rest, request for visitation from a clergyperson, reading her Bible, and statement, "I don't feel I can make a decision about this."

Expected Outcome. The client will make an informed choice about the outcome of the current pregnancy within 1 week of when the results of the amniocentesis are known.

(continued)

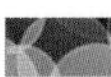

NURSING CARE PLAN 14-1 A Client Undergoing Amniocentesis to Diagnose a Possible Fetal Genetic Disorder (continued)

Interventions	Rationales
Acknowledge the client's distress.	Empathy demonstrates awareness of the client's emotional state.
Convey an accepting nonjudgmental attitude.	Trust enhances the open expression of feelings.
Offer referrals to pro-choice and right-to-life groups and organizations that provide information about the disorder that may affect the client's child.	Consulting others helps to clarify issues and decreases feelings of helplessness.
Encourage the client to discuss concerns with other significant people.	Sharing concerns with others helps the client to perceive conflicts more realistically and facilitates implementation of a subsequent plan.
Suggest that the client compose a written list of the advantages and disadvantages to possible choices before the return appointment.	Identifying the pros and cons of alternatives is the first step in formulating a decision.
Give verbal recognition for efforts made to reach a solution.	Acknowledgment improves the client's ability to cope with the burden of a difficult decision.
Support the client's decision even if it is not your personal choice.	Clients have the right to autonomy and self-determination.

Evaluation of Expected Outcome

Client makes a decision with support of significant others to continue pregnancy carrying a fetus that will have cystic fibrosis.

CRITICAL THINKING EXERCISES

1. Discuss how the procedure for a sigmoidoscopy or another test or examination may differ if performed on an outpatient basis rather than in a hospital.
2. How might diminished mentation (the capacity to understand), reduced strength and stamina, and pain affect the performance of a diagnostic examination or test?
3. How might a pelvic examination be different if the person being examined is a victim of rape?
4. How would you respond to a client who is uncertain about having a lumbar puncture because of a fear of paralysis from trauma to the spinal cord?

NCLEX-STYLE REVIEW QUESTIONS

1. Which of the following indicates that a client needs more teaching before a sigmoidoscopy?
   1. The client says an anesthetic will be given before the examination.
   2. The client says a light meal is allowed the evening before the examination.
   3. The client says a flexible scope will be inserted into the rectum.
   4. The client says prescribed medications may be taken in the morning.
2. Which nursing action is essential before performing a chest roentgenogram (X-ray)?
   1. Make sure that the client does not eat food.
   2. Remove the client's metal necklace.
   3. Have the client swallow contrast dye.
   4. Administer a dose of pain medication.
3. Which of the following instructions is most appropriate if a specimen for a Pap (Papanicolaou) test will be obtained at the time of a pelvic examination?
   1. Do not douche for several days before your appointment.
   2. Stop using any and all forms of contraception temporarily.
   3. Drink at least 1 quart of liquid 1 hour before your appointment.
   4. Take a mild laxative the night before your scheduled appointment.
4. Which of the following actions are correct when measuring a client's capillary blood glucose? Select all that apply.
   1. Plan to perform the test 1 hour before a meal.
   2. Check that the test strip code matches the one programmed in the glucometer.
   3. Have the client wash his or her hands with soap and water before the test.
   4. Puncture the central pad of the thumb or fingers with the lancet.
   5. Cover the test spot on the test strip completely with a drop of blood.
5. When assisting with a pelvic examination during which a Pap smear will be obtained, place the following steps in the order in which they are performed. Use all the statements.
   1. Hand the examiner a brush applicator.
   2. Apply a chemical fixative to the specimen slide.
   3. Place the client in a lithotomy position.
   4. Lubricate the examiner's gloved fingers.
   5. Provide the examiner with a vaginal speculum.

SKILL 14-1 Assisting With a Pelvic Examination

Suggested Action	Reason for Action
ASSESSMENT	
Determine the identity of the client on whom the examination will be performed.	Prevents errors.
Determine whether a Pap test is needed.	Indicates the need for additional equipment and supplies.
Find out whether the client has had a pelvic examination before.	Provides a basis for teaching.
Ask whether the client is currently menstruating or has had intercourse within the last 48 hours.	Blood, semen, and lubricant are three substances that obscure and distort cells, making it difficult to determine whether they are atypical and interfering with the microscopic examination of collected specimens. The examiner may wish to delay obtaining a specimen.
Inquire whether the client has douched or used vaginal hygiene products in the last 24 hours.	Suggests a need to reschedule the Pap test because an adequate sample of cells and secretions may not be available.
Ask the client's age, date of the last menstrual period, number of pregnancies and live births, and description of symptoms such as bleeding or drainage, itching, or pain.	Provides data to determine the possibility of pregnancy, to compare cellular specimens with hormonal activity, and to provide clues as to possible pathology and the need for additional tests.
Determine if and what type of birth control the client is using if she is premenopausal. For oral contraceptives, identify the name of the drug and the dosage.	Correlates the influence of prescribed hormones on cellular specimens.
Ask menopausal women whether they are taking hormone replacement, and the brand name and dosage.	Correlates the influence of prescribed hormones on cellular specimens.
Observe for impaired strength or joint limitation.	Suggests the need to modify the examination position.
PLANNING	
Explain the procedure and give the client an opportunity to ask questions.	Tends to reduce anxiety.
Provide an examination gown and direct the client to empty her bladder.	Facilitates palpation of the uterus and ovaries.
Place a **speculum** (a metal or a disposable plastic instrument for widening the vagina), gloves, examination light, lubricant, and the following materials for the Pap smear: long soft applicators and spatula and at least three glass slides, a chemical fixative, and a container for holding the slides on the counter or on a tray in the examination room (Fig. A).	Promotes efficient time management. Metal specula (plural of speculum) are reused after sterilization. Select an appropriate size according to the individual client.

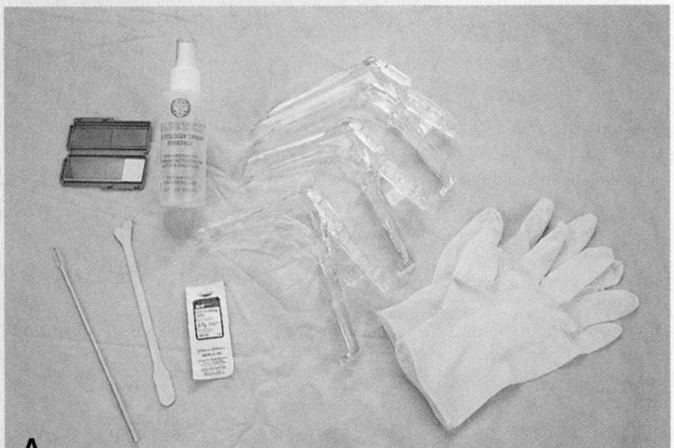

A

Equipment used for a pelvic examination.

Suggested Action	Reason for Action
(The liquid-based cytology [ThinPrep Pap Test], an alternative technique of specimen preservation approved by the US Food and Drug Administration, eliminates using slides; instead it involves rinsing the collection tool within a liquid transport medium.)	
Mark one slide with an E for endocervical, another with a C for cervical, and the last with a V for vaginal.	Identifies the location from which the specimens are taken; *endocervical* means inside the cervix. The cervix is the lower portion of the uterus, or womb.

(continued)

Assisting With a Pelvic Examination (continued)

PLANNING (CONTINUED)

Action	Rationale
Arrange for a female nurse to be with the client during the examination, especially if the examiner is a man.	Reduces the potential for claims of sexual impropriety.
Plan to assist with the collection of the vaginal and cervical secretions for the Pap test before the examiner proceeds to palpate the internal organs.	Prevents lubricant used during palpation from interfering with a microscopic examination of the specimens.

IMPLEMENTATION

Action	Rationale
Place the client's legs in stirrups to facilitate a lithotomy position (Fig. B); use an alternative position, such as Sims' or dorsal recumbent, if the client is disabled.	Provides access to the vagina

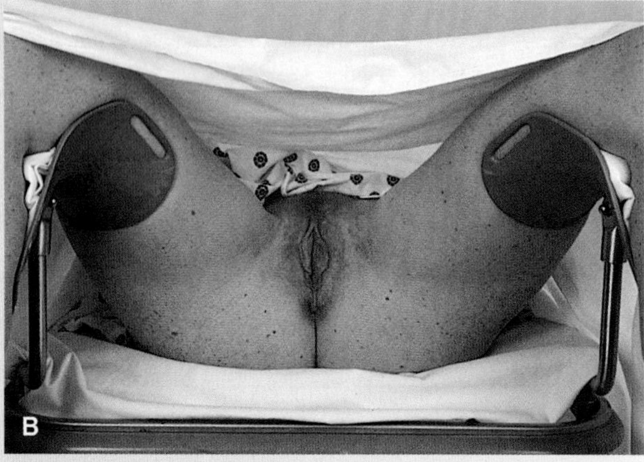

Lithotomy position.

Action	Rationale
Cover the client with a cotton or paper drape.	Maintains modesty and privacy.
Introduce the examiner to the client if the two are strangers.	Tends to reduce anxiety.
Fold back the drape just before the examination begins.	Exposes the genitalia while minimizing client exposure.
Direct the examination light from behind the examiner's shoulder toward the vaginal opening.	Illuminates the area, facilitating inspection.
Wet the speculum with warm water; if a Pap smear will not be obtained, apply water-soluble lubricant to the speculum blades.	Eases and provides comfort during insertion.
Prepare the client to expect the momentary insertion of the speculum. Explain that she will hear a loud click as it locks in place.	Tends to reduce anxiety and aids in relaxation.
Hand the examiner a soft-tipped applicator, spatula, and brush applicator in that order.	Facilitates collection of secretions for the Pap smear.
Hold the slide marked E so that the examiner can roll or slide the specimen across the slide; follow a similar pattern as the second and third samples are collected from the cervix and vagina (see Fig. C).	Deposits intact cells and secretions according to their source; excessive manipulation of the cells while being obtained or applied to the slide can make normal cells look like atypical cells.

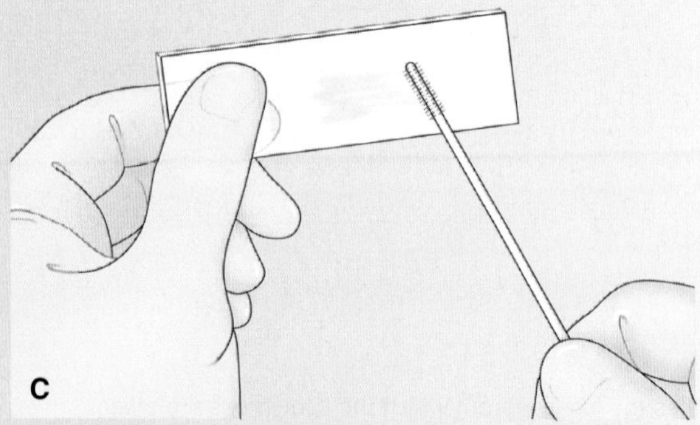

Transferring secretions to a glass slide.

Action	Rationale
Position the lined receptacle so the examiner can dispose of the collection device and the speculum after use.	Controls the spread of microorganisms.

(continued)

Assisting With a Pelvic Examination (continued)

IMPLEMENTATION (CONTINUED)

Place each slide in a chemical fixative solution or spray it with a similar chemical (see Fig. D).	Preserves the integrity of the specimens; a delay in applying a fixative leads to air drying, distortion of cells, and loss of details in the nucleus, thus making it difficult to determine whether cells are atypical.

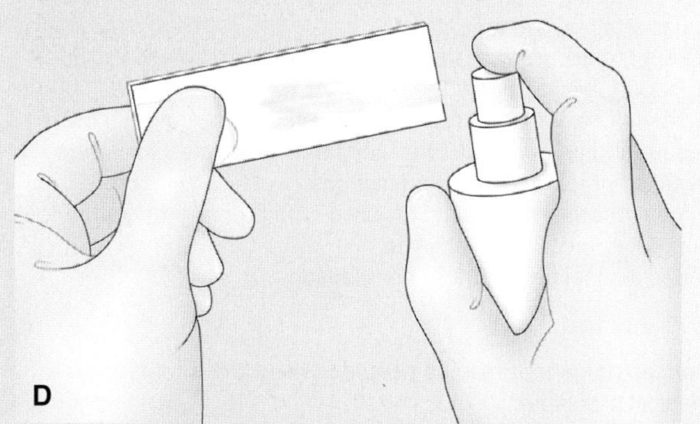

Preserving the specimen.

If using the liquid-based cytology technique, immerse the sampling device in the container of solution, cap it, and discard the tool.	Disperses the cells and breaks up blood, mucus, and nondiagnostic debris.
Lubricate the gloved fingers of the examiner's dominant hand and prepare the client for an internal vaginal (and in some cases, rectal) examination.	Reduces friction; keeps the client informed of the progress of the examination.
Don gloves and clean the skin of lubricant when the examination is completed; then, remove the gloves.	Prevents the transmission of microorganisms; promotes comfort and hygiene.
Wash hands or perform hand antisepsis with an alcohol rub (see Chap. 10).	Reduces microorganisms on the hands.
Lower both feet simultaneously from the stirrups and assist the client to sit up.	Reduces strain on abdominal and back muscles.
Assist the client from the room after she has dressed.	Maintains client safety.

Evaluation

- Client demonstrated understanding of the purpose for the examination.
- Client assumed and was maintained in a satisfactory position for examination.
- Client privacy, comfort, and safety were maintained.
- Specimens were collected, identified, and preserved.

Document

- Date and time
- Pertinent preassessment data, if any
- Type of examination, including any specimens collected
- Examiner and/or location
- Condition of the client after the examination
- Disposition of specimens

SAMPLE DOCUMENTATION

Date and Time Taken to examination room by wheelchair for pelvic examination by Dr. Wood. Able to assume lithotomy position without difficulty. Smears of endocervical, cervical, and vaginal specimens obtained and sent to lab. Returned to room by wheelchair and assisted into bed. ———————— SIGNATURE/TITLE

SKILL 14-2 Assisting With a Sigmoidoscopy

Suggested Action	Reason for Action
ASSESSMENT	
Identify the client on whom the examination will be performed.	Prevents errors.
Check for a signed consent form.	Provides legal protection.
Ask the client to describe the procedure.	Indicates the accuracy of the client's understanding and provides an opportunity to clarify the explanation.
Inquire about the client's current symptoms and family history of significant diseases.	Provides information about the purpose for performing the procedure and an opportunity for reinforcing the need for future regular sigmoidoscopic examinations.
Ask for a description of the client's dietary and fluid intake and bowel cleansing protocol and results.	Indicates whether the client complied with proper preparation for the procedure.
Assess the client's vital signs and obtain other physical assessments according to agency policy, such as weight or bowel sounds.	Provides a baseline for future comparisons.
Ask for an allergy history and a list of medications being taken.	Influences drugs that may be prescribed and alerts staff to other medical problems.
PLANNING	
Direct the client to undress, don an examination gown, and use the restroom.	Facilitates the examination and gives the client an opportunity to empty the bowel and bladder again.
Prepare for the examination by placing a sigmoidoscope (Fig. A), gloves, gown, mask, goggles, lubricant, suction machine, and containers for biopsied tissue in the examination room.	Promotes efficient time management.

A

Flexible sigmoidoscope.

Suggested Action	Reason for Action
Check that the light at the end of the sigmoidoscope and the suction equipment are operational.	Avoids delay, inconvenience, and discomfort once the examination is in progress.
IMPLEMENTATION	
Help the client to assume a Sims' position if a flexible sigmoidoscope will be used, or a knee—chest position if a rigid sigmoidoscope, which is less common, is used.	Facilitates passage of the scope; an endoscopic table may be used in lieu of a self-maintained knee—chest position.
Cover the client with a cotton or paper drape.	Maintains modesty and privacy.
Introduce the examiner to the client if the two are strangers.	Tends to reduce anxiety.
Lubricate the examiner's gloved fingers.	Reduces discomfort when the fingers are used to dilate the anal and rectal sphincters.
Prepare the client for the introduction of the examiner's fingers, followed by the insertion of the sigmoidoscope.	Tends to reduce anxiety by keeping the client informed of each step and the progress being made.
Acknowledge any discomfort that the client may be experiencing; explain that it should be short-lived.	Indicates that the nurse empathizes with the client's distress.
Inform the client if, and before, suction is used, air is introduced, or a sample of tissue is obtained.	Prepares the client for unexpected sensations or temporary increase in discomfort.
Open the specimen container, cover the specimen with preservative, and recap the container.	Prevents the loss and decomposition of the specimen.

(continued)

Assisting With a Sigmoidoscopy (continued)

IMPLEMENTATION (CONTINUED)

Action	Rationale
Inform the client when the scope will be withdrawn.	Keeps the client informed of progress.
Don gloves and clean the skin of lubricant and stool after the examination is completed; remove the gloves.	Prevents the transmission of microorganisms; promotes comfort and hygiene.
Wash hands or perform hand antisepsis with an alcohol rub (see Chap. 10).	Reduces microorganisms.
Assist the client from the room to an area where his or her clothing is located or provide a clean gown.	Maintains client safety and dignity.
Explain that there may be slight abdominal discomfort until the instilled air has been expelled and that the client may observe some rectal bleeding if a biopsy was taken.	Provides anticipatory health teaching.
Stress that if severe pain occurs or bleeding is excessive, the client should notify the physician.	Identifies significant data to report.
Advise that the client may consume food and fluids as desired.	Clarifies dietary guidelines.
Clean the sigmoidoscope and any other soiled equipment according to agency and infection control guidelines.	Prevents the transmission of microorganisms.
Restore order and cleanliness to the examination room; restock supplies.	Prepares the room for future use.
Complete the laboratory requisition form, label the specimen, and ensure that the specimen is transported to the laboratory for analysis.	Facilitates microscopic examination.

Evaluation

- Client demonstrated understanding of the purpose for the examination.
- Appropriate dietary and bowel preparations were carried out.
- Client assumed required position.
- Comfort and safety were maintained.
- Postprocedural instructions were given.
- Specimen was preserved, identified, and delivered appropriately.

Document

- Date and time
- Pertinent preassessment data, if any
- Type of examination and specimen collected, if any
- Examiner and/or location
- Condition of the client after the examination
- Instructions provided
- Disposition of specimens

SAMPLE DOCUMENTATION

Date and Time Arrived ambulatory for routine sigmoidoscopic examination. No current symptoms, no known allergies. Takes atenolol (Tenormin) for hypertension. Last dose was @0700. BP 142/90 in right arm while sitting. T–98.2; P–90; R–22. Bowel sounds active in all four quadrants. Has eaten lightly this morning and self-administered two enemas last night with good results and one this morning with very little stool expelled. Placed in Sims' position for examination. Biopsy omitted. Instructed to resume eating and taking fluid as desired. Explained that gas pains are possible and that walking about will help, but to notify Dr. Ross if the discomfort is prolonged or severe. Discharged ambulatory accompanied by wife. ———SIGNATURE/TITLE

SKILL 14-3 Using a Glucometer

Suggested Action	Reason for Action
ASSESSMENT	
Determine that a test using one or more control solutions has been performed on the glucometer since midnight in a health agency. Identify the client on whom the examination will be performed.	Determines that the glucometer is functioning accurately; complies with an agency's policies for quality assurance and prevents errors.
Find out whether the client has ever had a blood glucose level measured with a glucometer or whether the client has any questions.	Provides a basis for teaching.
Review previous blood glucose level and trends that may be obvious.	Helps evaluate the reliability of the assessed measurement when it is obtained.
Check to see whether insulin coverage has been ordered if glucose levels are higher than normal.	Aids in quickly reducing high blood glucose levels.
Check the date on the container of test strips; discard if the date has expired.	Determines whether test strips are still appropriate for use.
Discard unused test strips stored in a vial 4 months after they are opened.	Ensures accuracy.
Observe the code number on the container of test strips; compare it with the code number programmed into the glucometer (Fig. A).	Code numbers range from 1 to 16; if the numbers do not match, the meter number is changed.

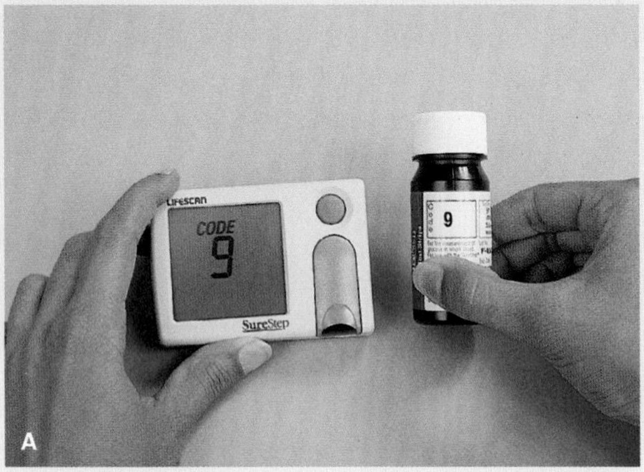

A

Comparing the code number on a test strip bottle to the glucometer code number. (Photo by B. Proud.)

Suggested Action	Reason for Action
Inspect the client's fingers and thumb for a nontraumatized area; also inspect the earlobes, which is an acceptable alternative.	Avoids secondary trauma.
PLANNING	
Test the machine's calibration with a control strip or solution supplied by the manufacturer if it has not been done since midnight.	Verifies the machine's accuracy.
Arrange care so that the test is performed approximately 30 minutes before a meal and at bedtime.	Ensures consistency in obtaining data and facilitates the detection of trends.
Collect the necessary equipment and supplies: a glucometer, lancets, a lancet holder, test strips, and gloves.	Promotes efficient time management.
IMPLEMENTATION	
Ask the client to wash his or her hands with soap and warm water and towel dry.	Reduces microorganisms on the skin; warmth dilates the capillaries and increases blood flow. Swabbing with alcohol is not necessary and can alter the results if not totally evaporated.
Turn on the machine; observe the last blood glucose reading, current test strip code, and the message "Insert strip."	Prepares the machine for testing the blood sample. The machine retains the last glucose measurement in its memory.
Place the notched end of one test strip into the holder with the test spot up.	Locates the strip in position for the application of blood.

(continued)

Using a Glucometer (continued)

IMPLEMENTATION (CONTINUED)

Assemble the lancet within the spring-loaded lancet holder (Fig. B).	Loads, holds the lancet in place, and prepares the lancet for a rapid thrust into the skin.

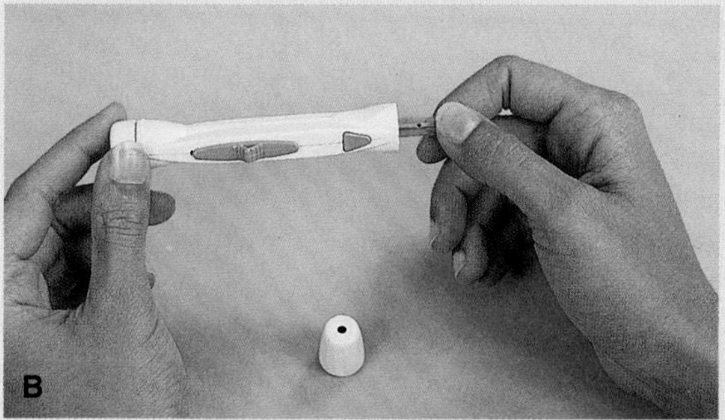

B Lancet insertion.

Don clean gloves after washing your hands or performing hand antisepsis with an alcohol rub (see Chap. 10).	Provides a barrier against contact with blood.
Select a nontraumatized side of a client's finger or thumb; avoid the central pads (Fig. C).	Avoids puncturing an area with sensitive nerve endings.

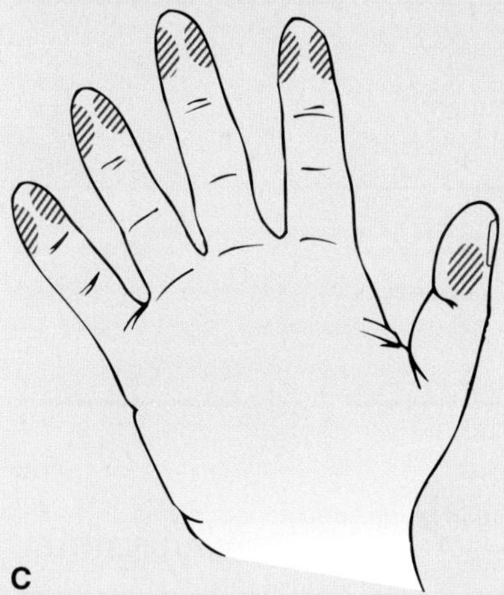

C Appropriate puncture sites.

Apply the lancet firmly to the side of the finger and press the release button.	Thrusts the lancet into the skin.
Release lancet and holder.	Opens a path for blood.
Hold the finger or thumb so that a large hanging drop of blood forms.	Uses gravity to aid in collecting blood.
Touch the hanging drop of blood to the test spot on the strip, making sure that the spot is completely covered and stays wet during the test (Fig. D).	Saturates the test spot to ensure accurate test results.

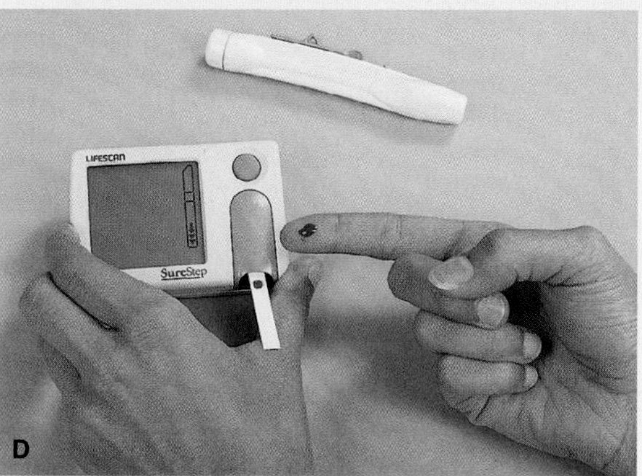

D One large drop of blood is placed in the center of the test strip. (Photo by B. Proud.)

(continued)

Using a Glucometer (continued)

IMPLEMENTATION (CONTINUED)

Listen for the meter to beep, followed by a series of beeps 45 seconds later.	Activates the timing mechanism.
Read the display on the meter after the series of beeps.	Identifies the client's blood glucose level.
Turn the machine off.	Extends the life of the battery.
Offer the client a Band-Aid or paper tissue.	Absorbs blood and controls bleeding.
Release the lancet into a puncture-resistant container.	Prevents the potential for a needlestick injury and transmission of blood-borne infectious microorganisms.
Clean the window of the glucometer and the hole of the test strip holder with a cotton swab or damp cloth to remove dirt, blood, or lint at least once a week.	Keeps the equipment free of debris that can impair light detection.
Remove gloves and immediately wash your hands or perform hand antisepsis with an alcohol rub (see Chap. 10).	Reduces microorganisms.
Remove equipment from the bedside if it does not belong to the client.	Facilitates the use of equipment that may be needed for other clients.
Store the test strips in a cool dry place at 37° to 85°F (1.7° to 30°C).	Prevents decomposition from heat and humidity.
Record the glucose measurement in the client's diabetic record.	Documents essential data.
Report the blood glucose level to the nurse in charge.	Communicates information for making treatment decisions.

Evaluation

- Client demonstrates understanding of the purpose for the examination.
- Adequate blood is obtained.
- Results are consistent with the client's present condition, previous trends, and concurrent treatment.
- Additional treatment is provided depending on glucose measurement.

Document

- Date and time
- Pertinent preassessment data, if any
- Results obtained when using the glucometer; in most agencies, the test data are recorded on a diabetic flow sheet rather than charted in narrative nursing notes
- Treatment provided based on abnormal test results

SAMPLE DOCUMENTATION

Date and Time Blood glucose level 210 mg/dL per glucometer. 5 units of Humulin R insulin given subcutaneously as coverage. —————————— SIGNATURE/TITLE

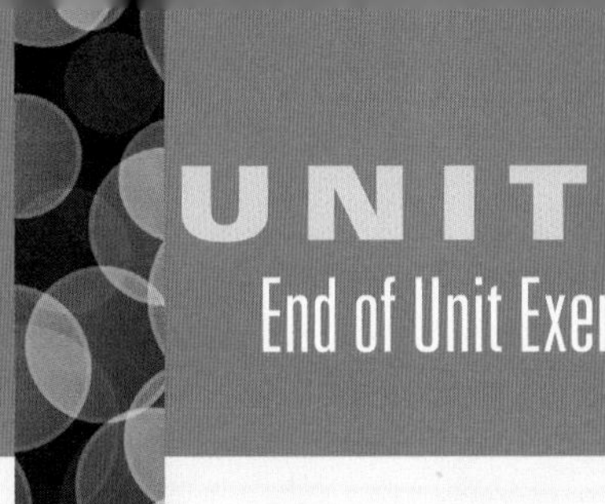

UNIT 4

End of Unit Exercises for Chapters 10, 11, 12, 13, and 14

Section I: Reviewing What You've Learned

Activity A: *Fill in the blanks by choosing the correct word from the options given in parentheses.*

1. ________________ bacteria exist without oxygen. (Aerobic, Anaerobic, Mycoplasmic)
2. Tinea corporis is a/an ________________ type of fungal infection. (intermediate, superficial, systemic)
3. Various anatomical and physiologic adaptations keep human body temperature within a narrow stable range regardless of environmental temperature; hence, humans are ________________. (heterothermic, homeothermic, poikilothermic)
4. A ________________ is the process of sending someone to another person or agency for special services. (discharge, referral, transfer)
5. Prolonged ________________ leads to brain damage or death. (apnea, dyspnea, orthopnea)
6. ________________ is a heart rate below 60 beats per minute. (Bradycardia, Palpitation, Tachycardia)
7. A/An ________________ is a crack in the skin, especially in or near mucous membranes. (abrasion, fissure, laceration)
8. ________________ sounds are located normally in the periphery of all the lung fields. (Bronchial, Bronchovesicular, Vesicular)
9. ________________ is a procedure for withdrawing fluid from the abdominal cavity. (Fluoroscopy, Paracentesis, Roentgenography)
10. The ________________ is the brain's temperature-regulating center that initiates processes that promote heat conservation and production. (cerebellum, hypothalamus, medulla)

Activity B: *Mark each statement as either T (True) or F (False). Correct any false statements.*

1. T____F____ A spore is a temporarily inactive microbe that can resist heat and destructive chemicals and survive without moisture.
2. T____F____ Some pathogens have tiny hairs called flagella that enable them to attach to the host's tissue and avoid expulsion.
3. T____F____ For every degree of Fahrenheit that temperature is elevated, heart and pulse rates increase 15 beats per minute.
4. T____F____ The apical heart rate can be counted by listening at the chest with a stethoscope.
5. T____F____ Orientation helps the client become familiar with and adapt to a new environment.
6. T____F____ The nurse performs light palpation by depressing tissue approximately 1 in. (2.5 cm) with the forefingers of one or both hands.
7. T____F____ Normal vision is the ability to read without prescription lenses printed letters that most people can see at a distance of 20 feet.
8. T____F____ Lordosis causes an increased curve in the thoracic area.
9. T____F____ A developing fetus is at increased risk for cellular damage from X-rays.
10. T____F____ Electroencephalography is an examination of the energy produced by stimulated muscles.

Activity C: *Write the correct term for each description below.*

1. Practices that decrease or eliminate infectious agents, their reservoirs, and their vehicles for transmission ________________
2. A haven in which microbes survive, grow, and reproduce ________________
3. Using atoms subjected to a strong electromagnetic field to produce an image ________________
4. A handheld probe used during an ultrasonography to project sound through the body's surface ________________
5. A pronounced lateral curvature of the spine ________________
6. An assessment technique used to listen to body sounds ________________
7. Rapid or deep breathing, or both, affecting the volume of air entering and leaving the lungs ________________
8. The termination of care from a health care agency ________________

Activity D: *1. Match the type of microorganism in Column A with its characteristics in Column B.*

Column A		Column B
1. ________________	Bacterium	A. Smallest microorganism known to cause infectious disease; visible only with an electron microscope
2. ________________	Virus	B. Protein that does not contain nucleic acid
3. ________________	Protozoan	C. Single-celled microorganism; may be round, rod-shaped, or spiral
4. ________________	Prion	D. Single-celled animal classified according to its ability to move

2. Match the terms indicating alterations in skin integrity in Column A with their descriptions in Column B.

Column A		Column B
1. ________________	Wound	A. Open crater-like area
2. ________________	Ulcer	B. Mark left by the healing of a lesion
3. ________________	Scar	C. Break in the skin

3. Match the positions used for physical examinations in Column A with their descriptions in Column B.

Column A		Column B
1. ________________	Dorsal recumbent position	A. The client lies on the left side with the chest leaning forward, the right knee bent toward the head, the right arm forward, and the left arm extended behind the body
2. ________________	Lithotomy position	B. The client rests on the knees and chest
3. ________________	Sims' position	C. The client reclines with the feet in metal supports called stirrups
4. ________________	Genupectoral position	D. The client reclines with the knees bent, the hips rotated outward, and the feet flat

Activity E: *1. Differentiate between medical and surgical asepsis.*

	Medical Asepsis	*Surgical Asepsis*
Definition		
Technique		
Methods of Obtaining Asepsis		

2. Differentiate between fever and hyperthermia.

	Fever	*Hyperthermia*
Definition		
Complications or Concerns		

3. Differentiate between the head-to-toe and the body-systems approaches to physical assessment.

	Head-to-Toe Approach	*Body-Systems Approach*
Definition		
Advantages		
Disadvantages		

Activity F: *Consider the following figure.*

1.

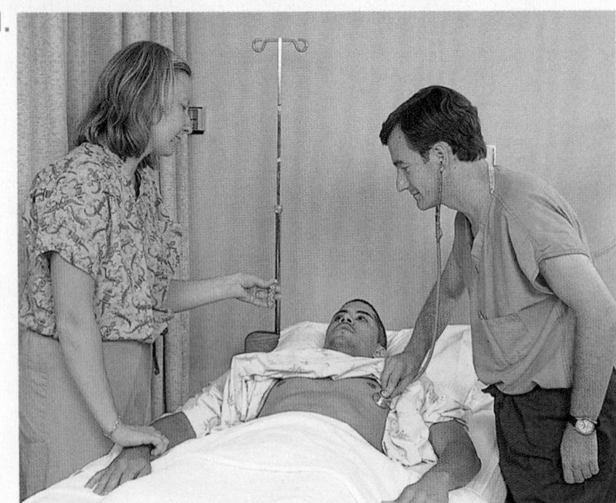

a. Identify the figure shown above.

b. Which of the two methods for assessing the pulse rate is more accurate? Why?

2.

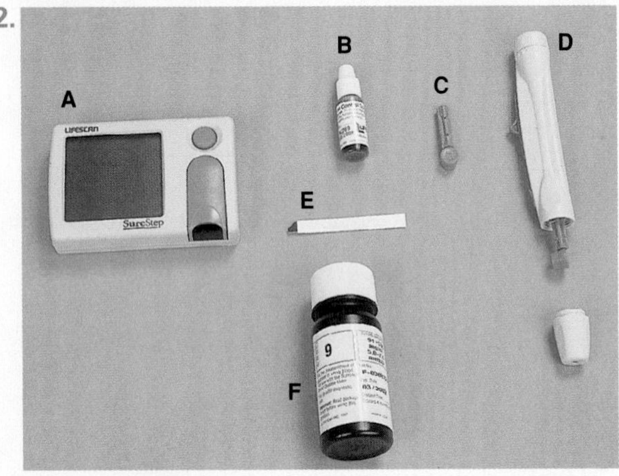

a. Identify the equipment shown in the figure.

b. What is this equipment used for?

Activity G: *A surgical scrub extensively removes transient microorganisms from the nails, hands, and forearms before an operative procedure. Write in the boxes provided below the correct sequence in which the nurse should perform the actions of a surgical scrub.*

1. Use friction to scrub all surfaces of the hands.
2. Use friction to lather the liquid cleanser.
3. Hold the hands and arms up and away from the body.
4. Put on a mask, hair, and shoe covers.
5. Rinse the lather while keeping the hands above the elbows.
6. Dry hands with a sterile towel.
7. Wet hands to the forearms.
8. Clean under each fingernail.

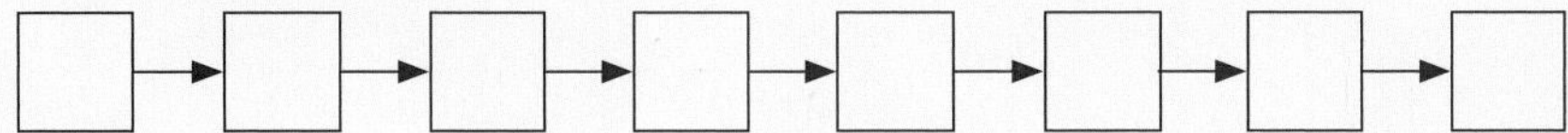

Activity H: *Answer the following questions.*

1. What is a nosocomial infection?

2. What are the six components of the chain of infection?

3. What is the purpose of a minimum data set (MDS)?

4. What are the nurse's duties when a client must be transferred within the same health care agency?

5. What are the phases of a fever?

6. What is postural hypotension?

7. Why is a physical assessment of the client upon admission to the health care facility important?

8. What is a Snellen eye chart?

9. How is a culture performed?

10. What is the purpose of a lumbar puncture or a spinal tap?

Section II: Applying Your Knowledge

Activity I: *Give rationales for the following questions.*

1. Why does the nurse pour out and discard a small amount of sterile solution before each use?

2. Why is it good practice for the nurse to remove chipped or peeling nail polish before working at a health care facility?

3. Why should the nurse have a second nurse's, supervisor's, or security person's signature on the envelope containing a client's secured valuables?

4. Why is it important for a nurse to measure a client's vital signs at regular intervals?

5. When should the nurse use clean gloves during nursing care?

6. Why should the nurse ensure that the client's garments are free of all metallic objects, such as hooks or medals, before a radiographic examination?

7. Why should the nurse drape the client during physical examinations?

8. Why is it better to assess skin turgor in the area over the chest in an elderly client?

Activity J: *Answer the following questions focusing on nursing roles and responsibilities.*

1. A nurse at an extended-care facility is caring for an elderly client with a hip fracture who has developed pulmonary congestion and respiratory distress during his stay.
   a. What could have caused the pulmonary congestion and respiratory distress?

   b. What care should the nurse take to prevent nosocomial infections at the facility?

2. A client at the health care facility is ready to give birth. A nurse is preparing to assist the obstetrician.
   a. What steps should the nurse follow before the procedure?

   b. What is the purpose of the previous steps?

3. A nurse at a health care facility is asked to proceed with admission procedures for a client scheduled for surgery.
   a. What is the nurse's responsibility during the admission of the client to the facility?
   b. What should the nurse include in the initial nursing care plan?

4. A nurse caring for a newborn at a health care facility is required to measure and document the baby's temperature at regular intervals.
   a. Which are the preferred routes for measuring the temperature of newborns or infants?
   b. Why do newborns and young infants tend to experience temperature fluctuations?

5. A child arrives at the clinic with complaints of pain in his right ear. A nurse is assisting the physician during the assessment.
   a. How does the nurse perform a gross examination of the ear?
   b. What kind of substance within the ear is considered normal?

6. A nurse is caring for a client who is to undergo an electrocardiography (ECG).
   a. How should the nurse explain to the client what to expect during the procedure?
   b. What are the nursing responsibilities for a client undergoing an ECG?

Activity K: *Think over the following questions. Discuss them with your instructor or peers.*

1. A nurse is caring for three different clients in a health care facility. The first is an immunosuppressed 68-year-old client undergoing chemotherapy. The second is a 40-year-old client with tuberculosis. The third is a teenager with a wound infection.
   a. What considerations are involved when caring for the older client undergoing chemotherapy?
   b. What techniques of asepsis should the nurse follow when caring for clients with infectious disorders?
2. A 34-year-old client with diabetes has undergone a foot amputation secondary to an untreated injury. Although the client is receiving occupational therapy and rehabilitation at the health care facility, he is severely depressed about the loss of his foot and its implications. He tells the nurse that he regrets his carelessness and fears that he will never be able to lead a normal life again. He has been very quiet and refuses to interact with his family. The client is to be discharged soon.
   a. What may be some special considerations for this client during discharge?
   b. What special referral services might be appropriate to help improve the client's condition?
   c. How can the nurse help the client deal with his loss?
3. A nurse employed in the rehabilitative care unit of a health care facility is required to measure the blood pressure of a severely obese client who is recovering from a motor vehicle collision. The client's right arm is in a cast. He has just returned to his room after actively exercising by ambulating in the hall.
   a. Should the nurse assess blood pressure soon after the client has exercised?
   b. What factors should be considered when using a sphygmomanometer to assess blood pressure in this client?
4. The nurse needs to perform a routine assessment for a client recovering from a head injury as directed by the primary health care provider. How can the nurse avoid making any subjective assessments of the client's mental status?

Section III: Getting Ready for NCLEX

Activity L: *Answer the following questions.*

1. A nurse is caring for a client scheduled for electromyography (EMG). Which of the following instructions should the nurse give the client regarding the procedure?
   a. Stay awake after midnight before the examination.
   b. Avoid cola beverages for 8 hours before the procedure.
   c. Pain will be felt if the electrode touches a terminal nerve in the area.
   d. Consult with the physician about withholding scheduled medications.
2. A nurse is caring for a client with an infection at a health care facility. What precautions should the nurse take after leaving the client's room? Select all that apply.
   a. Scrub the hands thoroughly, giving special attention to the nails.
   b. Use a wet towel to turn off faucets.
   c. Avoid touching any part of the sink or the faucets.
   d. Discard paper towels appropriately after drying the hands.
   e. Apply hand sanitizer to keep the hands free from odor.
3. During the physical assessment of a client, the nurse listens to lung sounds. How should the nurse document squeaking sounds caused by air moving through a narrowed passage in the lung?
   a. Crackle
   b. Gurgle
   c. Rub
   d. Wheeze

4. A fever generally goes through four distinct phases. Arrange the phases in the order in which they occur. Use all the options.
   a. Stationary
   b. Defervescence
   c. Invasion
   d. Prodromal

5. A nurse is assigned to measure and document the vital signs of a client recovering from an accident. The client is receiving intravenous medication in the right arm. The left arm and left lower leg are severely injured. Which of the following would be the best site for measuring the client's blood pressure?
   a. Right lower arm
   b. Right upper arm
   c. Left thigh
   d. Right thigh

6. During a physical assessment, the nurse taps the fingers against the client's abdomen. Which of the following techniques involves tapping or striking fingers on the client's body?
   a. Auscultation
   b. Palpation
   c. Percussion
   d. Observation

7. A nurse uses an alcohol rub after the physical assessment of each client. Which of the following is true about alcohol rubs?
   a. They remove dirt with organic material.
   b. They remove 80% of microorganisms.
   c. They can substitute for handwashing if the hands are visibly clean.
   d. They have a prolonged antiseptic effect after an initial use.

8. While taking a client's vital signs, the nurse identifies that the pulse is difficult to feel and easily obliterated with slight pressure. Which of the following is the most accurate description of the pulse?
   a. Thready
   b. Bounding
   c. Full
   d. Strong

UNIT 5
Assisting With Basic Needs

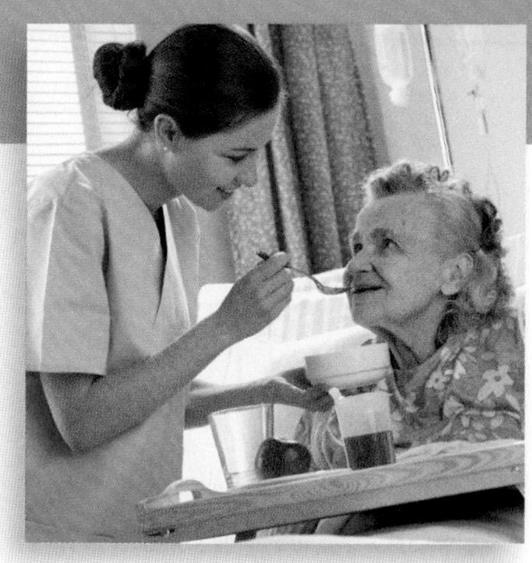

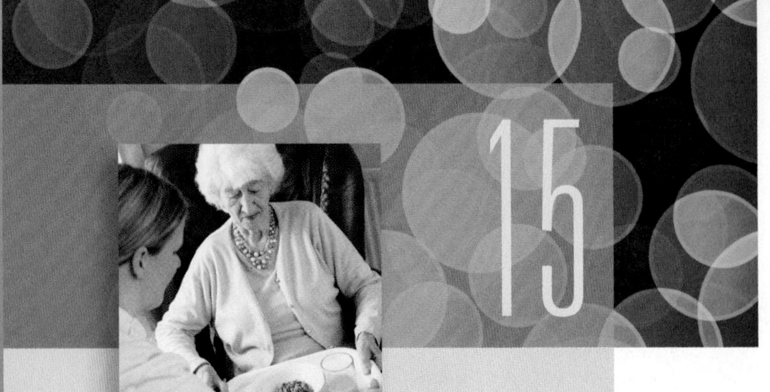

15 Nutrition

Words To Know

abdominal circumference
anorexia
anthropometric data
body mass index
cachexia
calorie
carbohydrates
cellulose
complete proteins
diet history
dysphagia
emaciation
emesis
eructation
essential amino acids
fats
fat-soluble vitamins
flatus
incomplete proteins
kilocalorie
lipoproteins
malnutrition
megadoses
metabolic rate
midarm circumference
minerals
nausea
nonessential amino acids
nutrition
obesity
projectile vomiting
protein
protein complementation
regurgitation
retching
saturated fats
triceps skinfold measurement
trans fats
unsaturated fats
vegans
vegetarians
vitamins
vomiting
vomitus
water-soluble vitamins

Learning Objectives

On completion of this chapter, the reader should be able to:

1. Define nutrition and malnutrition.
2. List six components of basic nutrition.
3. List at least five factors that influence nutritional needs.
4. Discuss the purpose and components of the MyPlate food guidelines.
5. Describe three facts available on nutritional labels.
6. Explain protein complementation.
7. Identify four objective assessments for determining a person's nutritional status.
8. Discuss the purpose of a diet history.
9. List five common problems that can be identified from a nutritional assessment.
10. Plan nursing interventions for resolving problems caused or affected by nutrition.
11. List seven common hospital diets.
12. Discuss four nursing responsibilities for meeting clients' nutritional needs.
13. Identify three facts a nurse must know about a client's diet.
14. Describe and demonstrate techniques for feeding clients.
15. Explain how to meet the nutritional needs of clients with visual impairment or dementia.
16. Discuss at least three unique aspects of nutrition that apply to older adults.

Healthy people, in general, are becoming increasingly selective about the quantity and quality of their daily food intake. In a country of affluence, Americans are both undernourished and overnourished. According to the Centers for Disease Control and Prevention (Ervin, 2009), 34% of adults meet the criteria for metabolic syndrome, which is characterized by obesity, abdominal fat, hypertension, and elevated blood glucose (insulin resistance) and fat levels.

Gerontologic Considerations

- Male and female adults who are 60 years and older are four times and six times more likely, respectively, than younger adults to have metabolic syndrome (Ervin, 2009).
- The escalating incidence of this syndrome indicates the critical need to control the epidemic of obesity in the United States.

This chapter includes information about normal nutrition for promoting health. It also provides suggestions that nurses may offer clients about what and how much to eat, the dangers of food fads and unsafe dieting, and techniques for managing the care of clients whose ability to eat, digest, absorb, or eliminate food is impaired.

OVERVIEW OF NUTRITION

Eating is a basic need. It is the mechanism by which nutrients are obtained. An optimal nutritional status provides (1) sufficient energy for daily activities, (2) maintenance and replacement of body cells and tissues, and (3) restoration of health following illness or injury. Because the type and amount of nutrients consumed affect health, it is important to understand basic **nutrition**, or the process by which the body uses food. Chronic, inadequate nutrition leads to **malnutrition** (a condition resulting from a lack of proper nutrients in the diet). Evidence of malnutrition is common among people living in poor, developing countries; however, it also occurs among people living in countries known for their affluence, like the United States. Examples of those in the United States at risk for an inadequate nutritional intake include the following:

- Older adults who are socially isolated or living on fixed incomes
- Homeless people
- Children of economically deprived parents
- Pregnant teenagers
- People with substance abuse problems, such as alcoholism
- Clients with eating disorders, such as anorexia nervosa and bulimia nervosa

Human Nutritional Needs

Increasing data support the connections between nutritional status and health and well-being. Consequently, an emphasis on improving nutrition to prevent and treat disease also is growing. All humans have basic nutritional needs. Through scientific study, researchers have determined standards for the recommended daily amounts of the following:

- Calories that provide the body with energy
- Proteins, carbohydrates, and fats that supply calories and are substances needed for the growth and repair of body structures
- Vitamins and minerals that do not supply calories but are essential for regulating and maintaining physiologic processes necessary for health
- Water, which is also necessary for life (discussed in Chapter 16)

Although standards have been established for the types and amounts of dietary components necessary to sustain health, individual nutritional needs are influenced by and may require adjustment according to the following:

- Age
- Weight and height
- Growth periods
- Activity
- Health status

Calories

Food is the source of energy for humans. Some nutrients produce more energy than others. By using a calorimeter, a device for measuring heat, the nutrients in food are burned in a laboratory and then analyzed to quantify their energy value.

The energy, or heat equivalent, of food is measured in calories. A **calorie** (cal) (the amount of heat that raises the temperature of 1 g of water by 1°C) is one way to express the energy value of food. Sometimes, the energy equivalent of food is expressed in **kilocalories** (kcal) (1,000 cal, or the amount of heat that raises the temperature of 1 kg of water by 1°C).

When proteins, carbohydrates, and fats are metabolized, they produce energy. Proteins yield 4 kcal/g, carbohydrates yield 4 kcal/g, and fats yield 9 kcal/g. Alcohol yields 7 kcal/g but is not considered an essential nutrient.

The number of calories a person needs depends on age, body size, physical condition, and physical activity. On average, healthy adult women require 1,600 to 2,400 cal/day and adult men require 2,000 to 3,000 cal/day; the lower end of the range is for sedentary individuals, whereas the higher end is for active individuals (U.S. Department of Agriculture, 2010). Unless the caloric intake includes an appropriate mix of proteins, carbohydrates, and fats, the person may be marginally nourished or malnourished. In other words, consuming 2,000 cal of chocolate, exclusive of any other food, is not adequate to sustain a healthy state! Fortunately, most foods contain a variety of nutrients, vitamins, and minerals.

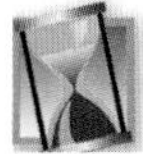

Gerontologic Considerations

- Older adults require fewer calories and, therefore, should be taught to select nutrient-dense foods such as meat, fruits, vegetables, dairy products, and whole-grain breads and cereals.

Proteins

Protein, a component of every living cell, is a nutrient composed of *amino acids*, or chemical compounds composed of nitrogen, carbon, hydrogen, and oxygen. Amino acids are responsible for building and repairing cells. Twenty-two amino acids have been identified so far. Of these, nine are referred to as **essential amino acids**, which are protein components that must be obtained from food because the body cannot synthesize them. **Nonessential amino acids** are protein components manufactured within the body; however, this term is misleading. "Nonessential" refers to the fact that these amino acids are not dependent on dietary intake, not that they are unnecessary for health.

The body uses proteins primarily to build, maintain, and repair tissue. The body spares protein from being used for energy as long as calories are available from carbohydrates and fats.

Dietary proteins are obtained from animal and plant food sources, which include milk, meat, fish, poultry, eggs, soy, legumes (peas, beans, and peanuts), nuts, and components of

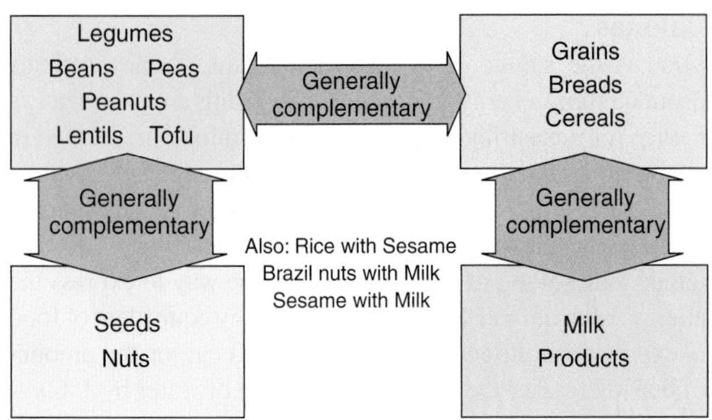

FIGURE 15-1 A complementary protein guide for meatless meals.

grains. Generally, animal sources provide **complete proteins** (proteins that contain adequate amounts and proportions of all the essential amino acids); plant sources contain **incomplete proteins** (proteins that contain insufficient quantities of one or more essential amino acids). **Protein complementation** (combining plant sources of protein) helps a person to acquire all essential amino acids from nonanimal sources (Fig. 15-1). Protein complementation is discussed later in relation to vegetarian diets.

Carbohydrates

Carbohydrates are nutrients that contain molecules of carbon, hydrogen, and oxygen, and are generally found in plant food sources. They are classified according to the number of sugar (saccharide) units they contain. Carbohydrates are subdivided into *monosaccharides, disaccharides,* and *polysaccharides* (starches).

Carbohydrates, the chief component of most diets, are the body's primary source for quick energy. In addition to providing calories, carbohydrates may contain fiber (complex polysaccharides that humans are unable to digest). **Cellulose** is a type of fiber in the stems, skins, and leaves of fruits and vegetables, which forms intestinal bulk to promote bowel elimination. Other types of fiber help lower serum cholesterol levels and delay the rise in serum glucose after eating.

Sources of carbohydrates include cereals and grains such as rice, wheat and wheat germ, oats, barley, corn, and corn meal; fruits and vegetables; and sweeteners. Milk is the only significant animal source of carbohydrates. Box 15-1 lists terms on food labels that identify ingredients that are, in essence, sugar. Foods containing added sugar as a major ingredient tend to supply calories but few, if any, other nutrients.

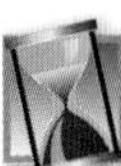

Gerontologic Considerations

■ Older adults often consume diets high in carbohydrates. Reasons include changes in taste; changes in the ability to prepare or obtain foods; or financial considerations of paying for medications, groceries, and living expenses on a fixed income.

Fats

Fats, nutrients that contain molecules composed of glycerol and fatty acids called *glycerides*, are part of a family of compounds known collectively as *lipids.* Depending on the number of fatty acids that make up a fat molecule, fats are referred to as monoglycerides, diglycerides, or triglycerides.

Fats are a concentrated energy source, supplying more than twice the calories per gram than either proteins or carbohydrates. Although fats are high in calories, they should not be eliminated from the diet. Fats provide energy and are necessary for many chemical reactions in the body. They are also necessary for the absorption of some vitamins. Fats also add flavor to food, and because they leave the stomach slowly, they promote a feeling of having satisfied appetite and hunger.

The following food sources contain fat: meat, fish, and poultry; butter, margarine, and vegetable oils; egg yolks; whole milk and cheese; peanut butter; salad dressings; avocados; chocolate; nuts; salty snacks; and most desserts.

Role of Cholesterol. Cholesterol is transported through the blood in molecules of **lipoproteins** (a combination of fats and proteins). Lipoproteins vary in their proportions of protein to cholesterol. The more protein a molecule contains, the higher is its density. High-density lipoprotein (HDL) is referred to as "good cholesterol," because the cholesterol is delivered to the liver for removal. Low-density lipoprotein is called "bad cholesterol" because the cholesterol is deposited within the walls of arteries, which can eventually result in cardiovascular disease.

Types of Fats. All fats in food are a mixture of saturated and unsaturated fats. **Saturated fats** are lipids that contain as much hydrogen as their molecular structure can hold and are generally solid. Saturated fats are the predominate type of fat in red meats, full fat dairy products, and palm and coconut oils. Cholesterol is only present in foods of animal origin, but the body also synthesizes cholesterol. **Unsaturated fats** are missing some hydrogen. They are a healthier form of fats and are liquid at room temperature or congeal slightly when refrigerated. Unsaturated fats are the predominate type

BOX 15-1 Label Ingredients That Represent Sugar

- Sucrose (table sugar)
- Fructose
- Glucose (dextrose)
- Brown sugar
- Corn sweetener
- Corn syrup
- High fructose corn syrup
- Fruit juice concentrate
- Honey
- Invert sugar
- Lactose
- Maltose
- Molasses
- Raw sugar
- Syrup
- Evaporated cane juice
- Malt

of fat in fish, poultry, nuts, and most plant oils, such as corn, safflower, olive, peanut, and soybean. **Trans fats** are unsaturated fats that have been *hydrogenated,* a process in which hydrogen is added to the fat. Hydrogenation changes the unsaturated fat to a more saturated form that remains solid at room temperature. An example includes the hydrogenation of vegetable oil to create margarine or shortening. Hydrogenation reduces the rate at which a fat becomes rancid, thus increasing the shelf life of food items that contain it (eg, cake mixes).

Health Risks Related to Fat and Cholesterol. Generally, Americans consume more fats than people do in most other countries. The relationship between fat consumption and obesity to disorders such as metabolic syndrome, heart disease, hypertension, diabetes, and some cancers is well documented. In an effort to improve national health, the Department of Health and Human Resources is continuing its initiative, *Healthy People 2020*. One goal the government advocates is for at least 50% of people 2 years and older to consume no more than 29.8% of their daily calories from fat; of that, less than 9.5% should be saturated fat.

Although the creation of trans fats has improved the marketing of convenience foods, health-concerned agencies like the American Heart Association (AHA, 2010) indicate that consumption of trans fats increases the risk for coronary heart disease. The U.S. Food and Drug Administration (FDA, 2010) now requires the listing of the amount of trans fatty acid content on food labels.

Health care providers use cholesterol and lipoprotein levels to assess clients' risks for cardiac and vascular diseases (Table 15-1). Cardiac risk also can be estimated by dividing the total serum cholesterol level, which should be less than 200 mg/dL, by the HDL level. A result greater than 5 suggests that a client has a potential for coronary artery disease.

TABLE 15-1 Cardiac Risk Associated With Blood Fat Levels

SUBSTANCE	VALUE	INTERPRETATION
Total cholesterol	<200 mg/dL	Desirable
	200–239 mg/dL	Borderline high
	≥240 mg/dL	High
Low-density lipoprotein	<100 mg/dL	Optimal
	100–129 mg/dL	Near optimal
	130–159 mg/dL	Borderline high
	160–189 mg/dL	High
	≥190 mg/dL	Very high
High-density lipoprotein	<40 mg/dL	Low
	40–59 mg/dL	Acceptable
	≥60 mg/dL	Optimal

Source: Adult Treatment Panel (ATPIII). (2001). *Clinical guidelines for cholesterol testing and management.* The National Cholesterol Education Program, a division of the National Heart, Lung, Blood Institute. (Online): http://rover.nhlbi.gov/guidelines/cholesterol/atp3_rpt.htm

Stop, Think, and Respond Box 15-1

Which client has the lowest cardiac risk factor?

- *Client A: Total cholesterol level is 224 mg/dL; HDL level is 38 mg/dL*
- *Client B: Total cholesterol level is 198 mg/dL; HDL level is 35 mg/dL*
- *Client C: Total cholesterol level is 210 mg/dL; HDL level is 55 mg/dL*

Minerals

Minerals (noncaloric substances in food that are essential to all cells) help regulate many of the body's chemical processes such as blood clotting and the conduction of nerve impulses. Table 15-2 lists some of the body's major and trace minerals, their chief functions, and common dietary sources.

As a national policy, specified amounts of certain minerals and vitamins are added to some processed foods. For example, enriched flour and bread contain thiamine, riboflavin, niacin, and iron to replace what is lost when the grain is ground into flour. Fortified foods have nutrients added that were either not naturally present in the food or were present in insignificant amounts.

TABLE 15-2 Common Dietary Minerals

MINERAL	CHIEF FUNCTIONS	COMMON DIETARY SOURCES
Sodium	Maintenance of water and electrolyte balance	Table salt Processed meat
Potassium	Maintenance of electrolyte balance Neuromuscular activity Enzyme reactions	Bananas Oranges Potatoes
Chloride	Maintenance of fluid and electrolyte balance	Table salt Processed meat
Calcium	Formation of teeth and bones Neuromuscular activity Blood coagulation Cell wall permeability	Milk Milk products
Phosphorus	Buffering action Formation of bones and teeth	Eggs Meat Milk
Iodine	Regulation of body metabolism Promotion of normal growth	Seafood Iodized salt
Iron	Component of hemoglobin Assistance in cellular oxidation	Liver Egg yolks Meat
Magnesium	Neuromuscular activity Activation of enzymes Formation of teeth and bones	Whole grains Milk Meat
Zinc	Constituent of enzymes and insulin	Seafood Liver

TABLE 15-3 Vitamins

VITAMIN	CHIEF FUNCTIONS	COMMON DIETARY SOURCES
A (Retinol) Not destroyed by ordinary cooking temperatures	Growth of body cells Promotion of vision, healthy hair and skin, and integrity of epithelial membranes Prevention of xerophthalmia, a condition characterized by chronic conjunctivitis	Animal fats: butter, cheese, cream, egg yolks, whole milk Fish liver oil and liver Dark green leafy vegetables; deep orange fruits and vegetables
B_1 (Thiamine) Not readily destroyed by ordinary cooking temperatures	Carbohydrate metabolism Functioning of the nervous system Normal digestion Prevention of beriberi, a condition characterized by neuritis	Fish Pork Lean meat and poultry Glandular organs Milk Whole, fortified, and enriched breads, cereals, and grains Peas, beans, and peanuts
B_2 (Riboflavin) Not destroyed by heat except in the presence of alkali	Formation of certain enzymes Normal growth Light adaptation in the eyes	Eggs Green leafy vegetables Lean meat Milk Whole grains Dried yeast
B_3 (Niacin)	Carbohydrate, fat, and protein metabolism Enzyme component Prevention of appetite loss Prevention of pellagra, a condition characterized by cutaneous, gastrointestinal, neurologic, and mental symptoms	Lean meat and liver Fish Peas, beans Whole-grain cereals Peanuts Yeast Eggs Liver
B_6 (Pyridoxine) Destroyed by heat, sunlight, and air	Healthy gums and teeth Red blood cell formation Carbohydrate, fat, and protein metabolism	Whole-grain cereals and wheat germ Vegetables Yeast Meat Bananas Blackstrap molasses
B_9 (Folic acid)	Protein metabolism Red blood cell formation Normal intestinal tract functioning	Green leafy vegetables Glandular organs Yeast
B_{12} (Cyanocobalamin)	Protein metabolism Red blood cell formation Healthy nervous system tissues Prevention of pernicious anemia, a condition characterized by decreased red blood cells	Liver and kidney Dairy products Lean meat Milk Saltwater fish and oysters
C (Ascorbic acid) Readily destroyed by cooking temperatures	Healthy bones, teeth, and gums Formation of blood vessels and capillary walls Proper tissue and bone healing Facilitation of iron and folic acid absorption Prevention of scurvy, a condition characterized by bleeding and abnormal bone and teeth formation	Citrus fruits and juices Tomatoes Berries Cabbage Green vegetables Potatoes
D (Calciferol) Relatively stable with refrigeration	Absorption of calcium and phosphorus Prevention of rickets, a condition characterized by weak bones	Fish liver oils, salmon, tuna Milk Egg yolks Butter Liver Oysters Formed in the skin by exposure to sunlight
E (Alpha-tocopherol) Heat stable in the absence of oxygen	Red blood cell formation Protection of essential fatty acids Important for normal reproduction in experimental animals (ie, rats)	Green leafy vegetables Wheat germ oil Margarine Brown rice
Pantothenic acid	Metabolism	Liver Egg yolks Milk

VITAMIN	CHIEF FUNCTIONS	COMMON DIETARY SOURCES
H (Biotin) Heat sensitive	Enzyme activity Metabolism of carbohydrates, fats, and proteins	Egg yolks Green vegetables Milk Liver and kidney Yeast
K (Menadione)	Production of prothrombin	Liver Eggs Green leafy vegetables Synthesized in the gastrointestinal tract by bacteria

Vitamins

Vitamins are chemical substances necessary in minute amounts for normal growth, the maintenance of health, and the functioning of the body (Table 15-3). They were originally named with letters; numbers were subsequently added to some letters as more vitamins were identified. Chemical names are now replacing the letter-number system of identification.

Water-soluble vitamins (B complex and C) are eliminated with body fluids and so require daily replacement. **Fat-soluble vitamins** (A, D, E, and K) are stored in the body as reserves for future needs.

With the exception of vitamin D, vitamin K (menadione), and biotin, the body does not manufacture vitamins. People can easily meet their vitamin requirements, however, by eating a variety of foods. Cooking, processing, and not refrigerating can deplete the content of some vitamins in food. Various commercially packaged foods such as margarine, milk, and flour have been vitamin enriched or fortified to promote health.

Generally, vitamin and mineral supplements are not necessary if a person eats a well-balanced diet. Consuming **megadoses** (amounts exceeding those considered adequate for health) of vitamins and minerals can be dangerous. Some athletes and people with terminal diseases choose to follow unconventional diets and take large doses of nutritional supplements. Athletes are motivated by a desire to alter their muscle mass, strength, and endurance; people with terminal diseases seek attempts for cure. Although various deficiency diseases develop from inadequate nutrition, no conclusive evidence at this time supports that consuming excessive nutrients, vitamins, or minerals is a safe substitute for healthy eating or works as a singular established treatment for disease.

Nutritional Strategies

Healthy People 2020, a national effort to improve the health of Americans, provides recommendations to enhance nutrition and weight status (Box 15-2). Other nutritional strategies include using the U.S. Department of Agriculture's MyPlate, referring to labels about nutrition on processed and packaged foods, and understanding standard definitions for the terms used on food labels.

MyPlate

MyPlate, introduced in 2011 by the U.S. Department of Agriculture, replaces the previously used *food pyramid* and *MyPyramid*. MyPlate is an improved simplified tool for promoting a healthful daily intake of food (Fig. 15-2). Its advantage is that the recommended percentages of consumed food from among five food group categories promote healthy nutrition. Nutritionists also advocate reducing salt consumption and substituting water for sugary beverages. Following MyPlate guidelines promotes the achievement of the dietary recommendations set by the U.S. Department of Health and Human Services and the U.S. Department of Agriculture's Dietary Guidelines for Americans (see Web Resources on thePoint).

Children, adolescents, pregnant women, and breast-feeding mothers require more servings per day of certain food groups, particularly the milk group. Recommenda-

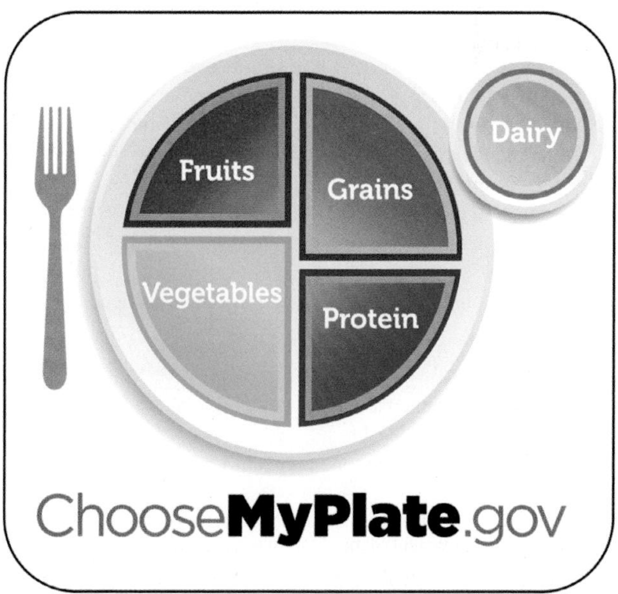

FIGURE 15-2 MyPlate is color-coded to show the five groups of foods that should be consumed each day in the following proportions: 30% grains, of which half are preferably whole grains; 30% vegetables; 20% fruits; 20% protein; which are accompanied by low-fat/nonfat milk or other reduced fat dairy products. (USDA, ChooseMyPlate.gov.)

BOX 15-2 Nutrition and Weight Status Objectives for Healthy People 2020

Healthier Food Access

Increase the number of states with nutrition standards for foods and beverages provided to preschool-aged children in child care.

Increase the proportion of schools that offer nutritious foods and beverages outside of school meals.

Increase the number of states that have state-level policies that incentivize food retail outlets to provide foods that are encouraged by the USDA's *Dietary Guidelines for Americans.*

Increase the proportion of Americans that have access to a food retail outlet that sells a variety of foods that are encouraged by the USDA's *Dietary Guidelines for Americans.*

Healthcare and Work Site Settings

Increase the proportion of primary care physicians who regularly measure the body mass index (BMI) of their patients.

Increase the proportion of physician office visits that include counseling or education related to nutrition or weight.

Increase the proportion of work sites that offer nutrition or weight management classes or counseling.

Reduce the proportion of children and adolescents who are considered obese.

Prevent inappropriate weight gain in youth and adults.

Food Insecurity

Eliminate very low food security (a state in which people have access at all times to sufficient, safe, nutritious food to maintain a healthy and active life) among children.

Reduce household food insecurity and, in doing so, reduce hunger.

Food and Nutrient Consumption

Increase the contribution of fruits to the diets of the population aged 2 years and older.

Increase the variety of vegetables to the diets of the population aged 2 years and older.

Increase the contribution of whole grains to the diets of the population aged 2 years and older.

Reduce consumption of calories from solid fats and added sugars in the population aged 2 years and older.

Reduce consumption of saturated fat in the population aged 2 years and older.

Reduce consumption of sodium in the population aged 2 years and older.

Increase consumption of calcium in the population aged 2 years and older.

Iron Deficiency

Reduce iron deficiency among young children and females of childbearing age.

Reduce iron deficiency among pregnant females.

U.S. Department of Health and Human Services. (2010). Healthy People 2020, Nutrition and Weight Status. http://www.healthypeople.gov/2020/topicsobjectives2020/overview.aspx?topicid=29, accessed March 1, 2011.

tions for specific populations can be accessed at the Web site for the Department of Health and Human Resources: Dietary Guidelines for Americans (see Web Resources on thePoint).

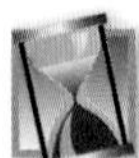

Gerontologic Considerations

■ Some older adults have difficulty obtaining and preparing nutritious meals because of socioeconomic barriers such as low income and an inability to get to the grocery store. In addition, appropriate food storage (including food expiration dates, proper storage temperature, and access to cupboards if arthritic changes are present) should be evaluated.

Stop, Think, and Respond Box 15-2

Using MyPlate, what percentage of whole grains should an adult consume each day?

Nutritional Labeling

Nutritional information has appeared on food labels since 1974. Today, all packages of fresh meat and poultry must provide printed disease prevention guidelines. There have also been major changes in the way nutritional information is provided on approximately 90% of processed and packaged food labels (Fig. 15-3). The labels identify the amounts of each nutrient per serving, which is identified in household measurements. To interpret the information accurately, however, consumers must become familiar with a variety of terms, such as daily value (DV). DVs are calculated in percentages based on standards set for total fat, saturated fat,

Nutrition Facts

Serving Size 1/2 cup (114g)
Servings Per Container 4

Amount Per Serving	
Calories 90	Calories from Fat 30
	% Daily Value*
Total Fat 3 g	5
Saturated Fat 0 g	0
Trans Fat 1 g	
Cholesterol 0 mg	0
Sodium 300 mg	13
Total Carbohydrate 13 g	4
Dietary Fiber 3 g	12
Sugars 3 g	
Protein 3 g	

Vitamin A 80%	•	Vitamin C 60%
Calcium 4%	•	Iron 4%

* Percent Daily Values are based on a 2,000 cal diet. Your daily values may be higher or lower depending on your caloric needs:

		Calories 2,000	2,500
Total Fat	Less than	65 g	80 g
Sat Fat	Less than	20 g	25 g
Cholesterol	Less than	300 mg	300 mg
Sodium	Less than	2,400 mg	2,400 mg
Total Carbohydrate		300 g	375 g
Fiber		25 g	30 g

Calories per gram:
Fat 9 • Carbohydrate 4 • Protein 4

FIGURE 15-3 A sample label with nutritional information (Taylor, 2010).

cholesterol, sodium, carbohydrate, and fiber in a 2,000-cal diet. The standards are as follows:

- Total fat: less than 65 g
- Saturated fat: less than 20 g
- Cholesterol: less than 300 mg
- Sodium: less than 2,400 mg
- Total carbohydrate: 300 g
- Dietary fiber: 25 g

People consuming diets of more or less than 2,000 cal must adjust the percentage of DVs. The required calculation may be difficult for the average consumer. An expanded table showing the DV equivalents for both a 2,000- and a 2,500-cal diet appears on some, but not all, food labels. Because the requirements for vitamins and minerals do not depend on calories, those amounts are uniform to all consumers.

Additional regulations affect food labels. For example, the federal Nutrition Labeling and Education Act requires companies to comply with standard definitions if they use health-related claims such as "low-fat" on their labels (Box 15-3).

NUTRITIONAL PATTERNS AND PRACTICE

Influences on Eating Habits

Most people learn their eating habits early in life. Cultural (Fig. 15-4), economic, emotional, and social variables influence the kinds of food a person consumes and his or her eating habits. Some influential factors include the following:

- Food preferences acquired during childhood
- Established patterns for meals
- Attitudes about nutrition

BOX 15-3 Regulations for Labeling Terms

- *Calorie-free:* <5 cal
- *Low calorie:* ≤40 cal
- *Reduced calorie:* at least 25% fewer calories than the standard product
- *Light or "lite":* one third fewer calories or 50% less fat than the regular product
- *Fat-free:* <0.5 g fat; example: skim milk
- *Low fat:* ≤3 g fat; example: 1% milk
- *Reduced fat:* at least 25% less fat than the regular product; for example: 2% milk
- *Cholesterol-free:* <2 mg cholesterol and ≤2 g saturated fat
- *Low cholesterol:* ≤20 mg cholesterol and ≤2 g saturated fat
- *Sugar-free:* <0.5 g sugar
- *Fruit drink/beverage:* <100% fruit juice
- *Imitation:* new food that resembles a traditional food and contains less protein or less of any essential vitamin or mineral than the traditional food; example: imitation cheese

Figures per serving.

Food and Drug Administration. Guidance for industry: A food labeling guide. Washington, DC: FDA, 2011. http://www.fda.gov/Food/GuidanceComplianceRegulatoryInformation/GuidanceDocuments/FoodLabelingNutition/FoodLabelingGuide, accessed November 30, 2011.

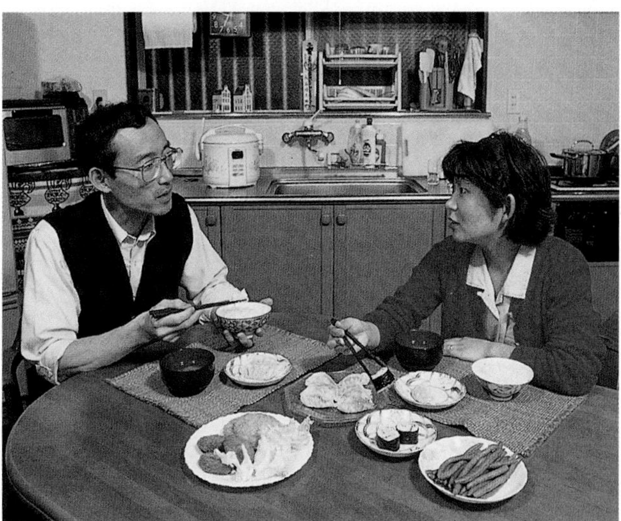

FIGURE 15-4 Cultural influences affect eating habits. (Copyright Charles Gupton/Stock Boston.)

- Knowledge of nutrition
- Income level
- Time available for food preparation
- Number of people in the household
- Access to food markets
- Use of food for comfort, celebration, or symbolic reward
- Satisfaction or dissatisfaction with body weight
- Religious beliefs

Vegetarianism

Vegetarians are people who restrict their consumption of animal food sources, modifying their diets for religious or personal reasons. Vegetarianism is practiced in various forms. For example, **vegans** rely exclusively on plant sources for protein. Semi-vegetarians exclude only red meat.

Overall, vegetarians have a lower incidence of colorectal cancer and fewer problems with obesity and diseases associated with a high-fat diet (American Dietetic Association, 2009; American Heart Association, 2010). Nevertheless, a vegan diet, unless skillfully planned, can be inadequate in protein, calcium, vitamins B_{12} and D, iron, zinc, and omega-3 fatty acids. Thus, it is helpful to teach vegans about protein complementation if they are unfamiliar with the practice. Protein complementation involves eating a variety of incomplete plant proteins over the course of the day to provide adequate amounts and proportions of all the essential amino acids present in animal protein sources (see Fig. 15-1 and Client and Family Teaching 15-1 for more information).

NUTRITIONAL STATUS ASSESSMENT

Because eating is a basic need, nurses must identify any current or potential client problems associated with nutrition. They obtain subjective information by asking clients focused questions on a diet history. Nurses gather objective data using physical assessment techniques.

Client and Family Teaching 15-1 Vegetarian Diets

The nurse teaches the vegetarian client and his or her family as follows:

- Plan menus 1 day or week at a time.
- Eat a wide variety of foods.
- Eat a variety of different plant proteins every day.
- Include fortified ready-to-eat cereals, soy foods, dried fruit, molasses, and dried peas for iron.
- Enhance absorption of iron by including a good source of vitamin C (eg, orange juice) with each meal.
- Use fortified ready-to-eat cereals and fortified soy milk to obtain vitamin B_{12}, vitamin D, and zinc.
- Choose calcium-fortified orange juice, fortified soy yogurt, milk, and tofu; and bok choy, broccoli, collards, kale, okra, and turnip greens for calcium.
- Select plant sources of omega-3 fatty acids, such as canola oil, ground flaxseed, walnuts, and soybeans.
- Select good sources of calcium such as broccoli, collard and mustard greens, kale, and tofu.
- Breast-feed infants, if possible.
- Consider taking cod liver oil as a source of vitamin D.
- Purchase meat analogues, products with the taste and appearance of meat, poultry, or fish that are made from textured vegetable protein. Such analogues are available in health food and grocery stores.
- Contact a Seventh-Day Adventist church, whose members practice vegetarianism, for information on sources for meatless products and food preparation classes.

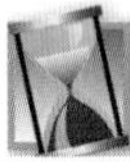

Gerontologic Considerations

- Medical conditions, adverse medication effects, functional impairments, and psychosocial conditions (eg, dementia, depression, social isolation) commonly affect the nutritional status of older adults.
- Oral and dental problems are common in older adults, which interfere with adequate nutrition. Encourage older adults to get dental care every 6 months and to practice good dental hygiene daily. Malfitting dentures may contribute to weight change.

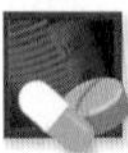

Pharmacologic Considerations

- Taking multiple medications increases the incidence of food–drug interactions. Some medications cause constipation, diarrhea, a loss of appetite, and other problems that interfere with nutrition. Teaching regarding medication dosage should include the potential side effects as well as the recommended timing of administration in relation to food intake. Also, over-the-counter (OTC) or herbal therapies can interfere with nutrient absorption.

Subjective Data

A **diet history** is an assessment technique for obtaining facts about a client's eating habits and factors that affect nutrition. The findings add to the database of nutritional information. Common components in a diet history include the following:

- The level of appetite
- Unintentional weight loss or gain of 10% in the past 6 months
- The number of meals the client eats per day
- Foods (in approximate household measurements) that the client has eaten in the previous 24 hours
- Time when the client generally eats meals
- Frequency with which the client eats meals alone
- Food likes, dislikes, allergies, intolerances, and cultural beliefs about food
- The amount of alcohol the client consumes daily or weekly
- Vitamin or mineral supplements the client takes routinely
- Any problems with eating, digestion, or elimination
- Special diets that have been medically prescribed or self-imposed
- The use of OTC drugs, such as antacids or laxatives
- Food supplements or restrictions and the reason for them
- The desire to improve nutritional intake or to gain or lose weight

Objective Data

The body is composed of water, fat, bone, and muscle. The nurse uses physical assessments and laboratory data, anthropometric data, and a person's body measurements to help determine a client's nutritional status.

Anthropometric Data

Anthropometric data are measurements pertaining to body size and composition. The nurse obtains them by measuring height and weight, calculating body mass index (BMI), and measuring midarm circumference, triceps skinfold thickness, and abdominal circumference. Eating disorder clinics and fitness centers use more sophisticated tests such as bioelectrical impedance analysis that calculate lean body mass, body fat, and total body water based on changes in conduction of an applied electrical current.

Obtaining the client's height and weight generally provides sufficient anthropometric data unless a severe nutritional problem is suspected or long-term therapy is anticipated. An actual weight, rather than the client's estimate, is essential. The nurse uses a standing, chair, or bed scale depending on the client's condition. He or she records the date and time, the type of scale, and the clothing the client wears. It is important to duplicate all these factors when taking subsequent weights for comparison. The nurse measures the client's height without shoes. A gross assessment tool using weight and height is shown in Figure 15-5.

	Healthy Weight						Overweight					Obese					
BMI	19	20	21	22	23	24	25	26	27	28	29	30	31	32	33	34	35
4'10"	91	96	100	105	110	115	119	124	129	134	138	143	148	153	158	162	167
4'11"	94	99	104	109	114	119	124	128	133	138	143	148	153	158	163	168	173
5'	97	102	107	112	118	123	128	133	138	143	148	153	158	163	168	174	179
5'1"	100	106	111	116	122	127	132	137	143	148	153	158	164	169	174	180	185
5'2"	104	109	115	120	125	131	136	142	147	153	158	164	169	175	180	186	191
5'3"	107	113	118	124	130	135	141	146	152	158	163	169	175	180	186	191	197
5'4"	110	116	122	128	134	140	145	151	157	163	169	174	180	186	192	197	204
5'5"	114	120	126	132	138	144	150	156	162	168	174	180	186	192	198	204	210
5'6"	118	124	130	136	142	148	155	161	167	173	179	186	192	198	204	210	216
5'7"	121	127	134	140	146	153	159	166	172	178	185	191	198	204	211	217	223
5'8"	125	131	138	144	151	158	164	171	177	184	190	197	203	210	216	223	230
5'9"	128	135	142	149	155	162	169	176	182	189	196	203	209	216	223	230	236
5'10"	132	139	146	153	160	167	174	181	188	195	202	209	216	222	229	236	243
5'11"	136	143	150	157	165	172	179	186	193	200	208	215	222	229	236	243	250
6'	140	147	154	162	169	177	184	191	199	206	213	221	228	235	242	250	258
6'1"	144	151	159	166	174	182	189	197	204	212	219	227	235	242	250	257	265
6'2"	148	156	164	171	179	186	194	202	210	218	225	233	241	249	256	264	272
6'3"	152	160	168	176	184	192	200	208	216	224	232	240	248	256	264	272	279

Height (rows) — Weight in Pounds

FIGURE 15-5 A tool for determining weight status. (NIH, 2005, http://www.health.gov/dietaryguidelines/dga2005/report/HTML/figure_e1.htm.)

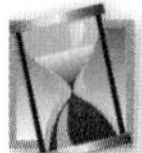

Gerontologic Considerations

■ Age-related changes are usually gradual; therefore, include evaluation of nutritional status in annual examinations or more frequently if indicated by weight gain or loss of 10% within 6 months or 5% within 1 month.

Body mass index (BMI) provides numeric data to compare a person's size in relation to established norms for the adult population. It is calculated using height and weight (Box 15-4).

Stop, Think, and Respond Box 15-3

Using the graph in Figure 15-5 and the formula in Box 15-4, what is your analysis of a person who is 5 ft 7 in. and weighs 185 lb?

Midarm circumference helps determine skeletal muscle mass. This technique, combined with other body measurements, helps assess a client's nutritional status. The measurement is based on the assumption that muscle usually is located in anatomic areas such as the biceps. When measuring midarm circumference:

- Use the nondominant arm
- Find the midpoint of the upper arm between the shoulder and the elbow
- Mark the midarm location
- Position the arm loosely at the client's side
- Encircle the arm with a tape measure at the marked position
- Record the circumference in centimeters

Triceps skinfold measurement adds additional data for estimating the amount of subcutaneous fat deposits (Fig. 15-6). The skinfold thickness measurement relates to total body fat. To measure triceps skinfold thickness:

- Use the same arm as for the midarm circumference measurement
- Grasp and pull the skin separate from the muscle at the previously marked location
- Place the calipers around the skinfold
- Record the measurement in millimeters

BOX 15-4 Body Mass Index Calculation and Interpretation

Calculation

1. Divide pounds by 2.2 = kilograms (kg).
2. Divide height in inches by 39.4 = meters (m).
3. Square the answer in step 2 by multiplying the number times itself.
4. Divide weight in kg by m^2.

INTERPRETATION	BMI
Underweight	<18.5
Normal	18.5–24.9
Overweight	25.0–29.9
Obese	30.0–34.9
Severely obese	35.0–39.9
Extremely obese	≥40

To calculate how much of the midarm circumference is actual muscle (midarm muscle circumference), multiply the triceps skinfold measurement by 0.314.

To interpret the significance of the midarm circumference measurement and triceps skinfold thickness, the nurse compares measurements with averages provided in standardized charts (Table 15-4). Skinfold thickness norms do not exist for adults older than 75 years.

Abdominal circumference is an indirect measurement of fatty (adipose) tissue that is distributed in and about the viscera of the abdomen. Accumulation of centrally located adipose tissue indicates a predisposition for diabetes and cardiovascular disease. To facilitate accuracy, the client should be (1) wearing underwear or light clothing to avoid including bulky fabric in the measurement, and (2) standing upright with the legs spread 10 to 12 in. apart. The tape measure should be placed around the client at the iliac crest of the pelvis without compressing the soft tissue, and read to the nearest quarter inch (Fig. 15-7). Increases or decreases in abdominal measurements correlate with changes in risk factors for diabetes and cardiovascular disease. Health risks increase for males whose abdominal circumference measures more than 40 in. and for females whose abdominal circumference is greater than 35 in. (National Heart, Lung, and Blood Institute, 2000).

TABLE 15-4 Anthropometric Measurements for Adults

MEASUREMENT	GENDER	NORMAL RANGE[a]
Midarm circumference	Male	29.3–17.6 cm
	Female	28.5–17.1 cm
Midarm muscle circumference	Male	25.3–15.2 cm
	Female	23.2–13.9 cm
Triceps skinfold	Male	12.5–7.3 mm
	Female	16.5–9.9 mm

[a]If measurements are below the lowest range for normal, nutritional support may be indicated.

Adapted from Jelliffe, D.B. (1986). *The assessment of the nutritional status of the community.* World Health Organization Monograph No. 53. Geneva: World Health Organization.

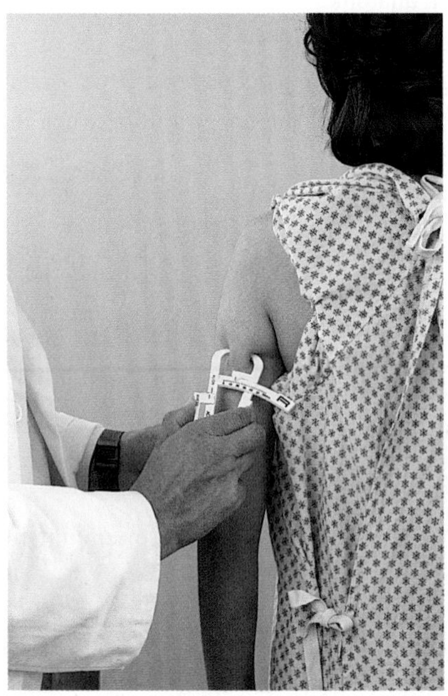

FIGURE 15-6 Measuring triceps skinfold thickness with calipers. (Photo by B. Proud.)

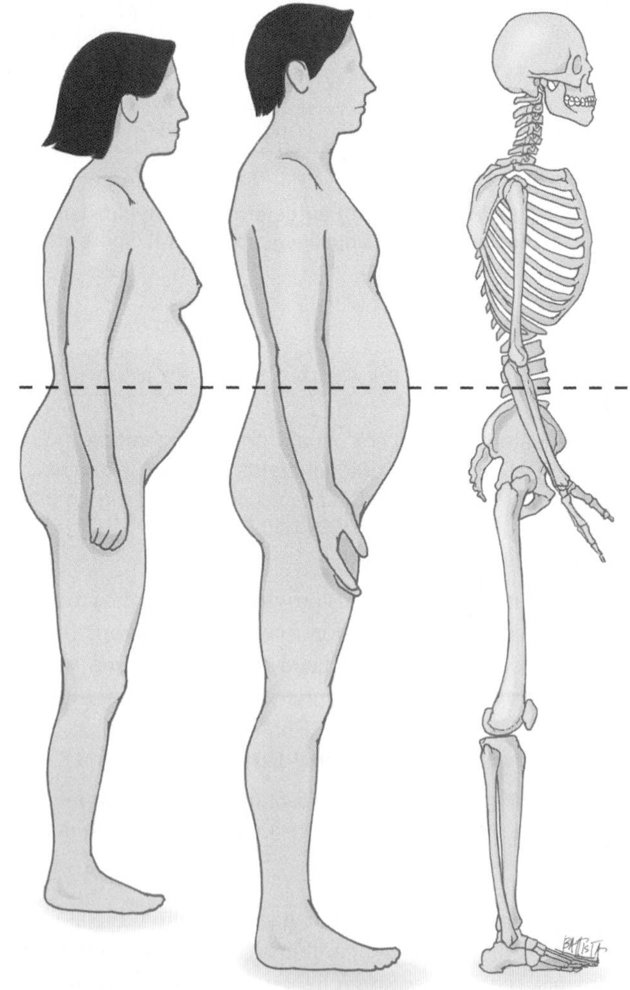

FIGURE 15-7 The location for measuring abdominal circumference in adults (Taylor, 2010).

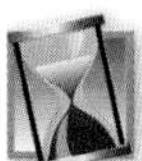

Gerontologic Considerations

■ The circumference of the abdomen may be a more accurate anthropometric measurement for older adults, but standardized norms have not been established for specific age groups.

Physical Assessment

In addition to anthropometric data, the nurse assesses the following in the client:

- General appearance
- Integrity of the mouth
- Condition of the teeth
- Ability to chew and swallow
- Gag reflex
- Characteristics of skin and hair
- Joint flexibility
- Hand strength
- Attention and concentration

Laboratory Data

Laboratory tests used in nutritional assessment include hemoglobin and hematocrit, glucose; serum albumin and transferrin levels that indicate protein status; and cholesterol, triglyceride, and lipoprotein levels that may reflect a need to adjust the amount of fat the client eats.

MANAGEMENT OF PROBLEMS INTERFERING WITH NUTRITION

Based on the assessment data, the nurse may identify one or more of the following nursing diagnoses:

- Imbalanced Nutrition: Less Than Body Requirements
- Imbalanced Nutrition: More Than Body Requirements
- Deficient Knowledge: Nutrition
- Self-Care Deficit: Feeding
- Impaired Swallowing
- Risk for Aspiration

If a nutritional problem is beyond the scope of independent nursing practice, the nurse consults with the physician. If the problem can be resolved through independent nursing measures, the nurse may proceed by collaborating with the dietitian, selecting the appropriate nursing interventions, and continuing to monitor the client to evaluate the effectiveness of the nursing care plan.

Obesity

Obesity is a condition in which a person's BMI equals or exceeds 30 or the triceps skinfold measurement exceeds 15 mm. Obesity indicates the need for healthy weight-reduction measures. Research (Mayo Clinic, 2009; National Institutes of Health, 2008, Vega et al., 2006) indicates that excess abdominal fat is a great health risk factor. An increased proportion of abdominal fat is associated with a higher incidence of heart and vascular disease, hypertension, and diabetes mellitus. Severely obese people are medically evaluated to determine whether there are physical etiologies for the disorder or health risks associated with a weight-loss program.

To lose 1 lb, the client must reduce his or her caloric intake by 3,500 cal/week. Thus, decreasing one's intake of food by 500 cal/day will produce a 1-lb weight loss per week. By omitting 1,000 cal/day, the person will lose 2 lb/week. Generally, a sustained loss of 1 to 2 lb/week is a healthy goal. The nurse advises clients trying to lose weight about healthy eating and the hazards of unsupervised weight-loss techniques such as fasting, fad diets, or diet drugs (see Client and Family Teaching 15-2).

Client and Family Teaching 15-2
Promoting Weight Loss

The nurse teaches the client who needs to lose weight and his or her family as follows:

- When using MyPlate, follow the food plan for the appropriate calorie allowance based on the individual's gender, age, and activity level.
- Count portions from each group based on MyPlate serving sizes:
  - *Grains—one slice of bread, 1 cup of ready-to-eat cereal, or a half-cup of cooked pasta, rice, or cooked cereal is a 1 oz equivalent*
  - *Vegetables—2 cups of raw leafy vegetables, 1 cup of other raw or cooked vegetables, or 1 cup of vegetable juice counts as 1 cup*
  - *Fruits—one cup of fruit or 100% fruit juice or half cup dried fruit counts as 1 cup*
  - *Milk—1 cup of milk or yogurt, 1.5 oz of natural cheese, or 2 oz of processed cheese counts as 1 cup*
  - *Meat and Beans—1 oz of lean meat, poultry, or fish, one-quarter cup of cooked dry beans, one egg, 1 tablespoon of peanut butter, or one-half oz of nuts or seeds equals 1 oz of meat*
- Use fats, oils, and sugar sparingly.
- Eliminate junk food (contributes calories but not much nutrition) and alcoholic beverages.
- Eat small but more frequent meals rather than three large meals per day. Any nutrients not used from large meals are stored as fat.
- Sit at the table to eat. Do not read or do other tasks while eating; distraction often fools the brain into thinking that food has not been consumed.
- Increase fiber in the diet from fresh fruits, vegetables, and whole grains. Fiber is not digested and may provide a full feeling without a large numbers of calories.
- Participate in some regular, active form of exercise. Exercise raises the **metabolic rate** (the speed at which the body uses calories) while suppressing appetite. Information on activity and exercise is located in Chapter 23.

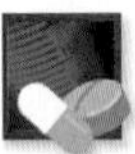

Pharmacologic Considerations

- Currently, the only FDA-approved medication for promoting weight loss or preventing weight gain following weight loss is orlistat (Xenical, and a reduced strength form called Alli). Weight loss occurs by decreasing the number of dietary calories by blocking the absorption of dietary fat. The action is a result of inhibiting the enzyme lipase. The function of lipase is to break down ingested fat into an absorbable form. The unabsorbed fat is excreted in stool. Due to a reduction in absorbed fat, it is essential to supplement fat-soluble vitamins 2 hours before or several hours after taking orlistat. There are several drug–drug interactions that can occur with drugs for diabetes and anticoagulants, for example. Some side effects include oily spotting of stool in underwear, flatulence, urgent bowel movements, and bowel incontinence.
- The Mayo Clinic (2010) reports that one can only expect modest weight loss when taking this drug. Modest weight loss is defined as 5 to 7 lb greater than diet and exercise after 1 year of taking Xenical or 3 to 5 lb with Alli.

Emaciation

Progressive or prolonged weight loss resulting in a BMI less than 16 can have serious consequences. **Emaciation** (excessive leanness) and **cachexia** (general wasting away of body tissue) are consistent with severe malnourishment. States of severe malnourishment require collaboration with a physician, who will prescribe measures to ensure the client's nutrition using gastric or enteral tube feedings or parenteral nutrition if oral intake is inadequate (see Chap. 29).

Independent nursing interventions, including client teaching, are appropriate for people who are approximately 10% below their ideal body weight. To gain 1 lb, a person must consume 3,500 cal more than his or her metabolic needs per week. This is best done gradually (see Client and Family Teaching 15-3).

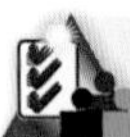

Client and Family Teaching 15-3 Promoting Weight Gain

The nurse teaches the client who needs to gain weight and his or her family as follows:

- Eat a variety of foods from MyPlate, but increase the number of servings or serving sizes.
- Eat small amounts frequently.
- Eat with others.
- Snack on high-calorie but nutritious foods such as hard cheese, milkshakes, and nuts.
- Disguise extra calories by fortifying foods with powdered milk, gravies, or sauces.
- Garnish food with cubed or grated cheese, diced meat, nuts, or raisins.
- Rest after eating.

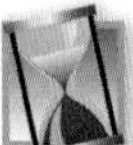

Gerontologic Considerations

- Psychosocial impairments such as dementia or depression interfere with food preparation, consumption, and enjoyment. An important initial sign of these changes may be weight loss.
- Homebound older adults may benefit from home-delivered meals. The nutrition of older adults who are isolated, depressed, or cognitively impaired may improve with participation in a group meal program. Home-delivered meals and group meal programs are widely available and are funded through the Older Americans Act. The National Eldercare Locator (800-667-1116) provides information.
- Refer low-income older adults to their local Council on Aging for assistance in obtaining food stamps.

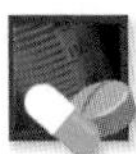

Pharmacologic Considerations

- There are many drugs whose side effects include weight gain. However, the drug megestrol (Megace) is prescribed for the primary purpose of promoting weight gain. Its prescription is generally reserved for clients who are cachectic (emaciated due to a serious illness like cancer or AIDS).

Anorexia

Anorexia (a loss of appetite) is associated with multiple factors: illness, altered taste and smell, oral problems, and tension and depression. Simple anorexia is generally a short-lived symptom that requires no medical or nursing intervention. Anorexia nervosa, a psychobiologic disorder, is associated with a 20% to 25% loss in previously stable body weight. No matter what the etiology, the nurse never ignores that a client is not eating. If food is uneaten, the nurse assesses for physiologic, emotional, cultural, or social etiologies that may be the contributing factors (see Nursing Guidelines 15-1).

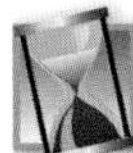

Gerontologic Considerations

- Diminished senses of smell and taste, which may occur with normal aging, can interfere with appetite and intake.
- When attempting to increase an older client's intake, nutritional supplements should be evaluated. Protein-based liquid supplements will not provide the needed fiber and should not be relied on as the main source of protein.
- Decreased exercise may lead to decreased appetite among sedentary older adults. Sitting exercises may be indicated if balance or functional abilities decline.

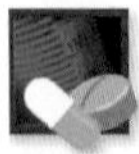

Pharmacologic Considerations

- Anorexic clients such as those with cancer may experience a stimulation in appetite by using medical marijuana, which can be purchased in states where it is legally available, or by taking its prescription form, dronabinol (Marinol), in states where possession of the natural marijuana plant is illegal.

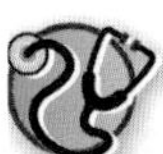

NURSING GUIDELINES 15-1

Overcoming Simple Anorexia

- Cater to the client's food preferences. *The client will more likely consume food he or she selects.*
- Serve nutrient-dense foods (foods loaded with calories). *They may compensate for a low intake of food.*
- Offer small servings of food frequently. *Eating small amounts frequently may result in a cumulative intake within acceptable nutritional levels.*
- Ensure that the client is rested before meals. *A lack of energy may overpower the desire to eat.*
- Provide an opportunity for oral hygiene before meals. *Mouth care stimulates salivation and potentiates the pleasure from eating.*
- Help the client to a sitting position. *Seeing food stimulates the appetite center; sitting also promotes access to the food.*
- Arrange for the client to eat with others. *Because eating is a social activity, the client may eat more when with a group.*
- Serve food attractively. *A visual presentation of food stimulates appetite.*
- Suggest adding spices and herbs to foods. *Intensifying flavors and aromas may stimulate a desire to eat; however, it may have the opposite effect as well. When experimenting, add new seasonings to small amounts of food.*
- Serve foods at their appropriate temperature. *The client may eat more food if hot foods are hot and cold foods are cold.*
- Serve cool, bland foods to clients with a mouth irritation. *Hot or spicy foods intensify the irritation of oral structures.*

Stop, Think, and Respond Box 15-4

How can the nurse make food and its presentation visually attractive to entice a client to eat?

Nausea

Nausea usually precedes vomiting and is produced when gastrointestinal sensations, sensory data, and drug effects stimulate a portion of the medulla that contains the vomiting center. Nausea may be associated with feeling faint or weak. Often, dizziness, perspiration, skin pallor, a rapid pulse rate, and headache are present. The nurse consults the physician when the measures presented in Nursing Guidelines 15-2 are unsuccessful for overcoming nausea. Prescribed medications may be necessary.

Once nausea is relieved, assisting the client to resume fluid intake and nourishment becomes a priority. The nurse starts this process gradually, offering sips of clear fluids first. If the client tolerates fluids, the nurse adds soft, bland foods in small amounts.

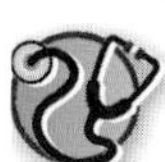

NURSING GUIDELINES 15-2

Relieving Nausea

- Check to see if something as simple as an annoying odor or sight is contributing to nausea. *Offensive sensory data can stimulate the vomiting center in the brain.*
- Assist the client to take deep breaths. *Distraction can overcome nausea by directing conscious attention away from the unpleasant sensation.*
- Limit the client's abrupt movements and activities. *Movement may shift gastrointestinal structures and their contents, intensifying stimulation of the vomiting center.*
- Limit the client's intake of food and fluid temporarily until nausea subsides. *Distention of the stomach is a common trigger of the vomiting center.*
- Avoid making negative comments about food. *Verbal comments create visual images that may cause psychogenic stimulation of the vomiting center.*

Vomiting

Vomiting (a loss of stomach contents through the mouth) commonly accompanies nausea. **Emesis** or **vomitus** (the substance that is vomited) is readily visible. **Retching** (the act of vomiting without producing vomitus) may occur if the stomach is empty. **Regurgitation** (bringing stomach contents to the throat and mouth without the effort of vomiting) occurs commonly among infants after eating. **Projectile vomiting** (vomiting that occurs with great force) is associated with certain disease conditions such as increased pressure in the brain or gastrointestinal bleeding. Nausea may be present, but it often is not (see Nursing Guidelines 15-3).

The nurse describes the emesis in the client's medical record. If possible, he or she measures the amount of emesis and records the volume. Documentation includes the amount, color, appearance, and any unusual odor such as the odor of fecal material or alcohol. If the characteristics of the emesis are unusual, the nurse saves a specimen for the physician to examine. If there are any doubts about whether to discard or save the emesis, it is best to check with a more experienced nurse.

The nurse always consults the physician when vomiting is prolonged. It may be necessary to administer prescribed medications for relief.

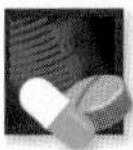

Pharmacologic Considerations

- Short-term bouts of nausea and vomiting can be treated with OTC nonprescription drugs such as Pepto-Bismol. Although prescription chlorpromazine (Thorazine) and prochlorperazine (Compazine) have been used for many years to relieve vomiting, many prescribers now are using drugs like metoclopramide (Reglan) and granisetron (Kytril) for a variety of conditions that are accompanied by vomiting, such as emesis due to cancer chemotherapy.

Stomach Gas

Gas in the stomach is primarily a result of swallowing air. It becomes a problem only when it accumulates. **Eructation** (belching) is a discharge of gas from the stomach through

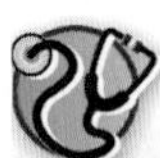

NURSING GUIDELINES 15-3

Managing the Care of a Vomiting Client

- Temporarily limit the client's food intake. *Adding contents to an already upset stomach may prolong episodes of vomiting.*
- Lean the client's head forward over a container or the toilet. *Tilting the chin toward the chest reduces the possibility that vomitus will enter the lungs.*
- Adjust light, sound, ventilation, and temperature to a comfortable level. *Minimizing sensory stimulation may reduce the urge to vomit.*
- Apply a cool washcloth to the client's forehead or back of the neck. *Increased perspiration and a clammy feeling to the skin may accompany vomiting.*
- Help the client rinse the mouth, offer mouthwash, or provide mouth care as soon as possible after vomiting. *Gastric acid is harmful to tooth enamel. Emesis usually produces an unpleasant aftertaste.*
- Turn a vomiting client who is unconscious or weak onto the abdomen or side. *Gravity helps emesis to drain from the mouth rather than remain in the throat, where the client could aspirate it into the lungs.*
- Use a suction machine to clear vomitus from the mouth and throat of a weak or unconscious client. *Suctioning pulls fluid from the oral cavity and airway, thus preventing choking and aspiration (see Chap. 36).*
- Provide firm support with the hands or a pillow to the abdominal incision if the client has had abdominal surgery. An abdominal binder also may help to support the incision (see Chap. 28). *Strong muscle contractions may pull on stitches and increase pain and discomfort.*
- Remove the container of emesis from the bedside as soon as possible. Provide ventilation to remove any lingering odors. *The appearance and odor of vomitus may stimulate more vomiting.*

the mouth. **Flatus** is gas formed in the intestine and released from the rectum when eructation does not occur. Nursing guidelines for relieving intestinal gas are discussed in Chapter 31 (see Nursing Guidelines 15-4).

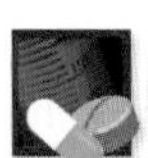

Pharmacologic Considerations

■ Avoiding gas-forming food in the diet is one of the first steps in preventing the accumulation of stomach and intestinal gas. However, there are several nonprescription products available for this purpose. For example, Beano contains an enzyme that breaks down vegetables containing polysaccharides that are difficult to digest and helps reduce the formation of gas in the colon. Another option is to take one of several products containing simethicone such as Gas-X, Flatulex, Mylicon, and Mylanta Gas.

MANAGEMENT OF CLIENT NUTRITION

Common Hospital Diets

Some common hospital diets include the following:

- Regular or general: allows unrestricted food selections
- Light or convalescent: differs from regular diet in preparation; typically omits fried, fatty, gas-forming, and raw foods and rich pastries
- Soft: contains foods soft in texture; is usually low in residue and readily digestible; contains few or no spices or condiments; provides fewer fruits, vegetables, or meats than a light diet
- Mechanical soft: resembles a light diet but is used for clients with chewing difficulties; provides cooked fruits and vegetables and ground meats

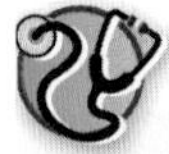

NURSING GUIDELINES 15-4

Preventing and Relieving Stomach Gas

- Suggest that the client chew food with the mouth closed. *Laughing and talking while eating increase the amount of swallowed air.*
- Advise against using a straw. *Each swallow of liquid also contains the air in the straw.*
- Advise against chewing gum and smoking cigarettes. *Chewing gum increases salivation and results in swallowing both secretions and air. The client actually may swallow a portion of inhaled cigarette smoke.*
- Limit or restrict foods that contain large volumes of air such as soufflés, yeast breads, and carbonated beverages. *Swallowing air trapped within food and drinking beverages that contain dissolved gas distend the stomach.*
- Recommend that when under stress, the client should avoid eating. *Emotions delay stomach emptying, which prevents the movement of gas to the intestine.*
- Propose walking if uncomfortable. *Activity helps gas to rise to its highest point in the stomach, making belching easier.*
- Consult with the physician about the use of medications that relieve gas accumulation. Instruct clients who purchase OTC drugs to follow label directions for their use. *Simethicone is an ingredient in several nonprescription antacids. Drugs containing simethicone facilitate the elimination of gas by reducing the surface tension of gas bubbles trapped in the gastrointestinal tract.*

- Full liquid: contains fruit and vegetable juices, creamed or blended soups, milk, ices, ice cream, gelatin, junket, custards, and cooked cereals
- Clear liquid: consists of water, clear broth, clear fruit juices, plain gelatin, tea, and coffee; may or may not include carbonated beverages
- Special therapeutic: consists of foods prepared to meet special needs, such as low in sodium, fat, calories, or fiber
- Most health care agencies have a dietitian who plans the meals and a centralized food service that prepares clients' meals

Nurses are generally responsible for ordering and canceling diets for clients, serving and collecting meal trays, helping clients to eat, and recording the percentage of food that clients eat. Nurses must know the type of diet prescribed for each client, the purpose for the diet, and its characteristics. They take care to ensure that clients receive the correct diet and that restricted foods are withheld.

Meal Trays

Meals are usually served at the bedside, but some health care institutions have dining rooms or cafeterias for ambulatory clients. Clients in nursing homes generally eat together in small groups unless they physically cannot. Nurses and dietary personnel work together to ensure that clients receive food at mealtimes and that trays are collected afterward. The nursing responsibilities for serving and removing trays are identified in Skill 15-1.

Feeding Assistance

Some clients need help with eating. Skill 15-2 provides suggested actions for feeding clients who can bite, sip, chew, and swallow but cannot cut food or use utensils for eating. Suggestions for helping clients with **dysphagia** (difficulty swallowing), for helping clients who are blind or have both eyes patched, and for promoting self-feeding in those with dementia (impairment of intellectual functioning) follow.

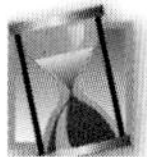

Gerontologic Considerations

- Older adults are likely to have chronic conditions such as arthritis and sensory impairments that affect their ability to meet their nutritional needs. Modifications such as plates with sides and large-handled utensils may help the older person maintain self-care ability in feeding.

Feeding the Client With Dysphagia

Nurses use the following techniques when caring for clients who have difficulty chewing and swallowing food:

- Always have equipment for oral and pharyngeal suctioning at the bedside (see Chap. 36).
- Remain with the client throughout eating when there is a potential for aspiration.
- If the client has a tracheostomy tube or endotracheal tube, make sure the cuff is inflated (see Chap. 36).
- Place the client in a sitting position.
- Ensure that the client is rested and that you have his or her attention.
- Give short, simple instructions to prompt the client to eat and swallow.
- Limit distracting stimuli; turn off the television and reduce or eliminate activities taking place in the area.
- Request a full liquid or mechanically soft diet for the client who has missing teeth or has recently had oral surgery.
- Provide small frequent meals if efforts to eat and swallow tire the client.
- Modify eating or feeding equipment to facilitate the client's safety and independence.
- Determine that the client has swallowed one portion of food before offering another.
- Encourage repeated swallowing attempts if there is wet, gurgly vocalization, a sign that food is in the esophagus and not the stomach.

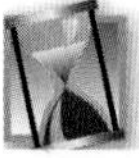

Gerontologic Considerations

- Dysphagia among older adults often results from neurologic conditions including stroke, esophageal disorders, or increased pressure from abdominal disorders. Swallowing studies may allow for the appropriate teaching of strategies to promote swallowing effectiveness.

Nursing Care Plan 15-1 is an example of how the nurse manages the care of a client who has a nursing diagnosis of impaired swallowing. This diagnostic category is defined in the NANDA-I taxonomy (2012, p. 178) as "abnormal functioning of the swallowing mechanism associated with deficits in oral, pharyngeal, or esophageal structure or function."

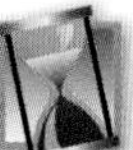

Gerontologic Considerations

- Dry mouth (xerostomia), a common problem in older adults and often results from medications or the effects of disease. It interferes with chewing, swallowing, and enjoying meals. Encourage people with dry mouth to drink adequate noncaffeinated and nonalcoholic beverages or to chew sugarless gum to promote salivation.
- Oral infections, poorly fitting dentures, or vitamin deficiencies can cause a painful or burning tongue, ulcers on the gums, or other difficulties that interfere with eating.

Feeding the Visually Impaired Client

When caring for clients who are temporarily or permanently sightless:

- Place a thick towel across the client's chest and over the lap.
- If the client can eat independently, consider using dishes with rims or bowls to prevent spilling.
- Arrange as much as possible to have finger foods (foods that may be eaten with the hands) prepared for the client.

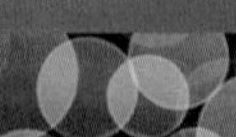

NURSING CARE PLAN 15-1 Impaired Swallowing

Assessment

- Note that if there is coughing, choking, or drooling from the mouth when the client swallows saliva, liquids, or food.
- Look for asymmetry of the mouth.
- Ask the client to extend the tongue; observe if it deviates from a midline position.
- Determine if the oral mucous membranes are moist or dry.
- Check for the gag reflex by stimulating the posterior oral pharynx with a cotton-tipped swab.
- Inspect the mouth and buccal cavities for retained food, the condition of the teeth, and evidence of tissue irritation, swelling, or injury.
- Observe the client's ability to understand and follow verbal instructions.
- Review the results of a fluoroscopic swallowing study as ordered by the physician.

Nursing Diagnosis. **Impaired swallowing** related to left hemiparesis secondary to cerebrovascular accident (stroke) as manifested by incomplete swallowing of food, occasional coughing while eating, and the statement, "I'm losing weight. I've almost given up trying to eat. I get more on me than in me since my stroke."

Expected Outcome. The client will swallow more effectively as evidenced by an empty mouth after each mastication and attempt at swallowing.

Interventions	Rationales
Maintain a suction machine, a suction catheter, and an oxygen mask at the bedside.	Equipment for suctioning the airway and improving oxygenation may be necessary if the airway becomes obstructed.
Place the client in a sitting position.	An upright position uses gravity to move food from the pharynx to the esophagus and stomach.
Provide oral hygiene before each meal.	Oral hygiene moistens the mouth, making it easier to swallow a bolus of food.
Request that the dietary department initially avoid dry foods such as crackers and sticky foods such as bananas.	Dry and sticky foods are more difficult for a client to masticate and swallow.
Request semisolid foods with some texture such as oatmeal, poached eggs, and mashed potatoes.	Semisolids are easier to swallow than liquids and watery pureed food.
Add a commercial thickener to oral liquids.	Thickeners create a consistency that the tongue can manipulate more easily against the pharynx.
Help the client load a spoon or fork with a 1/4 to 1/2 tsp of food.	Smaller amounts of food are more easily swallowed; the amount of food increases as the client demonstrates effective swallowing.
Place the food on the nonparalyzed (right) side of the mouth.	Chewing and swallowing require neuromuscular function.
Encourage the client to chew food thoroughly.	Chewing compresses food and mixes it with saliva to facilitate swallowing.
Instruct the client to lower the chin to the chest and swallow repeatedly without breathing in between.	A chin-to-chest position closes the pathway to the trachea and reduces the potential for aspiration. Repeated swallowing uses muscular contraction to move the food bolus into the esophagus.
Have the client raise the chin after swallowing efforts, clear the throat, and resume breathing.	Raising the chin, clearing the throat, and breathing improve ventilation.
Inspect the client's mouth after each swallowing attempt; encourage the client to do so as well by looking in the mouth with a handheld mirror.	Inspection helps identify retained food.
Have the client use the tongue or finger to sweep retained food from the cheek and repeat the swallowing technique; if the client is unsuccessful, apply finger pressure on the outside of the client's cheek.	Mechanical movement relocates the food to an area of the mouth where it can be manipulated and swallowed.
Keep the client in a sitting or semisitting position for at least a half hour.	The potential for aspiration is reduced once food leaves the stomach.

Evaluation of Expected Outcomes

- The client demonstrates techniques for clearing the mouth of food.
- The client swallows food completely.
- The client consumes sufficient calories to maintain weight.

- Describe the food and indicate its location on the tray.
- Guide the client's hand to reinforce the location of food and utensils.
- Prepare the food by opening cartons, cutting bite-size pieces, adding salt and pepper, buttering bread, and pouring coffee.
- Use the analogy of a clock when describing where the client may find food on the plate. For example, "The potatoes are at 3 o'clock."
- If the client needs to be fed, tell him or her what kind of food you are offering with each mouthful.
- Devise a system by which the client can indicate when he or she is ready for more food or drink, such as asking or raising a finger.

Do not rush the client; eating should be done at a leisurely pace.

Assisting the Client With Dementia

Dementia refers to the deterioration of previous intellectual capacity. It is a common problem among those with neurologic conditions such as Alzheimer's disease. These clients often can retain their ability to carry out activities of daily living, such as self-feeding, by maintaining attention and concentration and repeating actions. Therefore, the following are useful nursing actions:

- Have the same staff person help the client, if possible, to develop a rapport with the client and promote a continuity of care.
- Be consistent with the time and place for eating.
- Reduce or eliminate environmental distractions to promote concentration on the task at hand.
- Place the food tray close to the client, not the staff person, to communicate visually and spatially that the client is to eat the food.
- Remove wrappers, containers, and food covers to reduce confusion.
- Pour milk from the carton into a glass so that it is easily recognizable.
- Encourage the client's participation by offering finger foods and utensils to stimulate awareness and memory.
- Ensure that the client can see at least one other person who is also eating. This serves as a model for the desired behavior.
- Guide the hand with food to the client's mouth.
- Reinforce a desired response by praising, touching, and smiling at the client.
- Remain with the client. Do not begin feeding, leave, and then return because this interrupts the client's attention and concentration.

CRITICAL THINKING EXERCISES

1. Describe appropriate nursing actions if a client eats none or only some food served.

2. A client tells the nurse that she eats the following every day: cereal, milk, and banana for breakfast; a sandwich made with processed meat, mayonnaise, and a soft drink for lunch; a candy bar in the late afternoon; and meat, potatoes, a vegetable, and a glass of milk for supper. In the late evening, she snacks on potato chips. What recommendations would you make to improve this client's nutrition?

3. When a client reports experiencing nausea for the last few weeks, what questions would be appropriate for the nurse to ask to determine possible causes?

4. After calculating that a client's BMI is 32 and measured abdominal circumference is 42 in., what information is appropriate for the nurse to provide?

NCLEX-STYLE REVIEW QUESTIONS

1. When caring for a client whose oral mucous membranes are irritated and sore, which of the following items is best to withhold from the dietary tray?
   1. Tomato soup
   2. Lime gelatin
   3. Canned peaches
   4. Rice pudding

2. A nurse notes that a client coughs and chokes while eating. What initial nursing recommendation is best?
   1. Have the dietary department send baby foods from now on.
   2. Tell the client to chew his or her food very thoroughly.
   3. Advise the client to avoid drinking beverages with meals.
   4. Withhold milk and other dairy products in the future.

3. Which of the following is the best evidence that a client with anorexia as a result of cancer is responding to the nutritional regimen developed by the nurse and dietitian?
   1. The client remains alert.
   2. The client gains weight.
   3. The client feels hungry.
   4. The client is pain free.

4. When a client on a clear liquid diet asks for some nourishment, which of the following is appropriate for the nurse to provide?
   1. Milk
   2. Pudding
   3. Gelatin
   4. Custard

5. The nurse is most correct in recommending which of the following food sources of iron to a client with chronic anemia?
   1. Dairy products
   2. Citrus fruits
   3. Red meat
   4. Yellow vegetables

SKILL 15-1 Serving and Removing Meal Trays

Suggested Action	Reason for Action
ASSESSMENT	
Check on the usual time for meals.	Facilitates planning nursing care.
Determine which clients are undergoing tests or must have food withheld for some other reason.	Ensures that eating does not affect therapeutic outcomes.
Note the type of diet currently prescribed for each client.	Follows the client's therapeutic management plan.
Review the Kardex for information concerning clients' food allergies or food intolerances.	Reduces the potential for adverse reactions.
PLANNING	
Prepare clients so that they are ready to eat at the designated time.	Ensures food is served at its appropriate temperature.
Meet clients' needs for comfort, hygiene, and elimination before the meal arrives.	Promotes appetite and eating.
Help clients to a sitting position.	Assists ambulatory clients to a comfortable position.
IMPLEMENTATION	
Wash hands or perform hand antisepsis with an alcohol rub (see Chap. 10) before serving trays.	Prevents the transmission of microorganisms.
Deliver trays, one by one, as soon as possible.	Facilitates the enjoyment of eating through prompt delivery of food at its intended temperature.
Compare the name on the tray with the name on the client's identification bracelet, or ask the client to identify himself or herself by name.	Avoids dietary errors.
Place the tray in such a way that the client can see it.	Provides ease of access to food.
Uncover the food and check its appearance.	Ensures that the tray is complete, orderly, and tidy.
Assist the client, if necessary, to open cartons and prepare food.	Demonstrates consideration and facilitates independence.
Replace food that is objectionable or request special additional items from the dietary department.	Demonstrates respect for unique needs.
Before leaving the room, check whether the client has any further requests like an adjustment of pillows or donning eyeglasses.	Reduces inconveniences during meal time.
Make sure the signal cord is handy in case a need arises later.	Provides a means for summoning assistance.
Check the client's progress from time to time.	Indicates a willingness to provide assistance.
Remove the food tray after the client has finished eating.	Restores order and cleanliness to the environment.
Record the amount of fluid consumed from the dietary tray on the bedside flow sheet if the client's fluid intake is being monitored.	Ensures accurate fluid assessment.
Note the percentage of food that the client has eaten.[a]	Ensures documentation of dietary intake according to Joint Commission standards rather than vague terms such as *good, fair*, and *poor*.
Assist the client to brush and floss the teeth, if desired.	Removes food residue that may support microbial growth.
Place the client in a position of comfort.	Demonstrates care and concern.

Evaluation

- Client states that hunger is satisfied.
- Most food is consumed.

Document

Type of diet and percentage of food consumed

SAMPLE DOCUMENTATION[a]

Date and Time Ate 100% of mechanical soft diet with need for assistance. ———— SIGNATURE/TITLE

[a]Many agencies mandate that nurses should record the percentage of consumed food on a flow sheet or checklist. Nurses record other pertinent data within the medical record.

SKILL 15-2 Feeding a Client

Suggested Action	Reason for Action
ASSESSMENT	
Compare the dietary information on the Kardex with the medical record.	Ensures accuracy in therapeutic management.
Verify that food or fluids are not being temporarily withheld.	Prevents delaying or having to cancel diagnostic tests.
Determine whether the client's fluid intake is being measured.	Ensures the accurate documentation of data.
Assess the client to determine what or how much assistance is necessary.	Aids in identifying specific problems and selecting nursing interventions.
Review the medical record to see how well and how much the client has eaten during previous meals; note weight trends.	Helps to establish realistic goals and to evaluate progress.
Review the characteristics of the diet order.	Helps to determine whether the correct food is being served.
Analyze the purpose for the prescribed diet.	Assists in evaluating therapeutic responses.
Assess the client's needs for elimination or relief from pain, nausea, and fatigue.	Identifies unmet physiologic needs.
Check the medication record for drugs that must be administered before or with meals.	Facilitates optimal drug absorption and reduces drug side effects.
PLANNING	
Set realistic goals for how much food the client will eat and how much the client will participate with self-feeding.	Establishes criteria for evaluating client responses.
Select appropriate nursing measures to promote client comfort, such as administering an analgesic.	Helps resolve problems that, if ignored, may interfere with eating.
Complete priority responsibilities for assigned clients.	Allows a period of uninterrupted feeding.
Provide oral hygiene and handwashing before serving the tray.	Controls the transmission of microorganisms; promotes appetite and aesthetics.
Prepare medications that must be given before or with meals, or delegate that responsibility.	Coordinates drug and nutritional therapy.
Clear clutter and soiled articles from the eating area.	Promotes orderliness and a sanitary environment.
IMPLEMENTATION	
Wash hands or perform hand antisepsis with an alcohol rub (see Chap. 10) before preparing food.	Prevents the transmission of microorganisms.
Obtain or clean special utensils or containers that have been adapted for use by a client with a physical disability, for example a fork to which a hand grip has been attached.	Promotes independence and self-reliance.
Raise the head of the bed to a sitting position, or assist the client to a chair (Fig. A).	Promotes safety by facilitating swallowing.

Feeding a client.

Suggested Action	Reason for Action
Check that you serve the correct diet and tray to the correct client.	Indicates responsibility and accountability for therapeutic management.
Cover the client's upper chest and lap with a napkin or towel.	Protects bedclothes and linen.
Sit beside or across from client.	Promotes socialization and communication.
Uncover the food, open cartons, and season food.	Increases gastric secretions and motility.
Encourage the client to assist to the limit of his or her abilities.	Maintains or supports independence and self-care.
Avoid rushing.	Communicates a relaxed atmosphere while eating.
Collaborate with the client on which foods he or she desires before loading a fork or spoon.	Accommodates individual preferences.

(continued)

Feeding a Client (continued)

IMPLEMENTATION (CONTINUED)

Action	Rationale
Provide manageable amounts of food with each bite.	Prevents choking or airway obstruction.
For a client with a stroke, direct the food toward the nonparalyzed side of the mouth.	Places food in an area where there is feeling and muscle control for chewing and swallowing.
Give the client time to chew thoroughly and swallow.	Chewing aids digestion by grinding the food and mixing it with saliva and enzymes.
Let the client indicate when he or she is ready for more food or a sip of beverage.	Promotes an independent locus of control.
Talk with the client about pleasant subjects.	Combines eating with socialization.
Record fluid intake if the client's intake is being measured.	Documents essential assessment data.
Remove the tray and make the client comfortable. It is best for clients to remain sitting or semisitting for at least 30 min after eating unless there is a medical reason to do otherwise.	A sitting position prevents the reflux of stomach contents into the esophagus and reduces the potential for aspiration.
Offer the client an opportunity for oral hygiene.	Removes sugar and starches that support microbial growth and tooth decay.
Estimate the amount of food that the client has eaten.	Provides data for determining current and future nutritional needs.

Evaluation

- Client eats approximately 75% of meal.
- Client maintains body weight.
- Client participates at maximum capacity.

Document

- Type of diet
- Percentage of food consumed
- Tolerance of food
- Client's ability to participate
- Problems encountered with chewing or swallowing
- Approaches taken to resolve problems

SAMPLE DOCUMENTATION

Date and Time Stated "I'm full" after consuming 75% of full liquid diet. Unable to hold spoon or glass but could direct straw into mouth. ——— SIGNATURE/TITLE

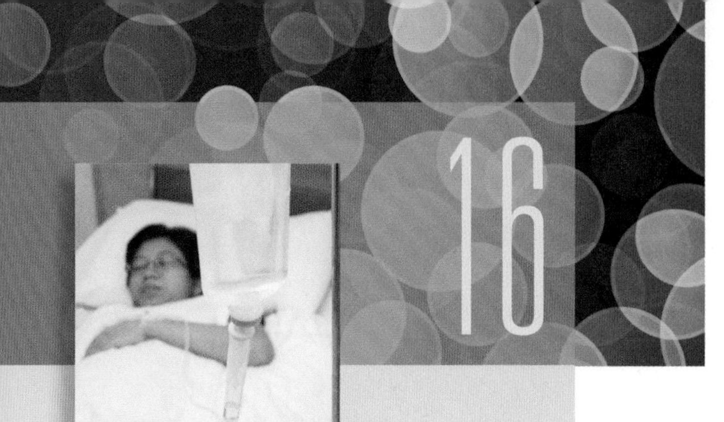

16 Fluid and Chemical Balance

Words To Know

active transport
air embolism
anions
blood substitutes
cations
circulatory overload
colloids
colloid solutions
colloidal osmotic pressure
crystalloid solutions
dehydration
drop factor
edema
electrochemical neutrality
electrolytes
emulsion
extracellular fluid
facilitated diffusion
filtration
fluid imbalance
hydrostatic pressure
hypertonic solution
hypervolemia
hypoalbuminemia
hypotonic solution
hypovolemia
infiltration
infusion pump
intake and output
intermittent venous access device
interstitial fluid
intracellular fluid
intravascular fluid
intravenous fluids
ions
isotonic solution
needleless systems
nonelectrolytes
osmosis
oxygen therapeutics
parenteral nutrition
passive diffusion
peripheral parenteral nutrition
phlebitis
ports

Learning Objectives

On completion of this chapter, the reader should be able to:

1. Name four components of body fluid.
2. List five physiologic transport mechanisms for distributing fluid and its constituents.
3. Name 10 assessments that provide data about a client's fluid status.
4. Describe three methods for maintaining or restoring fluid volume.
5. Describe four methods for reducing fluid volume.
6. List six reasons for administering intravenous (IV) fluids.
7. Differentiate between crystalloid and colloid solutions, and give examples of each.
8. Explain the terms isotonic, hypotonic, and hypertonic when used in reference to IV solutions.
9. List four factors that affect the choice of tubing used to administer IV solutions.
10. Name three techniques for infusing IV solutions.
11. Discuss at least five criteria for selecting a vein when administering IV fluid.
12. List seven complications associated with IV fluid administration.
13. Discuss two purposes for inserting an intermittent venous access device.
14. Identify three differences between administering blood and crystalloid solutions.
15. Name at least five types of transfusion reactions.
16. Explain the concept of parenteral nutrition.

Body fluid is a mixture of water, chemicals called electrolytes and nonelectrolytes, and blood cells. Water, the vehicle for transporting the chemicals, is the very essence of life. Because water is not stored in any great reserve, daily replacement is the key to maintaining survival. This chapter discusses the mechanisms for maintaining fluid balance and restoring fluid volume and the components in body fluid.

BODY FLUID

Water

Depending on age and gender, the human body comprises approximately 45% to 75% water. Body water normally is supplied and replenished from three sources: drinking liquids, consuming food, and metabolizing

Words To Know (continued)
pulmonary embolus
third-spacing
thrombus formation
total parenteral nutrition
venipuncture
volumetric controller

nutrients. Once the water is absorbed, it is distributed among various locations, called compartments, within the body.

Fluid Compartments

Body fluid is located in two general compartments. **Intracellular fluid** (fluid inside cells) represents the greatest proportion of water in the body. The remaining body fluid is **extracellular fluid** (fluid outside cells). Extracellular fluid is further subdivided into **interstitial fluid** (fluid in the tissue space between and around cells) and **intravascular fluid** (the watery plasma, or serum, portion of blood) (Fig. 16-1). The percentage of water in these compartments varies according to age and gender (Table 16-1).

Electrolytes

Electrolytes are chemical compounds, such as sodium and chloride, that possess an electrical charge when dissolved, absorbed, and distributed in body fluid. They are obtained from dietary sources of food and beverages, but may be provided through pharmaceutical supplements for clients who are not eating or cannot do so, or lose electrolytes because of an altered state of health. They are essential for maintaining cellular, tissue, and organ functions. For example, electrolytes affect fluid balance and complex chemical activities such as muscle contraction and the formation of enzymes, acids, and bases (see discussion of minerals in Chap. 15).

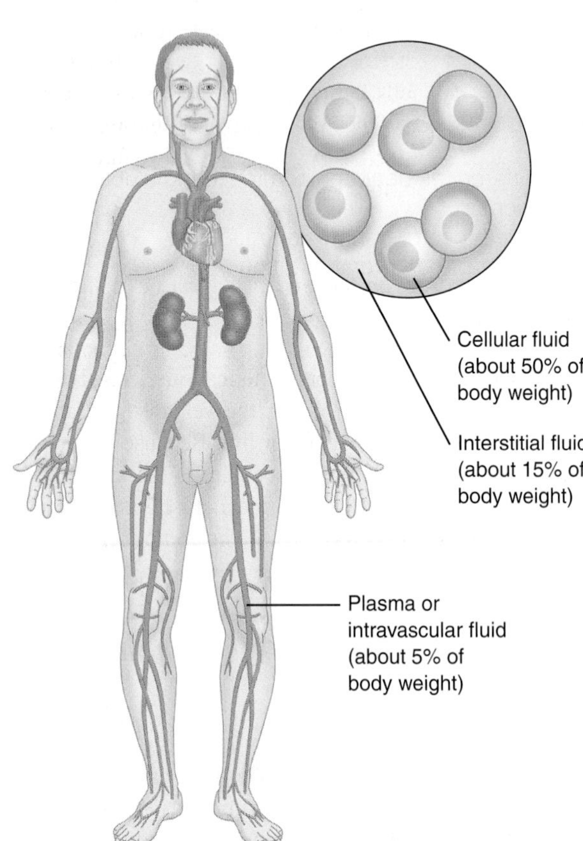

FIGURE 16-1 The average distribution of body fluid.

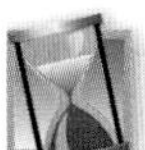

Gerontologic Considerations

- Mobility limitations, cognitive impairments, and an impaired ability to perform activities of daily living can lead to fluid and electrolyte deficits in older adults who cannot maintain adequate food and fluid intake independently.

Collectively, electrolytes are called **ions** (substances that carry either a positive or a negative electrical charge). **Cations** (electrolytes with a positive charge) and **anions** (electrolytes with a negative charge) are present in equal amounts overall, but their distribution varies in each body fluid compartment (Table 16-2). For example, more potassium ions are present inside the cells than outside.

Electrolytes are measured in the serum of blood specimens, and the amount is reported in milliequivalents (mEq). When one or more cations or anions become excessive or deficient, an electrolyte imbalance occurs. Significant imbalances can lead to dangerous physiologic problems. In many situations, electrolyte imbalances accompany changes in fluid volumes.

Nonelectrolytes

Nonelectrolytes are chemical compounds that remain bound together when dissolved in a solution and do not possess an

TABLE 16-1 Percentages of Body Fluid According to Age and Gender

FLUID COMPARTMENT	INFANTS (%)	ADULT MEN (%)	ADULT WOMEN (%)	ELDERLY (%)
Intravascular	4	4	5	5
Interstitial	25	11	10	15
Intracellular	48	45	35	25
Total	77	60	50	45

TABLE 16-2 Major Serum Electrolytes

ELECTROLYTE	CHEMICAL SYMBOL	CATION/ANION	NORMAL SERUM LEVEL (mEq/L)	PREDOMINANT COMPARTMENT
Sodium	Na	Cation	135–148	ECF
Potassium	K	Cation	3.5–5.0	ICF
Chloride	Cl	Anion	90–110	ECF
Phosphate	PO_4	Anion	1.7–2.6	ICF
Calcium	Ca	Cation	2.1–2.6	ICF
Magnesium	Mg	Cation	1.3–2.1	ICF
Bicarbonate	HCO_3	Anion	22–26	ICF

ECF, extracellular compartment; ICF, intracellular compartment.

electrical charge. The chemical end products of carbohydrates, proteins, and fat metabolism–namely glucose, amino acids, and fatty acids–provide a continuous supply of nonelectrolytes.

In the absence of metabolic disease, a stable amount of nonelectrolytes circulate in body fluid as long as a person consumes adequate nutrients. Deficiency states occur when body fluid is lost or when the ability to eat is compromised.

Blood

On average, blood consists of 3 L of plasma, or fluid, and 2 L of blood cells for a total circulating volume of 5 L. Blood cells include erythrocytes, or red blood cells; leukocytes, or white blood cells; and platelets, also known as thrombocytes. For every 500 red blood cells, there are approximately 30 platelets and 1 white blood cell (Fischbach & Dunning, 2008).

Any disorder that alters the volume of body fluid, whether it is fluid retention or loss, also affects the plasma volume of blood. Examples include chronic bleeding or hemorrhage, infection, chemicals or conditions that destroy the blood cells once they have been produced, and disorders that affect the bone marrow's production of blood cells. Deficits in either fluid or cell volume are treated by administering fluid, whole blood or packed cells, or individual blood components.

Fluid and Electrolyte Distribution Mechanisms

Although fluid compartments are identified separately, water and the substances dissolved therein continuously circulate throughout all areas of the body. Physiologic transport mechanisms such as osmosis, filtration, passive diffusion, facilitated diffusion, and active transport govern the movement and relocation of water and substances within body fluid (Fig. 16-2).

Osmosis

Osmosis helps regulate the distribution of water by controlling the movement of fluid from one location to another. Under the influence of osmosis, water moves through a semipermeable membrane like those surrounding body cells, capillary walls, and body organs and cavities, from an area where the fluid is more dilute to another area where the fluid is more concentrated (see Fig. 16-2A). Once the fluid is of equal concentration on both sides of the membrane, the transfer of fluid between compartments does not change appreciably except volume for volume.

The presence and quantity of colloids on either side of the semipermeable membrane influence osmosis. **Colloids** are undissolved protein substances such as albumin and blood cells within body fluids that do not readily pass through membranes. Their very presence produces **colloidal osmotic pressure** (the force for attracting water) that influences fluid volume in any given fluid location.

Filtration

Filtration regulates the movement of water and substances from a compartment where the pressure is higher to one where the pressure is lower. It is another mechanism that influences fluid distribution. The force of filtration is referred

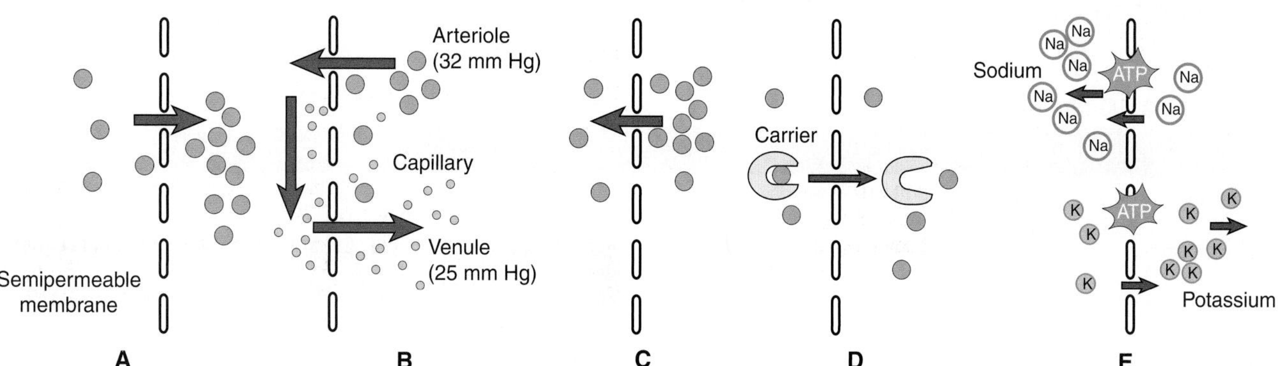

FIGURE 16-2 A. Osmosis. **B.** Filtration. **C.** Passive diffusion. **D.** Facilitated diffusion. **E.** Active transport. ATP, adenosine triphosphate.

to as **hydrostatic pressure** (the pressure exerted against a membrane). For example, because of contraction of the left ventricle, the fluid pressure is higher at the arterial end of a capillary than at the venous end. Consequently, fluid and dissolved substances are forced into the interstitial compartment at the capillary's arterial end. Water is then reabsorbed from the interstitial fluid in comparable amounts at the venous end of the capillary because of colloidal osmotic pressure (see Fig. 16-2B). Filtration also governs how the kidney excretes fluid and wastes and then selectively reabsorbs water and substances that need to be conserved.

Passive Diffusion

Passive diffusion is the physiologic process in which dissolved substances, such as electrolytes and gases, move from an area of higher concentration to an area of lower concentration through a semipermeable membrane (see Fig. 16-2C). It occurs without an expenditure of energy—hence the word *passive.* Passive diffusion facilitates **electrochemical neutrality** (an identical balance of cations with anions) in any given fluid compartment. Like osmosis, passive diffusion remains fairly static once equilibrium is achieved.

Facilitated Diffusion

Facilitated diffusion is the process in which certain dissolved substances require the assistance of a carrier molecule to pass from one side of a semipermeable membrane to the other (see Fig. 16-2D). It also regulates chemical balance. Facilitated diffusion distributes substances from an area of higher concentration to one that is lower. Glucose is an example of a substance distributed by facilitated diffusion. Insulin is the carrier substance for glucose.

Active Transport

Active transport, a process of chemical distribution that requires an energy source, involves a substance called *adenosine triphosphate* (ATP) (see Fig. 16-2E). ATP provides energy to drive dissolved chemicals against the concentration gradient. In other words, it allows chemical distribution from an area of low concentration to one that is higher—the opposite of passive diffusion.

An example of active transport is the *sodium–potassium pump system* on cellular membranes, which regulates the movement of potassium from lower concentrations in the extracellular fluid into cells where it is more highly concentrated. It also moves sodium, which has a lower concentration within the cells, to extracellular fluid where it is more abundant.

Fluid Regulation

In healthy adults, fluid intake generally averages approximately 2,500 mL/day, but it can range from 1,800 to 3,000 mL/day with a similar volume of fluid loss (Table 16-3). Normal mechanisms for fluid loss are urination, bowel elimination, perspiration, and breathing. Losses from the skin in areas other than where sweat glands are located and from the vapor in exhaled air are referred to as *insensible losses* because they are, for practical purposes, unnoticeable and unmeasurable.

Under normal conditions, several mechanisms maintain a match between fluid intake and output. For example, as body fluid becomes concentrated, the brain triggers the sensation of thirst, which then stimulates the person to drink. As fluid volume expands, the kidneys excrete a proportionate volume of water to maintain or restore proper balance.

There are circumstances, however, in which oral intake or fluid losses are altered. Therefore, nurses assess clients for signs of fluid deficit or excess, particularly in those prone to fluid imbalances (Box 16-1).

FLUID VOLUME ASSESSMENT

Nurses assess fluid status using a combination of a physical assessment (Table 16-4) and a measurement of intake and output volumes.

Intake and output (I&O) is one tool to assess fluid status by keeping a record of a client's fluid intake and fluid loss over a 24-hour period. Agencies often specify the types of clients that are placed automatically on I&O; generally, they include the following:

- Clients who have undergone surgery until they are eating, drinking, and voiding in sufficient quantities
- Clients receiving IV fluids
- Clients receiving tube feedings
- Clients with some type of wound drainage or suction equipment

TABLE 16-3 Daily Fluid Intake and Losses

SOURCES OF FLUID		MECHANISMS OF FLUID LOSS	
Oral liquids	1,200–1,500 mL/day	Urine	1,200–1,700 mL/day
Food	700–1,000 mL/day	Feces	100–250 mL/day
Metabolism	200–400 mL/day	Perspiration	100–150 mL/day
		Insensible losses:	
		Skin	350–400 mL/day
		Lungs	350–400 mL/day
Total	2,100–2,900 mL/day	**Total**	2,100–2,900 mL/day
Average intake	2,500 mL/day	**Average loss**	2,500 mL/day

BOX 16-1 Conditions That Predispose to Fluid Imbalances

Fluid Deficit
- Starvation
- Impaired swallowing
- Vomiting
- Gastric suction
- Diarrhea
- Laxative abuse
- Potent diuretics
- Hemorrhage
- Major burns
- Draining wounds
- Fever and sweating
- Exercise and sweating
- Environmental heat and humidity

Fluid Excess
- Kidney failure
- Heart failure
- Rapid administration of IV fluid or blood
- Administration of albumin
- Corticosteroid drug therapy
- Excessive intake of sodium
- Pregnancy
- Premenstrual fluid retention

- Clients with urinary catheters until it can be determined that output is adequate or they are voiding well after removal of the catheter
- Clients undergoing diuretic drug therapy

In addition, many agencies allow nurses to independently order an I&O assessment for clients who have or are at risk for a fluid imbalance problem. The nurse discontinues the nursing order when the assessment is no longer indicated but consults with the physician if it has been medically ordered.

TABLE 16-4 Signs of Fluid Imbalance

ASSESSMENT	FLUID DEFICIT	FLUID EXCESS
Weight	Weight loss ≥2 lb/24 hr	Weight gain ≥2 lb/24 hr
Blood pressure	Low	High
Temperature	Elevated	Normal
Pulse	Rapid, weak, thready	Full, bounding
Respirations	Rapid, shallow	Moist, labored
Urine	Scant, dark yellow	Light yellow
Stool	Dry, small volume	Bulky
Skin	Warm, flushed, dry Poor skin turgor	Cool, pale, moist Pitting edema
Mucous membranes	Dry, sticky	Moist
Eyes	Sunken	Swollen
Lungs	Clear	Crackles, gurgles
Breathing	Effortless	Dyspnea, orthopnea
Energy	Weak	Fatigues easily
Jugular neck veins	Flat	Distended
Cognition	Reduced	Reduced
Consciousness	Sleepy	Anxious

Each agency has a specific I&O form kept at the bedside so that nurses can conveniently record the type of fluid and amounts that are consumed and lost throughout the day (Fig. 16-3). The nurse subtotals the amounts at the end of each shift or more frequently in critical care areas. He or she documents the grand total in a designated area in the medical record, for example, on the graphics sheet with other vital sign information.

Fluid Intake

Fluid intake is the sum of all fluid volume that a client consumes or is instilled into the client's body, including the following:

- All the liquids a client drinks
- The liquid equivalent of melted ice chips, which is half of the frozen volume
- Foods that are liquid by the time they are swallowed, such as gelatin, ice cream, and thin cooked cereal
- Fluid infusions such as IV solutions
- Fluid instillations such as those administered through feeding tubes or tube irrigations

Fluid volumes are recorded in milliliters (mL). The approximate equivalent for 1 oz is 30 mL, a teaspoon is 5 mL, and a tablespoon is 15 mL. Packaged beverage containers such as milk cartons usually indicate the specific fluid volume on the label. Hospitals and nursing homes commonly identify the volume equivalents contained in the cups, glasses, and bowls used to serve food and beverages from the dietary department (Box 16-2). If an equivalency chart is not available, the nurse uses a calibrated container (Fig. 16-4) to measure specific amounts; estimated volumes are considered inaccurate.

BOX 16-2 Volume Equivalents for Common Containers

CONTAINER	VOLUME (mL)
Teaspoon	5
Tablespoon	15
Juice glass	120
Drinking glass	240
Coffee cup	210
Milk carton	240
Water pitcher	900
Paper cup	180
Soup bowl	200
Cereal bowl	120
Ice cream cup	120
Gelatin dish	90

24 HOUR INTAKE/OUTPUT RECORD

DATE 2-17	WEIGHT 137#	TIME 0700	TYPE OF WEIGHT ☒ STANDING ☐ CHAIR ☐ BED
CVP READING: TIME READING	TIME READING	TIME READING	

INTAKE 7-3 SHIFT

Time	Oral	IV	Piggyback	Blood	Tube/Feed
0730	100	600 ↓			
0900			50		
1130	240				
1300			50		
8 HR TOTAL	340	600	100		
				8° GRAND TOTAL	1040

OUTPUT 7-3 SHIFT

Time	Irrig.	Urine	NG	Emesis	Other	Tube	Tube	BM
0700		250						
0800				100				
1200		300						
1400		400						
		950		100				
							8° GRAND TOTAL	1050

INTAKE 3-11 SHIFT

Time	Oral	IV	Piggyback	Blood	Tube/Feed
1600	30				
1700		600 ↓	50		
1730	30				
2000	100				
8 HR TOTAL	160	600	50		
				8° GRAND TOTAL	810

OUTPUT 3-11 SHIFT

Time	Irrig.	Urine	NG	Emesis	Other	Tube	Tube	BM
1530				50				
1800		200						
2200		300						
		500		50				
							8° GRAND TOTAL	550

INTAKE 11-7 SHIFT

Time	Oral	IV	Piggyback	Blood	Tube/Feed
0030	30	600 ↓			
8 HR TOTAL	30	600			
				8° GRAND TOTAL	630
				24° GRAND TOTAL	2480

OUTPUT 11-7 SHIFT

Time	Irrig.	Urine	NG	Emesis	Other	Tube	Tube	BM
0100		300						
0400		200						
0600		100						
		600						
							8° GRAND TOTAL	600
							24° GRAND TOTAL	2200

FORM 96 (9/92) CIRRUS 3025

24 HOUR INTAKE / OUTPUT RECORD

FIGURE 16-3 Intake and output volumes are recorded throughout a 24-hour period and subtotaled at the end of each 8-hour shift.

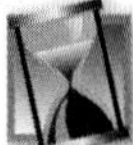

Gerontologic Considerations

■ Dehydration in older adults may be a consequence or indicator of abuse or neglect.

■ Older adults may need to be encouraged to drink fluids, even at times when they do not feel thirsty, because age-related changes may diminish the sensation of thirst.

■ Older adults may consume more fluid if the nurse offers it, rather than if the nurse asks the older adult if he or she would like a drink. Offering a small amount of liquid hourly throughout the day will assist in keeping oral mucosa moist and providing hydration needs. Types of fluid and temperature preferences (which may vary at different times of the day) should be determined.

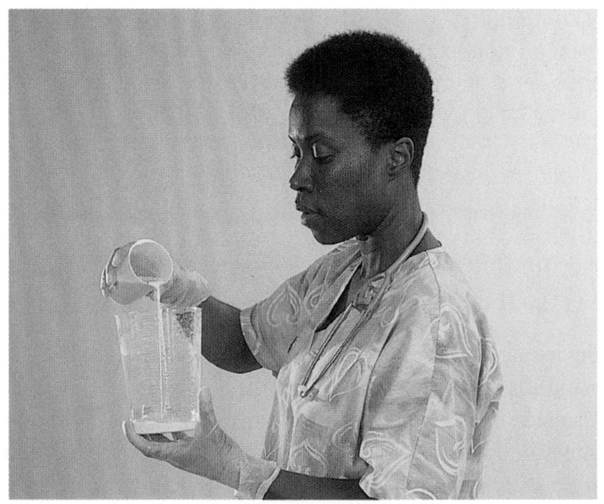

FIGURE 16-4 Calibrated containers used to measure liquid volumes. (Photo by B. Proud.)

- To maintain adequate consumption of nutrients, it is best to offer fluids to older adults at times other than meals. Distending the stomach with liquids creates a sensation of satiety (fullness) and reduces the consumption of food.
- When older adults must fast before certain procedures, emphasize the need to increase oral fluid intake in the hours before beginning fluid restrictions to prevent dehydration.
- Encourage older adults to drink noncaffeinated beverages because of the diuretic effect of caffeine or to replace the volume of caffeinated beverages by consuming the same volume of noncaffeinated fluids per day.

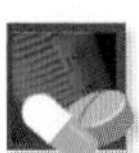

Pharmacologic Considerations

- Diuretic medications, often prescribed for adults with cardiovascular disorders, increase the risk for fluid and electrolyte imbalances. Laxatives, enemas, antihistamines, or tricyclic antidepressants may also alter fluid and electrolyte balance.

Stop, Think, and Respond Box 16-1

Use Box 16-2 to calculate the volume of fluid intake for the following: a glass of orange juice, a half-pint carton of milk, a bowl of tomato soup, a dish of lime gelatin, a cup of coffee, a 100-mL infusion of IV antibiotic solution.

Fluid Output

Fluid output is the sum of liquid eliminated from the body, including the following:

- Urine
- Emesis (vomitus)
- Blood loss
- Diarrhea
- Wound or tube drainage
- Aspirated irrigations

In cases in which an accurate assessment is critical to a client's treatment, the nurse weighs wet linens, pads, diapers, or dressings and subtracts the weight of a similar dry item. An estimate of fluid loss is based on the equivalent: 1 lb (0.47 kg) = 1 pint (475 mL).

Client cooperation is needed for accurate I&O records. Therefore, the nurse informs clients whose I&O volumes are being recorded about the purpose and goals for fluid replacement or restrictions and the ways they can assist in the procedure (Client and Family Teaching 16-1). Suggested actions for maintaining an I&O record are provided in Skill 16-1.

COMMON FLUID IMBALANCES

Fluid imbalance is a general term describing any of several conditions in which the water content of the body is not in the proper volume or location within the body. It can be life-threatening. Common fluid imbalances include hypovolemia, hypervolemia, and third-spacing.

Hypovolemia

Hypovolemia refers to a low volume of extracellular fluid. If untreated, it may result in **dehydration** (a fluid deficit in both extracellular and intracellular compartments). Mild dehydration is present when there is a 3% to 5% loss of body weight; moderate dehydration is associated with a 6% to 10% loss of body weight; and severe dehydration, a life-threatening

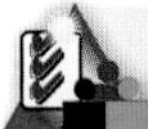

Client and Family Teaching 16-1
Recording Intake and Output

The nurse teaches the client or family as follows:

- Write down the amount or notify the nurse whenever oral fluid is consumed.
- Use a common household measurement, such as 1 glass or cup, to describe the volume consumed, or refer to an equivalency chart.
- Do not let a staff person remove a dietary tray until the fluid amounts have been recorded.
- Do not empty a urinal or urinate directly into the toilet bowl.
- Make sure that a measuring device is in the toilet bowl if the bathroom is used for voiding (Fig. 16-5).
- If a urinal needs to be emptied, call the nurse or empty its contents into a calibrated container.
- Use a container such as a bedpan or bedside commode if diarrhea occurs. Notify the nurse to measure the contents before it is emptied.
- If vomiting occurs, use an emesis basin rather than the toilet.

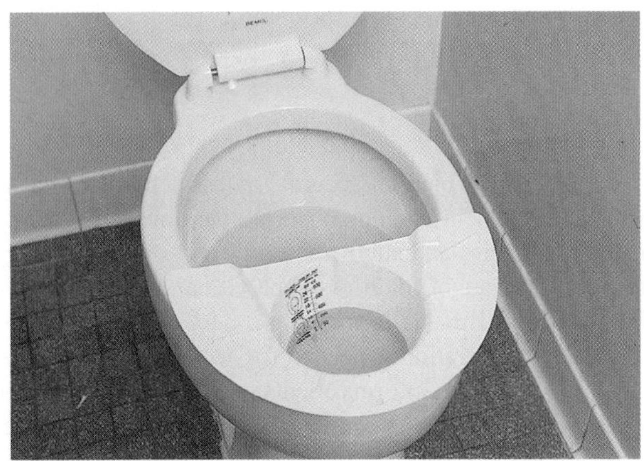

FIGURE 16-5 Urine is collected in a calibrated container sometimes referred to as a "hat". (Photo by B. Proud.)

emergency, occurs with a loss of more than 9% to 15% of body weight. In addition to weight loss, dehydration is evidenced by decreased skin turgor.

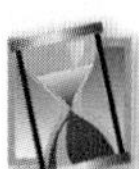

Gerontologic Considerations

■ Skin elasticity diminishes with aging as subcutaneous fat deposits decrease. Therefore, an assessment of skin turgor over the sternum is essential. Additional indicators of dehydration in older adults include mental status changes; increases in pulse and respiration rates; a decrease in blood pressure; dark, concentrated urine with a high specific gravity; dry mucous membranes; warm skin; furrowed tongue; low urine output; hardened stools; and elevated hematocrit, hemoglobin, serum sodium, and blood urea nitrogen.

■ Older adults may restrict their fluid intake under the mistaken notion that this will reduce urinary incontinence. This practice actually contributes to the problem by increasing bladder irritability and increases the risks for urinary tract infection, postural hypotension, falls, and injuries. An assessment of fluid and electrolyte imbalances is important for any older adult who has a change in mental status.

Causes of fluid volume deficits include the following:

- Inadequate fluid intake
- Fluid loss in excess of fluid intake
- Translocation of large volumes of intravascular fluid to the interstitial compartment or to areas with only potential spaces such as the peritoneal cavity, pericardium, and pleural space

Fluid balance is restored by treating the cause of hypovolemia, increasing oral intake, administering IV fluid replacements, controlling fluid losses, or a combination of these measures (see Nursing Guidelines 16-1).

Hypervolemia

Hypervolemia means a higher-than-normal volume of water in the intravascular fluid compartment and is another example of a fluid imbalance. **Edema** develops when excess fluid is distributed to the interstitial space (Fig. 16-6). When fluid accumulates in dependent areas of the body (those influenced by gravity), the tissue pits (forms indentations) when compressed (see Chap. 13). Edema does not usually occur unless there is a 3 L excess in body fluid. Hypervolemia can lead to **circulatory overload** (severely compromised heart function) if it remains unresolved.

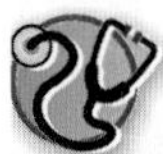

NURSING GUIDELINES 16-1

Increasing Oral Intake

- Explain to the client the reasons for increasing consumption of oral fluids. *Knowledge facilitates client cooperation.*
- Compile a list of the client's preferences for beverages. *Involving the client facilitates individualized collaboration with the dietary department.*
- Obtain a variety of beverages on the client's list. *Catering to client preferences promotes compliance.*
- Develop a schedule for providing small portions of the total fluid volume over a 24-hour period. *Scheduling ensures that the final goal is reached by meeting short-term goals.*
- Plan to provide the bulk of the projected fluid intake at times when the client is awake. *Providing a higher proportion of fluid during waking hours avoids disturbing sleep.*
- Offer verbal recognition and frequent feedback, or design a method for demonstrating the client's progress; for example, a bar graph or pie chart. *Positive reinforcement encourages compliance and maintains goal-directed efforts.*
- Keep fluids handy at the bedside and place them in containers the client can handle. *Availability and convenience promote compliance.*
- Vary the types of fluid, serving glass, or container frequently. *Variety reduces boredom and maintains interest in working toward the goal.*
- Serve fluids in small containers and in small amounts. *Small portions avoid overwhelming the client.*
- Ensure that fluids are at an appropriate temperature. *Palatability promotes pleasure and enjoyment.*
- Include gelatin, popsicles, ice cream, and sherbet as alternatives to liquid beverages (if allowed). *Varying the liquid's consistency and techniques for consumption offers an alternative to items that are sipped from a glass.*

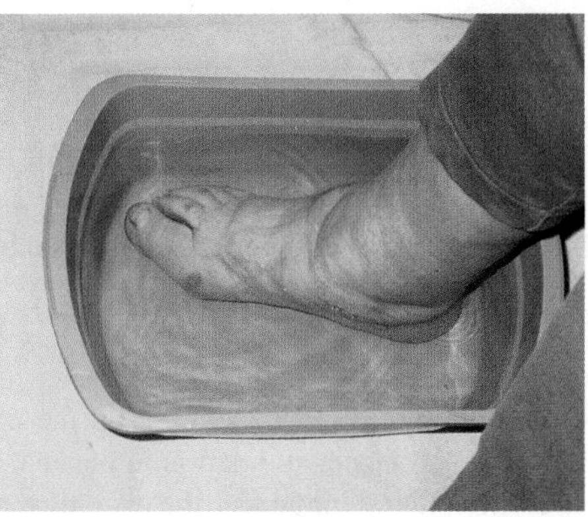

FIGURE 16-6 Foot care is very important for the client with edema. The edema and reddened areas can easily break down.

Control of edema is an important nursing priority. Fluid balance is restored by the following:

- Treating the disorder contributing to the increased fluid volume
- Restricting or limiting oral fluids
- Reducing salt consumption (Box 16-3)
- Discontinuing IV fluid infusions or reducing the infusing volume
- Administering drugs that promote urine elimination
- Using a combination of these interventions

See Nursing Guidelines 16-2.

Third-Spacing

Third-spacing is the movement of intravascular fluid to nonvascular fluid compartments, where it becomes trapped and useless. It generally is manifested by tissue swelling or fluid that accumulates in a body cavity such as the peritoneum (Fig. 16-7). Third-spacing is associated commonly with disorders in which albumin levels are low. Causes of **hypoalbuminemia** (a deficit of albumin in the blood) include liver disease, chronic kidney disease, and disorders in which capillary and cellular permeability are altered such as burns and severe allergic reactions.

Depletion of fluid in the intravascular space may lead to hypotension and shock; thus, fluid therapy becomes critical. The priority is to restore the circulatory volume by providing IV fluids, sometimes in large volumes at rapid rates. Blood transfusions or the administration of albumin by IV infusion also are used to restore colloidal osmotic pressure and to pull the trapped fluid back into the intravascular space. When this occurs, clients who were previously hypovolemic can suddenly become hypervolemic. The nurse closely monitors clients who receive albumin replacement for signs of circulatory overload.

BOX 16-3 Foods High in Salt (Sodium)

- Processed meats such as frankfurters and cold cuts
- Smoked fish
- Frozen egg substitutes
- Peanut butter
- Dairy products, especially hard cheese
- Powdered cocoa or hot chocolate mixes
- Canned vegetables, especially sauerkraut
- Pickles
- Tomato and tomato-vegetable juice
- Canned soup and bouillon
- Boxed casserole mixes
- Baking mixes
- Salted snack foods
- Seasonings such as ketchup, gravy mixes, soy sauce, monosodium glutamate, pickle relish, tartar sauce

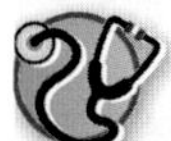

NURSING GUIDELINES 16-2

Restricting Oral Fluids

- Explain the purpose for the restrictions. *Knowledge facilitates client cooperation.*
- Identify the total amount of fluid the client may consume, using measurements with which the client is familiar. *An explanation helps the client to understand the extent of the restrictions.*
- Work out a plan for distributing the permitted volume over a 24-hour period with the client. *Including the client in planning promotes cooperation.*
- Ration the fluid so that the client can consume beverages between meals as well as at mealtimes. *Distributing opportunities to drink fluid helps minimize thirst.*
- Avoid sweet drinks and foods that are dry or salty. *This reduces thirst and the desire for fluid.*
- Serve liquids at their proper temperature. *This demonstrates concern for the client's pleasure and enjoyment.*
- Offer ice chips as an occasional substitute for liquids. *Ice chips appear to contain more liquid than they actually do, and holding them within the mouth prolongs the time over which the fluid is consumed.*
- Provide water or other fluid in a plastic squeeze bottle or spray atomizer. *These devices provide only a small volume of fluid.*
- Help the client with frequent oral hygiene. *Oral hygiene relieves thirst, moistens oral mucous membranes, and prevents drying and chapping of lips.*
- Allow the client to rinse his or her mouth with water but not swallow it. *Rinsing reduces thirst and keeps the mouth moist.*

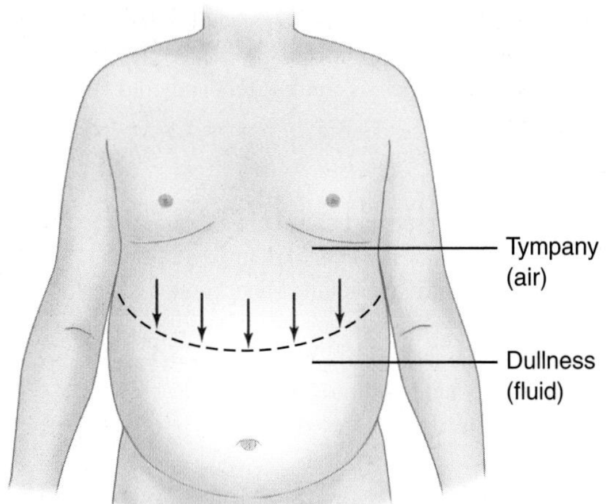

FIGURE 16-7 Fluid accumulation within the peritoneal cavity. Dullness on percussion indicates fluid, whereas tympany indicates air.

INTRAVENOUS FLUID ADMINISTRATION

Policies and practices vary concerning how much responsibility practical/vocational nurses assume with IV fluid therapy. The discussion that follows is provided to meet the needs of those nurses who have been trained and have demonstrated competencies for administering IV fluids.

Intravenous fluids are solutions infused into a client's vein to:

- Maintain or restore fluid balance when oral replacement is inadequate or impossible
- Maintain or replace electrolytes
- Administer water-soluble vitamins
- Provide a source of calories
- Administer drugs (see Chap. 35)
- Replace blood and blood products

Types of Solutions

There are two types of IV solutions: crystalloid and colloid. **Crystalloid solutions** are made of water and other uniformly dissolved crystals such as salt and sugar. **Colloid solutions** are made of water and molecules of suspended substances such as blood cells and blood products (such as albumin).

Crystalloid Solutions

Crystalloid solutions are classified as isotonic, hypotonic, and hypertonic (Table 16-5), depending on the concentration of dissolved substances in relation to plasma. The concentration of the solution influences the osmotic distribution of body fluid (Fig. 16-8).

Isotonic Solutions. An **isotonic solution** contains the same concentration of dissolved substances normally found in plasma. It generally is administered to maintain fluid balance in clients who may not be able to eat or drink for a short period. Because of its equal concentration, an isotonic solution does not cause any appreciable redistribution of body fluid.

Hypotonic Solutions. A **hypotonic solution** contains fewer dissolved substances than normally found in plasma. It is administered to clients with fluid losses in excess of fluid intake, such as those who have diarrhea or vomiting. Because hypotonic solutions are dilute, the water in the solution passes through the semipermeable membrane of blood cells, causing them to swell. This temporarily increases blood pressure as it expands the circulating volume. The water also passes through capillary walls and becomes distributed within other body cells and the interstitial spaces. Hypotonic solutions, therefore, are an effective way to rehydrate clients experiencing fluid deficits.

TABLE 16-5 Types of Crystalloid Intravenous Solutions

SOLUTION	COMPONENTS	SPECIAL COMMENTS
Isotonic Solutions		
0.9% saline, also called normal saline	0.9 g of sodium chloride/100 mL of water	Amounts of sodium and chloride are physiologically equal to those found in plasma.
5% dextrose and water, also called D_5W	5 g of dextrose (glucose/sugar)/100 mL of water	Isotonic when infused but the glucose metabolizes quickly, leaving a solution of dilute water.
Ringer's solution or lactated Ringer's	Water and a mixture of sodium, chloride, calcium, potassium, bicarbonate, and in some cases lactate	Electrolyte replacement in amounts similar to those found in plasma. The lactate, when present, helps maintain acid–base balance.
Hypotonic Solutions		
0.45% sodium chloride, also called half-strength saline	0.45 g of sodium chloride/100 mL of water	Smaller ratio of sodium and chloride than found in plasma, causing it to be less concentrated in comparison.
5% dextrose in 0.45% saline	5 g of dextrose and 0.45 sodium chloride/100 mL of water	A quick source of energy from sugar, leaving a hypotonic salt solution.
Hypertonic Solutions		
10% dextrose in water, also called $D_{10}W$	10 g of dextrose/100 mL of water	Twice the concentration of glucose as in plasma.
3% saline	3 g of sodium chloride/100 mL of water	Dehydration of cells and tissues from the high concentration of salt in the plasma.
20% dextrose in water	20 g of dextrose/100 mL water	Rapid increase in the concentration of sugar in the blood, causing a fluid shift to the intravascular compartment.

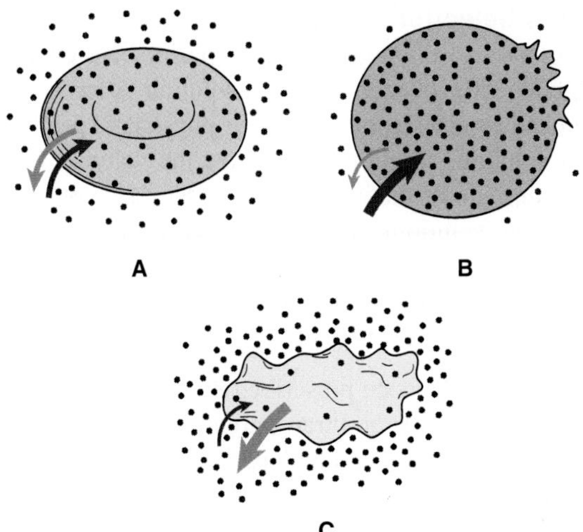

FIGURE 16-8 A. Isotonic solutions. **B.** Hypotonic solutions. **C.** Hypertonic solutions.

Hypertonic Solutions. A **hypertonic solution** is more concentrated than body fluid and draws cellular and interstitial water into the intravascular compartment. This causes cells and tissue spaces to shrink. Hypertonic solutions are used infrequently except in extreme cases when it is necessary to reduce cerebral edema or to expand the circulatory volume rapidly.

Stop, Think, and Respond Box 16-2

Identify the net effect when the following IV solutions are infused: 0.45% sodium chloride, Ringer's solution, and 50% glucose.

Colloid Solutions

Colloid solutions are used to replace circulating blood volume because the suspended molecules pull fluid from other compartments. Examples are blood, blood products, and solutions known as plasma expanders.

Blood. Whole blood and packed cells are probably the most common colloid solutions. One unit of whole blood contains approximately 475 mL of blood cells and plasma plus 60 to 70 mL of preservative and anticoagulant (Smeltzer, et al., 2008). Packed cells have most of the plasma removed and are preferred for clients who need cellular replacement but do not need, or may be harmed by, the administration of additional fluid.

Most blood given to clients comes from public donors. In some cases, for example, when a person anticipates the potential need for blood in the near future or when procedures are used to reclaim blood from wound drainage, the client's own blood may be reinfused (see Chap. 27).

Blood Products. Several blood products are available for clients who need specific substances but do not need all the fluid or cellular components in whole blood (Table 16-6).

Blood Substitutes. **Blood substitutes** are fluids that when transfused carry and distribute oxygen to cells, tissues, and organs. Many practitioners feel blood substitutes should be more accurately called **oxygen therapeutics** because they do not replace all the functions of human blood.

Finding a safe blood substitute could have many advantages: (1) it would be an acceptable alternative for people, such as Jehovah's Witnesses, who object to receiving blood transfusions based on their religious beliefs, (2) the risks for blood-borne diseases, such as hepatitis and AIDS, and transfusion reactions from transfused human blood could be eliminated, (3) there would be a greater potential for saving the lives of military casualties in primitive locations, and (4) it could be used in disasters and major trauma cases while awaiting transfusable human blood.

Currently, oxygen therapeutics fall into two categories: *perfluorocarbons* (PFCs) and *hemoglobin-based oxygen carriers* (HBOCs). PFCs are solutions containing fluorine and carbon that have the potential to carry 50 times more oxygen than plasma (Whitehead, 2010). HBOCs are derived from three sources: hemoglobin (1) harvested from outdated human blood or (2) bovine (cattle) blood, and (3) cultured from bacteria in which the gene for human hemoglobin is inserted (recombinant technology), much like human insulin is produced.

Because PFCs have a smaller molecular size than red blood cells, it is possible that they could deliver oxygen-carrying molecules to blood vessels that have been narrowed as a result of blood clots, thus relieving impaired circulation after a stroke or heart attack. That same property could be

TABLE 16-6 Types of Blood Products

BLOOD PRODUCT	DESCRIPTION	PURPOSE FOR ADMINISTRATION
Platelets	Disk-shaped cellular fragments that promote coagulation of blood	Restores or improves the ability to control bleeding
Granulocytes	Types of white blood cells	Improves the ability to overcome infection
Plasma	Serum minus blood cells	Replaces clotting factors or increases intravascular fluid volume by increasing colloidal osmotic pressure
Albumin	Plasma protein	Pulls third-spaced fluid by increasing colloidal osmotic pressure
Cryoprecipitate	Mixture of clotting factors	Treats blood clotting disorders such as hemophilia

used to treat clients during a sickle cell crisis; their pain could be relieved by oxygenating tissues in which sickled red blood cells have obstructed blood flow. In addition, PFCs could prolong the preservation of organs for transplantation and could improve the oxygenation of cancer cells, making them more vulnerable to standard treatments.

PFCs are now in the second generation of development; use of first-generation PFCs has been placed on hold or abandoned because of safety issues. Oxycyte, a second-generation PFC is undergoing clinical trials. There are five HBOCs in clinical trials, most outside the United States. PolyHeme, an HBOC made from outdated human blood, is being tested in the United States. All of the oxygen therapeutics, and particularly the HBOCs, have been associated with adverse effects. Many believe that the best benefit to risk is to use them when blood is needed, but none is available (Moore, et al., 2009).

Plasma Expanders. Various nonblood solutions are used to pull fluid into the vascular space. Two examples are dextran 40 (Rheomacrodex) and hetastarch (Hespan). These two substances are polysaccharides—large, insoluble complex carbohydrate molecules. When mixed with water, they form colloidal solutions. Because the suspended particles cannot move through semipermeable membranes when given intravenously, they attract water from other fluid compartments. The desired outcome is to increase the blood volume and raise the blood pressure. Consequently, plasma expanders are used as economical and virus-free substitutes for blood and blood products when treating hypovolemic shock.

Preparation for Administration

Regardless of the prescribed solution, the nurse prepares the solution for administration, performs a venipuncture, regulates the rate of administration, monitors the infusion, and discontinues the administration when fluid balance is restored.

Solution Selection

IV solutions are commonly stored in plastic bags containing 1,000, 500, 250, 100, and 50 mL of solution. A few solutions are stocked in glass containers. The physician specifies the type of solution, additional additives, the volume (in mL), and the duration of the infusion. To reduce the potential for infection, IV solutions are replaced every 24 hours even if the total volume has not been completely instilled.

Before preparing the solution, the nurse inspects the container and determines that:

- The solution is the one prescribed by the physician.
- The solution is clear and transparent.
- The expiration date has not elapsed.
- No leaks are apparent.
- A separate label is attached, identifying the type and amount of other drugs added to the commercial solution.

Tubing Selection

All IV tubing consists of a spike for accessing the solution, a drip chamber for holding a small amount of fluid, a length of plastic tubing with one or more ports for adding IV medications (see Chap. 35), and a roller or slide clamp to regulate the rate of infusion (Fig. 16-9). The nurse then selects from several options:

- Primary (long) or secondary (short) tubing
- Vented or unvented tubing
- Microdrip (small drops) or macrodrip (large drops) chamber
- Unfiltered or filtered tubing
- Needle or needleless access ports

Primary Versus Secondary Tubing. Primary tubing is approximately 110 in. (2.8 m) and secondary tubing is 37 in. (94 cm) long. These measurements vary among manufacturers. Primary tubing is used when the tubing must span the distance from a solution that hangs several feet above the infusion site. Secondary tubing, which is shorter, is used to

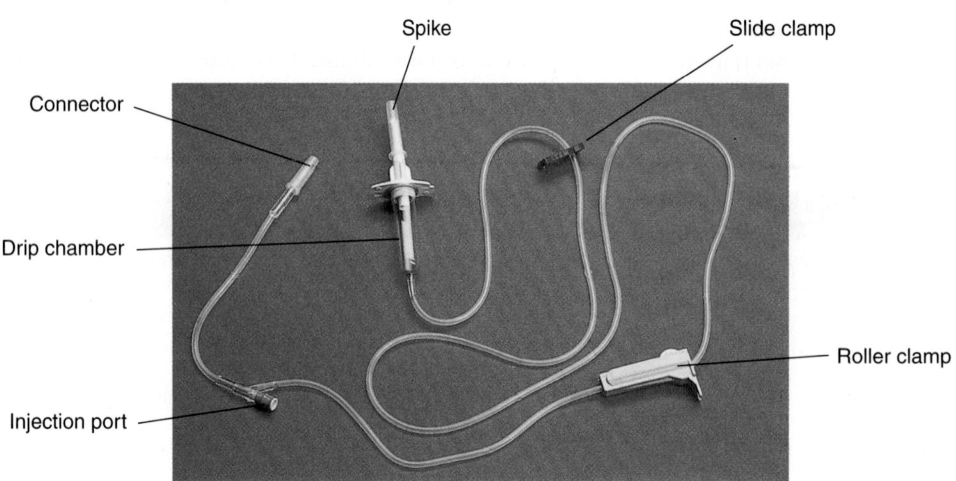

FIGURE 16-9 Basic intravenous tubing. (Courtesy of Abbott Laboratories, North Chicago, IL.)

administer smaller volumes of solution into a port within the primary tubing.

Vented Versus Unvented Tubing. Vented tubing draws air into the container, whereas unvented tubing does not (Fig. 16-10). The choice depends on the type of container in which the solution is packaged. Vented tubing is necessary for administering solutions packaged in rigid glass containers; if unvented tubing is inserted into a glass bottle, the solution will not leave the container. Plastic bags of IV solutions do not need vented tubing because the container collapses as the fluid infuses.

Drop Size. Drop size refers to the size of the opening through which the fluid is delivered into the tubing. The nurse determines whether it is more appropriate to use macrodrip tubing, which produces large drops, or microdrip tubing, which produces very small drops. When a solution infuses at a fast rate, such as 125 mL/hr, it is generally easier to count fewer, larger drops than many smaller ones. When the solution must infuse very precisely or at a slow rate, smaller drops are preferred.

Microdrip tubing, regardless of the manufacturer, delivers a standard volume of 60 drops/mL. Macrodrip tubing manufacturers, however, have not been consistent in designing the size of the opening. Therefore, the nurse must read the package label to determine the **drop factor** (number of drops/mL). Some common drop factors are 10, 15, and 20 drops/mL. The drop factor is important in calculating the infusion rate when it is instilled by gravity (eg, without an electronic infuser) and is discussed later in this chapter.

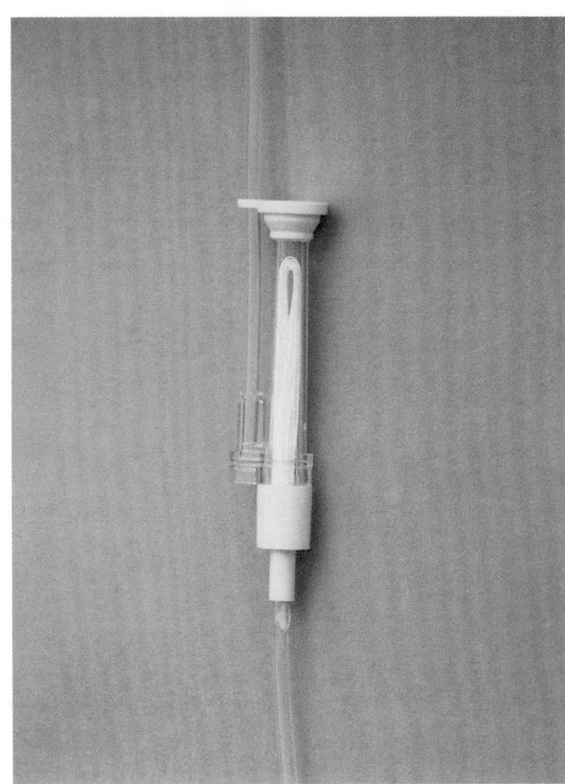

FIGURE 16-11 An in-line filter. (Photo by K. Timby.)

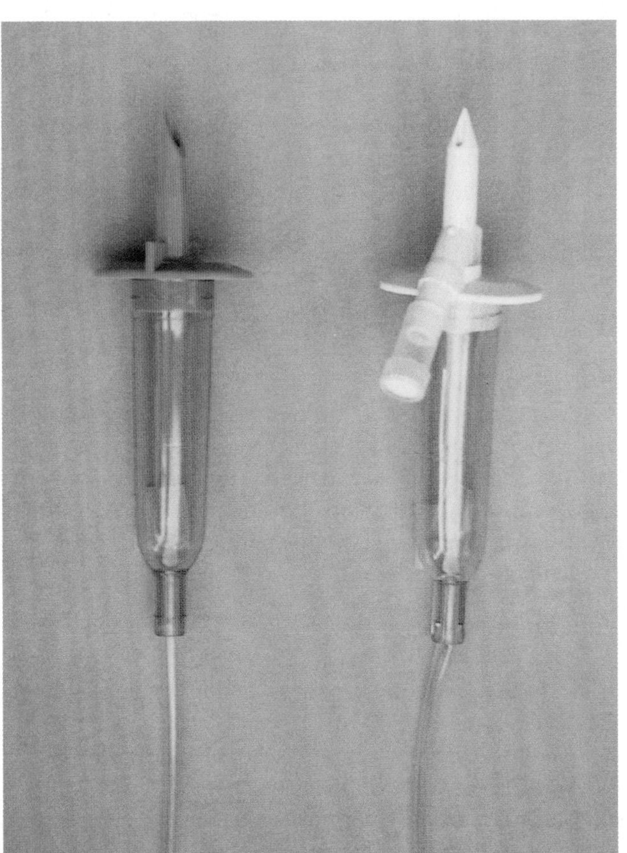

FIGURE 16-10 Unvented (*left*) and vented (*right*) tubing. (Photo by K. Timby.)

Filters. An in-line filter (Fig. 16-11) removes air bubbles as well as undissolved drugs, bacteria, and large substances. Filtered tubing generally is used when:

- Administering parenteral nutrition
- The client is at high risk for infection
- Infusing IV solutions to pediatric clients
- Administering blood and packed cells

Needle or Needleless Access Ports. Traditionally, the **ports** (sealed openings) in an IV tubing were designed for access with a needle. This method, however, contributes to the estimated 385,000 needle stick injuries among US health care workers each year (U.S. Department of Labor, 2008) and approximately 2 million annually worldwide (World Health Organization, 2005). To reduce the incidence of work-related injuries and the potential for infection with blood-borne pathogens, **needleless systems** (IV tubing that eliminates the need for access needles) are preferred.

With a needleless system, the nurse uses a blunt cannula to pierce the resealable port each time it is necessary to enter the tubing (Fig. 16-12; and see Chap. 35). A needleless access port can be pierced with a needle a limited number of

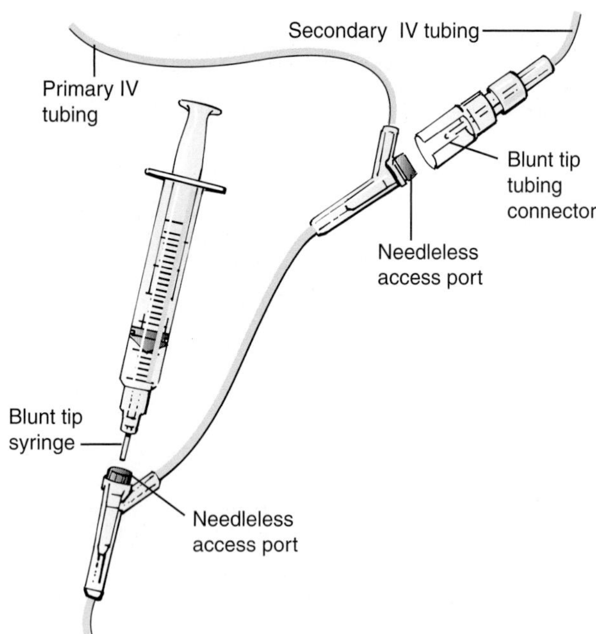

FIGURE 16-12 Needleless systems allow resealable ports to be punctured with a blunt tip syringe or secondary IV tubing connector.

times without altering its integrity, but a port that requires a needle for access cannot be punctured with a blunt cannula.

Infusion Techniques

IV infusions are administered either by gravity alone or with an infusion device–an electric or battery-operated machine that regulates and monitors the administration of IV solutions. The use of an infusion device may affect the type of tubing used.

Gravity Infusion

Generally, most basic types of tubing can be used for infusing a solution by gravity. The height of the IV solution rather than the tubing is the most important factor affecting gravity infusions.

To overcome the pressure within the client's vein, which is higher than atmospheric pressure, the solution is elevated at least 18 to 24 in. (45 to 60 cm) above the site of the infusion. The height of the solution affects the rate of flow: the higher the solution, the faster the solution infuses, and vice versa.

Electronic Infusion Devices

The two general types of electronic infusion devices are infusion pumps and volumetric controllers. Both are programmed to deliver a preset volume per hour. They trigger audible and visual alarms if the infusion is not progressing at the rate intended. They also sound an alarm when the infusion container is nearly empty, air is detected within the tubing, or an obstruction or resistance occurs in delivering the fluid.

Infusion Pumps. An **infusion pump** (an electronic infusion device that uses pressure to infuse solutions) requires special tubing that contains a device such as a cassette to create sufficient pressure to push fluid into the vein (Fig. 16-13). The machine adjusts the pressure according to the resistance it meets. This can be a disadvantage because if the catheter or needle within the vein becomes displaced, the pump continues to infuse fluid into the tissue until the machine's maximum preset pressure limit is reached.

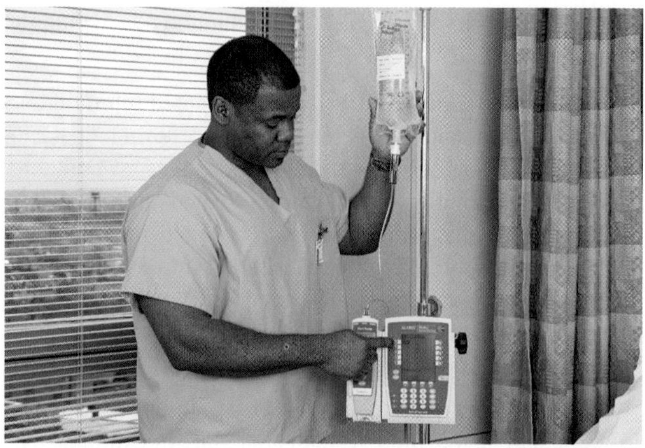

FIGURE 16-13 Special tubing with a cassette is inserted into the electronic infusion pump. (Photo by B. Proud.)

Volumetric Controllers. A **volumetric controller** (an electronic infusion device that instills IV solutions by gravity) mechanically compresses the tubing at a certain frequency to infuse the solution at a precise, preset rate. Volumetric controllers may or may not require special tubing.

Some models allow the nurse to program the infusion of more than one simultaneous infusion of solutions. In some cases, when one container of fluid finishes infusing, the controller automatically resumes infusing another solution. The solution and tubing are prepared before accessing the vein with a needle or catheter. Skill 16-2 describes how to prepare an IV solution for administration.

Venipuncture

Venipuncture (accessing the venous system by piercing a vein with a needle) is a nursing responsibility when a peripheral vein (one distant from the heart) is used. When performing a venipuncture, the nurse assembles the needed equipment, inspects and selects an appropriate vein, and inserts the venipuncture device.

Venipuncture Devices

Several devices are used to access a vein: a butterfly needle, an over-the-needle catheter (most common), or a through-the-needle catheter (Fig. 16-14).

Venipuncture devices are available in various diameters or gauges; the larger the gauge number, the smaller the diameter. The diameter of the venipuncture device always should be smaller than the vein into which it is inserted to reduce the potential for occluding blood flow. An 18-, 20-, or 22-gauge is the size most often used for adults.

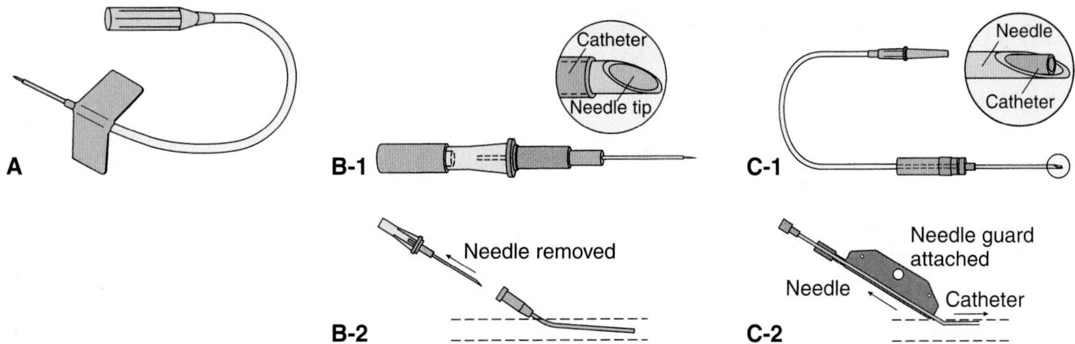

FIGURE 16-14 Venipuncture devices. **A.** A butterfly needle. **B-1.** An over-the-needle catheter. **B-2.** The needle removed. **C-1.** A through-the-needle catheter. **C-2.** A needle guard covers the tip of the needle, which remains outside the skin.

In addition to a device for puncturing the vein, the following items are needed: clean gloves, a tourniquet, antiseptic swabs to cleanse the skin, a transparent dressing to cover the puncture site, and adhesive tape to secure the venipuncture device and tubing. The use of antibiotic or antimicrobial ointment at the site varies; the nurse follows agency policy. An armboard may be needed to prevent the client from dislodging the venipuncture device.

Vein Selection

The veins in the hand and forearm are used most commonly for inserting a venipuncture device (Fig. 16-15); scalp veins are used for infants and small children (see Nursing Guidelines 16-3).

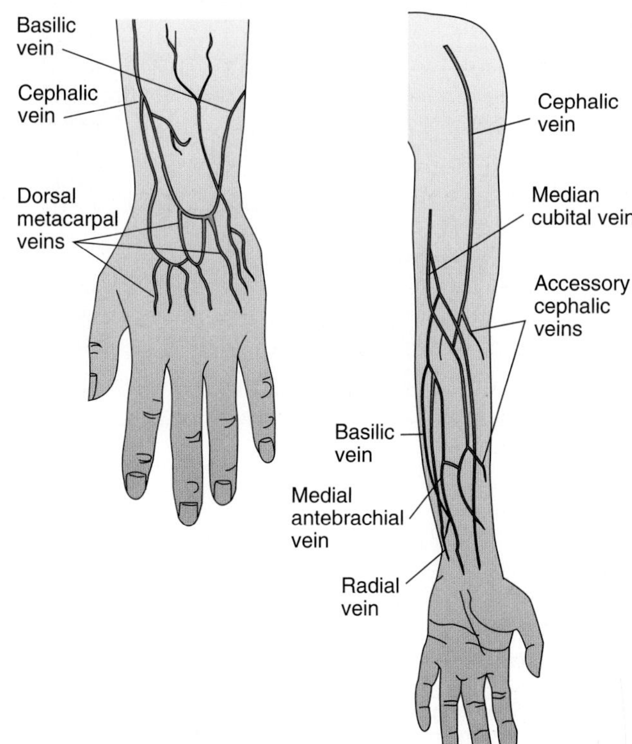

FIGURE 16-15 Potential venipuncture sites.

Once the general site is selected, the nurse applies a tourniquet to select a specific vein (Fig. 16-16). Box 16-4 identifies several techniques for promoting vein distention.

A blood pressure cuff can be substituted for a rubber tourniquet. Whichever technique is used, the radial pulse should be palpable to indicate that arterial blood flow is being maintained.

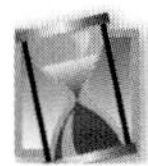

Gerontologic Considerations

- It may be possible and advantageous to avoid using a tourniquet when accessing a vein that is visually prominent on an older adult. Use of a tourniquet may result in bursting the vein, sometimes referred to as "blowing the vein," when it is punctured with a needle.

Venipuncture Device Insertion

Skill 16-3 describes the technique for inserting an over-the-needle catheter within a vein.

Infusion Monitoring and Maintenance

Once the venipuncture is performed and the solution is infusing, the nurse regulates the rate of infusion, assesses for complications, cares for the venipuncture site, and replaces equipment as needed.

Regulating the Infusion Rate

The nurse is responsible for calculating, regulating, and maintaining the rate of infusion according to the physician's

BOX 16-4 Techniques for Promoting Vein Distention

- Apply a tourniquet or blood pressure cuff tightly around the arm.
- Have the client make a fist and pump the fist intermittently.
- Tap the skin over the vein several times.
- Lower the client's arm to promote distal pooling of blood.
- Stroke the skin in the direction of the fingers.
- Apply warm compresses for 10 minutes to dilate veins, and then reapply the tourniquet.

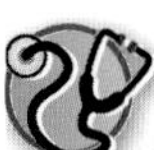

NURSING GUIDELINES 16-3

Selecting a Venipuncture Site

- Use veins on the nondominant side. *This reduces the potential for dislodging the device as a result of movement and use.*
- Do not use foot and leg veins. *Using foot and leg veins restricts mobility and increases the potential for blood clots.*
- If possible, do not use a vein on the side of previous breast surgery or in which vascular surgery has been performed for kidney dialysis. *Using such veins further compromises circulation and increases the potential for infection and poor healing.*
- Choose a vein in a location unaffected by joint movement. *A venipuncture device in such a location could become displaced more easily.*
- Look for a large vein if a large-gauge needle or catheter is necessary. *Matching the needle and vein size prevents compromising circulation.*
- Avoid using veins on the inner surface of the wrist. *This prevents pain and discomfort.*
- Look for a vein proximal to the current site or in the opposite hand or arm. *This promotes healing and decreases the risk of fluid leaking from the vein into the tissue.*
- Feel and look for a fairly straight vein. *It is easier to thread the device into a straight vein.*
- Do not use a vein that appears inflamed or if the skin over the area looks impaired in any way. *Use of such a site creates additional trauma.*

order. If an infusion device is used, the electronic equipment is programmed in milliliters per hour. If the solution is infused without an electronic infusion device (ie, by gravity), the rate is calculated in drops (gtt) per minute. Formulas for calculating infusion rates are provided in Box 16-5.

For gravity infusions, the nurse counts the number of drops falling into the drip chamber per minute. By adjusting the roller clamp, the number of drops is increased or decreased until the infusion rate matches the calculated rate. Thereafter, the nurse monitors the time strip on the side of the container at hourly intervals to ensure that the infusion is instilling at the prescribed rate.

Stop, Think, and Respond Box 16-3

Calculate the rate of infusion for the following two medical orders:

1. *Infuse 1,000 mL of 0.9% NaCl over 12 hours using an electronic infusion device.*
2. *Infuse 500 mL of 5% dextrose and 0.45% NaCl in 8 hours by gravity infusion; your tubing delivers 15 gtt/mL.*

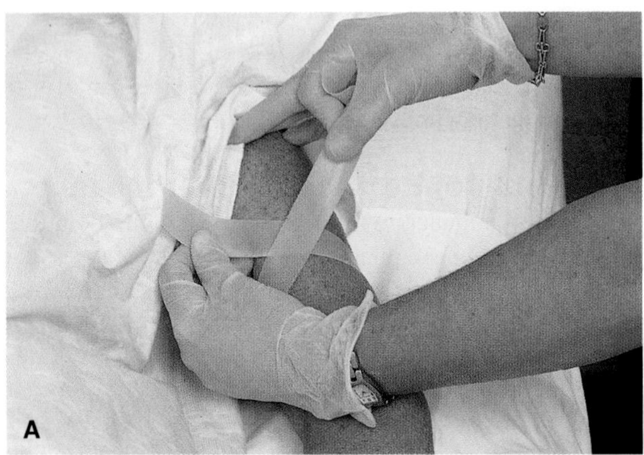

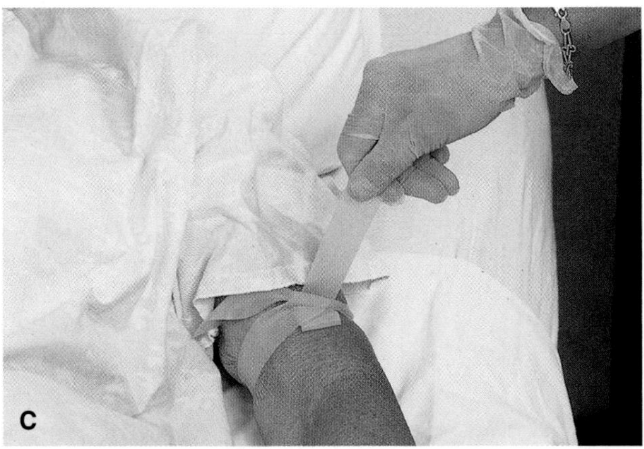

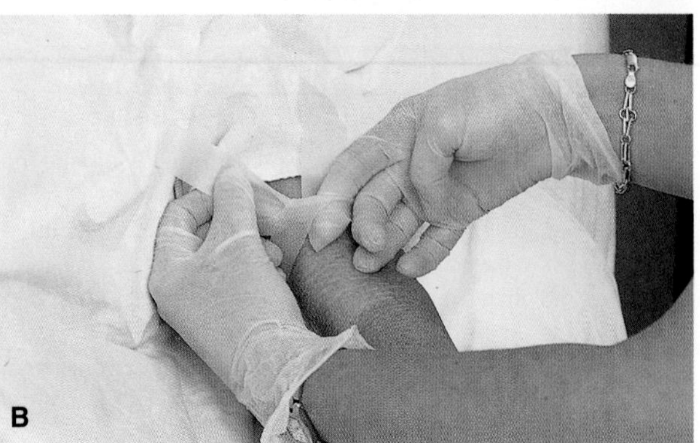

FIGURE 16-16 **A.** To apply a tourniquet, the ends are pulled tightly in opposite directions. **B.** Then one end is tucked beneath the other. **C.** This allows it to be released easily by pulling one of the free ends. (Photo by B. Proud.)

BOX 16-5 Formulas for Calculating Infusion Rates

When using an infusion device:

$$\frac{\text{Total volume in mL}}{\text{Total hours}} = \text{mL/hr}$$

When infusing by gravity:

$$\frac{\text{Total volume in mL}}{\text{Total time in minutes}} \times \text{drop factor}^{a} = \text{gtt/min}$$

Example:

$$\frac{1{,}000 \text{ mL}}{8 \text{ hr}} = 125 \text{ mL/hr}$$

$$\frac{1{,}000 \text{ mL}}{480 \text{ min}} \times 20 = 42 \text{ gtt/min}$$

[a]The macrodrip drop factor varies among manufacturers.

Assessing for Complications

Complications associated with the infusion of IV solutions (Table 16-7) are circulatory overload (an intravascular volume that becomes excessive), **infiltration** (the escape of IV fluid into the tissue), **phlebitis** (inflammation of a vein), **thrombus formation** (a stationary blood clot), **pulmonary embolus** (a blood clot that travels to the lung), infection (growth of microorganisms at the site or within the blood stream), and **air embolism** (a bubble of air traveling within the vascular system).

The minimum quantity of air that may be fatal to humans is not known. Animal research indicates that fatal volumes of air are much larger than the quantity present in the entire length of infusion tubing. The average infusion tubing holds about 5 mL of air, an amount not ordinarily considered dangerous. Clients, however, are often frightened when they see air in the tubing, and nurses make every effort to remove air bubbles (see Nursing Guidelines 16-4).

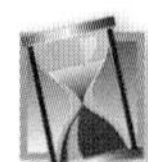

Gerontologic Considerations

- Nurses need to closely monitor the response of older adults to IV infusions who may be unable to tolerate volumes that may be safely administered to younger adults.

Caring for the Site

Because the venipuncture is a type of wound, it is important to inspect the site routinely. The nurse documents its appearance in the client's record. A common practice is to change the dressing over the venipuncture site every 24 to

TABLE 16-7 Complications of Intravenous (IV) Therapy

COMPLICATION	SIGNS AND SYMPTOMS	CAUSE(S)	ACTION
Infection	Swelling Discomfort Redness at site Drainage from site	Growth of microorganisms	Change site Apply antiseptic and dressing to previous site Report findings
Circulatory overload	Elevated blood pressure Shortness of breath Bounding pulse Anxiety	Rapid infusion Reduced kidney function Impaired heart contraction	Slow the IV rate Contact the physician Elevate the client's head Give oxygen
Infiltration	Swelling at the site Discomfort Decrease in infusion rate Cool skin temperature at the site	Displacement of the venipuncture device	Restart the IV Elevate the arm
Phlebitis	Redness, warmth, and discomfort along the vein	Administration of irritating fluid Prolonged use of the same vein	Restart the IV Report findings Apply warm compresses
Thrombus formation	Swelling Discomfort Slowed infusion	Stasis of blood at the catheter, needle tip, or vein	Restart the IV Report findings Apply warm compresses
Pulmonary embolus	Sudden chest pain Shortness of breath Anxiety Rapid heart rate Drop in blood pressure	Movement of a previously stationary blood clot to the lungs	Stay with the client Call for help Administer oxygen
Air embolism	Same as a pulmonary embolus	Failure to purge air from the tubing	Same as for a pulmonary embolus, but also place the client's head lower than the feet Position the client on his or her left side

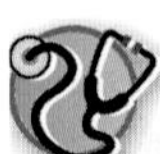

NURSING GUIDELINES 16-4

Removing Air Bubbles From IV Tubing

- Flush the line with IV solution before inserting the adaptor into the venipuncture device. *This action purges air from the tubing.*
- Tighten the roller clamp if small bubbles are observed. *This action prevents continued forward movement of the air.*
- Tap the tubing below the air bubbles (Fig. 16-17). *Doing so promotes upward movement of the air above the fluid in the drip chamber.*
- Milk the air in the direction of the drip chamber or filter, if one is incorporated within the tubing. *Doing so pushes the air physically to an area where it can be trapped or released.*
- Wrap the tubing around a circular object, like a pencil, starting below the trapped air. *This moves the air toward the drip chamber where it can escape from the liquid into the empty air space.*
- Insert the barrel of a syringe within a port below the air, and open the roller clamp. *This siphons fluid and air from the tubing as it passes by the bevel of the needle.*

72 hours, according to the agency's infection control policy (see Chap. 28).

Replacing Equipment

Solutions are replaced when they finish infusing or every 24 hours, whichever occurs first (Skill 16-4). IV tubing is changed every 72 hours, depending on agency policy, with some exceptions. Tubing used to instill parenteral nutrition is replaced daily. Tubing used to administer whole blood can be reused for a second unit if one unit is administered immediately after the other. Whenever tubing is changed, it is more convenient to replace both the solution and the tubing at the same time. Skill 16-5 describes how to replace just the tubing, which is generally more difficult.

Discontinuation of an Intravenous Infusion

IV infusions are discontinued when the solution has infused and no more is scheduled to follow. Skill 16-6 is a procedure for removing a venipuncture device when IV infusions are no longer needed. When the client needs occasional infusions of solutions or the administration of IV medications, the venipuncture is temporarily capped but kept patent with the use of an intermittent venous access device also known as a medication lock.

FIGURE 16-17 Removing air bubbles. **A.** Tapping the tubing may help air bubbles rise into the drip chamber. **B.** Twisting the tubing around a pencil or other object may displace air bubbles toward the drip chamber.

Insertion of an Intermittent Venous Access Device

An **intermittent venous access device** (a sealed chamber that provides a means for administering IV medications or solutions periodically; Fig. 16-18) is inserted into a venipuncture device. An intermittent peripheral venous access device also is called a "saline lock" because the chamber is filled and periodically flushed with sterile normal saline to prevent blood from clotting at the tip of the catheter or needle. Central venous catheters are usually kept patent by flushing the device with heparinized saline. Intermittent venous access devices are used when the client:

- No longer needs continuous infusions of fluid
- Needs intermittent administrations of IV medication
- May need emergency IV fluid or medications if his or her condition deteriorates

These devices are replaced when the venipuncture site is changed. Skill 16-7 describes how to insert an intermittent venous access device and ensure its patency. The use of a

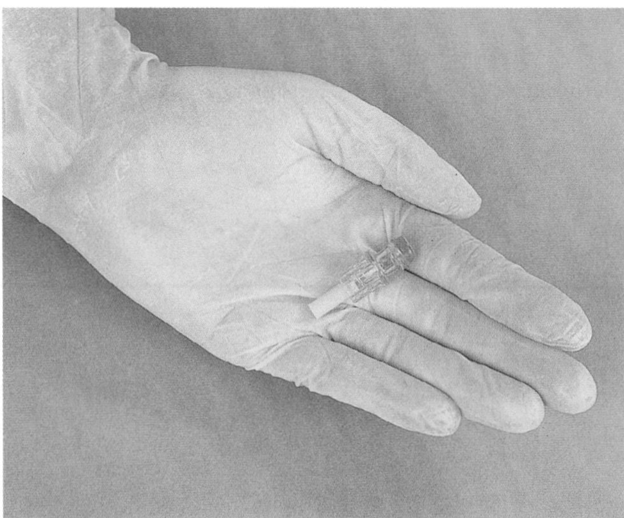

FIGURE 16-18 An intermittent venous access device. (Photo by B. Proud.)

medication lock when administering IV drugs is discussed in Chapter 35.

BLOOD ADMINISTRATION

Blood is collected, stored, and checked for safety and compatibility before it is administered as a transfusion.

Blood Collection and Storage

Blood donors are screened to ensure that they are healthy and will not be endangered by the temporary loss in blood volume. Refrigerated blood can be stored for 21 to 35 days, after which it is discarded.

Blood Safety

Once collected, the donated blood is tested for syphilis, hepatitis, and HIV antibodies to exclude administering blood that may transmit these blood-borne diseases. Blood that tests positive is discarded. Unfortunately, disease-carrying viruses may remain undetected if the antibodies have not reached a level high enough to be measured.

The U.S. Blood Safety Council, a division of the Department of Health and Human Services, has policies regarding potential hepatitis C infection by blood transfusions. All blood collection agencies must notify people who received blood before 1987 if the donation came from a donor who has tested positive for hepatitis C since 1990. This policy is being implemented to promote early diagnosis and treatment of infected but asymptomatic transfusion recipients.

The American Red Cross has a policy concerning blood donations to eliminate the potential transmission of neurologic infectious microorganisms known as *prions*. Prions cause various brain disorders, one of which is bovine spongiform encephalopathy ("mad cow disease") detected in people who live in the United Kingdom (UK). Because blood is one possible mode of transmitting prions from animals to humans and humans to humans, the collection of blood is banned from anyone who has lived in the UK for a total of 3 months or longer since 1980, lived anywhere in Europe for a total of 6 months since 1980, or received a blood transfusion in the UK (American Red Cross, 2005).

Blood Compatibility

There are several hundred differences among the proteins in the blood of a donor and a recipient. They can cause minor or major transfusion reactions. One of the most dangerous differences involves the antigens, or protein structures, on membranes of red blood cells. Antigens determine the characteristic blood group—A, B, AB, and O—and Rh factor. Rh positive means the protein is present; Rh negative means the protein is absent.

TABLE 16-8 Blood Groups and Compatible Types

BLOOD GROUPS	PERCENTAGE OF POPULATION	COMPATIBLE BLOOD TYPES
A	41%	A and O
B	9%	B and O
O	47%	O
AB	3%	AB, A, B, and O
Rh+	85% whites 95% African Americans	Rh+ and Rh–
Rh–	15% whites 5% African Americans	Rh– only

Before donated blood is administered, the blood of the potential recipient is typed and mixed, or cross-matched, with a sample of the stored blood to determine whether the two are compatible. To avoid an incompatibility reaction, it is best to administer the same blood group and Rh factor. Exceptions are listed in Table 16-8.

Type O blood is considered the universal donor because it lacks both A and B blood group markers on its cell membrane. Therefore, type O blood can be given to anyone because it will not trigger an incompatibility reaction when given to recipients with other blood types. Persons with type AB blood are referred to as universal recipients because their red blood cells have proteins compatible with types A, B, and O. Rh-positive persons may receive Rh-positive or Rh-negative blood because the latter does not contain the sensitizing protein. Rh-negative persons, however, should never receive Rh-positive blood.

Stop, Think, and Respond Box 16-4

Which blood type or types are compatible for clients who are blood types B (Rh) positive and O (Rh) negative?

Blood Transfusion

Before administering blood, the nurse obtains and documents the client's vital signs to provide a baseline for comparison should the client have a transfusion reaction. Each client who receives blood has a color-coded bracelet with identifying numbers that must correlate with those on the unit of blood. IV medications are never infused through tubing being used to administer blood.

Blood Transfusion Equipment

There are certain standards for the gauge of the catheter or needle and the type of tubing used to transfuse blood.

Catheter or Needle Gauge. Because blood contains cells in addition to water, it generally is infused through a 16- to 20-gauge—preferably an 18-gauge—catheter or needle. Using a smaller gauge increases the potential for prolonging the infusion beyond 4 hours, and 4 hours is the maximum safe period for administering one unit of blood.

Blood Transfusion Tubing. Blood is administered through tubing referred to as a Y-set (Fig. 16-19). Two branches are at the top of the tubing: one is used to administer normal saline solution and the other is used to administer blood. Normal saline (0.9% sodium chloride) is the only solution used when administering blood because other solutions destroy red blood cells. The two branches of the Y-set join above a filter that removes clotted blood and dead cell debris. The normal saline always is administered before the blood is hung and follows after the blood has been infused. It also is used during the infusion if the client has a transfusion reaction (Skill 16-8).

Transfusion Reactions

Life-threatening transfusion reactions generally occur within the first 5 to 15 minutes of the infusion, so the nurse or someone designated by the nurse usually remains with the client during this critical time. Because a transfusion reaction can occur at any time, however, nurses monitor clients frequently during a transfusion and instruct them to call for assistance if they feel any unusual sensations (Table 16-9).

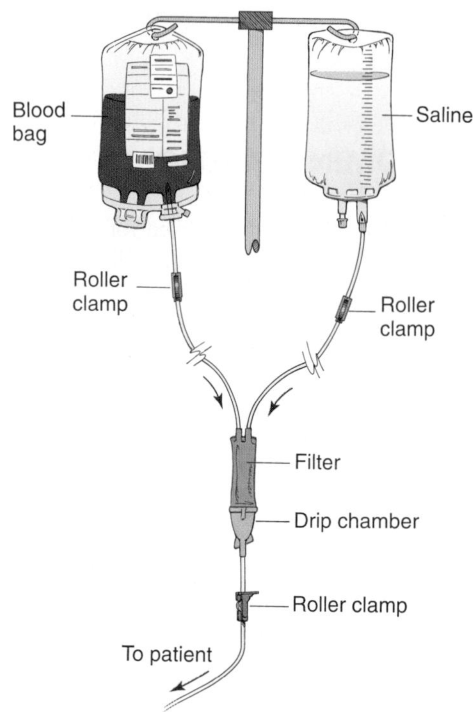

FIGURE 16-19 Blood transfusion tubing.

TABLE 16-9 Transfusion Reactions

TYPE OF REACTION	SIGNS AND SYMPTOMS	CAUSE(S)	ACTION
Incompatibility	Hypotension, rapid pulse rate, difficulty breathing, back pain, flushing	Mismatch between donor and recipient blood groups	Stop the infusion of blood Infuse saline at a rapid rate Call for assistance Administer oxygen Raise the feet higher than the head Be prepared to administer emergency drugs Send first urine specimen to laboratory Save the blood and tubing
Febrile	Fever, shaking chills, headache, rapid pulse, muscle aches	Allergy to foreign proteins in the donated blood	Stop the blood infusion Start the saline Check vital signs Report findings
Septic	Fever, chills, hypotension	Infusion of blood that contains microorganisms	Stop the infusion of blood Start the saline Report findings Save the blood and tubing
Allergic	Rash, itching, flushing, stable vital signs	Minor sensitivity to substances in the donor blood	Slow the rate of infusion Assess the client Report findings Be prepared to give an antihistamine
Moderate chilling	No fever or other symptoms	Infusion of cold blood	Continue the infusion Cover and make the client comfortable
Overload	Hypertension, difficulty breathing, moist breath sounds, bounding pulse	Large volume or rapid rate of infusion; inadequate cardiac or kidney function	Reduce the rate Elevate the head Give oxygen Report findings Be prepared to give a diuretic
Hypocalcemia (low calcium)	Tingling of fingers, hypotension, muscle cramps, convulsions	Multiple blood transfusions containing anticalcium agents	Stop the blood infusion Start saline Report findings Be prepared to give antidote (calcium chloride)

PARENTERAL NUTRITION

The term *parenteral* means "a route other than enteral or intestinal." Therefore, **parenteral nutrition** (nutrients such as protein, carbohydrate, fat, vitamins, minerals, and trace elements, administered intravenously) is provided by other than the oral route. Depending on the concentration of these substances, parenteral nutrition is administered through an IV catheter in a peripheral vein or through a catheter that terminates in a central vein near the heart.

Peripheral Parenteral Nutrition

Peripheral parenteral nutrition (an isotonic or hypotonic IV nutrient solution instilled in a vein distant from the heart) is not extremely concentrated and consequently can be infused through peripheral veins. It provides temporary nutritional support of approximately 2,000 to 2,500 cal daily. It can meet a person's metabolic needs when oral intake is interrupted for 7 to 10 days, or it can be used as a supplement during a transitional period as the client begins to resume eating.

Total Parenteral Nutrition

Total parenteral nutrition (TPN; a hypertonic solution of nutrients designed to meet almost all caloric and nutritional needs) is preferred for clients who are severely malnourished or may not be able to consume food or liquids for a long period. Box 16-6 lists clients who may benefit from TPN.

BOX 16-6 Candidates for Total Parenteral Nutrition

- Clients who have not eaten for 5 days and are not likely to eat during the next week
- Clients who have had a 10% or more loss of body weight
- Clients exhibiting self-imposed starvation (anorexia nervosa)
- Clients with cancer of the esophagus or stomach
- Clients with postoperative gastrointestinal complications
- Clients with inflammatory bowel disease in an acute stage
- Clients with major trauma or burns
- Clients with liver and renal failure

Because TPN solutions are extremely concentrated, they must be delivered to an area where they are diluted in a fairly large volume of blood. This excludes peripheral veins. TPN solutions are infused through a catheter inserted into the subclavian or jugular vein; the tip terminates in the superior vena cava. This type of a catheter is referred to as a central venous catheter (Fig. 16-20A). Sometimes a peripherally inserted central catheter is used; this long catheter is inserted into a peripheral arm vein, but its tip terminates in the superior vena cava (Fig. 16-20B) (see Nursing Guidelines 16-5).

Lipid Emulsions

An **emulsion** (a mixture of two liquids, one of which is insoluble in the other) can be administered parenterally. The combination allows a vehicle for administering lipids, or fat,

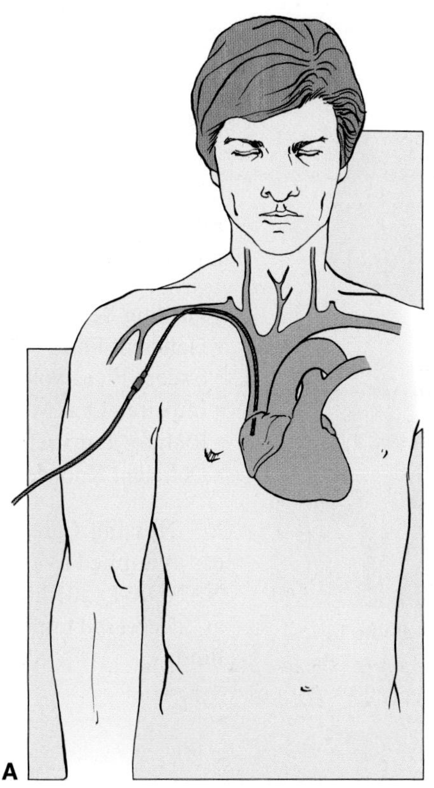

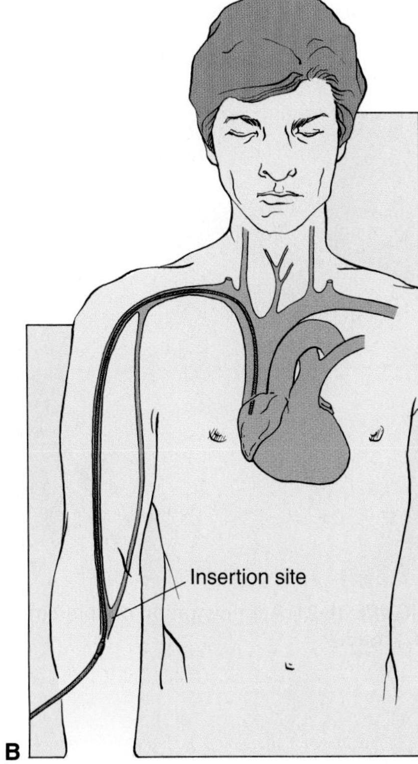

FIGURE 16-20 A. A central venous catheter inserted into the subclavian vein and threaded into the superior vena cava. **B.** A peripherally inserted central catheter with the distal tip in the superior vena cava.

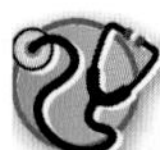

NURSING GUIDELINES 16-5

Administering TPN

- Weigh the client daily. *A record of the client's weight assists with monitoring his or her response to treatment.*
- Use tubing that contains a filter. *Filters absorb air and bacteria, two potential complications associated with the use of central venous catheters.*
- Change TPN tubing daily. *Doing so reduces the potential for infection.*
- Tape all connections in the tubing and central catheter. *Taping prevents accidental separation and reduces the potential for an air embolism.*
- Clamp the central catheter and have the client bear down whenever separating the tubing from its catheter connection. *This action prevents an air embolism.*
- Use an infusion device to administer TPN solution. *An infusion device monitors and regulates precise fluid volumes.*
- Infuse initial TPN solutions gradually (25 to 50 mL/hr). *Gradual administration allows time for physiologic adaptation.*
- Never increase the rate of infusion to make up for an uninfused volume unless the physician has been consulted. *Speeding up the infusion tends to increase blood glucose levels.*
- Monitor intake and especially urine output. *High blood glucose levels can trigger diuresis (increased urine excretion), resulting in output greater than intake.*
- Monitor capillary blood glucose levels (see Chap. 14). *Blood glucose may not be adequately metabolized without the additional administration of insulin.*
- Wean the client from TPN gradually. *Weaning prevents a sudden drop in blood glucose levels.*

which is often missing from parenteral nutritional solutions. A parenteral lipid emulsion is a mixture of water and fats in the form of soybean or safflower oil, egg yolk phospholipids, and glycerin.

Lipid solutions, which look milky white (Fig. 16-21), are given intermittently with TPN solutions. They provide additional calories and promote adequate blood levels of fatty acids. Lipid solutions are administered peripherally or in a port in the central catheter below the filter and close to the vein. If the lipid solution is squeezed or mixed with TPN solutions in larger volumes than those moving through the catheter, the lipid molecules tend to "break" and separate in the solution.

The client receiving an administration of lipids may have an adverse reaction within 2 to 5 hours of the infusion (Dudek, 2009). Common manifestations include fever, flushing, sweating, dizziness, nausea, vomiting, headache, chest and back pain, dyspnea, and cyanosis. Delayed reactions (up to 10 days later) are characterized by enlargement of the liver and spleen accompanied by jaundice, reduced white blood cell and platelet counts, elevated blood lipid levels, seizures, and shock.

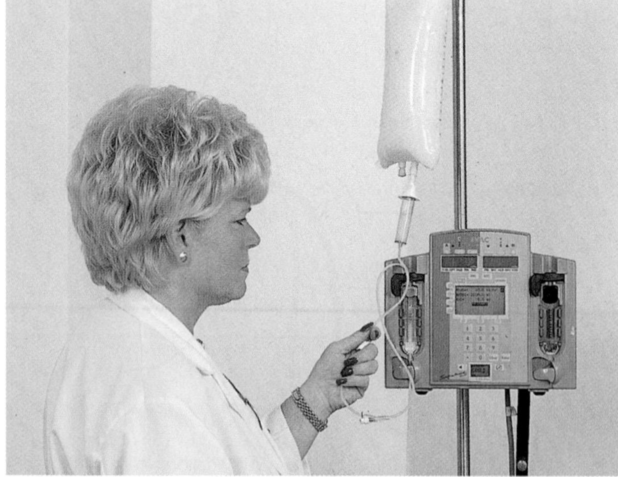

FIGURE 16-21 Administration of lipid emulsion. (Photo by B. Proud.)

NURSING IMPLICATIONS

Clients who have fluid, electrolyte, blood, and nutritional imbalances are likely to have one or more of the following nursing diagnoses:

- Feeding Self-Care Deficit
- Deficient Fluid Volume
- Excess Fluid Volume
- Impaired Oral Mucous Membrane
- Risk for Impaired Skin Integrity
- Deficient Knowledge

Nursing Care Plan 16-1 illustrates the nursing process as applied to a client with Deficient Fluid Volume. The NANDA-I (2012, p. 186) defines this diagnostic category as "decreased intravascular, interstitial, and/or intracellular fluid."

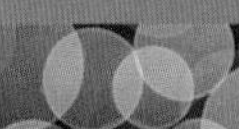

NURSING CARE PLAN 16-1 Deficient Fluid Volume

Assessment

- Monitor intake and output (I&O) each shift and total the sum every 24 hr.
- Assess for unusual loss of fluid via emesis, diarrhea, wound drainage, intestinal suction, blood loss, etc.
- Weigh the client consistently on the same scale, at the same time, and in similar clothing and compare the findings.
- Note the color and odor of urine.
- Check vital signs every 4 hr while the client is awake.
- Assess skin turgor over the sternum each shift.
- Note the color and warmth of the skin and the degree of moisture in the mucous membranes each shift.
- Ask the client to identify any thirst, weakness, or fatigue.
- Determine the client's level of consciousness and evidence of confusion or disorientation.
- Review laboratory data such as specific gravity of urine, hematocrit, and electrolyte concentration.

Nursing Diagnosis. **Deficient Fluid Volume** related to inadequate oral fluid intake and increased fluid loss as manifested by intake of 1,000 mL in previous 24 hr, urine output of 750 mL in previous 24 hr, dry oral mucous membranes, dark yellow urine with strong odor, oral temperature of 100°F, weak pulse rate of 100 beats/min, respiratory rate of 28 breaths/min, BP of 118/68 mm Hg, and dry skin that tents for more than 3 seconds.

Expected Outcome. The client's fluid volume will be adequate as evidenced by an oral intake of 1,500 to 3,000 mL in the next 24 hr (8/15) with a urine output nearly the same volume as oral intake.

Interventions	Rationales
Explain the need to increase oral fluid intake to the client and the process of recording the volume of fluid intake and output.	Teaching helps facilitate the client's cooperation in reaching the goal.
Place an I&O record form at the client's bedside.	Having a form for recording I&O promotes an accurate assessment.
Put a hat for collecting urine inside the bowl of the toilet; explain its purpose to the client.	Placing a device for collecting voided urine helps prevent accidental flushing of urine that needs to be measured.
Instruct the client to record fluids and amounts consumed and to remind nursing personnel to do likewise.	Periodic recording facilitates accuracy.
Ask the client to turn on the signal light after each use of the toilet or urinal.	Measuring urine output after each voiding and recording the amount ensure accuracy.
Compile a list of fluid likes and dislikes.	Catering to the client's personal preferences facilitates increasing oral fluid intake.
Provide a minimum of 100 to 200 mL of preferred oral fluid every hour over the next 16 hr (day and evening shifts).	An oral fluid intake of 100 mL/hr for 16 hr will meet the minimum target of 1,500 mL.
Offer oral fluid if the client awakens during the night, but avoid disturbing the client if asleep and if the oral intake from the previous shifts is adequate.	Ensuring sleep is a priority as long as the goals for fluid intake are met.
Request a regular diet from the dietary department that contains foods that are good sources of sodium such as milk, cheese, bouillon, and ham.	Sodium attracts water.

Evaluation of Expected Outcomes

- Total oral intake for 24 hr is 2,250 mL.
- Total urine output for 24 hr is 1,975 mL.
- Oral temperature is 98.2°F, pulse is 88 beats/min and strong, respirations are 18 breaths/min at rest, and BP is 128/84 mm Hg in right arm while lying down.
- Weight remains at admission weight of 157 lb.
- Urine is light yellow and free of strong odor.
- Oral mucous membranes are pink and moist.
- Skin is warm and elastic.
- The client is alert and oriented.
- The client is not thirsty, weak, or unusually fatigued.

CRITICAL THINKING EXERCISES

1. When calculating a client's I&O, you find that she has had a total 24-hour intake of 1,000 mL and output of 750 mL. What other assessment findings are you likely to observe?
2. A client whose oral intake is being limited to 1,000 mL/24 hours is experiencing thirst and asks for assistance in relieving his discomfort. What nursing actions could be taken?
3. While assessing a client's IV infusion that is instilling by gravity, you note that it is infusing at a significantly slower rate than when it was originally regulated. What actions are appropriate to take?
4. A client will be receiving a blood transfusion. The registered nurse who hangs the unit of blood and initiates the administration of the blood asks you to assess the client during its infusion. What assessments are appropriate to monitor?

NCLEX-STYLE REVIEW QUESTIONS

1. When the nursing care plan indicates that a client is to be weighed regularly, which is most important to consider?
   1. When the client was weighed before
   2. When the client last took a drink of fluid
   3. How much the client has eaten so far today
   4. Whether the client feels like being weighed
2. Which item in the following list, if identified by the client, is the best evidence that the client understands dietary restrictions for a low-sodium diet?
   1. Soy sauce
   2. Lemon juice
   3. Maple syrup
   4. Onion powder
3. When a client asks how a transfusion of packed red blood cells differs from the usual whole blood transfusion, which nursing explanation is most correct?
   1. A unit of packed red blood cells has the same number of red blood cells in less fluid volume.
   2. A unit of packed red blood cells contains more red blood cells in the same amount of fluid volume.
   3. A unit of packed red blood cells is less likely to cause an allergic transfusion reaction.
   4. A unit of packed red blood cells will stimulate the bone marrow to make more red blood cells.
4. If all the following units of blood are available, which is the nurse correct to refuse for a client with type A, Rh-positive blood because it is incompatible for this client?
   1. Type A, Rh negative
   2. Type O, Rh positive
   3. Type O, Rh negative
   4. Type AB, Rh positive
5. During the first 15 minutes of infusing a unit of blood, which of the following is most indicative that the client is experiencing a transfusion reaction?
   1. The client feels an urgent need to urinate.
   2. The client's blood pressure becomes low.
   3. Localized swelling develops at the infusion site.
   4. The skin is pale at the site of the infusing blood.

SKILL 16-1 Recording Intake and Output

Suggested Action	Reason for Action
ASSESSMENT	
Check the Kardex or listen in report to determine whether an assigned client is on I&O.	Ensures compliance with the plan for care.
Verify during the report how much IV fluid has been accounted for from any currently infusing solution.	Indicates the credited volume for calculating fluid intake at the end of the shift.
Review the nursing care plan for any previously identified fluid problem and nursing orders for specific interventions.	Promotes continuity of care.
Review the client's medical record and analyze trends in I&O, vital sign measurements, laboratory findings, and weight records.	Aids in analyzing trends in fluid status.
Perform a physical assessment to obtain data that reflect the client's fluid status (see Table 16-4).	Provides current data.
Inspect all tubings and drains to ensure they are patent (open).	Ensures that methods for instilling or removing fluids are functional.
Notice whether all suction containers or drainage containers were emptied at the end of the previous shift.	Ensures accurate record keeping.
Determine how much the client understands about I&O measurements, fluid intake goals, or fluid restrictions.	Verifies whether additional teaching is needed.
Look for a calibrated container and bedside I&O record.	Facilitates keeping accurate data.
Obtain a collection device for inside the toilet if the client has none and uses the toilet for urinary elimination.	Facilitates measuring voided urine.
Measure the amount of water in the client's bedside carafe at the beginning of the shift.	Provides a baseline for measuring fluid consumed in addition to that served at regular meal times.
PLANNING	
Place the client on I&O or plan to measure I&O if the client is at high risk for fluid imbalance or the assessment data suggest a problem.	Demonstrates safe and appropriate nursing care.
Identify the goal for fluid intake or restriction. A minimum of 1,000 mL in 8 hr is not unrealistic for a client in fluid deficit. An amount prescribed by the physician or an intake equal to the client's previous hourly output may be used as a guideline for fluid restrictions.	Provides a target for client care.
IMPLEMENTATION	
Explain or reinforce the purpose and procedures that will be followed for measuring I&O.	Facilitates client cooperation.
Record the volume for all fluids consumed from the dietary tray and other sources of oral liquids.	Contributes to accurate assessment records.
Make sure that all IV fluids or tube feedings are being administered at the prescribed rate.	Ensures compliance with medical therapy.
Ensure that the nurse who adds additional IV fluid containers also records the volume when the infusion is complete or replaced.	Ensures accurate record keeping.
Keep track of the fluid volumes used to irrigate drainage tubes or flush feeding tubes.	Ensures accurate record keeping.
Measure and record the volume of voided urine. Although urine is not considered a vehicle for the transmission of blood-borne microorganisms, gloves are worn as standard precautions.	Ensures accurate record keeping and reduces the transmission of microorganisms.

(continued)

Recording Intake and Output (continued)

IMPLEMENTATION (CONTINUED)

Action	Rationale
Measure and record the volume of urine collected in a catheter drainage bag near the end of the shift (Fig. A).	Ensures accurate record keeping.

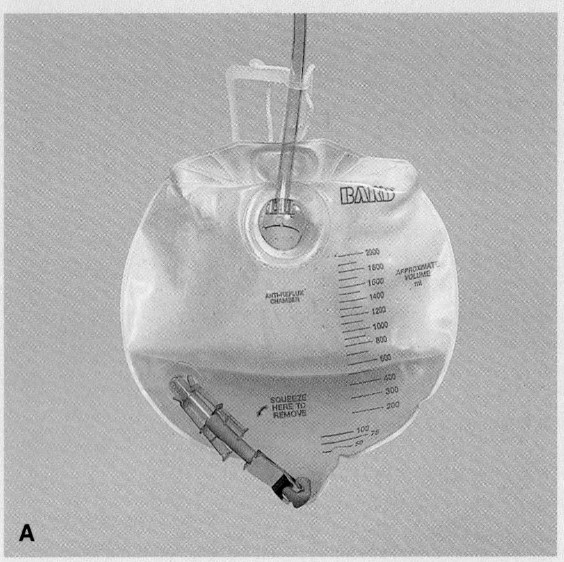

Urine drainage bag. (Photo by B. Proud.)

Action	Rationale
Wear gloves to measure liquid stool or other body fluids and record their measured amounts.	Prevents the transmission of microorganisms and provides assessment data.
Wash hands or perform hand antisepsis with an alcohol rub (see Chap. 10) after removing and disposing of the gloves.	Reduces the presence and potential transmission of microorganisms.
Check the volume remaining in currently infusing IV fluids; subtract the remaining volume from the credit provided at the beginning of the shift.	Ensures accurate assessment data.
Total all fluid intake volumes and all fluid output volumes for the current 8-hr shift; record the amounts.	Ensures accurate record keeping.
Compare the data to determine whether the I&O are approximately the same and if the goals for fluid intake or restrictions have been met.	Demonstrates concern for safe and appropriate care.
Report major differences in I&O to the nurse in charge or the client's physician.	Demonstrates concern for safe and appropriate care.
Review the plan of care and make revisions if the goals have not been met or if additional nursing interventions seem appropriate.	Demonstrates responsibility and accountability.
Report the I&O volumes, IV fluid credit amount, and any other pertinent data to the nurse who will be assuming responsibility for the client's care.	Demonstrates responsibility and accountability.

Evaluation

- Intake approximates output.
- Goals for fluid intake or restriction have been met.
- Significant data have been reported.
- The client's fluid status justifies continuing the care as planned, or the care plan has been revised.

Document

- Date and time
- Intake and output volumes for the previous 8 hours

SAMPLE DOCUMENTATION

Date and Time Fluid intake for the previous 8 hours is 1,200 mL and output is 1,000 mL. ——— SIGNATURE/TITLE

SKILL 16-2 Preparing Intravenous Solutions

Suggested Action	Reason for Action
ASSESSMENT	
Check the medical order for the type, volume, and projected length of fluid therapy.	Ensures accuracy and guides the selection of equipment.
Determine if the solution is in a bag or bottle and if the infusion will be administered by gravity or infusion device.	Affects the selection of tubing.
Review the client's medical record for information on the risk for infection.	Determines need for filtered tubing.
Read the label on the solution at least three times.	Helps prevent errors.
PLANNING	
Mark a time strip and attach it to the side of the container (see Fig. A).	Facilitates monitoring.

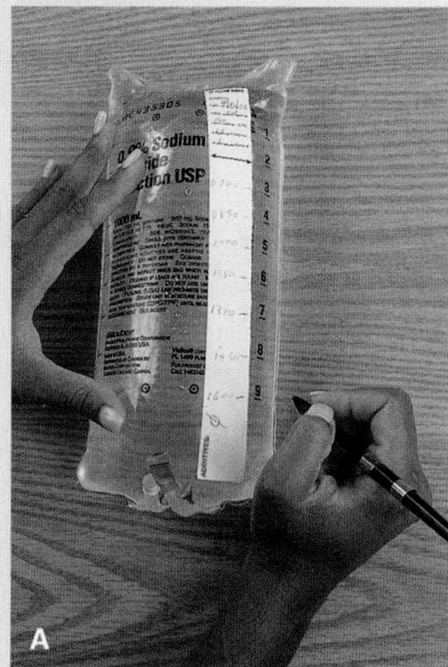

Marking a time strip. (Photo by B. Proud.)

Suggested Action	Reason for Action
IMPLEMENTATION	
Wash hands or perform hand antisepsis with an alcohol rub (see Chap. 10).	Reduces the transmission of microorganisms. 
Select the appropriate tubing and stretch it once it has been removed from the package.	Straightens the tubing by removing bends and kinks.
Tighten the roller clamp (see Fig. B).	Aids in filling the drip chamber.

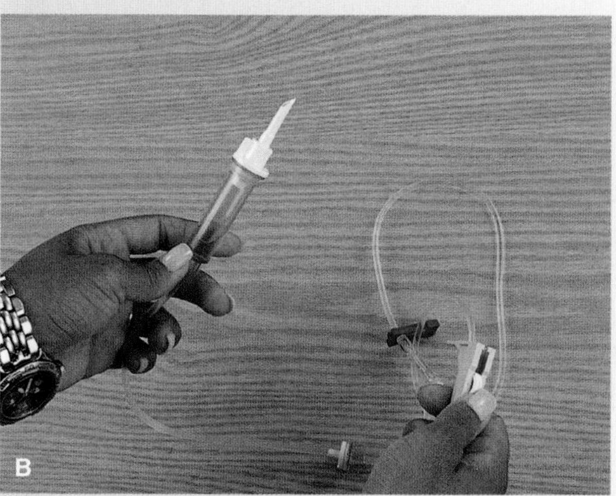

Tightening the roller clamp. (Photo by B. Proud.)

(continued)

Preparing Intravenous Solutions (continued)

IMPLEMENTATION (CONTINUED)

Remove the cover from the access port.	Provides access for inserting the spike.
Insert the spike by puncturing the seal on the container (see Fig. C).	Provides an exit route for fluid.

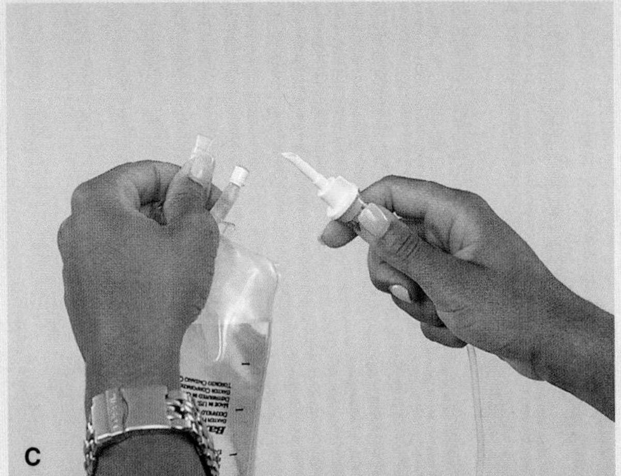

Inserting the spike. (Photo by B. Proud.)

Hang the solution container from an IV pole or suspended hook.	Inverts the container.
Squeeze the drip chamber, filling it no more than half full (see Fig. D).	Leaves space to count the drops when regulating the rate of infusion.

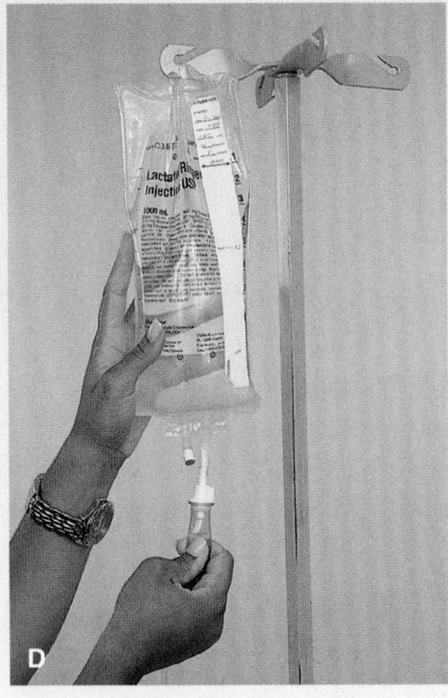

Squeezing the drip chamber. (Photo by B. Proud.)

Release the roller clamp.	Flushes air from the tubing.

(continued)

Preparing Intravenous Solutions (continued)

IMPLEMENTATION (CONTINUED)

Invert ports within the tubing as the solution approaches.	Displaces air that may be trapped in the junction.
Tighten the roller clamp when all the air has been removed.	Prevents a loss of fluid.
Attach a piece of tape or a label on the tubing giving the date, time, and your initials (see Fig. E).	Provides a quick reference for determining when the tubing needs to be changed.

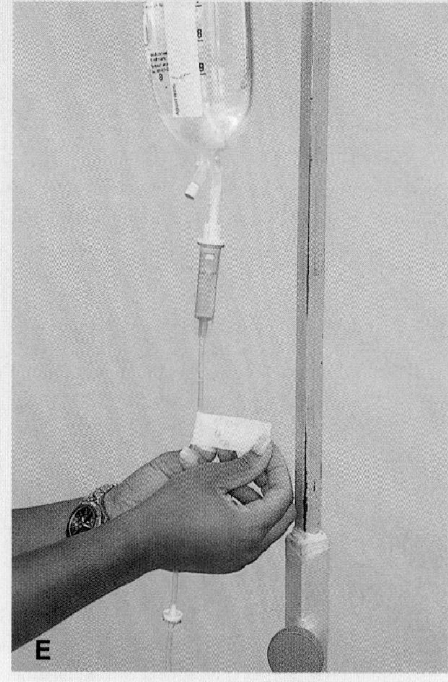

Attaching label on the tubing. (Photo by B. Proud.)

Take the solution and tubing to the client's room.	Facilitates administration.

Evaluation

- Solution and tubing are properly labeled.
- Tubing has been purged of air.

Document

- Date and time
- Type and volume of solution
- Rate of infusion once venipuncture has been performed
- Location of venipuncture site

SAMPLE DOCUMENTATION

Date and Time 1,000 mL of 5% D/W infusing at 125 mL/hr through IV in L. forearm. ———— SIGNATURE/TITLE

SKILL 16-3 Starting an Intravenous Infusion

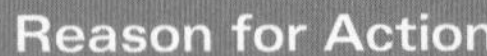

Suggested Action	Reason for Action
ASSESSMENT	
Check the identity of the client.	Prevents errors.
Review the client's medical record to determine whether there are any allergies to iodine or tape.	Influences supplies that will be used and modifications in the procedure.
Inspect and palpate several potential venipuncture sites (see Fig. A).	Provides an alternative if the first attempt is unsuccessful.
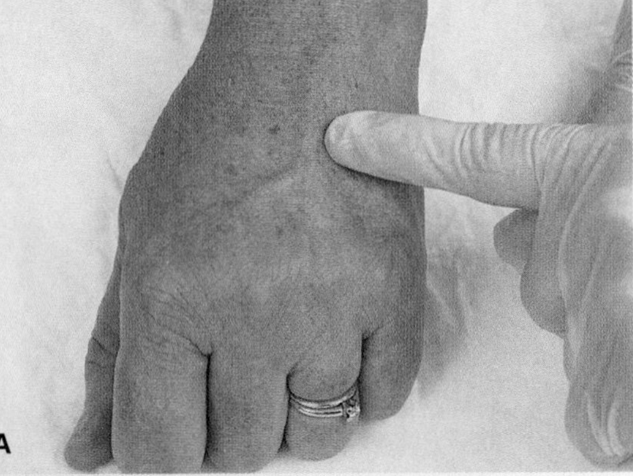 A	Palpating veins. (Photo by B. Proud.)
PLANNING	
Bring all the necessary equipment to the bedside.	Promotes organization and efficient time management.
Position the client on his or her back or in a sitting position.	Promotes comfort and facilitates inspection of the arm.
Place an absorbent pad beneath the hand or arm.	Prevents having to change the bed linen if the site bleeds.
Select a site most likely to facilitate the purpose for the infusion and comply with the criteria for vein selection.	Facilitates continuous fluid administration and minimizes potential complications.
Clip body hair at the site if it is excessive.	Facilitates visualization and reduces discomfort when adhesive tape is removed.
Apply topical anesthetic such as Numby Stuff™ or EMLA cream.	Provides local anesthesia to insertion site to minimize pain associated with a needle stick.
Tear strips of tape, open the package with the venipuncture device and transparent dressing, or place antiseptic ointment on an opened Band-Aid or gauze square, based on the agency's policy.	Saves time and ensures that the venipuncture device is not displaced once inserted. Transparent dressings facilitate site assessment. Use of a nontransparent cover and antimicrobial ointment is controversial and is dependent on agency policy.
IMPLEMENTATION	
Wash hands or perform hand antisepsis with an alcohol rub (see Chap. 10).	Reduces the number of microorganisms.
Apply a tourniquet or a blood pressure cuff 2 to 4 in. (5 to 10 cm) above the vein that will be used.	Distends the vein.
Use an antimicrobial solution such as Betadine and/or alcohol to cleanse the skin, starting at the center of the site outward 2 to 4 in. (see Fig. B).	Reduces the potential for infection.
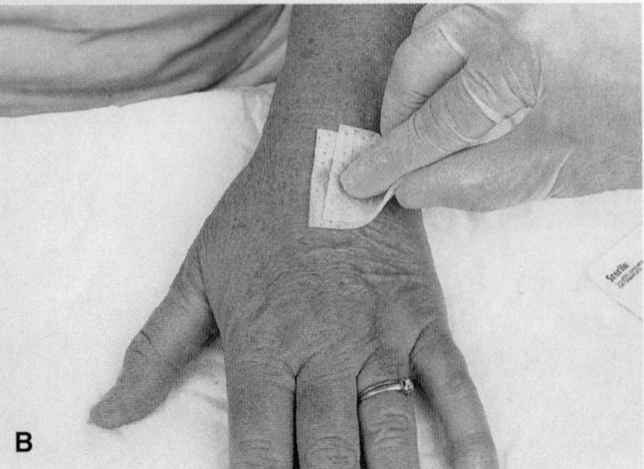 B	Swabbing the site. (Photo by B. Proud.)

(continued)

Starting an Intravenous Infusion (continued)

IMPLEMENTATION (CONTINUED)

Allow the antiseptic to dry. — Potentiates the effectiveness of antiseptic and prevents burning when the needle is inserted.

Don clean gloves. — Provides a barrier for blood-borne viruses.

Use the thumb to stretch and stabilize the vein and soft tissues about 2 in. (5 cm) below the intended site of entry (see Fig. C). — Helps straighten the vein and prevents it from moving around underneath the skin.

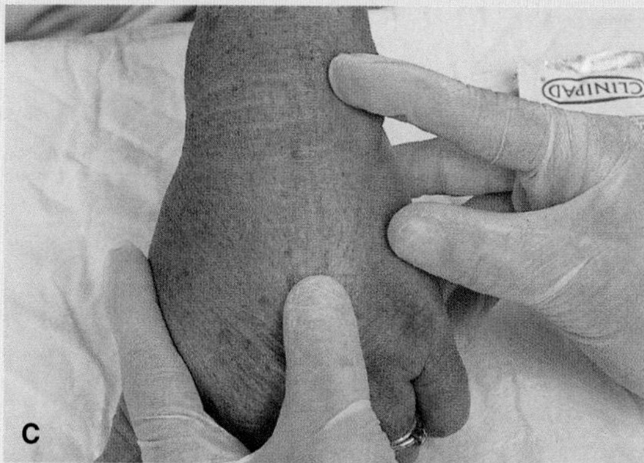

Stabilizing the vein. (Photo by B. Proud.)

Position the venipuncture device with the bevel up and at approximately a 45-degree angle above or to the side of the vein (see Fig. D). — Facilitates piercing the vein.

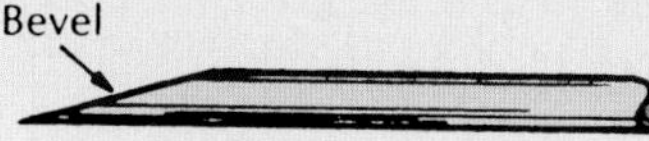

Placing the bevel up.

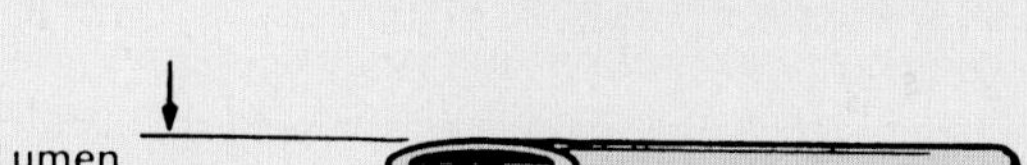

Warn the client just before inserting the needle. — Prepares the client for discomfort.

Feel for a change in resistance and look for blood to appear behind the needle. — Indicates the vein has been pierced.

Once blood is observed, advance the needle about ⅛ in. to ¼ in. (see Fig. E). — Positions the catheter tip within the inner wall of the vein.

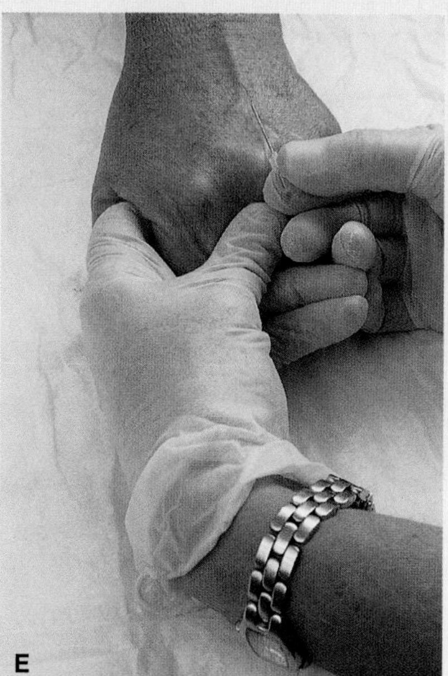

Advancing the needle tip. (Photo by B. Proud.)

(continued)

Starting an Intravenous Infusion (continued)

IMPLEMENTATION (CONTINUED)

Withdraw the needle slightly so that the tip is within the catheter.	Prevents puncturing the outside of the vein wall.
Slide the catheter into the vein until only the end of the infusion device can be seen.	Ensures full insertion of the catheter.
Release the tourniquet.	Reduces venous pressure and restores circulation.
Apply pressure over the internal tip of the catheter.	Limits blood loss.
Remove the protective cap covering the end of the IV tubing and insert it into the end of the venipuncture device.	Facilitates infusing the solution.
Release the roller clamp and begin infusing the solution slowly.	Clears blood from the venipuncture device before it can clot.
Remove gloves when there is no longer a potential for direct contact with blood.	Facilitates handling tape.
	Reduces the potential for infection.
Secure the catheter by criss crossing a piece of tape from beneath the tubing. Cover the site according to agency policy (see Fig. F).	Prevents catheter displacement.

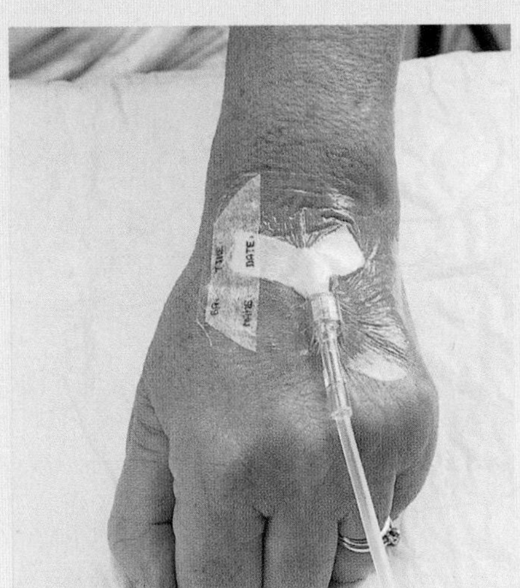

Stabilizing the catheter. (Photo by B. Proud.)

Apply additional strips of tape, taking care to loop and secure the tubing (see Fig. G).	Prevents tension on the tubing that may cause displacement.

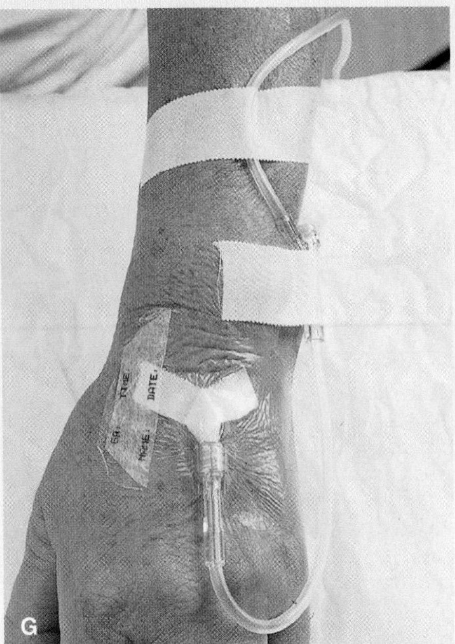

Securing the tubing. (Photo by B. Proud.)

(continued)

Starting an Intravenous Infusion (continued)

Suggested Action	Reason for Action
IMPLEMENTATION (CONTINUED)	
Write the date, time, gauge of the catheter, and your initials on the site dressing or the outer piece of tape.	Provides a quick reference for determining when the site must be changed.
Tighten or release the roller clamp to regulate the rate of fluid infusion.	Facilitates compliance with the medical order.

Evaluation

- A flashback of blood was observed before advancing the catheter.
- Minimal discomfort and blood loss occurred.
- Fluid is infusing at the prescribed rate.

Document

- Date and time
- Gauge and type of venipuncture device
- Site of venipuncture
- Type and volume of solution
- Rate of infusion

SAMPLE DOCUMENTATION

Date and Time No. 20 gauge over-the-needle catheter inserted into vein in L. forearm. 1,000 mL 0.9% saline infusing at 42 gtt/min. —————— SIGNATURE/TITLE

SKILL 16-4 Changing Intravenous Solution Containers

Suggested Action	Reason for Action
ASSESSMENT	
Assess the volume that remains in the infusing container and the rate at which it is infusing.	Helps establish when the solution will need to be replaced.
Check the medication record or physician's orders to determine what solution is to follow the current infusion.	Ensures compliance with the medical order.
PLANNING	
Obtain the replacement solution well in advance of needing it.	Ensures that the infusion will be uninterrupted.
Attach a time strip to the new container indicating the date, your initials, and the hourly infusion volumes.	Avoids having to complete this responsibility later.
Organize client care to change the container when the current infusion becomes low.	Demonstrates efficient time management.
IMPLEMENTATION	
Check the identity of the client.	Prevents errors.
Wash hands or perform hand antisepsis with an alcohol rub (see Chap. 10).	Reduces the transmission of microorganisms.
Tighten the roller clamp slightly or slow the rate of infusion on an infusion device.	Slows the rate of infusion so that the drip chamber remains filled with solution.
Remove the almost empty solution container from the suspension hook with the tubing still attached.	Facilitates separating the tubing from the container.
Invert the empty solution container and pull the spike free.	Prevents minor loss of remaining solution.
Deposit the empty bag in a lined waste receptacle.	Keeps the environment clean and orderly.
Remove the seal from the replacement solution container.	Provides access to the port.
Insert the spike into the port of the new container.	Provides a route for infusing fluid.
Hang the new container from the suspension hook on the IV standard or infusion device.	Restores height to overcome venous pressure.
Inspect for the presence of air within the tubing; remove it if present.	Reduces the potential for air embolism or an alarm from an infusion device detecting air.
Readjust the roller clamp or reprogram the infusion device to restore the prescribed rate of infusion.	Demonstrates compliance with the medical order.

(continued)

Changing Intravenous Solution Containers (continued)

Evaluation
- Solution container is replaced.
- Infusion continues.

Document
- Volume infused from previous container on I&O record
- Time, volume, type of solution, and signature on the medication record or wherever the agency specifies documenting the administration of IV solutions
- Condition of the client

SAMPLE DOCUMENTATION

Date and Time 1,000 mL lactated Ringer's instilling at 42 gtt/min. Dressing over venipuncture is dry and intact. No swelling or discomfort in the area of the infusing fluid. ———— SIGNATURE/TITLE

SKILL 16-5 Changing Intravenous Tubing

Suggested Action	Reason for Action
ASSESSMENT	
Determine the agency's policy for changing IV tubing.	Demonstrates responsibility for complying with infection control policies.
Check the date and time on the label attached to the tubing.	Determines the approximate time when the tubing must be changed.
Determine whether the solution container will need to be replaced before the time expires on the tubing.	Facilitates changing both the container and the tubing at the same time.
PLANNING	
Obtain appropriate replacement tubing and supplies for changing the dressing.	Ensures that equipment will be available and ready when needed.
Attach a new label to the tubing indicating the date and time the tubing is changed and your initials.	Provides a quick reference for determining when the tubing must be changed again.
IMPLEMENTATION	
Wash hands or perform hand antisepsis with an alcohol rub (see Chap. 10).	Reduces the transmission of microorganisms.
Tear strips of adhesive tape and prepare dressing materials and place them in a convenient location.	Facilitates dexterity later in the procedure.
Open the new package containing the tubing, stretch the tubing, and tighten the roller clamp.	Prepares the tubing for insertion into the solution container.
Remove the solution container from the suspension hook with the tubing still attached.	Facilitates separating the tubing from the container.
Invert the solution container and pull the spike free.	Prevents the minor loss of remaining solution.
Secure the spike to the IV pole with a strip of previously torn tape.	Facilitates continued infusion.
Insert the spike from the new tubing into the container of solution.	Provides a route for the fluid.
Squeeze the drip chamber to fill it half full, open the roller clamp, and purge the air from the tubing.	Prepares the tubing for use.
Remove the tape and dressing from the venipuncture site.	Provides access to the venipuncture device.
Don gloves.	Provides a barrier from contact with blood.
Tighten the roller clamp on the expired tubing.	Temporarily interrupts the infusion.
Stabilize the hub of the venipuncture device and separate the tubing from it.	Prevents accidental removal of the catheter or needle from the vein.
Remove the cap from the end of the new tubing and attach it to the end of the venipuncture device.	Connects the venipuncture device to the tubing without contaminating the tip of the tubing.
Continue to hold the venipuncture device with one hand while releasing the roller clamp on the new tubing.	Reestablishes the infusion.

(continued)

Changing IV Tubing (continued)

Suggested Action	Reason for Action
IMPLEMENTATION (CONTINUED)	
Replace the dressing on the venipuncture site and secure the tubing.	Covers the site and keeps the tubing and venipuncture device from being pulled out.
Readjust the rate of infusion.	Complies with the medical order.
Write the date, time, and your initials on the new dressing, and include the gauge of the venipuncture device and original date of insertion.	Provides a quick reference for determining future nursing responsibilities for infection control.
Dispose of the expired tubing in a lined receptacle.	Maintains a clean and orderly environment.

Evaluation

- Tubing is replaced.
- Solution continues to infuse at the prescribed rate.

Document

- Date and time
- Assessment findings of venipuncture site
- Dressing change

SAMPLE DOCUMENTATION

Date and Time No redness, swelling, or tenderness at venipuncture site in L. forearm. Dressing changed following replacement of IV tubing. ——— SIGNATURE/TITLE

SKILL 16-6 Discontinuing an Intravenous Infusion

Suggested Action	Reason for Action
ASSESSMENT	
Confirm that the physician has written an order to discontinue the infusion of IV fluid.	Demonstrates responsibility and accountability for carrying out medical orders.
Check the client's identity.	Prevents errors.
PLANNING	
Assemble necessary equipment, which includes clean gloves, sterile gauze, and tape.	Promotes organization and efficient time management.
IMPLEMENTATION	
Wash hands or perform hand antisepsis with an alcohol rub (see Chap. 10).	Reduces the spread of microorganisms.
Clamp the tubing and remove the tape that holds the dressing and venipuncture device in place.	Facilitates removal without leaking fluid.
Don gloves.	Prevents contact with blood.
Press a gauze square gently over the site where the venipuncture device enters the skin.	Helps absorb blood.
Remove the catheter or needle by pulling it out without hesitation following the course of the vein.	Prevents discomfort and injury to the vein.

(continued)

Discontinuing an Intravenous Infusion (continued)

IMPLEMENTATION (CONTINUED)

Action	Rationale
Apply pressure to the site of the venipuncture for 30 to 45 seconds while elevating the forearm (Fig. A).	Pressure and elevation control bleeding.

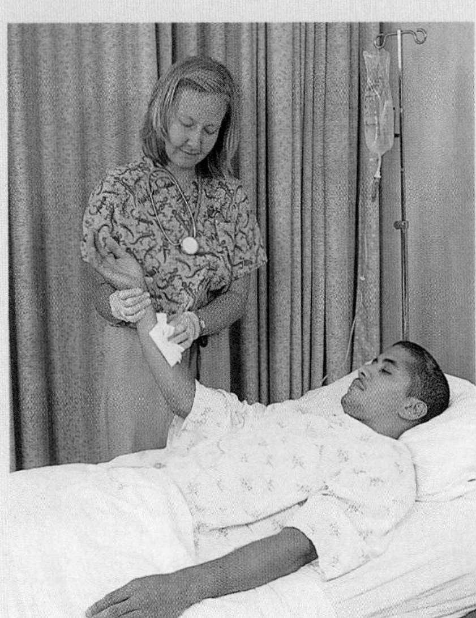

Applying pressure to the venipuncture site. (Photo by B. Proud.)

Action	Rationale
Secure the gauze with tape.	Acts as a dressing to reduce the potential for infection.
Dispose of the venipuncture device in a sharps container if it is a needle.	Prevents accidental needle-stick injuries and the transmission of blood-borne infectious microorganisms.
Enclose a catheter used for venipuncture within a glove as they are removed and discarded within a lined waste container.	Facilitates disposal and prevents contact with blood.
Wash hands or perform hand antisepsis with an alcohol rub (see Chap. 10) after glove disposal.	Removes transient microorganisms.
Encourage the client to flex and extend the arm or hand several times.	Helps the client to regain sensation and mobility.
Record the amount of intravenous fluid that the client received before discontinuing the infusion on the I&O sheet.	Contributes to an accurate record of fluid intake.
Document the time the infusion was discontinued and the condition of the venipuncture site.	Demonstrates responsibility and accountability for the client's care.

Evaluation

- Site appears free of inflammation.
- Bleeding is controlled.
- Discomfort is minimized or absent.
- Equipment is disposed in a manner to prevent injury and transmission of infection.

Document

- Date and time
- Condition of venipuncture site
- Volume of infused solution

SAMPLE DOCUMENTATION

Date and Time Infusion of Ringer's lactate discontinued per physician's order following administration of 1,000 mL. No. 22 gauge angiocatheter removed from left forearm. No redness, swelling, or drainage evident at site of venipuncture. Venipuncture site covered with a dry sterile dressing. ——— SIGNATURE/TITLE

SKILL 16-7 Inserting a Medication Lock

Suggested Action	Reason for Action
ASSESSMENT	
Confirm that the physician has written an order to discontinue the continuous infusion of IV fluid and insert a medication lock.	Demonstrates responsibility and accountability for carrying out medical orders.
Check the client's identity.	Prevents errors.
Inspect the site for signs of redness, swelling, or drainage.	Provides data indicating whether the site can be maintained or a new venipuncture should be performed.
Observe whether the infusion is instilling at the predetermined rate.	Indicates whether the vein and catheter are patent (open).
Determine whether the client understands the purpose and technique for inserting a medication lock.	Indicates the need for client teaching.
PLANNING	
Assemble necessary equipment, which includes the medication lock, syringe containing 2 mL of sterile normal saline (0.9% sodium chloride, depending on the agency's policy), alcohol swabs, gloves, and supplies for changing or reinforcing the dressing over the site.	Promotes organization and efficient time management.
IMPLEMENTATION	
Wash hands or perform hand antisepsis with an alcohol rub (see Chap. 10).	Reduces the spread of microorganisms.
Fill the chamber of the medication lock with saline solution.	Displaces air from the empty chamber.
Loosen the tape over the dressing to expose the connection between the hub of the catheter or needle and the tubing adapter; also remove the tape that is stabilizing the tubing to the client's arm.	Facilitates removing the tubing from the client.
Loosen the protective cap from the end of the medication lock.	Maintains sterility while preparing for the insertion of the lock.
Don clean gloves.	Provides a barrier from contact with blood.
Tighten the roller clamp on the tubing and stop the infusion pump or controller if one is being used.	Prevents leakage of fluid when the tubing is removed.
Apply pressure over the tip of the catheter or needle (see Fig. A).	Controls or prevents blood loss.

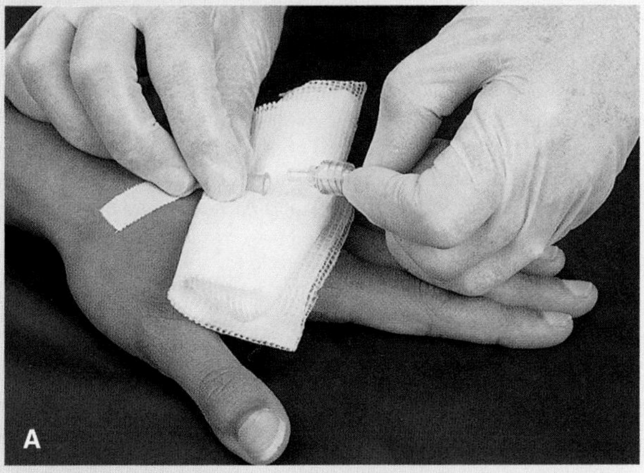

A

Applying pressure over the catheter tip. (Photo by B. Proud.)

Suggested Action	Reason for Action
Remove the tip of the tubing from the venipuncture device and insert the medication lock (see Fig. B).	Seals the opening in the catheter or needle.

(continued)

Inserting a Medication Lock (continued)

IMPLEMENTATION (CONTINUED)

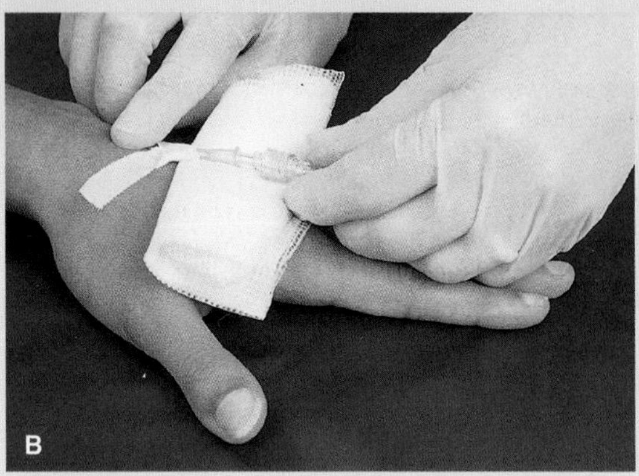

Inserting the device. (Photo by B. Proud.)

Action	Rationale
Screw the lock onto the end of the catheter or needle.	Stabilizes the connection.
Swab the rubber port on the medication lock with alcohol.	Cleanses the port.
Pierce the port with the blunt needleless adapter and gradually instill 2 mL of saline until the syringe is almost empty (see Fig. C).	Clears blood from the venipuncture device and lock before it can clot.

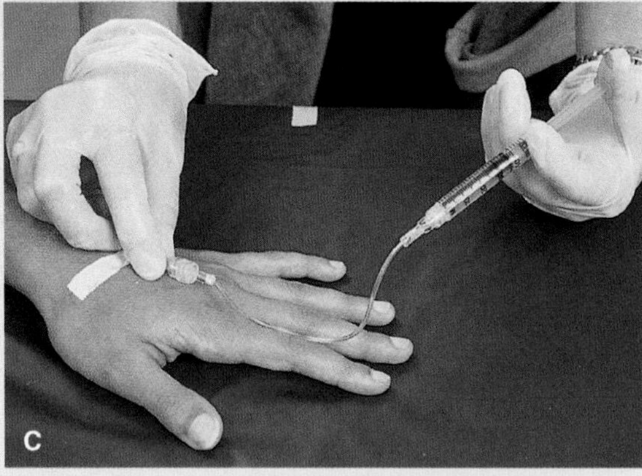

Instilling saline solution. (Photo by B. Proud.)

Action	Rationale
Begin to remove the syringe from the port as the last volume of solution is instilled; clamp or pinch the tubing, or press over the venipuncture device before removing a needleless adapter.	Continues the application of positive pressure (pushing effect) rather than negative pressure (pulling effect) during the time the syringe is removed. Negative pressure pulls blood into the catheter or needle tip, which may cause an obstruction.
Retape or secure the dressing.	Reduces the possibility that the lock and catheter may be accidentally dislodged.
Plan to flush the lock after each use or at least every 8 hours with 1 or 2 mL of flush solution depending on agency policy.	Ensures continued patency.

Evaluation

- Site appears free of inflammation.
- Patency is maintained.
- Flush solution instills easily.
- Device is stabilized.

Document

- Date and time
- Discontinuation of infusing solution
- Volume of infused IV solution
- Insertion of medication lock
- Volume and type of flush solution
- Assessment findings

SAMPLE DOCUMENTATION

Date and Time Infusion of 5% D/W discontinued. 700 mL of IV solution infused. Medication lock inserted into IV catheter in R. hand and flushed with 2 mL of normal saline. No redness, swelling, or discomfort at site. ——— SIGNATURE/TITLE

SKILL 16-8 Administering a Blood Transfusion

Suggested Action	Reason for Action
ASSESSMENT	
Check the client's identity.	Prevents errors.
Determine whether a special signed consent is required.	Complies with legal responsibilities.
Check the gauge of the current venipuncture device if an IV is infusing.	Indicates whether another venipuncture must be performed.
Review the medical record for results of type and cross-match.	Indicates whether blood is available in the blood bank.
Take temperature, pulse, respirations, and blood pressure within 30 minutes of obtaining blood.	Provides a baseline for comparison during the transfusion.
PLANNING	
Complete major nursing activities before starting the infusion of saline unless the blood must be given immediately.	Avoids disturbing the client once the blood is administered.
Plan to perform a venipuncture or start the infusion of saline just before obtaining the blood.	Prevents administering fluid unnecessarily.
Obtain necessary equipment including a 250-mL container of normal saline (0.9% NaCl) and a Y-set.	Complies with the standards of care for administering blood.
Tighten the roller clamp on one branch of the Y-tubing and the roller clamp below the filter.	Prepares the tubing for purging with saline.
Insert the unclamped branch of the Y-set into the container of saline; squeeze the drip chamber until it and the filter are half full.	Moistens the filter and fills the upper portion of the tubing with saline.
Release the lower clamp and flush air from the remaining section of tubing.	Reduces the potential for infusing a bolus of air.
IMPLEMENTATION	
Perform the venipuncture or connect the Y-set to the present venipuncture device if it is a 16–20 gauge.	Provides access to the venous circulation and ensures that blood will move freely through the catheter or needle.
Begin the infusion of saline.	Ensures that the site is patent and that there will be no delay once the unit of blood is obtained.
Go to the blood bank to pick up the unit of blood, making sure to take a form identifying the client.	Prevents mistaken identity when releasing the matched blood.
Double check the information on the blood bag with the cross-matched information on the lab slip with the blood bank personnel.	Prevents releasing the wrong unit of blood or blood that is not a compatible blood group and Rh factor.
Check that the blood has not passed the expiration date.	Ensures maximum benefit from the transfusion.
Inspect the container of blood and reject the blood if it appears dark black or has obvious gas bubbles inside.	Indicates deteriorated or tainted blood.
Plan to give the blood as soon as it is brought to the unit.	Demonstrates an understanding that blood must be totally infused within 4 hours after being released from the blood bank.
Rotate the blood, but do not shake or squeeze the container if the serum has separated from the cells.	Avoids damaging intact cells.
At the bedside, check the label on the blood bag with the numbers on the client's wristband with a second nurse; sign in the designated areas on the transfusion record.	Reduces the potential for administering incompatible blood.
Spike the container of blood.	Provides a route for administering the blood.
Tighten the roller clamp on the saline branch of the tubing and release the roller clamp on the blood branch.	Fills the tubing and filter with blood.
Regulate the rate of infusion at no more than 50 mL/hr for the first 15 minutes (check the drop factor to determine the rate in gtt/min).	Establishes a slow rate of infusion so that the nurse can monitor for and respond to signs of a transfusion reaction.
Increase the rate after the first 15 minutes to complete the infusion in 2 to 4 hours if a second assessment of vital signs is basically unchanged and no signs of a reaction have occurred.	Increases the rate of administration to infuse the unit within a safe period.
Assess the client at 15- to 30-minute intervals during the transfusion.	Ensures client safety.
Clamp the tubing from the blood and release the clamp on the saline when the blood has infused.	Flushes blood cells from the tubing.
Take vital signs one more time.	Documents the condition of the client at the completion of the blood administration.
Tighten the roller clamp below the filter when the tubing looks reasonably clear of blood.	Prevents leaking when the IV is discontinued.

(continued)

Administering a Blood Transfusion (continued)

IMPLEMENTATION (CONTINUED)

Don gloves.	Provides a barrier from contact with blood.
Loosen the tape covering the venipuncture site and remove the catheter, or remove the blood tubing and reconnect the previously infusing solution.	Discontinues the infusion or restores previous fluid therapy.
Apply a dressing or Band-Aid over the venipuncture site if the IV is discontinued.	Prevents infection.
Dispose of the blood container and tubing according to agency policy.	Blood is a biohazard and requires special bagging to ensure that others will not accidentally come in direct contact with the blood.

Evaluation

- Entire unit of blood is administered within 4 hours.
- Client demonstrates no evidence of transfusion reaction
- Reactions have been minimized by appropriate interventions.
- Infusion is discontinued or previous orders are resumed.

Document

- Venipuncture procedure, if initiated for the administration of blood
- Preinfusion vital signs
- Names of nurses who checked armband and blood bag container
- Time blood administration began
- Rate of infusion during first 15 minutes and remaining period of time
- Signs of reaction, if any, and nursing actions
- Periodic vital sign assessments
- Time blood infusion completed
- Volume of blood and saline infused

SAMPLE DOCUMENTATION

Date and Time No. 18 gauge over-the-needle catheter inserted into L. forearm and connected to 250 mL of 0.9% saline infusing at 21 mL/hr. T—98°F (tympanic), P—90, R—22, BP 116/64 in R. arm while lying flat. One unit of type O+ whole blood No.684381 obtained from the blood bank and checked by E. Rogers, RN, and D. Baker, RN. Blood bag and wrist band information found to be compatible. Blood infusing at 50 mL/hr for 15 minutes. Rate increased to 125 mL/hr during remainder of infusion. Blood transfusion completed at 1,600. No evidence of transfusion reaction. T—98°F (tympanic), P—86, R—20, BP 122/70 in R. arm at end of transfusion. Total of 100 mL of saline and 500 mL of blood infused before IV discontinued. ———— SIGNATURE/TITLE

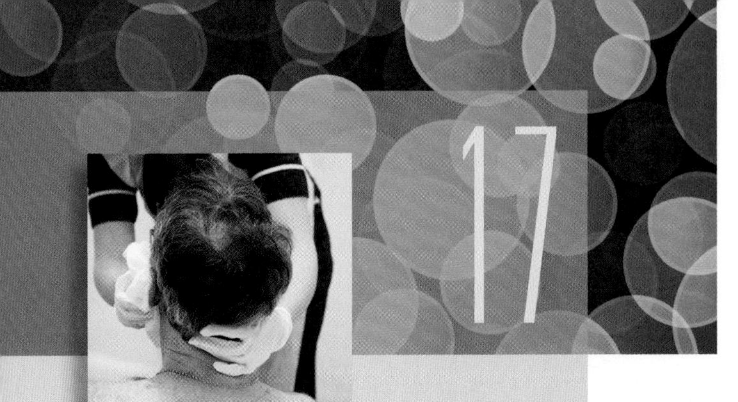

Hygiene

Words To Know

bag bath
bed bath
bridge
caries
cuticles
dentures
gingivitis
hygiene
integument
ophthalmologist
optometrist
oral hygiene
partial bath
perineal care
periodontal disease
plaque
podiatrist
sordes
tartar
towel bath

Learning Objectives

On completion of this chapter, the reader should be able to:

1. Define hygiene.
2. Name five hygiene practices that most people perform regularly.
3. Give two reasons why a partial bath is more appropriate than a daily bath for older adults.
4. List at least three advantages of towel or bag baths.
5. Name two situations in which shaving with a safety razor is contraindicated.
6. Name three items recommended for oral hygiene.
7. Identify two methods to prevent the chief hazard when providing oral hygiene to an unconscious client.
8. Describe two techniques for preventing damage to dentures during cleaning.
9. Describe two methods for removing hair tangles.
10. Name two types of clients for whom nail care is provided with extreme caution.
11. Name four visual and hearing devices.
12. List two alternatives for clients who cannot insert or care for their own contact lenses.
13. Discuss four reasons for sound disturbances experienced by people who wear hearing aids.
14. Describe an infrared-listening device.

Hygiene means those practices that help in promoting health through personal cleanliness. People foster hygiene through activities such as bathing, performing oral care, cleaning and maintaining fingernails and toenails, and shampooing and grooming hair. Hygiene also includes care and maintenance of devices such as eyeglasses and hearing aids to ensure continued and proper function. Hygiene practices and needs differ according to age, inherited characteristics of the skin and hair, cultural values, and the state of health.

This chapter provides suggestions to nurses for carrying out hygiene practices when providing client care. Principles that refer to the client's environment, such as bed-making skills, are discussed in Chapter 18.

THE INTEGUMENTARY SYSTEM

The word **integument** (covering) refers to the collective structures that cover the surface of the body and its openings. Most hygiene practices are based on maintaining or restoring a healthy integumentary system, which includes the skin, mucous membranes, hair, and nails. Because the

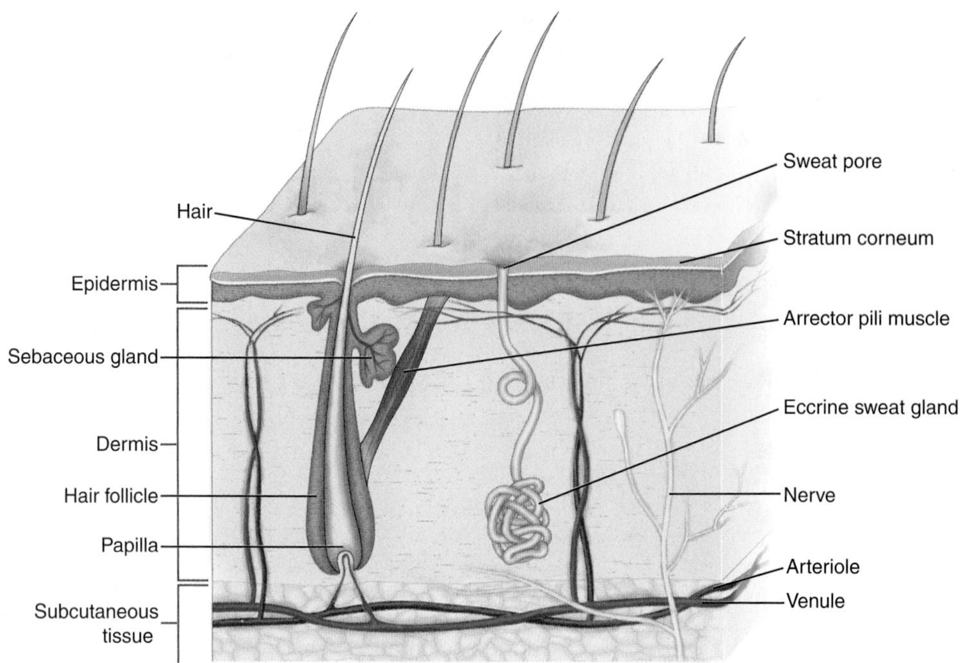

FIGURE 17-1 A cross-section of the skin.

mouth, or oral cavity (which is lined with mucous membrane), contains teeth, this chapter also discusses this accessory structure.

Skin

The skin consists of the epidermis, dermis, and subcutaneous layer (Fig. 17-1). The *epidermis,* or outermost layer, contains dead skin cells that form a tough protein called keratin. Keratin protects the layers and structures within the lower portions of the skin. The cells in the epidermis are shed continuously and replaced by the *dermis,* or true skin, which contains most of the secretory glands (Table 17-1). The *subcutaneous layer* separates the skin from skeletal muscles. It contains fat cells, blood vessels, nerves, and the roots of hair follicles and glands.

Skin structures carry out the following functions:

- Protect inner body structures from injury and infection
- Regulate body temperature
- Maintain fluid and chemical balance
- Provide sensory information such as pain, temperature, touch, and pressure
- Assist in converting precursors to vitamin D when exposed to sunlight

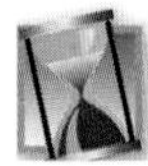

Gerontologic Considerations

■ Benign skin lesions such as *seborrheic keratoses* (tan to black raised areas on the trunk) and *senile lentigines* (brown, flat patches on the face, hands, and forearms) are common in older adults.

Mucous Membranes

The mucous membranes are continuous with the skin. They line body passages such as the digestive, respiratory, urinary, and reproductive systems. Mucous membranes also line the conjunctiva of the eye. Goblet cells in the mucous membranes

TABLE 17-1 Types of Skin Glands

GLAND	LOCATION	SECRETION	PURPOSE
Sudoriferous	Throughout the dermis and subcutaneous layers, especially in the axilla and groin	Sweat	Regulate body temperature Excrete body waste
Ceruminous	Ear canals	Cerumen	Perform protective functions; cerumen has antimicrobial properties
Sebaceous	Throughout the dermis	Sebum	Lubricate skin and hair
Ciliary	Eyelids	Sweat and sebum	Protect lid margin and lubricate eyelash follicles

secrete *mucus,* a slimy substance that keeps the membranes soft and moist.

Hair

Each hair is a thread of keratin. Hair is formed from the cells at the base of a single follicle. Although hair covers the entire body, its amount, distribution, color, and texture vary considerably according to location and among males and females, infants and adults, and ethnic groups.

In addition to contributing to a person's unique appearance, hair basically helps prevent heat loss. As heat escapes from the skin, it gets trapped in the air between the hairs. The contraction of small arrector pili muscles around hair follicles, commonly described as goose bumps, further generates body heat.

Sebaceous glands in the hair follicles release sebum, an oily secretion that adds weight to the shafts of hair, causing them to flatten against the skull. Oily hair further attracts dust and debris.

The texture, elasticity, and porosity of hair are inherited characteristics influenced by the amount of keratin and sebum produced. To alter the basic genetically inherited structure, some people use chemicals to curl, relax, or lubricate their hair.

Nails

Fingernails (Fig. 17-2) and toenails also are made of keratin, which in concentrated amounts, gives them their tough texture. Fingernails and toenails provide some protection to the digits. Normal nails are thin, pink, and smooth. The free margin ordinarily extends from the end of each finger or toe, and the skin around the nails is intact. Changes in the shape, color, texture, thickness, and integrity of the nails provide evidence of local injury or infection and even systemic diseases (see Chap. 13).

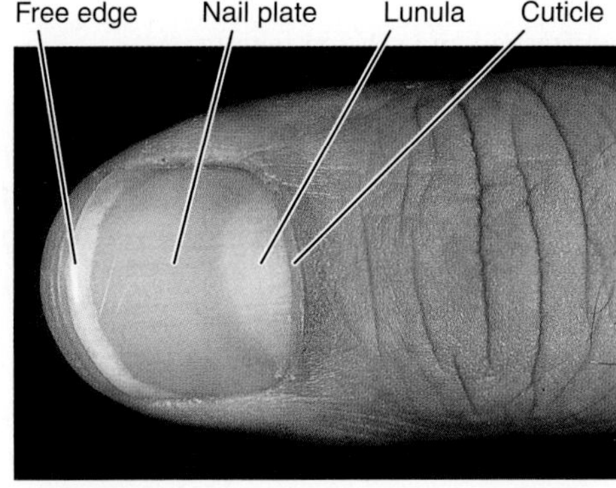

A External nail structures

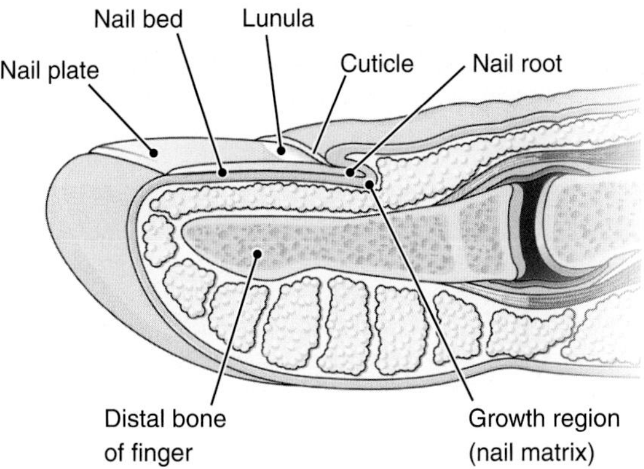

B Internal and external nail structures

FIGURE 17-2 The external and cross-sectional views of a nail. **A.** External nail structures. **B.** Internal and external nail structures.

Teeth

Teeth, the enamel of which is a keratin structure, are present beneath the gums at birth. The exposed portion of each tooth is referred to as the crown; the portion within the gum is the root (Fig. 17-3).

The teeth begin to erupt at about 6 months of age and continue to do so for 2 or 2½ more years. As the jaw grows, the *deciduous teeth* (baby teeth) are replaced by *permanent teeth.* Adults have 28 to 32 permanent teeth, depending on whether the third molars (wisdom teeth) are present.

Healthy teeth are firmly fixed within the gums. Their alignment, which is related to jaw structure, generally is a result of heredity. Although the teeth are white originally, they become discolored from chronic consumption of coffee or tea, tobacco use, or certain drugs such as tetracycline antibiotics taken during childhood.

The integrity of the teeth largely depends on the person's oral hygiene practices, diet, and general health. Saliva, which moistens food and begins the digestive processes, tends to keep the teeth clean and inhibits bacterial growth. The accumulation of food debris, especially sugar, and **plaque** (a substance composed of mucin and other gritty substances in saliva) supports the growth of mouth bacteria. The combination of sugar, plaque, and bacteria may eventually erode the tooth enamel, causing **caries** (cavities).

Tartar (hardened plaque) is more difficult to remove and may lead to **gingivitis** (inflammation of the gums). Pockets of gum inflammation promote **periodontal disease,** a condition that results in the destruction of the tooth-supporting structures and bones that make up the jaw.

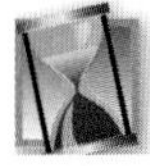

Gerontologic Considerations

- Tooth loss is common in older adults as a result of periodontal disease.

HYGIENE PRACTICES

The integument contains many secretory glands that produce odors and attract debris, and the teeth are prone to decay if uncared for. Therefore, hygiene measures are beneficial for maintaining personal cleanliness and healthy integumentary structures. Although hygiene practices vary widely, most Americans routinely perform bathing, shaving, brushing teeth, shampooing, and caring for nails.

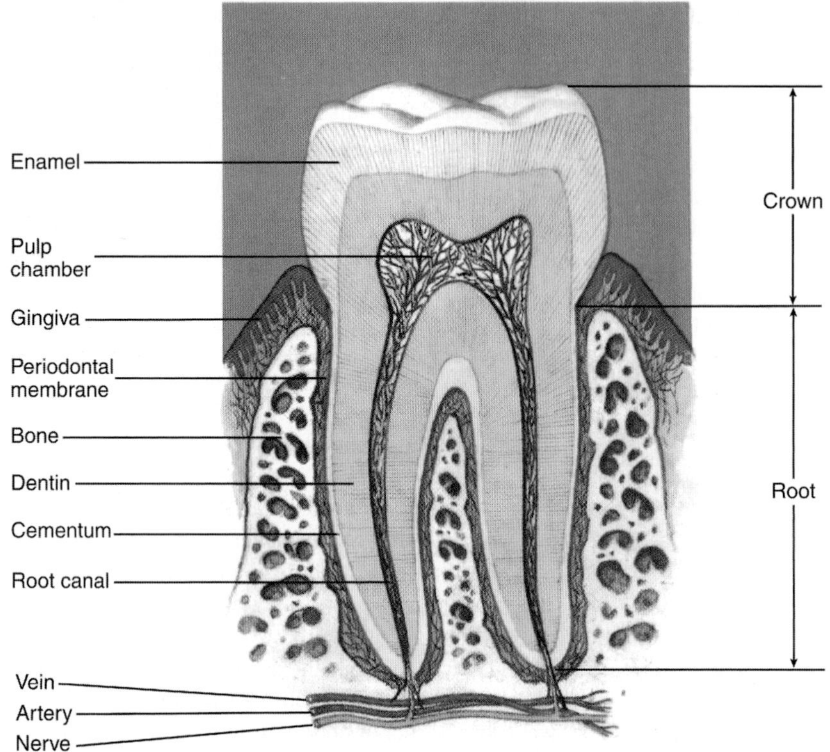

FIGURE 17-3 A cross-section of a tooth. (From Cohen B. [2010] *Medical terminology: An illustrated guide* [4th ed.]. Philadelphia: Lippincott Williams & Wilkins.)

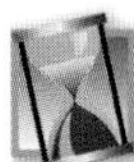

Gerontologic Considerations

■ Poor hygiene and grooming in older adults are often signs of visual impairment, functional changes, dementia, depression, abuse, or neglect.

Bathing

Bathing is a hygiene practice in which a person uses a cleansing agent such as soap and water to remove sweat, oil, dirt, and microorganisms from the skin. Although restoring cleanliness is the primary objective, bathing has several other benefits:

- Eliminating body odor
- Reducing the potential for infection
- Stimulating circulation
- Providing a refreshed and relaxed feeling
- Improving self-image

In addition to bathing for hygiene purposes, other types of bathing serve different functions (Table 17-2). In general, however, most bathing is done in a tub or shower, at a sink, or at the bedside.

Stop, Think, and Respond Box 17-1

How might a nurse respond to a client who believes that daily bathing is unnecessary or even unhealthy?

Tub Bath or Shower

If the safety risks are negligible and there are no contraindications, the nurse encourages clients to bathe independently in a tub or shower (Skill 17-1). Most hospitals and nursing

TABLE 17-2 Therapeutic Baths

TYPE	DESCRIPTION	PURPOSE
Sitz bath	Immersion of the buttocks and perineum in a small basin of continuously circulating water	Removes blood, serum, stool, or urine Reduces local swelling Relieves discomfort
Sponge bath	Applications of tepid water to the skin	Reduces a fever
Medicated bath	Soaking or immersing in a mixture of water and another substance, such as baking soda (sodium bicarbonate), oatmeal, or cornstarch	Relieves itching or a rash
Whirlpool bath	Warm water that is continuously agitated within a tub or tank	Improves circulation Increases joint mobility Relieves discomfort Removes dead tissue

homes equip bathing facilities with various rails and handles to promote client safety.

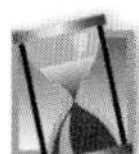

Gerontologic Considerations

- To reduce the risk of falls in older adults when bathing, nonskid strips on the floor of tubs and showers are helpful. Grab bars should be placed at arm level and within reach of the dominant hand.
- A tub or shower seat is an important safety measure for adults who have mobility limitations or difficulty maintaining balance.
- Diminished ability to sense temperature changes may occur with aging. The temperature of bath water should be checked with the wrist before immersing older adults.
- Long-handled bath sponges or hand held shower attachments help older adults with limited range of motion maintain independence.
- Older adults should use soap sparingly because it is extremely drying to the skin. A mild, superfatted, nonperfumed soap such as Castile, Dove, Tone, or Basis may be preferable.
- Because older adults have thin skin, decreased skin elasticity, and increased fragility of blood vessels in the dermis, gentle patting motions rather than harsh rubbing motions should be used when drying the skin.
- One should thoroughly inspect the feet of older adults for ulcerations or other lesions of which they are unaware.

Partial Bath

A daily bath or shower is not always necessary—in fact, for older adults, who perspire less than younger adults and are prone to dry skin, frequent washing with soap further depletes oil from the skin. Therefore, partial or less frequent bathing sometimes is appropriate. A **partial bath** means washing only those body areas that are subject to greatest soiling or that are sources of body odor: generally, the face, hands, axillae, and perineal area. Partial bathing is done at a sink or with a basin at the bedside.

Sometimes the *perineum,* the area around the genitals and rectum, requires special or frequent cleansing in addition to bathing. **Perineal care** (peri-care; techniques used to cleanse the perineum) is especially important after a vaginal delivery or gynecologic or rectal surgery so that the impaired skin remains as clean as possible. It is also appropriate whenever male or female clients have bloody drainage, urine, or stool collected in this area.

When providing perineal care, nurses must:

- Prevent direct contact between themselves and any secretions or excretions; this is generally accomplished by wearing clean gloves (see Standard Precautions in Chap. 22).
- Cleanse so that secretions and excretions are removed from less soiled to more soiled areas.

These principles help prevent the transfer of infectious microorganisms to the nurse and to uncontaminated areas on or within the client (Skill 17-2).

Stop, Think, and Respond Box 17-2

What suggestions can you make to promote the dignity of clients who need nursing assistance with perineal care?

Bed Bath

Clients who cannot take a tub bath or cannot shower independently may be given any one of three types of baths: a bed bath, a towel bath, or a bag bath. During a **bed bath** (washing with a basin of water at the bedside), the client may actively assist with some aspects of bathing. Skill 17-3 explains how to give a bed bath (also see Nursing Guidelines 17-1).

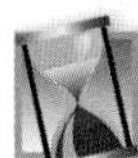

Gerontologic Considerations

- Bath oils can be added to a water basin when administering a bed bath to an older adult. Oils are not used in showers or bathtubs, however, because they increase the risk of falls.
- It is best to avoid the use of skin care products containing alcohol or perfumes when caring for older adults because they tend to aggravate dry skin conditions, cause allergic reactions, and over time, lotions may be a medium for bacterial growth.
- Increasing oral fluid intake or adding humidity to the air reduces the discomfort of dry skin experienced by older adults.

Some agencies use two variations of the traditional bed bath—the towel bath and the bag bath—because they save time and expense. Box 17-1 lists their advantages.

Towel Bath

With a **towel bath,** the nurse uses a single large towel to cover and wash a client. It requires a towel or bath sheet measuring 3 × 7.5 ft but no basin or soap. The nurse prefolds and moistens the towel or bath sheet with approximately one-half gallon (2 L) of water heated to 105° to 110°F (40° to 43°C) and 1 oz (30 mL) of no-rinse liquid cleanser. He or she unfolds the towel so that it covers the client and uses a separate section to wipe each part of the body, beginning at the feet and moving upward. The nurse folds the soiled areas of the towel to the inside as he or she bathes each area and allows the skin to air-dry for 2 to 3 seconds. After washing the front side of the body, the nurse positions the client on the side and repeats the procedure. He or she unfolds the towel so that the clean surface covers the client. The nurse bathes the client's back, and then the buttocks. When the towel bath is complete, the nurse changes the bed linens.

Bag Bath

A **bag bath** involves the use of a commercially packaged kit with 8 to 10 premoistened, disposable cloths in a plastic bag or container and is another form of a bed bath. The cloths contain a no-rinse *surfactant* (a substance that reduces

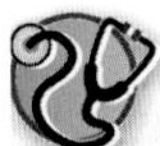

NURSING GUIDELINES 17-1

Bathing Clients

- Ask the client if he or she uses special soap, lotion, or other hygiene products. *Determining the client's preferences individualizes care.*
- Wear gloves if there is any potential for direct contact with blood, drainage, or other body fluid. *Gloves reduce the potential for acquiring an infection.*
- Keep the client covered during the bath. *Covering the client demonstrates respect for modesty.*
- Wash cleaner areas of the body first and dirtier areas last. *This reduces the spread of microorganisms.*
- Encourage the client to participate at whatever level is appropriate. *Participation promotes independence and self-esteem.*
- Monitor the client's tolerance of activity. *If activity becomes too strenuous, it should be discontinued and resumed later.*
- Inspect the body during washing for skin disorders (see Table 17-3). *Bathing provides an excellent opportunity for physical assessment.*
- Communicate with the client and use the occasion to do informal health teaching. *Talking demonstrates respect for the client as a person rather than an object being washed; teaching promotes health.*
- Wash one part of the body at a time. *Exposing only one part prevents chilling.*
- Place a towel under the part of the body being washed. *A towel absorbs moisture.*
- Use firm but gentle strokes. *Gentle strokes avoid friction that can damage the skin.*
- Wash and dry well between folds of skin. *Effective washing removes debris and microorganisms from areas where they are apt to breed.*
- Keep the washcloth wet, but not so wet that it drips. *This demonstrates concern for the client's comfort.*
- Wash more soiled areas, such as the anus, last. *Doing so prevents transferring microorganisms to cleaner areas of the body.*
- Remove all soap residues. *This prevents drying of the skin and possible itching.*
- Dry the skin after it has been rinsed. *Drying the skin prevents chilling.*
- Replace the water as it cools. *Using warm water shows concern for the client's comfort.*
- Apply an emollient lotion to the skin after bathing. *A lotion restores lubrication to the skin.*

surface tension between the skin and surface contaminants) and an *emollient/humectant* (a substance that attracts and traps moisture in the skin), but no soap. The nurse warms the container and its contents in a microwave or warming unit or sets them in a container of warm water before use. At the bedside, the nurse uses a separate cloth to wash each part of the client's body. Rinsing is not required. Air-drying circumvents the need for a towel.

Stop, Think, and Respond Box 17-3

Which method of bathing (shower, tub bath, bed/towel/bag bath) is appropriate for (1) a 75-year-old woman with arthritis of the hips; (2) a 60-year-old man with frequent seizures; (3) a 65-year-old man who becomes short of breath with exertion; and (4) a 72-year-old woman recovering from pneumonia? Explain the reasons for your answers.

Shaving

Shaving removes unwanted body hair. In the United States, most men shave their face daily, and most women shave their axillae and legs regularly. The nurse respects personal or cultural differences and asks each client about his or her preferences before assuming otherwise.

Shaving is accomplished with an electric or a safety razor. In some circumstances, use of a safety razor is contraindicated (Box 17-2), and an electric or battery-operated

BOX 17-1 Advantages of Towel or Bag Baths

- Reduce the potential for skin impairment because the nonrinsable cleanser lubricates rather than dries the skin
- Prevent the transmission of microorganisms that may be growing in wash basins
- Reduce the spread of microorganisms from one part of the body to another because separate cloths or regions of the towel are used
- Preserve the integrity of the skin because friction is not used while drying the skin
- Promote self-care among clients who may lack the strength or dexterity to wet, wring, and lather a washcloth
- Save time compared to conventional bathing
- Promote comfort because the moist towel or cloths are used so quickly, and they are warmer when applied

BOX 17-2 Contraindications to Using a Safety Razor

Use of a safety razor is contraindicated for clients:

- Receiving anticoagulants (drugs that interfere with clotting)
- Receiving thrombolytic agents (drugs that dissolve blood clots)
- Taking high doses of aspirin
- With blood disorders such as hemophilia
- With liver disease who have impaired clotting
- With rashes or elevated or inflamed skin lesions on or near the face
- Who are suicidal

TABLE 17-3 Examples of Integumentary Disorders

CONDITION	DESCRIPTION	CLIENT TEACHING
Acne	Inflammation of sebaceous glands and hair follicles on the face, upper chest, and back	Keep the face clean Refrain from touching or squeezing lesions Avoid the use of oily cosmetics
Contact dermatitis	Allergic sensitivity evidenced by red skin rash and itching	Avoid scratching or wearing clothing made of irritating fibers, such as wool Use tepid water and hypoallergenic or glycerin soap when bathing Pat the skin dry; do not rub
Furuncle (boil)	Raised pustule, usually in the neck, axillary, or groin area that feels hard and painful	Keep hands away from the infected lesion Use separate face cloth and towels from the rest of the family; launder personal bath items in hot water and bleach Wash hands thoroughly before and after applying medication to the skin
Psoriasis	Noninfectious chronic skin disorder that appears as elevated silvery scales that shed over elbows, knees, trunk, and scalp; acute episodes occur between periods of relief	Follow medical regimen, which may be lifelong Be wary of advertised remedies that promise a cure or quick relief, because they rarely do
Pediculosis (lice infestation)	Brown crawling insects that move over the scalp and skin and deposit yellowish-white eggs on hair shafts including pubic area; skin bite causes itching	Inspect the skin carefully as adult lice move quickly from light Look for eggs (nits) on hairs ¼ in. to ½ in. from the scalp or skin surface Do not share clothing, combs, and brushes; lice are spread by direct contact Use a pediculicide (chemical that kills lice), in addition to a lice comb and manual removal Do not use hair conditioner: it coats the hair and protects the nits
Scabies	Infestation with an itch mite that burrows within the webs and sides of fingers, around arms, axilla, waist, breast, lower buttocks, and genitalia	Bathe thoroughly in the morning and at night Apply prescribed medication after bathing Don clean clothes after bathing Avoid skin-to-skin contact with uninfected people
Tinea capitis, pedis, corporis, and cruris	Fungal infection in the scalp, feet, body, or groin that appears as a ring or cluster of papules or vesicles that cause itching, become scaly, cracked, and sore	Use separate bathing and grooming articles Keep body areas dry, especially in folds of skin Wear clothing that promotes evaporation of perspiration
Skin cancer	Newly pigmented growth or change in existing skin lesion, especially where skin is chronically exposed to sun	See a physician for examination and possible biopsy Avoid direct sun exposure between 10 AM and 4 PM Recommend using a sunscreen with an SPF ≥15 Wear a wide-brimmed hat on sunny days Do not use artificial tanning facilities
Fungal nail infection	Thick, yellowed, rough-appearing toenails or fingernails that can spread from one nail to others	Consult a physician about prescription drugs, which are approximately 50% effective Wear leather shoes, and alternate pairs to reduce damp shoe conditions Be aware that unsanitary utensils used in the application of artificial fingernails can spread the fungus Seek professional nail care from a podiatrist
Candidiasis	Yeast infection of the mouth or vagina; oral candidiasis appears as white patches or red spots on the tongue, gums, or throat; vaginal candidiasis appears as a thick, cottage cheese-like discharge that causes itching and burning	Follow directions for oral or topical antifungal medications Swish antifungal mouth rinses, retain the solution in the mouth as long as possible, and then swallow the rinse Avoid simple sugars and alcohol because they promote the growth of yeast Eat yogurt that contains live *Lactobacillus acidophilus* to restore a balance of helpful to harmful microbes

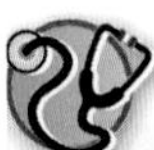

NURSING GUIDELINES 17-2

Shaving Clients

- Prepare a basin of warm water, soap, a face cloth, and a towel. *These supplies are necessary for wetting, rinsing, and lathering the face (or other area that requires shaving).*
- Wash the skin with warm, soapy water. *Washing removes oil, which helps raise hair shafts.*
- Lather the skin with soap or shaving cream. *Use of soap or shaving cream reduces surface tension as the razor is pulled across the skin.*
- Start at the upper areas of the face (or other area that requires shaving) and work down (see Fig. 17-4). *This progression provides more control of the razor.*
- Pull the skin taut below the area to be shaved. *This evens the level of the skin.*
- Pull the razor in the direction of hair growth. *Shaving with the hair reduces the potential for irritation.*
- Use short strokes. *They provide more control of the razor.*
- Rinse the razor after each stroke or as hair accumulates. *Rinsing keeps the cutting edge of the razor clean.*
- Rinse the remaining soap or shaving cream from the skin. *Rinsing reduces the potential for drying the skin.*
- Apply direct pressure to areas that bleed, or apply alum sulfate (styptic pencil) at the site of bleeding. *Pressure or alum helps to promote clotting.*
- Apply aftershave lotion, cologne, or cream to the shaved area if the client desires it. *The alcohol in lotion and cologne reduces and retards microbial growth in the tiny abrasions caused by the razor; cream restores oil to the skin.*

razor is used. When the client cannot shave, the nurse assumes responsibility for this hygiene practice (see Nursing Guidelines 17-2 and Fig. 17-4).

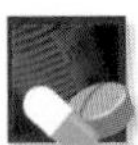

Pharmacologic Considerations

- Anticoagulants—even daily low-dose aspirin therapy—increase the potential for bleeding. An electric shaver may be substituted for a safety razor.

Oral Hygiene

Oral hygiene consists of those practices used to clean the mouth, especially brushing and flossing the teeth. Dentures and bridges also require special cleaning and care.

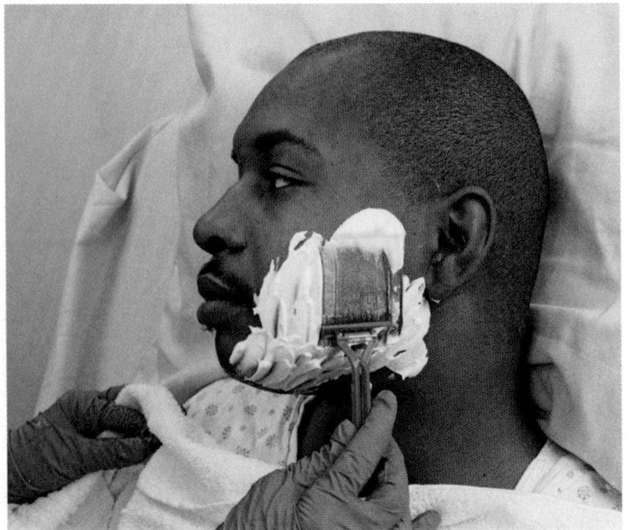

FIGURE 17-4 Shaving a client's face.

Tooth Brushing and Flossing

Clients who are alert and physically capable generally attend to their own oral hygiene. For clients confined to a bed, the nurse assembles the necessary items—a toothbrush, toothpaste, a glass of water, an emesis basin, and floss.

Most dentists recommend using a soft-bristled or electric toothbrush and toothpaste twice a day. For the advantages of electric toothbrushes, see Box 17-3. Flossing removes plaque and food debris from the surfaces of teeth that a manual or electric toothbrush may miss. The choice of unwaxed or waxed floss is personal. Waxed floss is thicker and more difficult to insert between teeth; unwaxed floss frays more quickly.

Although conscientious oral hygiene does not prevent dental problems completely, it reduces the incidence of tooth and gum disease. Therefore, clients need to learn how to maintain the structure and integrity of their natural teeth (see Client and Family Teaching 17-1 and Fig. 17-5).

BOX 17-3 Advantages of Electric Toothbrushes

- Last longer than manual toothbrushes
- Promote a full 2 min of toothbrushing with a built-in timer
- Remove 30% more plaque than manual toothbrushing
- Have a higher reduction of gingivitis compared with manual toothbrushing
- Decrease gingival trauma and gum recession because of less force used in brushing
- Facilitate self-care among clients with disabilities or reduced manual dexterity

Electric vs. manual toothbrushes. (2008). http://tips4dentalcare.com/2008/07/29/electric-vs-manual-toothbrushes. Accessed March 9, 2010.

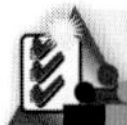

Client and Family Teaching 17-1
Reducing Dental Disease and Injuries

The nurse teaches the client or family as follows:

- Brush and floss the teeth as soon as possible after each meal, using the following techniques:
- Moisten the toothbrush and apply toothpaste.
- Hold a manual toothbrush at a 45-degree angle to the teeth.
- Brush the front and back of all teeth from gum line toward crown, using circular motions (see Fig. 17-5).
- Brush back and forth over the chewing surfaces of the molars.
- Rinse the mouth periodically to flush loosened debris.
- Wrap an 18-inch length of floss around the middle fingers of each hand.
- Slide the floss between two teeth until it is next to the gum.
- Move the floss back and forth.
- Repeat flossing with new sections of the floss until all the teeth have been flossed including the outer surface of the last molar.
- Use a tartar-control toothpaste or rinse containing fluoride.
- If brushing is impossible, rinse the mouth with water after eating.
- Use a battery-operated oral irrigating device, which uses pulsating jets of water to flush debris from teeth, bridges, or braces.
- Eat fewer sweets such as soft drinks containing sugar, candy, gum that contains fructose or another form of sugar, pastries, and sweet desserts.
- Eat more raw fruits and vegetables that naturally remove plaque and other food as they are chewed.
- Eat two or three servings of dairy products per day to provide calcium.
- If antacids are used, select ones with calcium.
- Use frozen orange juice concentrate fortified with calcium.
- Do not use the teeth to open packages or containers.
- Use scissors rather than the teeth to cut thread.
- Do not chew ice cubes or crushed ice.
- Avoid chewing unpopped or partially popped kernels of popcorn.
- Have dental checkups at least every 6 months.

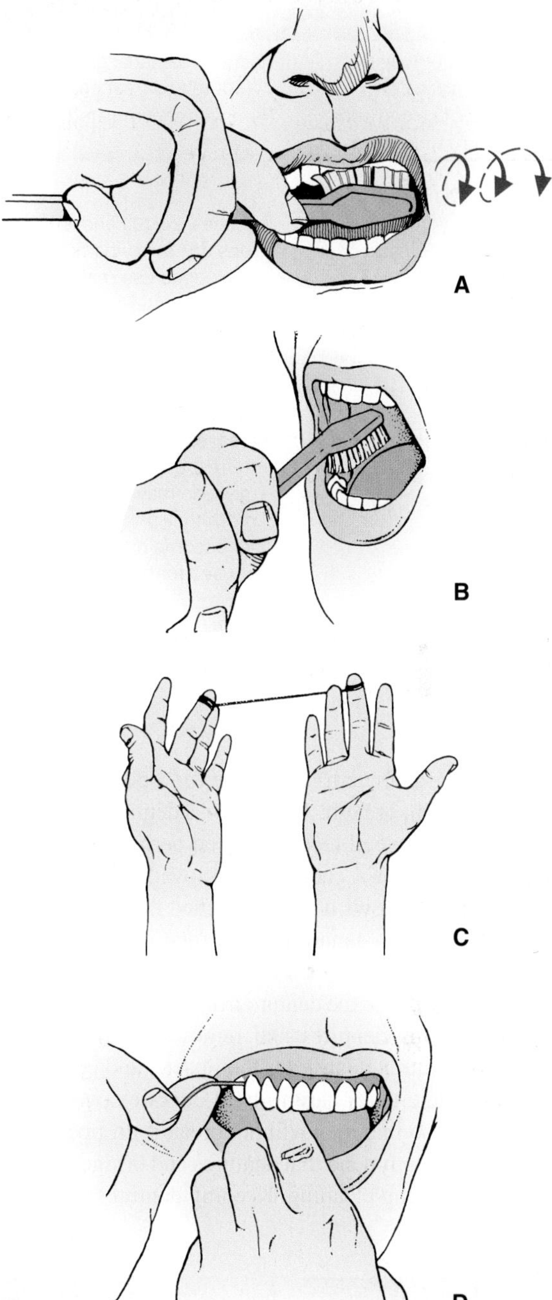

FIGURE 17-5 A. Brushing toward the crown of the teeth. **B.** Rinsing the mouth. **C.** Using floss. About 1¼ in. of approximately 18 in. of wrapped floss is used at any one time. **D.** Inserting floss between the teeth.

Oral Care for Unconscious Clients

Oral hygiene cannot be neglected because the client is unconscious. In fact, because unconscious clients are not salivating in response to seeing, smelling, and eating food, they need oral care even more frequently than conscious clients. **Sordes** (dried crusts containing mucus, microorganisms, and epithelial cells shed from the mucous membrane) are common on the lips and teeth of unconscious clients.

Toothbrushing is the preferred technique for providing oral hygiene to unconscious clients (Skill 17-4). Clients who are not alert, however, are at risk for aspirating (inhaling) saliva and liquid oral hygiene products into their lungs. Aspirated liquids predispose clients to pneumonia. Therefore, the nurse uses special precautions to avoid getting fluid in the client's airway.

In addition to toothbrushing, the nurse moistens and refreshes the client's mouth with oral swabs. He or she uses various substances for oral hygiene depending on the circumstances and assessment findings for each client (Table 17-4).

TABLE 17-4 Optional Substances for Oral Care

SUBSTANCE	USE
Antiseptic mouthwash diluted with water	Reduces bacterial growth in the mouth and freshens breath
Equal parts of baking soda and table salt in warm water, or baking soda mixed with normal saline	Removes accumulated secretions
One part of hydrogen peroxide to 10 parts of water	Releases oxygen and loosens dry, sticky particles; prolonged use may damage tooth enamel
Milk of magnesia	Reduces oral acidity; dissolves plaque, increases flow of saliva, and soothes oral lesions
Lemon and glycerin swabs	Increases salivation and refreshes the mouth; glycerin may absorb water from the lips and cause them to become dry and cracked if used for more than several days
Petroleum jelly	Lubricates lips

Denture Care

Dentures (artificial teeth) substitute for a person's lower or upper set of teeth, or both. A **bridge**—a dental appliance that replaces one or several teeth—is fixed permanently to other natural teeth so that it cannot be removed, or it is fastened with a clasp that allows it to be detached from the mouth.

For clients who cannot remove their own dentures, the nurse dons gloves and uses a dry gauze square or clean face cloth to grasp and free the denture from the mouth (Fig. 17-6). He or she cleans dentures and removable bridges with a toothbrush, denture cleanser or toothpaste, and cold or tepid water. The nurse takes care to hold dentures over a plastic basin or towel so that they will not break if dropped.

Dentists recommend that dentures and bridges remain in place except during cleaning. Keeping dentures and bridges out for long periods permits the gum lines to change, affecting the fit. If a nurse removes a client's bridge or dentures during the night, he or she stores them in a covered cup. Plain water is used most often to cover dentures when they are not in the mouth, but some add mouthwash or denture cleanser to the water.

Stop, Think, and Respond Box 17-4

Compare independent oral hygiene performed by a client and that administered by a nurse. How are they similar; how are they different?

Hair Care

Sometimes, clients need assistance with grooming or shampooing their hair.

Hair Grooming

The following are recommendations for grooming a client's hair:

- Try to use a hairstyle the client prefers.
- Brush the hair slowly and carefully to avoid damaging the hair.
- Brush the hair to increase circulation and distribution of sebum.
- Use a wide-toothed comb, starting at the ends of the hair rather than from the crown downward if the hair is matted or tangled.
- Apply a conditioner or alcohol to loosen tangles.
- Use oil on the hair if it is dry. Many preparations are available, but pure castor oil, olive oil, and mineral oil are satisfactory.
- Braid the hair to help prevent tangles.
- If hair loss occurs from cancer therapy or some other disease or medical treatment, provide the client with a turban or baseball cap.
- Avoid using hairpins or clips that may injure the scalp.
- Obtain the client's or family's permission before cutting the hair if it is hopelessly tangled and cutting seems to be the only solution to provide adequate grooming.

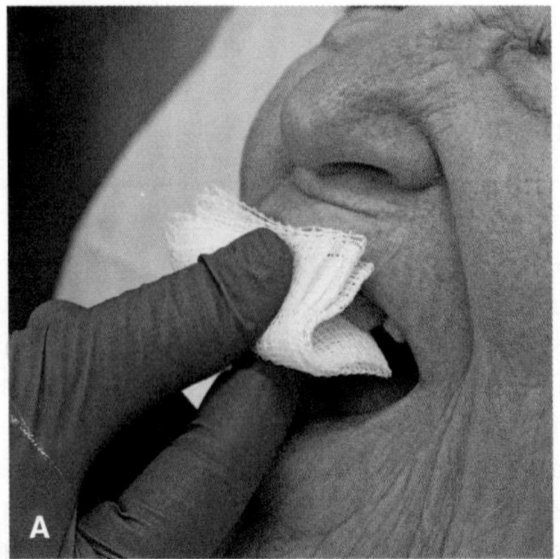

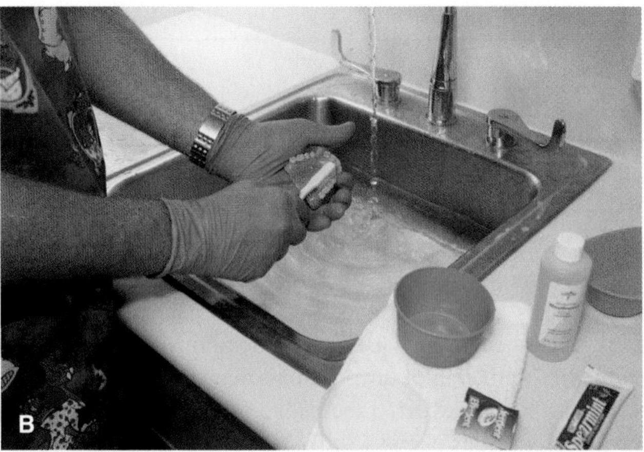

FIGURE 17-6 A. Removing an upper denture. **B.** Cleaning dentures.

Shampooing

Hair should be washed as often as necessary to keep it clean. A weekly shampoo is sufficient for most people, but shampooing more or less often will not damage the hair.

Long-term health care facilities often employ beauticians and barbers, but if professional services are unavailable, the nurse or delegated nursing staff member shampoos the client's hair (Skill 17-5). Dry shampoos, which are applied to the hair as a powder, aerosol spray, or foam, are available for occasional use. The nurse applies the cleaning agent to the hair, massages it thoroughly to distribute, and brushes or towels it from the hair afterward.

Nail Care

Nail care involves keeping the fingernails and toenails clean and trimmed. Clients who have diabetes, impaired circulation, or thick nails are at risk for vascular complications secondary to trauma. The services of a **podiatrist** (a person with special training in caring for feet) are often indicated. It is best to check with the client's physician before cutting fingernails or toenails.

If there are no contraindications, the nurse cares for the client's nails as follows:

- Soak the hands or feet in warm water to soften the keratin and loosen trapped debris. (Fig. 17-7).
- Clean under the nails with a wooden orange stick or other sturdy but blunt instrument.
- Push **cuticles** (thin edge of skin at the base of the nail) downward with a soft towel.
- Use a handheld electric rotary file made by Dremel or some other company or an emery board to reduce the length of long fingernails or toenails.
- Avoid sharp or jagged points that may injure the adjacent skin.

To keep the skin and nails soft and supple, the nurse applies lotion or an emollient cream after bathing and nail care. If foot perspiration is a problem, he or she uses a prescribed antifungal, deodorant powder. Because impaired skin, especially on the feet, is often slow to heal and is susceptible to infection, the nurse immediately reports any abnormal assessment findings. To avoid injuring the feet, clients should wear sturdy slippers or clean socks and supportive shoes.

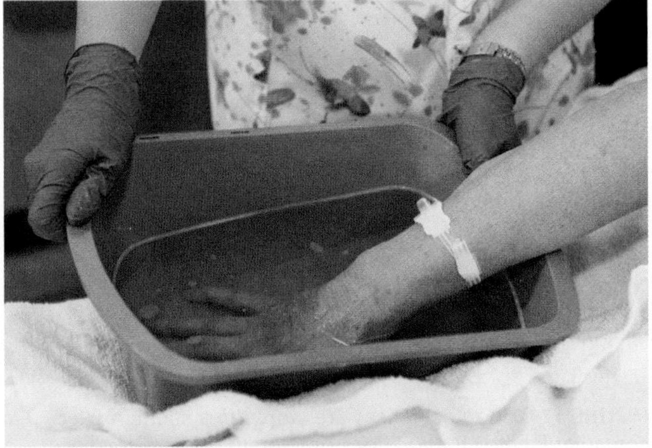

FIGURE 17-7 Soaking a hand before proceeding with nail care.

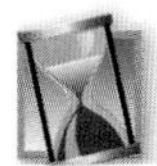

Gerontologic Considerations

- Older adults should be encouraged to purchase sturdy shoes and to replace or repair them as they become worn to prevent skin and nail impairment in the lower extremities.

VISUAL AND HEARING DEVICES

Eyeglasses and hearing aids improve communication and socialization. Both represent a considerable financial investment. If they become damaged or broken, the temporary loss deprives clients of full sensory perception. Therefore, they should be well maintained and safely stored when not in use.

Although eyeglasses and hearing aids are not body structures, they are worn in close contact with the body for long periods. Consequently, they tend to collect secretions, dirt, and debris that may interfere with their function and use. Therefore, the nurse cares for these devices at the same time that he or she provides other hygiene measures.

Eyeglasses

Prescription lenses are made of glass or plastic. Plastic lenses weigh much less but are more easily scratched. Glass lenses are more likely to break if dropped. When not in use, eyeglasses are stored in a soft case or rested on the frame.

The nurse cleans glass and plastic lenses as follows:

- Hold the eyeglasses by the nose or ear braces.
- Run tepid water over both sides of the lenses (hot water damages plastic lenses).
- Wash the lenses with soap or detergent.
- Rinse with running tap water.
- Dry with a clean, soft cloth such as a handkerchief. Do not use paper tissues because some contain wood fibers, and pulp can scratch the lenses.

Some prefer to use a commercial glass cleaner, but this is not necessary.

Contact Lenses

A contact lens is a small plastic disk placed directly on the cornea. Clients usually wear contact lenses in both eyes, but some clients who have had cataract surgery on one eye wear a single contact lens or a single contact lens and eyeglasses. The nurse should not assume that someone who wears eyeglasses does not use a contact lens, and vice versa.

Several types of contact lenses are available: hard, soft, or gas permeable (Fig. 17-8). All contact lenses, even disposable types, need removal for cleaning, eye rest, and disinfection. People who are not conscientious about following a routine for contact lens care risk infection, eye abrasion, and permanent damage to the cornea.

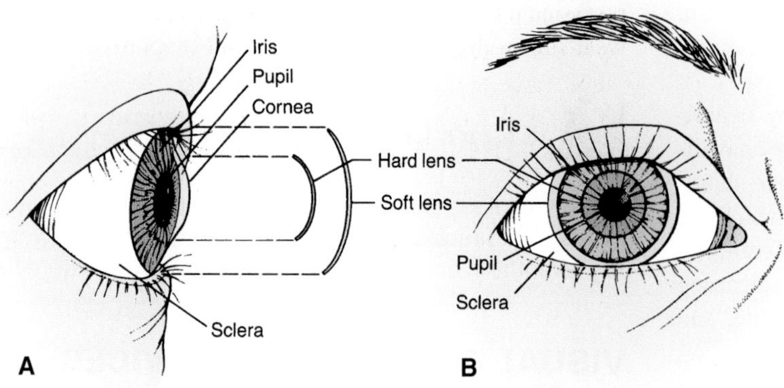

FIGURE 17-8 The location and size of hard and soft contact lenses. **A.** Side view. **B.** Front view.

When caring for a client who wears contact lenses, the nurse asks the client to remove and insert the lenses and to care for them according to his or her established routine. For clients who cannot do so, the nurse may assist with the removal of the lenses or should consult the client's **ophthalmologist** (a medical doctor who treats eye disorders) or **optometrist** (a person who prescribes corrective lenses) about alternatives to promote adequate vision and safety. Some people, when ill, resume wearing eyeglasses temporarily, use a magnifying glass, or do without any visual aid.

Contact Lens Removal

Before removing contact lenses, the nurse obtains an appropriate storage container. Commercial containers are available. Because the lens prescriptions may differ for each eye, the nurse labels the container "left" and "right." The nurse elevates the client's head and places a towel over the chest to prevent loss or damage to the contact lenses. The technique for removing soft contact lenses is different than for hard contact lenses.

To remove a soft contact lens, the nurse moves the lens from the cornea to the sclera by sliding it into position with a clean, gloved finger as the client looks upward (Fig. 17-9). When repositioning the lens, he or she compresses the lid margins together toward the lens. Compression bends the pliable lens, allowing air to enter beneath it. The air releases the lens from the surface of the eye. The nurse then gently grasps the loosened lens between thumb and forefinger for removal. Soft lenses dry and crystallize if exposed to air, so the nurse immediately places them in a soaking solution in the storage container (Fig. 17-10).

To remove a hard contact lens, the blink method is the most common technique. The nurse positions and

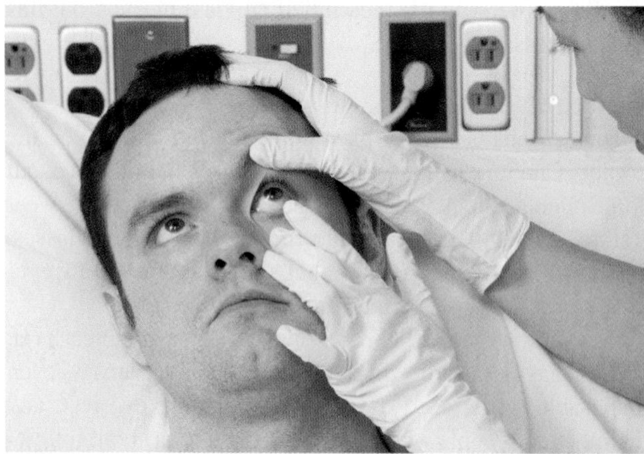

FIGURE 17-9 The nurse removes a soft contact lens from the client's eye.

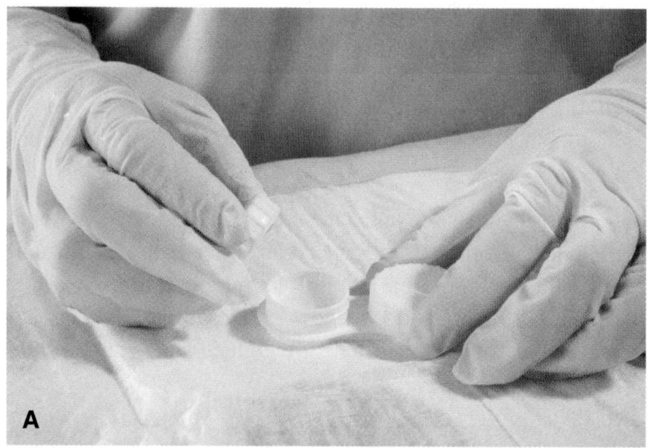

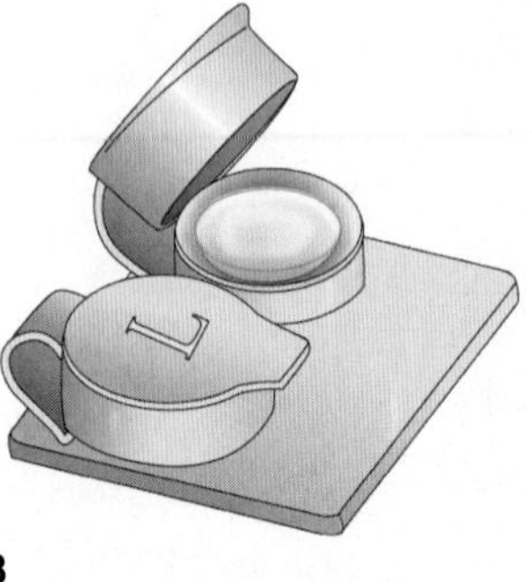

FIGURE 17-10 Contact lenses are stored in a solution-filled container labeled R and L for right versus left lens, respectively.

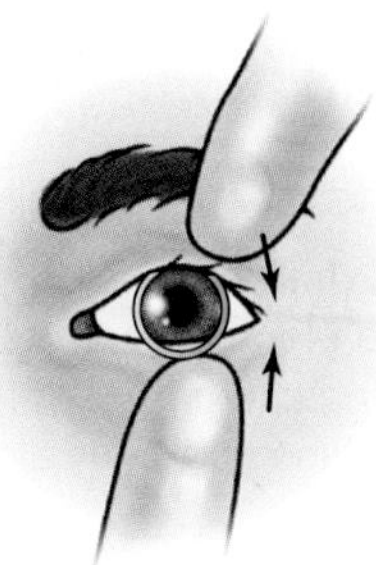

FIGURE 17-11 Moving the eyelids toward one another loosens the hard contact lens from the cornea surface when the client blinks.

prepares the client similarly as for removing soft contact lenses, leaving the lens in place on the cornea. He or she places the thumb and a finger on the center of the upper and lower lids (Fig. 17-11). The nurse applies slight opposing pressure to the lids while instructing the client to blink, which separates the hard lens from the cornea. If the blink method is unsuccessful, the nurse places an ophthalmic suction cup on the lens and, with gentle suction, lifts the lens from the eye. After removal, the nurse soaks the lenses in the storage container.

Artificial Eyes

An artificial eye is a plastic shell that acts as a cosmetic replacement for the natural eye. There is no way to restore vision once the natural eye is removed. The artificial eye and the socket into which it is placed need occasional cleaning. If the client cannot care for the artificial eye, the nurse removes it by depressing the lower eyelid until the lid margin is wide enough to allow the artificial eye to slide free. The nurse irrigates the eye socket with water or saline before reinserting the artificial eye.

Hearing Aids

There are four types of hearing aids:

- In-the-ear devices are small, self-contained aids that fit in the outer ear.
- Canal aids fit deep within the ear canal and are largely concealed. Because of their small size, they may be difficult to remove and adjust.
- Behind-the-ear devices consist of a microphone and an amplifier worn behind the ear that delivers sound to an internal receiver.
- Body-aid devices use electrical components enclosed in a case carried somewhere on the body to deliver sound through a wire connected to an ear mold receiver (Fig. 17-12).

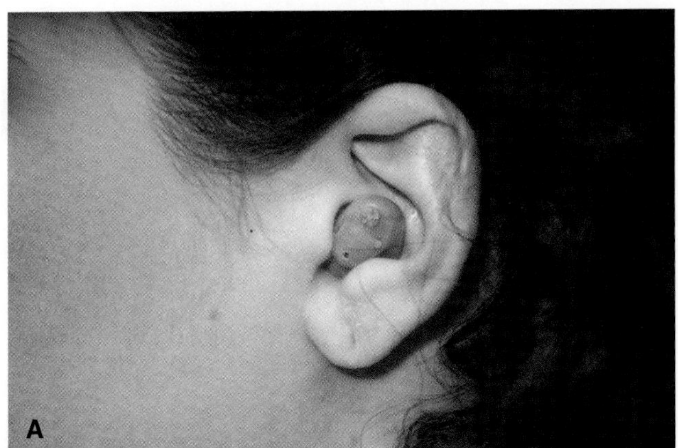

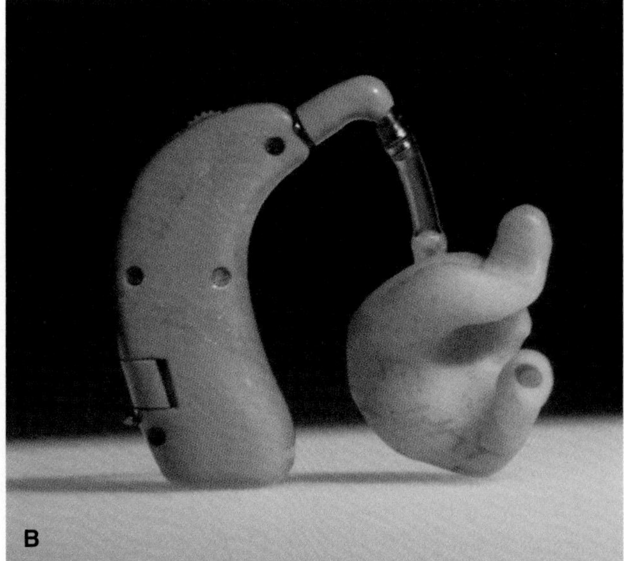

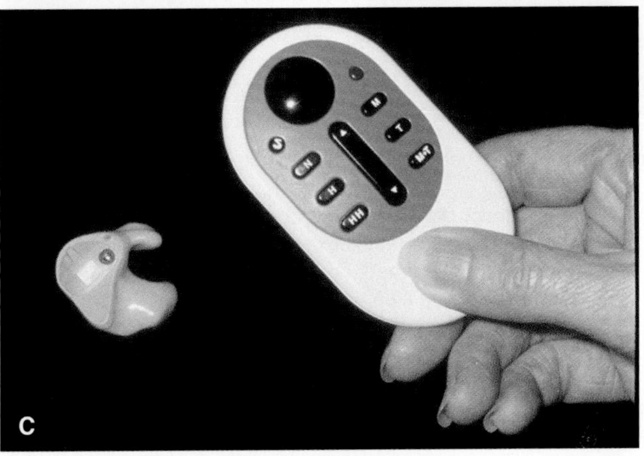

FIGURE 17-12 Examples of hearing aids: in-the-ear (**A**), behind-the-ear (**B**), and one whose volume, pitch, and noise reduction can be controlled by a handheld remote control (**C**).

In-the-ear and behind-the-ear models are most common. Hearing aids for the right ear will be marked with an R or will have a red dot; hearing aids for the left ear will be marked with an L or will have a blue dot.

Behind-the-ear models can be attached to an eyeglass frame. Use of body aids is most common for those with severe hearing loss or those who cannot care for a small device. Hearing aids are powered by small mercury or zinc batteries that need to be replaced after 100 to 200 hours of use.

Most clients insert and remove their own hearing aids, but the nurse may need to assess and troubleshoot problems that develop (Table 17-5). Clients and their families need to know how to maintain the hearing aid (Client and Family Teaching 17-2).

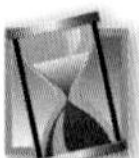

Gerontologic Considerations

- Older adults are more susceptible to impacted cerumen (ear wax)—a common cause of hearing loss. Over-the-counter eardrops such as Debrox are used to prevent and treat this condition. Irrigation of the ear with body-temperature tap water followed by instillation of a drying agent such as 70% alcohol may be necessary to remove impacted cerumen.

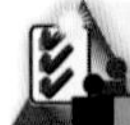

Client and Family Teaching 17-2 Maintaining a Hearing Aid

The nurse teaches the client and family as follows:

- Keep a supply of extra batteries on hand.
- Avoid exposing the electrical components to extreme heat, water, cleaning chemicals, or hair spray.
- Wipe the outer surface of a body aid or behind-the-ear case occasionally.
- Clean cerumen that has become embedded in the earpiece with a special instrument that comes with the hearing aid. If this is not available, use a thin needle as a substitute (Ellis & Bentz, 2007).
- Turn the hearing aid off when not in use to prolong the life of the battery.
- Check the battery before inserting a hearing aid by slowly turning the volume to high, placing a hand over the hearing aid, and listening for feedback (Lippincott's Visual Encyclopedia of Clinical Skills, 2009).
- Store the hearing aid in a safe place where it will not fall or become lost.

TABLE 17-5 Troubleshooting Hearing Aid Problems

PROBLEM	POSSIBLE CAUSES	ACTION
Reduced or absent sound	Weak or dead battery	Test and replace battery
	Incorrect battery position	Match the positive pole of the battery to the positive symbol in the case
	Cracked tubing leading to the receiver	Repair tubing
	Broken wire between body aid and receiver	Repair wire
	Accumulation of cerumen in the ear	Clean the ear
	Cerumen plugging the receiver	Remove cerumen with an instrument called a wax loop, or by using the tip of a pin, or the needle on a syringe
	Ear congestion from an upper respiratory infection	Consult the physician about administering a decongestant
	Damaged electrical components	Have the device inspected by a person who services hearing aids
Shrill noise, called *feedback*, caused by conditions that return sound to the microphone	Malposition or failure to insert the receiver fully in the ear	Remove and reinsert
	Kinked receiver tubing	Remove and untwist
	Excessive volume	Reduce volume control
	Hearing aid left on while removed from the ear	Turn hearing aid off or replace it in the ear
Garbled sound	Poor battery contact	Check battery for correct size; make sure the battery compartment is closed; clean metal contact points with an emery board
	Dirty components	Clean with a soft cloth
	Debris in the on/off switch	Move the switch back and forth several times
	Corroded battery	Remove and replace
	Cracked case	Repair or replace

Infrared Listening Devices

Infrared listening devices (IRLDs) resemble earphones attached to a handheld receiver. They are an alternative to conventional hearing aids. An IRLD converts sound into infrared light and sends it through a wall- or ceiling-mounted receiver to the person wearing the listening device. The light is converted back into an auditory stimulus. People who need help hearing lectures, television, or live performances may use an IRLD. Some geriatric centers are installing IRLDs in rooms used for social and recreational activities.

One advantage of an IRLD over a conventional hearing aid is that an IRLD reduces background noise, which is a common reason people give for not wearing their hearing aids. A disadvantage is that IRLDs cannot be used outdoors, in rooms that contain many windows, or in rooms that are brightly lit because infrared light jams the signal, causing audio interference.

NURSING IMPLICATIONS

Clients who require assistance with personal hygiene may have a variety of nursing diagnoses:

- Bathing Self-Care Deficit
- Dressing Self-Care Deficit
- Activity Intolerance
- Risk for Impaired Skin Integrity

Nursing Care Plan 17-1 is for a client with a nursing diagnosis of Bathing Self-Care Deficit, defined in the NANDA-I taxonomy (2012, p. 250) as "impaired ability to perform or complete bathing activities for self."

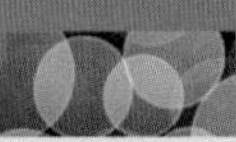

NURSING CARE PLAN 17-1 Bathing Self-Care Deficit

Assessment

- Observe client's motor skills, strength, and coordination to determine the extent to which he or she can perform hygiene skills.
- Determine if the client's mental status is sufficient to follow directions, complete tasks required for hygiene, and ensure safety.
- Assess client's level of endurance to accomplish hygiene activities such as changes in respiratory and heart rate, increased blood pressure, pain, or fatigue when performing self-care.

Nursing Diagnosis. **Bathing Self-Care Deficit** related to an inability to use hands secondary to bilateral arm fractures sustained from a fall as manifested by inability to use two hands for self-care due to short arm cast on dominant arm and traction with suspension applied to nondominant arm.

Expected Outcome. The client will receive assistance with bathing and oral hygiene on a daily and prn (as needed) basis.

Interventions	Rationales
Administer a daily bed bath at a convenient time for the client.	Scheduling hygiene according to the client's preference and avoiding conflicts with other components of care and treatment meets the client's individualized needs and avoids unnecessary interruptions.
Use castile soap that the client prefers, soft-bristled toothbrush, and fluoride toothpaste.	Demonstrates organization and respect for the client's personal choices.
Let the client use the arm in the cast to dry areas of the skin that can be reached after the nurse has washed them.	Facilitates participation in care and maintains self-esteem.
Turn the client toward the arm in traction when bathing the client's back and buttocks.	Avoids disturbing the alignment of the arm in traction.
Apply the client's deodorant and body lotion located in the bedside cabinet after bathing is completed.	Demonstrates respect for the client's choices in hygiene products; ensures a feeling of well-being and confidence in social interactions.
Assist the client to don a hospital gown that has sleeves that fasten with snaps.	Facilitates covering the arm suspended in traction.
Help the client to perform oral hygiene by wrapping and taping a washcloth around the handle of the toothbrush.	Promotes self-care with modifications for using the toothbrush.

Evaluation of Expected Outcomes

- The client's hygiene needs for bathing and oral care are completed.
- The client assists with hygiene needs to the extent possible.
- The client states, "I feel so much better about seeing my doctor and visitors after I've gotten cleaned up in the morning."

CRITICAL THINKING EXERCISES

1. You have been assigned to two clients: a 75-year-old woman who is unconscious after a stroke and a 38-year-old male mechanic being treated for an ulcer. How do their hygiene needs differ?
2. You are responsible for inspecting long-term care facilities such as nursing homes. What criteria should health care agencies meet in relation to bathing facilities and hygiene policies to receive a positive evaluation?
3. Explain why attending to shaving, oral hygiene, and nail care are important to families of those being cared for in a long-term care facility.
4. What strategies might a nurse use for meeting the hygiene needs of a client who refuses to bathe and perform oral care?

NCLEX-STYLE REVIEW QUESTIONS

1. When a health nurse visits the home of a family being treated for pediculosis (head lice), which of the following items should the nurse discourage?
   1. Pediculicide shampoo
   2. Fine-toothed comb
   3. Hair conditioner
   4. Warm tap water
2. When examining the skin of a client with psoriasis, the nurse is most likely to observe:
   1. Weeping skin lesions on the trunk of the body
   2. Red skin patches covered with silvery scales
   3. Fluid-filled blisters surrounded by crusts
   4. A red rash containing pus-filled lesions
3. When a client develops pruritus (itching skin), which nursing measure is best for relieving the client's discomfort?
   1. Use a medicated bath with oatmeal or cornstarch.
   2. Apply extra wool blankets to the bed for warmth.
   3. Give frequent showers or tub baths.
   4. Rub the skin dry after bathing.
4. A client experiences a shrill noise, known as feedback, from a hearing aid. What are some possible causes for the nurse to check? Select all that apply.
   1. Incorrect battery position
   2. Malposition within the ear
   3. Accumulation of cerumen
   4. Kinked receiver tubing
   5. Excessive volume
5. When shaving a male client with a safety razor, which of the following nursing actions is correct?
   1. Start at the neck working upward.
   2. Pull the razor in the direction of hair growth.
   3. Use long strokes with the razor.
   4. Replace the razor after each use.

SKILL 17-1 Providing a Tub Bath or Shower

Suggested Action	Reason for Action
ASSESSMENT	
Check the Kardex or nursing care plan for hygiene directives.	Ensures continuity of care.
Assess the client's level of consciousness, orientation, strength, and mobility.	Provides data for evaluating the client's ability to carry out hygiene practices independently.
Check for gauze dressings, plaster cast, or electrical or battery-operated equipment; determine whether they can be protected with waterproof material or are safe if they become wet.	Maintains the client's safety and ensures integrity of treatment devices.
Determine if and when any laboratory or diagnostic procedures are scheduled.	Aids in time management.
Check the occupancy, cleanliness, and safety of the tub or shower (Fig. A).	Helps organize the plan for care.

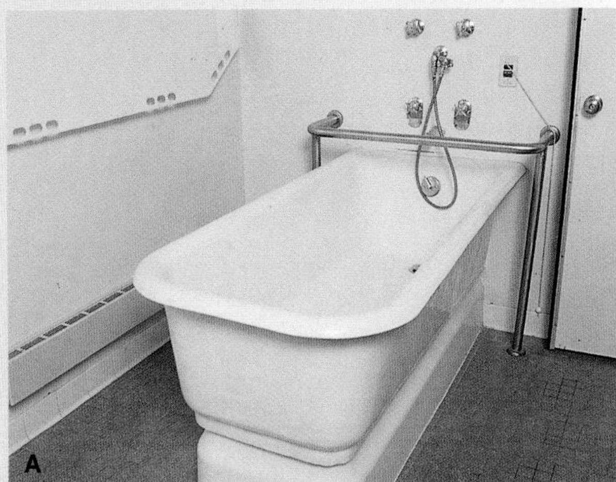

A Tub and shower equipped for client safety. (Photo by B. Proud.)

Suggested Action	Reason for Action
PLANNING	
Clean the tub or shower if necessary.	Reduces potential for spreading microorganisms.
Consult with the client about a convenient time for tending to hygiene needs.	Promotes client cooperation and participation in decision making.
Assemble supplies: floor mat, towels, face cloth, soap, clean pajamas, or gown.	Demonstrates organization and efficient time management.
IMPLEMENTATION	
Escort the client to the shower or bathing room.	Shows concern for the client's safety.
Demonstrate how to operate the faucet and drain.	Ensures the client's safety and comfort.
Fill the tub approximately halfway with water 105°–110°F (40°–43°C) or adjust the shower to a similar temperature if the client cannot operate the faucet.	Demonstrates concern for the client's safety and comfort.
Place a "Do Not Disturb" or "In Use" sign on the outer door.	Ensures privacy.
Help the client into the tub or shower if he or she needs assistance by: • Placing a chair next to the tub • Having the client swing his or her feet over the edge of the tub • Asking the client to lean forward, grab a support bar, and raise the buttocks and body until he or she can fully enter the tub	Reduces the risk of falling.

(continued)

Providing a Tub Bath or Shower (continued)

IMPLEMENTATION (CONTINUED)

Have the client sit on a stool or seat in the tub or shower if the client will have difficulty exiting the tub or may become weak while bathing (Fig. B).	Ensures safety.

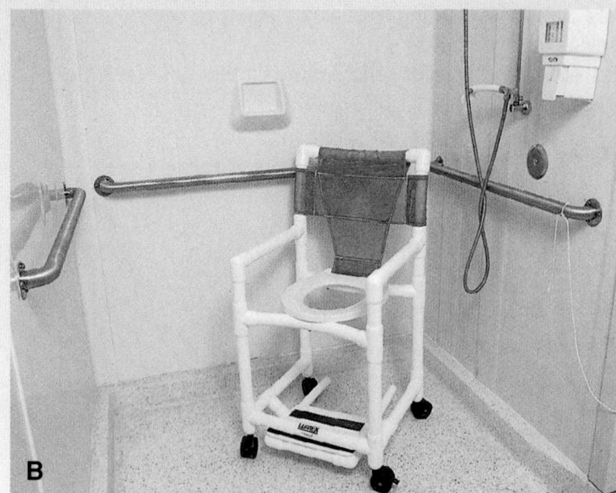

Shower chair. (Photo by B. Proud.)

Show the client how to summon help.	Promotes safety.
Stay close at hand.	Ensures proximity in case the client needs assistance.
Check on the client frequently by knocking on the door and waiting for a response.	Shows respect for privacy yet concern for safety.
Escort the client to his or her room after the bath or shower.	Demonstrates concern for safety and welfare.
Clean the tub or shower with an antibacterial agent; dispose of soiled linen in its designated location.	Reduces the spread of microorganisms and demonstrates concern for the next person to use the tub or shower.
Remove the "In Use" sign from the door.	Indicates that the bathing room is unoccupied.

Evaluation

- Client is clean.
- Client remains uninjured.

Document

- Date and time
- Tub bath or shower

SAMPLE DOCUMENTATION[a]

Date and Time Tub bath taken independently. ———————— SIGNATURE/TITLE

[a]Generally, nurses document routine hygiene measures on a checklist, but for teaching purposes an example of narrative charting has been provided.

SKILL 17-2 Administering Perineal Care

Suggested Action	Reason for Action
ASSESSMENT	
Inspect the client's genital and rectal areas.	Provides data for determining if perineal care is necessary.
PLANNING	
Wash hands or perform hand antisepsis with an alcohol rub (see Chap. 10).	Reduces the spread of microorganisms.
Gather gloves, soap, water, and clean clothes or antiseptic wipes, or a container of cleansing solution in a squeeze bottle, and several towels or absorptive pads.	Provides a means of removing debris and microorganisms.
Explain the procedure to the client.	Reduces anxiety and promotes cooperation.
Pull the privacy curtain.	Demonstrates respect for modesty.
Place the client in a dorsal recumbent position and cover with a bath blanket (Fig. A).	Provides access to the perineum.

A

Positioning and draping the client. (Photo by B. Proud.)

Suggested Action	Reason for Action
Pull and fan-fold the top linen to the foot of the bed while the client holds the top of the blanket.	Maintains client modesty and keeps upper linen clean and dry.
For a female client, place a disposable pad beneath the buttocks or place the client on a bedpan; for a male client, place a disposable pad under the penis and beneath the buttocks.	Helps to absorb liquid that may drip during cleansing.
IMPLEMENTATION	
Bend the female client's knees and spread her legs.	Exposes area for cleansing.
Put on gloves.	Prevents contact with blood, secretions, or excretions.
Wash the outer folds of the labia and then separate the folds of the labia and wash from the pubic area toward the anus (Figs. B and C).	Cleanses in a direction from less soiled to more soiled; prevents reintroducing microorganisms into previously cleaned areas.

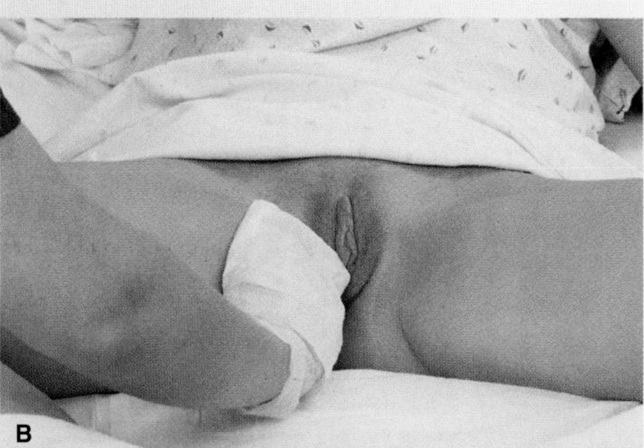

Cleansing the outer labia.

(continued)

Administering Perineal Care (continued)

IMPLEMENTATION (CONTINUED)

C

Cleansing the inner labia toward the anus.

Action	Rationale
Never go back over an area that you already have cleaned.	Avoids resoiling already clean areas.
Use a clean area of the cloth or a separate antiseptic wipe for each stroke.	
Wash debris on the outside of a urinary catheter, if one exists, especially where it is in contact with mucous membrane and genital tissue.	Reduces the number and growth of microorganisms that may ascend to the bladder.
Squeeze the antiseptic solution container, if one is used, starting at the upper areas of the labia down toward the anus (Fig. D).	Ensures that the solution will drain toward more soiled body areas; prevents reintroducing microorganisms into previously cleaned areas.

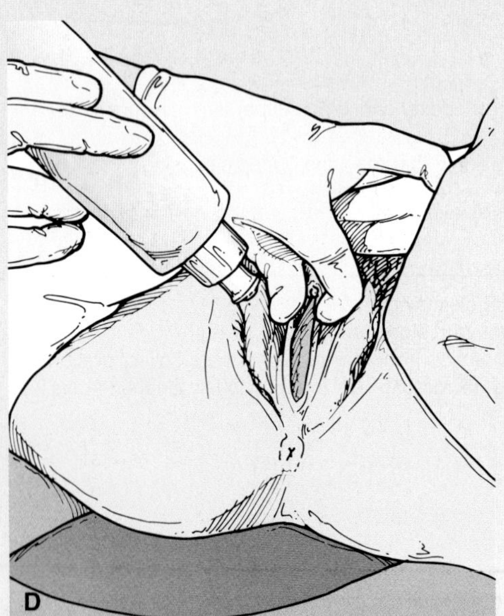

Rinsing the perineum.

Action	Rationale
For males, grasp the penis; if the client is uncircumcised, retract the foreskin.	Facilitates removing debris and secretions that may be trapped beneath the fold of skin.
Clean the tip of the penis using circular motions (Fig. E). Never go back over an area that you already have cleaned.	Keeps the urethral opening clean.
Replace the foreskin.	Prevents trauma.

(continued)

Administering Perineal Care (continued)

IMPLEMENTATION (CONTINUED)

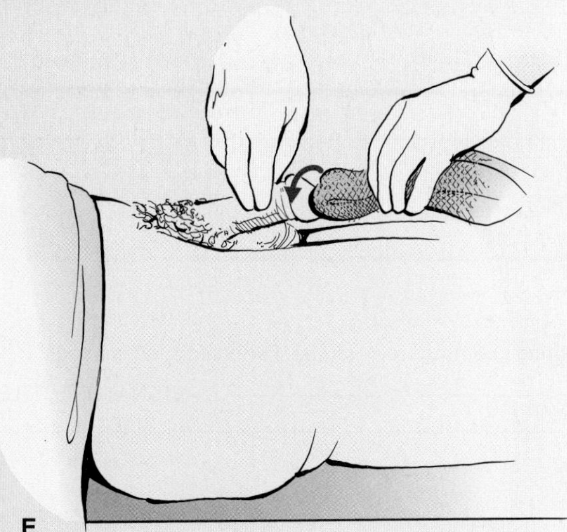

Cleansing the glans penis.

Wipe the shaft of the penis toward the scrotum (Fig. F).	Keeps microorganisms and debris from the urethral opening.

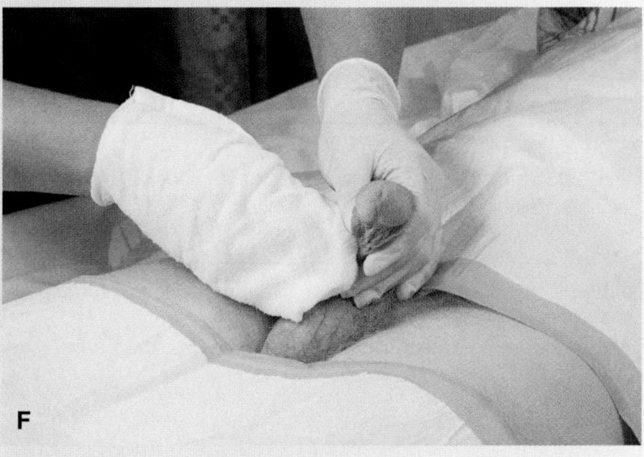

Cleansing the shaft of the penis.

Spread the legs and wash the scrotum.	Removes debris where it may be trapped and harbor microorganisms.
Pat the skin dry with a towel.	Removes excess moisture.
Turn the client to the side and wash from the perineum toward the anus.	Cleans in a direction toward more soiled body areas.
Rinse and pat the skin dry.	Prevents skin irritation from soap residue and retained moisture; a warm, dark, moist environment contributes to fungal skin infections.
Apply a clean absorbent perineal pad to clients who are menstruating or have other types of vaginal or rectal drainage.	Promotes cleanliness and reduces contact between the skin and moist drainage.
Remove damp towels, place an absorbent disposable pad beneath the client if drainage is excessive, and cover the client with bed linen.	Restores comfort; protects linen from soiling.
Deposit wet cloths, soiled wipes, and towels in an appropriate container.	Controls the spread of microorganisms.
Empty and rinse the bedpan.	Controls the spread of microorganisms.
Remove gloves and wash hands or perform hand antisepsis with an alcohol rub (see Chap. 10).	Reduces the spread of microorganisms.
Attend to the client's comfort and safety.	Demonstrates concern for the client's welfare.

(continued)

Administering Perineal Care (continued)

Evaluation
- Genital, perineal, and rectal areas are clean and dry.
- Cleansing has been from less to more soiled areas of the body.
- There has been no direct contact with drainage, secretions, or excretions.
- Soiled articles have been properly disposed.

Document
- Date and time
- Care provided
- Description of drainage and tissue

SAMPLE DOCUMENTATION

Date and Time Peri-care provided to remove moderate bloody drainage coming from vagina. Perineal tissue is intact.
———————— SIGNATURE/TITLE

SKILL 17-3 Giving a Bed Bath[a]

Suggested Action	Reason for Action
ASSESSMENT	
Check the Kardex or nursing care plan for hygiene directives.	Ensures continuity of care.
Inspect the skin for signs of dryness, drainage, or secretions.	Provides data for determining whether a complete or partial bath is appropriate.
PLANNING	
Consult with the client to determine a convenient time for tending to hygiene needs.	Promotes client cooperation; allows client participation in decision making.
Assemble supplies: bath blanket, towels, face cloths, soap, wash basin, clean pajamas or gown, clean bed linen, other hygiene articles such as deodorant or antiperspirant, and a razor for males.	Demonstrates organization and efficient time management.
IMPLEMENTATION	
Wash hands or perform hand antisepsis with an alcohol rub (see Chap. 10).	Reduces the spread of microorganisms.
Pull the privacy curtain.	Demonstrates respect for modesty.
Raise the bed to an appropriate height.	Reduces muscle strain on the back when providing care.
Remove extra pillows or positioning devices and place the client on his or her back.	Prepares the client for washing the anterior body surface.
Cover the client with a bath blanket.	Shows respect for the client's modesty and provides warmth.
Remove the client's gown.	Facilitates washing the client.
While the client holds the top of the bath blanket, pull and fan-fold the top linen to the bottom of the bed, or remove the linen, fold it, and lay it on a chair.	Keeps linen, which may be reused, clean.
If linen is too soiled for reuse, place it in a laundry hamper.	Reduces the spread of microorganisms.
Hold dirty linen away from contact with your uniform.	Reduces the spread of microorganisms.
Fill a basin with 105°–110°F (40°–43°C) water; place the basin on the overbed table.	Provides comfortably warm water for bathing within easy access.

(continued)

Giving a Bed Bath[a] (continued)

IMPLEMENTATION (CONTINUED)

Wet the washcloth and fold it to fashion a mitt (Fig. A).	Keeps water from dripping from the margins of the cloth.

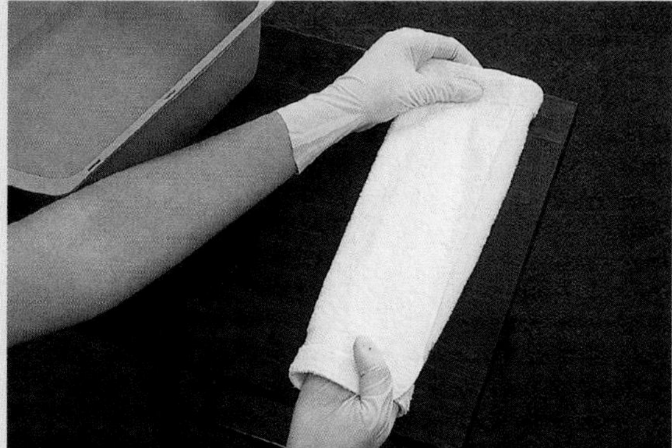

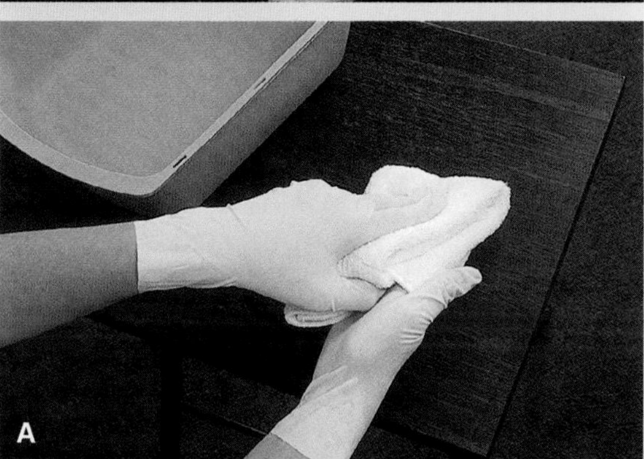

Straightening washcloth before folding into mitt.

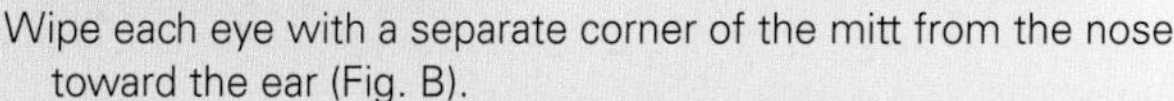
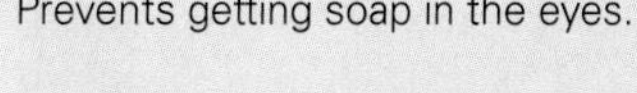

Wipe each eye with a separate corner of the mitt from the nose toward the ear (Fig. B).	Prevents getting soap in the eyes.

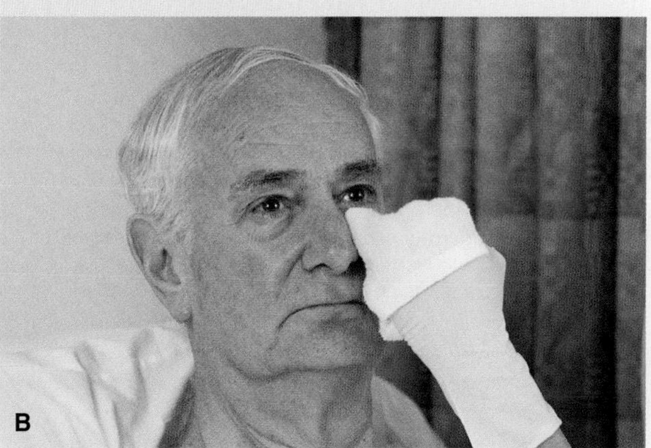

Wiping the eyes.

Lather the wet washcloth with soap and finish washing the face.	Removes oil, sweat, and microorganisms.
Rinse the washcloth and remove soapy residue from the face, then dry well.	Prevents drying the skin.

(continued)

Giving a Bed Bath[a] (continued)

IMPLEMENTATION (CONTINUED)

Bathe each of the client's arms separately; the axillae may be included now or when the chest is washed (Fig. C).

Cleanses soiled material and keeps the client from becoming too chilled.

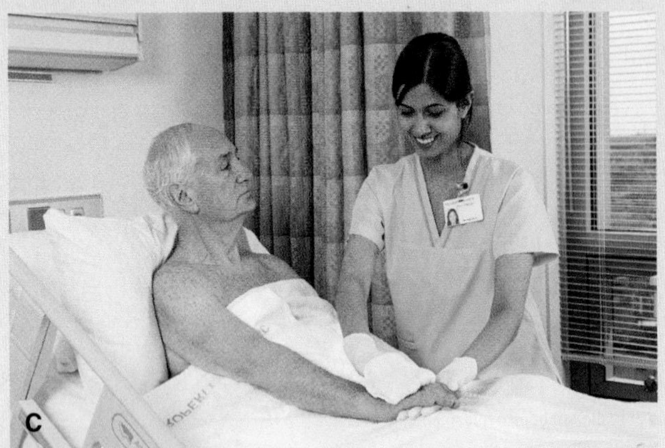

Washing the arm.

Offer to apply deodorant or antiperspirant after washing the axillae.

Demonstrates respect for the client's usual hygiene practices; reduces perspiration and body odor.

Place each hand in the basin of water as you wash it (Fig. D).

Facilitates more thorough washing than just using the washcloth.

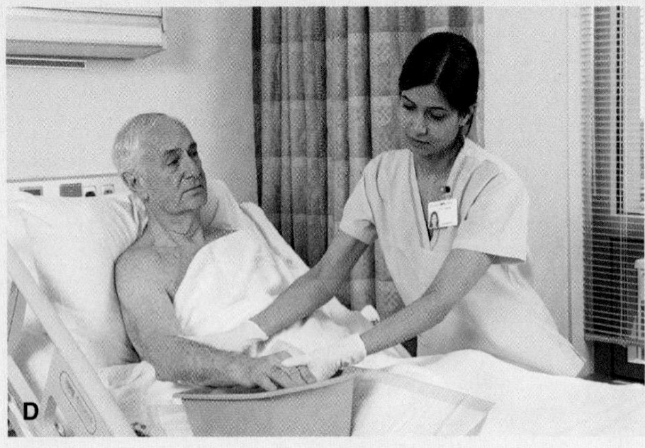

Soaking the hand in a basin.

Discard and replace the water in the basin; rinse the washcloth well or replace it with a clean one.

Eliminates debris, microorganisms, and soap residue and increases the warmth of the water in preparation for washing cleaner areas of the body.

Wash the chest, abdomen, each leg, and then the feet following the steps described for the upper body (Fig. E).

Follows the principle of washing from cleaner to more soiled areas.

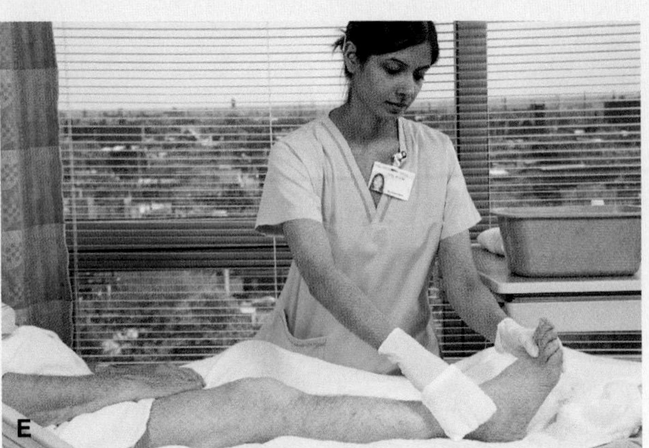

Washing a leg.

(continued)

Giving a Bed Bath[a] (continued)

IMPLEMENTATION (CONTINUED)

Help the client onto his or her side.	Repositions the client so you can bathe the posterior of the body.
Change the water and bathe the client's back. (Fig. F)	Allows washing to begin at a cleaner area on the posterior aspect of the body.

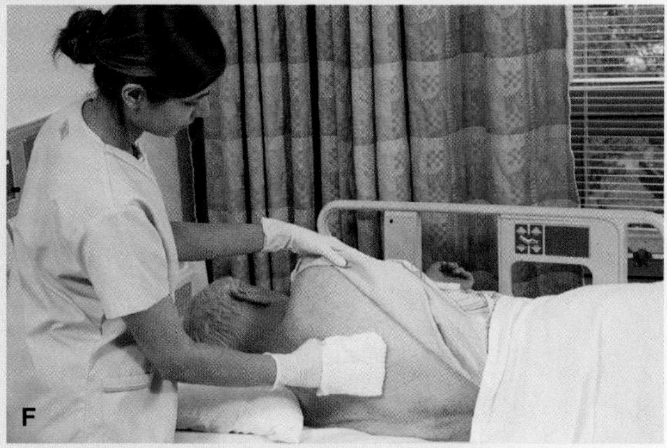

Washing the back.

Offer to apply lotion and provide a back rub.	Improves circulation and relaxes the client.
Don gloves and wash the buttocks, genitals, and anus last. Dry thoroughly.	Reduces the potential for contact with lesions or drainage that may contain infectious microorganisms. Prevents moisture accumulation.
Discard the water and wipe the basin dry.	Controls growth and spread of microorganisms.
Remove gloves and help the client to don a fresh gown.	Restores comfort and modesty.

Evaluation

- Client is completely bathed.
- Client experiences no discomfort or intolerance of activity.

Document

- Date and time
- Type and extent of hygiene
- Client response
- Assessment findings observed during bath

SAMPLE DOCUMENTATION[b]

Date and Time Complete bed bath given. Client could wash face and genitals independently. Skin is intact. No dyspnea noted during bath. ——— SIGNATURE/TITLE

[a]The nurses depicted here are wearing gloves; however, gloves are not necessary when giving a bath, unless there is a risk of infectious contact.
[b]Generally, nurses document routine hygiene measures on a checklist, but for teaching purposes an example of narrative charting has been used.

SKILL 17-4 Giving Oral Care to Unconscious Clients

Suggested Action	Reason for Action
ASSESSMENT	
Check the nursing care plan about the frequency of oral hygiene.	Maintains continuity of care.
Inspect the client's mouth.	Helps to determine equipment and supplies needed.
Look for oral hygiene supplies that may be at the client's bedside already.	Controls costs.
PLANNING	
Arrange to brush the client's teeth once per shift and to provide additional oral care at least every 2 hours if necessary.	Promotes a schedule for removing plaque and microorganisms and moistening and refreshing the mouth.
Assemble the following equipment: toothbrush, toothpaste, suction catheter, water, bulb syringe, padded tongue blade, emesis basin, towel or absorbent pad, and gloves. Some agencies may stock a toothbrushing device connected directly to a suction catheter (Fig. A).	Promotes organization and efficient time management.

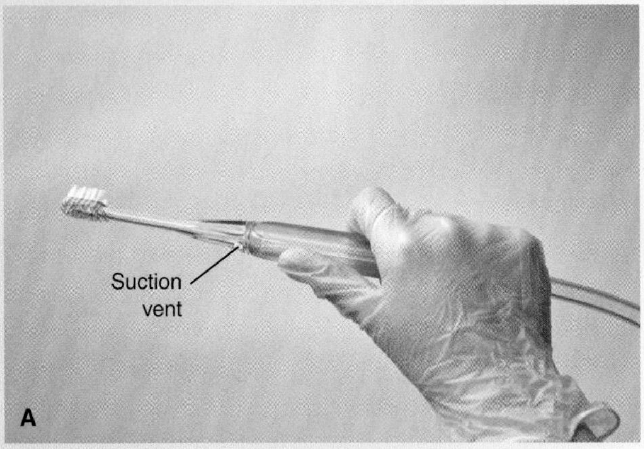

Toothbrushing device with suction catheter.

Suggested Action	Reason for Action
IMPLEMENTATION	
Explain to the client what you are about to do.	Reduces anxiety if the client has the cognitive capacity to understand.
Position the client on the side with the head slightly lowered.	Prevents liquids from draining into the airway.
Place a towel beneath the head.	Absorbs liquids.
Connect a Yankeur suction tip or catheter to a portable or wall-mounted suction source.	Promotes safety.
Spread toothpaste over a moistened toothbrush.	Prepares the toothbrush for use.
Don gloves.	Prevents direct contact with blood or microorganisms in the mouth.
Use a tongue blade or lower the client's chin to open the mouth and separate the teeth	Serves as a safe substitute for the nurse's fingers.
Brush all tooth surfaces with the toothbrush (Fig. B).	Removes plaque and microorganisms.

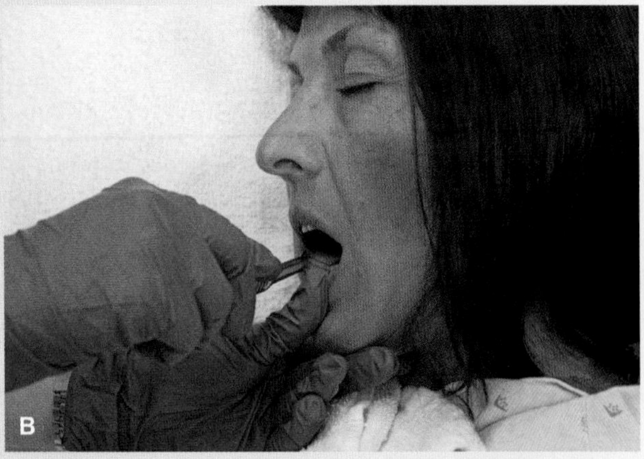

With the head lowered, the teeth are brushed.

(continued)

Giving Oral Care to Unconscious Clients (continued)

IMPLEMENTATION (CONTINUED)

Instill water and suction the mouth with a bulb syringe (Fig. C).

Removes loosened debris.
Reduces the potential for aspiration.

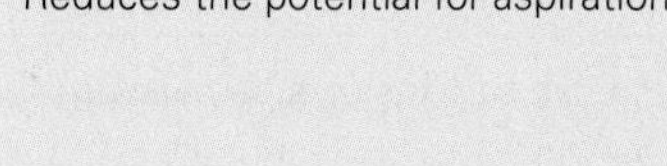

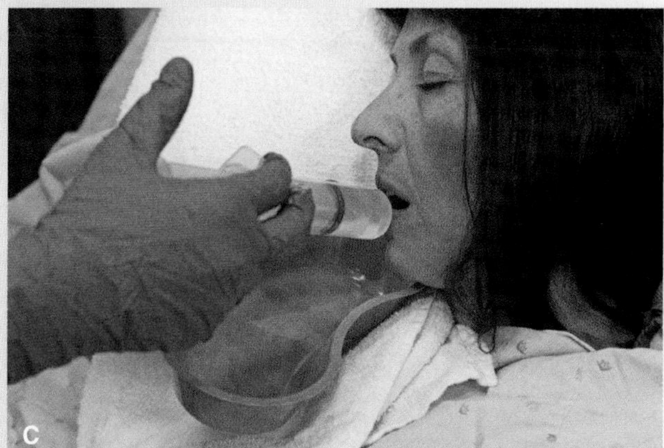

Rinsing the mouth while keeping the head lowered.

Suction the rinsing solution with a Yankeur suction device (Fig. D)

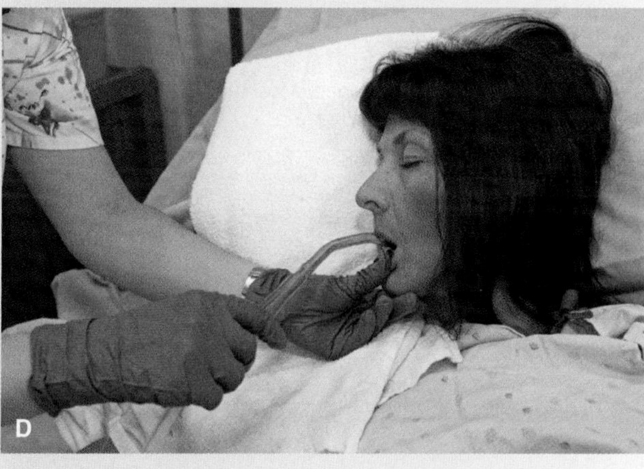

Suctioning fluid from the mouth.

Clean and store oral hygiene supplies.

Restores cleanliness and order to the client's environment.

Remove wet towel and gloves; restore client to a position of comfort and safety.

Demonstrates concern for the client's dignity and welfare.

Evaluation

- The teeth are clean.
- The oral mucosa is smooth, pink, moist, and intact.
- Safety is maintained.

Document

- Date and time
- Assessment findings if significant
- Type of oral care
- Unusual events such as choking and nursing action that was taken
- Outcome of any nursing action

SAMPLE DOCUMENTATION[a]

Date and Time Teeth brushed and mouth rinsed. Liquid suctioned from the mouth using a Yankeur suction catheter. No choking during oral care. Lung sounds are clear bilaterally. ———————— SIGNATURE/TITLE

[a]Generally, the nurse documents routine hygiene measures on a checklist, but for teaching purposes an example of narrative charting has been used.

SKILL 17-5 Shampooing Hair

Suggested Action	Reason for Action
ASSESSMENT	
Inspect the client for oily and limp hair or signs of accumulating secretions or lesions on the scalp.	Provides data to determine the need for shampooing and what supplies may be appropriate to use.
Assess for respiratory symptoms, pain, or other conditions that increase or contribute to activity intolerance.	Aids in establishing priorities for care.
Determine if and when medical treatments or tests are scheduled.	Ensures that hygiene measures will not interrupt therapeutic or diagnostic procedures.
Discuss the types of products available for shampooing.	Facilitates individualized care.
PLANNING	
Collaborate with the client on the time of day that is best for shampooing.	Involves the client in decision making.
Assemble equipment, which may include shampoo, conditioner, hair oil treatment, towels, a water pitcher, and a shampoo basin or trough.	Promotes organization and efficient time management.
IMPLEMENTATION	
Close the door to the room and pull the privacy curtain.	Reduces the potential for chilling and promotes respect for privacy.
Remove the pillow and protect the upper area of the bed with towels; cover the client's chest and shoulders with a towel.	Absorbs moisture.
Don gloves if any open lesions are on or near the head.	Prevents direct contact with blood or secretions.
Wet the hair thoroughly and apply shampoo. (Fig. A).	Dilutes and distributes the shampoo.

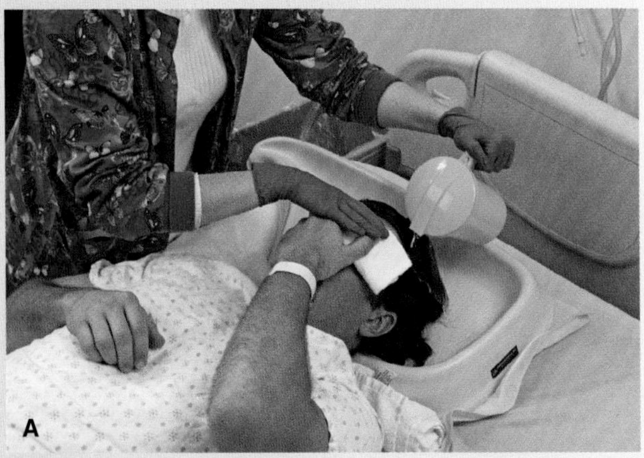

A

Shampooing the hair using a shampoo trough.

Suggested Action	Reason for Action
Work the shampoo into a lather.	Facilitates cleansing throughout the hair.
Rinse the hair with water.	Removes oil and shampoo from the hair.
Apply conditioner if requested and available.	Relaxes the hair and reduces tangles.
Wrap the head with a dry towel and fluff the hair.	Absorbs water and shortens the drying time.
Remove and discard gloves when there is no threat for direct contact with blood or secretions.	Facilitates hair care.
Comb, braid, or style the hair according to the client's preference.	Promotes self-esteem.
Clean and store shampooing supplies.	Restores cleanliness and order to the client's environment.

(continued)

Shampooing Hair (continued)

Evaluation

The hair is clean and dry.

Document

- Date and time
- Assessment findings
- Type of care
- Response of the client

SAMPLE DOCUMENTATION

Date and Time Scalp and hair appear oily. Skin is intact. Bed shampoo provided. Hair dried, combed, and styled in braids. Scalp is clean and intact. No evidence of chilling, fatigue, or discomfort during shampoo. States, "I feel so much better." ———— SIGNATURE/TITLE

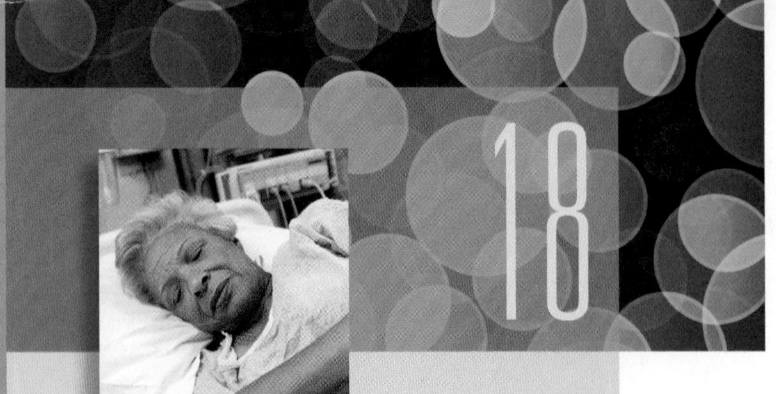

18 Comfort, Rest, and Sleep

Words To Know

apnea
bruxism
cataplexy
circadian rhythm
climate control
comfort
drug tolerance
environmental psychologist
humidity
hypersomnia
hypersomnolence
hypnogogic hallucinations
hypnotic
hypopnea
hypoxia
insomnia
jet lag
massage
mattress overlay
melatonin
microsleep
multiple sleep latency test
narcolepsy
nocturnal enuresis
nocturnal polysomnography
occupied bed
parasomnia
photoperiod
phototherapy
progressive relaxation
relative humidity
rest
restless legs syndrome
sedative
sleep
sleep apnea/hypopnea syndrome
sleep diary
sleep paralysis
sleep rituals
sleep–wake cycle disturbance
somnambulism
stimulants
sundown syndrome
sunrise syndrome
thermoregulation
tranquilizer
unoccupied bed
ventilation

Learning Objectives

On completion of this chapter, the reader should be able to:

1. Differentiate between comfort, rest, and sleep.
2. Describe four ways to modify the client environment to promote comfort, rest, and sleep.
3. List four standard furnishings in each client room.
4. State at least five functions of sleep.
5. Describe the two phases of sleep and their differences.
6. Describe the general trend in sleep requirements as a person ages.
7. Name 10 factors that affect sleep.
8. List four categories of drugs that affect sleep.
9. Name four techniques for assessing sleep patterns.
10. Describe four categories of sleep disorders.
11. Discuss at least five techniques for promoting sleep.
12. Name two nursing measures that promote relaxation.
13. Discuss unique characteristics of sleep among older adults.

Comfort (a state in which a person is relieved of distress) facilitates **rest** (a waking state characterized by reduced activity and mental stimulation) and **sleep** (a state of arousable unconsciousness). One factor that contributes to comfort is a safe, clean, and attractive environment.

This chapter addresses measures for ensuring that the setting for client care promotes a sense of well-being. It includes measures for maintaining the order and cleanliness of the client's bed and room and describes nursing interventions that facilitate rest and sleep.

CLIENT ENVIRONMENT

The term *environment*, as used here, refers to the room where the client receives nursing care and its furnishings. In a broader sense, however, the health care facility's location and design involve many other subtle elements that influence the consumer's overall impression of the institution.

Most clients are unaware of the thoughts and considerations that go into their surroundings. Accessible parking, lighting inside and outside of the physical plant, landscaping, barriers that reduce traffic noise, and signage that helps clients find their way around the building create a positive appeal among those in need of health care.

Client Rooms

Client rooms resemble bedrooms but are no longer the bare, white, sterile environments of a few decades ago. Thanks to **environmental**

psychologists (specialists who study how the environment affects behavior and well-being), client rooms are now brighter, more colorful, and tastefully decorated. The wall and floor treatments, lighting, and mechanisms for maintaining climate control are practical and conducive to comfort.

Walls

Blue and colors with blue tints, such as mauve and light green, promote relaxation, so these color schemes are preferred within health care settings and client rooms. If these colors are not used exclusively, they are integrated into wallpaper trim and decorative accessories such as framed pictures. The art often depicts country scenes and peaceful images.

Floors

Because noise interferes with comfort, the hallways and work stations are carpeted in most agencies. The floors in client rooms have tile or linoleum surfaces to facilitate the cleaning of spills.

Lighting

Adequate lighting, both natural and artificial, is important to the comfort of clients and nursing personnel. Newer buildings have large window areas, atriums, skylights, and enclosed courtyards to facilitate exposure to sunlight as a technique for reducing stress.

Bright artificial light facilitates nursing care but is not conducive to client comfort. Therefore, most client rooms have multiple lights in various locations with adjustable intensity. Dim light and darkness promote sleep; however, injuries are more likely in dark and unfamiliar environments. Therefore, client rooms have adjustable window blinds and night lights near the floor.

Climate Control

Climate control refers to mechanisms for maintaining temperature, humidity, and ventilation. It is a method of promoting physical comfort.

Temperature and Humidity

Most clients are comfortable when the room temperature is 68° to 74°F (20° to 23°C). Newer buildings provide thermostats in each room so that the temperature can be adjusted to suit the client.

Humidity (the amount of moisture in the air) and **relative humidity** (the ratio between the amount of moisture in the air and the greatest amount of water vapor the air can hold at a given temperature) affect comfort. At a relative humidity of 60%, the air contains 60% of its potential water capacity. A relative humidity of 30% to 60% is comfortable for most clients.

If the environmental temperature becomes greater than the skin temperature, evaporation is the only mechanism for regulating body temperature. Evaporation is reduced when humidity levels rise because air that is almost or fully saturated with water cannot absorb additional moisture. Therefore, instead of evaporating, sweat accumulates and drips from the skin. Many agencies are air-conditioned. Electric fans and dehumidifiers are not always an adequate substitute but may be used if air conditioners are not available. In buildings where the air is dry, a humidifier or a cool mist machine can add moisture to the environment. Clients who have ineffective **thermoregulation** (the ability to maintain stable body temperature) may feel hot or cold even when the temperature and humidity are optimal.

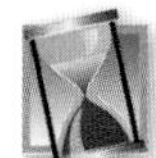

Gerontologic Considerations

- Older adults tend to prefer warmer room temperatures because of decreased subcutaneous fat deposits. Those with cognitive impairment, however, may feel that environmental temperatures are uncomfortably warm or cool, even when the temperature is comfortable for others.

Ventilation

At home, methods of **ventilation** (the movement of air) include opening windows or using ceiling fans. In hospitals and nursing homes, however, open windows are a fire and safety hazard, and ceiling fans spread infectious microorganisms. Consequently, ventilation usually occurs through a system of air ducts that circulate air in and out of each client room.

Poorly ventilated rooms and buildings tend to smell badly. Removing soiled articles, emptying bedpans and urinals, and opening privacy curtains and room doors help reduce odors. An alternative is to use an air freshener or deodorizer; generally, however, scented sprays substitute one odor for another, and ill clients usually find any strong smell disagreeable. Nurses should be conscientious about their own body and oral hygiene, refrain from wearing overpowering perfume, and avoid smelling of cigarette smoke.

Room Furnishings

Manufacturers of hospital furnishings attempt to design equipment that is both attractive and practical (Fig. 18-1).

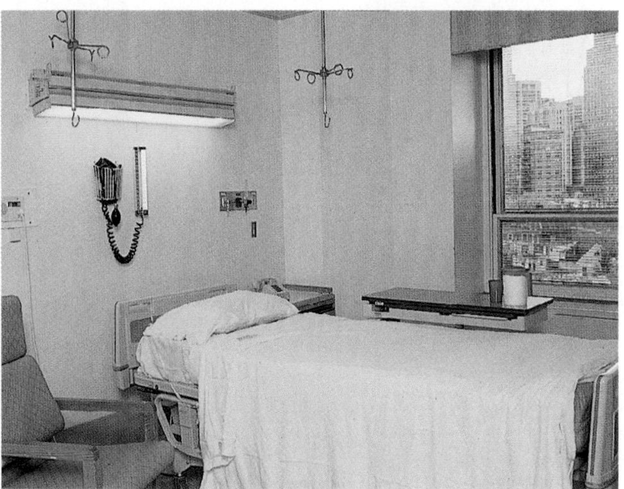

FIGURE 18-1 Typical hospital room furnishings. (Photo by B. Proud.)

The bed and its components—the mattress and pillows, chairs, overbed table, and bedside stand—must be safe, durable, and comfortable.

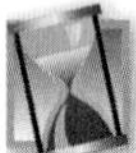

Gerontologic Considerations

■ Older adults who move to institutional settings, such as nursing homes or assisted living facilities, are usually more comfortable with their own bed furnishings and personal mementos and belongings.

Bed

Hospital beds are adjustable; that is, the height and position of the head and knees can be changed either electronically or manually. Adjusting the bed promotes comfort, enables self-care, and facilitates a therapeutic position (see Chap. 23). Hospital beds usually remain in their lowest position except when clients are receiving nursing care or during a change of bed linens. Skill 18-1 describes how to make an **unoccupied bed** (changing the linens when the bed is empty).

Full or half side rails are attached to the bed frame. There is controversy as to whether raised side rails are a risk or benefit because some clients climb over them rather than seek nursing assistance. Side rails are considered a form of physical restraint in long-term care facilities, and their use must be justified (Omnibus Budget Reconciliation Act of 1987; see Chap. 19).

Some beds have removable headboards (Fig. 18-2). This facilitates resuscitation efforts if the client experiences respiratory or cardiac arrest. Removing the headboard gives the code team responders better access for airway intubation. Placing the headboard under the client's upper body allows more effective cardiac compression than is possible on a mattress.

Mattress. Many people equate the comfort of a bed with the quality of the mattress. A good mattress adjusts to the shape of the body while supporting it. A mattress that is too soft alters the alignment of the spine, causing some people to awaken feeling sore from muscle and joint strain.

Hospital mattresses generally consist of tough materials that will withstand long-term use. Because mattresses are washed but not sterilized between uses, they are covered with a waterproof coating that withstands cleaning with strong antimicrobial solutions.

Occasionally, **mattress overlays** (layers of foam or other devices placed on top of the mattress; Fig. 18-3) are used to promote comfort or to keep the skin intact (see Chap. 23). Box 18-1 lists clients for whom a mattress overlay or therapeutic mattress of foam, gel, air, or water is appropriate.

Pillows. Pillows are primarily used for comfort, but they are also used to elevate a part of the body, relieve swelling, promote breathing, or help maintain a therapeutic position (see Chap. 23). Pillows are stuffed with foam, kapok (a mass of silky fibers), or feathers.

Bed Linen

The linens used for most hospital beds includes the following:

- Mattress pad
- Bottom sheet that is sometimes fitted
- Optional draw sheet that is placed beneath the client's hips
- Top sheet
- Blanket, depending on the client's preference
- Spread
- Pillowcase

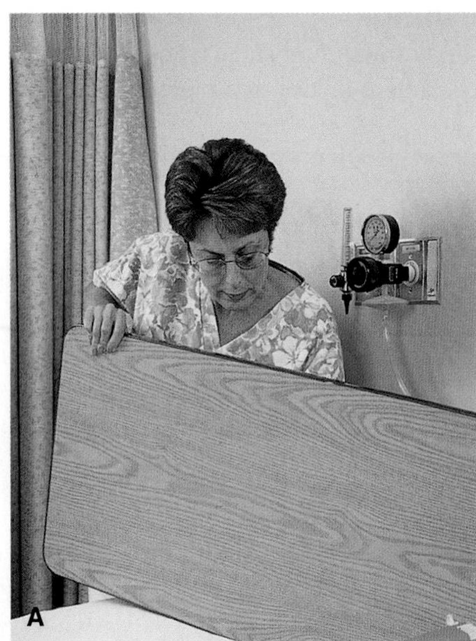

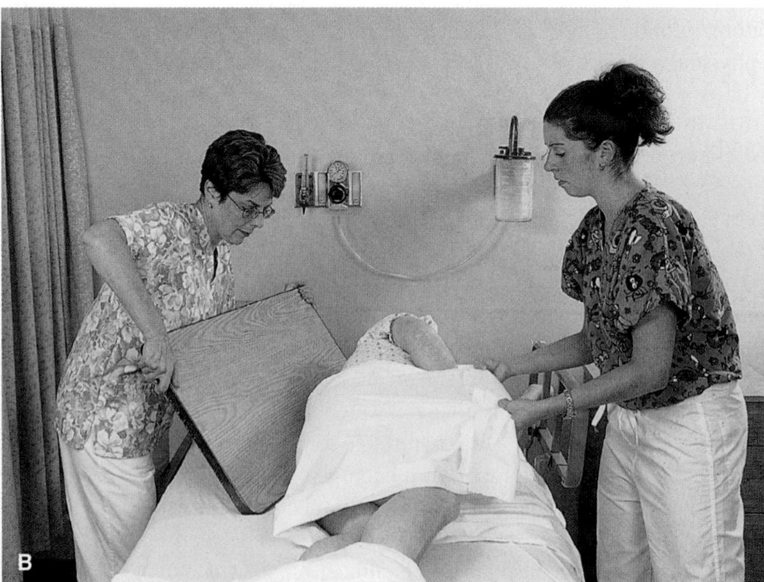

FIGURE 18-2 A. The nurse removes the headboard from a standard hospital bed. **B.** The nurse places the headboard beneath a client before resuscitation. (Photo by B. Proud.)

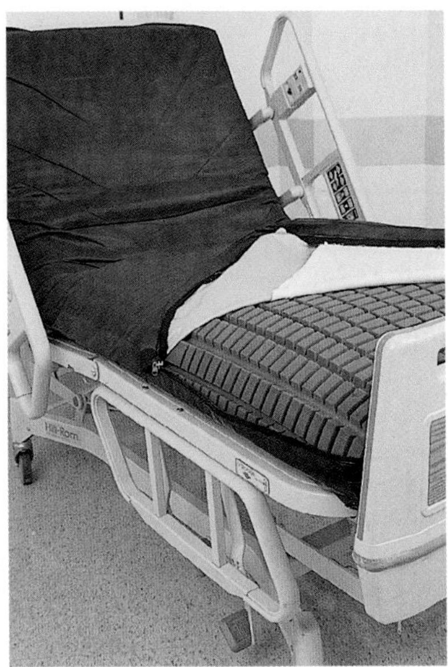

FIGURE 18-3 A waterproof mattress cover protects the mattress overlay. (Photo by B. Proud.)

Some hospitals use printed sheets to provide a more homelike atmosphere.

To control expenses, bed linen may not be changed every day, but any wet or soiled linen is changed as frequently as necessary. Sometimes, folded sheets or disposable, absorbent pads are placed between the client and the bottom sheet to avoid the need to change the entire bed when linen becomes soiled. Skill 18-2 explains how to make an **occupied bed** (changing the linens while the client remains in bed).

Stop, Think, and Respond Box 18-1

List situations when it would be appropriate to change some linens when providing client care and other situations in which it is more appropriate to change all linens.

Privacy Curtain

A privacy curtain is a long fabric partition mounted from the ceiling. It can be drawn completely around each client's bed. The privacy curtain preserves the client's dignity and modesty whenever it is necessary to examine or expose him or her for care. It is also used to shield a client from observation while using a urinal or bedpan.

BOX 18-1 Client Criteria for a Mattress Overlay or a Therapeutic Mattress

- Complete immobility
- Limited mobility
- Impaired skin integrity
- Inadequate nutritional status
- Incontinence of stool, urine, or both
- Altered tactile perception
- Compromised circulatory status

Overbed Table

An overbed table is a portable, flat platform positioned over the client's lap. The height of the table is adjustable depending on whether the bed is in a high or low position. The overbed table makes it convenient for the client to eat while in bed and to perform personal hygiene or other activities requiring a flat surface. Nurses also use the overbed table to hold equipment when providing client care. Most overbed tables have a concealed compartment that may contain a mounted mirror and a place for personal items (hairbrush, comb, cosmetic bag, razor, or book).

Bedside Stand

A bedside stand is actually a small cupboard. It usually contains a drawer for personal items and two shelves. The upper shelf is used to store the client's bath basin, soap dish, soap, and a kidney-shaped basin called an "emesis basin." The lower shelf is used to store a bedpan, urinal, and toilet paper. The elimination utensils are kept separate from the hygiene supplies to reduce the transmission of microorganisms. A carafe of water and a drinking container are placed atop the bedside stand.

Chairs

Generally, there is at least one chair per client in each room. Hospital chairs usually are straight-backed to facilitate good postural support. The best sitting position is when the hips, knees, and ankles are all at 90-degree angles. There may be one upholstered chair in each client room. Although upholstered chairs are more comfortable, some clients find it difficult to rise from them.

SLEEP AND REST

No matter how comfortable the physical environment or how attractive and homelike the furnishings, failure to promote rest and sleep may sabotage or prolong recuperation. Although sleep requirements vary, alterations in sleep patterns can have serious physical and emotional consequences. Family members, especially spouses, may experience sleep disturbances if someone snores, wakes up during the night, or wanders.

Functions of Sleep

In addition to promoting emotional well-being, sleep enhances various physiologic processes. Although the exact mechanisms are not totally understood, the restorative functions of sleep can be inferred from the effects of sleep

BOX 18-2 Effects of Chronic Sleep Deprivation

- Reduced physical stamina
- Altered comfort, such as headaches and nausea
- Impaired coordination, especially of fine motor skills
- Loss of muscle mass and weight
- Increased susceptibility to infection
- Slower wound healing
- Decreased pain tolerance
- Poor concentration
- Impaired judgment
- Unstable moods
- Suspiciousness

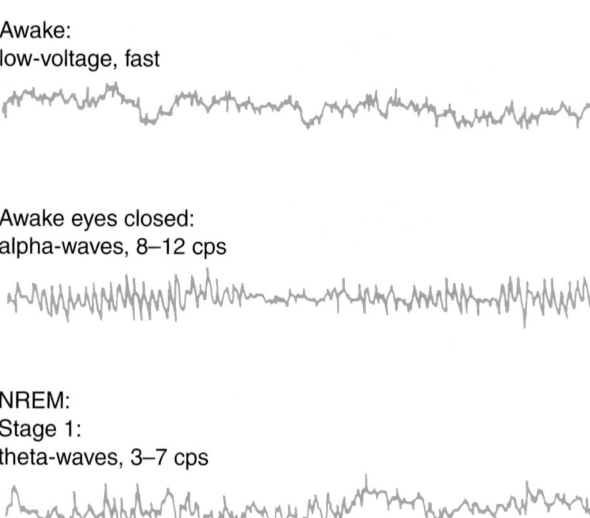

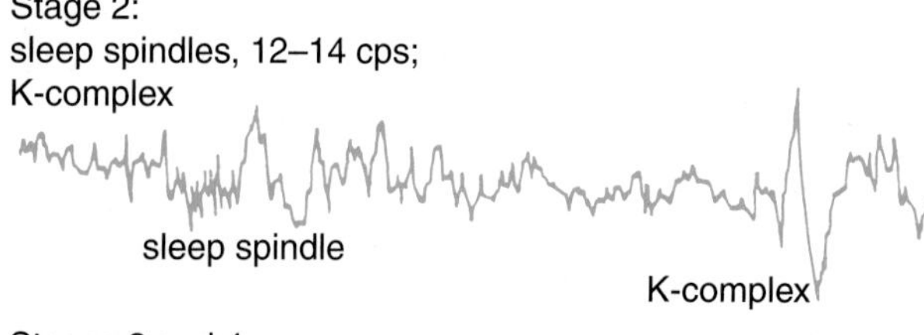

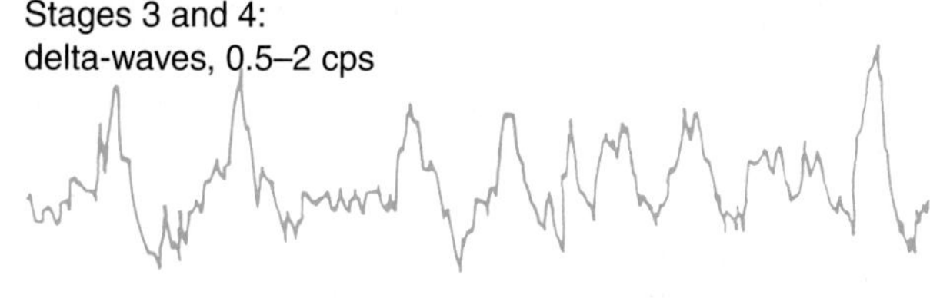

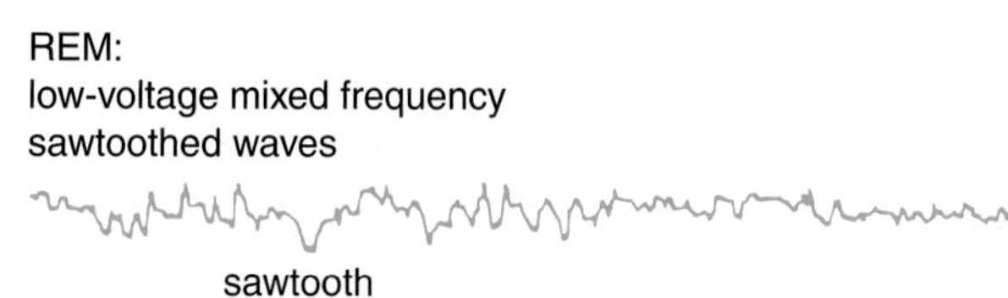

FIGURE 18-4 Characteristic electroencephalogram waveforms by sleep stage. cps, cycles per second. (From Craven, R.F., & Hirnle, C.J. [2008]. *Fundamentals of nursing: Human health and function* [6th ed.]. Philadelphia, PA: Lippincott Williams & Wilkins.)

deprivation (Box 18-2). Sleep is believed to play a role in the following:

- Reducing fatigue
- Stabilizing mood
- Improving blood flow to the brain
- Increasing protein synthesis
- Maintaining the disease-fighting mechanisms of the immune system
- Promoting cellular growth and repair
- Improving the capacity for learning and memory storage

Sleep Phases

Sleep is divided into two phases: nonrapid eye movement (NREM) sleep and rapid eye movement (REM) sleep. These names derive from the periods during sleep when eye movements are either subdued or energetic.

NREM sleep, which progresses through four stages, is also called "slow wave sleep" because during this phase electroencephalographic waves appear as progressively slower oscillations. The REM phase of sleep is referred to as *paradoxical sleep* because the electroencephalographic waves appear similar to those produced during periods of wakefulness (Fig. 18-4), but it is the deepest stage of sleep. Thus, NREM sleep is characterized as quiet sleep and REM sleep as active sleep.

Sleep Cycles

During sleep, people alternate between NREM and REM phases (Table 18-1). NREM sleep normally precedes REM sleep, the phase during which most dreaming occurs. Although the time spent in any one phase or stage varies according to age and other variables, most people cycle between stages 2, 3, and 4 of NREM to REM phases four to six times during the night.

Sleep Requirements

Sleep requirements vary among different age groups. The need for sleep decreases from birth to adulthood, although individuals vary (Table 18-2). Although an average of 7 to 9 hours of sleep is a requirement from adolescence through old age, 20% of Americans report sleeping less than 6 hours a night, an increase from the 13% reporting the same a decade ago (National Sleep Foundation, 2009a).

With age, the time spent in stages 3 and 4 of NREM decreases, whereas periods of REM sleep increase (Fig. 18-5). According to the National Sleep Foundation (2009b), older adults sleep more on weeknights, but younger adults sleep more on weekends. Older adults nap more than younger adults, a fact that may be attributed to daytime inactivity or reduced mental stimulation.

TABLE 18-1 Characteristics of Sleep Phases

SLEEP PHASE	LENGTH	FEATURES
NREM	50–90 min	Deep, restful, dreamless sleep
Stage 1	A few minutes	Light sleep, easily aroused Gradual reduction in vital signs
Stage 2	10–20 min	Deeper relaxation Can be awakened with effort
Stage 3	15–30 min	Early phase of deep sleep Snoring Relaxed muscle tone Little or no physical movement Difficult to arouse
Stage 4	15–30 min; shortens toward morning	Deep sleep Sleepwalking, sleep talking, and bedwetting may occur
REM	20-min average; lengthens toward morning	Darting eye movements Very difficult to awaken Vivid, colorful, emotional dreams Loss of muscle tone; jaw relaxes; tongue may fall to the back of the throat Vital signs fluctuate Irregular respirations Pauses in breathing for 15–20 sec Absence of snoring Muscle twitching Gastric secretions increase Men may have erections

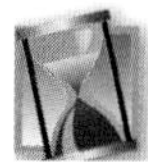

Gerontologic Considerations

- Older adults often report feeling tired, complain of sleep problems, and spend more time in bed without actually sleeping.
- Short daytime naps and rest periods, usually less than 2 hours in duration, can restore energy for an older adult without interfering with nighttime sleep. However, 7 to 9 hours of sleep within a 24-hour period is the usual total amount of sleep required by older adults. Therefore, expectations for the number of sleep hours during the night must be adjusted according to the amount of daytime sleep.
- Boredom may be a cause of daytime napping. Working with older adults to determine meaningful diversions may actually help with nighttime sleep, when naps are diminished.

TABLE 18-2 Sleep Requirements

AGE	TOTAL SLEEP TIME	PERCENTAGE IN REM
Newborn	16–20 hr/day	50
3 months–1 year	14–15 hr/day	35
Toddler	12 hr/night plus 1 or 2 naps	No data
Preschool	9–12 hr/night	No data
5–6 years	11 hr/night	20
6–11 years	10–11 hr/night	No data
11 years	9 hr/night	No data
Adolescent	7–9 hr/night	25
Adult	7–9 hr/night	20–25
Elderly	7–9 hr/night	13–15

Factors Affecting Sleep

Both the quantity and the quality of sleep decreases with age. According to the Division of Sleep Medicine at Harvard Medical School (2007), older adults suffer disproportionately from chronic sleep deprivation. The latter finding is not surprising because older adults awaken more frequently during the night for several reasons: pain; smaller bladder capacity, which results in an increased need to urinate; dementia-related sleep problems; side effects from medications such as diuretics; and diminished production of neurochemicals, such as melatonin, that promote sleep. Other factors not related to age also affect the amount and quality of a person's sleep (Table 18-3).

TABLE 18-3 Factors Affecting Sleep

SLEEP-PROMOTING FACTORS	SLEEP-SUPPRESSING FACTORS
Darkness, dim light	Sunlight, bright light
Consistent sleep schedule	Inconsistent sleep schedule
Secretion of melatonin	Suppression of melatonin
Familiar sleep environment	Strange sleep environment
Optimal warmth and ventilation	Cold, hot, stuffy room
Performance of sleep rituals	Disturbance of sleep rituals
Sedative, hypnotic drugs	Stimulant drugs
Depression	Depression, anxiety, worry
Relaxation	Activity
Satiation	Hunger, thirst
Proteins containing L-tryptophan	Protein-deficient diets
Excessive alcohol consumption	Metabolism of alcohol
Comfort	Pain, nausea, full bladder
Quiet	Noise
Effortless breathing	Difficulty breathing

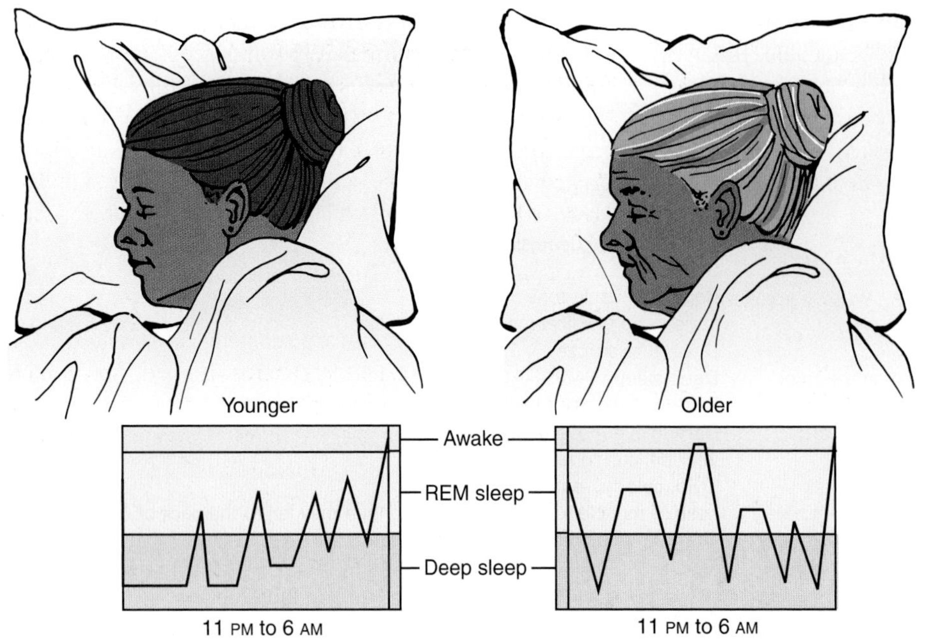

FIGURE 18-5 The time spent in REM and NREM sleep is different in younger adults than in older adults.

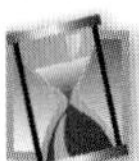

Gerontologic Considerations

■ Using night lights rather than bright room lights is preferred if an older adult arises during the night. Bright lights stimulate the brain and interfere with efforts to resume sleep.

Light

Daylight and darkness influence the sleep–wake cycle. **Circadian rhythm** (phenomena that cycle on a 24-hour basis) is a term derived from two Latin words: *circa* (about) and *dies* (day). Thus, drowsiness and sleep correlate with the circadian rhythm of the setting sun and night. Wakefulness corresponds with sunrise and daylight.

Researchers (Rosenthal et al., 1984) have suggested that the cycles of wakefulness followed by sleep are linked to a photosensitive system involving the eyes and the pineal gland in the brain (Fig. 18-6). Without bright light, the pineal gland secretes **melatonin** (a hormone that induces drowsiness and sleep); light triggers the suppression of melatonin secretion.

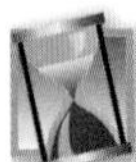

Gerontologic Considerations

■ The older adult's established pattern and circadian rhythms may not correspond to schedules of institutional settings. Modifications in established institutional routines may be needed to accommodate individual differences.

Activity

Activity, especially exercise, increases fatigue and the need for sleep. Activity appears to increase both REM and NREM sleep, especially the deep sleep of NREM stage 4. When physical activity occurs just before bedtime, however, it has a stimulating rather than a relaxing effect.

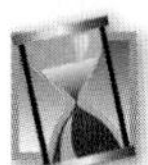

Gerontologic Considerations

■ Older adults with limited mobility may sleep better if they participate in chair or water exercises during the day.

Environment

Most people sleep best in their usual environment; they develop a preference for a particular pillow, mattress, and blankets. They also tend to adapt to the unique sounds where they live, such as traffic, trains, and the hum of appliance motors or furnaces.

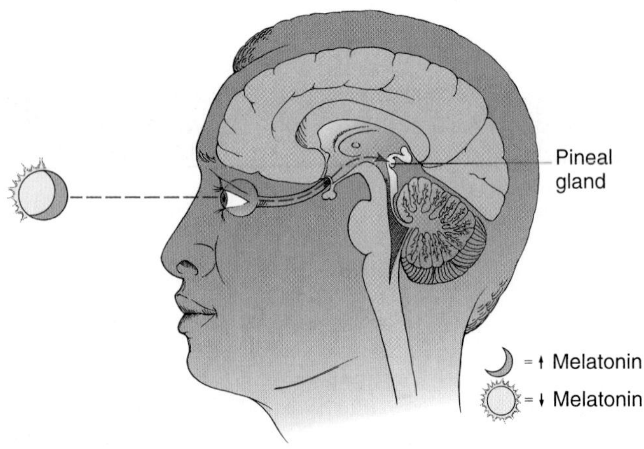

FIGURE 18-6 A photosensitive light system influences the sleep–wake cycle.

In addition, **sleep rituals** (habitual activities performed before retiring) induce sleep. Examples include eating a light snack, watching television, reading, and performing hygiene. Therefore, alterations in the environment or the activities performed before bedtime—such as occur during vacation or in the hospital—negatively affect a person's ability to fall and remain asleep.

Motivation

When a person has no particular reason to stay awake, sleep generally occurs easily. But if the desire to remain awake is strong, such as when a person wishes to participate in something interesting or important, the desire to sleep can be overcome.

Emotions and Moods

Depressive disorders are classically associated with an inability to sleep or the tendency to sleep more than usual. Also, emotions such as anger, fear, anxiety, and dread interfere with sleep. All are more than likely the result of changes in the types and amounts of neurotransmitters that affect the sleep–wake center in the brain.

Sometimes sleeplessness is conditioned—that is, anticipating sleeplessness, a characteristic pattern of some chronic insomniacs, actually reinforces it (a self-fulfilling prophecy). The expectation that the onset of sleep will be difficult increases the person's anxiety. The anxiety then floods the brain with stimulating chemicals that interfere with relaxation, a prerequisite for natural sleep.

Food and Beverages

Hunger or thirst interferes with sleep. The consumption of particular foods and beverages also may promote or inhibit the ability to sleep.

Sleep is facilitated by a chemical known as L-tryptophan, found in protein foods such as milk and dairy products. The recommendation to drink warm milk to induce sleep may have originally been an anecdotal observation of its **hypnotic** (sleep-producing) effect. L-tryptophan is also present in poultry, fish, eggs, and, to some extent, plant sources of protein such as legumes.

Alcohol is a depressive drug that promotes sleep, but it tends to reduce normal REM and deep-sleep stages of NREM sleep. As alcohol is metabolized, stimulating chemicals that were blocked by the sedative effects of the alcohol surge forth from neurons, causing early awakening. Beverages containing caffeine, a central nervous system stimulant, cause wakefulness. Caffeine is present in coffee, tea, chocolate, and most cola drinks.

Illness

Stress, anxiety, and discomfort accompany almost any illness, which can alter normal sleep patterns. In the hospital, other factors that contribute to sleep loss or fragmentation include being aroused by noise from equipment, awakened for nursing activities, and disturbed by unfamiliar sounds such as loud talking, elevators, dietary carts, and housekeeping equipment.

Several medical disorders involve symptoms that are aggravated at night or can disturb sleep. For example, ulcers tend to be more painful during the night because hydrochloric acid increases during REM sleep. In fact, pain of any kind is more distressing when there are few distractions. Conditions worsened by lying flat in bed, such as some cardiac, respiratory, and musculoskeletal disorders, contribute to sleeplessness.

Drugs

Caffeine and alcohol, which have already been discussed, are nonprescription drugs that affect sleep. Some prescribed drugs also can promote or interfere with sleep. **Sedatives** and **tranquilizers** (drugs that produce a relaxing and calming effect) promote rest, a precursor to sleep. Hypnotics are drugs that induce sleep. **Stimulants** (drugs that excite structures in the brain) cause wakefulness (Table 18-4).

Some sedatives and hypnotics have a paradoxical effect when administered to older adults: they tend to produce restlessness and wakefulness instead of sleep. Also, people who chronically take sedative and hypnotic drugs tend to develop **drug tolerance** (a diminished effect from the drug at its usual dosage range). Without realizing the danger, these people may increase the dose of the drug or the frequency of its

TABLE 18-4 Drugs That Affect Sleep

DRUG CATEGORY	DRUG FAMILY	EXAMPLE	ADVERSE REACTIONS
Sedatives	Barbiturates	phenobarbital (Luminal)	Sleepiness, lethargy, slowed respiratory rate, agitation, confusion
	Antihistamines	diphenhydramine (Benadryl)	Sleepiness, dizziness, slowed reaction time, impaired coordination
	Antipsychotics	haloperidol (Haldol)	Sleepiness, postural hypotension, abnormal facial and mouth movements, stiff gait, dry mouth
Tranquilizers	Benzodiazepines	alprazolam (Xanax)	Sleepiness, dry mouth, constipation, slowed heart rate, hypotension, liver damage
Hypnotics	Barbiturates	pentobarbital (Nembutal)	Same as phenobarbital, daytime drowsiness
	Nonbarbiturates	temazepam (Restoril)	Dizziness, lethargy during the day
Stimulants	Amphetamines	dextroamphetamine (Dexedrine)	Insomnia, restlessness, anorexia, rapid heart rate
	Amphetamine-like	methylphenidate (Ritalin)	Nervousness, insomnia, rash, anorexia, nausea

administration to achieve the same effect first experienced at a lower dose. Increasing the dose or frequency has potentially life-threatening consequences.

The abrupt discontinuation of sedatives, tranquilizers, and hypnotics produces a period of intense stimulation that interferes with sleep.

Some drugs that increase the formation of urine, such as diuretics, may awaken those who take them with a need to empty the bladder. For this reason, diuretics generally are administered early in the morning so that the peak effect has diminished by bedtime.

SLEEP ASSESSMENT

Many people blame inadequate sleep for daytime fatigue, or they underestimate the actual time they sleep. Nurses can obtain a more accurate sleep pattern assessment through sleep questionnaires, sleep diaries, polysomnographic evaluation, and a multiple latency sleep test.

Questionnaires

Several questionnaires have been developed to help identify sleep patterns. They are either designed to obtain specific information or are unstructured to give the person more freedom to respond. Nurses can gather data during interviews, or clients can answer the questions independently in the form of a self-reporting assessment.

Examples of questions for the client include the following:

- When you think about your sleep, what kinds of impressions come to mind?
- Does anything about your sleep bother you?
- Do you fall asleep at inappropriate times?
- Do you wake feeling rested?
- How long does it take you to fall asleep?
- Do you feel stiff and sore in the morning?
- Have you been told that you stop breathing while asleep?
- Do you fall asleep during physical activities?
- What do you do to help yourself sleep well?

Examples of questions for members of the client's household include the following:

- Does the client snore or gasp for air when sleeping?
- Does the client kick or thrash around while sleeping?
- Does the client sleepwalk?

Sleep Diary

A **sleep diary** is a daily account of sleeping and waking activities. The client or personnel compile the information in a sleep disorder clinic. The client notes the times he or she sleeps, describes daily activities during each 15-minute waking period, completes a 24-hour log of consumed food and beverages, and notes when he or she takes any medications. These self-kept diaries generally cover a 2-week period.

Although sleep diaries and questionnaires such as the Pittsburgh Sleep Quality Index and the Epworth Sleepiness Scale are inexpensive and simple to compile, they can vary in accuracy and reliability (Smyth, 2008, 2009). Therefore, sleep assessments include other objective diagnostic techniques for gathering data to ensure the accurate identification of sleep disorders and their etiologies.

Nocturnal Polysomnography

Nocturnal polysomnography is a diagnostic assessment technique in which a client is monitored for an entire night's sleep to obtain physiologic data. It generally takes place in a sleep disorder clinic, but it is now possible to conduct the study at the client's home; a technician monitors a computerized recording system up to 60 ft. away.

Dime-sized sensors attached to the head and body (Fig. 18-7) record the following:

- Brain waves
- Eye movements
- Muscle tone
- Limb movement
- Body position
- Nasal and oral airflow
- Chest and abdominal respiratory effort
- Snoring sounds
- Oxygen level in the blood

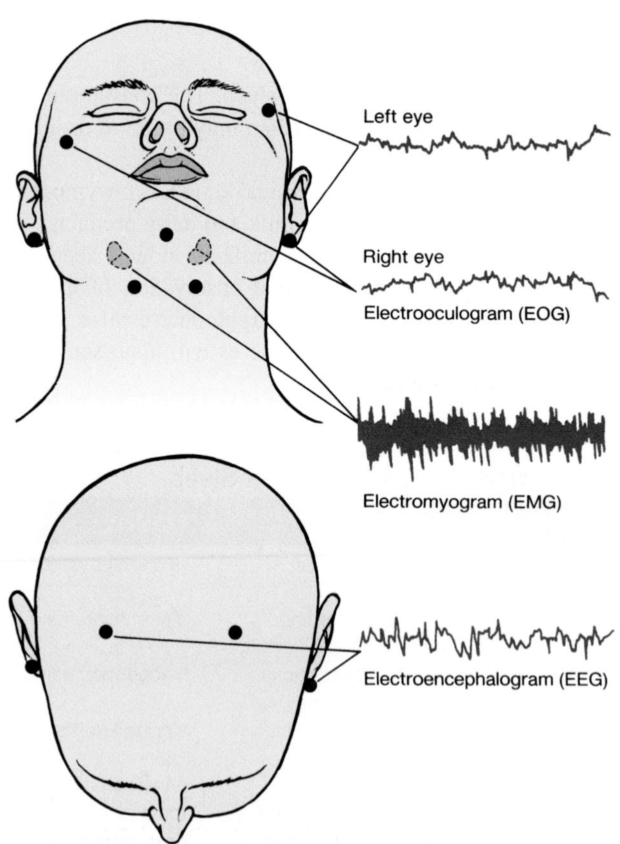

FIGURE 18-7 Providers evaluate normal sleep patterns and sleep disorders by collecting physiologic data.

The diagnostic data are compared with the patterns and characteristics of normal sleep cycles to help diagnose sleep disorders.

Multiple Sleep Latency Test

A **multiple sleep latency test** (an assessment of daytime sleepiness) is another helpful study. The person undergoing this test is asked to take a daytime nap at 2-hour intervals while attached to sensors similar to those used in polysomnography. The client is allowed to nap for about 20 minutes. The nap periods are repeated four or five times throughout the day.

Clients who have certain sleep disorders causing daytime sleepiness have a short latency period—that is, they fall asleep in less than 5 minutes. Most well-rested persons take an average of 15 minutes before they experience the onset of daytime sleep.

Experiencing early REM sleep is also a pathologic finding that can be detected during a multiple sleep latency test. A REM period normally does not occur for at least 1 hour and after cycling through the first four stages of NREM. Therefore, REM should not occur during a 20-minute test nap.

SLEEP DISORDERS

About 40 million Americans have some type of sleep disorder, the most common being insomnia, followed by sleep apnea. An additional 20 to 30 million have intermittent sleep-related problems (National Institute of Neurological Disorders and Stroke, 2007). Many of those affected do not seek treatment. Most problems are short-lived, but some sleep disorders are both chronic and serious.

There are four categories of sleep disorders: insomnia, hypersomnia, sleep–wake cycle disturbance, and parasomnia.

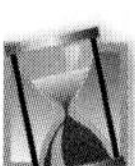

Gerontologic Considerations

- Insomnia and hypersomnia are often manifestations of depression among older adults.

Insomnia

Insomnia means difficulty in falling asleep, awakening frequently during the night, or awakening early. It results in feeling unrested the next day. Almost everyone has had insomnia, and most cases resolve in less than 3 weeks. According to the American Psychiatric Association (2000), insomnia is considered a sleep disturbance if it occurs over at least 1 month. Although chronic insomnia can be treated with hypnotic drugs, it is helpful to start treatment with nonpharmacologic interventions (see Client and Family Teaching 18-1).

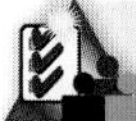

Client and Family Teaching 18-1
Promoting Sleep

The nurse teaches the client or the family as follows:

- Resist napping during the day.
- Use the bed and bedroom just for sleeping.
- Perform sleep rituals.
- Go to bed and get up at approximately the same time, even on weekends or days off.
- If you cannot get to sleep for more than 20 to 30 minutes, get out of bed and do something else such as reading.
- Try a bedtime relaxation tape that plays soothing music, sounds of nature, or a constant background sound (white noise).
- Exercise regularly during the day but not late in the evening.
- Avoid alcohol, nicotine, and caffeine.
- Eat dairy products and other proteins daily.
- Modify the temperature and ventilation in the bedroom according to personal preferences.
- Use earplugs or eyeshades to reduce environmental noise or light.
- Avoid using nonprescription or prescription sleeping pills unless they have been recommended by a physician. Hypnotics should be used only on a short-term basis.
- Try drinking chamomile tea, which some claim improves sleep.
- Follow label directions on any medications.
- If a diuretic drug is prescribed, take it early in the morning.

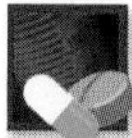

Pharmacologic Considerations

- The National Institute of Neurological Disorders and Stroke (2006) recommends that sleep disorders in older adults be managed without hypnotic medications, which tend to have paradoxical effects in older adults (ie, a stimulating effect or mental changes).
- Although hypnotic medications may be effective initially, tolerance usually develops sometimes within a few days; therefore, their use is not recommended for longer than 2 weeks. Hypnotic medications reduce REM sleep and may cause older adults to have nightmares and other sleep cycle disturbances for several weeks after discontinuation.
- Many hypnotic medications, particularly those with a very long half-life such as flurazepam (Dalmane), tend to cause daytime drowsiness and increase the risk for falls. Examples of hypnotics with shorter half-lives that are better tolerated by older adults include triazolam (Halcion), temazepam (Restoril), zolpidem (Ambien), or zaleplon (Sonata).

Hypersomnia

Hypersomnia is a sleep disorder characterized by feeling sleepy despite getting normal sleep. Two conditions of hypersomnia are sleep apnea/hypopnea syndrome and narcolepsy.

Sleep Apnea/Hypopnea Syndrome

Apnea (the cessation of breathing) and **hypopnea** (hypoventilation) are concomitant forms of hypersomnia: **sleep**

apnea/hypopnea syndrome. In this disorder, the sleeper stops breathing or breathing slows for 10 seconds or longer five or more times per hour (Rowley, 2009). This is discussed further in Chapter 21.

During the apneic or hypopneic periods, ventilation decreases and blood oxygenation drops. The accumulation of carbon dioxide and the fall in oxygen cause brief periods of awakening throughout the night. This disturbs the normal transitions and periods of NREM and REM sleep. Consequently, clients with sleep apnea/hypopnea syndrome feel tired after having slept, or worse, their symptoms may cause a heart attack, stroke, or sudden death from **hypoxia** (decreased cellular oxygenation) of the heart, brain, and other organs.

The incidence of sleep apnea is highest among older adults, especially obese men who snore. Methods to reduce apneic episodes include sleeping in other than the supine position, losing weight, and avoiding substances that depress respirations such as alcohol or sleeping medications. In severe cases, clients wear a continuous positive airway pressure (CPAP) mask (see Chap. 21) that keeps the alveoli inflated during sleep. Surgery on the tonsils, uvula, pharynx, tongue, or epiglottis is another treatment option when conservative measures are ineffective.

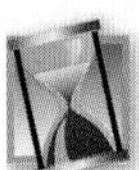

Gerontologic Considerations

- Older adults may need an evaluation for sleep apnea if morning headaches or frequent nighttime awakenings occur.

Narcolepsy

Narcolepsy is characterized by the sudden onset of daytime sleep, a short NREM period before the first REM phase, and pathologic manifestations of REM sleep. This disabling condition should not be confused with **hypersomnolence**, which is excessive sleeping for long periods, as in Washington Irving's 1819 American folk story, *Rip Van Winkle.*

Although the diagnosis of narcolepsy generally requires a multiple sleep latency test and polysomnography, its symptoms help distinguish it from other conditions that cause sleepiness. For example, the sleepiness of narcolepsy is accompanied by the following:

- **Sleep paralysis**—the person cannot move for a few minutes just before falling asleep or awakening
- **Cataplexy**—a sudden loss of muscle tone triggered by an emotional change such as laughing or anger
- **Hypnogogic hallucinations**—a dream-like auditory or visual experiences while dozing or falling asleep
- **Automatic behavior**—the performance of routine tasks without full awareness or later memory of having done them

Many older adults experience a decrease in the severity of narcoleptic symptoms after 60 years of age (National Institute of Neurologic Disorders and Stroke, 2006). If untreated, the client may become involved in a motor vehicle crash or occupational accident. Prescribed stimulant drugs, such as methylphenidate (Ritalin) or amphetamine (Adderall), help improve alertness. Antidepressants reduce the symptoms associated with atypical REM sleep.

Sleep–Wake Cycle Disturbances

A **sleep–wake cycle disturbance** results from a sleep schedule that involves daytime sleeping and interferes with biologic rhythms. Changes in the intensity of light trigger sleeping. When exposure to light comes at an atypical time, the sleep–wake cycle is desynchronized. Sleep–wake cycle disorders occur among shift workers, jet travelers, and those diagnosed with seasonal affective disorder, a cyclical mood disorder believed to be linked to diminished exposure to sunlight.

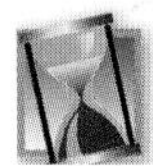

Gerontologic Considerations

- Some older adults with cognitive impairment develop **sundown syndrome** (the onset of disorientation as the sun sets) (Box 18-3). Others develop **sunrise syndrome** (early-morning confusion) associated with inadequate sleep or the effects of sedative and hypnotic medications.

Shift Work

Those who work evening or night shifts or who switch from one shift to another are especially prone to unsynchronized sleep–wake cycles. The indoor lighting to which most shift workers are exposed is not bright enough to suppress melatonin; consequently, many shift workers fight to stay awake. Some experience **microsleep**, which is unintentional sleep lasting 20 to 30 seconds. Statistics show that shift workers are more prone to errors and accidents from sleepiness (Harrington, 2001; National Institute for Occupational Safety and Health [NIOSH], 2004). Most people who work night shifts never completely adapt to the reversal of day and night activities, no matter how long the pattern is established.

BOX 18-3 Characteristics of Sundown Syndrome

- Alert and oriented during the day
- Onset of disorientation as the sun sets
- Disorganized thinking
- Restlessness
- Agitation
- Perseveration (ruminating over the same repetitive thought)
- Wandering

Jet Travel

Jet travel causes a sudden change in the currently established **photoperiod** (the number of daylight hours) to which a person is accustomed. Consequently, travelers often describe having **jet lag**, or emotional and physical changes experienced when arriving in a different time zone. Many travelers have difficulty falling or staying asleep, but jet lag is more transient than shift work. Some travelers re-establish normal sleep–wake cycles, but it takes at least 1 day for each time zone that is crossed when traveling east, slightly less when traveling west.

Seasonal Affective Disorder

Seasonal affective disorder is characterized by depression, hypersomnolence, a lack of energy when awake, increased appetite accompanied by cravings for sweets, and weight gain. The symptoms begin during darker winter months and disappear as daylight hours increase in the spring. In some ways, the disorder resembles the hibernation patterns in bears and other animals.

Some suggest that seasonal affective disorder results from excessive melatonin. To counteract the symptoms, **phototherapy** (a technique for suppressing melatonin by stimulating light receptors in the eye) is prescribed. The artificial light used in phototherapy is at least 2,000 to 2,500 lux, the equivalent of the bright light measured on a sunny spring day. Clients use the lights for 2 to 6 hours each day to simulate the number of daylight hours during sunnier months (Box 18-4). Phototherapy usually relieves symptoms within 3 to 5 days, but symptoms tend to recur in the same amount of time if a client abruptly discontinues phototherapy.

Parasomnia

Parasomnias are conditions associated with activities that cause arousal or partial arousal, usually during transitions in NREM periods of sleep. They are not life-threatening, but they disturb others in the household—most significantly, the bed partner. Some examples of parasomnias include the following:

- **Somnambulism** (sleepwalking)
- **Nocturnal enuresis** (bedwetting)
- Sleep talking
- Nightmares and night terrors
- **Bruxism** (grinding of the teeth)
- **Restless legs syndrome** (movement typically in the legs [but occasionally in the arms or other body parts] to relieve disturbing skin sensations)

Restless legs syndrome, also known as nocturnal myoclonus, may be the most disabling parasomnia. The symptoms keep the person awake or prevent continuous sleep. Eventually, sleep deprivation affects the person's life, damaging work productivity and personal relationships. Medical etiologies, such as iron deficiency, kidney failure, and peripheral nerve pathology, can mimic the manifestations of restless legs syndrome. Once these conditions are diagnostically eliminated, the condition is confirmed with polysomnography.

Conservative treatments for parasomnias include safety measures for sleepwalkers (stair gates, security locks on doors and windows), mouth devices for bruxism, lifestyle changes, nutritional support, and good sleep hygiene. In severe cases, drug therapy is used.

BOX 18-4 Components of Phototherapy

To relieve the symptoms of seasonal affective disorder, the client:

- Initiates a schedule of full-spectrum[a] light exposure beginning in October and November
- Removes eyeglasses or contact lenses that have ultraviolet filters
- Sits within 3 ft. of the artificial light for approximately 2 hours soon after awakening from sleep
- Glances at the light periodically but may engage in other activities such as reading or handiwork
- Repeats the exposure to light after sundown (to simulate extending the daylight hours) up to a cumulative time of 3 to 6 hours a day
- Continues the pattern of light exposure until spring

[a]Full-spectrum light simulates the energy of bright natural sunlight.

NURSING IMPLICATIONS

After assessing client comfort and sleep patterns and the accompanying symptoms, nurses identify one or more nursing diagnoses that require interventions:

- Fatigue
- Impaired bed mobility
- Disturbed sleep pattern
- Sleep deprivation
- Relocation stress syndrome
- Risk for injury
- Impaired gas exchange

Nursing Care Plan 18-1 is an example of how the nursing process has been used to develop a plan of care for a client with Insomnia, defined in the NANDA-I taxonomy (2012, p. 217) as a "disruption in amount and quality of sleep that impairs functioning."

Several sleep-promoting nursing measures, such as maintaining sleep rituals, reducing the intake of stimulating chemicals, promoting daytime exercise, and adhering to a regular schedule for retiring and awakening, have already been discussed. Two additional beneficial methods are assisting the client with progressive relaxation exercises and providing a back massage.

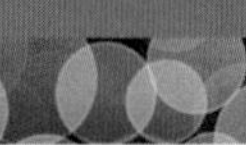

NURSING CARE PLAN 18-1 Insomnia

Assessment

- Ask the client to rate his or her quality of sleep using a numeric scale of 10 indicating severe disturbance to 0 indicating satisfactory.
- Identify sleep aids including medications, alcohol, and sleep rituals and lifestyle practices, such as excessive consumption of caffeine, that may interfere with sleep.
- Inquire about the client's usual time for retiring and awakening without an alarm clock.
- Have the client keep a diary for several days of:
  - Bedtime
  - Approximate time for onset of sleep
  - Number of times awakened during sleep and reason for awakening
  - Time of awakening in the morning
  - Number and length of daytime naps
- Compare collected data with age-related norms.
- Seek information from his or her sleep partner regarding symptoms of disorders manifested during sleep, such as snoring interrupted by a period of apnea, unusual movement, or sleepwalking.
- Consult with the family regarding the client's level of stress, emotional stability, attention, work endurance, and incidence of work-related or driving accidents.

Nursing Diagnosis. **Insomnia** related to excessive neurostimulation secondary to anxiety over slow recovery from illness as evidenced by statement, "I'd rate the quality of my sleep at 5. It seems that it takes forever to fall asleep. It's been 2 weeks since I've gotten more than 4 hours of sleep. I worry constantly that I'll never go home again," and need for barbiturate hypnotic that is repeated each night.

Expected Outcome. The client will sleep within 30 minutes of going to bed and remain asleep for a minimum of 7 hours within 5 days (by 3/15).

Interventions	Rationales
Have the client retire at 2100 each evening and arise at 0730 each morning regardless of the duration or quality of sleep.	Retiring and arising at a consistent time helps to develop a sleep–wake pattern.
Allow naps only in early morning.	More REM sleep occurs during early morning than afternoon naps. Increasing REM will improve a feeling of rest and well-being.
Limit naps to less than 90 minutes.	Short naps promote longer sleep cycles during the night, which in turn contributes to additional REM periods of sleep.
Avoid disturbing the client at night within 100-minute blocks of sleep.	The duration of a complete cycle of NREM and REM sleep is approximately 70–100 minutes four or five times a night.
Reduce or eliminate the client's intake of caffeine.	Caffeine is a central nervous system stimulant that interferes with relaxation and sleep.
Encourage moderate exercise for at least 20 minutes three times a day but no later than 1930.	Regular exercise promotes sleep but may overstimulate a person if performed close to bedtime.
Provide milk, yogurt, vanilla pudding, custard, or some other dairy product at approximately 2030.	Dairy products are a good source of L-tryptophan, which promotes sleep.
Delay administering sleeping medication and give a back massage at bedtime.	Massage promotes relaxation, which is a precursor to sleep. Sleep medications can interfere with REM sleep and may cause daytime drowsiness.

Evaluation of Expected Outcomes

- The client was observed to fall asleep in 30–45 minutes.
- The client experienced uninterrupted sleep for 3 hours.
- The client's total duration of sleep was 6–7 hours.

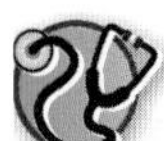

NURSING GUIDELINES 18-1

Facilitating Progressive Relaxation

- Select a room that is quiet, private, and dimly lit. *Such a setting reduces stimulation of the arousal center in the brain, which responds to noise, bright lights, and activity.*
- Encourage the client to assume a comfortable position; this usually involves lying down or sitting. *Sitting or lying down provides external support for the body, which facilitates muscle relaxation.*
- Advise the client to avoid talking and instead listen to the suggestions that will follow. *Advising the client to take a passive role reduces performance anxiety (a worry about appearing incompetent or foolish).*
- Instruct the client to close the eyes and consciously focus on breathing. *Closing the eyes blocks visual stimuli; focusing on breathing helps to turn the client's attention away from distracting thoughts and feelings.*
- Tell the client to inhale deeply through the nose and exhale slowly out the mouth. Repeat the activity several times. *This breathing oxygenates the blood and brain and reduces the heart rate.*
- Tell the client to tighten the muscles in an area of the body, such as the foot, and hold the position for at least 5 seconds. *Tightening a muscle depletes the level of stimulating neurotransmitters.*
- Direct the client to relax the tensed muscles and focus on the pleasant feeling. *Focusing on the pleasant feeling directs the cortex's attention to the desired outcome and raises the client's awareness.*
- Proceed with sequence after sequence of muscle contraction followed by relaxation until all muscle groups in the body have been exercised. *Continued tensing and relaxation leads to higher planes of relaxation.*
- Continue suggesting throughout that the client focus on how relaxed or weightless he or she feels. *These verbal cues reinforce relaxation.*
- Tell the client that as you reach zero after counting backward from 10, he or she can begin to move. *This provides a gradual end to the relaxation period.*

Progressive Relaxation

Progressive relaxation is a therapeutic exercise in which a person actively contracts then relaxes muscle groups to break the worry–tension cycle that interferes with relaxation (see Nursing Guidelines 18-1).

Clients can learn to perform progressive relaxation exercises independently using self-suggestion. Some clients eventually omit the muscle contraction phase and go directly to progressive relaxation of muscle groups.

Back Massage

Massage (stroking the skin) promotes two desired outcomes: it relaxes tense muscles and improves circulation (Skill 18-3). Nurses perform massage using various stroking techniques (Table 18-5). Stimulating strokes are omitted if the purpose is to relax the client.

Stop, Think, and Respond Box 18-2

Describe techniques for maximizing the positive effects of a back massage.

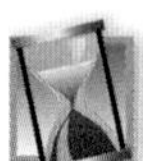

Gerontologic Considerations

- Sleep may be promoted among older adults with any of the following relaxation techniques before bedtime: imagery, meditation, deep breathing, soothing music, body or foot massage, chair rocking, reading nonstimulating materials, or watching nonstimulating television programs.

TABLE 18-5 Massage Techniques

TECHNIQUE	DESCRIPTION	METHOD
Effleurage	To skim the surface	The hands are used to make a circular pattern using long strokes over the massaged area.
Pétrissage	To knead	The skin is lifted and compressed or pulled in opposing directions.
Frôlement	To brush	The skin is lightly touched with the fingertips.
Tapotement	To tap	The skin is lightly struck with the sides of the hands.
Vibration	To set in motion	The skin is moved rhythmically with open or cupped palms, causing the tissue to quiver.
Friction	To rub	The skin is pulled from opposite directions using the thumbs and fingers.

CRITICAL THINKING EXERCISES

1. What items in the health care environment would you find important in supporting your comfort, rest, and sleep?
2. What actions could a nurse take to promote sleep among clients in a hospital or other types of health care facility such as a nursing home?
3. Discuss possible effects of suffering from or living with a person who has a sleep disorder.
4. Explain why nursing interventions that promote sleep may be preferable to administering a medication that promotes sleep.

NCLEX-STYLE REVIEW QUESTIONS

1. When observing an unlicensed nursing assistant make an occupied bed, which of the following actions indicates a need for further learning?
   1. The assistant loosens all the linen under the client.
   2. The assistant wears gloves to remove soiled linen.
   3. The assistant keeps the bed in a low position.
   4. The assistant rolls the client to the far side of the bed.
2. When making an unoccupied bed of a client who has been incontinent of stool, which action is essential?
   1. The nurse discards all linen.
   2. The nurse dons clean disposable gloves.
   3. The nurse uses a fitted bottom sheet.
   4. The nurse puts a blanket over the top sheet.
3. To help a client suffering from insomnia, which plan for nursing care is best?
   1. Administer a prescribed hypnotic drug each night.
   2. Try to duplicate the client's pattern of sleep rituals.
   3. Have the client exercise for 30 minutes at bedtime.
   4. Suggest the client go to bed earlier than the usual time.
4. Which of the following are aseptic practices that are appropriate when making an unoccupied bed? Select all that apply.
   1. Raise the bed to a high position.
   2. Loosen the bed linen from the mattress.
   3. Place clean linen on a chair.
   4. Hold soiled linen away from the uniform.
   5. Place soiled linen directly into a hamper.
5. When observing a sleeping client, which of the following suggests that the client is in REM sleep? Select all that apply.
   1. Muscle twitching
   2. Snoring
   3. Little physical movement
   4. Darting movement beneath the eyelids
   5. Talking while asleep

SKILL 18-1 Making an Unoccupied Bed

Suggested Action	Reason for Action
ASSESSMENT	
Check the Kardex or nursing care plan to determine the client's activity level.	Determines if the client can be out of bed during bedmaking.
Inspect the linen for moisture or evidence of soiling.	Indicates what and how much linen must be changed and if gloves are appropriate when removing soiled linen.
PLANNING	
Plan to change the linen after the client's hygiene needs have been met.	Reduces the potential for wetting or soiling the clean linen.
Wash hands or perform hand antisepsis with an alcohol rub (see Chap. 10). Use gloves if there is a potential for direct contact with blood, stool, or other body fluids.	Reduces the transmission of microorganisms.
Bring necessary bed linen to the room.	Demonstrates organization and efficient time management.
Place the clean linen on a clean, dry surface such as the seat or back of a chair (Fig. A).	Reduces transmission of microorganisms to clean supplies.

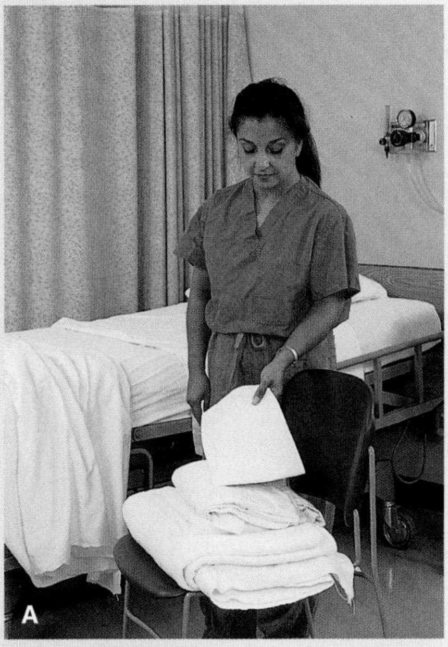

A

Arranging clean bed linen. (Photo by B. Proud.)

Suggested Action	Reason for Action
Assist the client from the bed.	Facilitates bedmaking.
IMPLEMENTATION	
Raise the bed to a high position and lower the side rails.	Prevents postural and muscular strain.
Remove equipment attached to the bed linens, such as the signal cord and drainage tubes, and check for personal items.	Avoids breakage, spills, or loss of personal items.
Loosen the bed linen from where it has been tucked under the mattress.	Facilitates removal or retightening.
Fold any linen that may be reused and place it on a clean surface.	Promotes efficiency and orderliness.

(continued)

Making an Unoccupied Bed (continued)

IMPLEMENTATION (CONTINUED)

Don gloves, if necessary, and roll linen that will be replaced so that the soiled surface is enclosed (Fig. B).

Gloves are a standard precaution to provide a barrier between the nurse and blood or body fluids; gloves are unnecessary if linen does not contain blood or body fluid. Rolling linen with the soiled side inward reduces contact with sources of microorganisms.

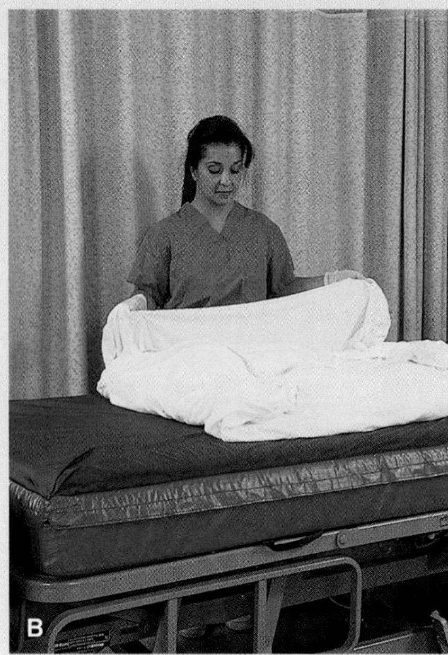

Enclosing soiled side of linen. (Photo by B. Proud.)

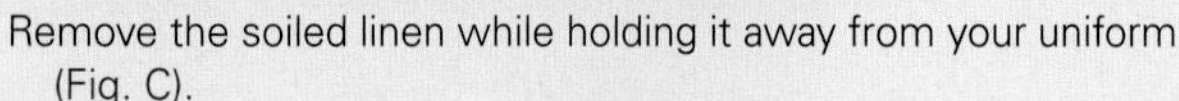

Remove the soiled linen while holding it away from your uniform (Fig. C).

Prevents transferring microorganisms to your uniform and then to other clients.

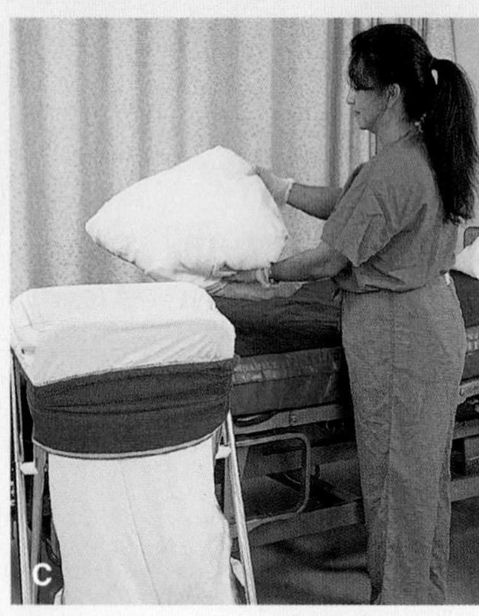

Avoiding contact with uniform. (Photo by B. Proud.)

(continued)

Making an Unoccupied Bed (continued)

IMPLEMENTATION (CONTINUED)

Place the soiled linen directly into a pillowcase, laundry hamper, or self-made pouch from one of the removed sheets (Fig. D). *Do not place the soiled linen on the floor.* — Keeps the soiled linen from being further contaminated.

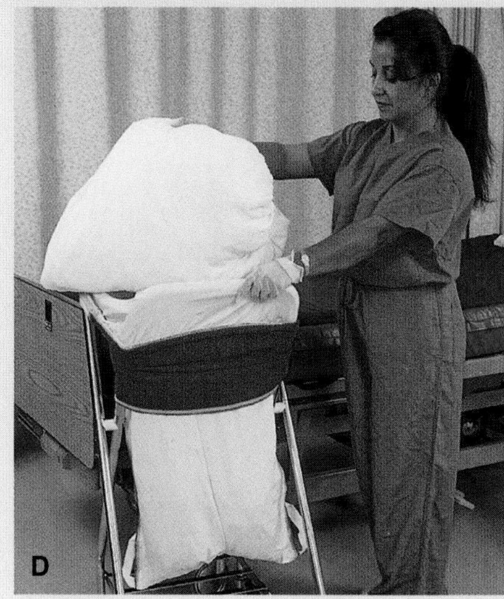

Placing soiled linen in hamper. (Photo by B. Proud.)

Remove gloves and wash hands or perform hand antisepsis with an alcohol rub (see Chap. 10) once contact with body secretions is no longer likely. — Facilitates use of the hands.

Reposition the mattress so it is flush with the headboard. — Provides maximum foot room.

Tighten any linen that will be reused. — Removes wrinkles, which promotes client comfort.

If the bottom sheet needs changing, center the longitudinal fold and open the layers of folded linen to one side of the bed. — Reduces postural strain.

If using a flat sheet, make sure the flat edge of the hem is flush with the edge of the mattress at the foot end. — Prevents skin pressure and irritation.

If using a flat sheet, tuck the upper portion under the mattress. Make a mitered or square corner at the top of the bed. — Anchors the bottom sheet.

If using a fitted sheet, position the upper and lower corners of the mattress within the contoured corners of the sheet (Fig. E).

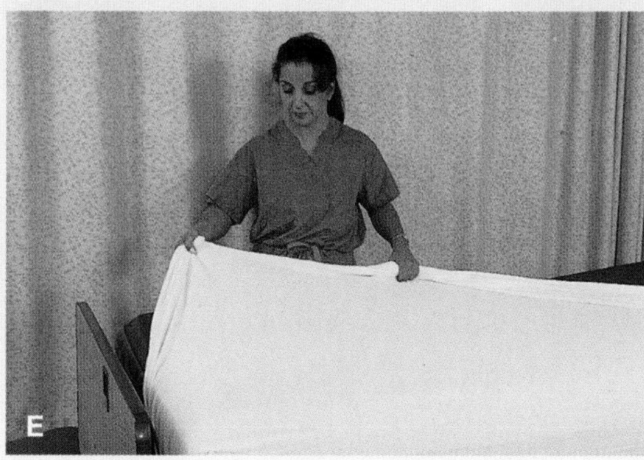

Stretching the fitted sheet taut. (Photo by B. Proud.)

(continued)

Making an Unoccupied Bed (continued)

IMPLEMENTATION (CONTINUED)

If the client is apt to soil the linen with urine or stool, fold a flat sheet horizontally with the smooth edge of the hem toward the foot of the bed and tuck it in place approximately where the buttocks will be. Do the same if a draw sheet is available (Fig. F).

Reduces the need to change all the bottom linen.

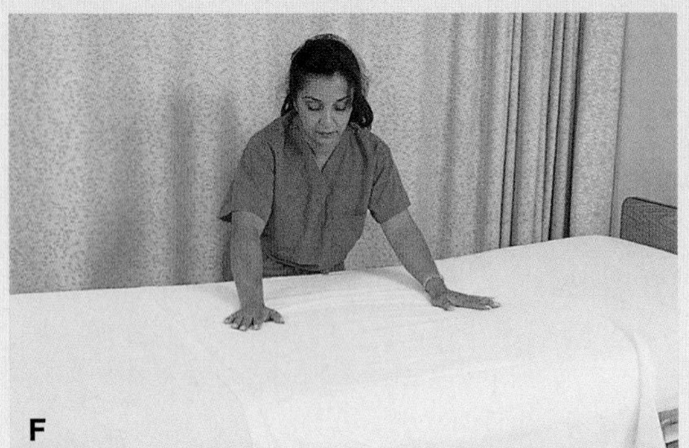

F

Smoothing the draw sheet before securing it snugly under the mattress. (Photo by B. Proud.)

Position the top linen on one half of the bed at this time. Move to the other side of the bed, pull the linen taut, and tuck the free edges beneath the mattress.

Saves time by reducing the number of moves around the bed.

Alternatively, wait until you have secured all the bottom linen to position the top sheet.

Secures and smooths the bottom linens.

Center the top sheet and unfold it to one side, leaving sufficient length at the top to make a fold over the spread.

Provides a smooth edge next to the client's neck.

Add blankets if the client wishes.

Demonstrates concern for the client's comfort.

Cover the top sheet with the spread if desired. Tuck the excess linen at the foot of the bed under the bottom of the mattress and finish the sides with a mitered or square corner (Fig. G).

Secures the top linen.

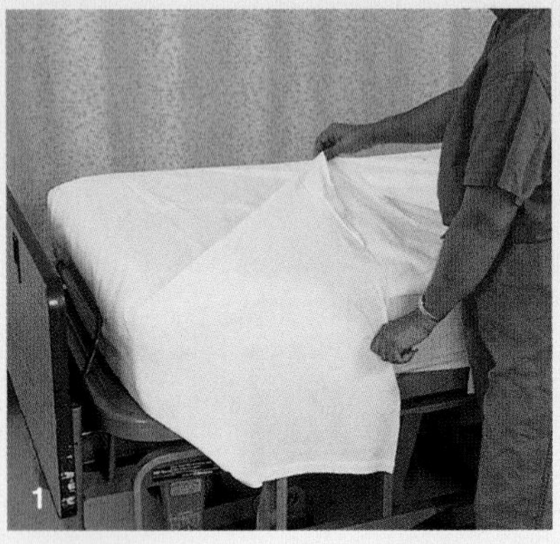

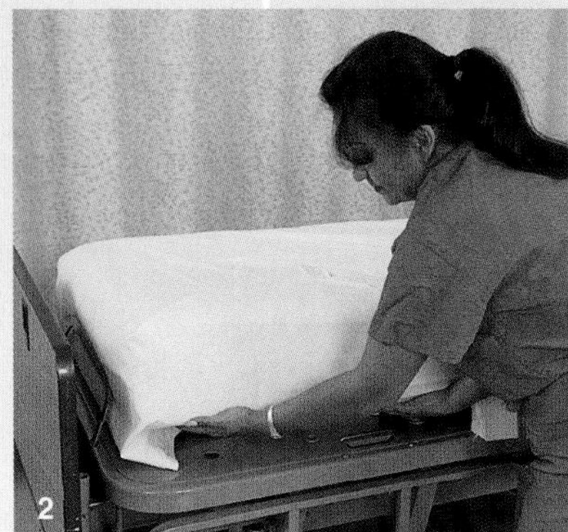

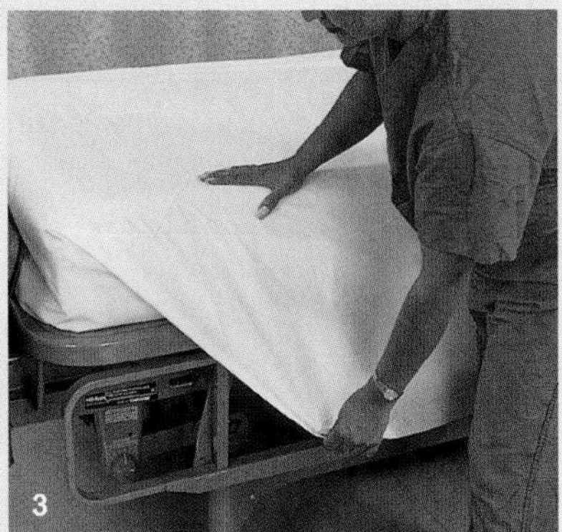

G 1 2 3

(1) Folding the edge of the top sheet back onto itself. (2) Tucking the edge hanging from the bed under the mattress. (3) Pulling the top sheet taut. (Photo by B. Proud.)

(continued)

Making an Unoccupied Bed (continued)

IMPLEMENTATION (CONTINUED)

Smooth the top sheet (Fig. H).

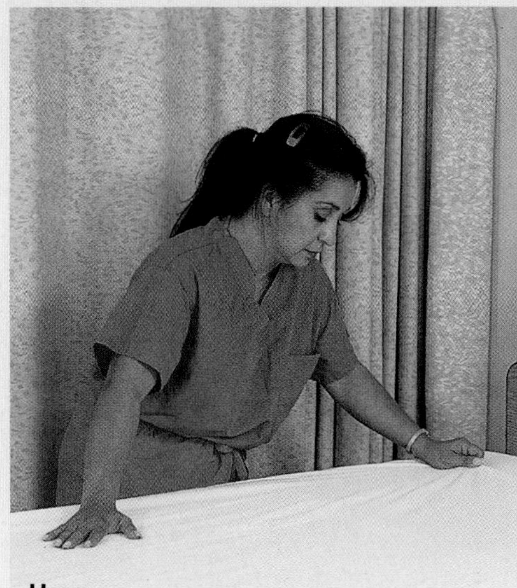

Smoothing the top sheet. (Photo by B. Proud.)

Gather the pillowcase as you would hosiery and slip the case over the pillow (Fig. I).

Prevents contact between the pillow and your uniform.

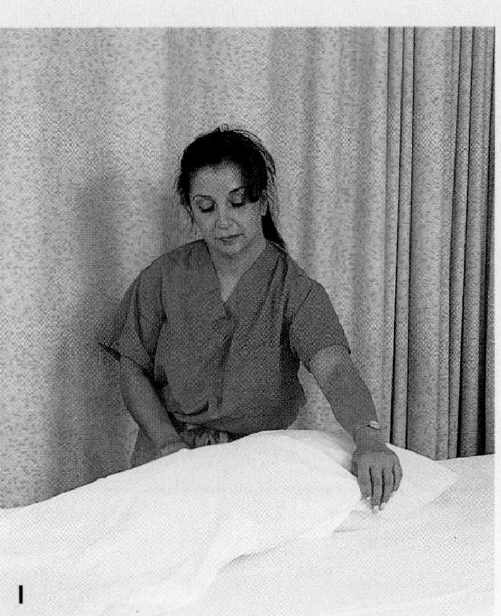

Covering the pillow. (Photo by B. Proud.)

Place the pillow at the head of the bed with the open end away from the door and the seam of the pillowcase toward the headboard.

Presents a tidy view of the room from the hallway; prevents pressure on the skin around the head and neck.

(continued)

Making an Unoccupied Bed (continued)

IMPLEMENTATION (CONTINUED)

Fan-fold or pie-fold the top linen toward the foot of the bed (Fig. J). — Facilitates returning to bed.

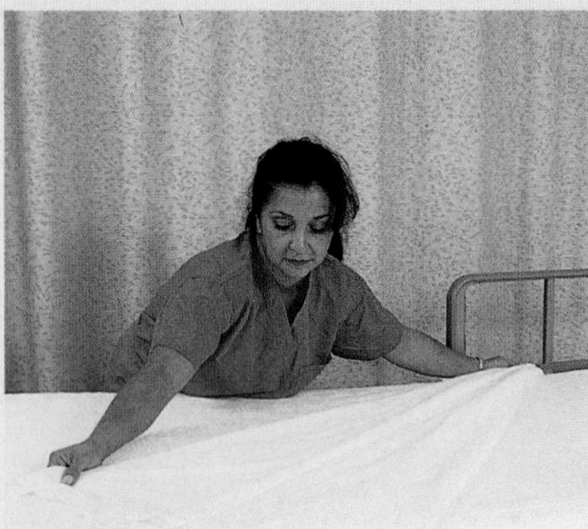

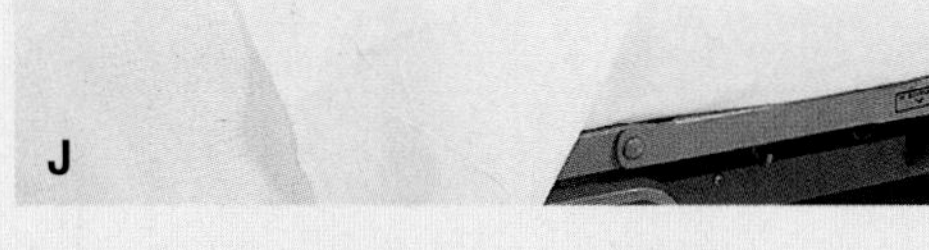

Prefolding the linen. (Photo by B. Proud.)

Secure the signal device on or to the bed. — Ensures that the client can receive nursing assistance.

Adjust the bed to a low position. — Enables the client to return to bed.

Wash hands or perform hand antisepsis with an alcohol rub (see Chap. 10). — Reduces the transmission of microorganisms.

Evaluation

- The bed is clean and dry.
- The linen is free of wrinkles.
- The environment is orderly.
- The client feels comfortable.

Document

- Date and time
- Characteristics of drainage, if present
- Any unique measures taken to ensure client comfort

SAMPLE DOCUMENTATION

Date and Time Menses established. Bed linen changed while shower taken. Given a supply of sanitary napkins. Absorbent pad placed over bottom sheet. —— SIGNATURE/TITLE

SKILL 18-2 Making an Occupied Bed

Suggested Action	Reason for Action
ASSESSMENT	
Check the Kardex or nursing care plan to confirm that the client must remain in bed.	Demonstrates compliance with the care plan.
Assess the client's level of consciousness, physical strength, breathing pattern, heart rate, and blood pressure.	Indicates a need for bedrest if abnormal findings are noted, whether it has been prescribed or not.
Inspect the linen for moisture or evidence of soiling.	Indicates what and how much linen must be changed and if gloves are appropriate when removing soiled linen.
Determine who might be available to assist if the client is too weak or unable to cooperate.	Avoids postural or muscular injury and ensures the client's comfort and safety.
PLANNING	
Plan to change the linen after the client's hygiene needs have been met.	Reduces the potential for wetting or soiling the clean linen.
Wash hands or perform hand antisepsis with an alcohol rub (see Chap. 10). Use gloves if there is a potential for direct contact with blood, stool, or other body fluids.	Reduces the transmission of microorganisms.
Bring necessary bed linen to the room.	Demonstrates organization and efficient time management.
Place the clean linen on a clean, dry surface such as the back of a chair.	Reduces the transmission of microorganisms to clean supplies.
IMPLEMENTATION	
Explain what you plan to do.	Informs the client and promotes cooperation.
Raise the bed to a high position.	Prevents postural and muscular strain.
Cover the client with a bath blanket or leave the top sheet loosened but in place.	Maintains warmth and demonstrates respect for modesty.
Fold the top sheet or spread if it will be reused and place it on a clean surface.	Promotes efficiency and orderliness.
Unfasten equipment attached to the bottom linen and check for personal items.	Avoids breakage, spills, or loss of personal items.
Loosen the bed linen from where it has been tucked under the mattress.	Facilitates removal or retightening.
Lower the rail on the side of the bed where you are standing and roll the client toward the opposite side rail.	Provides room for making the bed while ensuring the client's safety.
Roll the soiled bottom sheets as close to the client as possible.	Facilitates removal.
Proceed to unfold and tuck the bottom sheet and drawsheet on the vacant side of the bed, as described in Skill 18-1 (Fig A).	Remakes half of the bed with clean linen.

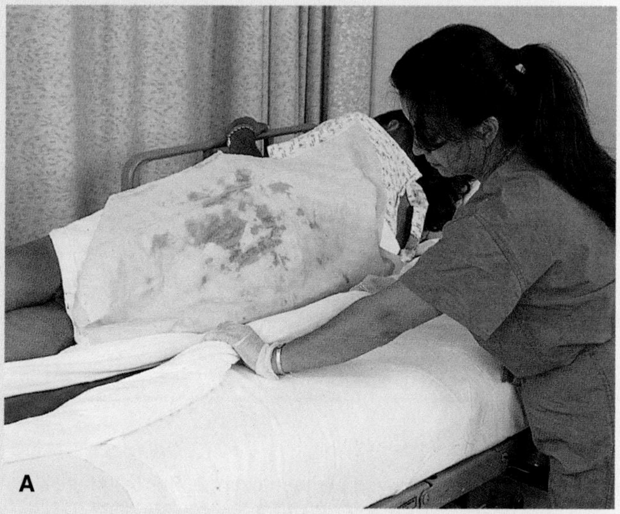

A

Changing linen on half of the bed. (Photo by B. Proud.)

Suggested Action	Reason for Action
Fold the free edges of the sheet under the folded portion of the soiled sheets.	Keeps the clean sheet from becoming soiled; facilitates pulling the sheets from under the client.
Raise the side rail and move to the opposite side of the bed.	Prevents postural and muscular strain.

(continued)

Making an Occupied Bed (continued)

IMPLEMENTATION (CONTINUED)

Action	Rationale
Lower the side rail in your new position and help the client to roll over the mound of sheets.	Helps reposition the client on the clean side of the bed.
Pull the soiled laundry close to the edge of the bed and the clean linen close beside it.	Reduces the mound of linen in the center of the bed.
Remove the soiled linen and place it into a pillowcase or pouch that is off the floor.	Keeps the soiled linen from becoming further contaminated.
Pull the clean bottom sheet until it is unfolded from beneath the client (Fig. B).	Promotes client comfort.

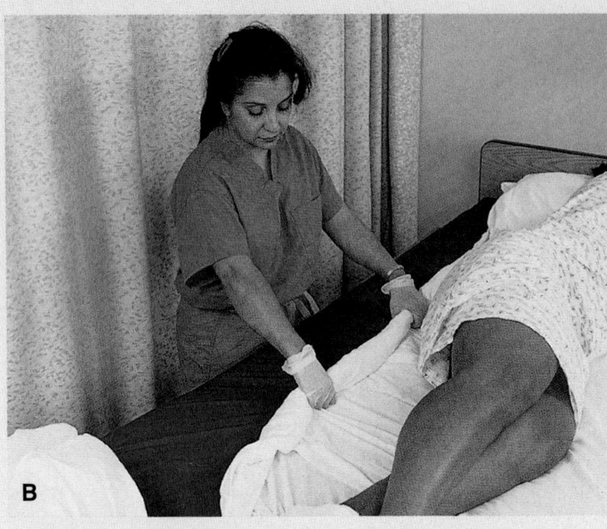

Pulling the clean linen through. (Photo by B. Proud.)

Action	Rationale
Miter or square the upper corner of the sheet; pull and tuck the free edges under the mattress.	Secures the clean sheets.
Assist the client to the middle of the bed.	Ensures comfort and safety.
Straighten or replace the top sheet, blankets, and spread; remove and replace the pillowcase if necessary.	Restores comfort and orderliness to the environment.
Reposition the client according to the therapeutic regimen or comfort.	Demonstrates compliance with the care plan; shows concern for client comfort.
Lower the height of the bed and raise the remaining side rail if appropriate.	Reduces the potential for injury.
Dispose of the soiled linens in a laundry hamper outside of the room.	Restores order to the room and ensures that the linens will be collected for laundering.
Wash hands or perform hand antisepsis with an alcohol rub (see Chap. 10).	Reduces the transmission of microorganisms.

Evaluation

- The bed is clean and dry.
- The linen is free of wrinkles.
- The environment is orderly.
- The client feels comfortable.

Document

- Date and time
- Characteristics of drainage, if present
- Measures taken to ensure client comfort.

SAMPLE DOCUMENTATION

Date and Time Unresponsive even to painful stimuli. Complete bed bath given followed by linen change. Repositioned on L side with head at a 45-degree elevation. Full side rails raised. Bed in low position. — SIGNATURE/TITLE

SKILL 18-3 Giving a Back Massage

Suggested Action	Reason for Action
ASSESSMENT	
Observe if the client is still awake 30 minutes after retiring for sleep.	Indicates a delay in the usual onset of sleep.
Determine if the client is experiencing pain, has a need for bladder or bowel elimination, is hungry, is too warm or cold, or has any other physical or environmental problem that may be easily overcome.	Eliminates all but psychophysiologic etiologies as the cause for sleeplessness.
Check the medical record to determine if the client has any condition that would contraindicate a backrub, such as fractured ribs or a back injury.	Demonstrates concern for the client's safety and comfort.
Ask the client if he or she would like a back massage.	Allows the client an opportunity to participate in decision making.
PLANNING	
Obtain lotion or an alternative substance such as alcohol or powder if the client's skin is oily.	Demonstrates organization and efficient time management.
Use gloves if there are any open, draining lesions on the skin.	Provides a barrier against blood-borne microorganisms.
Reduce environmental stimuli such as bright lights and loud noise.	Decreases stimulation of the wake center in the brain.
IMPLEMENTATION	
Pull the privacy curtain around the client's bed.	Demonstrates respect for modesty.
Raise the bed to an appropriate height to avoid bending at the waist.	Reduces back strain.
Wash hands or perform hand antisepsis with an alcohol rub (see Chap. 10); don gloves if appropriate.	Reduces the spread of microorganisms.
Help the client to lie on the abdomen or side, and untie the hospital gown or remove it completely.	Provides access to the back.
Instruct the client to breathe slowly and deeply in and out through an open mouth.	Promotes ventilation and relaxation.
Squirt a generous amount of lotion into your hands and rub them together.	Warms the lotion.
Place the entire surface of the hands on either side of the lower spine and move them upward over the shoulders and back again using long, continuous strokes. Repeat the stroke pattern several times (Fig. A).	Uses *effleurage* to promote relaxation.

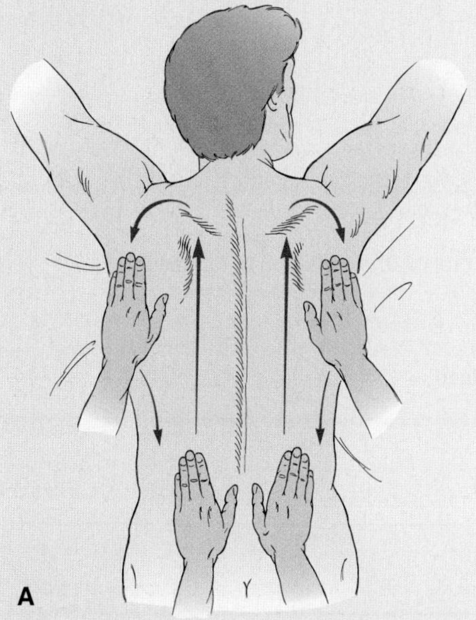

A

Effleurage (example 1).

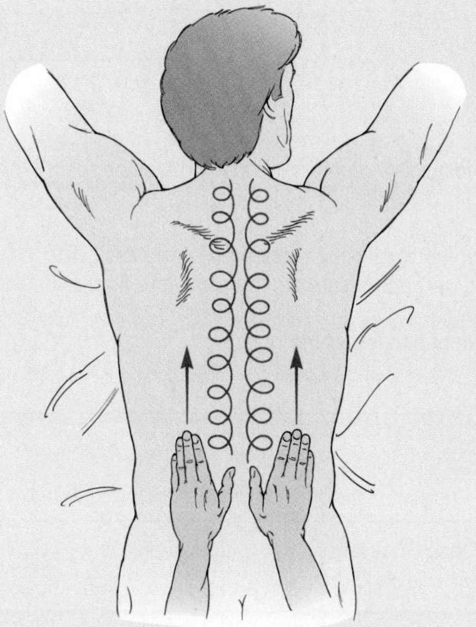

Effleurage (example 2).

Suggested Action	Reason for Action
Apply firmer pressure with the upstroke and lighter pressure during the downstroke.	Enhances relaxation by alternating pressure and rhythm.
Make smaller circular strokes up and down the length of the back with the thumbs.	Improves blood flow and removes chemicals that accumulate in contracted muscles.

(continued)

Giving a Back Massage (continued)

IMPLEMENTATION (CONTINUED)

Lift and gently compress tissue with the fingers, starting at the base of the spine and ending at the neck and shoulder areas (Fig. B). — Uses *pétrissage* to increase blood circulation.

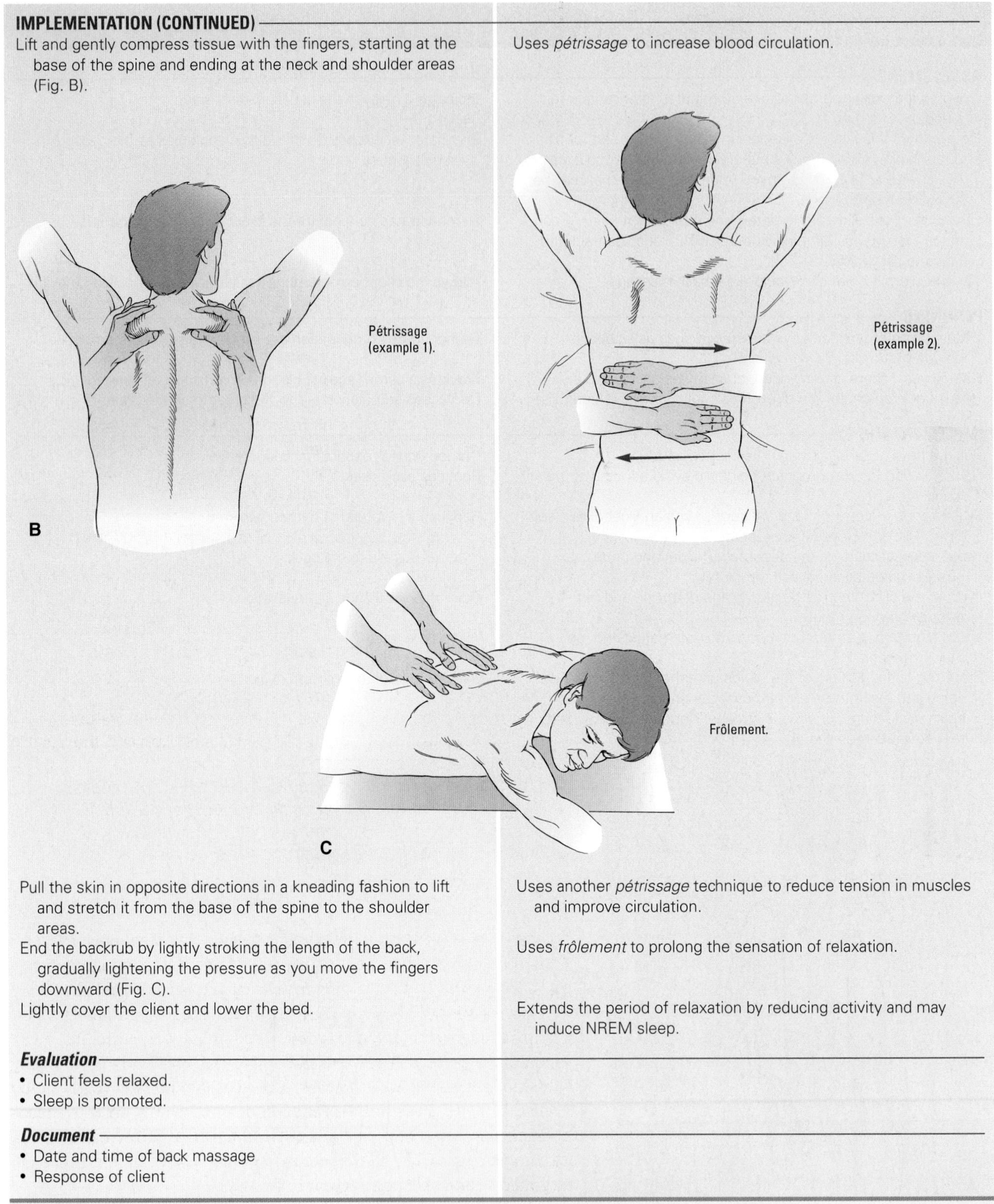

Pull the skin in opposite directions in a kneading fashion to lift and stretch it from the base of the spine to the shoulder areas. — Uses another *pétrissage* technique to reduce tension in muscles and improve circulation.

End the backrub by lightly stroking the length of the back, gradually lightening the pressure as you move the fingers downward (Fig. C). — Uses *frôlement* to prolong the sensation of relaxation.

Lightly cover the client and lower the bed. — Extends the period of relaxation by reducing activity and may induce NREM sleep.

Evaluation

- Client feels relaxed.
- Sleep is promoted.

Document

- Date and time of back massage
- Response of client

SAMPLE DOCUMENTATION

Date and Time Unable to sleep. Assisted to bathroom to void. Light snack of graham crackers and milk provided. Back massaged for 10 minutes. Observed to be sleeping 20 minutes later. ——————— SIGNATURE/TITLE

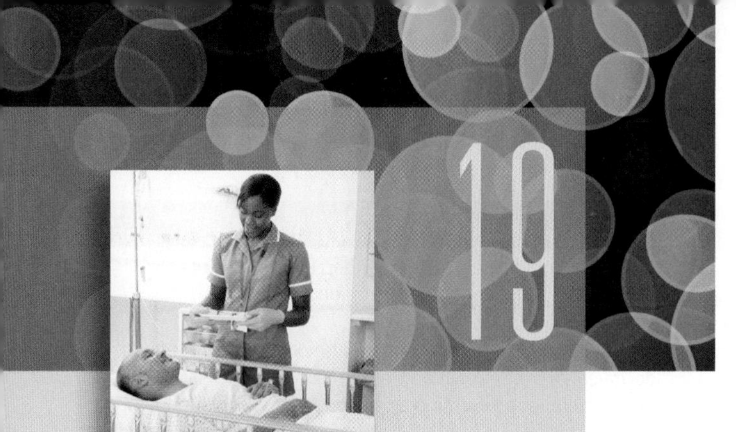

19 Safety

Words To Know

asphyxiation
chemical restraints
drowning
electrical shock
environmental hazards
fire plan
latex-safe environment
latex sensitivity
macroshock
microshock
National Patient Safety Goals
physical restraints
poisoning
restraint alternatives
safety
thermal burn

Learning Objectives

On completion of this chapter, the reader should be able to:

1. Discuss the purpose of the National Patient Safety goals and methods for implementing them.
2. Give an example of one common injury that predominates during each developmental stage (infancy through older adulthood).
3. Name six injuries that result from environmental hazards.
4. Identify at least two methods for reducing latex sensitization.
5. List four areas of responsibility incorporated into most fire plans.
6. Describe the indications for using each class of fire extinguishers.
7. Discuss five measures for preventing burns.
8. Name three common causes of asphyxiation.
9. Discuss two methods for preventing drowning.
10. Explain why humans are susceptible to electrical shock.
11. Discuss three methods for preventing electrical shock.
12. Name at least six common substances associated with poisonings.
13. Discuss four methods for preventing poisonings.
14. Discuss the benefits and risks of using physical restraints.
15. Explain the basis for enacting restraint legislation and the Joint Commission's accreditation standards.
16. Differentiate between a restraint and a restraint alternative.
17. Give at least four criteria for applying a physical restraint.
18. Describe two areas of concern during an accident.
19. Explain why older adults are prone to falling.

Safety (measures that prevent accidents or unintentional injuries) is a major nursing responsibility. The Joint Commission considers safety a priority when caring for clients and began establishing **National Patient Safety Goals** in 2003. The purpose of these goals is to help health care organizations obtain and retain their accreditation by demonstrating safe and effective care of the highest quality by reducing the risk of adverse client outcomes. The goals are revised yearly based on the recommendations of the Patient Safety Advisory Group to reduce the incidences of deaths and injuries among those being cared for in health agencies (Table 19-1). Methods of implementing the goals are integrated within skills that appear in this text.

Most hospital deaths and injuries are attributed to medication errors and adverse medication effects, infections, and surgical errors (Starfield, 2000). If identified and ranked by the National Center for Health Statistics, deaths from hospital errors, excluding preventable deaths due to medical treatments outside of hospitals, would be between the fifth and eighth leading cause of death (Woo et al., 2008). Such findings validate

TABLE 19-1 Summary of National Patient Safety Goals 2009–2010

GOAL	IMPLEMENTATION
Prevent infection	Follow handwashing and hand antisepsis guidelines recommended by the Centers for Disease Control and Prevention or the World Health Organization. Use evidence-based practices to prevent and treat infections. Promote influenza and pneumococcal immunizations among institutionalized older adults.
Identify patients/clients correctly	Use at least two methods for identification (for example, the client's name and date of birth) prior to administering medications or performing a treatment such as a blood transfusion.
Improve staff communication	Use only approved abbreviations and symbols. Contact appropriate health care providers promptly when a client's health status changes. Inform the appropriate person quickly about important test results. Repeat or read back verbal and phone orders. Discuss a client's care with a subsequent caregiver prior to a transfer.
Use medicines safely	Label all medications that are not already labeled in syringes, cups, and basins; be especially cautious with clients who take medications that thin the blood. Confirm that any new medication or medication prescribed in small amounts or for a short time is appropriate to take with current medications. Provide a list of the client's current medications to the physician, client, family, and next caregiver prior to the client's discharge.
Identify clients with safety risks	Assess clients who are at risk for falls, suicide, and fires from oxygen administration, and institute precautionary measures.
Prevent pressure ulcers	Determine which clients are at risk for pressure ulcers, develop a plan for their prevention, and reassess periodically.
Prevent surgical errors	Mark the body part intended for surgery; include the client's participation. Perform a "time out" to check the client and required documents immediately before a surgical procedure begins.
Involve clients in their care	Inform clients how to report safety issues.

Adapted from The 2009 National Patient Safety Goals. http://www.jointcommission.org/NR/rdonlyres/40A7233C-C4F7-4680-80CDFD5F62CF/09_NPSG_HAP_gp.pdf; 2010 National Patient Safety Goals. http://www.jointcommission.org/GeneralPublic/NPSG/10_npsgs.htm.

the conclusion that receiving health care is an extreme risk to a person's safety. This chapter examines factors that place people at risk for injuries, environmental hazards in homes and health care facilities, and nursing measures that keep clients safe.

AGE-RELATED SAFETY FACTORS

No age group is immune to accidental injury. Distinct differences among age groups exist, however, because of varying levels of cognitive function and judgment, activity and mobility, and degree of supervision, as well as the design of and safety devices within physical surroundings.

Infants and Toddlers

Infants rely on the safety consciousness of their adult caretakers. They are especially vulnerable to injuries resulting from falling off changing tables or being unrestrained in automobiles. Toddlers are naturally inquisitive and more mobile than infants and fail to understand the dangers that accompany climbing. Consequently, they are often the victims of accidental poisoning, falls down stairs or from high chairs, burns, electrocution from exploring outlets or manipulating electric cords, and drowning.

School-Aged Children and Adolescents

School-aged children are physically active, which makes them prone to play-related injuries. Many adolescents suffer sports-related injuries because they participate in physically challenging activities—sometimes without adequate protective equipment—before their musculoskeletal systems can withstand the stress. Adolescents also tend to be impulsive and take risks as a result of poor judgment and peer pressure.

Adults

Adults are at risk for injuries from ignoring safety issues, fatigue, sensory changes, and effects of disease. The types of injuries that young, middle-aged, and older adults incur depend on their social, developmental, and physical differences (Table 19-2).

ENVIRONMENTAL HAZARDS

Environmental hazards are potentially dangerous conditions in the physical surroundings. Examples in the home and health care environment include latex sensitization, thermal burns, asphyxiation, electrical shock, poisoning, and falls.

TABLE 19-2 Age-Related Factors Affecting Adult Safety

ADULT GROUP	CONTRIBUTING FACTORS	COMMON TYPES OF INJURIES
Young adults	Alcohol and drug abuse Emancipation from parental supervision Naiveté about workplace hazards	Motor vehicle collisions Boating accidents Head and spinal cord injuries Eye injuries, chemical burns, traumatic amputations, and soft tissue and back injuries
Middle-aged adults	Failure to use safety devices Overexertion and fatigue Disregard for use of seat belts and car safety harnesses Lack of expertise in performing home maintenance or repairs	Physical trauma (see previous) Burns and asphyxiation related to nonfunctioning smoke, heat, and carbon monoxide detectors
Older adults	Visual impairment Urinary urgency Postural hypotension Reduced coordination Impaired mobility Inadequate home maintenance Mental confusion Impaired temperature regulation	Falls Poisoning/medication errors Hypothermia and hyperthermia Scalds and burns

Latex Sensitization

Increasing numbers of people are developing **latex sensitivity** (allergic response to the proteins in latex). Latex, a natural rubber sap whose origin is a species of tree indigenous to Brazil, is a component of many household items, such as balloons, envelope glue, erasers, and carpet backing, as well as health care products. Health-related sensitization is partly the result of repeated exposure to latex in medical gloves and other equipment (Box 19-1). Clients predisposed to latex sensitivity include those with a history of asthma and allergies to other substances, multiple surgeries, and recurring medical procedures.

Types of Latex Reactions

Sensitization follows latex exposure through the skin, mucous membranes, inhalation, ingestion, injection, or wound management. The two forms of allergic reactions to latex or the chemicals used in its manufacture are as follows:

- Contact dermatitis, a delayed localized skin reaction that occurs within 6 to 48 hours and lasts for several days
- Immediate hypersensitivity, an instantaneous or fairly prompt systemic reaction manifested by swelling, itching, respiratory distress, hypotension, and death in severe cases

BOX 19-1 Common Items Containing Latex

Medical gloves	Intravenous injection ports
Band-Aids	Nondisposable sheet protectors
Bulb syringes	Stethoscope tubing
Medication vial stoppers	Tourniquets
Urinary catheters	Elastic (Jobst) stockings
Condoms	Mattress covers
Wound drains	Dental bands
Endoscopes	Blood pressure cuffs and tubing

Sensitized people also can develop a cross-reaction to fruits and vegetables such as avocados, bananas, almonds, peaches, kiwi, tomatoes, and others because the molecular structure of latex and other plant substances is similar.

Safeguarding Clients and Personnel

One of the best techniques for preventing latex sensitization and allergic reactions is to minimize or eliminate latex exposure. Health care agencies now provide personnel with more than one type of glove (Table 19-3). If they use latex gloves, nurses should avoid using oil-based hand creams or lotions and should wash their hands thoroughly after removing gloves to reduce the transfer of latex proteins to others and to other objects in the environment. Other measures to protect clients and personnel include the following:

- Obtaining an allergy history, and a sensitivity to latex in particular
- Flagging the chart and room door and attaching an allergy-alert identification bracelet on latex-sensitive clients
- Assigning clients with a latex allergy to a private room or **latex-safe environment** (room stocked with latex-free equipment and wiped clean of glove powder)
- Stocking a latex-safe cart containing synthetic gloves and latex-free client care and resuscitation equipment in the room of a client sensitive to latex
- Communicating with personnel in other departments so that they use nonlatex equipment and supplies during diagnostic or treatment procedures
- Reporting allergic events and their possible cause promptly to the agency's administration; administrators are required to report injuries, serious illnesses, or deaths from unsafe equipment to the U.S. Food and Drug Administration
- Referring sensitized clients to latex allergy support groups
- Recommending that latex-sensitive clients wear a Medic-Alert bracelet at all times

TABLE 19-3 Types of Medical Gloves

TYPE	ADVANTAGES	DISADVANTAGES
Latex		
Powdered latex	Inexpensive Elastic Adequate barrier against blood-borne pathogens	Releases latex protein allergen into the air via powder
Low-powder latex	Less potential for airborne distribution of latex and chemical proteins	Unproven ability to prevent sensitization
Powder-free latex	Reduced sensitization of nonallergic individuals from lack of airborne distribution of latex allergen	Deposits latex protein on surface environment, causing symptoms in sensitized individuals Slightly more expensive than powdered latex gloves
Low-protein latex	Less latex protein	No significant evidence that use eliminates sensitization
Nonlatex		
Vinyl—powder and powder-free	Similar strength of latex gloves Cost approximately the same as powdered latex gloves	Less durable and more likely to leak than latex Recommend changing after 30 minutes to maintain barrier protection
Nitrile	Better resistance to tears, punctures, and chemical disintegration than latex or vinyl gloves	Possible contact dermatitis from chemicals contained in nitrile More expensive than latex or vinyl
Neoprene	Fit, strength, and barrier protection similar to latex	Contains potentially allergic chemicals More expensive than nitrile gloves
Thermoplastic elastomer	Strength and protection similar or superior to latex	Free of latex or chemical allergens Most expensive of all gloves

- Advising latex-sensitive clients to notify their employer's health officer about the allergy in case of a future claim for worker's compensation or a legal case concerning discrimination in the workplace

Burns

A **thermal burn** is a skin injury caused by flames, hot liquids, or steam and is the most common form of burn. Burns also result from contact with caustic chemicals such as lye, electric wires, or lightning.

Burn Prevention

Because many adults become complacent about safety hazards, the nurse reviews burn-prevention measures with clients being treated for thermal-related accidents (see Client and Family Teaching 19-1).

Exits must be identified, lighted, and unlocked. Most fire codes require that public buildings, including hospitals and nursing homes, have a functioning sprinkler system. Sprinkler systems help control fires and limit structural damage.

Fire Plans

To prevent or limit burn injuries in a health care setting, all employees must know and follow the agency's **fire plan** (procedure followed for a possible or actual fire). Compliance with the fire plan is a major component of the Joint Commission's inspection. Every accredited health care agency must demonstrate and document that staff members have been trained in the following five areas:

- Specific roles and responsibilities at and away from the fire's point of origin
- Use of the fire alarm system
- Roles in preparing for building evacuation
- Location and proper use of equipment for evacuation or transporting clients to areas of refuge
- Building compartmentalization procedures for containing smoke and fire (National Fire Protection Agency, 2006)

To obtain the Joint Commission's accreditation, staff members on each shift also must participate in fire drills, the frequency of which must be identified in the agency's fire plan.

Fire Management

The National Fire Protection Association, whose Life Safety Code is the basis for the Joint Commission's management standards, recommends using the acronym RACE to identify the basic steps to take when managing a fire:

R—Rescue
A—Alarm
C—Confine (the fire)
E—Extinguish

Most health care agencies incorporate these concepts by including the following actions in their fire plans:

- Evacuate clients from the room with the fire.
- Inform the switchboard operator of the fire's location. He or she will alert personnel over the public address system and notify the fire department.
- Return to the nursing unit when an alarm sounds; do not use the elevator.
- Clear the halls of visitors and equipment.

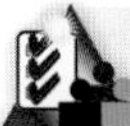

Client and Family Teaching 19-1 Burn Prevention

The nurse teaches the client or the family the following:

- Change the batteries in smoke, heat, and carbon monoxide detectors at least every year.
- Equip the home with at least one fire extinguisher.
- Develop an evacuation plan (and an alternate escape route) and a place for family members to meet after exiting a burning home.
- Practice the evacuation plan periodically.
- Keep all windows and doors barrier free.
- Identify the location of exits when staying in a hotel.
- Dispose of rags that have been saturated with solvents.
- Keep items away from the pilot lights on the furnace, water heater, or clothes dryer.
- Avoid storing gasoline, kerosene, turpentine, or other solvents.
- Go to public fireworks displays rather than igniting them at home.
- Never smoke when sleepy or around oxygen equipment.
- Use safety matches rather than a lighter; children are less capable of using matches.
- Buy clothing, especially sleepwear, made from natural or flame-resistant fabrics.
- Never run if clothing is on fire; instead stop, drop, and roll.
- Do not overload electrical outlets or circuits.
- Set thermostats on hot water heaters to less than 120°F (48.8°C).
- Keep cords to coffee pots, electric frying pans, or other small cooking appliances above the reach of young children.
- Follow label directions about the use of gloves when using chemicals.
- Flush chemicals with copious amounts of water if they come in contact with skin.
- Go inside if the weather is threatening or you see lightning.
- If you are inside a burning building:
  - Feel if the surface of a door is hot before opening it.
  - Close doors behind you.
  - Crawl on the floor if the room is smoke-filled.
  - Use stairs rather than elevators.
  - Never go back inside, regardless of whom or what has been left there.
  - Go to a neighbor's home to call the fire department or 911 operator.

- Close the doors to client rooms and stairwells as well as fire doors between adjacent units. Wait for further directions.
- Place moist towels or bath blankets at the threshold of doors if smoke is escaping.
- Use an appropriate fire extinguisher if necessary.

Rescue and Evacuation

The first priority is to rescue clients in the immediate vicinity of the fire. Nurses lead those who can walk to a safe area and close the room and fire doors after exiting. Nursing personnel evacuate those who cannot walk using a variety of techniques (Fig. 19-1).

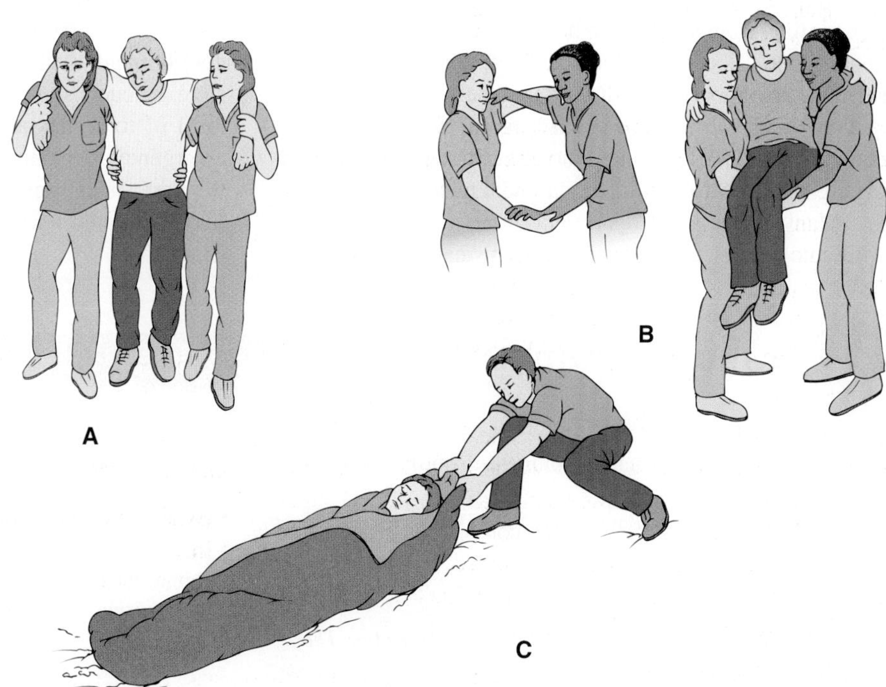

FIGURE 19-1 Evacuation of clients. **A.** Human crutches—rescuers secure a weak but ambulatory client's arm and waist. **B.** Seat carry—rescuers interlock arms and carry a nonambulatory client. **C.** Body drag—rescuer drags an unconscious victim or one who cannot assist on a blanket or sheet.

TABLE 19-4 Types of Fire Extinguishers

TYPE	SYMBOL	CONTENTS	USE
Class A	A	Water under pressure	Burning paper, wood, and cloth
Class B	B	Carbon dioxide	Fires caused by gasoline, oil, paint, grease, and other flammable liquids
Class C	C	Dry chemicals	Electrical fires
Class ABC (combination extinguisher)	A B C	Graphite	Fires of any kind

Fire Extinguishers

There are four types of fire extinguishers (Table 19-4). Each type is labeled. Nurses must know the type of extinguisher that is appropriate for the burning substance and how to use it (see Nursing Guidelines 19-1).

Asphyxiation

Asphyxiation (an inability to breathe) can result from airway obstruction (see Chap. 37), drowning, or inhalation of noxious gases such as smoke or carbon monoxide (CO).

Smoke Inhalation

Smoke can be more deadly than fire. Almost all health care facilities have banned cigarette smoking; consequently, smoke inhalation now accounts for far fewer deaths. However, when a fire occurs, regardless of its location or cause, smoke inhalation results in 50% to 80% of the deaths rather than burns (Holstege, 2007; Fig. 19-2).

Despite efforts to ban smoking, there continues to be a risk for fires from smoking in health care facilities and other nonresidential locations. Some attribute this to the fact that secretive smokers tend to discard smoldering cigarette butts quickly in order to avoid being discovered. Home fires, on the other hand, often occur when smokers fall asleep with a burning cigarette or when children play with matches or lighters.

Many homes and apartment buildings are equipped with smoke detectors. Some people dismantle their smoke detector, however, when it begins to emit an audible alarm signaling low battery power, and they fail to replace the batteries.

Carbon Monoxide

CO, an odorless gas, is released during the incomplete combustion of carbon products such as fossil fuels (eg, kerosene, natural gas, wood, and coal; substances commonly used to heat homes). When inhaled, CO binds with hemoglobin and interferes with the oxygenation of cells. Without adequate ventilation, the consequences can be lethal.

Because CO can be present even without smoke, CO detectors should be installed in all homes, and fire department personnel should investigate alarms. Without detectors, victims may be unaware of the presence of CO and may attribute their symptoms to the flu (Box 19-2). As their condition deteriorates, they become confused and lapse into a coma, followed by death.

If a person is suspected of being poisoned by CO, initial treatment requires getting the victim out of the present environment. If moving the person out of doors is impossible, rescuers should open windows and doors to reduce the level of toxic gas and promote adequate ventilation. Once emergency personnel arrive, they administer oxygen. In the case of extremely high blood levels of CO, the victim may be treated with hyperbaric (high-pressure) oxygen (see Chap. 21).

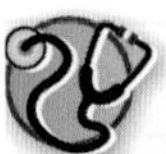

NURSING GUIDELINES 19-1

Using a Fire Extinguisher

- Know the location of each type of fire extinguisher. *Doing so minimizes response time.*
- Free the extinguisher from its enclosure. *The extinguisher must be removed for use.*
- Remove the pin that locks the handle. *The pin must be removed for use.*
- Aim the nozzle near the edge, not the center, of the fire. *The chemical will contain the fire.*
- Move the nozzle from side to side. *Doing so increases the effectiveness of fire control.*
- Avoid skin contact with the contents of the fire extinguisher. *The chemicals in the extinguisher can cause injury.*
- Return the extinguisher to the maintenance department. *The extinguisher will be replaced or refilled for future use.*

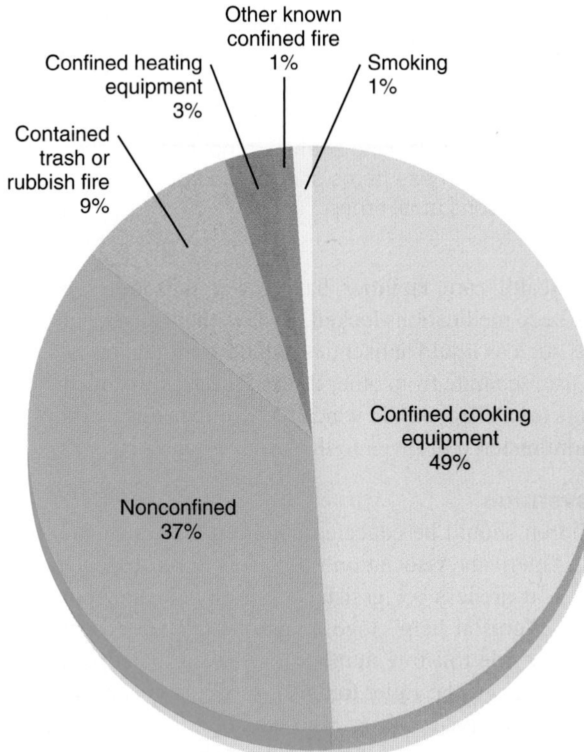

FIGURE 19-2 Fire statistics as collected by the National Fire Protection Association. (From Flynn, J. [2009]. *Structure fires in medical, mental health, and substance abuse facilities.* National Fire Protection Association. Accessed March 15, 2010, from http://www.nfpa.org/assets/files/PDF/MentalHealthExecSum.pdf)

Drowning

Drowning is a condition in which fluid occupies the airway and interferes with ventilation. It can occur in swimmers and nonswimmers alike. Accidental drownings occur during water activities such as fishing, boating, swimming, and water skiing. Some incidents are linked to alcohol abuse, which tends to interfere with judgment and promotes risk taking. Other victims overestimate their stamina.

Drownings also can occur at home or in health care environments. Young children can drown if left momentarily in a bathtub or if they have access to a swimming pool. Swimming pools should be fenced and locked, and children should never be left unattended in a bathtub or pool.

Although the potential for drowning in a health care institution is statistically remote, it can happen. Therefore, nurses should never leave any helpless or cognitively impaired client, young or old, alone in a tub of water regardless of its depth.

Victims of cold-water drownings are more likely to be resuscitated because the cold lowers their metabolism, thus conserving oxygen (see Chap. 12). Prevention, however, is far better:

- Learn to swim.
- Never swim alone.
- Wear an approved flotation device.
- Do not drink alcohol when participating in water-related sports.
- Notify a law enforcement officer if boaters appear unsafe.

Resuscitation

Cardiopulmonary resuscitation (CPR), if begun immediately, may be lifesaving for a victim of asphyxiation or drowning. Current CPR certification is generally an employment requirement for nurses. Many hospitals teach new parents how to administer CPR (Fig. 19-3).

Electrical Shock

Electrical shock (the discharge of electricity through the body) is a potential hazard wherever there are machines and electrical equipment. The body is susceptible to electrical shock because it is composed of water and electrolytes, both of which are good conductors of electricity. A conductor is a substance that facilitates the flow of electrical current; an insulator is a substance that contains electrical currents so they do not scatter. Electric cords are covered with rubber or some other insulating substance.

Macroshock is a harmless distribution of low-amperage electricity over a large area of the body. It feels like a slight tingling. **Microshock** is low-voltage but high-amperage distribution of electricity. A person with intact skin usually does not feel microshock because intact skin offers resistance or acts as a barrier between the electrical current and the water

BOX 19-2 Symptoms of Carbon Monoxide Poisoning

Nausea	Confusion
Vomiting	Shortness of breath
Headache	Cherry-red skin color
Dizziness	Loss of consciousness
Muscle weakness	

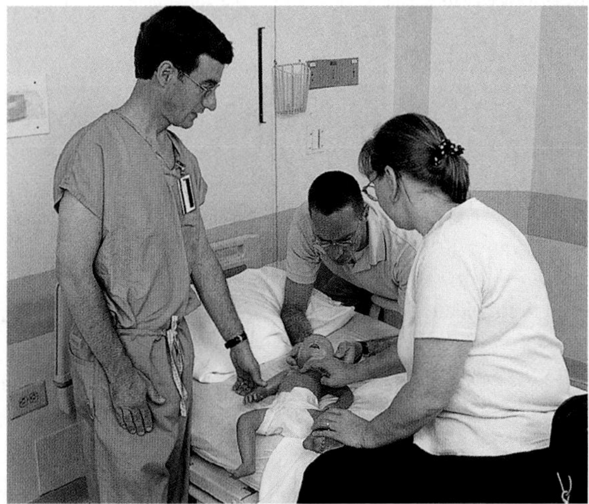

FIGURE 19-3 Parents being taught cardiopulmonary resuscitation as part of discharge planning. (Photo by B. Proud.)

and electrolytes within. If the skin is wet or its integrity is impaired, however, the electrical current can be fatal, especially if delivered directly to the heart.

Use of grounded equipment reduces the potential for electrical shock. A *ground* diverts leaking electrical energy to the earth. Grounded equipment can be identified by the presence of a three-pronged plug.

In addition to using grounded equipment, other safety measures to prevent electrical shock include the following:

- Never use an adaptor to bypass a grounded outlet.
- Make sure all outlets and switches have cover plates.
- Plug all machines used for client care into outlets within 12 ft. of one another or within the same cluster of wall outlets.
- Unplug machines if they are no longer necessary.
- Discourage clients from resting electric hair dryers, curling irons, or razors on or near a sink that contains water.
- Do not use a machine that has a frayed or cracked cord or a plug with exposed wires.
- Grasp the plug, not the cord, to remove it from an outlet.
- Do not use extension cords.
- Report macroshocks to the engineering department.
- Clean liquid spills as soon as possible.
- Stand clear of the client and bed during cardiac defibrillation.

Poisoning

Poisoning is injury caused by the ingestion, inhalation, or absorption of a toxic substance. These are more common in homes than in health care institutions, although medication errors could be considered a form of poisoning (see Chap. 32). Preventing medication errors is addressed in the National Patient Safety Goals for keeping people safe in health care agencies. Medication safety is discussed in more depth in Unit 9, Medication Administration. Accidental poisonings usually occur among toddlers and commonly involve substances located in bathrooms or kitchens (Box 19-3). Many children treated for accidental poisoning have a repeat episode.

BOX 19-3 Common Substances Associated With Childhood Poisonings

Drugs: Aspirin, acetaminophen, vitamins with iron, antidepressants, sedatives, tranquilizers, antacid tablets, diet pills, and laxatives

Cleaning agents: Bleach, toilet bowl or tank disks, detergents, and drain cleaners

Paint solvents: Turpentine, kerosene, and gasoline

Heavy metals: Lead paint chips

Chemical products: Glue, shoe polish, antifreeze, and insecticides

Cosmetics: Hair dye, shampoo, and nail polish remover

Plants: Mistletoe berries, rhubarb leaves, foxglove, and castor beans

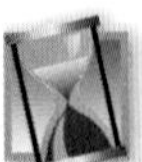

Gerontologic Considerations

■ Older adults with cognitive impairments need protection from accidental ingestion of toxic substances, such as medications and cleaning agents, in households and institutional settings. These items should be kept in secure, locked locations at all times.

Health care facilities have fewer poisonings because they keep medications locked. By law, they must keep chemicals such as liquid antiseptics, which are intended for external use, separate from other drugs. Nevertheless, medication errors (see Chap. 32), in which the wrong medication or dose is administered or given to the wrong client, persist.

Prevention

Children should be educated about the hazards of poisons. The American Association of Poison Control Centers promotes awareness for assistance with accidental poisoning with a "poison help" logo (Fig. 19-4). The logo provides a nationwide toll-free number that, when dialed, automatically connects the caller to the closest poison control center. Nurses and pharmacists who are certified specialists in poison information answer emergency calls around the clock. All nurses can teach parents and others how to reduce the risk of poisoning in the home (see Client and Family Teaching 19-2). Adults who have trouble remembering or who cannot administer their own medications safely can use containers prefilled by a responsible person (Fig. 19-5).

Treatment

Initial treatment for a victim of suspected poisoning involves maintaining breathing and cardiac function. After that, rescuers attempt to identify what was ingested, how much, and when. Definitive treatment depends on the substance, the client's condition, and if the substance is still in the stomach. For ingestions of commercial products containing multiple ingredients, the poison control center is consulted. Otherwise, treatment follows the decision tree in Figure 19-6.

Falls

Falls, more than any other injury discussed thus far, are the most common accident experienced by older adults and

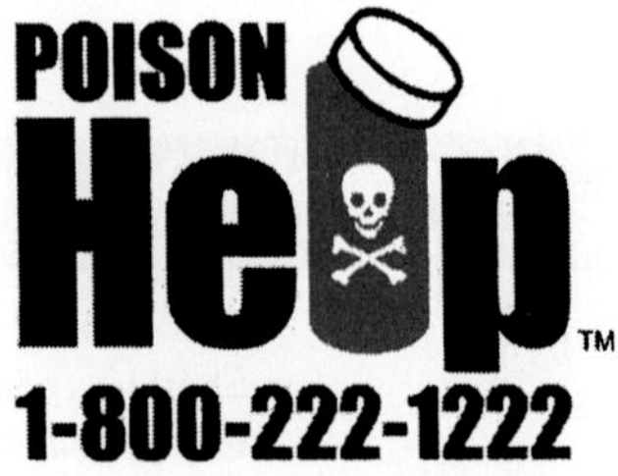

FIGURE 19-4 The toll-free number provides immediate access to an expert at a poison center with answers to questions about poisons and poisonings.

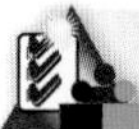

Client and Family Teaching 19-2
Preventing Childhood Poisoning

The nurse teaches the parents or the caretakers the following:

- Install child-resistant latches on cupboard doors.
- Request childproof caps on all prescription medications.
- Buy chemicals and nonprescription drugs with tamper-proof lids.
- Never transfer a toxic substance to a container usually used for storing food.
- Do not refer to medications as "candy," and do not tell children they taste "yummy."
- Do not keep drugs in your purse.
- Remind grandparents or babysitters to "childproof" their homes.
- Remove toxic houseplants from the home.
- Keep the home well ventilated when using an aerosol or another substance that leaves lingering fumes in the air.

have the most serious consequences for this age group. More than one third of adults aged 65 years and older fall each year in the United States; falls are the most common cause of nonfatal injuries and hospital admissions for trauma. According to statistics from 2009, of those people who fell, more than 433,000 required hospitalization, and nearly 16,000 died (National Center for Injury Prevention and Control, 2009). Most falls among older adults occur at home. Common injuries include those to the head, wrist, spine, and hip. Half of all clients hospitalized after falling are transferred to a nursing care facility (Tideiksaar, 2010). Many who survive a fall suffer years of disability, impaired mobility, and pain.

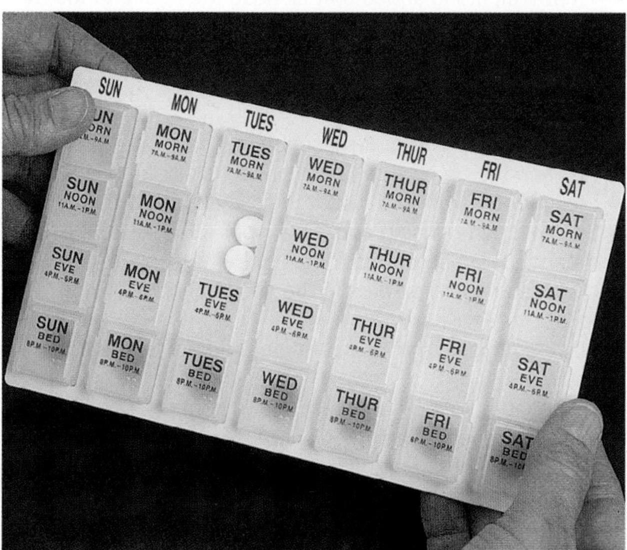

FIGURE 19-5 A pill organizer may help reduce the incidence of medication overdoses. (Photo by B. Proud.)

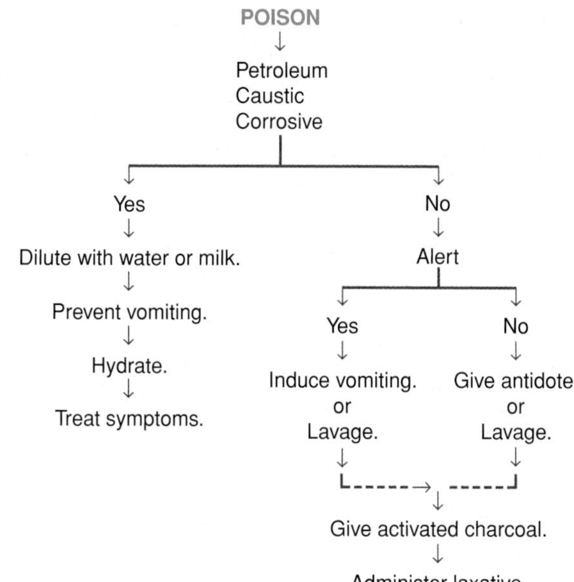

FIGURE 19-6 Decision tree for treating ingested poisons.

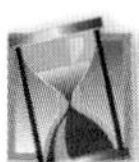

Gerontologic Considerations

■ Osteoporosis (loss of bone mass) increases the risk of fractures, especially in older women. Osteoporotic fractures may occur with little or no trauma and even without a fall.

■ Older adults who have had a previous fall or have a history of falling are more likely to fall again and often exhibit a characteristic gait attributed more to being overly cautious than a result of a prior injury. Fear of falling can significantly limit mobility, which may actually increase the risk for falls.

■ Practical methods such as assessing risk factors for falls and teaching fall management should be initiated. Placing beds at low heights may diminish risks from falls.

Contributing Factors

Older adults are more prone to falls for several reasons. Many have age-related changes such as visual impairments and disorders affecting gait, balance, and coordination. Some take medications that lower blood pressure, causing them to feel dizzy on rising. Others have urinary urgency and rush to reach the toilet. Other social and environmental factors also contribute to the risk of falling. For example, older adults often wear slippers to accommodate swollen feet. Although slippers are more comfortable, less expensive, and less tiring to put on than shoes, they do not offer much support or traction. Clutter may accumulate around the house if the older adult lacks the energy to clean or does not want to discard old items.

For hospitalized older adults, the risk for falls rises. They are in an unfamiliar environment. They must rely on nursing assistance for mobility, and such assistance may not be prompt. Medications and altered health status may cause temporary confusion and poor judgment.

Risk Factors	Risk Points	Score
Confusion/disorientation	+4	
Depression	+2	
Altered elimination (incontinence, nocturia, frequency)	+1	
Dizziness/vertigo	+1	
Sex = male	+1	
Antiepileptics (any prescribed)	+2	
Benzodiazepines (any prescribed)	+1	
Get-up-and-go (rising from chair) test:		
Able to rise in a single movement	0	
Pushes up, successful in one attempt	+1	
Multiple attempts, but successful	+3	
Unable to rise without assistance	+4	
	FINAL RISK SCORE =	*

* KEY: >5, High risk for falling

FIGURE 19-7 The Hendrich Fall Risk Tool. (Original research in Hendrich, A., Nyhuis, A., Kippenbrock, T., & Soja, M. E. [1995]. Hospital falls: Development of a predictive model for clinical practice. *Applied Nursing Research,* 8[3], 129–139. Used with permission of Ann Hendrich, MSN, RN, Methodist Hospital, Indianapolis, IN.)

Assessment

Determining which clients are at higher risk can prevent some falls. Identifying at risk clients and preventing falls also is a National Patient Safety Goal (see Table 19-1). Accredited hospitals and long-term care agencies use assessment tools to determine which clients need fall-prevention protocols (Fig. 19-7).

Prevention

Different fall-prevention approaches are used in the home and in health care facilities. Measures for preventing falls are modified based on the client's circumstances (see Client and Family Teaching 19-3).

Older adults should keep a list of emergency numbers posted by the phone. Those who live alone may want to become part of a daily phone tree in which someone investigates if an older adult does not call in or answer a call. Personal response services are also available in which the subscriber wears a wireless, waterproof pendant with a button that he or she can use to summon help in an emergency. Activating the button places a call to the manufacturer's emergency response center; once connected, the user can carry on a two-way hands-free conversation. The center directs calls for assistance to predetermined people such as family, neighbors, the physician, or emergency personnel. If the user cannot communicate, the center dispatches emergency personnel to the user's location.

Client and Family Teaching 19-3
Preventing Falls

The nurse teaches the client or the family as follows:

- Keep the environment well lit.
- Install and use handrails on stairs inside and outside the home.
- Place a strip of light-colored adhesive tape on the edge of each stair for visibility.
- Remove scatter rugs.
- Keep extension cords next to the wall.
- Do not wax floors.
- Wear well fitting shoes that enclose the heel and toe of the foot and have nonskid soles.
- Keep pathways clutter free.
- Wear short robes without cloth belts that may loosen and trip the client.
- Use a cane or walker if prescribed.
- Replace the tip on a cane as it wears down.
- Stay indoors when the weather is icy or snowy.
- Sit down when using public transportation, even if it means asking someone for his or her seat.
- Install and use grab bars in the shower and near the toilet.
- Place a nonskid mat or decals on the floor of the tub or shower.
- Use soap-on-a-rope or a suspended container of liquid soap to prevent slipping on a loose soap bar.
- Use a flashlight or nightlight when it is dark.
- Make sure that pets are not underfoot.
- Mop up spills immediately.
- Use long-handled tongs rather than climbing on a chair to reach high objects.

RESTRAINTS

In health care agencies, fall prevention measures are necessary for identified clients. The use of restraints, however, is closely regulated. **Physical restraints** are methods that immobilize or reduce the ability of a client to freely move his or her arms, legs, body, or head. **Chemical restraints** are medications that are not a standard treatment or dosage for the client's condition but rather are used to manage a client's behavior or freedom of movement. These are generally warranted to manage violent or self-destructive behavior that jeopardizes the immediate physical safety of the client, staff, or others. Physical restraint devices that may be used for client safety include those that protect a client from falling out of bed or permit the client to participate in activities without the risk of physical harm (The Joint Commission, 2009).

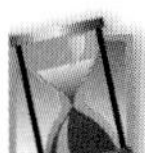

Gerontologic Considerations

- Wandering is not a justification for restraining clients. Older adults who are confused or otherwise cognitively impaired, without an awareness or appreciation for personal safety, may need alternative precautions to prevent wandering. Helpful devices include placing a specially designed net with a stop sign across the exit doorway with Velcro, using bells over doors to alert caregivers, or disguising an exit door by covering it with a curtain or wallpaper that blends in with the surrounding environment. Several different types of monitors, identification bracelets (that include a phone number), and alerting/alarm devices are available for use with older adults at risk for wandering.
- Special environments may be designed so that the hallways form a circle around the nursing stations, allowing the older adult to walk, yet remain in view of the nursing staff, rather than having exit doors placed at the ends of hallways.
- Caregivers should be aware that early identification is necessary so that proper precautions can be initiated. Daily documentation of what a person is wearing is helpful should the client wander and need to be identified.
- The Alzheimer's Association (1-800-272-3900) sponsors a program called "Safe Return," which facilitates the reporting and return of people with cognitive impairments who become lost. Local police departments may provide a service of digital photography of the older adult and coded identification bracelets. The photos and identification codes are stored in the computers maintained by the police department for identification of an adult found wandering. Clients with dementia may also be fitted with a global positioning satellite (GPS) device to facilitate locating a missing person.

Although the use of restraints may be intended to prevent falls and other injuries, in many cases, their risks outweigh their benefits. Restrained clients become increasingly confused; suffer chronic constipation, incontinence, and infections such as pneumonia and pressure ulcers; and experience a progressive decline in their ability to perform activities of daily living. Restrained clients are more likely to die during their hospital stay than those who are not restrained.

It is unethical and a violation of the Joint Commission's standards to use physical or chemical restraints for disciplinary reasons or to compensate for limited personnel.

BOX 19-4 OBRA Legislation Addressing Restraints

The Omnibus Reconciliation Act (OBRA) of 1987 specifies that:

The resident (patient) has the right to be free from any physical restraints imposed or psychoactive drug administered for purposes of discipline or convenience, and not required to treat the resident's (patient's) medical symptoms. . . . Restraints may only be imposed to ensure the physical safety of the resident or other residents and only upon the written order of a physician that specifies the duration and the circumstances under which the restraints are to be used (except in emergency situations which must be addressed in the facility's restraint policy).

Restraints must be the last intervention used after trying all other measures to solve the problem. Nurses must take measures to protect the restrained client's health, safety, dignity, rights, and well-being.

Legislation

After research studies revealed the widespread use of physical restraints in long-term care facilities, federal legislation known as the Nursing Home Reform Law was incorporated in the Omnibus Budget Reconciliation Act (OBRA) in 1987 (Box 19-4). Compliance with the law has been mandatory since 1990.

Accreditation Standards

The Joint Commission followed the lead of OBRA legislation by developing restraint and seclusion standards in 1991. They continue to revise these standards, which differ for nonpsychiatric and psychiatric institutions; the most recent revision occurred in 2009. The standards address three areas: agency restraint protocol, medical orders, and client monitoring and documentation of nursing care.

Restraint Protocol

A *protocol* is a plan or set of steps to follow when implementing an intervention. During a Joint Commission inspection, the accrediting team examines an agency's protocol for restraint use that the medical staff has approved. The protocol must identify the criteria that justify the application and discontinuation of restraints. Nonphysical interventions, such as reorienting a person to place and circumstances, or "time-out," which involves removing the client from the immediate environment to a quiet room, is preferred. In the case of a client attempting to remove an endotracheal tube that facilitates mechanical ventilation, personnel must first attempt less restrictive measures, such as having someone sit with the client.

Medical Orders

A physician must write a restraint order, or a nurse must obtain one from a physician by telephone. If a physician is unavailable, a registered nurse who has knowledge, training, and experience in the techniques that necessitate the use of restraints may initiate restraint use based on appropriate assessment of the client.

If need for a restraint used to protect the physical safety of a nonviolent or nondestructive client is ongoing, the physician must renew the medical order according to the agency's protocol.

Monitoring and Documentation

The client's chart must contain documented evidence of frequent and regular nursing assessments of the restrained client's vital signs; circulation; skin condition or signs of injury; psychological status and comfort; and readiness for discontinuing restraint. In addition, the nurse must record nursing care concerning toileting, nutrition, hydration, and range of motion while the client is restrained. The documented care must reflect the agency's established protocol. The nurse also promptly communicates with the client's family regarding the need for restraints and notes the time in the documentation. When the assessment findings indicate that the client has improved, the nurse must legally and ethically remove the restraint.

Restraint Alternatives

Agencies are being challenged to implement interventions that protect clients from injury while ensuring their freedom, mobility, and dignity. The intent of both the OBRA legislation and the Joint Commission standards is to promote **restraint alternatives** (protective or adaptive devices that promote client safety and postural support but that the client can release independently) and, eventually, restraint-free client care.

Restraint alternatives are generally appropriate for clients who tend to need repositioning to maintain their body alignment or improve their independence and functional status. Some examples include seat inserts or gripping materials that prevent sliding, support pillows, seat belts or harnesses with front-releasing Velcro or buckle closures, and commercial or homemade tilt wedges (Fig. 19-8). If the client is unaware of or cannot release the restraint alternative, it is considered a restraint.

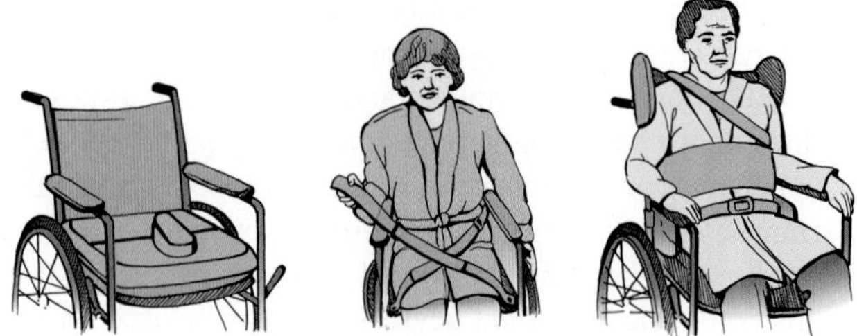

FIGURE 19-8 Examples of restraint alternatives.

Other supplementary measures also may reduce the need for restraints. Personnel are encouraged to improve gait training, provide physical exercise, reorient clients, encourage assistive ambulatory devices such as walkers and hall rails, and use electronic seat and bed monitors that sound an alarm when clients get up without assistance. Before considering the use of physical restraints, the nurse observes and documents the client's response to other alternatives. When clients are in a wheelchair, nurses must position them correctly (Table 19-5).

Use of Restraints

When the use of restraints is justified, nurses and the personnel they supervise must demonstrate continued competency in their safe application. Skill 19-1 explains how to apply restraints and use them appropriately.

Stop, Think, and Respond Box 19-1

List some methods for avoiding a lawsuit when restraints are necessary.

TABLE 19-5 Basic Wheelchair Positioning Principles

STRUCTURE	FRONT VIEW	SIDE VIEW
Head	Head/neck centered over trunk midline	Head/ear centered over hip
Shoulders	Level in horizontal line	Top of shoulder over hip
Trunk	Sternum perpendicular to center of pelvis	Spine perpendicular to hip
Pelvis	Top of hip level in horizontal line	Lumbar curve preserved
Thighs	Knee level in horizontal line	Hip and knee level in horizontal line
Knees	Knees not touching; legs perpendicular to floor	Knees bent 90 degrees; edge of seat 3 in. from knee crease
Feet	Great toes and fifth toes level in horizontal line	Heel and forefoot positioned on footplate; ankle in neutral position

Available from Posey Co. J.T., & Arcadia, CA. *Positioning in wheelchairs,* http://www.posey.com/Products/Positioning-In-Wheelchairs_8509.aspx.

NURSING IMPLICATIONS

Nurses must recognize safety hazards and identify clients at the greatest risk for injury. Once they gather and analyze the data, they may identify several nursing diagnoses:

- Risk for Latex Allergy Response
- Risk for Injury
- Risk for Trauma
- Impaired Walking
- Disturbed Sensory Perception
- Acute Confusion
- Chronic Confusion
- Impaired Environmental Interpretation Syndrome
- Impaired Home Maintenance

Nursing Care Plan 19-1 gives sample interventions for a client with a nursing diagnosis of Risk for Injury, defined in the NANDA-I taxonomy (2012, p. 430) as a state in which a person is "at risk for injury as a result of environmental conditions interacting with the individual's adaptive and defensive resources."

Despite appropriate assessments and plans for preventing injuries, accidents still occur. When they do, the nurse's first concerns are the safety of the client and the potential for allegations of malpractice. Therefore, if an accident occurs, the nurse takes the following actions:

- Checks the client's condition immediately
- Calls for help if the client is in danger
- Begins resuscitation measures if necessary
- Comforts and reassures the client
- Avoids moving the client until safe to do so
- Reports the accident and assessment findings to the physician
- Completes an incident report as soon as the client is stabilized (see Chap. 3)

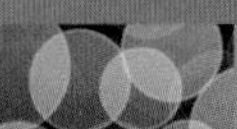

NURSING CARE PLAN 19-1 Risk for Injury

Assessment

- Note evidence of altered mental status.
- Determine signs of impaired mobility, balance, and coordination.
- Take vital signs and document postural changes in blood pressure.
- Consult drug references for medications that cause sensory or motor effects or deficits.
- Check the client's use of an ambulatory aid such as crutches, canes, or a walker.
- Communicate with the client regarding self-assessment of functional status.

Nursing Diagnosis. **Risk for Injury** related to impaired mobility and postural hypotension as evidenced by a difference of 20 mm Hg in systolic pressure when lying and standing (135/85 lying; 115/80 standing), previous fall that resulted in a fractured hip, inconsistent use of walker, and client's statement, "I've had some near-falls at home since my surgery. I get dizzy when I hurry and my feet get all tangled up."

Expected Outcome. The client will remain free of injury throughout the duration of care.

Interventions	Rationales
Assess blood pressure (BP) lying and standing daily at 0800.	Determines effects of postural changes on BP regulation.
Keep the bed in a low position.	Facilitates safety when relocating from the bed to a chair or to ambulate.
Reinforce the need to use the call signal.	Obtaining assistance with ambulation reduces the potential for falling.
Assist the client to a sitting position until dizziness passes before standing.	Given time, baroreceptors for regulating BP can adjust to accommodate for venous pooling.
Keep the walker within reach at all times.	Enhances the possibility that the client will use the ambulatory aid.
Help to put on nonskid shoes or slippers and glasses for ambulation.	Footwear with traction and support and maximizing vision help reduce the risk for falling.

Evaluation of Expected Outcomes

- Ambulation is delayed briefly until dizziness has passed.
- Client is assisted with nonskid slippers and glasses before ambulating.
- Client ambulates with assistance and the use of a walker.
- No falls occur.

CRITICAL THINKING EXERCISES

1. What rationale would you give as the reason the Joint Commission identified National Patient Safety Goals as a criterion for compliance with accreditation?
2. If someone you know is contemplating a career in nursing, but is hesitant because of a latex allergy, what information would you offer?
3. When discharging an older adult to the care of a family member, what safety measures are appropriate to include in the discharge instructions?
4. Without resorting to the use of restraints, how can you prevent falls in a client with an unsteady gait?

NCLEX-STYLE REVIEW QUESTIONS

1. When examining an unconscious client, which assessment finding is most indicative of carbon monoxide poisoning?
   1. Bilaterally dilated pupils
   2. Cherry-red skin color
   3. Smoky odor to clothing
   4. Rapid, irregular pulse rate
2. During the orientation of an unlicensed nursing assistant, which of the nurse's descriptions of a restraint alternative is most accurate?
   1. It fastens behind the client.
   2. It is made of cloth or nylon.
   3. The client must be able to release the device.
   4. The client must give consent for its application.
3. When providing health teaching to caregivers of older adults, the nurse is most correct in identifying which of the following as the greatest safety issue?
   1. Chemical poisoning
   2. Thermal burns
   3. Electrical shock
   4. Accidental falls
4. Which of the following nursing actions is best to implement initially when discovering an alert person who has ingested too much prescribed medication?
   1. Induce vomiting
   2. Administer an antacid
   3. Transport the person to the emergency department
   4. Call the person's personal physician immediately
5. If a nurse determines that a physical restraint is necessary to maintain a client's safety, which of the following is essential?
   1. Obtaining a medical order for its use
   2. Notifying the nursing supervisor
   3. Administering a mild sedative
   4. Charging the client for the equipment

SKILL 19-1 Using Physical Restraints

Suggested Action	Reason for Action
ASSESSMENT	
Assess the client's physical and mental status for signs suggesting the need for safety.	Provides data for determining the need for physical protective restraints.
Consult with staff and the family on options other than restraints.	Supports the principle of using less restrictive approaches initially.
Observe the client's response to alternative measures.	Determines the need to revise the current plan for care.
Contact the physician for an order for the use of restraints.	Complies with the Joint Commission requirements.
Review the agency's restraint policy or procedure if unable to contact the physician.	Follows the standards for care.
Assess the client's skin and circulation.	Provides a baseline of information for future comparisons.
Inspect the restraint that will be used and avoid any that are in poor condition.	Ensures safety.
PLANNING	
Choose a restraint compatible with the client's size.	Prevents injury.
Approach the client slowly and calmly. Speak in a soft, controlled voice.	Reduces agitation.
Use the client's name and make eye contact.	Helps secure the client's attention.
Explain why a restraint is necessary.	Promotes understanding and cooperation.
Reassure the client that the restraints will be discontinued when the possibility for injury no longer exists.	Indicates the criteria for releasing restraints.
Plan to remove or loosen the restraints at times established by agency policy to assess circulation, provide joint mobility, give skin care, assist with elimination, offer food and fluids, and evaluate whether restraints are still needed.	Demonstrates attention to basic physiologic and safety needs; supports the principle that restraints are not applied longer than necessary.
IMPLEMENTATION	
Place the client in a position of comfort with proper body alignment.	Maintains functional position and reduces discomfort.
Protect any bony prominences or fragile skin that a restraint may injure.	Reduces or prevents injury.
Upper Extremity Restraints	
Apply mitts rather than wrist restraints, if possible (Fig. A).	Maintains freedom to move elbows and shoulders.

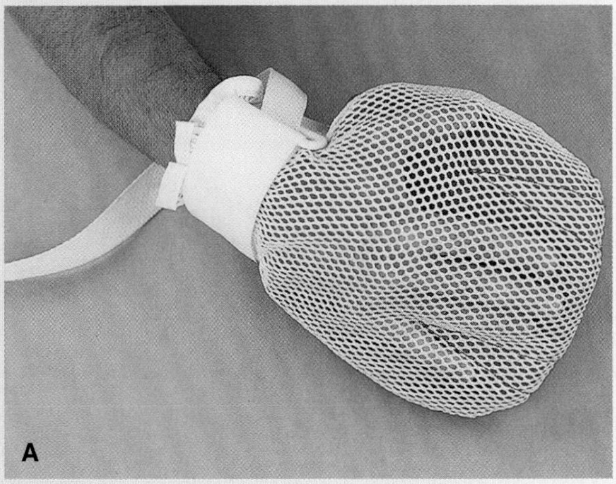

A

A netted hand mitt. (Photo by B. Proud.)

(continued)

Using Physical Restraints (continued)

IMPLEMENTATION (CONTINUED)

Use soft cloth restraints instead of stiff leather (Fig. B). — Promotes skin integrity.

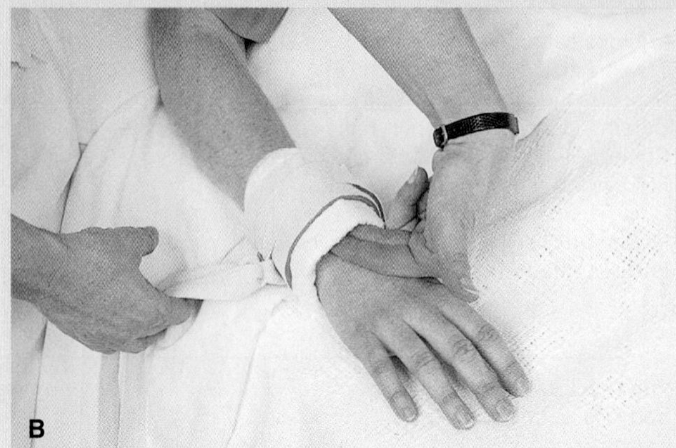

Soft wrist restraints are applied over padded bony prominences. Ensure that two fingers can be inserted between the restraint and the wrist. (Photo by B. Proud.)

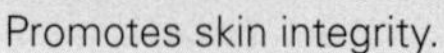

Provide as much length as possible without allowing the client to pull at tubes or other treatment devices. — Facilitates movement.

Wheelchair Restraints

Avoid back cushions if possible. — Creates the potential for slack if they become dislodged.

Make sure the client's hips are flush with the back of the chair. — Promotes good posture and skeletal alignment.

Apply belts snugly over the thighs with at least a 45-degree angle between the belt and knees (Fig. C). — Minimizes sliding up toward the ribs and compromising breathing.

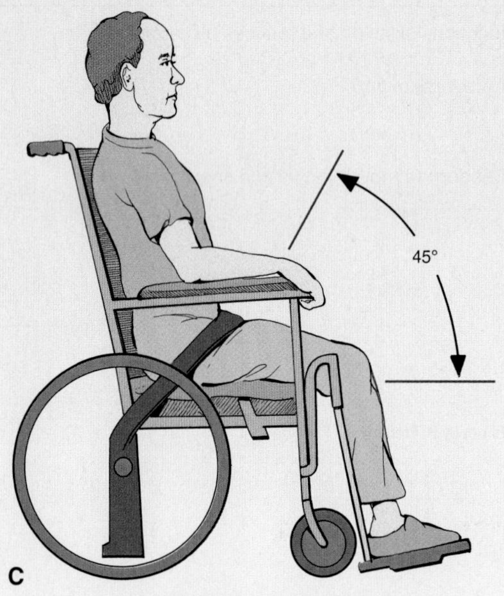

With the lap strap at a 45-degree angle to the knees, the hips are held toward the back of the chair.

Apply vests with Velcro or zipper closures at the back; use criss-crossing vests with front closures only on docile clients. — Keeps fasteners out of reach; prevents strangulation.

Support the feet on footrests. — Reduces pressure behind the knees and promotes blood circulation.

(continued)

Using Physical Restraints (continued)

IMPLEMENTATION (CONTINUED)

Action	Rationale
Tie restraints under the chair, not behind the back (Fig. D).	Prevents suffocation if the client should slide downward.

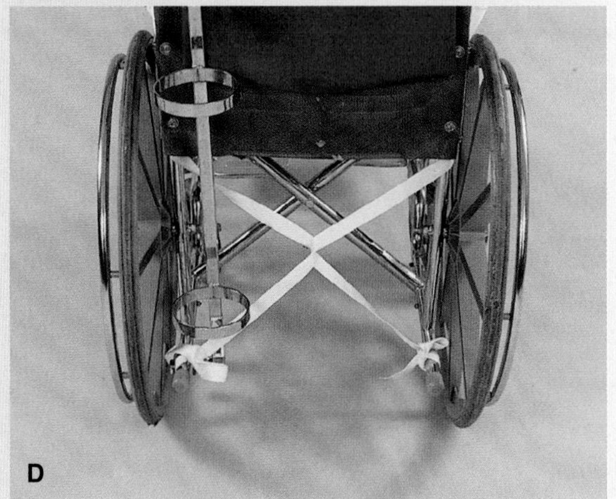

Restraint ties are secured beneath the chair. (Photo by B. Proud.)

Action	Rationale
Use a quick-release knot when tying any type of restraint (Fig. E).	Facilitates removal should the client's safety become compromised.

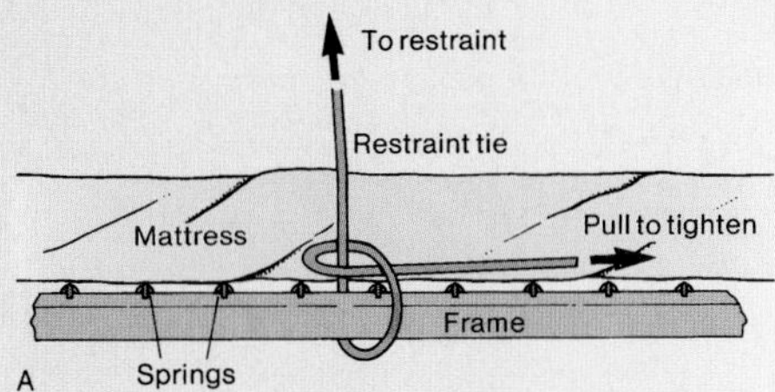

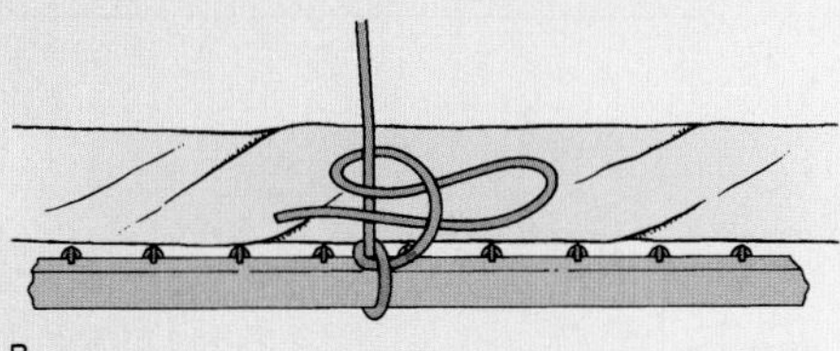

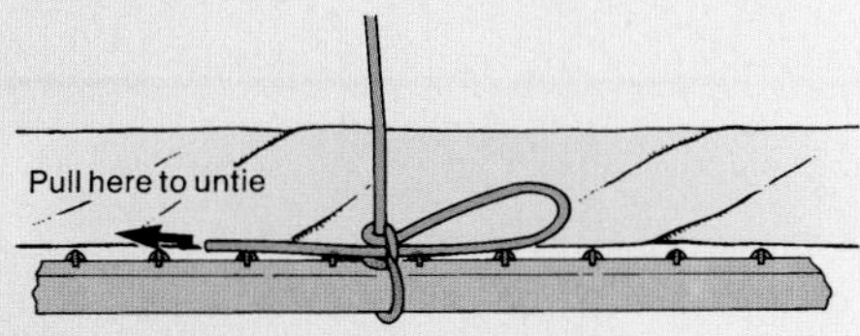

Follow the sequence in steps A, B, and C to tie a quick-release knot.

Action	Rationale
Keep the client in sight whenever restraints are used.	Aids in monitoring the client's safety.
Never restrain a client to a toilet.	Prevents drowning or falls.
Bed Restraints	
Position the client in the center of the mattress.	Allows maximum movement and proper body alignment.
Use full side rails and maintain them in an "up" position while the client is restrained.	Prevents injury from slipping between or below half rails.
Apply side rail covers or pad the rails with soft bath blankets if the client is extremely restless.	Reduces the potential for becoming caught or injured within the open spaces of the rails.
Apply jacket restraints snugly enough to prevent harm but not so tight as to constrict the chest and interfere with breathing.	Ensures ventilation.

(continued)

Using Physical Restraints (continued)

IMPLEMENTATION (CONTINUED)

Secure the straps to the moveable part of the bed frame, not the side rails or stationary frame (Fig. F)	Prevents sliding and chest compression.

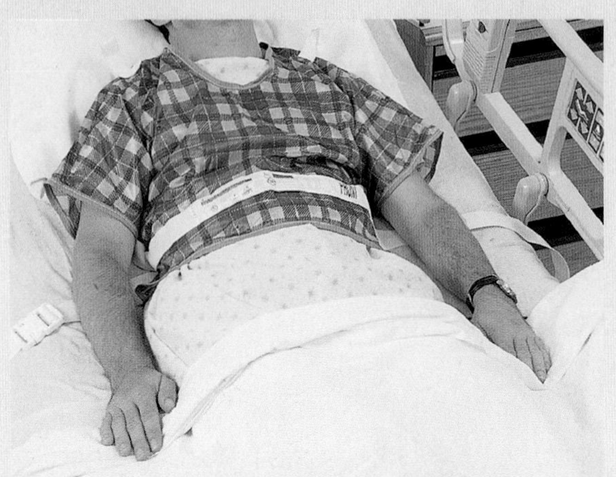

F

The restraint ties are secured to the moveable portion of the bed frame. (Photo by B. Proud.)

Monitor aggressive, agitated, or restless clients frequently.	Promotes client safety.

Evaluation

- Restraints are applied correctly.
- Client remains free of injury.
- Restraints are released according to policy.
- Basic needs are met.
- Restraints are discontinued when no longer needed.

Document

- Assessment findings that indicate a need for restraint
- Types of restraint alternatives and the client's response
- Condition of skin, circulation, sensation, and joint mobility before restraint application
- Type of restraint applied
- Communication with physician and responsible family member
- Frequency of release and assessment findings
- Nursing measures used to promote skin integrity and joint flexibility, and to meet nutritional and elimination needs
- Assessments indicating an ongoing need for restraints

SAMPLE DOCUMENTATION

Date and Time Pulling on urinary catheter. Reminded to leave catheter alone. Placed close to nursing station to allow quick intervention. Given a skein of yarn to wrap as a ball to distract client from catheter. Continues to tug at catheter. Catheter is patent, but urine now appears bloody. Order obtained for soft cloth wrist restraints. Skin over wrists is intact, no edema, full mobility, fingers are warm and pink, can differentiate sharp from dull sensation. Restraints secured to arms of wheelchair. Daughter notified of need to use restraints at this time and concurs with treatment plan. ——— SIGNATURE/TITLE

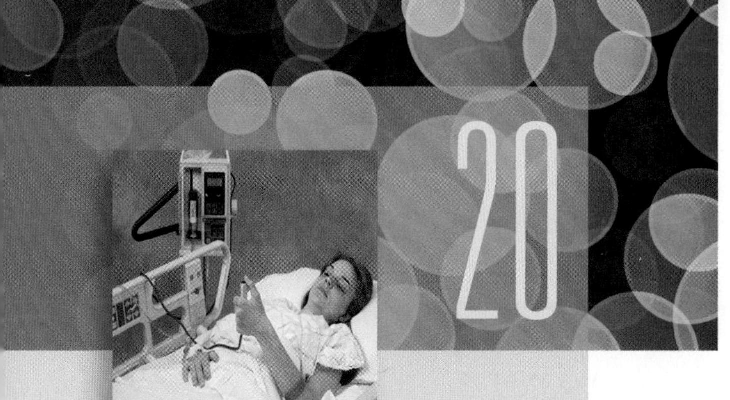

20 Pain Management

Words To Know

acupressure
acupuncture
acute pain
adjuvants
alternative medical therapy
analgesic
biofeedback
bolus
chronic pain
controlled substances
cordotomy
cutaneous pain
distraction
endogenous opioids
equianalgesic dose
fifth vital sign
hypnosis
imagery
intractable pain
intraspinal analgesia
loading dose
malingerer
meditation
modulation
neuropathic pain
nociceptors
nonopioids
opioids
pain
pain management
pain threshold
pain tolerance
patient-controlled analgesia (PCA)
perception
percutaneous electrical nerve stimulation (PENS)
placebo
referred pain
relaxation
rhizotomy
somatic pain
suffering
transcutaneous electrical nerve stimulation (TENS)
transduction
transmission
visceral pain

Learning Objectives

On completion of this chapter, the reader should be able to:

1. Give a general definition of pain.
2. List four phases in the pain process.
3. Explain the difference between pain perception, pain threshold, and pain tolerance.
4. Discuss how endogenous opioids reduce pain transmission.
5. Name at least five types of pain.
6. Give at least three characteristics that differentiate acute pain from chronic pain.
7. List five components of a basic pain assessment.
8. Name four common pain-intensity assessment tools used by nurses.
9. Identify at least three occasions when it is essential to perform a pain assessment and document assessment findings.
10. Name four physiologic mechanisms for managing pain.
11. Give three categories of drugs used alone or in combination to manage pain.
12. Identify two surgical procedures used when other methods of pain management are ineffective.
13. List at least five nondrug, nonsurgical methods for managing pain.
14. Discuss the most common reason why clients request frequent administrations of pain-relieving drugs.
15. Define addiction.
16. Discuss how fear of addiction affects pain management.
17. Define placebo and explain the basis for its positive effect.

Pain is probably the major cause of physical distress among clients. According to the American Pain Society (2004), clients "should have access to the best pain relief that can safely be provided." This chapter provides information about pain and techniques for pain relief.

PAIN

Pain is an unpleasant sensation usually associated with disease or injury. It causes physical discomfort and also is accompanied by **suffering**, which is the emotional component of pain. Because there is no effective method for validating or invalidating pain, Margo McCaffery (1968), a nursing expert on pain, defines pain as being "whatever the person says it is, and existing whenever the person says it does." Understanding how pain is produced and perceived is essential to finding mechanisms for

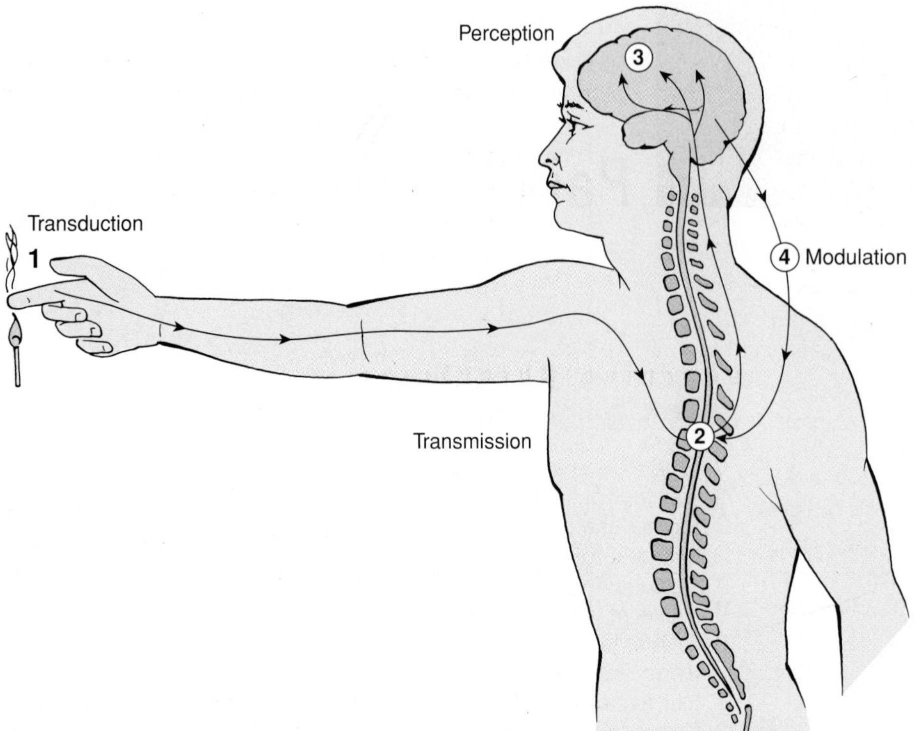

FIGURE 20-1 The phases of pain.

pain relief. Extensive research is being conducted to discover more about pain transmission, types of pain, and the management of pain.

The Process of Pain

The process by which people experience pain occurs in four phases: transduction, transmission, perception, and modulation (Fig. 20-1).

Transduction

Transduction refers to the conversion of chemical information at the cellular level into electrical impulses that move toward the spinal cord. Transduction begins when injured cells release chemicals such as substance P, prostaglandins, bradykinin, histamine, and glutamate. These chemicals excite **nociceptors** (a type of sensory nerve receptors activated by noxious stimuli) located in the skin, bones, joints, muscles, and internal organs (Fig. 20-2).

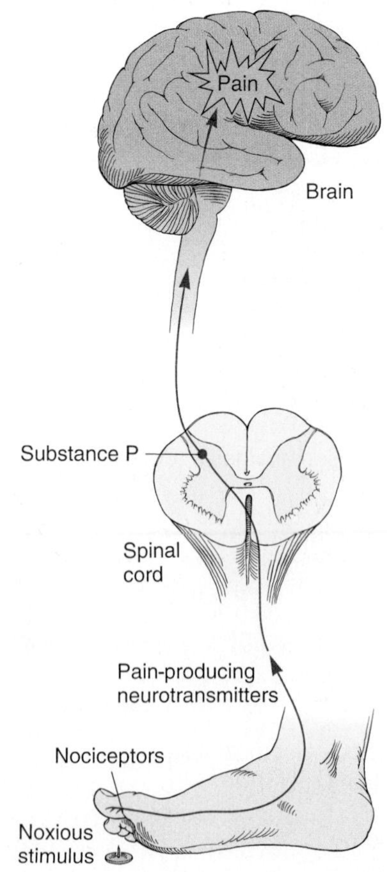

FIGURE 20-2 Pain transmission pathway.

Transmission

Transmission is the phase during which stimuli move from the peripheral nervous system toward the brain. Transmission occurs when peripheral nociceptors form synapses with neurons within the spinal cord that carry pain impulses and other sensory information such as pressure and temperature changes via fast and slow nerve fibers. *A-delta fibers*, which are large myelinated fibers, carry impulses rapidly at a rate of approximately 5 to 30 meters per second (m/sec) (Porth & Matfin, 2008). Impulses through the fast pain pathway result in sharp, acute initial sensations like those felt when touching a hot iron. The result is that the person almost immediately withdraws from the pain-provoking stimulus. Following the fast transmission, impulses from small unmyelinated fibers known as *C-fibers* carry impulses at a slower rate of 0.5 to 2 m/sec. They are responsible for the throbbing, aching, or burning sensation that persists after the initial discomfort.

With the help of substance P, pain impulses move to sequentially higher levels in the brain, such as the reticular activating system, thalamus, cerebral cortex, and limbic system. Prostaglandin, a chemical released from injured cells, speeds up the transmission. As the pain impulses are transmitted, pain receptors become increasingly sensitized. This finding helps explain the clinical observation that established pain is more difficult to suppress.

When pain impulses reach the thalamus within the brain, two responses occur. First, the thalamus transmits the message to the cortex, where the location and severity of the injury are identified. Second, it notifies the nociceptors that the message has been received and that continued transmission is no longer necessary. A malfunction in this secondary process may be one reason why chronic pain lingers.

Perception

Perception (the conscious experience of discomfort) occurs when the **pain threshold** (the point at which sufficient pain-transmitting stimuli reach the brain) is reached. Once pain is perceived, structures within the brain determine its intensity, attach meaningfulness to the event, and provoke emotional responses.

Pain thresholds tend to be the same among healthy people, but each person tolerates or bears the sensation of pain differently. **Pain tolerance** (the amount of pain a person endures) is influenced by genetics; learned behaviors specific to gender, age, and culture (see Chap. 6); and other biopsychosocially unique factors such as current anxiety level, past pain experiences, and overall emotional disposition (Mayo Clinic, 2009).

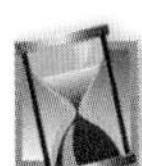

Gerontologic Considerations

- Data related to age-associated changes in pain perception, sensitivity, and tolerance are conflicting. Therefore, it is a dangerous assumption to believe that older adults are less sensitive to pain stimuli. Older adults may experience needless suffering or undertreatment as a result of this assumption.
- Older adults with depression, chronic conditions, or high levels of stress usually have diminished pain tolerance because they have less energy to cope with pain.
- Older adults may endure pain for several reasons. They may not want to be perceived as a nuisance or a complainer, may believe that pain is expected with aging or indicates weakness, may fear tests or becoming addicted to pain medication, or may believe that they are suffering from a serious illness.

Modulation

Modulation is the last phase of pain impulse transmission during which the brain interacts with the spinal nerves in a downward fashion to subsequently alter the pain experience. At this point, the release of pain-inhibiting neurochemicals reduces the painful sensation. Examples of such neurochemicals include endogenous opioids (discussed later in this chapter), gamma-aminobutyric acid (GABA), and others.

Research is being conducted to develop new types of pain-modulating drugs. Current efforts are being directed at medications that (1) occupy cell receptors for neurotransmitters like acetylcholine and serotonin, (2) block glutamate receptors and peptides (protein compounds) like tachykinin-neurokinin and substance P, and (3) reduce cytokines (a type of immune system protein) that trigger pain by promoting inflammation; and other scientific endeavors to discover new methods for relieving pain without the unwanted side effects of current analgesics (Pain—Hope Through Research, 2009).

Pain Theories

Several theories attempt to explain how pain is transmitted and reduced. No one theory is all-encompassing.

A hypothesis for how the perception of pain is diminished involves **endogenous opioids** (naturally produced morphine-like chemicals). The endogenous opioids–*endorphins*, *dynorphins*, and *enkephalins*–reduce pain. Two neurotransmitters, serotonin and norepinephrine, stimulate their release (see Chap. 5). When endogenous opioids are released, they are thought to bind to sites on the nerve cell's membrane that block the transmission of pain-conducting neurotransmitters such as substance P and prostaglandins (Fig. 20-3).

Types of Pain

Not all pain is exactly the same. Five types of pain have been described according to the source (cutaneous, visceral, and neuropathic) or duration (acute and chronic).

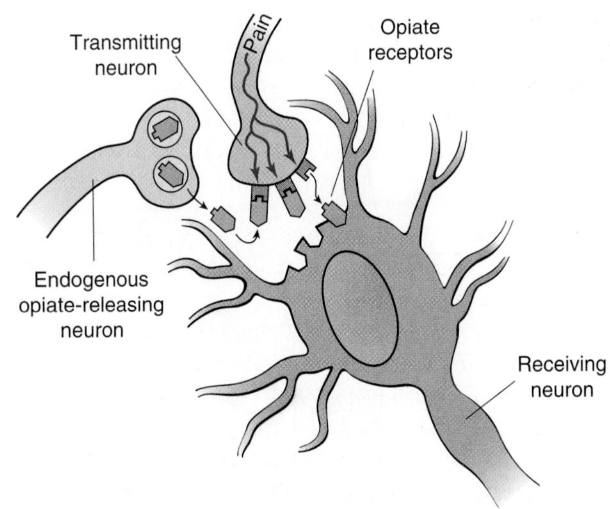

FIGURE 20-3 Mechanism of pain transmission and interference.

Cutaneous Pain

Cutaneous pain, discomfort that originates at the skin level, is a commonly experienced sensation resulting from some form of trauma. The depth of the trauma determines the type of sensation felt. Damage confined to the epidermis produces a burning sensation. At the dermis level, pain is localized and superficial. Subcutaneous tissue injuries produce an aching, throbbing pain. **Somatic pain** (discomfort generated from deeper connective tissue) develops from injury to structures such as muscles, tendons, and joints.

Visceral Pain

Visceral pain (discomfort arising from internal organs) is associated with disease or injury. It is sometimes referred or poorly localized. **Referred pain** (discomfort perceived in a general area of the body, usually away from the site of stimulation) is not experienced in the exact site where an organ is located (Fig. 20-4). Other autonomic nervous system symptoms such as nausea, vomiting, pallor, hypotension, and sweating may accompany visceral pain.

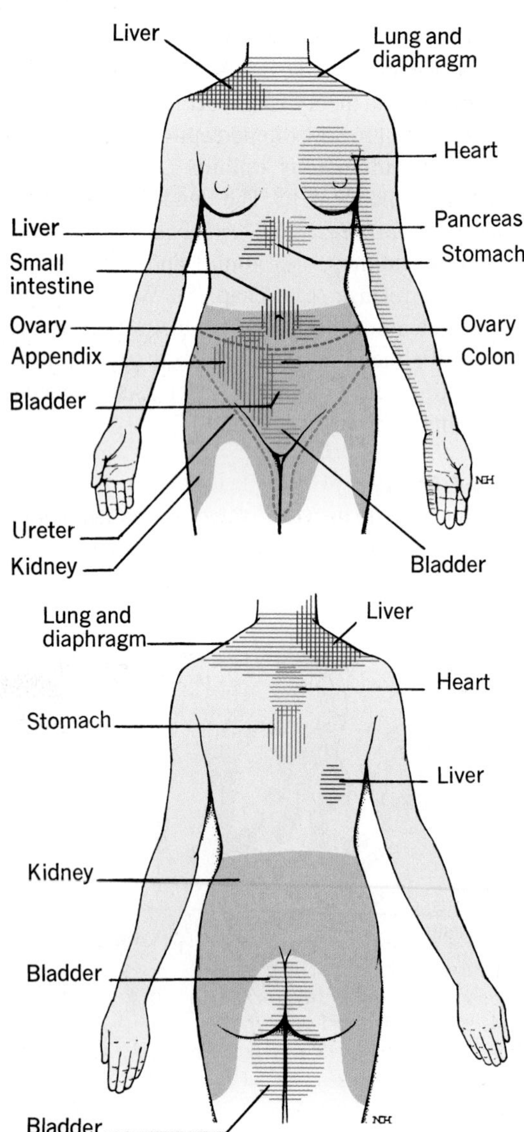

FIGURE 20-4 Areas of referred pain.

Neuropathic Pain

Neuropathic pain (pain with atypical characteristics) is also called functional pain. This type of pain often is experienced days, weeks, or even months after the source of the pain has been treated and resolved (Copstead-Kirkhorn & Banasik, 2010). This has led some to speculate that the transduction circuitry is dysfunctional, allowing pain stimuli to continue in the absence of injury or disease.

One example of neuropathic pain is *phantom limb pain* or *phantom limb sensation*, in which a person with an amputated limb perceives that the limb still exists and feels burning, itching, and deep pain in tissues that have been surgically removed. Some researchers believe that the pain associated with fibromyalgia is a pain processing disorder caused by the disruption in the way the body perceives and communicates pain (Roan, 2005).

Acute Pain

Acute pain (discomfort that has a short duration) lasts for a few seconds to less than 6 months. It is associated with tissue trauma, including surgery or some other recent identifiable etiology. Although severe initially, acute pain eases with healing and eventually disappears. The gradual reduction in pain promotes coping with the discomfort because there is a reinforcing belief that the pain will disappear in time. Both acute and chronic pain result in physical and emotional distress and can be intermittent (incorporating periods of relief), but that is where the similarities end.

Chronic Pain

The characteristics of **chronic pain** (discomfort that lasts longer than 6 months) are almost totally opposite from those of acute pain (Table 20-1). The longer the pain exists, the more far-reaching its effects on the sufferer (Box 20-1). Other people begin to show negative reactions to the chronic pain sufferer, such as the following:

- Saying they are tired of hearing about the pain
- Ignoring the sufferer's concerns and complaints

BOX 20-1 Quality-of-Life Activities Affected by Chronic Pain

- Exercising
- Working around the house
- Sleeping
- Enjoying hobbies and leisure time
- Socializing
- Walking
- Concentrating
- Having sex
- Maintaining relationships with family and friends
- Working a full day
- Caring for children

TABLE 20-1 Characteristics of Acute and Chronic Pain

ACUTE PAIN	CHRONIC PAIN
Recent onset	Remote onset
Symptomatic of primary injury or disease	Uncharacteristic of primary injury or disease
Specific and localized	Nonspecific and generalized
Severity associated with the acuity of the injury or disease process	Severity out of proportion to the stage of the injury or disease
Favorable response to drug therapy	Poor response to drug therapy
Requires less and less drug therapy	Requires more and more drug therapy
Diminishes with healing	Persists beyond the healing stage
Suffering is decreased	Suffering is intensified
Associated with sympathetic nervous system responses such as hypertension, tachycardia, restlessness, and anxiety	Absence of autonomic nervous system responses; manifests depression and irritability

- Getting angry
- Suggesting that the pain has a psychological basis
- Telling the person he or she is using the pain to manipulate others for selfish purposes
- Criticizing the person for using drugs "as a crutch"
- Suggesting that the person is addicted to pain medication (American Chronic Pain Association, 2004)

PAIN ASSESSMENT STANDARDS

The American Pain Society has proposed that pain assessment is the **fifth vital sign**. In other words, the nurse checks and documents the client's pain every time he or she assesses the client's temperature, pulse, respirations, and blood pressure. In August 1999, The Joint Commission established Pain Assessment and Management Standards with which all accredited health care organizations must comply. Aspects incorporated in the Joint Commission standards include the following:

- Everyone cared for in an accredited hospital, long-term care facility, home health care agency, outpatient clinic, or managed care organization has the right to an assessment and management of pain.
- Pain is assessed using a tool appropriate for the person's age, developmental level, health condition, and cultural identity. Refer to Table 20-2 for pain-related information that is included in an initial comprehensive pain assessment.
- Pain is assessed regularly throughout the health care delivery.
- Pain is treated in the health care agency, or the client is referred elsewhere.
- Health care workers are educated regarding pain assessment and management.
- Clients and their families are educated about effective pain management as an important part of care.
- The client's choices regarding pain management are respected.

To comply with the established standards of care, the nurse assesses pain whenever he or she considers it appropriate and routinely in the following circumstances:

- When the client is admitted
- Whenever the nurse takes vital signs
- At least once per shift when pain is an actual or potential problem

TABLE 20-2 Components of a Comprehensive Pain Assessment[a]

COMPONENT	FOCUS OF ASSESSMENT
Intensity	Rating for present pain, worst pain, and least pain using a consistent scale
Location	Site of pain or identifying mark on a diagram
Quality	Description in client's own words
Onset	Time the pain began
Duration	Period that pain has existed
Variations	Pain characteristics that change
Patterns	Repetitiveness or lack thereof
Alleviating factors	Techniques or circumstances that reduce or relieve the pain
Aggravating factors	Techniques or circumstances that cause the pain to return or escalate in intensity
Present pain management regimen	Approaches used to control the pain and results and effectiveness
Pain management history	Past medications or interventions and response; manner of expressing pain; personal, cultural, spiritual, or ethnic beliefs that affect pain management
Effects of pain	Alterations in self-care, sleep, dietary intake, thought processes, lifestyle, and relationships
Person's goal for pain control	Expectations for level of pain relief, tolerance, or restoration of functional abilities
Physical examination of pain	Assessment of structures that relate to the site of pain

[a]If clients have pain in more than one area, assessment data are collected for each.

- When the client is at rest and when involved in a nursing activity
- After each potentially painful procedure or treatment
- Before implementing a pain-management intervention, such as administering an **analgesic** (a pain-relieving drug) and again 30 minutes later

PAIN ASSESSMENT DATA

A basic or brief pain assessment includes the client's description of the *onset*, *quality*, *intensity*, *location*, and *duration* of the pain (Table 20-3). Nurses also ask about symptoms that accompany the pain and what, if anything, makes it better or worse. During an admission assessment, the nurse also asks questions such as:

- What activities are you unable to do because of pain?
- Do you ever take pain medication? If so, when?
- What are the names and dosages of pain medicine you take?
- What nondrug methods, such as rest, do you use to relieve your pain?
- How does your pain change with self-treatment?
- What are your preferences for managing your pain?
- What pain level is an acceptable goal for you if total pain relief is not possible?

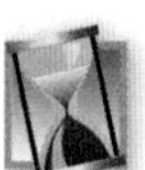

Gerontologic Considerations

■ Chronic illnesses and disease increase the risk for pain for older people. Multiple chronic conditions (eg, peripheral vascular disease, diabetic neuropathies, orthopedic problems, cancer) can contribute to the pain. Pain often goes underreported among older adults because of many factors. For example, the older person may believe that pain is a normal part of aging, may be a punishment for past actions, may result in a loss of independence, or may indicate that death is near, or that nothing can be done about it.

When caring for clients, especially those who are often underassessed and undertreated (Box 20-2), the nurse observes for behavioral signs that are common nonverbal indicators of pain, such as moaning, crying, grimacing, guarded position, increased vital signs, reduced social interactions, irritability, difficulty concentrating, and changes in eating and sleeping. Autonomic nervous system responses such as tachycardia, hypertension, dilated pupils, perspiration, pallor, rapid and shallow breathing, urinary retention, reduced bowel motility, and elevated blood glucose levels may be apparent. Clients with chronic pain are not as likely to manifest autonomic nervous system responses.

BOX 20-2 Underassessed and Undertreated Pain Populations

- Infants
- Children younger than 7 years of age
- Culturally diverse clients
- Clients who are mentally challenged
- Clients with dementia (diminished brain function)
- Clients who are hearing or speech impaired
- Clients who are psychologically disturbed

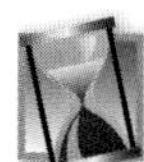

Gerontologic Considerations

■ Regardless of its source, pain is one of the most common complaints of older people, who are more likely to have atypical presentations of pain.

■ Older adults with cognitive impairment may not be able to complain of pain or discomfort. Changes in mental status or behavior are primary manifestations of pain in people with dementia. When assessing pain in older adults, attention should be focused on how the pain or discomfort interferes with activities of daily living and quality of life.

■ Astute assessment of behavior changes such as increased pulse, respiration, restlessness, agitation, and wandering may provide the only clues to pain in older adults with cognitive or expressive changes.

PAIN INTENSITY ASSESSMENT TOOLS

There is no perfect way for determining whether pain exists and how severe it is. Because no machines or laboratory tests can measure pain, nurses are limited to the subjective

TABLE 20-3 Basic Components of Pain Assessment

CHARACTERISTIC	DESCRIPTION	EXAMPLES
Onset	Time or circumstances under which the pain became apparent	After eating, while shoveling snow, during the night
Quality	Sensory experiences and degree of suffering	Throbbing, crushing, agonizing, annoying
Intensity	Magnitude of pain	None, slight, mild, moderate, severe; or numeric scale from 0–10
Location	Anatomic site	Chest, abdomen, jaw
Duration	Time span of pain	Continuous, intermittent, hours, weeks, months

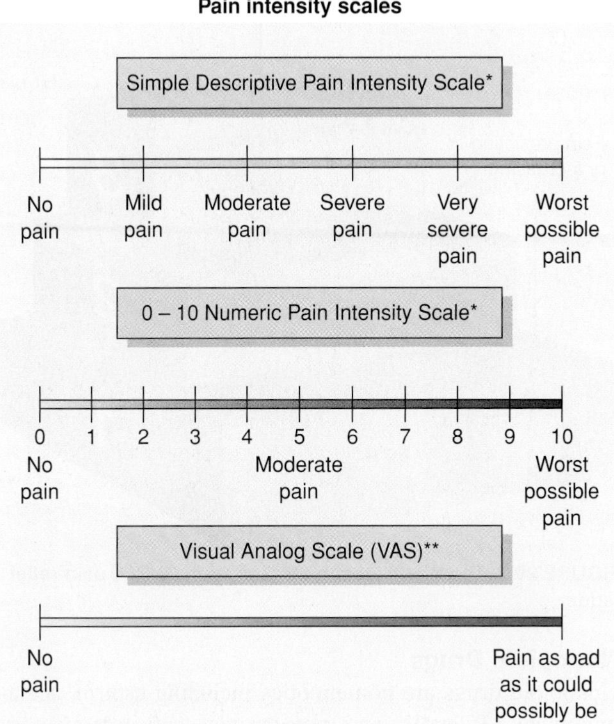

FIGURE 20-5 Pain assessment tools: word scale (*top*), numeric scale (*middle*), and linear scale (*bottom*).

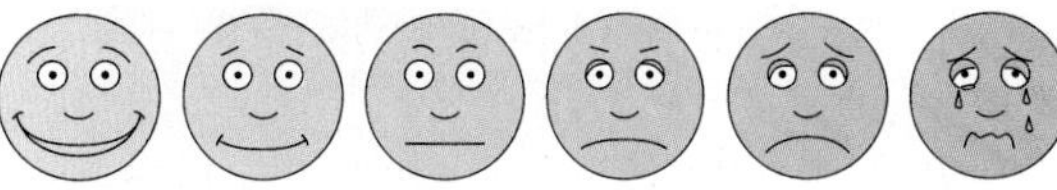

FIGURE 20-6 The Wong-Baker FACES Pain Rating Scale. Instructions: Explain to the person that each face is for a person who feels happy because he or she has no pain (hurt) or for a person who feels sad because he or she has some or a lot of pain. Face 0 is very happy because he or she does not hurt at all. Face 1 hurts just a little bit. Face 2 hurts a little more. Face 3 hurts even more. Face 4 hurts a whole lot. Face 5 hurts as much as you can imagine, although you do not have to be crying to hurt this bad. Ask the person to choose the face that best describes how he or she is feeling. Rating scale is recommended for persons aged 3 years and older. (From Wong, D. L., Hockenberry-Eaton, M., Wilson D., Winkelstein, M. L., Ahmann, E., & DiVito-Thomas, P. A. [1999]. *Whaley & Wong's nursing care of infants and children* [6th ed., p. 1153]. St. Louis: Mosby. Copyrighted by Mosby-Year Book, Inc. Reprinted by permission.)

information that only clients can provide. Individual characteristics, family, culture, and ethnicity influence tolerance and expression of pain.

Nurses generally use one of the four simple assessment tools to quantify a client's pain intensity: a numeric scale, a word scale, a linear scale (Fig. 20-5), and a picture scale (Fig. 20-6). Clients identify how their pain compares with the choices on the scale.

One scale is not better than another. A numeric scale is the most commonly used tool when assessing adults. The Wong-Baker FACES scale is best for children or clients who are culturally diverse or mentally challenged. Children as young as 3 years can use the FACES scale. Regardless of the assessment tool used, many clients underrate or minimize their pain intensity.

PAIN MANAGEMENT

Because of the wide variety of types of pain and effects on lifestyle and personal relationships, management of the client's pain is a priority. Despite the fact that the client is the only reliable source for quantifying pain, nurses are not consistent in responding to clients' reports of pain because of personal biases.

Treatment Biases

According to McCaffery and Ferrell (1999), nurses sometimes delay pain-relieving measures because "[they] expect someone in severe pain to *look* as if he hurts." Neither behaviors nor physiologic data, however, are irrefutable indicators of pain. Responses to pain and coping techniques are learned, and clients may express them in a variety of ways. If a client's expressions of pain are incongruent with the nurse's expectations, pain management may not be readily forthcoming. Consequently, the client's pain may be undertreated.

Pain Management Techniques

Pain management (techniques for preventing, reducing, or relieving pain) is a major focus for quality improvement programs in health care agencies. The American Pain Society, working with the Agency for Health Care Policy and Research (a division of the Department of Health and Human Services), has developed *Standards for the Relief of Acute Pain and Cancer Pain* (Box 20-3). The objective of this collaborative effort is to improve how pain is assessed and controlled. The original effort has been expanded to include the assessment and treatment of pain in all client populations.

Most techniques for managing pain fall into one of the four general physiologic categories (Table 20-4).

Drug Therapy

Drug therapy, either alone or in combination with other therapeutic measures, is the cornerstone of pain management. The World Health Organization (WHO, 2010) recommends following a three-tiered drug approach based on the pain intensity and the client's response to therapy (Fig. 20-7). The original target of the WHO's analgesic ladder in 1996 was to address methods for relieving pain from cancer. Nevertheless, the principles continue to be applicable for managing pain from cancer as well as other causes of pain (American

BOX 20-3 Standards for the Relief of Acute Pain and Cancer Pain

Standard I
Acute and cancer pain are recognized and effectively treated.

Standard II
Information about analgesics is readily available.

Standard III
Patients are informed on admission, both orally and in writing, that effective pain relief is an important part of their treatment, that their communication of unrelieved pain is essential, and that health professionals will respond quickly to their reports of pain.

Standard IV
Explicit policies for use of advanced analgesic technologies are defined.

Standard V
Adherence to standards is monitored by an interdisciplinary committee.

Reprinted with permission from American Pain Society. (2008). *Principles of analgesic use in the treatment of acute pain and chronic cancer pain* (6th ed.) Skokie, IL: Author.

Pain Society, 2005). It is the WHO's belief that if the recommendations for pain management are followed, 80% to 90% of clients will be free of pain (WHO, 2009).

Using a tiered approach, physicians prescribe one or more of the following classes of drugs: **nonopioids** (nonnarcotic drugs), **opioids** (narcotic drugs), and **adjuvants** (drugs that assist in accomplishing the desired effect of a primary drug). The choice of drug, its dose, and the timing of medication administration are critical in achieving optimal pain relief.

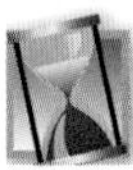

Gerontologic Considerations

■ Adverse effects of analgesics, even over-the-counter products, often are more pronounced in older adults. Common adverse effects include confusion, disorientation, gastritis, constipation, urinary retention, blurred vision, and gastrointestinal bleeding.

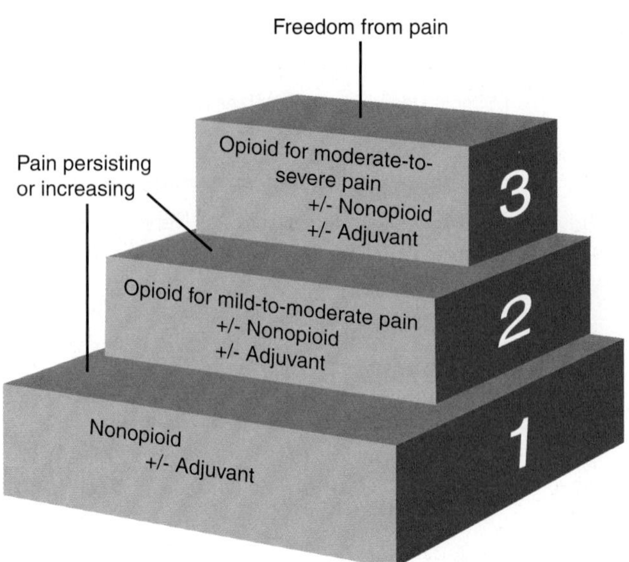

FIGURE 20-7 The World Health Organization (WHO) pain relief ladder.

Nonopioid Drugs

Nonopioid drugs are nonnarcotics including aspirin, acetaminophen (Tylenol), and nonsteroidal anti-inflammatory drugs (NSAIDs) such as ibuprofen (Motrin, Advil, Nuprin), ketoprofen (Orudis KT), and naproxen sodium (Naprosyn, Aleve). These drugs relieve pain by altering neurotransmission peripherally at the site of injury.

Another category of nonopioid drugs is the cyclooxygenase-2 (COX-2) inhibitors. COX is an enzyme: COX-1 protects the gastrointestinal tract and urinary system, and COX-2 promotes the production of pain-transmitting and inflammatory chemicals such as prostaglandins. The inhibition of COX-2 results in pain relief. COX-2 inhibitors are believed to be superior to older NSAIDs, which suppress both COX-1 and COX-2 enzymes. Inhibiting COX-2 to a greater extent than COX-1 causes fewer undesirable gastric side effects. However, all COX-2 inhibitors with the exception of celecoxib (Celebrex) have been withdrawn from prescription use either voluntarily by the manufacturing drug company or by the U.S. Food and Drug Administration because there have been cardiac-related deaths among some users.

Most nonopioids are very effective at relieving pain caused by inflammation. The exception is acetaminophen, which has limited anti-inflammatory activity; however, it is

TABLE 20-4 Approaches to Pain Management

APPROACH	INTERVENTION	EXAMPLES
Interrupting pain-transmitting chemicals at the site of injury	Local anesthetics, anti-inflammatory drugs	Procaine, lidocaine, aspirin, ibuprofen, acetaminophen, naproxen, indomethacin
Altering transmission at the spinal cord	Intraspinal anesthesia and analgesia, neurosurgery	Epidural, caudal, rhizotomy, cordotomy, sympathectomy
Substituting sensory stimuli for pain-producing stimuli	Cutaneous stimuli	Massage, acupuncture, acupressure, heat, cold, therapeutic touch, electrical stimulation
Blocking brain perception	Narcotics, nondrug techniques	Morphine, codeine, hypnosis, imagery, distraction

still an effective analgesic. Almost all of the NSAIDs cause gastrointestinal irritation and bleeding, so they should be given with food.

Opioid Drugs

When pain is no longer controlled with a nonopioid, the nonopioid is combined with an opioid; for example, aspirin with codeine or acetaminophen with codeine or an adjuvant drug, which is discussed later. Opioids (synthetic narcotics) and opiate analgesics, narcotics containing opium or its derivatives, are **controlled substances** (drugs whose prescription and dispensing are regulated by federal law because they have the potential for being abused). Examples include the following:

- Morphine sulfate
- Codeine sulfate
- Meperidine (Demerol)
- Fentanyl (Duragesic, Sublimaze)

Narcotics interfere with central pain perception (at the brain) and generally are reserved for treating moderate and severe pain. They are administered primarily by the oral, rectal, transdermal, or parenteral (injected) route. Opioids and opiates cause sedation, nausea, constipation, and respiratory depression.

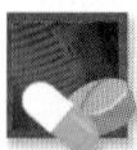

Pharmacologic Considerations

- Normeperidine, a metabolite of meperidine, is a potent convulsant, especially in persons who are not able to break down or excrete the drug properly. Therefore, some physicians are less apt to prescribe it.
- Fentanyl is 100 times as potent as morphine. It is currently one of the most widely prescribed synthetic opioids because of the various choices in methods of administration. One of the most popular methods of administration is a transdermal patch, which is especially useful for controlling chronic pain. Another form of fentanyl that is available is a buccal soluble film that dissolves almost immediately when it makes contact with the mucosa of the cheek. Some clients prefer a fentanyl lozenge in a berry-flavored lollipop that dissolves slowly for transmucosal absorption.

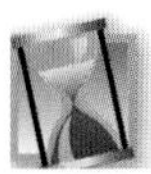

Gerontologic Considerations

- Physiologic changes in older adults such as decreased gastric acid production, decreased gastrointestinal motility, changes in body fat ratio, and changes in organ function (eg, decreased liver blood flow and decreased glomerular filtration rate) affect drug absorption, metabolism, and excretion. Medication may be absorbed more slowly from the intramuscular route in older adults, resulting in delayed onset of action, prolonged duration, and altered absorption with potential for toxicity. Dermal, oral, and sublingual routes may be more effective.
- Older adults have increased sensitivity to narcotics. Initial dosing should be at lower levels (begin with half of the recommended dose) and titrated to the most effective dose. "Start low, go slow" is a rule of thumb for analgesic administration.

Because of an exaggerated fear of causing addiction, narcotics tend to be underprescribed even if clients can benefit from their use. When they are used, treatment biases lead some nurses to administer the lowest dosage of a prescribed range or to delay administration until the maximum time between dosages has elapsed. Consequently, many clients experience inadequate pain management, which contributes to long-term suffering and disability. In addition, unrelieved pain can lead to pneumonia due to shallow breathing, suppressed coughing, and reduced movement. Psychological effects of unrelieved pain include anxiety, depression, and despair, even to the point of suicide.

Patient-Controlled Analgesia

Patient-controlled analgesia (PCA) is an intervention that allows clients to self-administer narcotic pain medication through use of an infusion device (Fig. 20-8). PCA is used primarily to relieve acute pain after surgery, but this technology is finding its way into the home health arena where nonhospitalized clients with cancer are using it.

PCA has several advantages to both clients and nurses:

- Pain relief is rapid because the drug is delivered intravenously.
- Pain is kept within a constant tolerable level (Fig. 20-9).
- Less drug is actually used because small doses continuously control the pain.
- Clients are spared the discomfort of repeated injections.
- Anxiety is reduced because the client does not wait for the nurse to prepare and administer an injection.
- Side effects are reduced with smaller individual dosages and lower total dosages.
- Clients tend to ambulate and move more, reducing the potential for complications from immobility.

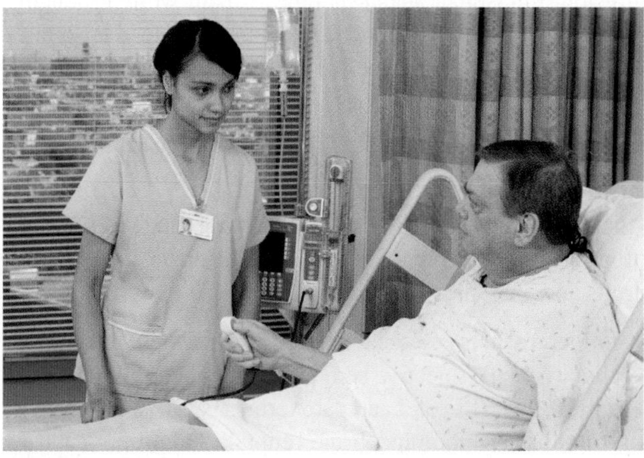

FIGURE 20-8 Patient-controlled analgesia.

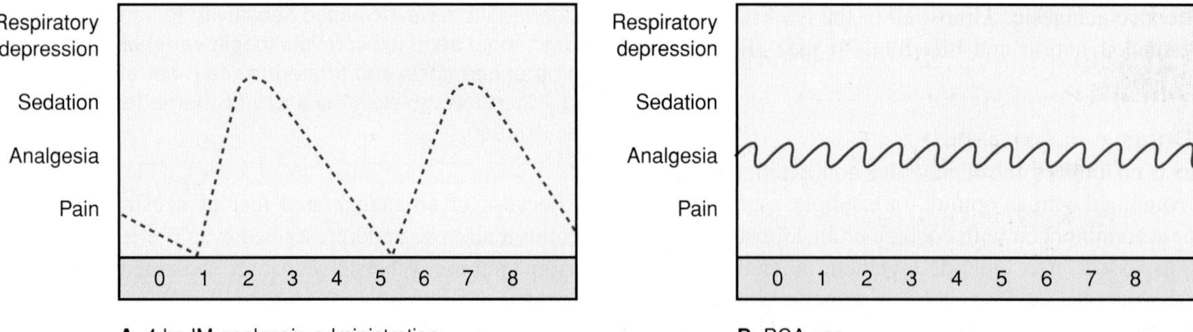

FIGURE 20-9 Pain is less effectively controlled and produces more side effects with intramuscular (IM) analgesia **(A)** than with patient-controlled analgesia (PCA) **(B)**. (Adapted from Harmer, M., Rosen, M., Vickers, M. D. Eds. [1985]. *Patient-controlled analgesia.* St. Louis: CV Mosby.)

- Clients take an active role in their pain management.
- The nurse is free to carry out other nursing responsibilities.

The nurse programs the infusion device so that the client can receive a **bolus** or **loading dose** (a larger dose of drug administered initially or when pain is exceptionally intense) and additional lower doses at frequent intervals depending on the client's level of discomfort (Skill 20-1). Once a dose is delivered, the client cannot administer another dose for a specified amount of time; this period, known as a lockout, prevents overdoses.

Stop, Think, and Respond Box 20-1

Discuss appropriate nursing actions when a client uses the maximum doses of drug with a PCA infuser.

Intraspinal Analgesia

Intraspinal analgesia is a method of relieving pain by instilling a narcotic or local anesthetic through a catheter into the subarachnoid or epidural space of the spinal cord. It is another technique for managing pain. The intraspinal analgesic is administered several times per day or as a continuous low-dose infusion. Intraspinal analgesia relieves pain while producing minimal systemic drug effects. In clients who need long-term analgesia, the use of intraspinal analgesia diminishes the risk for injuring the subcutaneous tissue with repeated injections that may eventually lessen drug absorption.

Adjuvant Drugs

Analgesic drugs are combined with a wide range of adjuvant drugs to improve pain control. The categories of adjuvant drugs and examples of each are as follows:

- Antidepressants: tricyclic antidepressants such as amitriptyline (Elavil); selective serotonin reuptake inhibitors such as fluoxetine (Prozac) and paroxetine (Paxil), and selective serotonin and norepinephrine reuptake inhibitors such as duloxetine (Cymbalta).
- Anticonvulsants: carbamazepine (Tegretol), gabapentin (Neurontin)
- *N*-methyl-D-aspartate (NMDA) receptor antagonists: dextromethorphan, ketamine (Ketalar)
- Nutritional supplements such as glucosamine

Each category of adjuvant drugs acts by different mechanisms. The antidepressants may produce their analgesic-enhancing effect by increasing norepinephrine and serotonin levels, augmenting the release of endorphins. Anticonvulsants are believed to inhibit the transmission of pain by regulating and potentiating the inhibitory neurotransmitter GABA (see Chap. 5). NMDA drugs interfere with the function of nociceptive nerve fibers, perhaps blocking the release of substance P, its nerve-sensitizing properties, and other inflammatory chemicals. Those who favor **alternative medical therapy** (treatment outside the mainstream of traditional medicine) contend that glucosamine slows the breakdown of joint cartilage and promotes its regeneration, relieving pain associated with joint diseases.

Adjuvant drugs are never used as a first-line treatment for pain. When they are used as combination drug therapy, however, the dose of the primary drug can often be decreased. With a lowered opioid dosage, for instance, the client will have less sedation and fewer undesirable side effects.

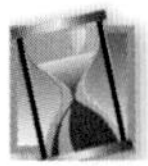

Gerontologic Considerations

- Although the administration of low doses of antidepressants, anticonvulsants, or stimulants may enhance the effectiveness of analgesics for older adults, these agents also increase the risk for adverse effects and drug interactions.

Botulinum Toxin Therapy

Botulinum toxin (Botox) is an agent made from the bacterium *Clostridium botulinum*, which is found in soil and water. Of the seven types of neurotoxins it produces, botulinum type A (BTX-A) has been approved to treat painful musculoskeletal conditions and various types of headaches.

When injected directly into a muscle, the toxin blocks the action of acetylcholine. Under normal conditions, acetylcholine, a neurotransmitter, causes skeletal muscle contraction when it is released at the synapses of motor nerves. Blocking acetylcholine results in temporary paralysis of the injected muscle. When muscles are paralyzed, spasms and nociceptive transduction are inhibited, resulting in pain relief. The effect is local and specific rather than systemic and lasts 2 to 6 months or more (Childers, 2009; M.D. Anderson Cancer Center, 2009). Injections must be repeated to continue the therapeutic effect. The duration of each injection's effect tends to become shorter over time. Clinical resistance may result from the development of neutralizing BTX-A antibodies.

Those who are candidates for botulinum toxin therapy may experience local pain, bruising, or infection at the injection site. The muscle weakness may be somewhat disturbing to some; a few develop new patterns of pain. Because this type of therapy has been approved only since 1989 and increasingly used since 1997, the long-term risks and benefits are still being compiled.

Surgical Approaches

Intractable pain (pain unresponsive to other methods of pain management) can be relieved with surgery. Rhizotomy and cordotomy are neurosurgical procedures that provide pain relief.

Rhizotomy refers to the surgical sectioning of a nerve root close to the spinal cord. It prevents sensory impulses from entering the spinal cord and traveling to the brain. Generally, more than one nerve needs to be sectioned to achieve the desired result. Chemical rhizotomy, which uses alcohol or phenol, and percutaneous rhizotomy, which uses radiofrequency waves, are nonsurgical alternatives for destroying nerve fibers. **Cordotomy** refers to surgical interruption of pain pathways in the spinal cord. It is accomplished by cutting bundles of nerves. Although both procedures interrupt the sensation of pain, they also inhibit the perception of pressure and temperature in the area supplied by the nerves. Consequently, there is a greater risk for undesirable secondary effects.

Nondrug and Nonsurgical Interventions

Several additional interventions can be used to help manage pain. Some independent nursing measures include education, imagery, distraction, relaxation techniques, and applications of heat or cold. Other interventions, such as transcutaneous electrical nerve stimulation (TENS), acupuncture and acupressure, percutaneous electrical nerve stimulation (PENS), biofeedback, and hypnosis, require collaboration with people who have specialized training and expertise. The latter interventions are more likely to be used for clients with chronic pain or those for whom acute pain management techniques have been unsuccessful or are contraindicated.

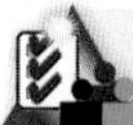

Client and Family Teaching 20-1
Pain and Its Management

The nurse teaches the client and the family as follows:

- Ask the doctor what to expect from the disorder or its treatment.
- Discuss pain-control methods that have worked well or not so well before.
- Talk with the doctor and nurses about any concerns you have about pain medicine.
- Identify any drug allergies you have.
- Inform the doctor and nurses about other medicines you take, in case they may interact with pain medications.
- Help the doctor and nurses measure your pain on a pain scale by stating the number or word that best describes the pain.
- Ask for or take pain-relieving drugs when pain begins or before an activity that causes pain.
- Set a pain-control goal such as having no pain worse than 4 on a scale of 0 to 10.
- Inform the doctor and nurses if the pain medication is not working.
- Perform simple techniques such as abdominal breathing and jaw relaxation to increase comfort.
- Consult with the doctor or nurses about using cold or hot packs or other nondrug techniques to enhance pain control.

Education

Educating clients about pain and methods of pain management supports the principle that clients who assume an active role in their treatment achieve positive outcomes sooner than others (see Client and Family Teaching 20-1). It may be unrealistic for clients to expect to be totally pain-free, but they should not have to endure severe pain.

Imagery

Imagery means using the mind to visualize an experience and sometimes is referred to as intentional daydreaming. The person chooses images based on pleasant memories. In *guided imagery*, the nurse or another person suggests the image to use, such as a walk in the woods, and describes the sensory experiences in great detail. Tape recordings for guided imagery and relaxation (discussed later) are also available, but the subject matter and descriptions can become boring when played repeatedly. Some prefer to use taped sounds of nature, making it easy to conjure different images each time.

Physiologically, the process of imagery produces an alteration in consciousness that allows the client to forget uncomfortable sensory experiences such as pain. Some believe that imagery stimulates the visual portion of the brain's cortex, located in the right hemisphere, where abstract concepts and creative activities occur (Fig. 20-10). While the person is imaging, neurotransmitters are released that calm the body physically and promote emotional well-being.

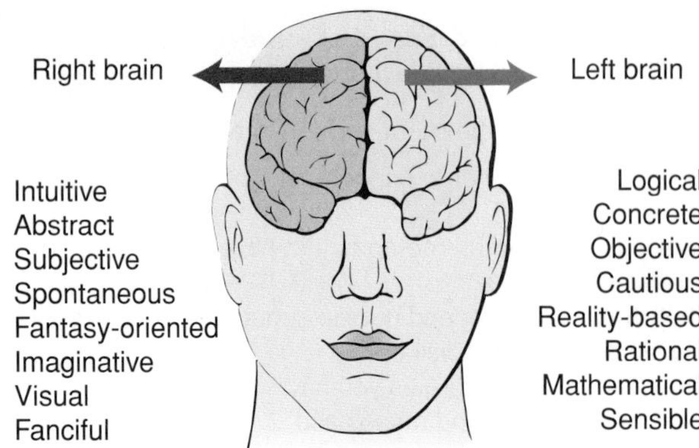

FIGURE 20-10 Right hemispheric functions are used during imagery and meditation.

Meditation

Meditation involves concentrating on a word or idea that promotes tranquility and is similar to imagery except the subject matter tends to be more spiritual. Sometimes meditation involves silent repetition of a word such as "love" or "peace," a prayer, or a statement that reflects a strong personal or religious belief. Those who use this technique successfully tend to experience a relaxed state with lowered blood pressure and pulse rates.

Distraction

Distraction is the intentional diversion of attention to switch the person's focus from an unpleasant sensory experience to one that is neutral or more pleasant. The distraction occurs in the "here and now": it is not imagined. Examples include talking with someone, watching television, participating in a hobby, and listening to music. The mind can attend to only one stimulus at a time; while the person is occupied with the diversional activity, the brain is blocked from perceiving painful stimuli.

Relaxation

Relaxation is a technique for releasing muscle tension and quieting the mind, which helps reduce pain, relieve anxiety, and promote a sense of well-being. Consciously relaxing breaks the circuit among neurons that are overloading the brain with distressing thoughts and painful stimuli (see Client and Family Teaching 20-2 for a procedure clients can learn for relaxation).

Client and Family Teaching 20-2
Relaxation

The nurse teaches the client and family as follows:

- Assume a comfortable position, either sitting or lying down.
- Close your eyes and clear your mind.
- Let the chair or bed effortlessly support your body.
- Become aware of how your body feels.
- Take deep abdominal breaths.
- Focus on the rhythm of your breathing.
- Relax with each breath in and out.
- Tighten and then release muscles in sequential parts of your body such as the toes, feet, lower legs, thighs, and buttocks. Progress toward the face and scalp.
- Visualize healing energy flowing from your feet through your head. Release your worries and discomfort as it passes through.
- Let yourself sleep, if possible.
- At the end of the session, wake up or begin to move gradually.

Heat and Cold

Applications of heat or cold (thermal therapy) are well established techniques for relieving pain. In some locations of practice, nurses must obtain permission from the physician before applying heat or cold.

Pain caused by an injury is best treated initially with cold applications (ice bag or chemical pack). The cold reduces localized swelling and promotes vasoconstriction decreasing the circulation of pain-producing chemicals. Many believe that cold applications relieve pain faster and sustain pain relief longer. Heat applications (hot water bottle, rice bag [cloth bag containing uncooked rice that is heated in the microwave], or moist packs) are placed over a painful area 24 to 48 hours after the injury.

Thermal applications, whether hot or cold, are never used longer than 20 minutes at any one time (see Chap. 28). The skin is always protected with an insulating layer such as a cloth or a towel. The client should never go to sleep while a hot or cold pack is in place, and hot and cold applications are contraindicated in areas of the body where circulation or sensation is impaired.

Menthol (Icy Hot, Heet, BenGay) and capsaicin (Zostrix), compounds found in red pepper, are chemicals sometimes applied topically. Both increase blood flow in the area of application, creating a warm or cool feeling that lasts for several hours.

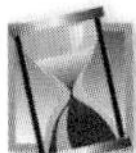

Gerontologic Considerations

- To ensure safety, it is important to assess the condition of the skin and cognitive level of older adults prior to using topical application of heat or cold.

Transcutaneous Electrical Nerve Stimulation

Transcutaneous electrical nerve stimulation (TENS), a medically prescribed pain management technique that delivers bursts of electricity to the skin and underlying nerves, is an intervention implemented by nurses (Skill 20-2). The client perceives the electrical stimulus, generated by a battery-powered stimulator, as a pleasant tapping, tingling, vibrating, or buzzing sensation. TENS is used intermittently for 15 to 30 minutes or longer whenever the client feels a need for it.

For some time, clients with chronic pain have used TENS, but currently, surgical clients also are using it. Reports of its effectiveness range from "useless" to "fantastic."

No one is sure exactly how TENS works. Supposedly, the transmission of electrical stimuli over larger myelinated nerves takes precedence over the transmission of pain-producing stimuli to the brain. Others believe that TENS stimulates the body to release endogenous opioids, and still others suggest that its effectiveness is based on the power of suggestion.

TENS is a nonnarcotic, noninvasive method without harmful side effects. It is contraindicated in pregnant women because its effect on the unborn fetus has not been determined. Clients with cardiac pacemakers (especially the demand type), clients prone to an irregular heartbeat, and clients with previous heart attacks are not candidates for TENS.

Stop, Think, and Respond Box 20-2

Give some reasons that a person may object to using a TENS unit for pain management.

Acupuncture and Acupressure

Acupuncture is a pain management technique in which long, thin needles are inserted into the skin; **acupressure** is a technique that involves tissue compression rather than needles to reduce pain. Both are based on ancient traditions of Chinese medicine and have been demonstrated to prevent or relieve pain. Their exact analgesic mechanisms, however, are not completely understood. Some speculate that these techniques stimulate the body's production of endogenous opioids or that the twisting and vibration of the needles and the pressure applied are forms of cutaneous stimuli that interfere with pain-transmitting neurochemicals. Others believe that the pain relief is a result of a placebo effect (see later discussion); however, combining acupuncture with conventional treatment has shown better results than with conventional treatment alone. Acupuncture and acupressure are becoming more accepted as legitimate forms of pain therapy in the United States (National Center for Complementary and Alternative Medicine, 2009).

Percutaneous Electrical Nerve Stimulation

One of the newer innovations in acute and chronic pain management is **percutaneous electrical nerve stimulation** (PENS), a pain management technique involving a combination of acupuncture needles and TENS. Acupuncture-like needles are inserted into the soft tissue at the site of pain, and an electrical stimulus is conducted through the needles (Fig. 20-11). Percutaneous neuromodulation therapy is an investigational variation of PENS, the difference being that the needle-like filaments are of different lengths and are placed in anatomic landmarks rather than at the site of pain.

PENS is considered superior to TENS in providing pain relief because the needles are located closer to nerve endings. PENS therapy is administered three times a week for 30 minutes for 4 or more weeks. Sustained analgesia for a period of time can be obtained by performing PENS for at least 8 weeks (Yokoyama et al., 2004; Johnson & Martinson, 2007). The technique has been successful in research trials on clients with low back pain, pain caused by the spread of cancer to bones, shingles (acute herpes zoster viral infection), diabetic neuropathy, and migraine headaches.

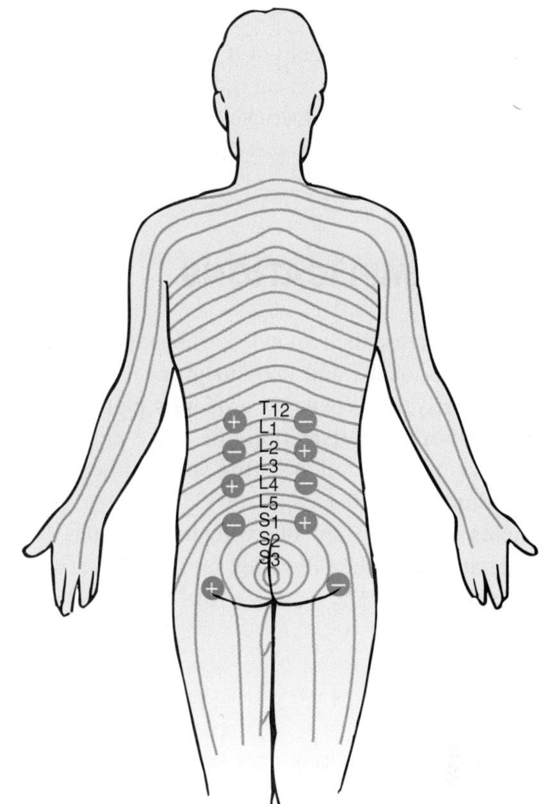

FIGURE 20-11 With percutaneous electrical nerve stimulation (PENS) therapy, five pairs of electrical stimulating leads (alternating positive and negative current) are connected to needles inserted into the lumbar and sacral regions of the spine.

Biofeedback

With **biofeedback**, a client learns to control or alter a physiologic phenomenon (eg, pain, blood pressure, headache, heart rate and rhythm, seizures) as an adjunct to traditional pain management. Initially, the client is connected to a physiologic sensing instrument such as a pulse oximeter or an electromyography machine. The instrument produces a visual or audible signal that correlates with the person's heart rate, skin temperature, or muscle tension. The client is encouraged to reduce or extinguish the signal using whatever mechanism he or she can—generally by physically relaxing. The feedback from the machine demonstrates to the client how well he or she is accomplishing the goal. Eventually, clients can learn to control their symptoms without the assistance of the equipment, using self-suggestion alone.

Hypnosis

Hypnosis is a therapeutic technique in which a person enters a trance-like state resulting in an alteration in perception and memory. During hypnosis, the suggestion is made that the person's pain will be eliminated or that the client will experience the sensation in a more pleasant way.

Although self-hypnosis is possible, more often, hypnosis is induced with the help of a hypnotherapist. Hypnotherapists receive special clinical training; their professional organizations include the American Society of Clinical Hypnosis and the International Society for Medical and Psychological Hypnosis.

NURSING IMPLICATIONS

Nurses must increase their knowledge about pain, take every client's pain seriously, and implement measures for treating pain effectively. Whenever a client's pain is not controlled to his or her satisfaction, the nurse pursues better goal achievement by collaborating with pain experts (see Nursing Guidelines 20-1).

Clients with pain are likely to have various nursing diagnoses, including the following:

- Acute Pain
- Chronic Pain
- Anxiety
- Fear
- Ineffective Coping
- Deficient Knowledge

Nursing Care Plan 20-1 is an example of how a nurse can follow the steps in the nursing process when planning the care of a client with Acute Pain, a nursing diagnosis defined in the NANDA-I taxonomy (2012, p. 478) as "an unpleasant sensory and emotional experience arising from actual or potential tissue damage or described in terms of such damage (International Association for the Study of Pain); sudden or slow onset of any intensity from mild to severe with an anticipated or predictable end and a duration of less than 6 months."

Addiction

One of the leading factors interfering with adequate pain management is the fear of addiction. The American Pain Society (2008) defines addiction as "a pattern of compulsive drug use characterized by a continued craving for an opioid and the need to use the opioid for effects other than pain relief." Statistics indicate that the fear of addiction is greater than the reality.

Nurses often assume that a client's desire to experience the drug's pleasant effects motivates his or her desire for frequent doses of narcotics. What may be happening is that the prescribed dose or frequency of administration is not controlling the pain, a phenomenon that occurs as clients develop drug tolerance. Nurses may undertreat the pain or may convince the physician to prescribe a placebo.

Placebos

A **placebo** is an inactive substance or treatment used as a substitute for an analgesic drug or conventional therapeutic

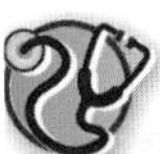

NURSING GUIDELINES 20-1

Managing Pain

- Never doubt the client's description of pain or need for relief. *Bias on the nurse's part may lead to withholding prescribed medication or undertreating the symptoms.*
- Follow the written medical orders for administering pain medications. *This practice demonstrates compliance with nurse practice acts.*
- Administer pain-relieving drugs as soon as the need becomes evident. *Prompt administration of drugs reduces the client's suffering.*
- Consult the physician if the current drug therapy is not controlling the client's pain. *Consulting with the physician demonstrates client advocacy.*
- Collaborate with the physician to develop several pain-management options involving combinations of drugs, alternative routes of administration, and different dosing schedules. *Developing options individualizes pain management.*
- Support the formation of an interdisciplinary pain management team (physicians, surgeons, nurses, pharmacists, anesthesiologists, physical therapists, massage therapists, and so forth) who can be consulted on hard-to-manage pain problems. *Such a group makes available the expertise of a variety of practitioners.*
- Administer pain medication before an activity that produces or intensifies pain. *This timing prevents pain, which is much easier than treating it.*
- When the client's pain is continuous, administer analgesic drugs on a scheduled basis rather than irregularly. *Giving the drugs regularly controls pain when it is at a lower intensity.*
- Monitor for drug side effects such as respiratory depression, decreased levels of consciousness, nausea, vomiting, and constipation. *Careful monitoring demonstrates concern for the client's safety and comfort.*
- Consult the professional literature or experts on the **equianalgesic dose** (an oral dose that provides the same level of pain relief as a parenteral dose). *This prevents undertreatment of pain because of changes in drug absorption or drug metabolism.*
- Change the client's position, elevate a swollen limb to reduce swelling, loosen a tight dressing, and assist the client with bowel or bladder elimination. *These measures reduce factors that intensify the pain experience.*
- Implement independent and prescribed nondrug interventions, such as client teaching, imagery, meditation, distraction, and TENS, as additional techniques for pain management. *These techniques reduce mild-to-moderate pain when used alone or potentiate pain management when combined with drug therapy.*
- Allow rest periods between activities. *Exhaustion reduces the client's ability to cope with pain.*

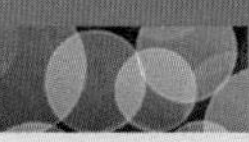

NURSING CARE PLAN 20-1 Acute Pain

Assessment

- Determine the source of the client's pain; when it began; its intensity, location, characteristics; and related factors such as what makes the pain better or worse.
- Ask how the client's pain interferes with life such as diminishing the person's ability to meet his or her own needs for hygiene, eating, sleeping, activity, social interactions, emotional stability, concentration, and so on.
- Identify at what level the client can tolerate pain.
- Measure the client's vital signs.
- Note pain-related behaviors such as grimacing, crying, moaning, and assuming a guarded position.
- Perform a physical assessment, taking care to gently support and assist the client to turn as various structures are examined. Use light palpation in areas that are tender. Show concern when assessment techniques increase the client's pain. Postpone nonpriority assessments until the client's pain is reduced.

Nursing Diagnosis. **Acute pain** related to cellular injury or disease as manifested by the statement, "I'm in severe pain," rating pain at a 10 using a numeric scale, pointing to the lower left abdominal quadrant, describing the pain as being "continuous and throbbing that started this morning" without any known cause.

Expected Outcome. The client will rate the pain intensity at his tolerable level of "5" within 30 minutes of implementing a pain management technique.

Interventions	Rationales
Assess the client's pain and its characteristics at least every 2 hours while awake and 30 minutes after implementing a pain management technique.	Prompt interventions prevent or minimize pain.
Modify or eliminate factors that contribute to pain such as a full bladder, uncomfortable position, pain-aggravating activity, excessively warm or cool environment, noise, and social isolation.	Multiple stressors decrease tolerance of pain.
Determine the client's choice for pain relief techniques from among those available.	Doing so encourages and respects the client's participation in decision making.
Administer prescribed analgesics or alternative pain management techniques promptly.	Suffering contributes to the pain experience; eliminating delays in nursing responses can reduce suffering.
Advocate on the client's behalf for doses of prescribed analgesics or the addition of adjuvant drug therapy if pain is not satisfactorily relieved.	The Joint Commission standards mandate nurses and other health care workers to facilitate pain relief for all clients.
Administer a prescribed analgesic before a procedure or activity that is likely to result in pain or intensify pain that already exists.	Prophylactic interventions facilitate keeping pain within a manageable level.
Plan for periods of rest between activities.	Fatigue and exhaustion interfere with pain tolerance.
Reassure the client that there are many ways to moderate the pain experience.	Suggesting that there are additional untried options reduces frustration or despair that there is no hope for pain relief.
Assist the client to visualize a pleasant experience.	Imaging interrupts pain perception.
Help the client to focus on deep breathing, relaxing muscles, watching television, putting a puzzle together, or talking to someone on the telephone.	Diverting attention to something other than pain reduces pain perception.
Apply warm or cool compresses to a painful site.	Flooding the brain with alternative sensory stimuli interrupts impulses that transmit pain.
Gently massage a painful area or the same area on the opposite side of the body (contralateral massage).	Massage promotes the release of endorphins and enkephalins that moderate the sensation of pain.
Promote laughter by suggesting that the client relate a humorous story or watch a video or comedy program of his or her choice.	Laughter releases endorphins and enkephalins that promote a feeling of well-being.

Evaluation of Expected Outcomes

- The client reports that pain is gone or at a tolerable level.
- The client perceives the pain experience realistically and copes effectively.
- The client can participate in self-care activities without undue pain.

measure. Placebos can relieve pain, especially when clients have confidence in their health care providers. The trust a client has in the nurse or physician probably has more to do with the efficacy of placebos than any other factor. Consequently, it is wrong to assume that a client whose pain is relieved with placebos is addicted or is a **malingerer** (someone who pretends to be sick or in pain). Using deception and withholding pain medication are considered unethical (American Pain Society, 2005).

CRITICAL THINKING EXERCISES

1. Describe factors that can intensify pain.

2. How would you respond to a coworker who feels that a client is "faking" pain to receive medication?

NCLEX-STYLE REVIEW QUESTIONS

1. When a nurse observes that a client with upper abdominal pain is curled in a fetal position and rocking back and forth, which action would help most to further assess the client's pain?

1. Determine whether the client can stop moving.
2. Ask the client to rate the pain from 0 to 10.
3. Observe whether the client is perspiring heavily.
4. Give the client a prescribed pain-relieving drug.

2. What type of pain is a client with an amputated arm experiencing who states, "I know my arm is not there, but I feel it throbbing?"

1. Referred pain
2. Phantom pain
3. Visceral pain
4. Cutaneous pain

3. A nurse can expect that acute pain may have which of the following effects on the client's vital signs?

1. The temperature may be elevated.
2. The pulse rate may be rapid.
3. The respiratory rate may be slow.
4. The blood pressure may fall.

4. Which of the following is the best action for a hospice nurse to take to provide maximum pain relief when caring for a client with terminal cancer?

1. Give analgesic medication whenever the client requests it.
2. Administer pain medication every 3 hours as prescribed.
3. Ask the physician to prescribe a high dose of pain medication.
4. Give pain medication when the client's pain is severe.

5. Which of the following categories of medications would be considered adjuvants? Select all that apply.

1. Nonsteroidal anti-inflammatory drugs (NSAIDS)
2. Botulinum toxin
3. Antidepressants
4. Anticonvulsants
5. Opioids (narcotics)

SKILL 20-1 Preparing a Patient-Controlled Analgesia (PCA) Infuser

Suggested Action	Reason for Action
ASSESSMENT	
Check the written medical order for the use of a PCA infusion device, the prescribed drug, the initial loading dose, the dose per self-administration, and the lockout interval.	Provides data for programming the infusion device.
Check the client's wristband.	Prevents medication errors.
Obtain two forms of identification such as asking the client's name and date of birth.	Supports the Joint Commission's National Patient Safety Goal for identifying clients correctly.
Assess what the client understands about PCA.	Indicates the type and amount of teaching that must be provided.
Check that the currently infusing intravenous (IV) solution is compatible with the prescribed analgesic.	Avoids incompatibility reactions.
PLANNING	
Obtain the following equipment: the infuser, the PCA tubing, and the prefilled medication container.	Promotes organization and efficient time management.
Plug the power cord into the electrical wall outlet.	Prolongs the life of the battery.
Explain the equipment and how it functions.	Reduces anxiety and promotes independence.
IMPLEMENTATION	
Wash hands or perform hand antisepsis with an alcohol rub (see Chap. 10).	Reduces the transmission of microorganisms.
Attach the PCA tubing to the assembled syringe (Fig. A).	Provides a pathway for delivering the medication.

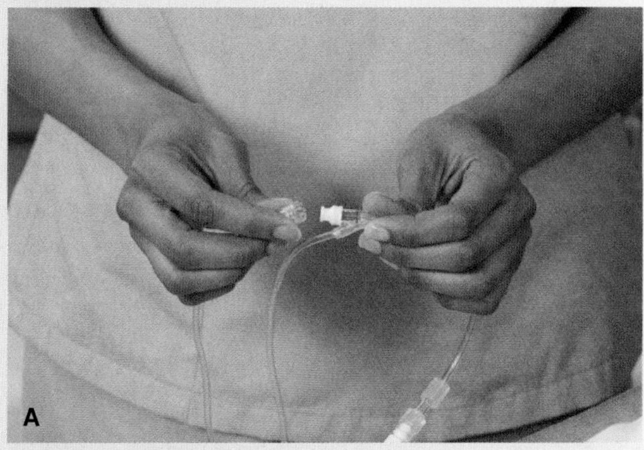

Connecting the tubing. (Photo by B. Proud.)

Suggested Action	Reason for Action
Open the cover or door of the infuser and load the syringe into its cradle (Fig. B).	Stabilizes the syringe within the infuser.

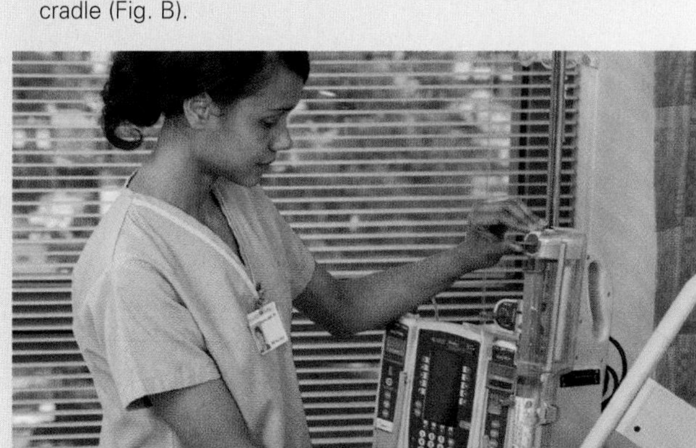

Loading the syringe within the PCA machine. (Photo by B. Proud.)

Suggested Action	Reason for Action
Fill the PCA tubing with fluid.	Displaces air from the tubing.
Connect the PCA tubing to the IV tubing.	Facilitates intermittent administration of medication.
Assess the client's pain.	Provides data from which to evaluate the drug's effectiveness.

(continued)

Preparing a Patient-Controlled Analgesia (PCA) Infuser (continued)

IMPLEMENTATION (CONTINUED)

Set the volume for the prescribed loading dose (Fig. C).

Administers a slightly larger dose of the drug to establish a reduced level of pain rather quickly.

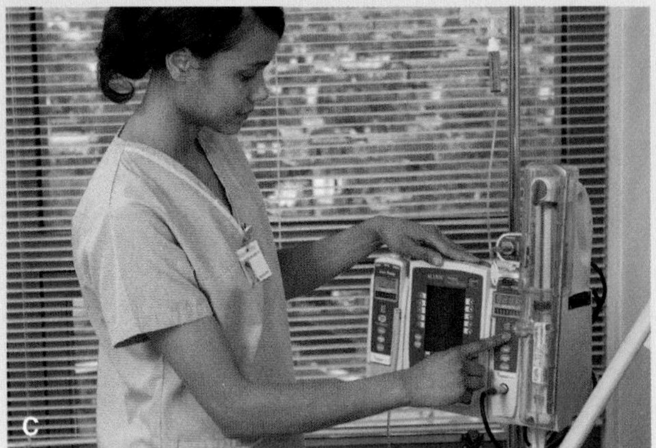

Setting the loading dose. (Photo by B. Proud.)

Program the infuser according to the individual dose and lockout period.

Prevents overdosing.

Close the security door and lock it with a key (Fig. D).

Prevents tampering.

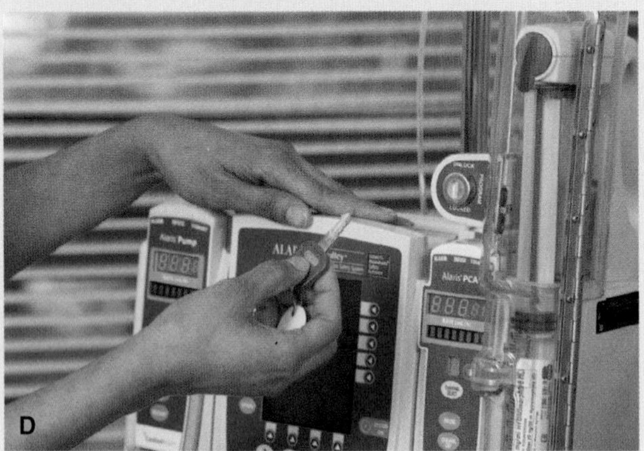

Locking the infuser within the PCA machine. (Photo by B. Proud.)

Instruct the client to press and release the control button each time pain relief is needed (Fig. E).

Educates the client on how to operate the equipment.

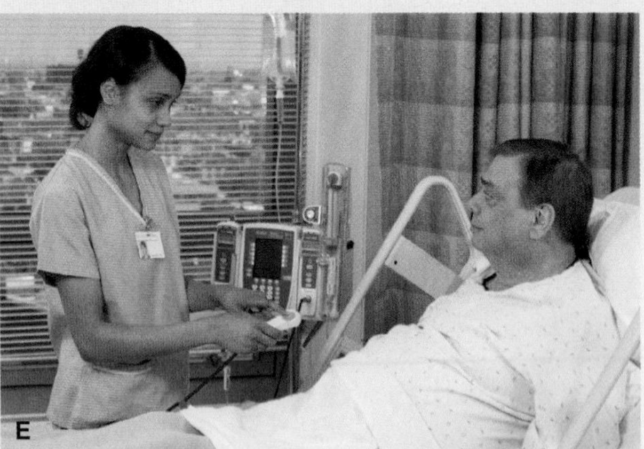

Explaining the use of the PCA infuser. (Photo by B. Proud.)

Explain that a bell will sound when the infuser delivers medication.

Provides sensory reinforcement that the machine is working.

Assess the client's pain at least every 2 hours.

Complies with standards of care.

Replace the medication syringe when it becomes empty.

Maintains continuous pain management.

Change the primary IV solution container every 24 hours.

Complies with infection control policies.

(continued)

Preparing a Patient-Controlled Analgesia (PCA) Infuser (continued)

Evaluation

- The client self-administers pain medication.
- The client's pain is controlled within a tolerable level.

Document

- Date and time
- Volume and type of analgesic solution
- Name of analgesic drug
- Initial pain assessment
- Loading dose
- Individual dose and time schedule
- Reassessments of pain
- Total volume self-administered per shift

SAMPLE DOCUMENTATION

Date and Time A 30 mL syringe of saline with 30 mg of morphine sulfate inserted into a PCA pump. Describes pain around abdominal incision as continuous and stabbing. Rates the pain at a level of 7 on a scale of 0–10. Loading dose of 2 mg administered. Infuser programmed to deliver 0.1 mL—the equivalent of 0.1 mg—at no more than 10-minute intervals. Rates pain at a level of 5 within 10 minutes after loading dose. Instructed and observed to self-administer a subsequent dose. —————— SIGNATURE/TITLE

SKILL 20-2 Operating a Transcutaneous Electrical Nerve Stimulation (TENS) Unit

Suggested Action	Reason for Action
ASSESSMENT	
Check the written medical order for providing the client with a TENS unit.	Demonstrates collaboration with the medical management of client care.
Ask the physician or physical therapist about the best location for electrode placement. Some possible variations are as follows: • On or near the painful site • On either side of an incision • Over cutaneous nerves • Over a joint	Optimizes pain management by individualizing electrode placement.
Read the client's history to determine whether there are any conditions for which the use of a TENS unit is contraindicated.	Demonstrates concern for client safety.
Check the client's wristband, ask the client to identify himself or herself, and state his or her date of birth.	Prevents errors and ensures proper client identification.
Assess what the client understands about TENS.	Indicates the type and amount of teaching that the nurse must provide.
PLANNING	
Obtain the TENS unit and two to four self-adhesive electrodes (Fig. A).	Promotes organization and efficient time management.

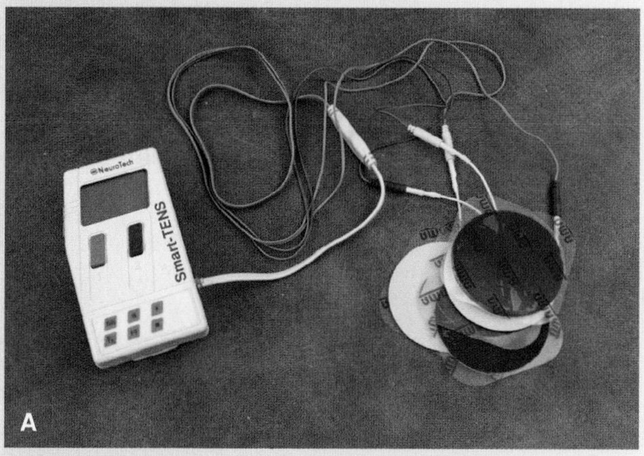

TENS unit.

(continued)

Operating a Transcutaneous Electrical Nerve Stimulation (TENS) Unit (continued)

PLANNING (CONTINUED)

Explain the equipment and how it functions. — Reduces anxiety and promotes independence.

Establish a goal with the client for the level of pain management desired. — Aids in evaluating the effectiveness of the intervention.

IMPLEMENTATION

Wash hands or perform hand antisepsis with an alcohol rub (see Chap. 10). — Reduces the transmission of microorganisms.

Peel the backing from the adhesive side of the electrodes. — Facilitates skin contact.

Position each electrode flat against the skin (Fig. B). — Enhances contact with the skin for maximum effectiveness.

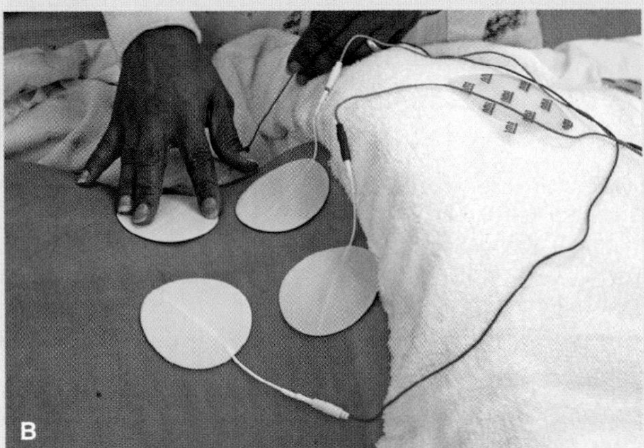

Applying electrodes.

Space the electrodes at least the width of one from the other. — Prevents the potential for burning caused by close proximity of the electrodes.

Make sure the settings on the TENS unit are off. — Prevents premature stimulation to the skin.

Attach the cord(s) from the electrodes to the outlet jack(s) on the TENS unit, much like a headset connects with a radio. — Completes the circuitry from the electrodes to the battery-operated power unit.

Turn the amplitude (intensity) knob on to the lowest setting and assess whether the client can feel a tingling, buzzing, or vibrating sensation. — Helps acquaint the client with the sensation that the TENS unit produces.

Gradually increase the intensity to the point at which the client experiences a mild or moderately pleasant sensation (Fig. C). — Adjusts intensity according to the client's response—a high intensity does not always provide the most pain relief; in fact, it may cause discomfort, muscle contractions, or itching.

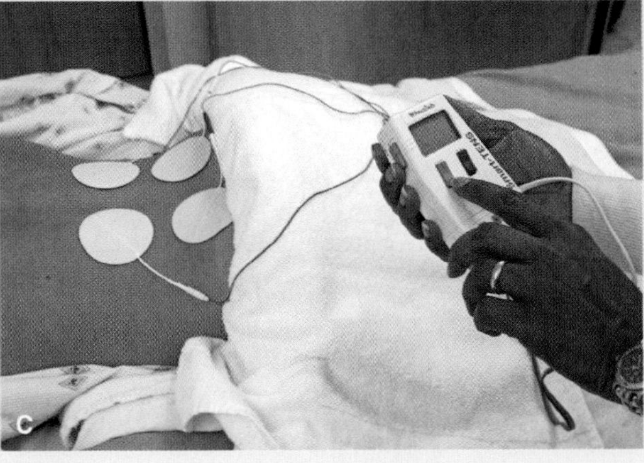

Adjusting the TENS settings.

Set the rate (pulses per second) at a low rate and increase upward; a rate of 80–125 pulses per second is a conventional setting. — Adjusts the frequency of stimuli according to the client's comfort and tolerance.

Set the pulse width (the duration of each pulsation); a pulse width of 60–100 microseconds usually is used for acute pain, but 220–250 microseconds at higher amplitudes may be necessary for chronic or intense pain. — Provides wider and deeper stimulation as the pulse width increases.

(continued)

Operating a Transcutaneous Electrical Nerve Stimulation (TENS) Unit (continued)

IMPLEMENTATION (CONTINUED)

Turn the unit off when a sufficient level of pain relief occurs and turn it back on when pain reappears.	Tests whether or not the TENS unit may be sufficient for intermittent rather than continuous use.
Turn the unit off and remove the cord from the outlet jacks before bathing the client.	Reduces hazards from potential contact of electrical equipment with water.
Remove the electrode patches periodically to inspect the skin; reapply electrodes if they become loose.	Aids in skin assessment.
Slightly change the position of the electrodes if skin irritation develops.	Promotes skin integrity.
Replace or recharge the batteries as needed.	Maintains function of the unit.

Evaluation

- Pain is managed at the goal set by the client.
- Activity is increased.
- Less pain medication is required.
- Emotional outlook is improved.

Document

- Date and time
- Initial pain assessments
- Location of electrodes
- Power settings
- Length of time TENS unit is in use
- Reassessments of pain 30 minutes after application of unit and at least once per shift
- Time when TENS is stopped or discontinued

SAMPLE DOCUMENTATION

Date and Time Rates pain intensity as "10" on a scale from 0 to 10. Pain is described as "piercing" and continuous. Points to lower spine when asked to identify location of pain. Electrodes placed to the immediate R. and L. of the lumbosacral vertebrae. TENS unit initially set at a rate of 80 pulses per second and a pulse width of 60 microseconds. Used for 30 minutes, at which time rated pain at "moderate." Rate increased to 100 pulses per second with a pulse width of 150. ——— SIGNATURE/TITLE

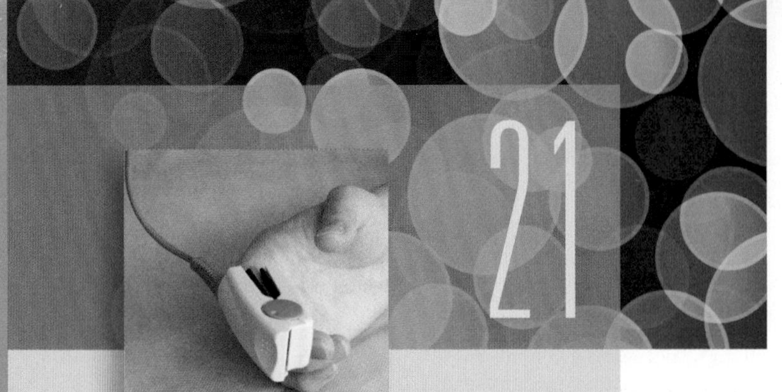

Oxygenation

Words To Know

apnea
arterial blood gas
CPAP mask
diaphragmatic breathing
expiration
face tent
flowmeter
Fowler's position
fraction of inspired oxygen
humidifier
hyperbaric oxygen therapy
hypercarbia
hypoxemia
hypoxia
incentive spirometry
inspiration
liquid oxygen unit
nasal cannula
nasal catheter
nonrebreather mask
orthopneic position
oxygen analyzer
oxygen concentrator
oxygen tent
oxygen therapy
oxygen toxicity
partial rebreather mask
pulse oximetry
pursed-lip breathing
respiration
simple mask
stent
surfactant
tension pneumothorax
tidaling
T-piece
tracheostomy collar
transtracheal catheter
ventilation
Venturi mask
water-seal chest tube drainage

Learning Objectives

On completion of this chapter, the reader should be able to:

1. Explain the difference between ventilation and respiration.
2. Differentiate between external and internal respiration.
3. Name two methods for assessing the oxygenation status of clients at the bedside.
4. List at least five signs of inadequate oxygenation.
5. Name two nursing interventions that can be used to improve ventilation and oxygenation.
6. Identify four items that may be needed when providing oxygen therapy.
7. Name four sources for supplemental oxygen.
8. List five common oxygen delivery devices.
9. Discuss two hazards related to the administration of oxygen.
10. Describe two additional therapeutic techniques that relate to oxygenation.
11. Discuss at least two facts concerning oxygenation that affect the care of older adults.

Oxygen, which measures approximately 21% in the Earth's atmosphere, is essential for sustaining life. Each cell of the human body uses oxygen to metabolize nutrients and produce energy. Without oxygen, cell death occurs rapidly.

This chapter describes the anatomic and physiologic aspects of breathing, techniques for assessing and monitoring oxygenation, types of equipment used in oxygen therapy, and skills needed to maintain respiratory function. Techniques for airway management, such as suctioning and other methods for maintaining a patent airway, are presented in Chapter 36.

ANATOMY AND PHYSIOLOGY OF BREATHING

The elasticity of lung tissue allows the lungs to stretch and fill with air during **inspiration** (breathing in) and return to a resting position after **expiration** (breathing out). **Ventilation** (the movement of air in and out of the lungs) facilitates **respiration** (the exchange of oxygen and carbon dioxide). External respiration takes place at the most distal point in the airway between the alveolar–capillary membranes (Fig. 21-1). Internal respiration occurs at the cellular level by means of hemoglobin and body cells. For people without respiratory disease, increased blood levels of carbon dioxide and hydrogen ions trigger the stimulus to breathe, both chemically and neurologically.

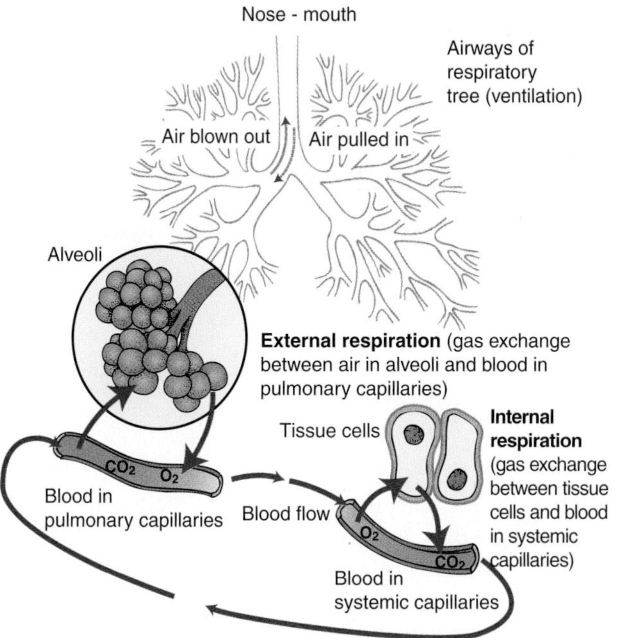

FIGURE 21-1 External and internal respiration.

Ventilation results from pressure changes within the thoracic cavity produced by the contraction and relaxation of respiratory muscles (Fig. 21-2). During inspiration, the dome-shaped diaphragm contracts and moves downward in the thorax. The intercostal muscles move the chest outward by elevating the ribs and sternum. This combination expands the thoracic cavity. Expansion creates more chest space, causing the pressure within the lungs to fall below that in the atmosphere. Because air flows from an area of higher pressure to one of lower pressure, air is pulled in through the nose, filling the lungs. When there is an acute need for oxygen, additional muscles known as accessory muscles of respiration (the pectoralis minor and sternocleidomastoid) contract to assist with even greater chest expansion.

During expiration, the respiratory muscles relax, the thoracic cavity decreases, the stretched elastic lung tissue recoils, intrathoracic pressure increases as a result of the compressed pulmonary space, and air moves out of the respiratory tract. A person can forcibly exhale additional air by contracting abdominal muscles such as the rectus abdominis, transverse abdominis, and external and internal obliques.

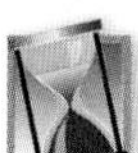

Gerontologic Considerations

- Reduced gas exchange and efficiency in ventilation are the major age-related changes in the respiratory system.
- Age-related structural changes affecting the respiratory system in older adults include the following: respiratory muscles become weaker and the chest wall becomes stiffer as a result of calcification of the intercostal cartilage, kyphoscoliosis, and arthritic changes to costovertebral joints; the ribs and vertebrae lose calcium; the lungs become smaller and less elastic; alveoli enlarge; and alveolar walls become thinner.
- Functional changes to the respiratory system include diminished coughing and gag reflexes, increased use of accessory muscles for breathing, diminished efficiency of gas exchange in the lungs, and increased mouth breathing and snoring.
- Some changes in lung volumes occur, resulting in a slight decrease in overall efficiency and increased energy expenditure by older adults. Older adults experience no change in the volume of air in the lungs after maximal inhalation (known as total lung capacity) as a result of using accessory muscles to breathe.

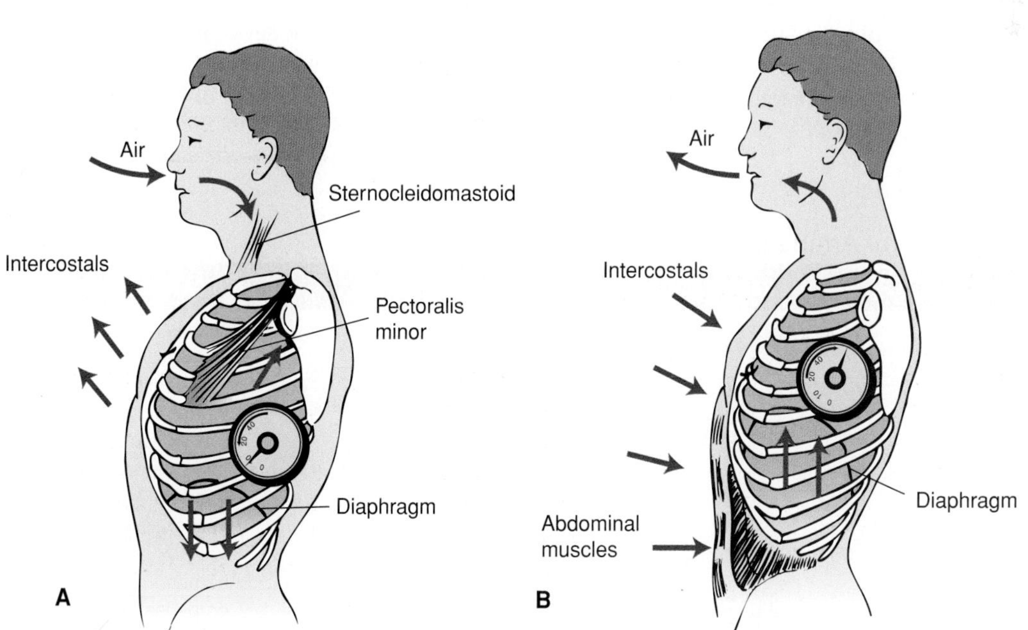

FIGURE 21-2 Ventilation and thoracic pressure changes. **A.** Inspiration. **B.** Expiration.

ASSESSING OXYGENATION

The nurse can determine the quality of a client's oxygenation by collecting physical assessment data, monitoring arterial blood gases, and using pulse oximetry. A combination of these helps to identify signs of **hypoxemia** (insufficient oxygen within arterial blood) and **hypoxia** (inadequate oxygen at the cellular level).

Physical Assessment

The nurse physically assesses oxygenation by monitoring the client's respiratory rate, observing the breathing pattern and effort, checking chest symmetry, and auscultating lung sounds (see Chap. 13). Additional assessments include recording the heart rate and blood pressure, determining the client's level of consciousness, and observing the color of the skin, mucous membranes, lips, and nail beds (Box 21-1).

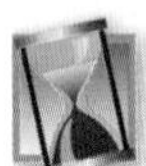

Gerontologic Considerations

- Careful assessment of older adults who demonstrate restlessness or confusion is imperative to differentiate signs of inadequate oxygenation accurately from signs of early delirium or dementia.

Arterial Blood Gases

An **arterial blood gas** (ABG) assessment is a laboratory test using arterial blood to assess oxygenation, ventilation, and acid–base balance. It measures the partial pressure of oxygen dissolved in plasma (PaO_2), the percentage of hemoglobin saturated with oxygen (SaO_2), the partial pressure of carbon dioxide in plasma ($PaCO_2$), the pH of blood, and the level of bicarbonate (HCO_3) ions (Table 21-1). Arterial blood is preferred for sampling because arteries have greater oxygen content than veins and are responsible for carrying oxygen to all cells. Initial and subsequent ABGs are ordered to assess the client in acute respiratory distress or to evaluate the progress of a client receiving medical treatment.

In most situations, a laboratory technician and the nurse collaboratively collect arterial blood. The nurse notifies the laboratory of the need for the blood test, records pertinent assessments on the laboratory request form and in the client's chart, prepares the client, assists the laboratory technician who obtains the specimen, and implements measures for preventing complications after the arterial puncture. In emergencies, a nurse who is trained in performing arterial punctures may obtain the specimen (see Nursing Guidelines 21-1).

BOX 21-1 Common Signs of Inadequate Oxygenation

- Decreased energy
- Restlessness
- Rapid, shallow breathing
- Rapid heart rate
- Sitting up to breathe
- Nasal flaring
- Use of accessory muscles
- Hypertension
- Sleepiness, confusion, stupor, coma
- Cyanosis of the skin (mucous membranes in dark-skinned clients), lips, and nail beds

Pulse Oximetry

Pulse oximetry is a noninvasive, transcutaneous technique for periodically or continuously monitoring the oxygen saturation of blood (Skill 21-1). A pulse oximeter is composed of a photodetector sensor, a red and infrared light emitter, and a microprocessor. The device is attached to a finger, toe, earlobe, or the bridge of the nose using spring-tension or adhesive. The sensor detects the amount of light absorbed by hemoglobin.

TABLE 21-1 Values for Arterial Blood Gases

COMPONENT	NORMAL RANGE	ABNORMAL FINDINGS	INDICATION OF ABNORMAL FINDINGS
pH	7.35–7.45	<7.35	Acidosis
		>7.45	Alkalosis
PaO_2	80–100 mmHg	60–80 mmHg	Mild hypoxemia
		40–60 mmHg	Moderate hypoxemia
		<40 mmHg	Severe hypoxemia
		>100 mmHg	Hyperoxygenation
$PaCO_2$	35–45 mmHg	<35 mmHg	Hyperventilation
		>45 mmHg	Hypoventilation
SaO_2	95%–100%	<95%	Hypoventilation
			Anemia
HCO_3	22–26 mEq	<22 or >26 mEq	Compensation for acid–base imbalance

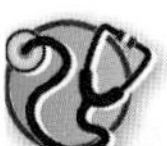

NURSING GUIDELINES 21-1

Assisting With an ABG

- Perform the Allen test before the arterial puncture by doing the following:
  - Flex the client's elbow and elevate the forearm where the arterial puncture will be made.
  - Compress the radial and ulnar arteries simultaneously (see Fig. 21-3A).
  - Instruct the client to open and close the fist until the palm of the hand appears blanched.
  - Release pressure from the ulnar artery while maintaining pressure on the radial artery (see Fig. 21-3B).
  - Observe whether the skin flushes or remains blanched.
  - Release pressure on the radial artery.

The Allen test determines if the hand has an adequate ulnar arterial blood supply should the radial artery become damaged or occluded. The radial artery should not be punctured if the Allen test shows absent or poor collateral arterial blood flow as evidenced by continued blanching after pressure on the ulnar artery has been released. Alternative sites include the brachial, femoral, or dorsalis pedis arteries.

- Keep the client at rest for at least 30 minutes before obtaining the specimen unless the procedure is an emergency. *Because an ABG reflects the client's status at the moment of blood sampling, activity can transiently lower oxygen levels in the blood and lead to an incorrect interpretation of the test results.*
- Record the client's current temperature, respiratory rate, and level of activity if other than resting. *Increased metabolism and activity affect cellular oxygen demands. Therefore, the data help in interpreting the results of laboratory findings.*
- Record the amount of oxygen the client is receiving at the time of the test (either room air or prescribed amount) and ventilator settings. *This information helps to determine if oxygen therapy is necessary or aids in evaluating its current effectiveness.*
- Hyperextend the wrist over a rolled towel. *Hyperextension brings the radial artery nearer the skin surface to facilitate penetration.*
- Comfort the client during the puncture. *An arterial puncture tends to be painful unless a local anesthetic is used.*
- After obtaining the specimen, expel all air bubbles from it. *Doing so ensures that the only gas in the specimen is that contained in the blood.*
- Rotate the collected specimen. *Rotation mixes the blood with the anticoagulant in the specimen tube, ensuring that the blood sample will not clot before it can be examined.*
- Place the specimen on ice immediately. *Blood cells deteriorate outside the body, causing changes in the oxygen content of the sample. Cooling the sample slows cellular metabolism and ensures more accurate test results.*
- Apply direct manual pressure to the arterial puncture site for 5–10 minutes. *Arterial blood flows under higher pressure than venous blood. Therefore, prolonged manual pressure is necessary to control bleeding.*
- Cover the puncture site with a pressure dressing composed of several 4 × 4 in. gauze squares and tape. *Tight mechanical compression provides continued pressure to reduce the potential for arterial bleeding.*
- Assess the puncture site periodically for bleeding or formation of a hematoma (collection of trapped blood) beneath the skin. *Periodic inspection aids in the early identification of arterial bleeding, which can lead to substantial blood loss and discomfort.*
- Report the laboratory findings to the prescribing physician as soon as they are available. *Collaboration with the physician assists in making changes in the treatment plan to improve the client's condition.*

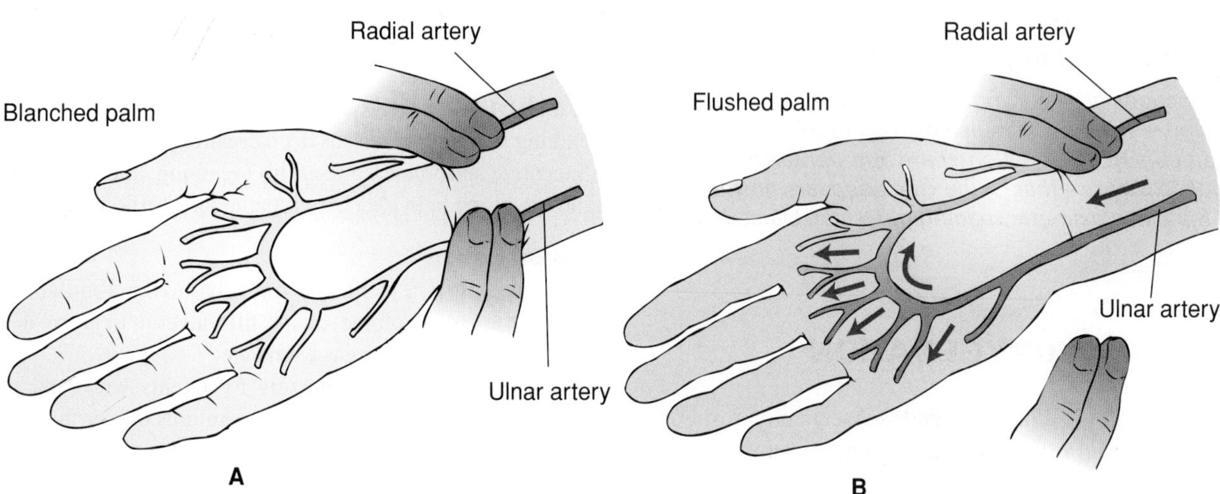

FIGURE 21-3 A. Simultaneous compression of radial and ulnar arteries. **B.** Pressure on the ulnar artery is released.

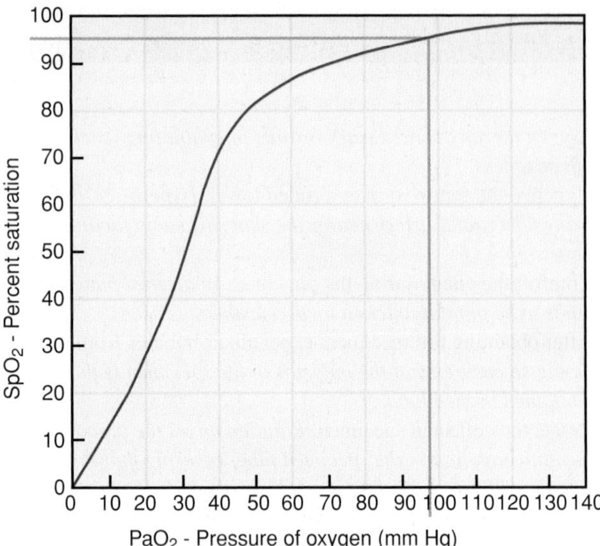

FIGURE 21-4 Draw a line from the SpO_2 in the left column across the graph to the point at which it intersects the curve. Use the numeric scale at the bottom to calculate the PaO_2. In this example, with an SpO_2 of 95%, the PaO_2 is approximately 98 mmHg.

TABLE 21-2 Factors That Interfere With Accurate Pulse Oximetry

FACTOR	CAUSE	REMEDY
Movement of the sensor	Tremor Restlessness Loss of adhesion	Relocate sensor to another site Replace sensor or tape in place
Poor circulation at the sensor site	Peripheral vascular disease Edema Tourniquet effect from taped sensor Vasoconstrictive drug effects	Change the sensor location or type of sensor Loosen or change sensor location
Barrier to light	Nail polish Thick toenails Acrylic nails	Discontinue use temporarily Remove polish Relocate sensor Remove acrylic nails
Extraneous light	Direct sunlight Treatment lights	Cover sensor with a towel
Hemoglobin saturation with other substances	Carbon monoxide poisoning	Discontinue use temporarily

The microprocessor then computes the information and displays it on a monitor at the bedside. The measurement of oxygen saturation when obtained by pulse oximetry is abbreviated and recorded as SpO_2 to distinguish it from the SaO_2 measurement obtained from arterial blood.

Based on the oxygen–hemoglobin dissociation curve (Fig. 21-4), it is possible to infer the PaO_2 from the pulse oximetry measurement. The normal SpO_2 is 95% to 100%. A sustained level of less than 90% is cause for concern. If the SpO_2 remains low, the client needs oxygen therapy. Various factors, however, affect the accuracy of the displayed information (Table 21-2). Troubleshooting the equipment, performing current physical assessments, and obtaining an ABG help to confirm the significance of the displayed findings.

Stop, Think, and Respond Box 21-1

What actions are appropriate if a client appears to be hypoxemic, but the pulse oximeter indicates a normal SpO_2? What action(s) are appropriate if the opposite occurs—that is, the client appears normal but the pulse oximeter reading gives you cause for concern?

PROMOTING OXYGENATION

Many factors affect ventilation and, subsequently, respiration (Table 21-3). Positioning and teaching breathing techniques are two nursing interventions frequently used to promote oxygenation. Adhesive nasal strips can be used to improve oxygenation by reducing nasal airway resistance and improving ventilation.

Positioning

Unless contraindicated by their condition, clients with hypoxia are placed in high **Fowler's position** (an upright seated position; see Chap. 23). This position eases breathing by allowing the abdominal organs to descend away from the diaphragm. As a result, the lungs have the potential to fill with a greater volume of air.

As an alternative, clients who find breathing difficult may benefit from a variation of Fowler's position called the **orthopneic position**. This is a seated position with the arms supported on pillows or the arm rests of a chair, and the client leans forward over the bedside table or a chair back (Fig. 21-5). The orthopneic position allows room for maximum vertical and lateral chest expansion and provides comfort while resting or sleeping.

Breathing Techniques

Breathing techniques such as deep breathing with or without an incentive spirometer, pursed-lip breathing, and diaphragmatic breathing help clients to breathe more efficiently.

Deep Breathing

Deep breathing is a technique for maximizing ventilation. Taking in a large volume of air fills alveoli to a greater capacity, thus improving gas exchange.

Deep breathing is therapeutic for clients who tend to breathe shallowly, such as those who are inactive or in pain. To encourage deep breathing, the client learns to take in as much air as possible, hold the breath briefly, and exhale slowly. In some cases, it is helpful to use an incentive spirometer; however, deep breathing alone, if performed effectively, is sufficiently beneficial.

TABLE 21-3 Factors Affecting Oxygenation

FACT	NURSING IMPLICATION
Adequate respiration depends on a minimum of 21% oxygen in the environment and normal function of the cardiopulmonary system.	Clients with cardiopulmonary disorders require more than 21% oxygen to maintain adequate oxygenation of blood and cells.
Breathing can be voluntarily controlled.	Assist clients who are hyperventilating to slow the rate of breathing; teach clients to perform pursed-lip breathing to exhale more completely.
Clients with chronic lung diseases are stimulated to breathe by low blood levels of oxygen, called "the hypoxic drive to breathe."	Giving high percentages of oxygen can depress breathing in clients with chronic lung disease. No more than 2–3 L oxygen is safe unless the client is mechanically ventilated.
Smoking causes increased amounts of inhaled carbon monoxide that compete and bond more easily than oxygen to the hemoglobin.	Clients who smoke have a greater potential for compromised gas exchange and acquiring chronic pulmonary and cardiac diseases.
Nicotine increases the heart rate and constricts arteries.	Teach people who do not smoke never to start. Identify products that are available, such as nicotine skin patches and gum, which can help smokers.
Pregnant women who smoke have a risk for low-birth-weight infants because low blood oxygenation affects fetal metabolism and growth.	Promote smoking cessation for pregnant women who are addicted to nicotine.
Pulmonary secretions within the airway and fluid within the interstitial space between the alveoli and capillaries interfere with gas exchange.	Encourage coughing, deep breathing, turning, and ambulating to keep alveoli inflated and the airway clear. Antibiotics, diuretics, and drugs that improve heart contraction reduce fluid within the lungs.
Gas exchange is increased by maximum lung expansion and compromised by any condition that compresses the diaphragm, such as obesity, intestinal gas, pregnancy, and an enlarged liver.	Assist clients to sit up to lower abdominal organs away from the diaphragm. Encourage weight loss, expulsion of gas via ambulation and bowel elimination, and assist with removing abdominal fluid by paracentesis (see Chap. 14) to improve breathing.
Activity and emotional stress increase the metabolic need for greater amounts of oxygen.	Provide rest periods and teach stress reduction techniques such as muscle relaxation to promote maintenance of blood oxygen levels.
Pain associated with muscle movement around abdominal and flank surgical incisions decreases the incentive to breathe deeply and cough forcefully.	Teach and supervise deep breathing before surgery. Support the incision with a pillow and administer drugs that relieve pain to facilitate ventilation.

Incentive Spirometry

Incentive spirometry, a technique for deep breathing using a calibrated device, encourages clients to reach a goal-directed volume of inspired air. Although spirometers are constructed in different ways, all are marked in at least 100 mL increments and include some visual cue, such as elevation of lightweight balls, to show how much air the client has inhaled (Fig. 21-6). The calibrated measurement also helps the nurse to evaluate the effectiveness of the client's breathing efforts (see Client and Family Teaching 21-1).

Pursed-Lip Breathing

Pursed-lip breathing is a form of controlled ventilation in which the client consciously prolongs the expiration phase of breathing. This is another technique for improving gas exchange, which, if done correctly, helps clients eliminate more than the usual amount of carbon dioxide from the lungs. Pursed-lip breathing and diaphragmatic breathing are especially helpful for clients who have chronic lung diseases, such as emphysema, which are characterized by chronic hypoxemia and **hypercarbia** (excessive levels of

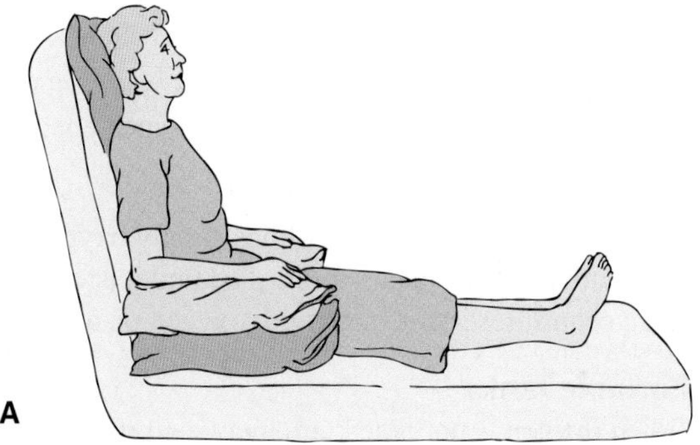

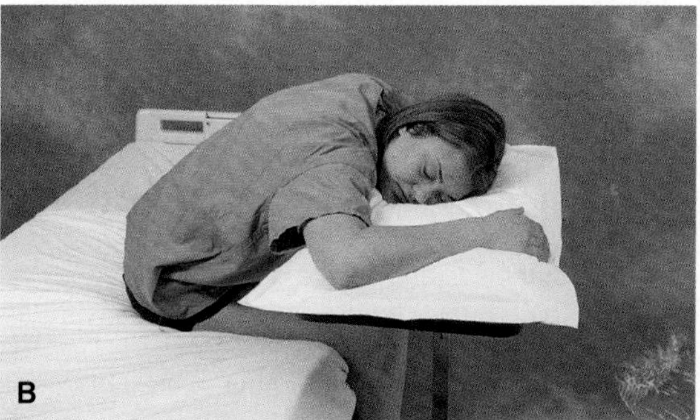

FIGURE 21-5 A. The orthopneic position. **B.** An alternative orthopneic position.

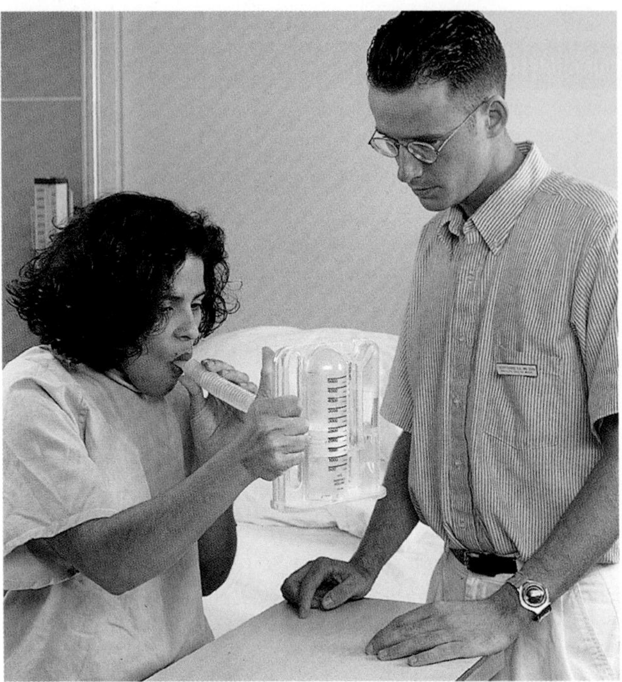

FIGURE 21-6 During deep inhalation, a ball rises in an incentive spirometer. (Courtesy of Swedish Hospital Medical Center.)

carbon dioxide in the blood). The client performs pursed-lip breathing as follows:

- Inhale slowly through the nose while counting to three
- Purse the lips as though to whistle
- Contract the abdominal muscles
- Exhale through pursed lips for a count of six or more

Expiration should be two to three times longer than inspiration. Not all clients can achieve this goal initially, but with practice the length of expiration can increase.

Diaphragmatic Breathing

Diaphragmatic breathing is breathing that promotes the use of the diaphragm rather than the upper chest muscles. It is used to increase the volume of air exchanged during inspiration and expiration. With practice, diaphragmatic breathing reduces respiratory effort and relieves rapid, ineffective breathing (see Client and Family Teaching 21-2).

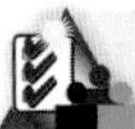

Client and Family Teaching 21-1 Using an Incentive Spirometer

The nurse teaches the client and the family as follows:

- Sit upright unless contraindicated.
- Identify the mark indicating the goal for inhalation.
- Exhale normally.
- Insert the mouthpiece, sealing it between the lips.
- Inhale slowly and deeply until the predetermined volume has been reached.
- Hold the breath for 3–6 seconds.
- Remove the mouthpiece and exhale normally.
- Relax and breathe normally before the next breath with the spirometer.
- Repeat the exercise 10–20 times per hour while awake or as prescribed by the physician.

Client and Family Teaching 21-2 Diaphragmatic Breathing

The nurse teaches the client and the family as follows:

- Lie down with knees slightly bent.
- Place one hand on the abdomen and the other on the chest.
- Inhale slowly and deeply through the nose while letting the abdomen rise more than the chest.
- Purse the lips.
- Contract the abdominal muscles and begin to exhale.
- Press inward and upward with the hand on the abdomen while continuing to exhale.
- Repeat the exercise for 1 full minute; rest for at least 2 minutes.
- Practice the breathing exercises at least twice a day for a period of 5–10 minutes.
- Progress to doing diaphragmatic breathing while upright and active.

Nasal Strips

Adhesive nasal strips, available commercially in drug stores, are used to reduce airflow resistance by widening the breathing passageways of the nose. Increasing the nasal diameter promotes easier breathing. Common users of nasal strips are people with ineffective breathing as well as athletes, whose oxygen requirements increase during sustained exercise. Another use for nasal strips is to reduce or eliminate snoring.

OXYGEN THERAPY

When positioning and breathing techniques are inadequate for keeping the blood adequately saturated with oxygen, oxygen therapy is necessary. **Oxygen therapy** is an intervention for administering more oxygen than is present in the atmosphere to prevent or relieve hypoxemia. It requires an oxygen source, a flowmeter, in some cases an oxygen analyzer or humidifier, and an oxygen delivery device.

Oxygen Sources

Oxygen is supplied from any one of four sources: wall outlet, portable tank, liquid oxygen unit, or oxygen concentrator.

Wall Outlet

Most modern health care facilities supply oxygen through a wall outlet in the client's room. The outlet is connected to a large central reservoir filled with oxygen on a routine basis.

Portable Tanks

When oxygen is not piped into individual rooms or if the client needs to leave the room temporarily, oxygen is provided

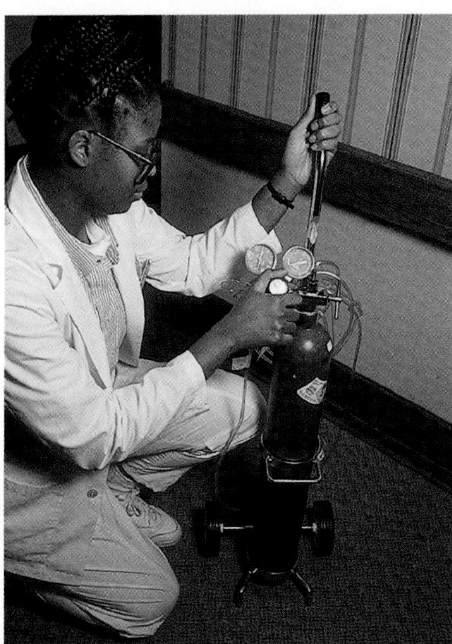

FIGURE 21-7 A portable oxygen tank.

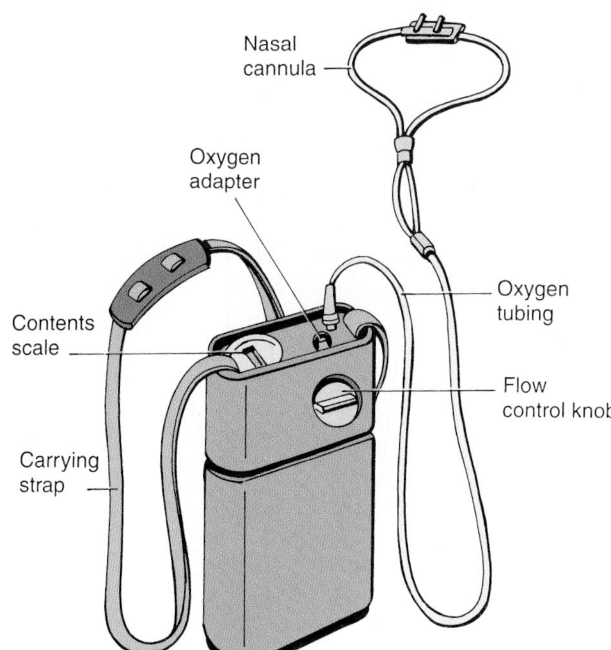

FIGURE 21-8 A liquid oxygen unit.

in portable tanks resembling steel cylinders (Fig. 21-7) that hold various volumes under extreme pressure. A large tank of oxygen contains 2,000 lb of pressure per square inch. Therefore, tanks are delivered with a protective cap to prevent accidental force against the tank outlet. Any accidental force applied to a partially opened outlet could cause the tank to take off like a rocket, with disastrous results. Therefore, oxygen tanks are transported and stored while strapped to a wheeled carrier.

Before oxygen is administered from a portable tank, the tank is "cracked," a technique for clearing the outlet of dust and debris. Cracking is done by turning the tank valve slightly to allow a brief release of pressurized oxygen. The force causes a loud hissing noise, which may be frightening. Therefore, it is best to crack the tank away from the client's bedside.

Liquid Oxygen Unit

A **liquid oxygen unit** is a device that converts cooled liquid oxygen to a gas by passing it through heated coils (Fig. 21-8). Ambulatory clients at home primarily use these small, lightweight, portable units because they allow greater mobility inside and outside the house. Each unit holds approximately 4 to 8 hours' worth of oxygen. Potential problems include that liquid oxygen is more expensive, the unit may leak during warm weather, and frozen moisture may occlude the outlet.

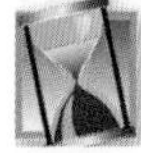

Gerontologic Considerations

- Older adults who require home oxygen need encouragement to continue socializing with others outside the home to prevent feelings of isolation and depression.

Oxygen Concentrator

An **oxygen concentrator** is a machine that collects and concentrates oxygen from room air and stores it for client use. To do so, the concentrator uses a substance called "zeolite" within two absorbing chambers. The machine compresses atmospheric air and diverts it into a chamber containing zeolite. The zeolite absorbs nitrogen from the air, leaving nearly pure oxygen, which is stored in the second chamber. When the nitrogen-absorbing chamber becomes saturated, the machine releases nitrogen back into the atmosphere, and the process repeats itself, providing a constant supply of oxygen (Fig. 21-9).

An oxygen concentrator eliminates the need for a central reservoir of piped oxygen or the use of bulky tanks that must be constantly replaced. This type of oxygen source is used in home health care and long-term care facilities primarily because of its convenience and economy.

Although it is more economical than oxygen supplied in portable tanks, the device increases the client's electric bill. Other disadvantages are that it generates heat from its motor and that it produces an unpleasant odor or taste if the filter is not cleaned weekly. Also, it is best that clients have a secondary source of oxygen available in case of a power failure.

Equipment Used in Oxygen Administration

In addition to an oxygen source, other pieces of equipment used during the administration of oxygen are a flowmeter, oxygen analyzer, and humidifier.

Flowmeter

The flow of oxygen is measured in liters per minute (L/min). A **flowmeter** is a gauge used to regulate the amount of

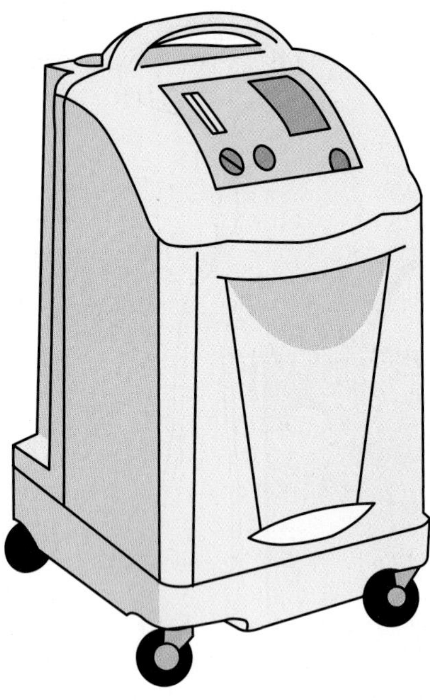

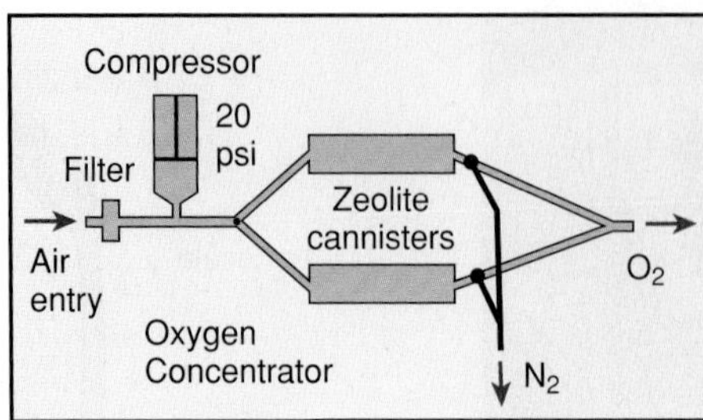

FIGURE 21-9 A portable oxygen concentrator extracts nitrogen and concentrates oxygen to enable clients who require oxygen therapy to travel about or maintain their lifestyle without the need for multiple tanks of oxygen.

oxygen delivered to the client and is attached to the oxygen source (Fig. 21-10). To adjust the rate of flow, the nurse turns the dial until the indicator is directly beside the prescribed amount.

The physician prescribes the concentration of oxygen, also called the **fraction of inspired oxygen** (FIO_2; the portion of oxygen in relation to total inspired gas), as a percentage or as a decimal (eg, 40% or 0.40). The prescription is based on the client's condition. The Joint Commission recommends that oxygen be prescribed as a percentage rather than in liters per minute (L/min) because, depending on the oxygen delivery device, liters per minute may provide different percentages of oxygen.

Oxygen Analyzer

An **oxygen analyzer** is a device that measures the percentage of delivered oxygen to determine whether the client is receiving the amount prescribed by the physician (Fig. 21-11). The nurse or respiratory therapist first checks the percentage of oxygen in the room air with the analyzer. If there is a normal mixture of oxygen and other gases in the environment, the analyzer indicates 0.21 (21%). When the analyzer is positioned near or within the device used to deliver oxygen, the reading should register at the prescribed amount (>0.21). If there is a discrepancy, the nurse adjusts the flowmeter to reach the desired amount. Oxygen analyzers are used most often when caring for newborns in isolettes, children in croup tents, and clients who are mechanically ventilated.

Humidifier

A **humidifier** is a device that produces small water droplets and may be used during oxygen administration because

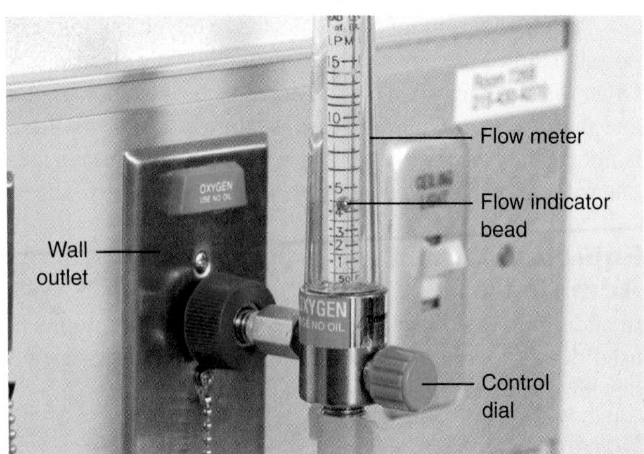

FIGURE 21-10 A flowmeter attached to a wall outlet for oxygen administration.

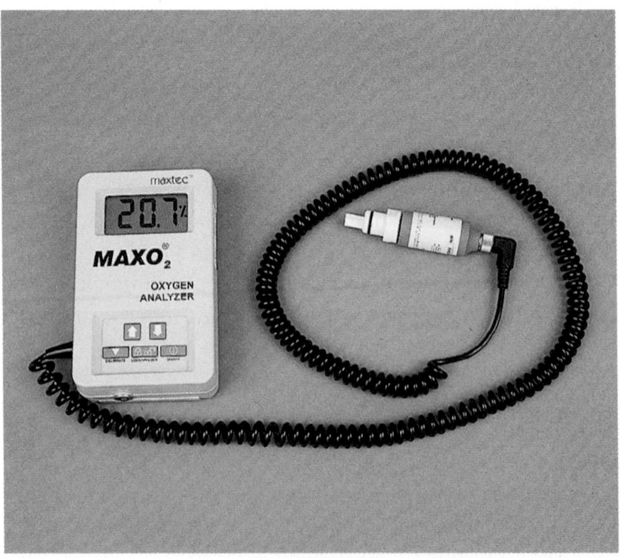

FIGURE 21-11 An oxygen analyzer. (Photo by B. Proud.)

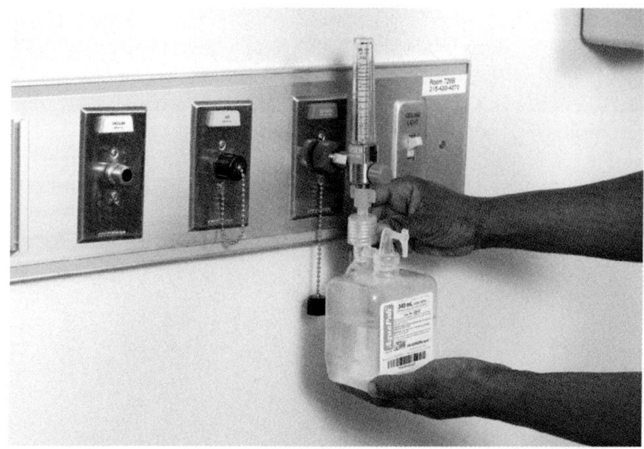

FIGURE 21-12 An oxygen humidifier attached to a flowmeter.

oxygen is drying to the mucous membranes. In most cases, oxygen is humidified only when more than 4 L/min is administered for an extended period. When humidification is desired, a bottle is filled with distilled water and attached to the flowmeter (Fig. 21-12). A respiratory therapist or nurse checks the water level daily and refills the bottle as needed.

Stop, Think, and Respond Box 21-2

Explain the difference between a flowmeter and an oxygen analyzer.

Common Delivery Devices

Common oxygen delivery devices include a nasal cannula, masks, a face tent, a tracheostomy collar, or a T-piece (Table 21-4). The device prescribed depends on the client's oxygenation status, physical condition, and amount of oxygen needed. Skill 21-2 describes how to administer oxygen by common delivery methods.

Nasal Cannula

A **nasal cannula** is a hollow tube with 1/2-in. prongs placed into the client's nostrils. It is held in place by wrapping the tubing around the ears and adjusting the fit beneath the chin. It provides a means of administering low concentrations of oxygen. Therefore, it is ideal for clients who are not extremely hypoxic or who have chronic lung diseases. High percentages of oxygen are contraindicated for clients with chronic lung disease because they have adapted to excessive levels of retained carbon dioxide and low blood oxygen levels stimulate their drive to breathe. Consequently, if clients with chronic lung disease receive more than 2 to 3 L of oxygen over a sustained period, their respiratory rate slows or even stops.

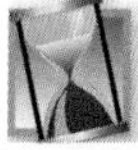

Gerontologic Considerations

- The skin behind the ears of older adults as well as others should be assessed for breakdown if oxygen administration equipment is secured by tubing or elastic.

Masks

Oxygen can be delivered using a simple mask, a partial rebreather mask, a nonrebreather mask, or a Venturi mask.

Simple Mask

A **simple mask** fits over the nose and mouth and allows atmospheric air to enter and exit through side ports. An elastic strap holds it in place. The simple mask, like other types of masks, allows for the administration of higher levels of oxygen than are possible with a cannula. A simple mask is sometimes substituted for a cannula when a client has nasal trauma or breathes through the mouth. When a simple mask is used, oxygen is delivered at no less than 5 L/min.

The efficiency of any mask is affected by how well it fits the face. Without a good seal, the oxygen leaks from the mask, thus diminishing its concentration. Other problems are associated with masks as well. All oxygen masks interfere with eating and make verbal communication difficult to understand. Also, some clients become anxious when their nose and mouth are covered because it creates a feeling of being suffocated. Skin care also becomes a priority because masks create pressure and trap moisture.

Partial Rebreather Mask

A **partial rebreather mask** is an oxygen delivery device through which a client inhales a mixture of atmospheric air, oxygen from its source, and oxygen contained within a reservoir bag. It provides a means for recycling oxygen and venting all the carbon dioxide during expiration from the mask. During expiration, the first third of exhaled air enters the reservoir bag. The portion of exhaled air in the reservoir bag contains a high proportion of oxygen because it comes directly from the upper airways; the gas in this area has not been involved in gas exchange at the alveolar level. Once the reservoir bag is filled, the remainder of exhaled air is forced from the mask through small ports. With a simple mask, some carbon dioxide always remains within the mask and is reinhaled.

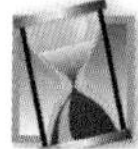

Gerontologic Considerations

- Older adults who have lost weight and subcutaneous fat in their cheeks or who are not wearing their dentures may not receive the prescribed amounts of oxygen by mask because of an inadequate facial seal.

Non-rebreather Mask

A **nonrebreather mask** is an oxygen delivery device in which all the exhaled air leaves the mask rather than partially entering the reservoir bag. It is designed to deliver an FIO_2 of 90% to 100%. This type of mask contains one-way valves that allow only oxygen from its source, as well as the oxygen in the reservoir bag, to be inhaled. No air from the atmosphere is inhaled. All the air that is exhaled is vented from the mask. None enters the reservoir bag. Obviously, clients for whom nonrebreather masks are used are those who require high concentrations of

(continued on page 451)

TABLE 21-4 Comparison of Oxygen Delivery Devices

DEVICE	COMMON RANGE OF ADMINISTRATION	ADVANTAGES	DISADVANTAGES
Nasal cannula	2–6 L/min FIO_2 24%–40%[a]	Is easy to apply; promotes comfort Does not interfere with eating or talking Is less likely to create a feeling of suffocation	Dries nasal mucosa at higher flows May irritate the skin at cheeks and behind ears Is less effective in some patients who tend to mouth breathe Does not facilitate administering high FIO_2 to hypoxic clients
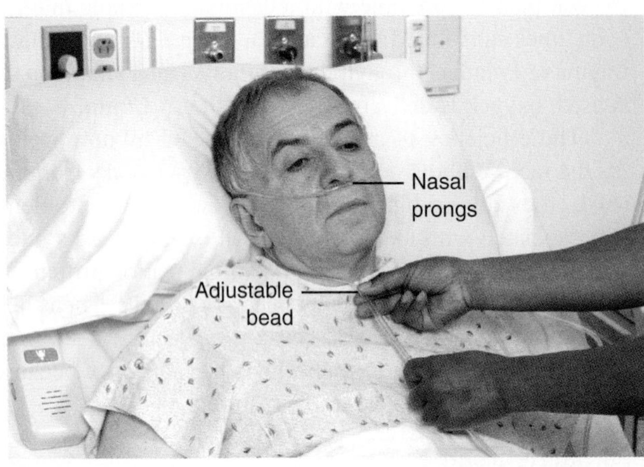 			
Masks			
Simple	5–8 L/min FIO_2 35%–50%[a]	Provides higher concentrations than possible with a cannula Is effective for mouth breathers or clients with nasal disorders	Requires humidification Interferes with eating and talking Can cause anxiety among those who are claustrophobic Creates a risk for rebreathing CO_2 retained within mask
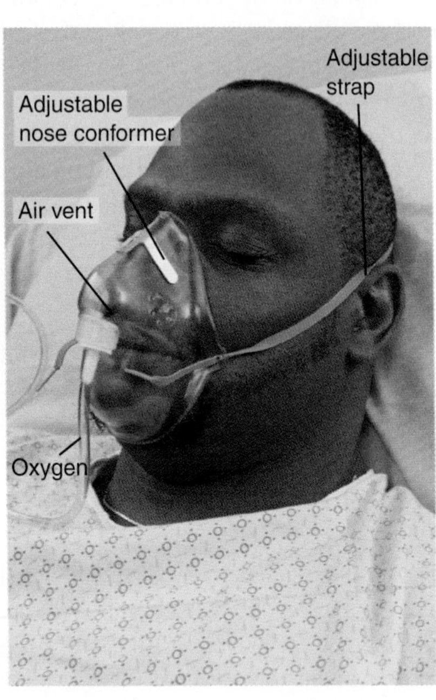 			

DEVICE	COMMON RANGE OF ADMINISTRATION	ADVANTAGES	DISADVANTAGES
Partial rebreather 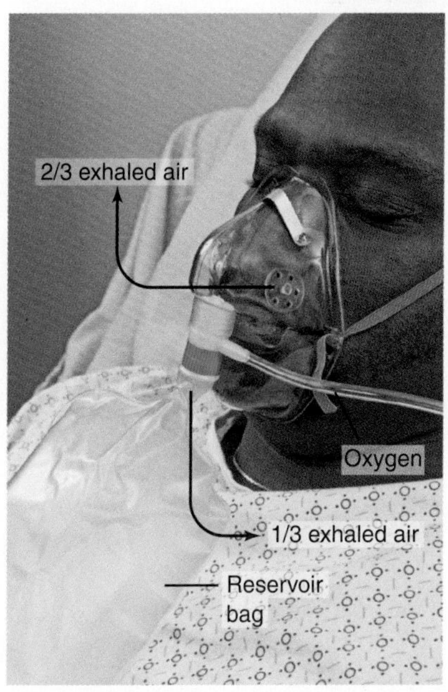 	6–10 L/min FIO_2 35%–60%[a]	Increases the amount of oxygen with lower liter flows	Requires a minimum of 6 L/min Creates a risk for suffocation Requires monitoring to verify that reservoir bag remains inflated at all times
Nonrebreather 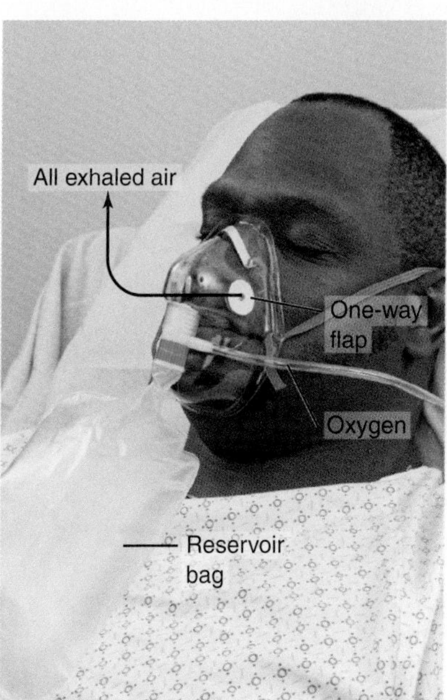 	6–10 L/min FIO_2 60%–90%[a]	Delivers highest FIO_2 possible with a mask 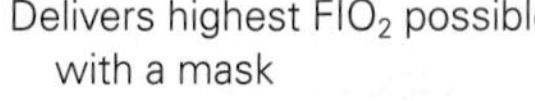	See partial rebreather mask Creates a risk for oxygen toxicity

(Table continues on page 450)

TABLE 21-4 Comparison of Oxygen Delivery Devices (continued)

DEVICE	COMMON RANGE OF ADMINISTRATION	ADVANTAGES	DISADVANTAGES
Venturi 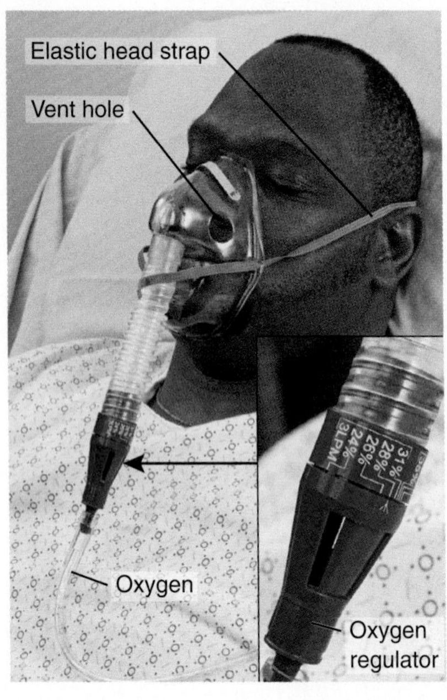 	4–8 L/min FIO_2 24%–40%[a]	Delivers FIO_2 precisely	Permits condensation to form in tubing, which diminishes the flow of oxygen
Face tent 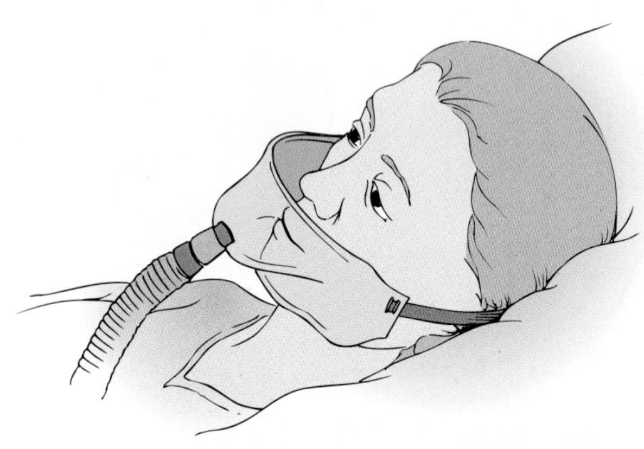	8–12 L/min FIO_2 30%–55%[a]	Provides a comfortable fit Is useful for clients with facial trauma and burns Facilitates humidification	Interferes with eating May result in inconsistent FIO_2, depending on environmental loss

DEVICE	COMMON RANGE OF ADMINISTRATION	ADVANTAGES	DISADVANTAGES
Tracheostomy collar	4–10 L/min FIO_2 24%–100%[a]	Facilitates humidifying and warming oxygen	Allows water vapor to collect in tubing, which may drain into airway
T-piece	4–10 L/min FIO_2 24%–100%[a]	Delivers any desired FIO_2 with high humidity	May pull on tracheostomy tube Allows humidity to collect and moisten gauze dressing

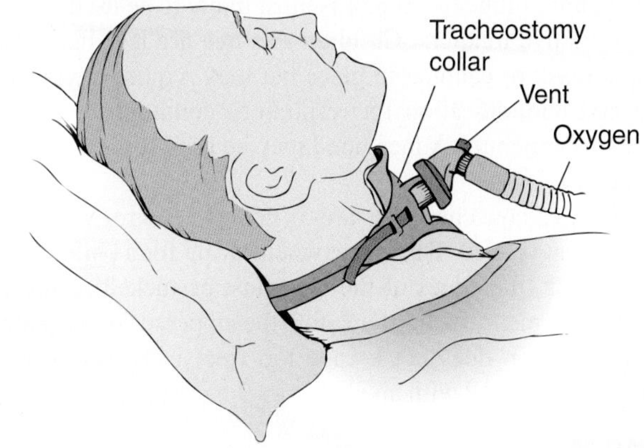

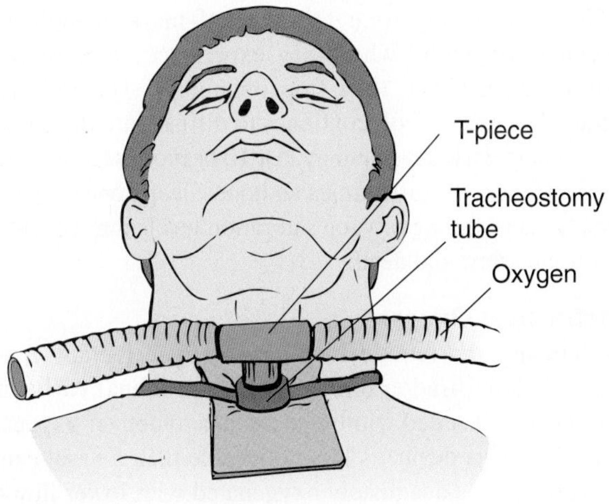

[a]Source: American Association for Respiratory Care (AARC).

oxygen. They are usually critically ill and may eventually need mechanical ventilation.

Humidification is not used when a mask with a reservoir bag is used, despite the high concentrations of oxygen. Also, clients with partial and nonrebreather masks are monitored closely to ensure that the reservoir bag remains partially inflated at all times.

Venturi Mask

A **Venturi mask** mixes a precise amount of oxygen and atmospheric air. Sometimes called a Venti mask, this mask has a large ringed tube extending from it. Adapters within the tube, which are color-coded or regulated by a dial system, permit only specific amounts of room air to mix with the oxygen. This feature ensures that the Venturi mask delivers the exact amount of prescribed oxygen. Unlike masks with reservoir bags, humidification can be added when a Venturi mask is used.

Face Tent

A **face tent** provides oxygen to the nose and mouth without the discomfort of a mask. Because the face tent is open and loose around the face, clients are less likely to feel claustrophobic. An added advantage is that a face mask can be used for clients with facial trauma or burns. A disadvantage is that the amount of oxygen clients actually receive may be inconsistent with what is prescribed because of environmental losses.

Tracheostomy Collar

A **tracheostomy collar** delivers oxygen near an artificial opening in the neck. It is applied over a tracheostomy–an opening into the trachea through which a client breathes (see Chap. 36). Because it bypasses the warming and moisturizing functions of the nose, a tracheostomy collar provides a means for both oxygenation and humidification. The moisture that collects, however, tends to saturate the gauze dressing around the tracheostomy, making it necessary to change it frequently.

T-Piece

A **T-piece** fits securely onto a tracheostomy tube or endotracheal tube. It is similar to a tracheostomy collar but is attached directly to the artificial airway. Although the gauze around the tracheostomy usually remains dry, the moisture that collects within the tubing tends to condense and may enter the airway during position changes if it is not drained periodically. Another disadvantage is that the weight of the T-piece, or its manipulation, may pull on the tracheostomy tube, causing the client to cough or experience discomfort.

Additional Delivery Devices

Other methods for delivering oxygen are used less commonly. Occasionally, oxygen is delivered by means of a nasal catheter, oxygen tent, transtracheal catheter, or continuous positive airway pressure (CPAP) mask.

Nasal Catheter

A **nasal catheter** is a tube for delivering oxygen that is inserted through the nose into the posterior nasal pharynx (Fig. 21-13). It is used for clients who tend to breathe through the mouth or experience claustrophobia when a mask covers their face. The catheter tends to irritate the nasopharynx; therefore, some clients find it uncomfortable. If a catheter is prescribed, the nurse secures it to the nose to avoid displacement and regularly cleans the nostril with a cotton applicator to remove dried mucus.

Oxygen Tent

An **oxygen tent** is a clear plastic enclosure that provides cooled, humidified oxygen. It is most likely to be used in the care of active toddlers. Children this age are less likely to keep a mask or cannula in place but may require oxygenation and humidification for respiratory conditions such as croup or bronchitis. A face hood may be used for less-active infants.

Oxygen concentrations are difficult to control when an oxygen tent is used. Therefore, when caring for a child in an oxygen tent, the edges of the tent must be tucked securely beneath the mattress; limit opening the zippered access ports so that oxygen does not escape too freely. Oxygen levels must be monitored with an analyzer.

CPAP Mask

A **CPAP mask** maintains positive pressure within the airway throughout the respiratory cycle (Fig. 21-14). It keeps the alveoli partially inflated even during expiration. The face mask is attached to a portable ventilator.

Clients generally wear this type of mask at night to maintain oxygenation when they experience sleep **apnea** (periods during which they stop breathing). The residual oxygen within the alveoli continues to diffuse into the blood during apneic episodes that may last 10 or more seconds and be as frequent as 10 to 15 times an hour. Sleep apnea is dangerous because falling oxygen saturation levels may precipitate cardiac arrest and death.

Transtracheal Oxygen

Some clients who require long-term oxygen therapy may prefer its administration through a **transtracheal catheter** (a hollow tube inserted within the trachea to deliver oxygen; Fig. 21-15). This device is less noticeable than a nasal cannula. The client is adequately oxygenated with lower flows, decreasing the costs of replenishing the oxygen source.

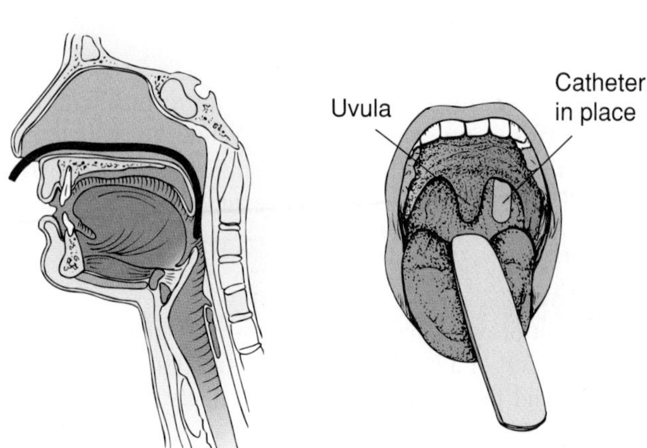

FIGURE 21-13 Nasal catheter placement.

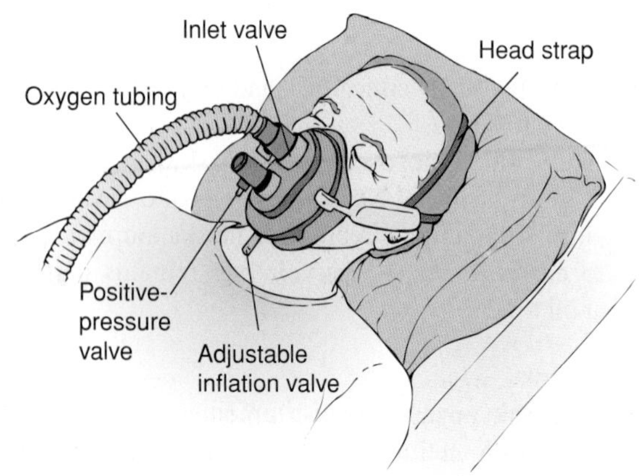

FIGURE 21-14 A CPAP mask.

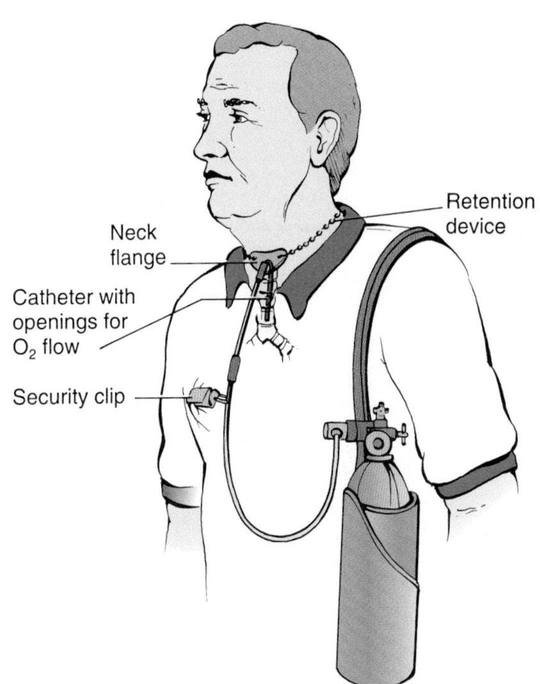

FIGURE 21-15 Transtracheal oxygen administration.

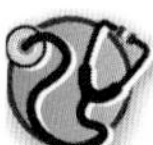

NURSING GUIDELINES 21-2

Administering Oxygen Safely

- Post "Oxygen in Use" signs wherever oxygen is stored or in use. *The sign warns others of a potential fire hazard.*
- Prohibit the burning of candles during religious rites. *Doing so eliminates a source of open flames.*
- Check that electrical devices have a three-pronged plug (see Chap. 19). *This type of plug provides a ground for leaking electricity.*
- Inspect electrical equipment for frayed wires or loose connections. *Inspection helps to prevent sparks or an uncontrolled pathway for electricity.*
- Avoid using petroleum products, aerosol products (such as hair spray), and products containing acetone (such as nail polish remover) where oxygen is used. *This measure prevents ignition of flammable substances.*
- Secure portable oxygen cylinders to rigid stands. *Doing so prevents the tank from rupturing.*

Before transtracheal oxygen is used, a **stent** (tube that keeps a channel open) is inserted into a surgically created opening and remains there until the wound heals. Thereafter, the stent is removed, and the catheter is inserted and held in place with a necklace-type chain. Clients learn how to clean the tracheal opening and catheter, a procedure performed several times a day. During cleaning, clients administer oxygen with a nasal cannula.

Stop, Think, and Respond Box 21-3

What evidence indicates that a client is well oxygenated?

Oxygen Hazards

Regardless of which device is used, oxygen administration involves potential hazards: first and foremost, oxygen's capacity to support fires, and second, the potential for oxygen toxicity.

Fire Potential

Oxygen itself does not burn, but it does support combustion; in other words, it contributes to the burning process. Therefore, it is necessary to control all possible sources of open flames or ungrounded electricity (see Nursing Guidelines 21-2).

Oxygen Toxicity

Oxygen toxicity means lung damage that develops when oxygen concentrations of more than 50% are administered for longer than 48 to 72 hours. The exact mechanism by which hyperoxygenation damages the lungs is not definitely known. One theory is that it reduces **surfactant**, which is a lipoprotein produced by cells in the alveoli that promotes elasticity of the lungs and enhances gas diffusion.

Once oxygen toxicity develops, it is difficult to reverse. Unfortunately, early symptoms are quite subtle (Box 21-2). The best prevention is to administer the lowest FIO_2 possible for the shortest amount of time.

RELATED OXYGENATION TECHNIQUES

Two additional techniques relate to oxygenation: a water-seal chest tube drainage system and hyperbaric oxygen therapy (HBOT).

Water-Seal Chest Tube Drainage

Water-seal chest tube drainage is a technique for evacuating air or blood from the pleural cavity, which helps to restore negative intrapleural pressure and reinflate the lung. Clients who require water-seal drainage have one or two chest tubes connected to the drainage system.

BOX 21-2 Signs and Symptoms of Oxygen Toxicity

- Nonproductive cough
- Substernal chest pain
- Nasal stuffiness
- Nausea and vomiting
- Fatigue
- Headache
- Sore throat
- Hypoventilation

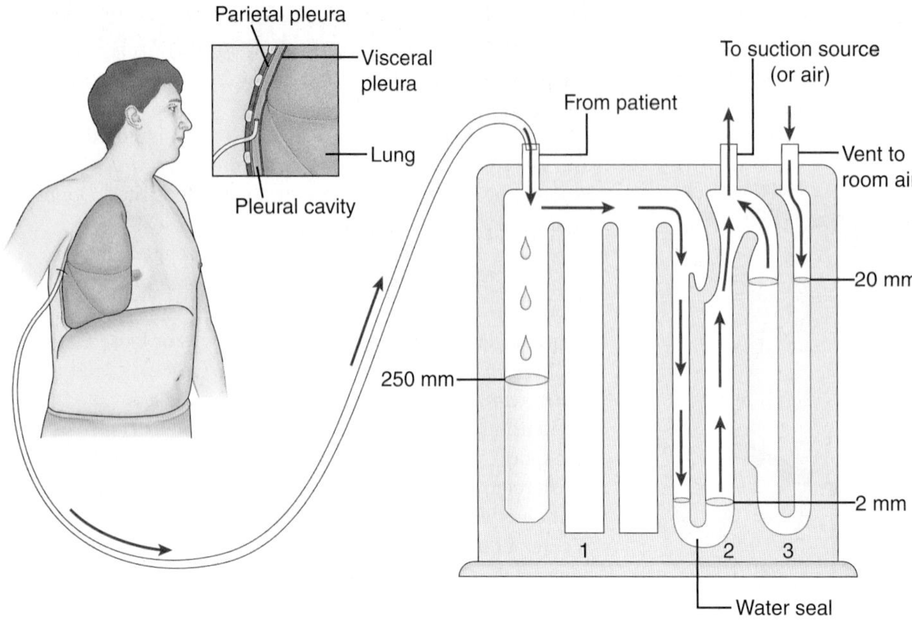

FIGURE 21-16 The three-chambered water-seal drainage system: (1) drainage collection chamber from the client, (2) the water-seal chamber, and (3) the suction control chamber attached to a source of suction and vented to room air.

Several companies provide equipment for water-seal drainage. All of these products consist of a three-chamber system (Fig. 21-16):

- One chamber collects blood or acts as an exit route for pleural air.
- A second compartment holds water that prevents atmospheric air from reentering the pleural space (hence the term "water seal").
- A third chamber, if used, facilitates the use of suction, which may speed the evacuation of blood or air.

One of the most important principles when caring for clients with water-seal drainage is that the chest tube must never be separated from the drainage system unless it is clamped. Even then, the tube is clamped for only a brief time. Additional nursing responsibilities are included in Skill 21-3.

Stop, Think, and Respond Box 21-4

Discuss how a collapsed lung affects oxygenation.

Hyperbaric Oxygen Therapy

Hyperbaric oxygen therapy (HBOT) consists of the delivery of 100% oxygen at three times the normal atmospheric pressure within an airtight chamber (Fig. 21-17). Treatments, which last approximately 90 minutes, are repeated over days, weeks, or months of therapy. Providing pressurized oxygen can deliver 15 times as much oxygen to tissues as can be obtained by breathing room air (Mayo Clinic, 2009). Providing clients with brief periods of breathing room air helps to prevent oxygen toxicity.

HBOT helps to regenerate new tissue at a faster rate; thus, its most popular use is for promoting wound healing. It also is used to treat carbon monoxide poisoning, gangrene associated with diabetes or other conditions of vascular insufficiency, decompression sickness experienced by deep-sea divers, anaerobic infections (especially in burn clients), and several other medical conditions.

NURSING IMPLICATIONS

Nurses assess the oxygenation status of clients on a day-by-day and a shift-by-shift basis. Therefore, it is not unusual to identify any one or several of the following nursing diagnoses among clients experiencing hypoxemia or hypoxia:

- Ineffective Breathing Pattern
- Impaired Gas Exchange
- Anxiety
- Risk for Injury (Related to Oxygen Hazards)

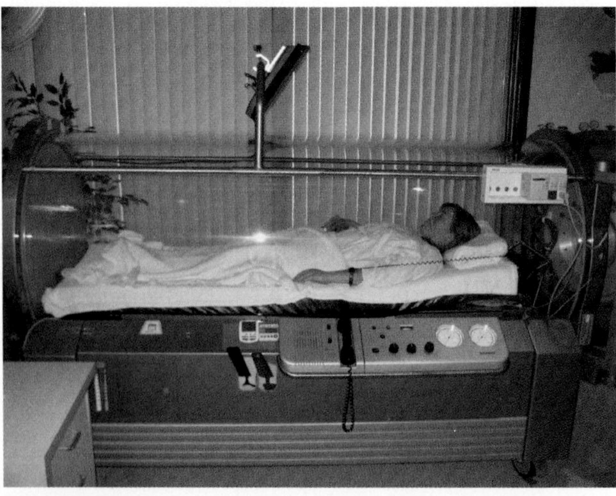

FIGURE 21-17 A hyperbaric oxygen chamber. (Photo courtesy of Moose Jaw Union Hospital, Saskatchewan, Canada.)

Abnormal assessment findings often lead to collaboration with the physician and the prescription for oxygen therapy. Nursing Care Plan 21-1 is one example of how the nursing process applies to a client with the nursing diagnosis of Ineffective Breathing Pattern. This diagnostic category is defined in the NANDA-I taxonomy (2012, p. 233) as "inspiration and/or expiration that does not provide adequate ventilation."

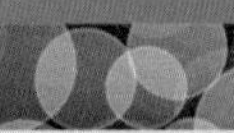

NURSING CARE PLAN 21-1 Ineffective Breathing Pattern

Assessment

- Determine the client's respiratory rate and effort.
- Check the radial or apical pulse rate.
- Measure the client's blood pressure.
- Note the client's level of consciousness and mental status.
- Assess for the evidence of a cough and its characteristics.
- Observe the use of accessory thoracic and abdominal muscles for breathing.
- Observe the client's chest contour.
- Inspect the skin, oral mucous membranes, and nail beds for signs of cyanosis.
- Palpate the client's abdomen for evidence of distention that could crowd the diaphragm.
- Note the client's body position, which may or may not facilitate breathing.
- Measure the client's SpO_2 with a pulse oximeter.
- Review the results of arterial blood gas measurements.
- Auscultate anterior, posterior, and lateral lung sounds.
- Ask the client to describe his or her current status of oxygenation.
- Perform a pain assessment.
- Inquire as to the client's medical history of respiratory disorders or other conditions that can affect ventilation.
- Identify the client's smoking history.
- Review the client's current medication history for drugs that can impair oxygenation.

Nursing Diagnosis. **Ineffective Breathing Pattern** related to the retention of carbon dioxide secondary to chronic pulmonary damage from long-term cigarette smoking as manifested by rapid, shallow breathing at 40 breaths per minute accompanied by the use of accessory muscles to breathe; frequent productive cough; history of smoking one to two packs of cigarettes daily for 30 years; barrel chest; diminished lung sounds bilaterally; and client's statements, "It seems so hard for me to get my breath. I can't work in my flower garden because I get winded when I try to do any gardening. I can't sleep lying down because I can't breathe except sleeping in a chair."

Expected Outcome. The client will demonstrate an effective breathing pattern by 5/10 as evidenced by a respiratory rate no greater than 32 while performing mild activity such as bathing face, arms, and chest.

Interventions	Rationales
Provide periods of rest between activities.	Rest decreases oxygen demand and facilitates maintenance or restoration of oxygen within blood.
Elevate the head of the bed up to 90 degrees.	Head elevation lowers abdominal organs by gravity and provides an increased area for chest expansion when the diaphragm contracts.
Teach how to perform diaphragmatic and pursed-lip breathing and practice same at least b.i.d.	Pursed-lip breathing decreases respiratory rate, increases tidal volume, decreases arterial CO_2, increases arterial oxygen, and improves exercise performance.
Provide a minimum of 2,000 mL of oral fluid per 24 hr.	Adequate hydration liquefies respiratory secretions and facilitates expectoration. Expectoration of sputum clears the airway and promotes ventilation.
Ensure a daily dietary intake of approximately 2,000–2,500 cal.	The act of breathing creates additional caloric demands for energy.
Administer oxygen per nasal cannula at 2 L/min as prescribed by the physician if SpO_2 falls below 90% and is sustained there.	Supplemental oxygen relieves hypoxemia. Administering 2–3 L/min prevents suppressing the hypoxic drive to breathe, experienced by clients with chronic respiratory diseases.
Explore nicotine cessation therapy with transdermal skin patches.	Transdermal nicotine skin patches reduce symptoms associated with nicotine withdrawal. The dose of nicotine can be reduced gradually to promote nicotine cessation.

Evaluation of Expected Outcomes

- Respiratory rate decreases from 34 to 26 when placed in high Fowler's position.
- SpO_2 increases from 86% to 90% with 2 L of oxygen per minute.
- The client demonstrates and performs pursed-lip breathing.
- The client consumes three cans of supplemental liquid nourishment, each of which has 350 cal, three times a day, to facilitate reaching a minimum caloric goal of 2,000 cal.
- Fluid intake for 24 hours is between 1,800 and 2,200 mL.
- Client expectorates copious volume of sputum.

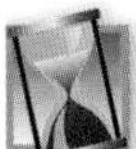

Gerontologic Considerations

■ Advise older adults to receive annual influenza immunizations and a pneumonia immunization after 65 years of age or earlier if there is a history of chronic illness. Current guidelines recommend a booster dose for older adults who received their initial pneumonia immunization 5 or more years ago.

CRITICAL THINKING EXERCISES

1. What levels of oxygen saturation and pulse rates are a cause for nursing concern and indicate a need for further assessment?

2. Discuss some differences between oxygen therapy in a health care setting and that in a home environment.

3. What health teaching would you provide to reduce potential problems with oxygenation?

4. What nursing actions may be appropriate if the alarm on a pulse oximeter sounds frequently because the sensor does not stay on a client's finger?

NCLEX-STYLE REVIEW QUESTIONS

1. When a client returns from surgery, which sign is an early indication that the client's oxygenation status is compromised?

1. The client's dressing is bloody.
2. The client becomes restless.
3. The client's heart rate is irregular.
4. The client reports being thirsty.

2. If a client is adequately oxygenated, in what range should a pulse oximeter identify as the SpO_2 measurement?

1. 80 to 100 mmHg
2. 95 to 100 mmHg
3. 80% to 100%
4. 95% to 100%

3. When administering oxygen with a partial rebreather mask, which of the following observations is most important to report to the respiratory therapy department?

1. Moisture accumulates inside the mask.
2. The reservoir bag collapses during inspiration.
3. The mask covers the mouth and nose.
4. The strap around the head is snug.

4. Which of the following oxygen flow rates is most appropriate for a client with emphysema, a chronic lung disease?

1. 2 L/min
2. 5 L/min
3. 8 L/min
4. 10 L/min

5. When the nurse monitors the water-seal chamber of a commercial chest tube drainage system that is draining by gravity, which finding suggests that the system is functioning appropriately?

1. The fluid rises and falls with respirations.
2. The fluid level is lower than when first filled.
3. The fluid bubbles continuously.
4. The fluid looks frothy white.

SKILL 21-1 Using a Pulse Oximeter

Suggested Action	Reason for Action
ASSESSMENT	
Assess potential sensor sites for quality of circulation, edema, tremor, restlessness, nail polish, or artificial nails (Fig. A) 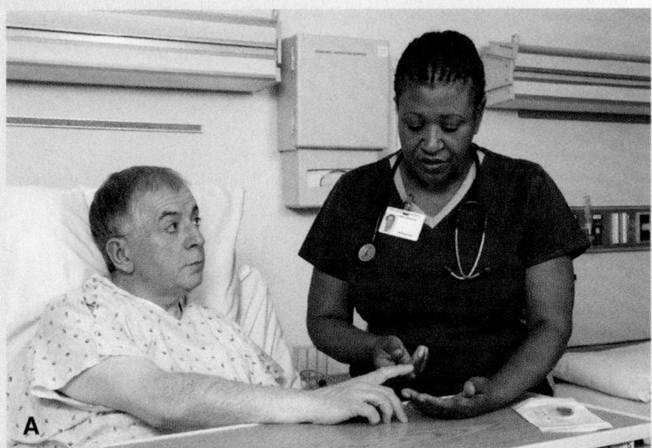	Determines where sensor is best applied. The finger is the preferred site, followed by the toe, earlobe, and bridge of the nose. Aids in controlling possible factors that might invalidate monitored findings. Assessing a sensor site.
Review the medical history for data indicating vascular or other pathology, such as anemia or carbon monoxide inhalation.	Suggests the potential for unreliable data. There must be adequate circulation, red blood cells, and oxygenated hemoglobin for reliable results.
Check prescribed medications for vasoconstrictive effects.	Impaired blood flow interferes with the accuracy of pulse oximetry.
Determine how much the client understands about pulse oximetry.	Indicates the need for and type of teaching; the best learning takes place when it is individualized.
PLANNING	
Explain the procedure to the client.	Reduces anxiety and promotes cooperation and a sense of security for coping with unfamiliar situations.
Obtain equipment.	Promotes organization and efficient time management, preventing wasted motion and repeating actions.
IMPLEMENTATION	
Wash hands or perform hand antisepsis with an alcohol rub (see Chap. 10).	Reduces the transmission of microorganisms.
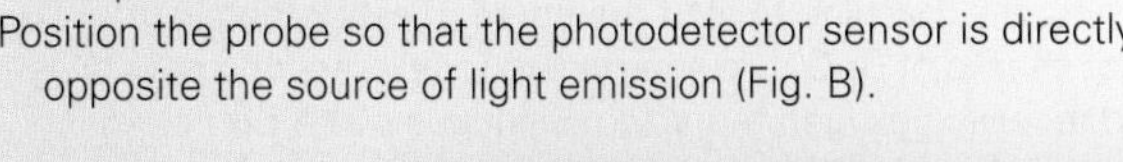 Position the probe so that the photodetector sensor is directly opposite the source of light emission (Fig. B). 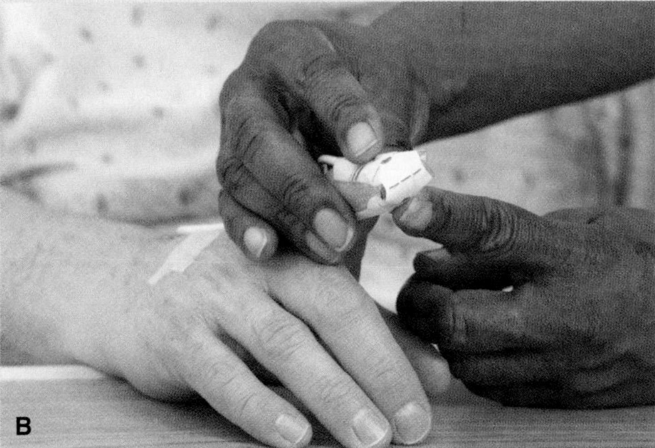	Ensures accurate monitoring; proper light and sensor alignment ensure accurate measurement of red and infrared light absorption by hemoglobin. Positioning the sensor.

(continued)

Using a Pulse Oximeter (continued)

IMPLEMENTATION (CONTINUED)

Attach the sensor cable to the machine (Fig. C).

Connects the sensor with the microprocessor to ensure proper function.

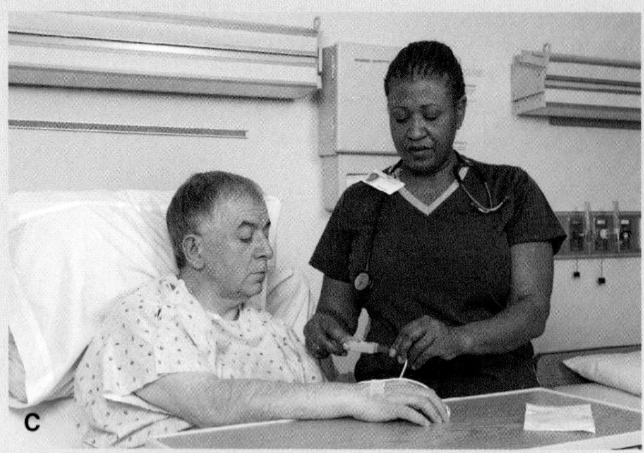

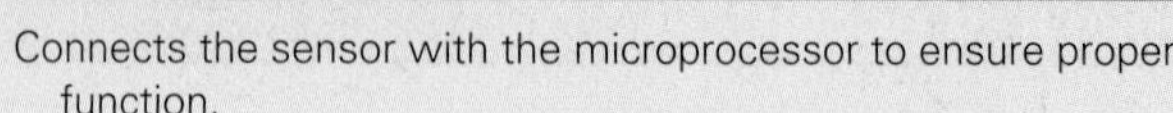

Connecting the sensing equipment.

Observe the numeric display, audible sound, and waveform on the machine (Fig. D).

Indicates that the equipment is functioning.

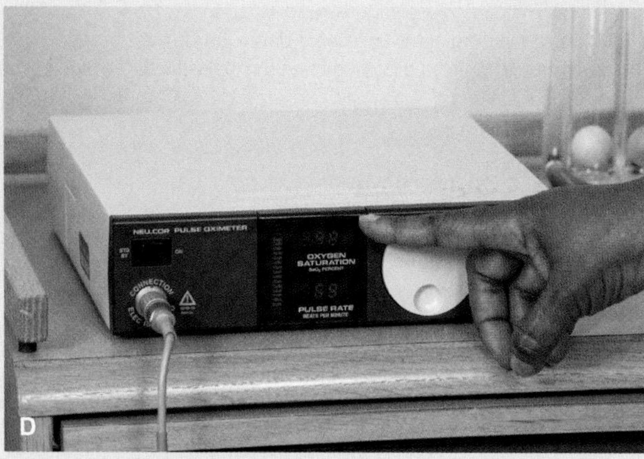

Checking the displayed data.

Set the alarms for saturation level and pulse rate according to the manufacturer's directions.

Programs the machine to alert the nurse to check the client. Spot checks of SpO_2 are appropriate for clients who are stable and receiving oxygen therapy; continuous pulse oximetry is recommended for clients who are unstable and may abruptly experience desaturation.

Move an adhesive finger sensor if the finger becomes pale, swollen, or cold; remove and reapply a spring-tension sensor every 2 hours.

Prevents vascular impairment and skin breakdown because pressure greater than 32 mm Hg leads to tissue hypoxia and cellular necrosis.

Evaluation

- SpO_2 measurements remain within 95%–100%.
- Client exhibits no evidence of hypoxemia or hypoxia.
- SpO_2 measurements correlate with SaO_2 measurements.

Document

- Normal SpO_2 measurements once a shift unless ordered otherwise
- Abnormal SpO_2 measurements when they are sustained
- Nursing measures to improve oxygenation if SpO_2 levels fall below 90% and are prolonged
- Person to whom abnormal measurements have been reported and outcome of communication
- Removal and relocation of sensor
- Condition of skin at sensor site

(continued)

Using a Pulse Oximeter (continued)

SAMPLE DOCUMENTATION

Date and Time SpO_2 remains constant at 95% to 98% with pulse rate that ranges between 80 and 92 bpm while receiving oxygen by nasal cannula at 4 L/min. Respirations unlabored. Skin under sensor is intact and warm. Nailbed beneath sensor is pink with capillary refill <2 seconds. Spring-tension sensor changed from L. index finger to R. index finger. ——— SIGNATURE/TITLE

SKILL 21-2 Administering Oxygen

Suggested Action	Reason for Action
ASSESSMENT	
Perform physical assessment techniques that focus on oxygenation.	Provides a baseline for future comparisons.
Monitor the SpO_2 level with a pulse oximeter.	Provides a baseline for future comparisons.
Check the medical order for the type of oxygen delivery device, liter flow or prescribed percentage, and whether the oxygen is to be administered continuously or only as needed.	Ensures compliance with the plan for medical treatment, because oxygen therapy is medically prescribed (except in emergencies).
Note whether a wall outlet is available or if another type of oxygen source must be obtained.	Promotes organization and efficient time management.
Determine how much the client understands about oxygen therapy.	Indicates the need for and the type of teaching that must be done.
PLANNING	
Obtain equipment, which usually includes a flowmeter, delivery device, and in some cases, a humidifier.	Promotes organization and efficient time management.
Contact the respiratory therapy department for equipment, if that is agency policy.	Follows interdepartmental guidelines; ensures nursing collaboration with various paraprofessionals to provide client care.
"Crack" the portable oxygen tank if that is the type of oxygen source being used.	Prevents alarming the client.
Explain the procedure to the client.	Decreases anxiety and promotes cooperation.
Eliminate safety hazards that may support a fire or explosion.	Demonstrates concern for safety because open flames, electrical sparks, smoking, and petroleum products are contraindicated when oxygen is in use.
IMPLEMENTATION	
Wash hands or perform hand antisepsis with an alcohol rub (see Chap. 10).	Reduces the transmission of microorganisms.
Assist the client to a Fowler's or alternate position.	Promotes optimal ventilation.
Attach the flowmeter to the oxygen source (Fig. A).	Provides a means for regulating the prescribed amount of oxygen.

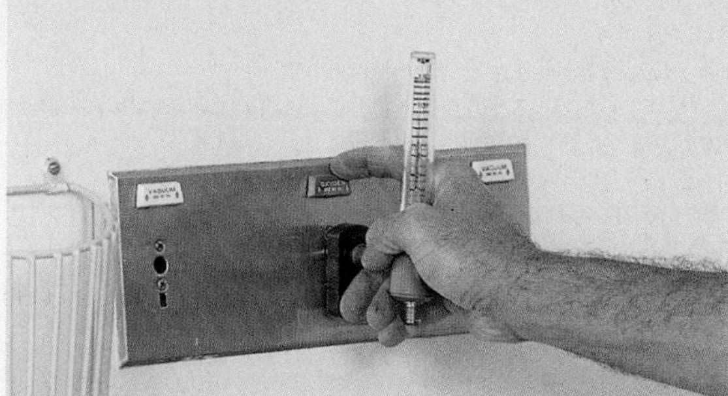

Attaching the flowmeter. (Photo by B. Proud.)

(continued)

Administering Oxygen (continued)

IMPLEMENTATION (CONTINUED)

Fill a humidifier bottle with distilled water to the appropriate level if administering 4 L/min or more.
Provides moisture because oxygen dries mucous membranes. The potential increases with the percentage being administered.

Connect the humidifier bottle to the flowmeter (Fig. B).
Provides a pathway through which moisture is added to the oxygen.

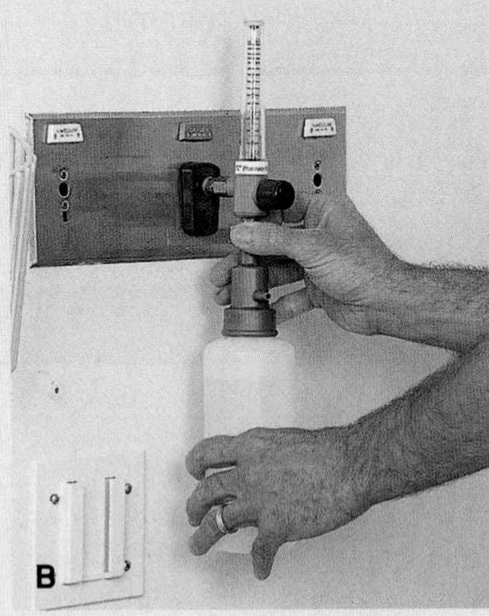

Connecting the humidification bottle. (Photo by B. Proud.)

Insert the appropriate color-coded valve or dial the prescribed percentage if a Venturi mask is being used.
Regulates the FIO_2.

Attach the distal end of the tubing from the oxygen delivery device to the flowmeter or humidifier bottle (Fig. C).
Provides a pathway for oxygen from its source to the client.

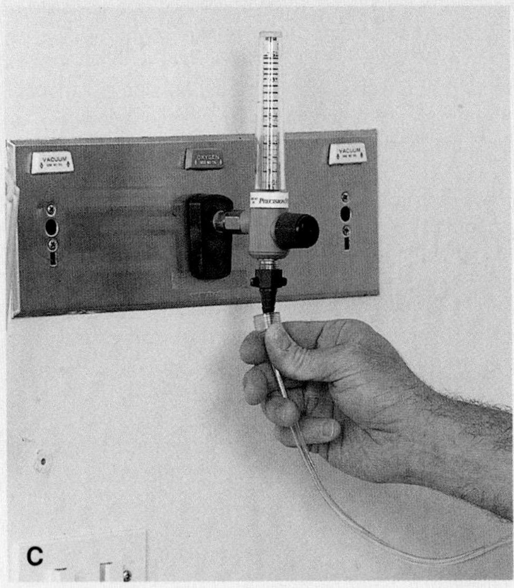

Attaching tubing from the delivery device. (Photo by B. Proud.)

Turn on the oxygen by adjusting the flowmeter to the prescribed volume.
Fills the delivery device with oxygen-rich air.

Note that bubbles appear in the humidifier bottle, if one is used, or that air is felt at the proximal end of the delivery device.
Indicates that oxygen is being released.

Make sure that if a reservoir bag is used, it is partially filled and remains that way throughout oxygen therapy.
Prevents asphyxiation and promotes high oxygenation. A reservoir bag must never become totally deflated during inhalation.

Attach the delivery device to the client.
Provides oxygen therapy.

Drain any tubing that collects condensation.
Maintains a clear pathway for oxygen and prevents accidental aspiration when turning a client.

Remove the oxygen delivery device and provide skin, oral, and nasal hygiene at least every 4–8 hours.
Maintains intact skin and mucous membranes; reduces the growth of microorganisms.

Reassess the client's oxygenation status every 2–4 hours.
Indicates how well the client is responding to oxygen therapy.

Notify the physician if the client manifests signs of hypoxemia or hypoxia despite oxygen therapy.
Demonstrates concern for the client's safety and well-being.

(continued)

Administering Oxygen (continued)

Evaluation

- Respiratory rate is 12–24 breaths per min at rest.
- Breathing is effortless.
- Heart rate is less than 100 bpm.
- Client is alert and oriented.
- Skin and mucous membranes are normal in color.
- SpO_2 is greater than or equal to 90%.
- FIO_2 and delivery device correspond to medical order.

Document

- Assessment data
- Percentage or liter flow of oxygen administration
- Type of delivery device
- Length of time in use
- Client's response to oxygen therapy

SAMPLE DOCUMENTATION

Date and Time Restless, pulse rate 120, resp. rate 32 with nasal flaring. Placed in high Fowler's position. SpO_2 at 85%–88%. Simple mask applied with administration of oxygen at 6 L/min. After 15 minutes of oxygen therapy is less agitated, pulse rate 100, respiratory rate 28, no nasal flaring noted. SpO_2 at 90%–92%. Oxygen continues to be administered. ———— SIGNATURE/TITLE

SKILL 21-3 Maintaining a Water-Seal Chest Tube Drainage System

Suggested Action	Reason for Action
ASSESSMENT	
Review the client's medical record to determine the condition that necessitated inserting a chest tube.	Indicates whether to expect air, bloody drainage, or both; any condition that causes an opening between the atmosphere and pleural space results in a loss of intrapleural negative pressure and subsequent lung deflation.
Determine if the physician has inserted one or two chest tubes (Fig. A).	Helps direct assessment; the usual sites for chest tubes are at the 2nd intercostal space in the midclavicular line and in the 5th to 8th intercostal spaces in the midaxillary line.

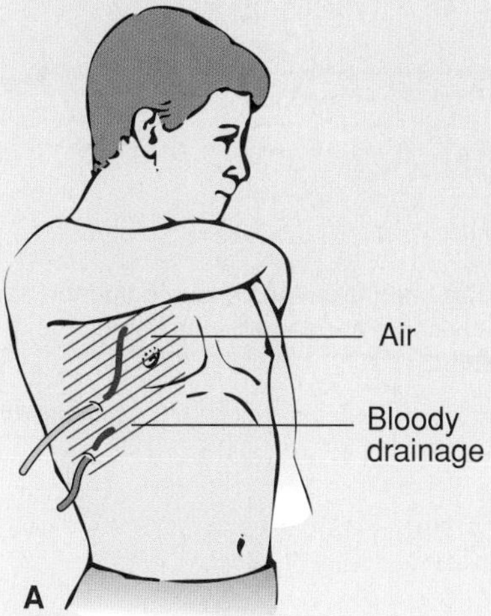

Determining whether the physician has inserted one or two chest tubes.

Suggested Action	Reason for Action
Note the date of chest tube(s) insertion.	Provides a point of reference for analyzing assessment data.
Check the medical orders to determine whether the drainage is being collected by gravity or with the addition of suction.	Provides guidelines for carrying out medical treatment; mechanical suction is used when there is a large air leak or potential for a large accumulation of drainage.

(continued)

Maintaining a Water-Seal Chest Tube Drainage System (continued)

PLANNING

Arrange to perform a physical assessment of the client and equipment as soon as possible after receiving the report. — Establishes a baseline and early opportunity for troubleshooting abnormal findings.

Locate a roll of tape and a container of sterile distilled water. — Facilitates efficient time management for general maintenance of the drainage system.

IMPLEMENTATION

Introduce yourself to the client and explain the purpose for the interaction. — Reduces anxiety and promotes cooperation.

Wash hands or perform hand antisepsis with an alcohol rub (see Chap. 10). — Reduces the transmission of microorganisms; conscientious handwashing is one of the most effective methods for preventing infection.

Check to see that a pair of hemostats (instruments for clamping) is at the bedside. — Facilitates checking for air leaks in the tubing or clamping the chest tube in the event the drainage system must be replaced to prevent the reentry of atmospheric air within the pleural space, thus maintaining lung expansion.

Turn off the suction regulator, if one is used, before assessing the client. — Eliminates noise that may interfere with chest auscultation.

Assess the client's lung sounds. — Provides a baseline for future comparison; because lung sounds cannot be heard in uninflated areas, lung sounds in previously silent areas indicates reexpansion.

Inspect the dressing for signs that it has become loose or saturated with drainage. — Indicates a need for changing the dressing.

Palpate the skin around the chest tube insertion site to feel and listen for air crackling in the tissues (Fig. B). — Indicates a subcutaneous air leak and an internal displacement of the drainage tube.

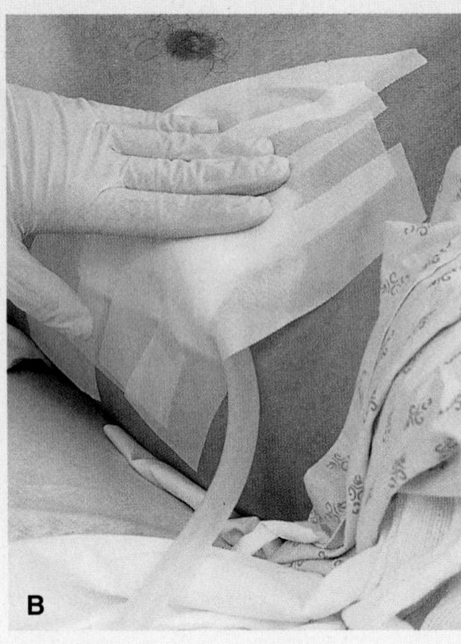

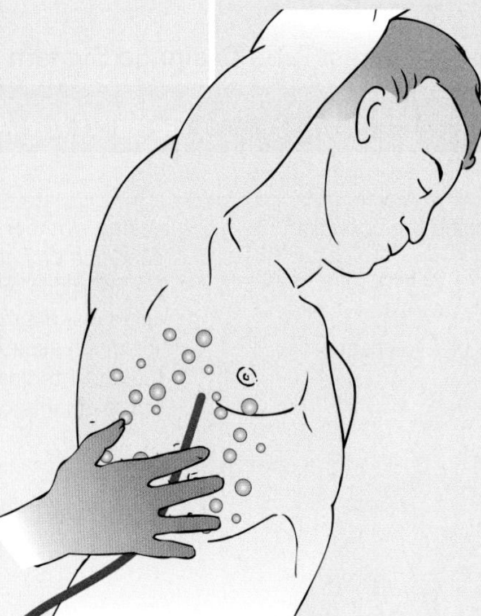

Palpating the skin around the chest tube insertion site to feel and listen for air crackling in the tissue. (Photo by B. Proud.)

Inspect all connections to determine that they are taped and secure. — Indicates appropriate care has been taken and ensures that the drainage system will not become accidentally separated.

Reinforce connections where the tape may be loose. — Prevents accidental separation.

(continued)

Maintaining a Water-Seal Chest Tube Drainage System (continued)

IMPLEMENTATION (CONTINUED)

Check that all tubing is unkinked and hangs freely into the drainage system (Fig. C).

Ensures the evacuation of air and bloody drainage because fluid cannot drain upward against gravity; neither air nor fluid can pass through a physical obstruction.

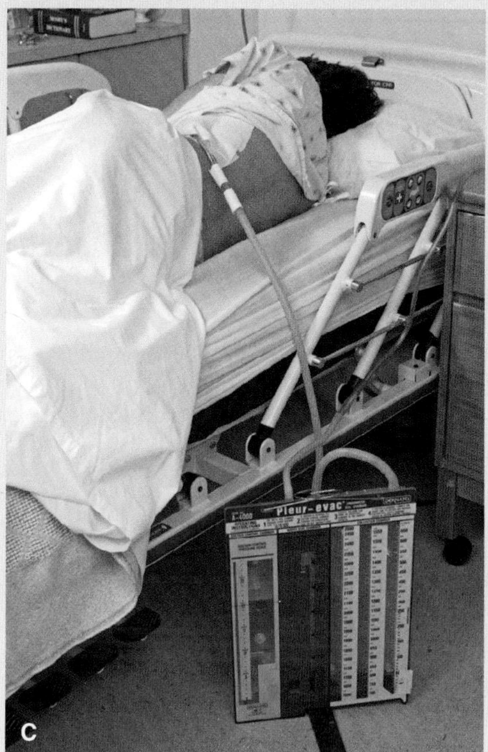

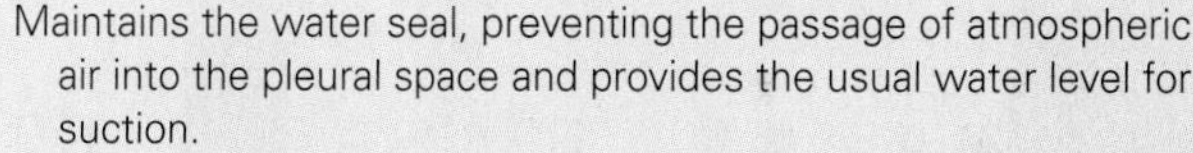
Keeping chest tubes unobstructed from the client to the drainage chamber.

Observe the fluid level in the water-seal chamber to see if it is at the 2-cm level and that the water in the suction chamber is at the 20-cm mark or the pressure prescribed by the physician (Fig. D).

Maintains the water seal, preventing the passage of atmospheric air into the pleural space and provides the usual water level for suction.

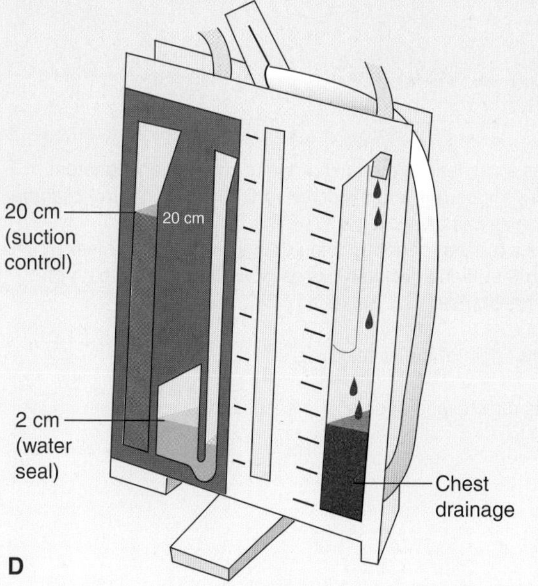

Noting water levels.

(continued)

Maintaining a Water-Seal Chest Tube Drainage System (continued)

IMPLEMENTATION (CONTINUED)

Add sterile distilled water to the 2-cm mark in the water-seal chamber or 20-cm mark to the suction control chamber if the fluid is below standard (Fig. E).

Two cm of water maintains the water seal; the 20-cm depth of water in the suction chamber determines the amount of negative pressure, *not* the pressure setting on the suction source.

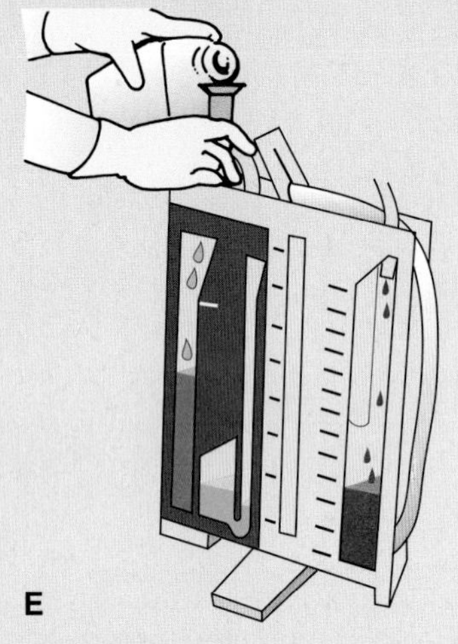

Adding water to the suction control chamber.

Note if the water is **tidaling** (the rise and fall of water in the water-seal chamber that coincides with respiration) (Fig. F).

Indicates that the tubing is unobstructed and the lung has not completely inflated; intrathoracic pressure changes during breathing cause the fluid to rise and fall.

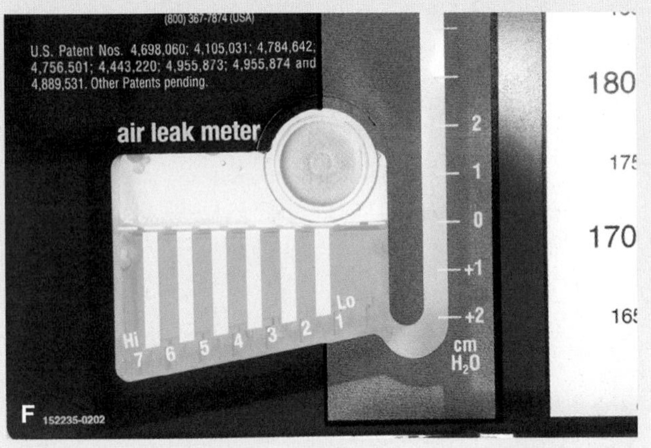

Watching for tidaling—movement of water up and down in the water-seal chamber.

Observe for continuous bubbling *in the water-seal chamber.*

Indicates an air leak in the tubing or at a connection; constant bubbling is normal and expected *in the suction control chamber* as long as it is used.

If constant bubbling is observed, clamp hemostats at the chest and within a few inches away; observe if the bubbling stops; continue releasing and reapplying the hemostats toward the drainage system until the bubbling stops.

Provides a means for determining the location of an air leak within the tubing because gas escapes through the path of least resistance.

Apply tape around the tube above where the last clamp was applied when the bubbling stopped.

Seals the origin of the air leak.

Regulate the wall suction so that it produces *gentle* bubbling.

Prevents rapid evaporation and unnecessary noise.

(continued)

Maintaining a Water-Seal Chest Tube Drainage System (continued)

IMPLEMENTATION (CONTINUED)

Observe the nature and amount of drainage in the collection chamber (Fig. G).	Provides comparative data; more than 100 mL/hr or bright-red drainage is reported immediately.

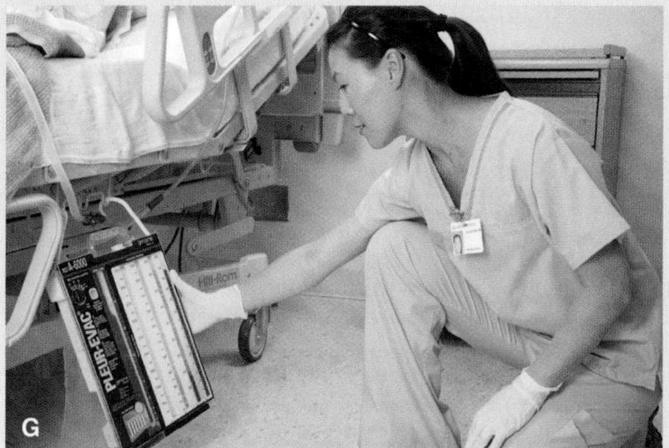

Observing drainage characteristics.

Keep the drainage system below chest level.	Maintains gravity flow of drainage.
Position the client to avoid compressing the tubing.	Facilitates drainage.
Curl and secure excess tubing on the bed.	Avoids dependent loops to facilitate drainage.
Milk the tubing, a process of compressing and stripping the tubing to move stationary clots, but only if necessary.	Creates extremely high negative intrapleural pressure; milking is never done routinely.
Encourage coughing and deep breathing at least every 2 hours while awake.	Promotes lung reexpansion because the mechanics of breathing and forceful coughing help evacuate air and fluid.
Instruct the client to move about in bed, ambulate while carrying the drainage system, and exercise the shoulder on the side of the drainage tube(s).	Prevents hazards of immobility and maintains joint flexibility with no danger to the client while the tube to the suction source is disconnected as long as the water seal remains intact.
Never clamp the chest tube for an extended period.	Predisposes to developing a **tension pneumothorax** (extreme air pressure within the lung when there is no avenue for its escape); clamping a chest tube *briefly* is safe, for example, when changing the entire drainage system.
If the tube and drainage system become separated, insert a separated chest tube within sterile water until it can be reattached and secured to the drainage system.	Provides a temporary water seal to prevent the entrance of atmospheric air, which can recollapse the lung.
Prevent air from entering the tube insertion site by covering it with a gloved hand or woven fabric if the tube is accidentally pulled out.	Reduces the amount of lung collapse.
Mark the drainage level on the collection chamber at the end of each shift (Fig. H).	Provides data about fluid loss without the risk of recollapsing the lung; *never* empty the drainage container.

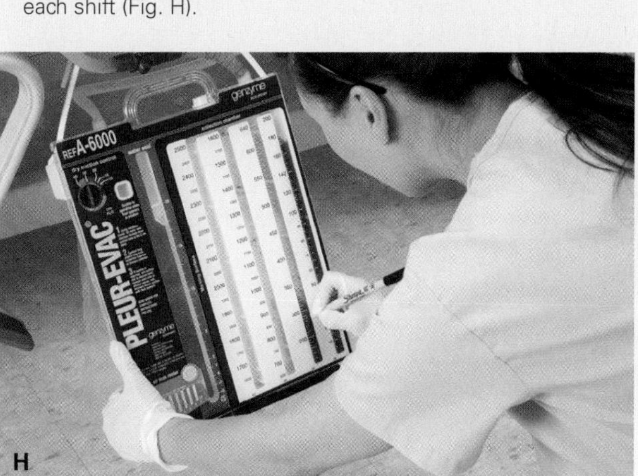

Marking the drainage level.

(continued)

Maintaining a Water-Seal Chest Tube Drainage System (continued)

Evaluation

- Client exhibits no evidence of respiratory distress.
- Dressing is dry and intact.
- Equipment is functioning appropriately.
- Water is at recommended levels.

Document

- Assessment findings
- Care provided
- Amount of drainage during period of care

SAMPLE DOCUMENTATION

Date and Time Upper and lower chest tubes connected to water-seal drainage system. Normal lung sounds heard throughout chest except in apex and base of left lung, where chest tubes are inserted. Tidaling still observed in water-seal chamber. 20 cm of suction maintained. Dark-red chest tube drainage measures a scant 50 mL. Ambulated in hall while disconnected from suction. Performed full range of motion with left shoulder. ——— SIGNATURE/TITLE

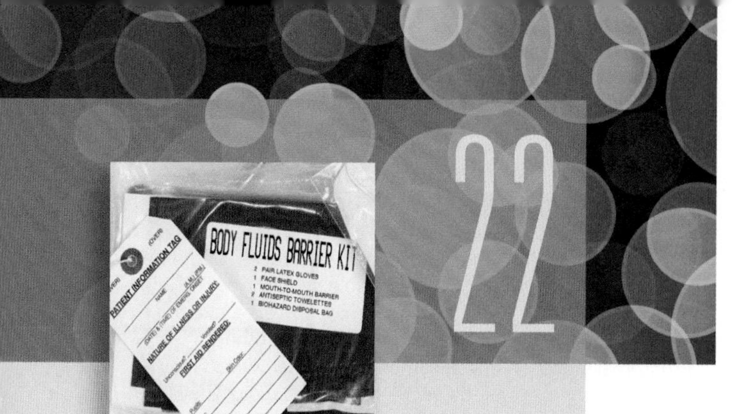

22

Infection Control

Words To Know

airborne precautions
colonization
contact precautions
double bagging
droplet precautions
hyperendemic infections
infection
infection control precautions
infectious diseases
N95 respirator
personal protective equipment
Powered Air Purifying Respirator
respiratory hygiene/cough etiquette
safe injection practices
standard precautions
transmission-based precautions

Learning Objectives

On completion of this chapter, the reader should be able to:

1. Explain the meaning of infectious diseases.
2. Differentiate between infection and colonization.
3. List five stages in the course of an infectious disease.
4. Define infection control measures.
5. Name two major techniques for infection control.
6. Identify three new elements of standard precautions.
7. Discuss situations in which nurses use standard precautions and transmission-based precautions.
8. Describe the rationale for using airborne, droplet, and contact precautions.
9. Explain the purpose of personal protective equipment (PPE).
10. Discuss the rationale for removing PPE in a specific sequence after caring for a client with an infection.
11. Explain how nurses perform double bagging.
12. List two psychological problems common among clients with infectious diseases.
13. Provide at least three teaching suggestions for preventing infections.
14. Discuss one unique characteristic of older adults in relation to infectious diseases.

Infectious diseases (diseases that spread from one person to another) are also called contagious or communicable diseases and community-acquired infections. They were once the leading cause of death, but that is no longer true because of vaccines, aggressive public health measures, and advances in drug therapy. Nevertheless, infectious diseases have not disappeared. In fact, the microorganisms that cause tuberculosis (TB), gonorrhea, and some forms of wound and respiratory infections have developed drug-resistant strains (see Chap. 10). Add to that the current public health problem with AIDS, an infectious disease spread by HIV in blood and some body fluids (Box 22-1), severe acute respiratory syndrome (SARS), and the potential for bird flu, and it is clear that humans have not won the war against pathogens.

This chapter discusses precautions that confine the reservoir of infectious agents and block their transmission from one host to another. To understand the concepts of infection control, it is important to understand the chain of infection (see Chap. 10) and the course of an infection.

INFECTION

Infection is a condition that results when microorganisms cause injury to a host. Infection differs from **colonization**, a condition in which

BOX 22-1 Facts and Myths About the Transmission of HIV

Facts

HIV is transmitted by:

- Having unprotected vaginal, anal, or oral sexual contact with an infected person
- Sharing needles or syringes with an infected person
- Acquiring a needle-stick injury with the blood of an infected person (see Chap. 34)
- Receiving transfusions of infected blood or blood products
- Being born to or breast-fed by an HIV-infected mother
- Having contact with the blood of an infected person through unsterilized equipment for ear piercing, tattooing, acupuncture, dental procedures, safety razors, or toothbrushes
- Contacting blood of an infected person through an open cut or splashes into the mucous membranes such as the eyes or inside of the nose
- Artificial insemination with infected semen
- Organ transplant taken from an HIV-infected donor

Myths

HIV is *not* transmitted by:

- Donating blood
- Being bitten by insects
- Sharing cups and eating utensils
- Inhaling droplets from sneezes or coughs
- Hugging, touching, or closed-mouth kissing an infected person
- Sharing telephones or computer keyboards
- Going to any public place with people infected with HIV
- Using public drinking fountains or toilet seats
- Swimming in pools

From Centers for Disease Control and Prevention. *HIV and its transmission.* Accessed April, 2010, from, http://www.cdc.gov/hiv/resources/factsheets/transmission.htm, last updated July 2007, accessed 4/10; Ten things everyone should know about HIV; Symptom checker. Accessed April 2010, from, http://symptomchecker.about.com/od/Diagnoses.hivaids.htm, last modified February 2005.

microorganisms are present, but the host does not manifest any signs or symptoms of infection. Regardless of whether the host is infected or colonized, the host can transmit pathogens and infectious diseases to others.

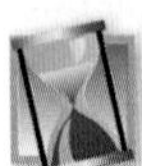

Gerontologic Considerations

■ Many long-term care residents, older hospitalized clients, and health care personnel are colonized with antibiotic-resistant bacteria, possibly with few or no symptoms.

Infections progress through distinct stages (Table 22-1). The characteristics and length of each stage may differ depending on the infectious agent. For example, the incubation period for the common cold is approximately 2 to 4 days before symptoms appear, but it may take months or years before a person infected with HIV demonstrates symptoms of AIDS.

TABLE 22-1 Course of Infectious Diseases

STAGE	CHARACTERISTIC
Incubation period	Infectious agent reproduces, but there are no recognizable symptoms. The infectious agent may, however, exit the host at this time and infect others.
Prodromal stage	Initial symptoms appear, which may be vague and nonspecific. They may include mild fever, headache, and loss of usual energy.
Acute stage	Symptoms become severe and specific to the tissue or organ that is affected. For example, TB is manifested by respiratory symptoms.
Convalescent stage	The symptoms subside as the host overcomes the infectious agent.
Resolution	The pathogen is destroyed. Health improves or is restored.

TB, tuberculosis.

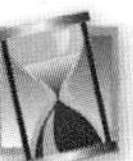

Gerontologic Considerations

■ Older clients are more susceptible to infections caused by diminished immune system functioning and inadequate nutrition and fluid intake.

■ Symptoms of infections tend to be subtle among older adults. Because older adults tend to have a lower "normal" or baseline temperature, a temperature in the normal range may actually be elevated for an older adult.

■ Infections are more likely to have a rapid course and life-threatening consequences once they become established. Common manifestations of infections in older adults include changes in behavior and mental status.

INFECTION CONTROL PRECAUTIONS

Infection control precautions are physical measures designed to curtail the spread of infectious diseases. They are essential when caring for clients. Infection control precautions require knowledge of the mechanisms by which an infectious disease is transmitted and the methods that will interfere with the chain of infection.

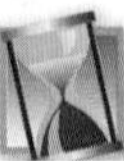

Gerontologic Considerations

■ Thinning, drying, and decreases in vascular supply to the skin predispose the older person to skin infections. Maintaining intact skin is an excellent first-line defense against acquiring infections.

■ Infections are often transmitted to vulnerable older adults through equipment reservoirs such as indwelling urinary catheters, humidifiers, and oxygen equipment or through incisional sites such as those for intravenous tubing, parenteral nutrition, or tube feedings. Use of proper aseptic techniques is essential for preventing the introduction of microorganisms. A daily assessment for any signs of infection is imperative.

- Older adults, family caregivers/members in close contact with older people, and all personnel in health care settings should obtain annual immunizations against influenza. Those who are 65 years and older and younger people with chronic diseases should receive an initial dose of the pneumococcal vaccine.
- Visitors with respiratory infections need to wear a mask or avoid contact with older adults in their home or long-term care settings until their symptoms have subsided. In addition to a mask, frequent and thorough hand hygiene can help prevent the transfer of organisms.
- Health care workers who are ill should take sick leave rather than exposing susceptible clients to infectious organisms.

Under the auspices of the Centers for Disease Control and Prevention (CDC), the Healthcare Infection Control Practices Advisory Committee (2007) has continued to recommend guidelines for two major categories of infection control precautions: standard precautions and transmission-based precautions.

Standard Precautions

Standard precautions are measures for reducing the risk of microorganism transmission from both recognized and unrecognized sources of infection. Health care personnel follow standard precautions when caring for all clients, regardless of the suspected or confirmed infection status (Box 22-2). This precautionary system combines methods previously known as *universal precautions* and *body substance isolation.* The use of standard precautions reduces the potential for transmitting infectious agents in blood, body fluids, secretions, and excretions (except sweat), nonintact skin, mucous membranes, and equipment or items in the client's environment that may contain transmissible infectious agents whether or not they contain visible blood. Health care personnel follow standard precautions when caring for all clients in all settings in which health care is delivered. Standard precautions include hand hygiene, use of gloves, a gown, a mask, eye protection or a face shield, and safe injection practices (see Chap. 34). The type of **personal protective equipment** (PPE) used is determined by the nature of the client interaction and the extent of anticipated blood, body fluid, or pathogen exposure.

A sign that alerts health care workers may be posted in various areas of the health care agency (Fig. 22-1).

New Standard Precaution Recommendations

The CDC has identified three new standard precautions for infection control. They include respiratory hygiene/cough etiquette, safe injection practices, and practices for special lumbar puncture procedures.

Respiratory Hygiene/Cough Etiquette

Respiratory hygiene/cough etiquette (Fig. 22-2) refers to infection control measures used at the first point of an encounter with clients, family, or friends of persons with signs of illness suggesting an undiagnosed transmissible respiratory infection. It includes:

- Covering the mouth/nose with a tissue when coughing; coughing or sneezing into an upper sleeve or elbow is another alternative when a tissue is unavailable.
- Disposing of used tissues promptly.

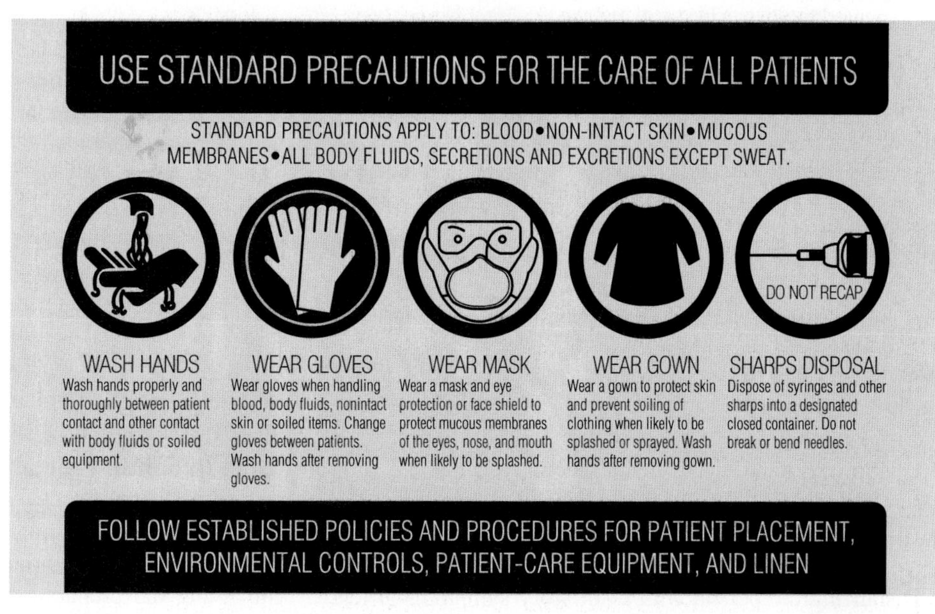

FIGURE 22-1 A Sign that identifies standard precautions.

BOX 22-2 Standard Precautions

Hand Hygiene
- Use an alcohol-based product or plain (nonantimicrobial) soap for routine hand hygiene.
- Perform hand hygiene after touching blood, body fluids, secretions, excretions, and contaminated items, whether or not gloves are worn.
- Perform hand hygiene immediately after gloves are removed, between client contacts, and when otherwise indicated; perform hand hygiene between tasks and procedures on the same client to prevent cross-contamination of different body sites.
- Use an antimicrobial agent or a waterless antiseptic agent to control outbreaks or **hyperendemic infections** (infections that are highly infectious in all age groups).

Gloves
- Wear clean, nonsterile gloves that fit snugly around the wrist when touching blood, body fluids, secretions, excretions, and contaminated items; latex or nitrile gloves are preferred for clinical procedures that require manual dexterity or involve more than brief client contact.
- Change gloves between tasks on the same client after contact with material that may contain a high concentration of microorganisms and before touching portable computer keyboards or other mobile equipment that is transported from room to room.
- Remove gloves and perform hand hygiene immediately before caring for another client.

Mask, Eye Protection, Face Shield
- Wear a mask and eye protection (goggles), or face shield to protect the eyes, nose, and mouth when there is a likelihood that splashes or sprays of blood, body fluids, secretions, or excretions will occur; eyeglasses and contact lenses are not adequate for eye protection.
- Obtain a user-seal check (also called a "fit check") to minimize air leakage around the facepiece of a respirator; reuse of a particulate respirator by the same person is acceptable as long as the respirator is not damaged or soiled, the fit is not compromised by change in shape, and the respirator has not been contaminated with blood or body fluids.

Gown
- Wear a clean, nonsterile gown that covers the arms and body from neck to mid thigh or below when there is a likelihood that splashes or sprays of blood, body fluids, secretions, or excretions will occur.
- Remove a soiled gown promptly and perform hand hygiene.

Client-Care Equipment
- Locate containers for used disposable or reusable PPE at a site that is convenient for the removal and disposal of contaminated materials.
- Handle equipment soiled with blood, body fluids, secretions, and excretions so as to prevent the transfer of microorganisms to oneself, others, or the environment.
- Ensure that soiled reusable equipment is cleaned and disinfected or sterilized before another subsequent use.
- Discard soiled single-use equipment properly.

Environmental Control
- Ensure that procedures for the routine cleaning and disinfection of environmental surfaces, beds, bed rails, bedside equipment, and other frequently touched surfaces are carried out.

Linen
- Handle, transport, and process soiled linen in such a way as to prevent exposure to oneself, others, and the environment.

Occupational Health and Blood-Borne Pathogens
- Prevent injuries when using needles, scalpels, and other sharp devices.
- Never recap used needles.
- Use either a one-handed "scoop" method or a mechanical device for covering a needle.
- Place all disposable sharp items in a puncture-resistant container as close to the location of use as possible; transport reusable syringes and needles in a puncture-resistant container for reprocessing.
- Use mouthpieces, resuscitation bags, or other ventilation devices as an alternative to mouth-to-mouth resuscitation methods in areas where the need for resuscitation is predictable.

Client Placement
- Place potentially infectious clients in a private room whenever possible.
- Consult with an infection control professional concerning alternatives if a private room is not available.
- Place a client who contaminates the environment, who does not—or cannot be expected to—assist in maintaining appropriate hygiene or environmental control in a private room.

Adapted from Centers for Disease Control and Prevention. (2007). *2007 Guidelines for isolation precautions: Preventing transmission of infectious agents in healthcare settings*. Accessed April 12, 2010, from http://www.cdc.gov/ncidod/dhqp/pdf/isolation2007.pdf.

- Performing hand hygiene after contact with respiratory secretions.
- Using a surgical mask on a coughing client who can tolerate this measure.
- Distancing the person with respiratory symptoms at least 3 ft. from others in common waiting areas.

Safe Injection Practices

Safe injection practices are infection control measures that prevent the transmission of viral hepatitis B (HBV) and hepatitis C (HCV) through the use of aseptic techniques involving the preparation and administration of parenteral medications (see Chap. 34). Health care workers are advised

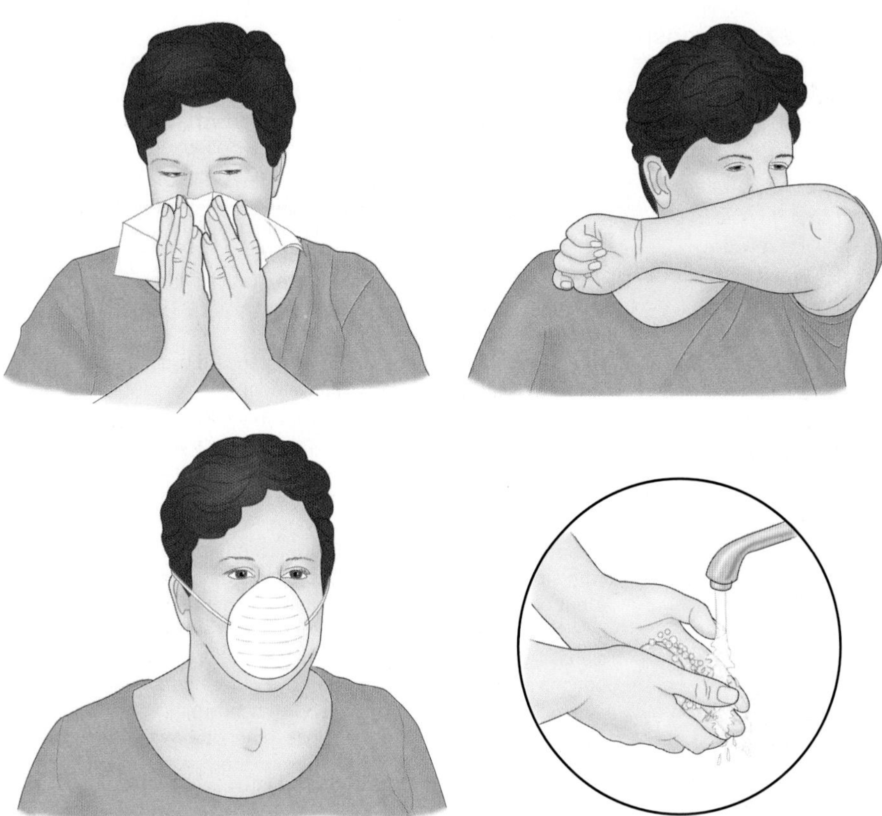

FIGURE 22-2 Techniques for preventing or reducing the spread of respiratory pathogens.

to (1) use a sterile, single-use, disposable syringe for each injection, (2) prevent the contamination of injection equipment and medication, and (3) use single-dose vials rather than multiple-dose vials when administering medications to multiple clients. Measures to handle needles and other sharp devices in a manner that avoids injury to the user and others who may encounter the device during or after a procedure continue to be a standard practice (see Chaps. 34 and 35).

Infection Control Practices for Special Lumbar Puncture Procedures

Lumbar puncture procedures are performed for a number of reasons such as performing a myeleogram, administering spinal and epidural anesthesia, placement of spinal catheters, and injecting medications within the spinal canal. Because there has been an increase in the incidence of bacterial meningitis most likely from respiratory droplet transmission at the time these procedures were performed, it is now recommended that the person performing the procedure wears a mask in addition to the usual protective equipment that is used.

Transmission-Based Precautions

Transmission-based precautions are measures for controlling the spread of highly transmissible or epidemiologically important infectious agents from clients when the known or suspected route(s) of transmission is (are) not completely interrupted using standard precautions alone. They are also called isolation precautions. The three types of transmission-based precautions are airborne precautions, droplet precautions, and contact precautions (Table 22-2). These three types replace the earlier categories of strict isolation, contact isolation, respiratory isolation, tuberculosis (AFB) isolation, enteric precautions, and drainage/secretion precautions. Health care personnel base the decision to use one or a combination of precautions on the mechanism of transmission of the pathogen. They use one or more categories of transmission-based precautions concurrently when diseases have multiple routes of transmission.

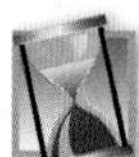

Gerontologic Considerations

- Older adults with cognitive impairment need more assistance with complying with infection control measures.

Transmission-based precautions are required for various lengths of time, depending on how long the risk of transmission of the infectious agent persists or for the duration of the illness. Personnel discontinue some precautions, with the exception of standard precautions, when culture or other laboratory findings document that the disease has been resolved, when a wound or lesion stops draining, after the initiation of effective therapy, or when state laws and regulations have dictated discontinuation. Sometimes personnel employ them throughout a client's treatment.

Airborne Precautions

Airborne precautions are measures that reduce the risk for transmitting pathogens that remain infectious over long

TABLE 22-2 Transmission-Based Precautions

TYPE OF PRECAUTION	CLIENT PLACEMENT	PROTECTION	EXAMPLES OF DISEASES
Airborne	Private room or in a room with a similarly infected client Negative air pressure[a] Six to 12 air changes per hour Discharge of room air to environment or filtered before being circulated	Follow standard precautions. Keep door closed; confine client to room. Wear a mask for trapping airborne pathogens, such as N95 respirator or Powered Air Purifying Respirator in the case of tuberculosis (TB). Place a mask on the client if transport is required.	Pulmonary TB Measles (rubeola) Chickenpox (varicella) Severe acute respiratory syndrome (SARS)
Droplet	Private room or in a room with a similarly infected client or one in which there are at least 3 ft. between other clients and visitors.	Follow standard precautions. Leave door open or closed. Wear a mask when entering the room depending on agency policy but always when within 3 ft. of the client. Place a mask on the client if transport is required.	Influenza Rubella Streptococcal pneumonia Meningococcal meningitis Whooping cough
Contact	Private room or in a room with similarly infected client or consult with an infection control professional if the previous options are not available	Follow standard precautions. Don gloves before entering the room. Change gloves during client care after contact with infective material that contains high concentrations of microorganisms. Remove gloves before leaving the room. Perform handwashing or perform an alcohol-based handrub with an antimicrobial agent immediately after removing gloves. Do not touch potentially contaminated surfaces or items in the immediate environment after glove removal and handwashing. Wear a gown when entering the room if there is the possibility that your clothing will touch the client, environmental surfaces, or items in the room, or if the client is incontinent or has diarrhea, an ileostomy, a colostomy, or wound drainage not contained by a dressing. Remove the gown before leaving the environment. Avoid transporting the client but, if transport is required, use precautions that minimize transmission. Clean bedside equipment and client care items daily. Use items such as a stethoscope, sphygmomanometer, and other assessment tools exclusively for the infected client; clean and disinfect them before use for another client.	Gastrointestinal, respiratory, skin, or wound infections that are drug resistant Gas gangrene Acute diarrhea Acute viral conjunctivitis Draining abscess

[a]Negative air pressure pulls air from the hall into the room when the door is opened, as opposed to positive air pressure, which pulls room air into the hall.

From Centers for Disease Control and Prevention. (2007). 2007 *Guidelines for isolation precautions: Preventing transmission of infectious agents in healthcare settings.* Accessed April 12, 2010, from http://www.cdc.gov/ncidod/dhqp/pdf/isolation2007.pdf

distances when suspended in the air (see Table 22-2). They block pathogens, 0.3 microns or smaller, that are present in the residue of evaporated droplets that remain suspended in the air, as well as those attached to dust particles.

TB is an example of a disease transmitted through the air. Caregivers must wear a specific type of mask when caring for clients with TB. An **N95 respirator**, which is individually fitted for each caregiver, can filter particles 1 micron (smaller than a millimeter) with an efficiency of 95% or more, provided the device fits the face snugly (Fig. 22-3A). A **Powered Air Purifying Respirator** (PAPR) is an alternative if a caregiver has not been fitted with an N95 respirator or has facial hair or a facial deformity that prevents a tight seal with an N95 respirator (Fig. 22-3B). A PAPR blows atmospheric air through belt-mounted air-purifying canisters to the facepiece through a flexible tube. A PAPR can also be used when rescuing victims exposed to hazardous chemicals or bioterrorist substances.

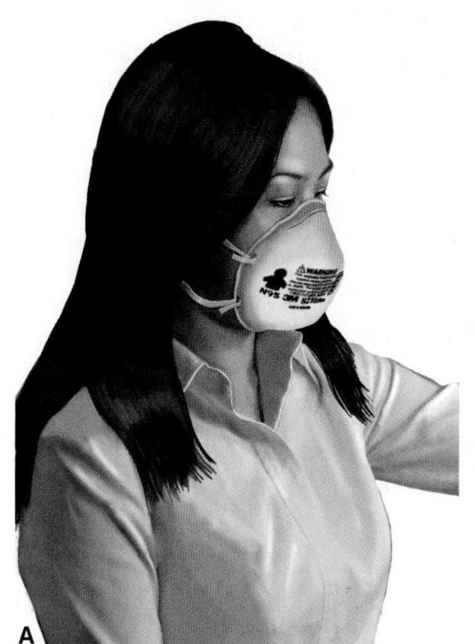
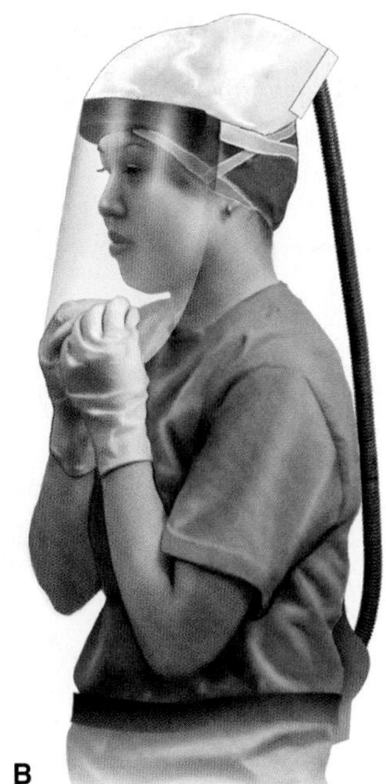

FIGURE 22-3 A. An N95 respirator must fit tightly around the mouth and nose with straps that attach it to the head. A secure seal is evidenced by a slight bulging on exhalation and slight collapse upon inhalation. **B.** A Powered Air Purifying Respirator uses a blower to remove contaminated air through a filter and supplies purified air to a facepiece.

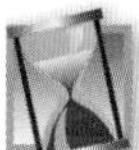

Gerontologic Considerations

■ The incidence of TB in community-living older adults is twice that of the general population (Miller, 2008). All long-term care facilities are required to test each resident on admission and each new employee for TB.

Droplet Precautions

Droplet precautions are measures that block infectious pathogens within moist droplets larger than 5 microns. They are used to reduce pathogen transmission from close contact (usually 3 ft. or less) with respiratory secretions or mucous membranes between infected persons or a person who is a carrier of a droplet-spread microorganism and others. Microorganisms carried on droplets commonly exit the body during coughing, sneezing, talking, and procedures such as airway suctioning (see Chap. 36) and bronchoscopy. Airborne precautions are not used because droplets do not remain suspended in the air.

Contact Precautions

Contact precautions are measures used to block the transmission of pathogens by direct or indirect contact. This is the final category of transmission-based precautions. Direct contact involves skin-to-skin contact with an infected or colonized person. Indirect contact occurs by touching a contaminated intermediate object in the client's environment. Additional precautions are necessary if the microorganism is resistant to antibiotics.

Some infectious diseases like chickenpox (varicella), smallpox (variola), and SARS require both airborne and contact precautions.

Stop, Think, and Respond Box 22-1

Which type of transmission precautions do health care personnel follow when caring for clients with the following medical diagnoses: (1) pulmonary TB, (2) streptococcal pneumonia, (3) an infected wound, (4) acute diarrhea, and (5) meningococcal meningitis?

INFECTION CONTROL MEASURES

Infection control measures involve the use of PPE (garments that block the transfer of pathogens from one person, place, or object to oneself or others) and techniques that serve as barriers to transmission (Fig. 22-4). Depending on the type of precautions used, nurses implement all or some of the following measures:

- Locating a client and equipping a room so as to confine pathogens to one area
- Using PPE such as cover gowns, face shields or goggles, cloth or paper masks or respirators (see Chap. 10), and gloves to prevent spreading microorganisms through direct and indirect contact
- Disposing of contaminated linen, equipment, and supplies in such a way that nurses do not transfer pathogens to others
- Using infection control measures to prevent pathogens from spreading when transporting laboratory specimens or clients

Client Environment

The client environment includes the room designated for the care of a client with an infectious disease and the equipment and supplies essential for controlling transmission of the pathogens.

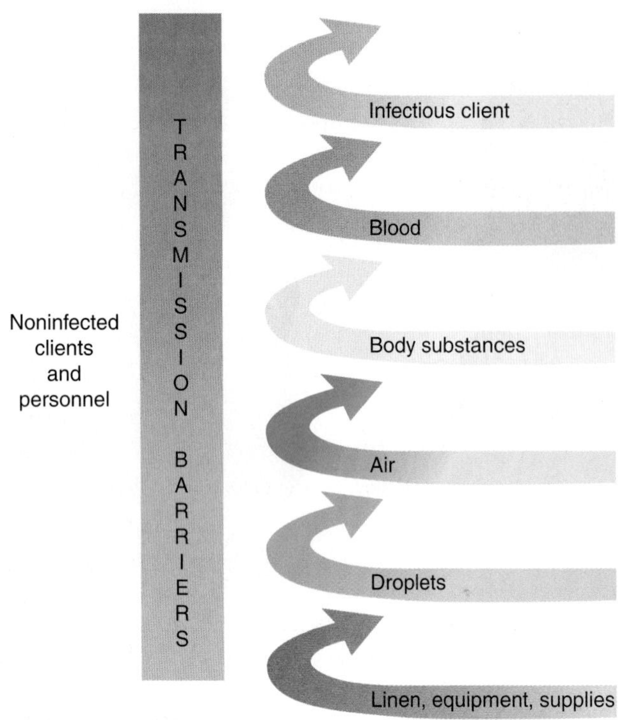

FIGURE 22-4 Blocking sources of infectious disease transmission.

Infection Control Room

Except when using standard precautions, most health care agencies assign infectious or potentially infectious clients to private rooms. Infection control personnel can offer alternatives if a private room is not available (see Table 22-2). They keep the door to the room closed to control air currents and the circulation of dust particles.

The room has a private bathroom so that personnel can flush contaminated liquids and biodegradable solids. A sink is also located in the room for handwashing.

Staff members post an instruction card on the door or nearby at eye level stating that isolation precautions are required (Fig. 22-5). Nurses are responsible for teaching visitors how to comply with the infection control measures.

In accord with the principles of medical asepsis, housekeeping personnel clean the infectious client's room last to avoid transferring organisms on the wet mop to other client areas. They deposit the mop head, if not disposable, with the soiled linen and wipe the mop handle with a disinfectant. They flush solutions used for cleaning down the toilet.

Equipment and Supplies

The infection control room contains the same equipment and supplies as any other hospital room, with a few modifications. A dedicated stethoscope and sphygmomanometer remain in the client's room whenever possible. This prevents the need to clean and disinfect these items each time they would need to be removed.

For the same reason, disposable thermometers are preferred. Personnel disinfect electronic or tympanic thermometers to make them safe for the next client. Items such as a container for soiled laundry (Fig. 22-6), lined waste containers, and liquid soap dispensers are also placed in the room.

Personal Protective Equipment

Infection control measures involve the use of one or more items for personal protection. PPE, also called "barrier garments" (Fig. 22-7), includes gowns, masks, respirators, goggles or face shields, and gloves (see Chap. 10). These items are located just outside the client's room or in an anteroom (Fig. 22-8).

Cover Gowns

Cover gowns are worn for two reasons: they prevent contamination of clothing and protect the skin from contact with blood and body fluids. When they are removed after direct care of the infectious client, they reduce the possibility of transmitting pathogens from the client, the client's environment, or contaminated objects. Many types of cover gowns exist, but all have the following common characteristics:

- They open in the back to reduce inadvertent contact with the client and objects.
- They have close-fitting wristbands to help avoid contaminating the forearms.
- They fasten at the neck and waist to keep the gown securely closed, thus covering all the wearer's clothing.

Nurses wear a cover gown only once and then discard it. They place discarded cloth gowns in the client's laundry

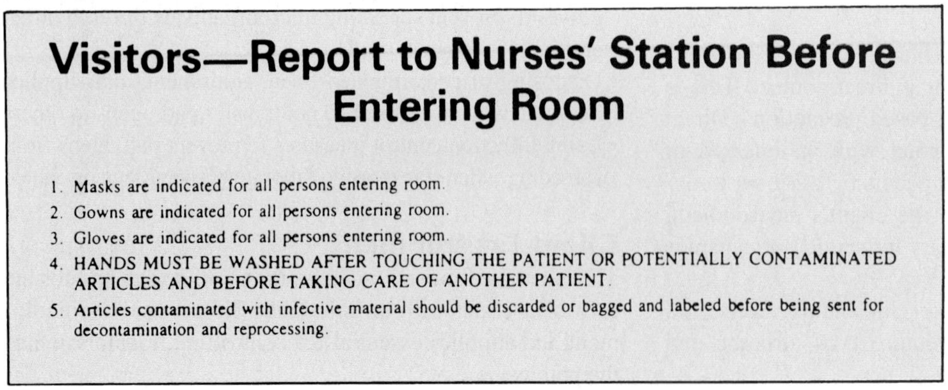

Visitors—Report to Nurses' Station Before Entering Room

1. Masks are indicated for all persons entering room.
2. Gowns are indicated for all persons entering room.
3. Gloves are indicated for all persons entering room.
4. HANDS MUST BE WASHED AFTER TOUCHING THE PATIENT OR POTENTIALLY CONTAMINATED ARTICLES AND BEFORE TAKING CARE OF ANOTHER PATIENT.
5. Articles contaminated with infective material should be discarded or bagged and labeled before being sent for decontamination and reprocessing.

FIGURE 22-5 A Door instructional card.

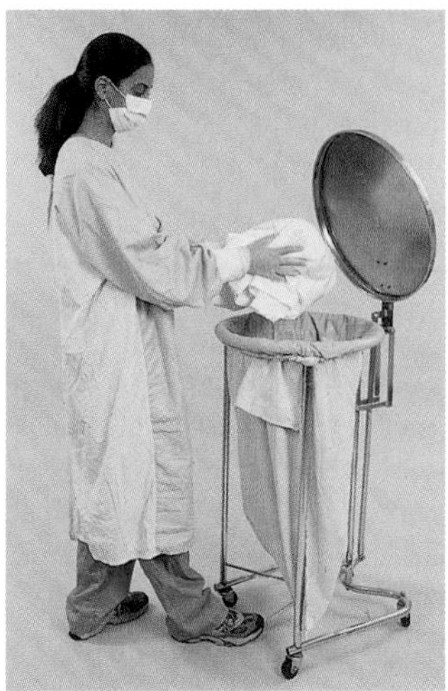

FIGURE 22-6 Containing soiled laundry. (Photo by B. Proud.)

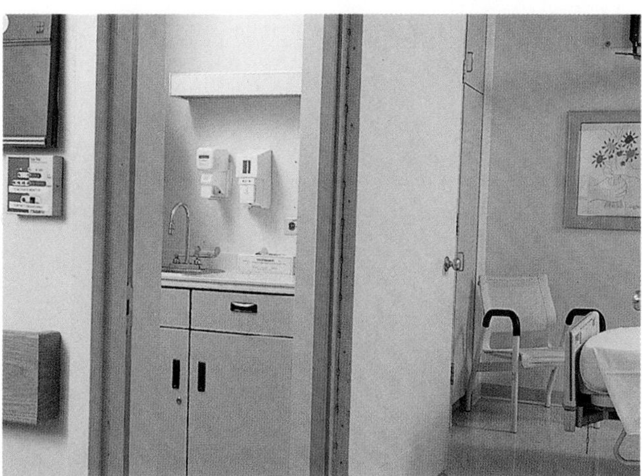

FIGURE 22-8 An anteroom outside the infection control room. (Photo by B. Proud.)

hamper, and remove them with the soiled linen. Cloth cover gowns are laundered before being used again. Disposable paper gowns are placed in a waste container and incinerated.

Face-Protection Devices

Depending on the mode of transmission of the pathogen, health care personnel wear a mask or respirator (see Chap. 10), goggles, or a face shield. They always apply these items before entering the client's room.

Gloves

Gloves are required when an infectious disease is transmitted by direct contact or contact with blood and body fluid substances. Health care personnel always don gloves before or immediately on entering the client's room. After one use, they are discarded.

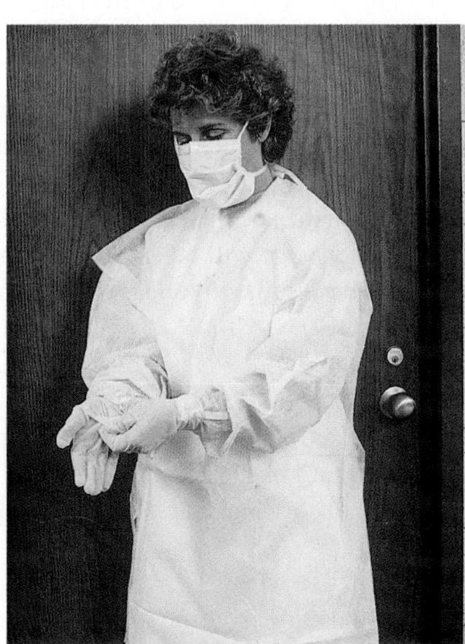

FIGURE 22-7 Donning personal protective equipment (PPE) helps prevent the transmission of infectious microorganisms. (Photo by B. Proud.)

Gloves are not a total and complete barrier to microorganisms. They are easily punctured and can leak; the potential for leakage increases with the stress of use.

Wearing gloves does not replace the need for hand antisepsis (see Chap. 10) after removal. Hands can be contaminated during glove removal, and microorganisms that were present on the hands before gloving grow and multiply rapidly in the warm, moist environment beneath the gloves.

Stop, Think, and Respond Box 22-2

What personal protective items would you expect to wear when managing the care of a client with a draining wound abscess?

Removing Personal Protective Equipment

Regardless of which garments they wear, nurses follow an orderly sequence for removing them (Skill 22-1). The goal is to leave the client's room without contaminating oneself or one's uniform. The procedure involves making contact between two contaminated surfaces or two clean surfaces. Nurses remove the garments that are most contaminated first, preserving the clean uniform underneath (Fig. 22-9).

Nurses can modify the technique to accommodate the removal of any combination of equipment. The most important nursing action is to perform thorough handwashing before leaving the client's room and before touching any other client, personnel, environmental surface, or client care items.

Disposing of Contaminated Linen, Equipment, and Supplies

Receptacles in the client's room are used to collect contaminated items. Soiled waste containers are emptied at the end of each shift or more often if their contents accumulate (Fig. 22-10). To avoid spreading pathogens, some items are double bagged.

Double bagging is an infection control measure in which one bag of contaminated items, such as trash or laundry, is

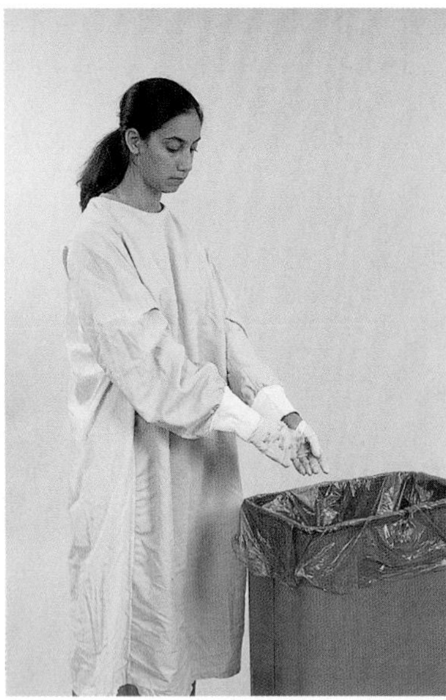

FIGURE 22-9 Removing and disposing the most contaminated garments first. (Photo by B. Proud.)

placed within another. This measure requires two people. One person bags the items and deposits the bag in a second bag held by another person outside of the client's room. The person holding the second bag prevents contamination by manipulating the bag underneath a folded cuff (Fig. 22-11).

The Centers for Disease Control and Prevention (2007) have relaxed their recommendation concerning double bagging. Their revised position is that one bag is adequate if the bag is sturdy and the articles are placed in the bag without contaminating the outside of the bag. Otherwise, double bagging is used.

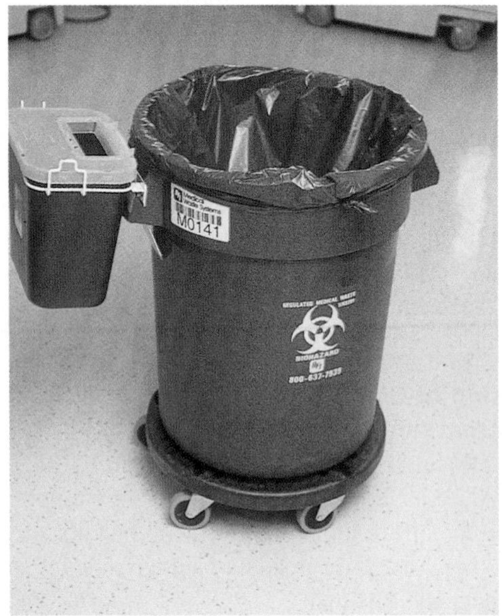

FIGURE 22-10 A waste container used for infectious waste. (Photo by B. Proud.)

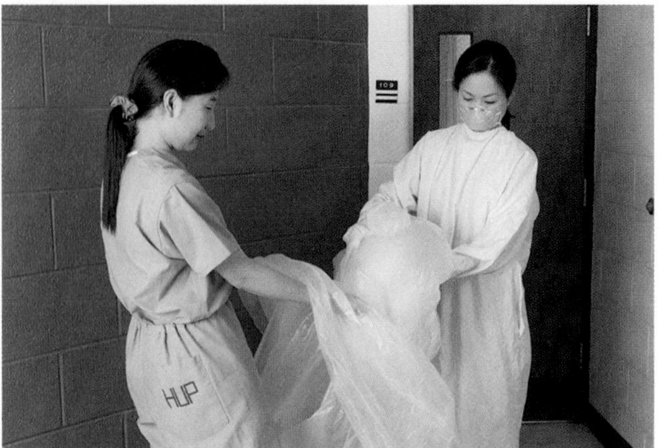

FIGURE 22-11 Double bagging technique.

Following the termination of transmission-based precautions, equipment that will be used again for other client care must first be thoroughly cleaned and disinfected.

Discarding Biodegradable Trash

Biodegradable trash is refuse that will decompose naturally into less complex compounds. It includes items such as unconsumed beverages, paper tissues, the contents of drainage collectors, urine, and stool. All these items can be flushed down the toilet in the client's room. Chemicals and filtration methods in sewage treatment centers are sufficient for destroying pathogens in human wastes.

Nurses place bulkier items in a lined trash container and remove them from the room by single or double bagging. They wrap moist items such as soiled dressings so that during their containment, flying or crawling insects cannot transfer pathogens. Eventually, the bag and its contents are destroyed by incineration, or they are autoclaved. Autoclaved items can be safely disposed of in landfills.

Removing Reusable Items

To reduce the need for disinfection of reusable items, disposable equipment and supplies such as plastic bedpans, basins, eating utensils, and paper plates and cups are used as much as possible. Following the termination of transmission-based precautions, equipment that will be used again for other client care must first be thoroughly cleaned, disinfected, and sterilized (see Chap. 10).

Delivering Laboratory Specimens

Specimens are delivered to the laboratory in sealed containers in a plastic biohazard bag. When the testing is complete, most specimens are flushed, incinerated, or sterilized.

Transporting Clients

Clients with infectious diseases may need to be transported to other areas such as the X-ray department. During transport, nurses use methods to prevent the spread of pathogens either directly or indirectly from the client. For example, to prevent the exit of pathogens from the client onto transport equipment, nurses line the surface of the wheelchair or stretcher with a clean sheet or bath blanket to protect the surface from direct client contact. They use a second sheet or blanket to cover as much of the client's body as possible during transport. The client wears a mask or particulate air filter respirator if the pathogen is transmitted by the airborne or droplet route. Any hospital personnel having direct contact with the client use PPE similar to that used in client care.

Interdepartmental coordination is important. The department to which the client is transported is made aware that the client has an infectious disease. This facilitates the expeditious care of the client and avoids unnecessary waiting in areas with other clients.

When the client returns, the nurse deposits the soiled linen in the linen hamper in the client's room, touching only the outside surface of the protective covers. Some agencies also spray or wash the transport vehicle with a disinfectant before reuse.

PYSCHOLOGICAL IMPLICATIONS

Although infection control measures are necessary, they often leave clients feeling shunned or abandoned. Clients with infectious diseases continue to need human contact and interaction, both of which are often minimal because of the elaborate precautions taken on entering and leaving the room. Fearful family and friends may avoid visiting, and clients are restricted from leaving their rooms. Measures are needed to relieve the client's feelings of isolation by providing social interaction and sensory stimulation.

Promoting Social Interaction

When transmission-based precautions are in effect, it is important to plan frequent contact with the client. Nurses encourage visitors to come as often as the agency's policies and the client's condition permit. They use every opportunity to emphasize that as long as visitors follow the infection control precautions, they are not likely to acquire the disease.

Combating Sensory Deprivation

Sensory deprivation results when a person experiences insufficient sensory stimulation or is exposed to sensory stimulation that is continuous and monotonous. The goal is to provide a variety of sensory experiences at intervals (see Nursing Guidelines 22-1).

NURSING IMPLICATIONS

Caring for clients with infectious diseases involves meeting their physical and emotional needs. Some frequently identified nursing diagnoses include the following:

- Risk for Infection
- Ineffective Protection
- Risk for Infection Transmission (not currently on the NANDA list)
- Impaired Social Interaction
- Social Isolation
- Risk for Loneliness
- Deficient Diversional Activity
- Powerlessness
- Fear

Nursing Care Plan 22-1 demonstrates how nurses apply the nursing process when caring for a client with the nursing diagnosis of Risk for Infection Transmission. The North American Nursing Diagnosis Association has not currently approved this diagnostic category, but Carpenito-Moyet (2010, p. 331) defines it as "a person at high risk for transferring an infectious agent to others."

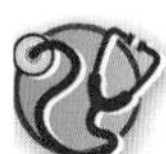

NURSING GUIDELINES 22-1

Providing Sensory Stimulation

- Move the bed to various places in the room or periodically rearrange the furnishings in the room. *Such a change provides a new perspective for the client.*
- Position the client so that he or she can look out the window. *Having something different to look at reduces boredom.*
- Encourage the client to use the telephone. *Telephone calls allow social interaction.*
- Communicate using the intercom system if entering the room is inconvenient. *This shows that the nurse is paying attention to the client.*
- Converse with the client about current world events. *Conversation stimulates the client's thought processes.*
- Help the client to select television or radio programs. *Watching television or listening to the radio engages the client's attention.*
- Change the location of equipment that produces monotonous sounds. *Changing the location will vary the volume or pitch of the noise.*
- Encourage the client to be active, within the confines of the room. *Activity provides a means of stimulation.*
- Encourage activities that the client can do independently such as reading, working crossword puzzles, playing solitaire, and putting picture puzzles together. *Such activities are diverting.*
- Offer a wide choice of foods with different flavors, temperatures, and textures. *Eating a variety of foods stimulates oral and olfactory sensations.*
- Use touch appropriately by giving a backrub or changing the client's position. *Touch produces tactile stimulation.*

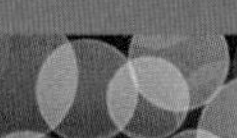

NURSING CARE PLAN 22-1 Risk for Infection Transmission

Assessment

- Monitor laboratory test findings for evidence of infection such as an elevated white blood cell count or the results of a culture indicating the growth of a pathogen.
- Check the client's temperature regularly and note if there is a persistent elevation.
- Inspect the skin, mucous membranes, wounds, sputum, urine, and stool for signs of purulent or unusual drainage.
- Listen for abnormal lung sounds, especially if the client has a cough.
- Inspect the area around invasive devices such as an intravenous catheter, wound drain, abdominal feeding tube, and so on.
- Ask whether the client has a decreased appetite, has lost weight, or feels weak and tired.
- Inquire about recent travel in a country or area where there has been an incidence of infectious disease or contact with others who have been ill lately.
- Ask about the client's immunization history.
- Read the results of a current skin test for tuberculosis or refer to a person who is certified to do so.

Nursing Diagnosis. **Risk for infection transmission** related to the airborne spread of the pathogen causing TB (positive TB test and suspicious chest X-ray).

Expected Outcome. The client will comply with infection control measures and accurately describe postdischarge drug therapy and medical follow-up by time of discharge.

Interventions	Rationales
Follow airborne transmission precautions until sputum culture is negative; follow standard precautions throughout the length of stay.	Airborne transmission precautions are the specified infection control measures for preventing the spread of TB to susceptible individuals. Nurses implement standard precautions during the care of all clients. Once sputum specimens are free of infectious microorganisms, the client will no longer require airborne transmission precautions.
Post infection control measures on the room door, but do not identify the name of the disease.	Posting instructions on the client's door informs personnel, family, and friends how to protect themselves from contact with organisms that can cause the infectious disease. Privacy regulations require that the client's health problem be kept confidential.
Wear a particulate air filter respirator during client care.	A particulate air filter respirator is more efficient than a cloth or paper mask because it can filter particles 0.3 micron in size with a minimum efficiency of 95%.
Teach the client to cover his or her nose and mouth with a paper tissue when coughing, sneezing, or laughing, and dispose of tissue in a paper bag.	A paper tissue collects moist respiratory secretions and decreases airborne transmission. Paper is disposable and is incinerated to destroy microorganisms present in secretions.
Directly observe the client taking prescribed drug therapy.	A combination of various medications can eliminate the infectious organism that causes TB when a client is compliant with drug therapy.
Explain the purpose of combination drug therapy and the need to continue its uninterrupted administration to avoid treatment failure and the development of a drug-resistant strain.	An informed and knowledgeable client promotes compliance.
Direct the client to provide a sputum specimen at the public health department within 2 to 3 weeks following discharge.	Continued monitoring of the client's sputum provides a means for evaluating whether the client is noninfectious and responding to treatment.
Recommend TB skin testing for close family members or friends.	TB is usually spread among those who have close contact with the infected person. Any person who previously had a negative skin test and now tests positive is placed on prophylactic drug therapy.

Evaluation of Expected Outcome

- The client remained in a private infection control room.
- The client used a paper tissue when coughing, sneezing, and talking.
- The client took all prescribed medications.
- The client's family and friends followed posted infection control instructions.
- The client's wife and children have received TB skin tests with negative results.
- The client verbalized how to self-administer his medications and the importance for remaining compliant.
- The client identified the date for a follow-up appointment with the Public Health Department for a repeat of sputum analysis.

Client and Family Teaching 22-1 Preventing Infections

The nurse teaches the client and the family as follows:

- Bathe daily and perform other forms of personal hygiene such as oral care.
- Keep the home environment clean and uncluttered.
- Use diluted household bleach (1:10 or 1:100) as a disinfectant.
- Obtain appropriate adult immunizations (tetanus vaccine at 10-year intervals, influenza vaccine yearly). A pneumococcal pneumonia immunization lasts a lifetime or revaccination is required every 5 years for extremely high-risk people.
- Investigate necessary vaccines, water purification techniques, and foods to avoid when traveling outside the United States.
- Practice a healthy lifestyle such as eating the recommended number of servings from the MyPlate nutrition guidelines (see Chap. 15).
- Perform frequent handwashing, especially before eating, after contact with nasal secretions, and after using the toilet.
- Use disposable tissues rather than a cloth handkerchief for nasal and oral secretions.
- Avoid sharing personal care items such as washcloths and towels, razors, and cups.
- Stay home from work or school when ill rather than exposing others to infectious pathogens.
- Assume the task of cooking if the family member who usually cooks is ill.
- Keep food refrigerated until use.
- Cook food thoroughly.
- Avoid crowds and public places during outbreaks of influenza.
- Follow infection control instructions when visiting hospitalized family members and friends.
- Comply with drug therapy when prescribed.

Nurses also play a pivotal role by teaching measures to prevent infection (see Client and Family Teaching 22-1).

CRITICAL THINKING EXERCISES

1. Give some reasons why controlling the spread of infectious diseases is difficult among children cared for in day-care centers.
2. Discuss some reasons why new cases of AIDS occur despite the fact that its mode of transmission is known.
3. What action(s) is/are appropriate to take if there are several residents in a long-term care facility who acquire an infection with a transmittable pathogen and there are not enough private rooms to relocate them?
4. If there is an outbreak in the community of H1N1 viral influenza A (swine flu), what measures might a long-term health care facility take to protect clients?

NCLEX-STYLE REVIEW QUESTIONS

1. When a nurse empties the secretions from a wound suction container, which of the following infection control measures is most important?
   1. Wear a mask
   2. Wear a gown
   3. Wear goggles
   4. Wear gloves
2. When a person comes to the emergency department with respiratory symptoms, which of the following infection control measures is appropriate to use initially?
   1. Contact precautions
   2. Airborne precautions
   3. Respiratory hygiene/cough etiquette
   4. Droplet precautions
3. When exiting the room of a client being cared for with contact precautions, what is the first step in removing personal protection items?
   1. Take off the mask or particulate air respirator
   2. Unfasten the waist tie at the back of the gown
   3. Unfasten the tie at the neck closure of the gown
   4. Remove gloves one at a time
4. What is the best advice the nurse can give to someone who is allergic to latex, yet must wear gloves for standard precautions?
   1. Rinse the latex gloves with running tap water before donning them
   2. Apply a petroleum ointment to both hands before donning latex gloves
   3. Eliminate wearing gloves, but wash both hands vigorously with alcohol afterward
   4. Wear two pairs of vinyl gloves when there is a potential for contact with blood or body fluid
5. Other than obtaining an immunization against influenza, what is the best advice the nurse can give to high-risk people to avoid acquiring this infection?
   1. Consume adequate vitamin C
   2. Avoid going to crowded places
   3. Dress warmly in cold weather
   4. Reduce daily stress and anxiety

SKILL 22-1 Removing Personal Protective Equipment

Suggested Action	Reason for Action
ASSESSMENT	
Determine which type of infection control precautions is being used.	Indicates whether garments must be removed and discarded within the room.
Note whether there are sufficient hand hygiene supplies, paper towels, a laundry hamper, and a lined waste receptacle within the room.	Provides a means for hand antisepsis and confining soiled garments and materials.
PLANNING	
Make sure that all direct care of the client has been completed.	Avoids having to don barrier garments a second time.
IMPLEMENTATION	
Untie the waist closure if it is fastened at the front of the cover gown; if it is secured on the backside, proceed with removing gloves.	The front of the cover gown is considered grossly contaminated.
Remove one glove by grasping at the wrist and pulling the glove inside out with a gloved hand (Fig. A).	Contains the contaminated surface inside the glove.
A	Removing the first glove.
Insert the fingers of the ungloved hand under the wrist of the remaining glove.	Reduces contact with the most contaminated surface of the gloves.
Pull the remaining glove inside out while holding the first removed glove (Fig. B)	Enfolds the contaminated surface inside the glove.
B	Removing the second glove.

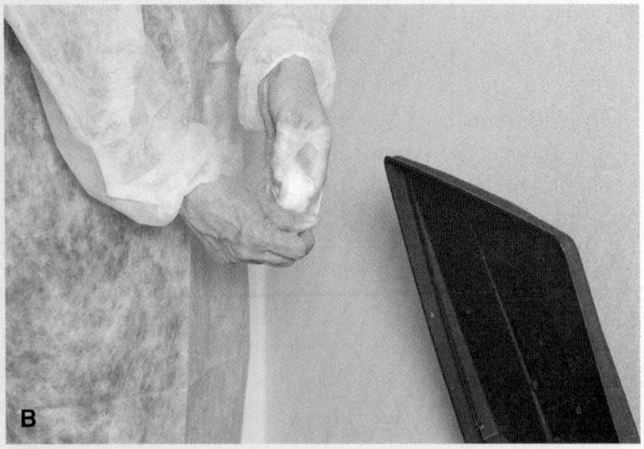

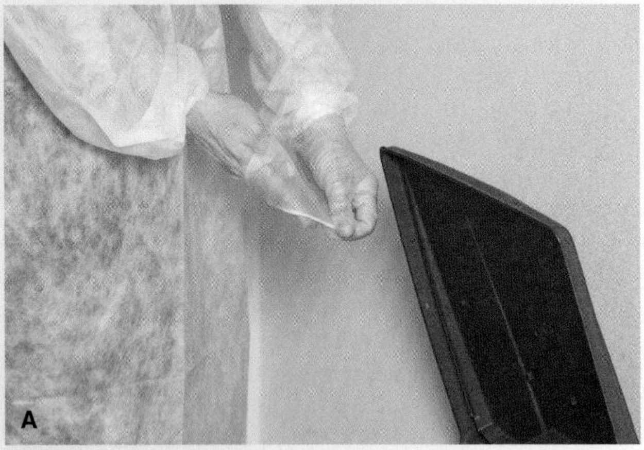

(continued)

Removing Personal Protective Equipment (continued)

IMPLEMENTATION (CONTINUED)

Action	Rationale
Wash hands or perform an alcohol-based hand rub (see Chap. 10).	Removes microorganisms from the surface of previously gloved hands.
Remove mask (see Chap. 10) or other disposable face-protection items by touching only the ties or elastic bands and discard them in the waste container (Fig. C).	The ties or other materials used to attach the mask or other face protection items are considered "clean" and can be touched with the bare hands; the surface covering the eyes and face are considered contaminated.

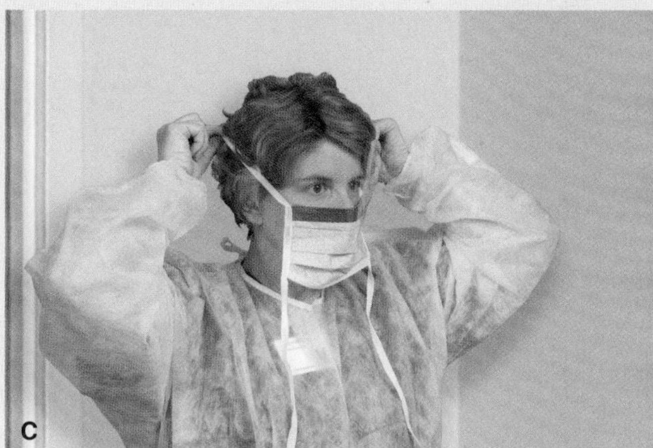

Unfastening ties.

Action	Rationale
Untie or unfasten the neck and then the back closure of the cover gown.	The back of the gown is considered less contaminated than the front and can be touched with the bare hands.
Remove the gown by inserting your fingers at the shoulder and pulling the gown forward to turn the gown inside out (Fig. D).	Prevents gross contamination of the hands with contaminated areas of the gown.

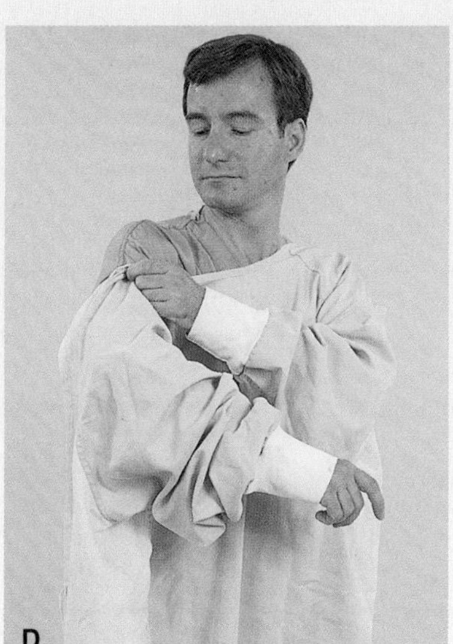

Removing a cover gown. (Photo by B. Proud.)

Action	Rationale
Fold the soiled side of the gown to the inside while holding it away from your uniform.	Prevents contamination of the hands and uniform.

(continued)

Removing Personal Protective Equipment (continued)

IMPLEMENTATION (CONTINUED)

Roll up the gown with the inner surface exposed and discard it in the waste container if it is made of paper. If the gown is made of cloth, discard it in the laundry hamper in the room (Fig. E).

Confines contaminated garments.

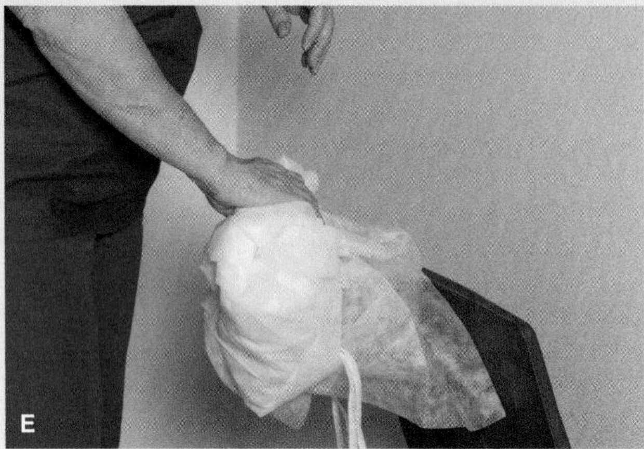

Discarding the cover gown.

Wash hands or perform an alcohol-based hand rub.

Removes microorganisms that may have been inadvertently transferred during face protection items and gown removal.

Use a clean paper towel to open the room door.

Protects clean hands from recontamination.

Discard the paper towel in the waste container in the client's room.

Confines contaminated material.

Leave the room, taking care not to touch anything.

Prevents recontamination.

Go directly to the utility room and perform hand antisepsis one final time.

Removes microorganisms; it is always safer to overdo than underdo any practice that controls the spread of pathogens.

Evaluation

- Appropriate PPE was worn.
- Garments were removed with the least contamination possible.
- Hand washing was performed appropriately.

Document

- Type of transmission-based precautions being followed
- Care provided
- Response of client

SAMPLE DOCUMENTATION

Date and Time Contact precautions followed. Assisted with bath while wearing gloves and gown. States, "I wish the door to my room could be left opened. It gets rather boring in here." Reinforced the purpose for keeping the door closed. ——— SIGNATURE/TITLE

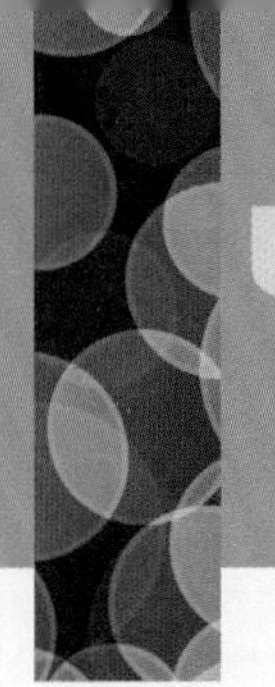

UNIT 5

End of Unit Exercises for Chapters 15, 16, 17, 18, 19, 20, 21, and 22

Section I: Reviewing What You've Learned

Activity A: *Fill in the blanks by choosing the correct word from the options given in parentheses.*

1. __________________ can result from a combination of sugar, plaque, and bacteria eroding the tooth enamel. (Caries, Gingivitis, Tartar)
2. A/an __________________ treats eye disorders medically and surgically. (ophthalmologist, optometrist, podiatrist)
3. __________________ is a waking state characterized by reduced activity and decreased mental stimulation. (Comfort, Rest, Sleep)
4. __________________ refers to disturbances in the sleep–wake cycle in which there is arousal or partial arousal, usually during transitions in NREM periods of sleep. (Hypersomnia, Insomnia, Parasomnia)
5. __________________ can result from airway obstruction, drowning, or inhalation of noxious gases such as smoke or carbon monoxide. (Asphyxiation, Macroshock, Poisoning)
6. A(n) __________________ is a substance that confines electrical currents so that they do not scatter. (conductor, ground, insulator)
7. __________________ is the conversion of chemical information at the cellular level into electrical impulses that move toward the spinal cord. (Perception, Transduction, Transmission)
8. __________________ pain is discomfort arising from diseased or injured internal organs. (Cutaneous, Neuropathic, Visceral)
9. __________________ is a loss of appetite associated with illness, altered taste and smell, oral problems, or tension and depression. (Anorexia, Cachexia, Nausea)
10. __________________, which commonly accompanies nausea, is the loss of stomach contents through the mouth. (Emesis, Regurgitation, Retching)
11. Electrolytes with a positive charge are called __________________. (anions, cations, ions)
12. __________________ is a fluid imbalance with an increased volume of water in the intravascular fluid compartment. (Hypervolemia, Hypoalbuminemia, Hypovolemia)
13. Insufficient oxygen in the arterial blood is called __________________. (hypocarbia, hypoxemia, hypoxia)
14. A caregiver should use __________________ to avoid infectious diseases transmitted by direct contact with a client's body, blood, or body substances. (gloves, hand lotion, towels)
15. __________________ is the intentional diversion of attention from an unpleasant sensory experience to one that is neutral or more pleasant. (Distraction, Imagery, Meditation)

Activity B: *Mark each statement as either T (True) or F (False). Correct any false statements.*

1. T____F____ The cells in the epidermis are shed continuously and replaced from the dermis.
2. T____F____ The contraction of small arrector pili muscles around hair follicles is commonly described as goose bumps.
3. T____F____ Sedatives produce a relaxing and calming effect in older clients, thus promoting rest.
4. T____F____ The EEG waves produced during REM sleep appear similar to those produced during wakefulness.

5. T____F____ Carbon dioxide is an odorless gas released during the incomplete combustion of fossil fuels commonly used to heat homes.

6. T____F____ A person with intact skin usually does not feel microshock.

7. T____F____ The Wong-Baker FACES scale can be used to assess pain in clients with language barriers.

8. T____F____ Adjuvant drugs are used as a first-line treatment for pain.

9. T____F____ Flatus is a discharge of gas from the stomach through the mouth.

10. T____F____ Dehydration is a fluid deficit in both the extracellular and intracellular compartments of the human body.

11. T____F____ Passive diffusion is an identical balance of cations with anions in any given fluid compartment.

12. T____F____ Pursed-lip breathing is a form of controlled ventilation in which the client consciously prolongs the expiration phase.

13. T____F____ Oxygen toxicity is lung damage that develops when oxygen concentrations of more than 20% are administered for longer than 24 hours.

14. T____F____ Infection control precautions are physical measures designed to curtail the spread of contagious diseases.

15. T____F____ When preparing to assist with a surgical or obstetric procedure, the nurse should perform a surgical scrub before applying a mask and hair cover.

Activity C: *Write the correct term for each description below.*

1. Practices that promote health through personal cleanliness ____________________
2. Dried crusts containing mucus, microorganisms, and epithelial cells shed from the mucous membrane ____________________
3. Sudden loss of muscle tone triggered by an emotional change, such as laughing or anger ____________________
4. Hormone secreted by the pineal gland in the absence of bright light ____________________
5. A condition in which fluid occupies the airway and interferes with ventilation ____________________
6. An inactive substance that resembles medication and can relieve symptoms, like pain, despite the absence of any active chemicals ____________________
7. Sensory nerve receptor activated by noxious stimuli ____________________
8. Anthropometric measurement that helps to determine a client's skeletal muscle mass ____________________
9. Fluid in the tissue space between and around cells ____________________
10. Naturally produced morphine-like chemicals that reduce pain ____________________

Activity D: *1. Match the terms related to nutrition in Column A with their descriptions in Column B.*

Column A	Column B
1. ____________________ Proteins	A. Noncaloric substances in food that are essential to all cells
2. ____________________ Carbohydrates	B. Nutrients that contain glyceride molecules and are collectively known as lipids
3. ____________________ Minerals	C. Nutrients composed of amino acids (chemical compounds containing nitrogen, carbon, hydrogen, and oxygen)
4. ____________________ Fats	D. Nutrients that include sugars and starches

2. Match the types of fire extinguishers in Column A with their uses in Column B.

Column A		Column B
1. ________________	Class A	A. Fires caused by gasoline, oil, paint, grease, and other flammable liquids
2. ________________	Class B	B. Fires caused by electricity
3. ________________	Class C	C. Fires of any kind
4. ________________	Class ABC	D. Fires caused by burning paper, wood, or cloth

3. Match the terms related to body fluids and chemical balance in Column A with their descriptions in Column B.

Column A		Column B
1. ________________	Venipuncture	A. Process by which body fluid is distributed from one location to another
2. ________________	Emulsion	B. Method of accessing the venous system by piercing a vein with a needle
3. ________________	Edema	C. Mixture of two liquids, one of which is insoluble in the other
4. ________________	Osmosis	D. Condition that develops when excess fluid is distributed to the interstitial space

Activity E: *1. Differentiate between crystalloid and colloid solutions.*

	Crystalloid Solution	Colloid Solution
Definition		
Effects		
Examples		

2. Differentiate between acute and chronic pain.

	Acute Pain	Chronic Pain
Duration		
Cause		
Site of pain		
Relief of pain		

3. Differentiate between inspiration and expiration.

	Inspiration	*Expiration*
Definition		
Process		
Additional muscles involved		

Activity F: *Consider the following figure.*

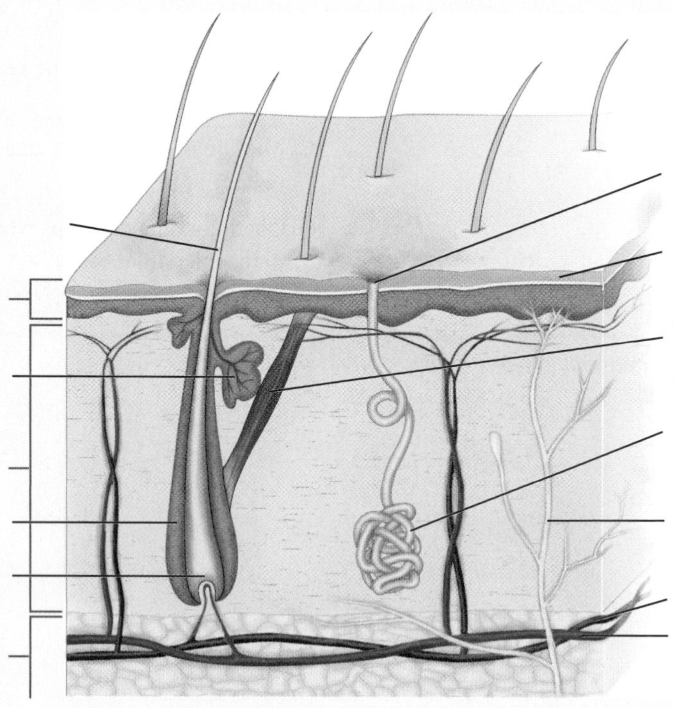

1. Identify and label the figure.

Activity G:

1. Pain is an unpleasant sensation usually associated with disease or injury. People experience pain in four phases. Write down in the boxes below the correct sequence of the phases in the pain process.
   a. Perception
   b. Transmission
   c. Modulation
   d. Transduction

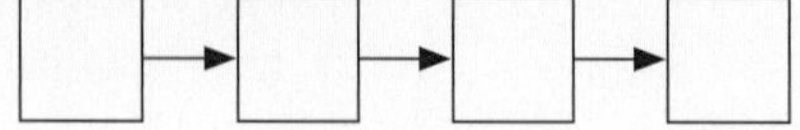

2. Incentive spirometry, a technique for deep breathing using a calibrated device, encourages clients to reach a goal-directed volume of inspired air. Write down in the boxes below the correct sequence for using an incentive spirometer.
   a. Hold the breath for 3 to 6 seconds.
   b. Sit upright unless contraindicated.
   c. Insert the mouthpiece, sealing it between the lips.
   d. Exhale normally.
   e. Relax and breathe normally before the next breath with the spirometer.
   f. Identify the mark indicating the goal for inhalation.
   g. Remove the mouthpiece and exhale normally.
   h. Inhale slowly and deeply until the predetermined volume has been reached.

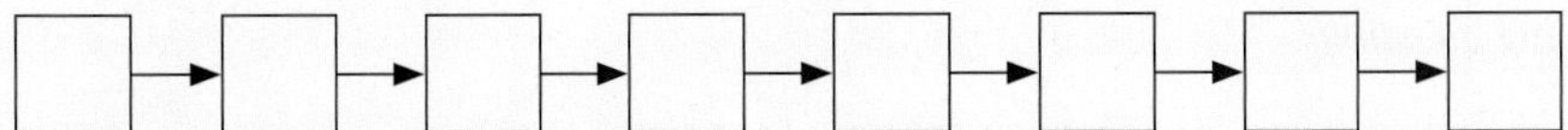

Activity H: *Answer the following questions.*

1. What is an infrared listening device?

2. How should the nurse care for a client's dentures?

3. What are the benefits of sleep?

4. What are the four categories of drugs that promote or interfere with sleep?

5. What is a thermal burn?

6. What are environmental hazards? Give examples.

7. What are the six nutritional components in food?

8. What are the seven common hospital diets?

9. What is parenteral nutrition?

10. What are the reasons for administering intravenous solutions?

11. Which two surgical procedures may be used when other methods of pain management are ineffective?

12. What is addiction?

13. Why are adhesive nasal strips used?

14. What are the uses and common characteristics of medical cover gowns?

Section II: Applying Your Knowledge

Activity I: *Give rationales for the following questions.*

1. Why is it important for the nurse to consult the client regarding a convenient time for a bath?

2. Why are diuretics administered early in the morning?

3. Why should the nurse suggest that the client with a disturbed sleep pattern reduce or eliminate caffeine intake?

4. Why are victims of cold-water drowning more likely to be resuscitated?

5. Why is high-density lipoprotein (HDL) referred to as good cholesterol?

6. Why do the plastic bags of intravenous solutions not need vented tubing?

7. When is it preferable to administer analgesic drugs on a scheduled basis?

8. Why is it important to use a humidifier when administering 4 L or more oxygen?

9. What is the purpose for implementing contact precautions during client care?

Activity J: *Answer the following questions focusing on nursing roles and responsibilities.*

1. A nurse is providing oral care for a client in a coma.
   a. What risks are involved in giving oral care to this client?

   b. What precautions should the nurse take when providing oral care for the client?

2. A nurse is caring for a client with a disturbed sleep pattern who cannot sleep for more than 4 hours most nights.
   a. What measures could the nurse take to promote the client's sleep?

   b. What methods could the nurse use to promote relaxation of the sleep-disturbed client's muscles and improve blood circulation?

3. A nurse is caring for a client who keeps tugging at the line being used for intravenous therapy.
   a. What should the nurse do before considering the use of any restraint?

   b. What are the nurse's responsibilities if a restraint is applied to the client?

4. A nurse is preparing to provide perineal care to a client who has given birth vaginally.
   a. What precautions should the nurse take when providing perineal care to the client?

   b. For what reasons would a sitz bath be beneficial to this client?

5. A client has been instructed to perform diaphragmatic breathing to reduce respiratory effort and relieve rapid, ineffective breathing. How should the nurse instruct this client to perform diaphragmatic breathing?

6. A nurse at an extended-care facility is using transmission-based precautions while caring for a client with acute diarrhea caused by an infectious microorganism.
   a. What transmission-based precautions should the nurse take when caring for this client?
   b. What actions should the nurse perform when discarding biodegradable trash from this client and his or her room?

7. A nurse at an extended-care facility is caring for a client having difficulty chewing and swallowing food.
   a. What kind of a diet is best for this client?
   b. What interventions should the nurse perform when feeding the client?

8. A nurse is caring for a client who has been ordered intravenous therapy.
   a. What actions should the nurse perform before preparing the intravenous solution?
   b. What technique will the nurse follow to remove air bubbles from the tubing?

Activity K: *Consider the following questions. Discuss them with your instructor or peers.*

1. A nurse is caring for an elderly client with Alzheimer's disease at an extended-care facility. Sometimes the client is alert and oriented; at other times, she is agitated or unaware of her surroundings. During periods of confusion and disorientation, the client needs assistance with activities of daily living and hygiene.
   a. How should the nurse assist the client with activities of daily living?
   b. What actions should the nurse take with respect to the client's hygiene?

2. A nurse is caring for a client who is to undergo surgery the following day. The client is anxious and cannot sleep.
   a. What interventions should the nurse perform to help the client relax?
   b. How can the nurse ensure that the client gets adequate sleep?

3. A fire erupts in the storeroom of the health care facility following an electrical short circuit. The storage area contains papers, books, and gauze dressing supplies. The fire spreads quickly toward the clients' rooms.
   a. How can the nurse ensure the safety of clients in this situation?
   b. What are the nurse's responsibilities during a fire?

4. A nurse is caring for a client who has undergone an amputation of the left leg and is experiencing pain at the severed site.
   a. What methods should the nurse use to divert the client's attention from the pain?
   b. What actions should the nurse perform when administering ordered drugs for pain relief?

5. During assessment of an adolescent in her first trimester of pregnancy, the nurse learns that the client smokes regularly. The client plans to care for the baby herself.
    a. What are the possible implications for the client's respiratory health and the health of the baby?
    b. What client teaching should the nurse provide?
6. A physician has ordered a transfusion to compensate for blood loss in a client following a severe accident.
    a. What procedures should the nurse perform before the blood transfusion?
    b. What actions should the nurse perform during the transfusion?
7. A nurse is required to clean and dress pressure ulcers on the feet of a client with restricted mobility.
    a. What actions should the nurse take to promote healing of the pressure ulcers?
    b. What precautions should the nurse take when changing this client's bed linens that contain serous drainage?

Section III: Getting Ready for NCLEX

Activity L: *Answer the following questions.*

1. Which of the following measures is most appropriate when cleaning plastic eyeglasses?
    a. Use paper tissue to clean the lenses.
    b. Rinse the lenses with running tap water.
    c. Immerse the lenses in hot soapy water.
    d. Allow the lenses to air dry.
2. A client with hypersomnolence related to seasonal affective disorder has been prescribed phototherapy. Which of the following points should the nurse include in the client teaching?
    a. Wear eyeglasses or contact lenses with ultraviolet filters.
    b. Sit 5 feet from the artificial light during phototherapy.
    c. Look at the artificial light continuously.
    d. Repeat exposure to artificial light up to 3 to 6 hours a day.
3. During a routine well child visit, the nurse needs to teach parents safety measures to prevent childhood poisoning. Which of the following should the nurse tell the parents?
    a. Discard old medications in the wastebasket.
    b. Tell the child that medication is sweet to help him or her take it.
    c. Keep the home ventilated when using aerosol sprays.
    d. Carry regular medications in purses.
4. A client with cancer is receiving patient-controlled analgesia (PCA). During the client teaching about the equipment, which of the following should the nurse tell the client?
    a. Pain relief is slow and long lasting.
    b. PCA requires less of the drug overall to control pain.
    c. Ambulation may be difficult.
    d. Complications from immobility may arise.
5. A nurse is caring for a client with hypoxia. What position should the nurse assist the client to assume to best facilitate improved breathing?
    a. Lie flat on the back.
    b. Sit with the bed inclined 15 degrees.
    c. Lie on the left side.
    d. Lean forward over the bedside table.

6. A nurse is caring for a client recovering from tuberculosis. What infection control interventions should the nurse follow? Select all that apply.
   a. Ask family members and friends to obtain a tuberculosis skin test.
   b. Ask the client to use paper tissues when coughing and then dispose of them.
   c. Keep the client's wheelchair or stretcher covered with a clean sheet.
   d. Read and analyze the client's latest skin test report for tuberculosis.
   e. Wear a particulate air filter respirator during client care.
7. A client who has been hospitalized and is recuperating from pneumonia is complaining of stomach gas. Which of the following interventions should the nurse perform? Select all that apply.
   a. Encourage walking if possible.
   b. Suggest drinking carbonated beverages.
   c. Provide a straw for drinking.
   d. Ask the client to avoid chewing gum.
   e. Remind the client to chew with the mouth closed.
8. Which of the following nursing interventions are appropriate for a client who is on fluid restrictions? Select all that apply.
   a. Suggest rinsing the mouth without swallowing water.
   b. Provide fluids in a plastic squeeze bottle or spray atomizer.
   c. Explain the need to restrict fluids in the diet.
   d. Encourage the intake of food with a moderately high salt content.

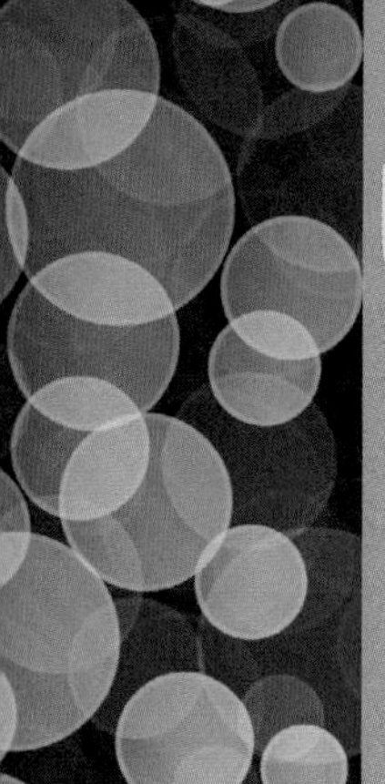

UNIT 6
Assisting the Inactive Client

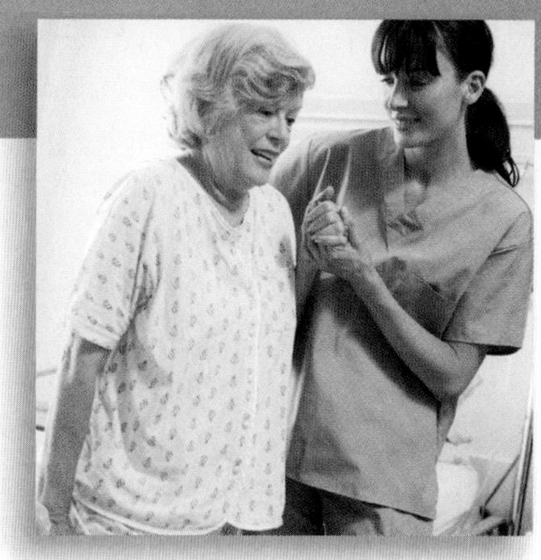

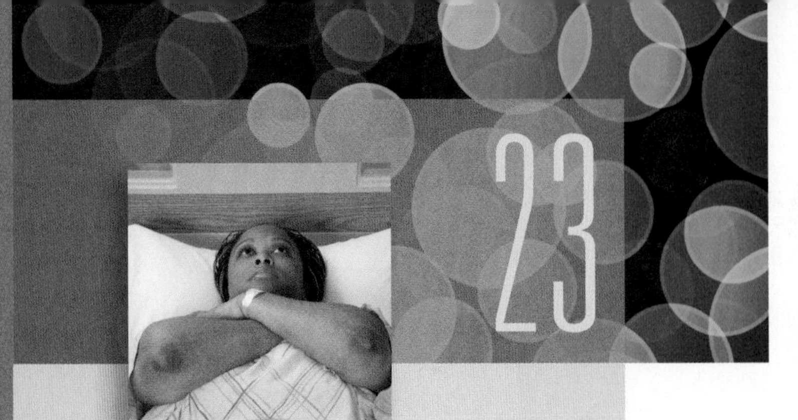

23 Body Mechanics, Positioning, and Moving

Words To Know

alignment
anatomic position
balance
bariatric client
base of support
bed board
body mechanics
center of gravity
contractures
disuse syndrome
energy
ergonomics
foot drop
Fowler's position
functional mobility
functional position
gravity
lateral oblique position
lateral position
line of gravity
muscle spasms
neutral position
posture
prone position
repetitive strain injuries
shearing
Sims' position
supine position
transfer

Learning Objectives

On completion of this chapter, the reader should be able to:

1. Identify characteristics of good posture in a standing, sitting, or lying position.
2. Describe three principles of correct body mechanics.
3. Explain the purpose of ergonomics.
4. Give at least two examples of ergonomic recommendations in the workplace.
5. Describe at least 10 signs or symptoms associated with the disuse syndrome.
6. Describe six common client positions.
7. Explain the purpose of five different positioning devices used for safety and comfort.
8. Name one advantage for each of three different pressure-relieving devices.
9. Discuss four types of transfer devices.
10. Give at least five general guidelines that apply to transferring clients.

Inactivity leads to deterioration of health. Multiple complications can occur among people with limited activity and movement (Table 23-1).

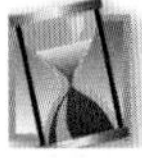

Gerontologic Considerations

- By the 7th or 8th decade of life, muscle strength, endurance, and coordination decline. Older adults need to maintain as much mobility as possible to prevent disability.
- The risk for social isolation among older adults increases as mobility is limited.

The consequences of inactivity are collectively referred to as **disuse syndrome** (signs and symptoms that result from inactivity). Nursing care activities such as positioning and moving clients reduce the potential for disuse syndrome. Nurses can become injured, however, if they fail to use good posture and body mechanics while performing these activities.

This chapter describes how to position and move clients to prevent complications associated with inactivity. It also discusses methods for protecting nurses from work-related injuries. Basic terms are defined in Table 23-2.

TABLE 23-1 Dangers of Inactivity

SYSTEMS	EFFECTS
Muscular	Weakness Decreased tone/strength Decreased size (atrophy)
Skeletal	Poor posture Contractures Foot drop
Cardiovascular	Impaired circulation Thrombus (clot) formation Dependent edema
Respiratory	Pooling of secretions Shallow respirations Atelectasis (collapsed alveoli)
Urinary	Oliguria (scanty urine) Urinary tract infections Calculi (stone) formation Incontinence (inability to control elimination)
Gastrointestinal	Anorexia (loss of appetite) Constipation Fecal impaction
Integumentary	Pressure sores
Endocrine	Decreased metabolic rate Decreased hormonal secretions
Central nervous	Sleep pattern disturbances Psychosocial changes

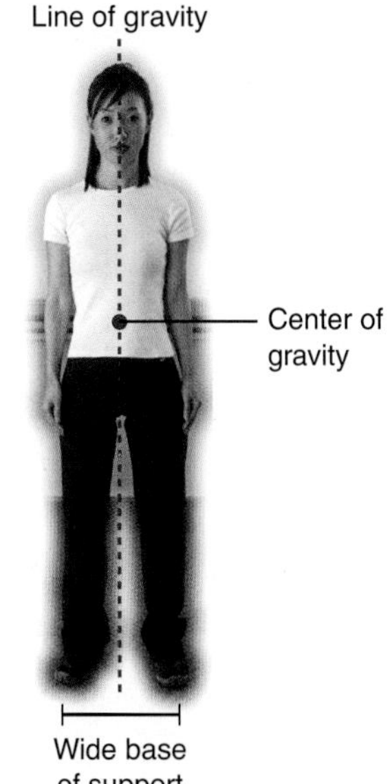

FIGURE 23-1 Good posture helps to align gravity through the center of the body. A wide stance provides a stable base for support.

MAINTAINING GOOD POSTURE

Posture (the position of the body, or the way in which it is held) affects a person's appearance, stamina, and ability to use the musculoskeletal system efficiently. Good posture, whether in a standing, sitting, or lying position, distributes gravity through the center of the body over a wide base of support (Fig. 23-1). Good posture is important for both clients and nurses.

When a person performs work while using poor posture, **muscle spasms** (sudden, forceful, and involuntary muscle contractions) often result. They occur more often when muscles are strained and forced to work beyond their capacity.

Standing

To maintain good posture in a standing position (Fig. 23-2):

- Keep the feet parallel, at right angles to the lower legs, and about 4 to 8 in. (10 to 20 cm) apart.
- Distribute weight equally on both feet to provide a broad base of support.

TABLE 23-2 Basic Terminology

TERM	DEFINITION AND EXAMPLE
Gravity	Force that pulls objects toward the center of the earth. The pull of gravity causes objects, such as an item dropped from the hand, to fall to the ground. It causes water to drain to its lowest level.
Energy	Capacity to do work. Energy is used to move the body from place to place. Energy is required to overcome the force of gravity.
Balance	Steady position with weight. A person falls when off balance.
Center of gravity	Point at which the mass of an object is centered. The center of gravity for a standing position is the center of the pelvis and about halfway between the umbilicus and the pubic bone.
Line of gravity	Imaginary vertical line that passes through the center of gravity. The line of gravity in a standing person is a straight line from the head to the feet through the center of the body.
Base of support	Area on which an object rests. The feet are the base of support when a person is in a standing position.
Alignment	Parts of an object being in proper relationship to one another. The body is in good alignment in a position of good posture.
Neutral position	The position of a limb that is turned neither toward nor away from the body's midline.
Anatomic position	Frontal and back views with arms at the sides and palms forward.
Functional position	Position in which an activity is performed properly and normally. In the hand, the wrists are slightly dorsiflexed between 20 and 35 degrees and the proximal finger joints are flexed between 45 and 60 degrees, with the thumb in opposition and in alignment with the pads of the fingers.

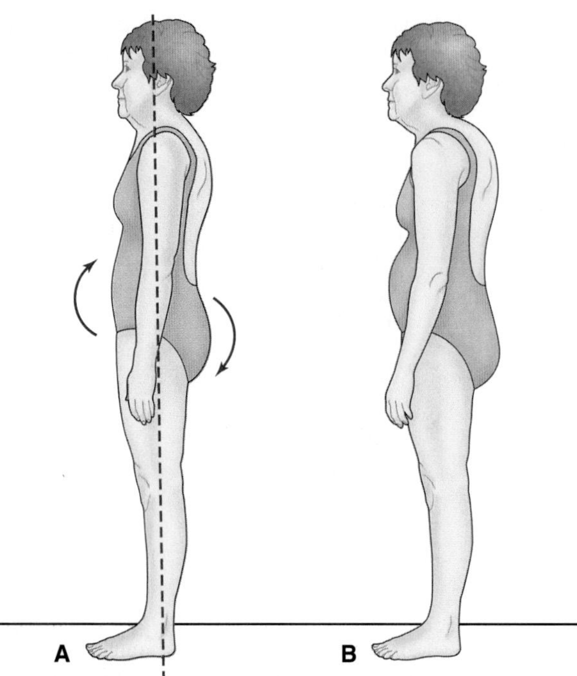

FIGURE 23-2 **A.** A good standing posture results when abdominal and gluteal muscles are contracted. **B.** A poor standing posture results when abdominal muscles are relaxed, causing altered body alignment.

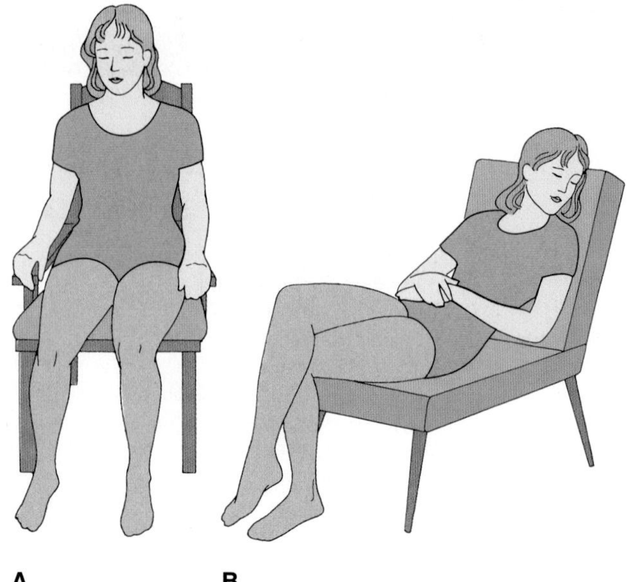

FIGURE 23-3 **A.** A correct sitting posture. **B.** An incorrect sitting posture. (Courtesy of Lowren West, New York, NY.)

- Bend the knees slightly to avoid straining the joints.
- Maintain the hips at an even level.
- Pull in the buttocks and hold the abdomen up and in to keep the spine properly aligned. This position supports the abdominal organs and reduces strain on both back and abdominal muscles.
- Hold the chest up and slightly forward and extend or stretch the waist to give internal organs more space and maintain good alignment of the spine.
- Keep the shoulders even and centered above the hips.
- Hold the head erect with the face forward and the chin slightly tucked.

Sitting

In a good sitting position (Fig. 23-3), the buttocks and upper thighs become the base of support. Both feet rest on the floor. The knees are bent, with the posterior of the knee free from the edge of the chair to avoid interfering with distal circulation.

Lying Down

Good posture in a lying position looks the same as in a standing position, except the person is horizontal (Fig. 23-4). The head and neck muscles are in a neutral position, centered between the shoulders. The shoulders are level, whereas the arms, hips, and knees are slightly flexed with no compression of the arms or legs under the body. The trunk is straight and the hips are level. The legs are parallel to each other with the feet at right angles to the leg.

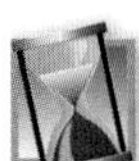
Gerontologic Considerations

■ Skeletal changes such as kyphosis, lordosis, or scoliosis change the older person's center of gravity. Also, pressure on cervical vertebrae from kyphotic changes while lying supine may be minimized by using a small towel roll or neck roll pillow.

BODY MECHANICS

The use of proper **body mechanics** (the efficient use of the musculoskeletal system) increases muscle effectiveness, reduces fatigue, and helps to avoid **repetitive strain injuries** (disorders that result from cumulative trauma to musculoskeletal

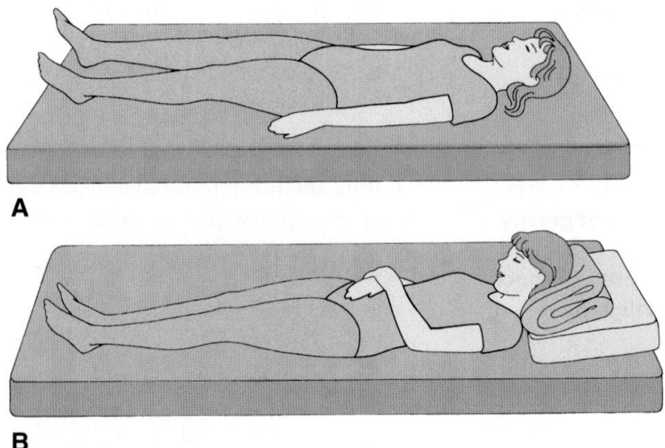

FIGURE 23-4 **A.** A correct lying posture. **B.** An incorrect lying posture. (Courtesy of Lowren West, New York, NY.)

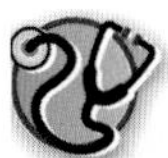

NURSING GUIDELINES 23-1

Using Good Body Mechanics

- Use the longest and strongest muscles of the arms and legs. *Use of these muscles provides the greatest strength and potential for performing work.*
- When lifting a heavy load, center it over the feet. *Such positioning creates a base of support.*
- Hold objects close to the body. *Doing so increases balance.*
- Bend the knees. *Bending the knees prepares the spine to accept the weight of the load.*
- Contract the abdominal muscles and make a long midriff. *Doing so protects the muscles of the abdomen and pelvis and prevents strain and injury to the abdominal wall.*
- Push, pull, or roll objects whenever possible rather than lifting them. *Lifting requires more effort.*
- Use body weight as a lever to assist with pushing or pulling an object. *This reduces muscle strain.*
- Keep feet apart for a broad base of support. *This stance lowers the center of gravity, which promotes stability.*
- Bend the knees and keep the back straight when lifting an object, rather than bending over from the waist with straight knees. *This stance makes best use of the longest and strongest body muscles and improves balance by keeping the weight of the object close to the center of gravity.*
- Avoid twisting and stretching muscles during work. *Twisting can strain muscles because the line of gravity is outside the body's base of support.*
- Rest between periods of exertion. *Resting promotes work endurance.*

structures). Basic principles of body mechanics are important regardless of a person's occupation or daily activities, but body mechanics alone will not necessarily reduce musculoskeletal injuries (see Nursing Guidelines 23-1).

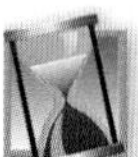

Gerontologic Considerations

■ An older person may be taught to use appropriate body mechanics, such as sitting in a chair to lift an object directly in front of it. Emphasize that the lifting of objects should be done only from directly in front to prevent pulling of lateral back muscles or vertebral disk compression.

ERGONOMICS

Using proper body mechanics is one component of preserving the integrity of the body, but body mechanics alone will not necessarily reduce musculoskeletal injuries. The other component is applying and implementing **ergonomics** (a specialty field of engineering science devoted to promoting comfort, performance, and health in the workplace). Ergonomics is used to improve the design of the work environment and equipment. The National Institute for Occupational Safety and Health (NIOSH), a division of the Centers for Disease Control and Prevention, requires employers to comply with many ergonomic recommendations. Examples include the following:

- Using assistive devices to lift or transport heavy items or clients.
- Using alternative equipment for tasks that require repetitive motions—for instance, telephone headsets or automatic staplers.
- Positioning equipment no more than 20 to 30 degrees away—about an arm's length—to avoid reaching or twisting the trunk or neck.
- Using a chair with good back support. A chair should be high enough so the user can place his or her feet firmly on the floor. There should be room for two fingers between the edge of the seat and the back of the knees. Arm rests should allow a relaxed shoulder position.
- Keeping the elbows flexed no more than 100 to 110 degrees, or use wrist rests to keep the wrists in a neutral position when working at a computer.
- Working under nonglare lighting.

Despite being taught principles of good body mechanics, health care workers, particularly nurses, are vulnerable to ergonomic hazards in the workplace as a direct consequence of (1) lifting heavy loads (ie, clients), (2) reaching and lifting with loads far from the body, (3) twisting while lifting, (4) unexpected changes in load demand during the lift, (5) reaching low or high to begin a lift, and (6) moving or carrying a load a significant distance (Fragala et al., 2005). Nursing personnel are among the occupational workers at the highest risk for musculoskeletal injuries (deCastro, 2004), a fact supported by the Department of Health and Human Services, which found that nurses experience 12.6 injuries per 100 full-time workers compared to 4.0 work-related injuries per 100 workers in mining, 7.9 in construction, and 8.1 in manufacturing (Pascale, 2007).

Because of the pervasiveness of the problem and its direct link to a shortage of employed nurses, the American Nurses Association (ANA) has taken an initiative to reduce injuries to nurses (and their clients) by recommending a "no lift policy," known as the *Handle With Care Campaign*, in the workplace. The campaign is an effort to reduce injuries through the use of assistive equipment and devices. Using assistive devices has many advantages (Box 23-1).

Health care agencies have already begun to implement the ANA guidelines. In 2009, two federal bills, H.R. 2381 and S. 1788, entitled Nurses and Healthcare Worker Protection Act of 2009 were introduced. The proposed legislation

BOX 23-1 Advantages of Assistive Devices

Nurses
- Lessens physical exertion during positioning, moving, and transferring clients
- Reduces musculoskeletal injuries
- Decreases sick or absentee time
- Lowers medical costs, pain, and suffering
- Decreases workman's compensation claims
- Maintains workforce of employed nurses

Clients
- Provides more security during repositioning and transfers from bed, chairs, toilets, stretchers
- Results in fewer handling mishaps and secondary injuries
- Relieves anxiety concerning safety
- Promotes comfort by reducing awkward or forceful manual handling
- Maintains dignity and self-esteem
- Promotes faster recovery

(Adapted from American Nurses Association. (2003). Handle with care campaign. Available at http://www.nursingworld.org/handlewithcare.)

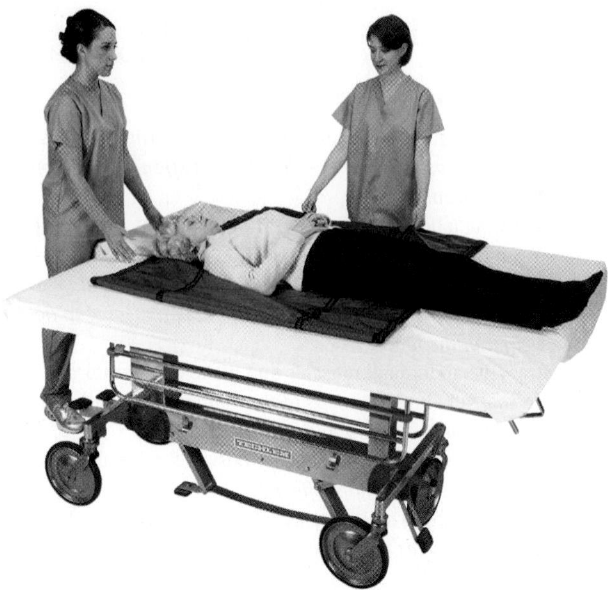

FIGURE 23-5 These nurses are using the Phil-e-slide Patient Handling System to transfer a client. (Photo courtesy of ErgoSafe Products, LLC. St. Louis, MO).

mandates safe patient/client movement for direct-care licensed nurses and other health care providers as a critical component in protecting health care workers and increasing patient/client safety (http://www.asphp.org/pdfs/SPH_Legislation_Update_March_2011.pdf). The congressional bills support methods to reduce risks associated with moving clients and evaluating alternatives or restricting manual lifting to emergency, life-threatening, or exceptional circumstances (Anderson, 2006). Voluntary changes in nursing practice, however, should not, and have not been delayed while waiting for federal legislative action; as of 2011, nine states have enacted safe client handling legislation.

POSITIONING CLIENTS

Good posture and body mechanics and ergonomically designed assistive devices are necessary when inactive clients require positioning and moving. An inactive client's position is changed to relieve pressure on bony areas of the body, promote **functional mobility** (an alignment that maintains the potential for movement and ambulation), and provide for therapeutic needs. General principles for positioning are as follows:

- Change the inactive client's position at least every 2 hours.
- Enlist the assistance of at least one other caregiver.
- Raise the bed to the height of the caregiver's elbow.
- Remove pillows and positioning devices.
- Unfasten drainage tubes from the bed linen.
- Use a low-friction fabric or gel-filled plastic sheet, roller sheet with handles, or a repositioning sling to slide, rather than to drag or lift, the client while turning or transferring from bed to a stretcher (Fig. 23-5).
- Turn the client as a complete unit to avoid twisting the spine.
- Place the client in good alignment with joints slightly flexed.
- Replace pillows and positioning devices.
- Support limbs in a functional position.
- Use elevation to relieve swelling or promote comfort.
- Provide skin care after repositioning.

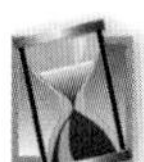

Gerontologic Considerations

- Older adults with cognitive impairment may have difficulty following directions regarding positioning and transferring. Instructions should be given using clear, simple words to make one request at a time. Demonstrations are very helpful in conveying the message if word recall is diminished. Photographs of the desired action may also be used.

Common Positions

Nurses commonly use six body positions when caring for bedridden clients: supine, lateral, lateral oblique, prone, Sims', and Fowler's (Fig. 23-6).

Supine Position

In the **supine position**, the person lies on his or her back. There are two primary concerns associated with the supine position: prolonged pressure, especially at the end of the spine, leads to skin breakdown; and gravity, combined with pressure on the toes from bed linen, creates a potential for **foot drop** (a permanent dysfunctional position caused by a shortening of the calf muscles and a lengthening of the opposing muscles on the anterior leg; Fig. 23-7). Foot drop hinders ambulation because it interferes with a person's ability to place the heel on the floor. The supine position,

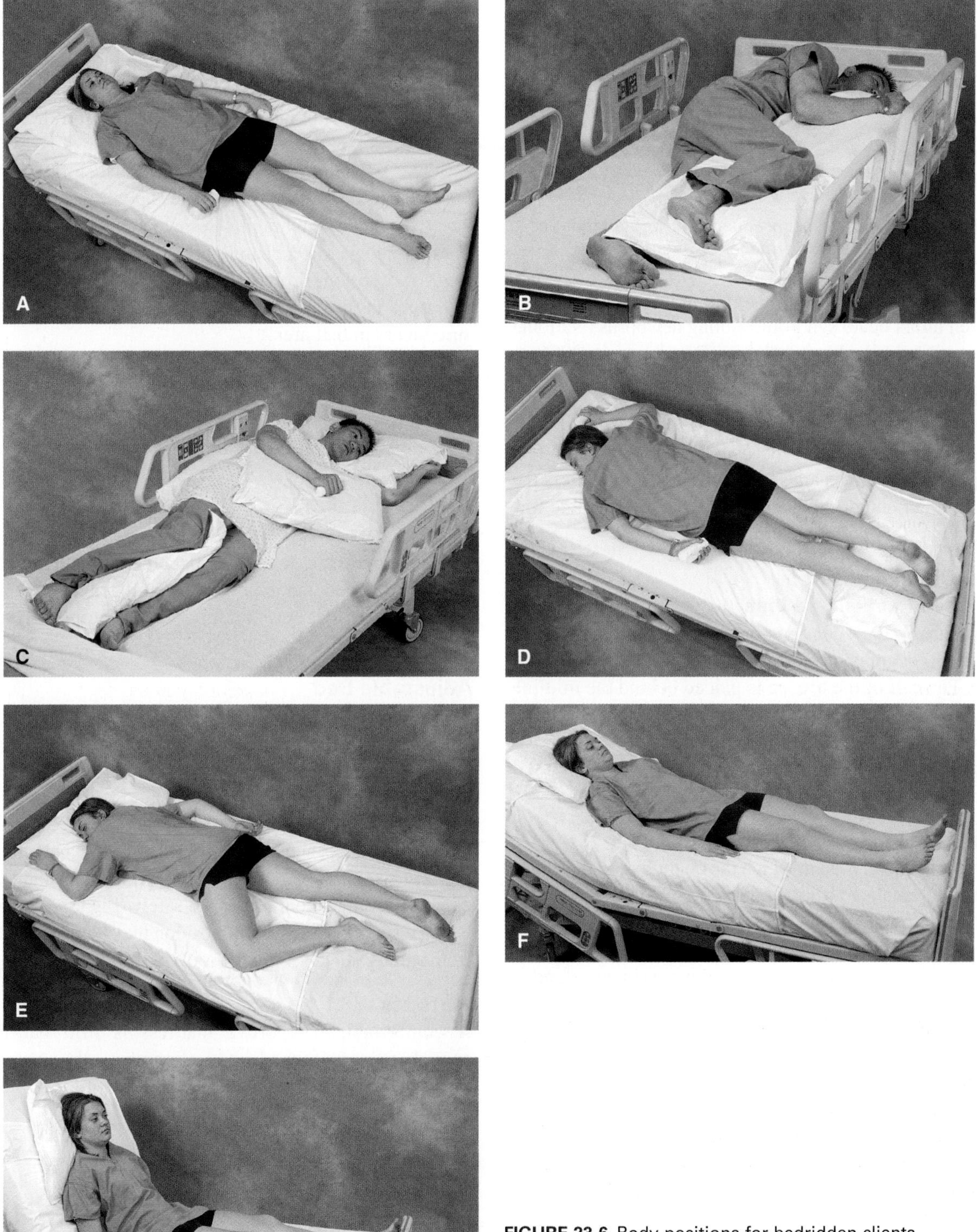

FIGURE 23-6 Body positions for bedridden clients. **(A)** The supine position. **(B)** The lateral position. **(C)** The lateral oblique position. **(D)** The prone position. **(E)** The Sims' position. **(F)** The low Fowler's position. **(G)** The high Fowler's position.

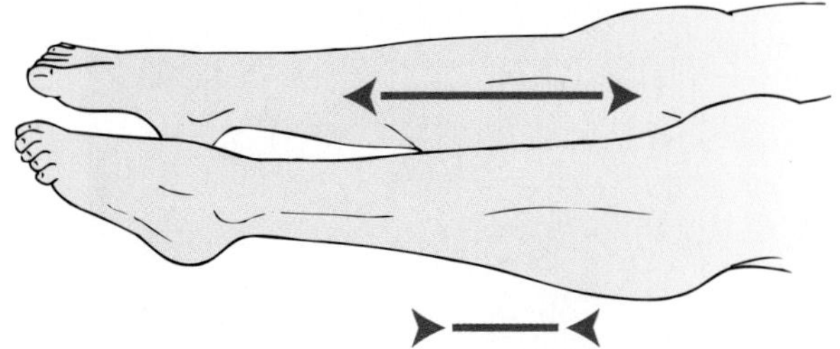

FIGURE 23-7 Foot drop is a consequence of weaked muscles for dorsiflexion resulting in permanent plantarflexion.

however, is recommended as a way to reduce the incidence of sudden infant death syndrome among newborns (National Institute of Child Health and Human Development, 2006).

Lateral Position

With the **lateral position** (a side-lying position), foot drop is of less concern because gravity does not pull down the feet as happens when clients are supine. Nevertheless, unless the upper shoulder and arm are supported, they may rotate forward and interfere with breathing.

Lateral Oblique Position

In the **lateral oblique position** (a variation of the side-lying position), the client lies on the side with the top leg placed in 30 degrees of hip flexion and 35 degrees of knee flexion. The calf of the top leg is placed behind the midline of the body on a support such as a pillow. The back is supported, and the bottom leg is in neutral position. This position produces less pressure on the hip than a strictly lateral position and reduces the potential for skin breakdown.

Prone Position

The **prone position** (one in which the client lies on the abdomen) is an alternative position for the person with skin breakdown from pressure ulcers (see Chap. 28). The prone position also provides good drainage from bronchioles, stretches the trunk and extremities, and keeps the hips in an extended position. The prone position has been found to improve arterial oxygenation in critically ill clients with adult respiratory distress syndrome who are mechanically ventilated, but does not necessarily result in higher rates of survival (Taccone et al., 2009). The prone position poses a nursing challenge for assessing and communicating with clients, however, and it is uncomfortable for clients with recent abdominal surgery or back pain, and interferes with eating.

Sims' Position

In **Sims' position** (a semi-prone position), the client lies on the left side with the right knee drawn up toward the chest. An arm is positioned along the client's back, and the chest and abdomen are allowed to lean forward. The Sims' position is also used for the examination of and procedures involving the rectum and vagina (see Chap. 14).

Fowler's Position

The **Fowler's position** (a semi-sitting position) makes it easier for the client to eat, talk, and look around. Three variations are common. In a *low Fowler's position*, the head and torso are elevated to 30 degrees. A *mid-Fowler's* or *semi-Fowler's position* refers to an elevation of up to 45 degrees. A *high Fowler's position* is an elevation of 60 to 90 degrees. The knees may not be elevated, but doing so relieves strain on the lower spine.

The Fowler's position is especially helpful for clients with dyspnea because it causes the abdominal organs to drop away from the diaphragm. Relieving pressure on the diaphragm allows the exchange of a greater volume of air. Sitting for a prolonged period, however, decreases blood flow to tissues in the coccyx area and increases the risk for pressure ulcers in that area.

Stop, Think, and Respond Box 23-1

Give one advantage and one disadvantage for the supine, lateral and lateral oblique, prone, Sims', and Fowler's positions.

Positioning Devices

Many devices are available to help maintain good body alignment in bed and to prevent discomfort or pressure. Any position, no matter how comfortable or anatomically correct, must be changed frequently.

Adjustable Bed

The adjustable bed (see Chap. 18) can be raised or lowered and allows the position of the head and knees to be changed. The high position facilitates the performance of nursing care. Raising the head of the bed helps the client to look around without twisting and bending. It also promotes drainage of the upper lobes of the lungs and prepares the client for eventually standing and walking. The low position enables an independent client to get in and out of the bed safely (Fig. 23-8). Placing a bed in a slight Trendelenburg position may help keep the client from sliding down toward the foot of the bed (Fig. 23-9).

Mattress

A comfortable, supportive mattress is firm but flexible enough to permit good body alignment. An unsupportive mattress promotes an unnatural curvature of the spine.

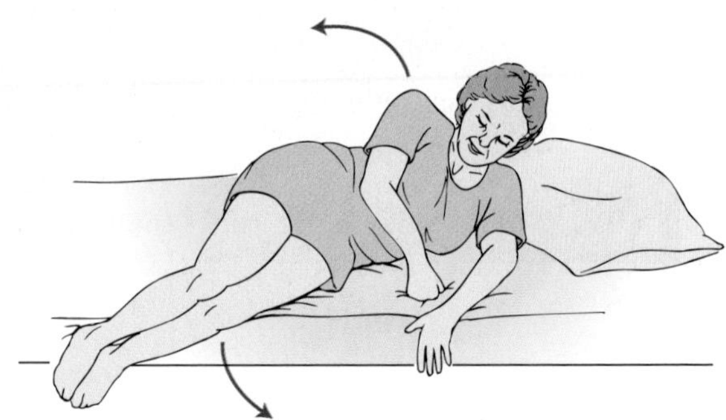

FIGURE 23-8 Grasping the mattress and pushing down with the other hand is an independent technique for sitting on the edge of the bed in preparation for ambulating.

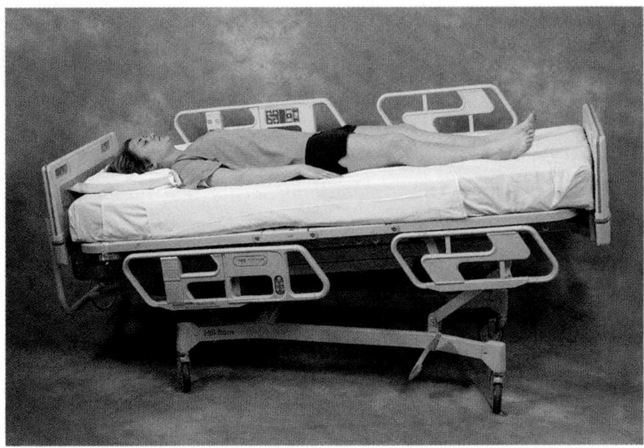

FIGURE 23-9 In the Trendelenburg position, the head is lower than the feet.

Bed Board

A **bed board** (a rigid structure placed under a mattress) provides additional skeletal support. Bed boards usually are made of plywood or some other firm material. The size varies with the situation. If sections of the bed (the head and foot) can be raised, the board must be divided into hinged sections. For home use, full bed boards can be purchased or made from sheets of plywood.

Pillows

Pillows are used to support and elevate a body part. Small pillows, such as contour pillows, triangular wedges, and bolsters, are ideal for supporting and elevating the head, extremities, and shoulders. For home use, oversized pillows are useful for elevating the upper part of the body if an adjustable bed is not available.

Roller Sheet

A roller sheet (also known as a slider sheet) that extends from the upper back to midthighs is a helpful positioning device. Some are designed with handles on either side. When made of substances that reduce friction, the roller sheets diminish the work of turning a client and avoid the potential for skin injuries. They are used to slide and roll, rather than to lift, the client. They help to move up clients in bed from a supine position in the center of the bed to the side of the bed, to turn clients to a lateral position, or to transfer clients from bed to a stretcher. A mechanical lift, which is discussed later, or a repositioning sling is recommended when major repositioning is required. The roller sheet is placed close to the sides of the client's body during repositioning (Fig. 23-10). Working as a team, nurses use the roller sheet to change the client to an alternate position while avoiding any stooping, reaching, or twisting. The sheet is removed after being used or kept dry and free of wrinkles to prevent skin breakdown.

Turning and Moving Clients

In some cases the client may be fully capable of assisting with turning or moving. The amount of client assistance

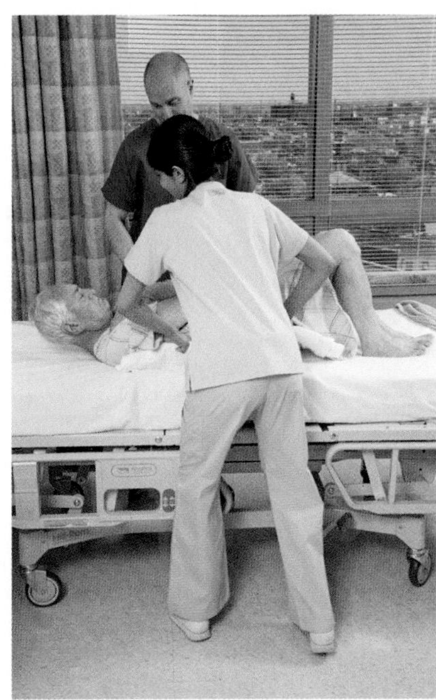

FIGURE 23-10 A roller sheet is used for turning, moving, and repositioning.

depends on factors such as size, weight, mental status, and strength.

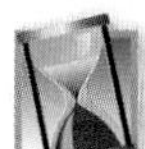

Gerontologic Considerations

- Elevated toilet seats with handrails may be helpful to allow older people to use arm muscles, rather than leg muscles, to assist with sitting and rising.
- Older adults require extra time and assistance during positioning, transferring, and ambulating. They may need modifications to positions because of limitations from pain or joint degeneration. Allow a few minutes for an older person's position changes, such as from supine to sitting or standing, to allow for compensatory changes in blood pressure, thus preventing orthostatic hypotension. Teach the client to wait until any dizziness has resolved before moving, thus decreasing the risk for falls.
- Older adults may fear falling and thus may limit their mobility. Handrails may be strategically placed to promote confidence in ambulation. In addition, placement of chairs near a frequent pathway in the home or institution allow for a "rest stop," thus increasing confidence in ambulation.

If all criteria suggest that the nurse and client can accomplish the task at hand, the nurse enlists the client's cooperation by explaining the plan and how the client can help. Assistive devices and additional caregivers are needed when turning or moving a client who cannot change from one position to another independently or who needs help doing so. Good turning and moving skills are important to prevent injury to the nurse and the client. Skill 23-1 describes the process of repositioning and moving clients.

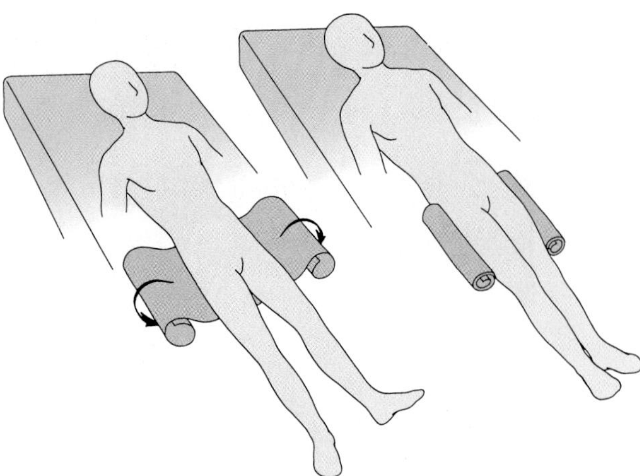

FIGURE 23-11 Placement of trochanter rolls.

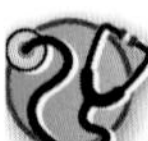

NURSING GUIDELINES 23-2

Using a Trochanter Roll

- Fold a sheet lengthwise in half or in thirds and place it under the client's hips. *The sheet will anchor the body in the correct position.*
- Place a rolled-up bath blanket or two bath towels under each end of the sheet that extends on either side of the client. *This provides support to the trochanters.*
- Roll the sheet around the blanket so that the end of the roll is underneath. *This action prevents unrolling.*
- Secure the rolls next to each hip and thigh. *The rolls prevent an external rotation of the hip.*
- Permit the leg to rest against the trochanter roll. *This position allows for normal alignment of the hips, preventing internal or external rotation.*

Trochanter Rolls

Trochanter rolls (Fig. 23-11) prevent the legs from turning outward. The trochanters are the bony protrusions at the head of the femur near the hip. Placing a positioning device at the trochanters helps to prevent the leg from rotating outward (see Nursing Guidelines 23-2).

Hand Rolls

Hand rolls (Fig. 23-12) are devices that preserve the client's functional ability to grasp and pick up objects. Hand rolls prevent **contractures** (permanently shortened muscles that resist stretching) of the fingers. They keep the thumb positioned slightly away from the hand and at a moderate angle to the fingers. The fingers are kept in a slightly neutral position rather than a tight fist. A rolled-up washcloth or a ball can be used as an alternative to commercial hand rolls. Hand rolls are removed regularly to facilitate movement and exercise.

Foot Boards, Boots, and Foot Splints

Foot boards, boots, and splints are devices that prevent foot drop by keeping the feet in a functional position (Fig. 23-13). Some commercial foot boards have supports that prevent the outward rotation of the foot and lower leg.

If the client is short and cannot reach a foot board, a foot splint is used. A foot splint allows for more variety in body positioning while maintaining the foot in a functional position. Some nurses have clients wear ankle-high tennis shoes while in bed to prevent foot drop. They remove the shoes regularly and give proper foot care.

If a foot splint or foot board is not available, the nurse can use a pillow and large sheet. He or she rolls the pillow in the sheet and twists the ends of the sheet before tucking it under the foot of the mattress. A pillow support does not provide the firmness of a board or splint, and the nurse replaces it as soon as possible with a sturdier device.

Stop, Think, and Respond Box 23-2

In addition to the usual hospital bed, what else will you obtain to facilitate moving and repositioning a client who is weak and cannot assist with positioning and turning?

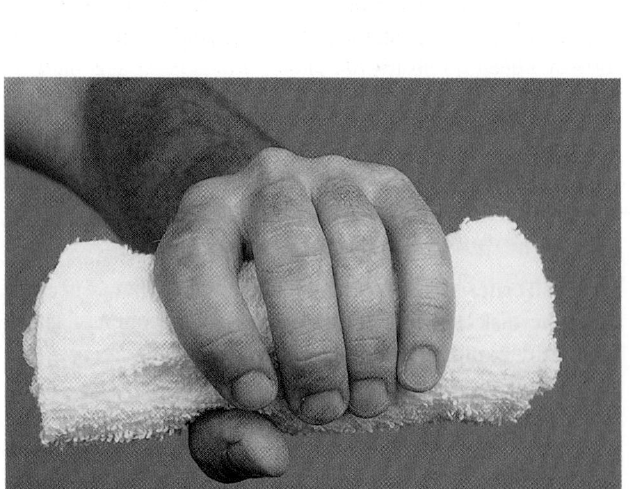

FIGURE 23-12 A hand roll. (Photo by B. Proud.)

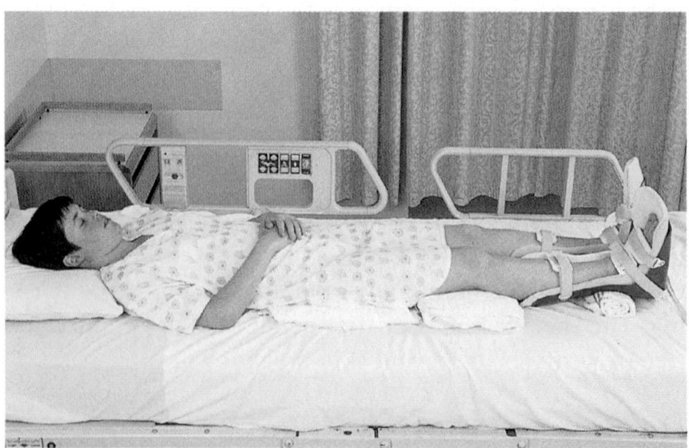

FIGURE 23-13 Protective boots to avoid foot drop. (Photo by B. Proud.)

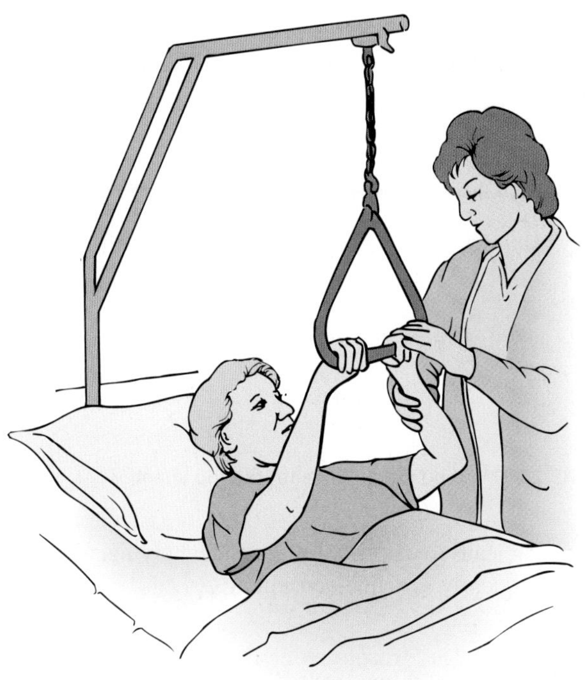

FIGURE 23-14 Using a trapeze to facilitate movement.

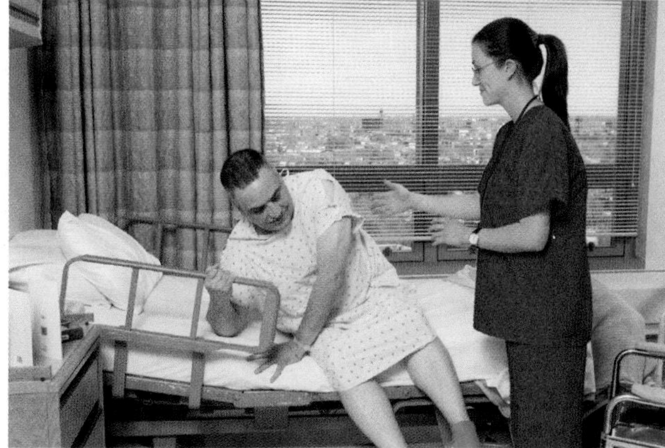

FIGURE 23-15 Using side rails to prepare for ambulation and to change position.

Trapeze

A trapeze is a triangular piece of metal hung by a chain over the head of the bed (Fig. 23-14). The client grasps the trapeze to lift the body and move about in bed. Unless arm movement or lifting is undesirable, a trapeze is an excellent device for helping a bedridden client to increase his or her activity.

PROTECTIVE DEVICES

Items such as side rails, mattress overlays, cradles, and specialty beds protect inactive clients from harm or complications.

Side Rails

Side rails (Fig. 23-15) are a valuable device to aid clients in changing their position and moving about while in bed. With side rails in place, the client can safely turn from side to side and sit up in bed. These activities help clients to maintain or regain muscle strength and joint flexibility.

Mattress Overlays

Mattress overlays are accessory items made of foam or containing gel, air, or water that nurses place over a standard hospital mattress. Nurses use mattress overlays to reduce pressure and restore skin integrity (see Chap. 28).

Foam and Gel Mattresses

Several types of foam mattresses, made of latex or polyethylene, are available. Foam acts like a layer of subcutaneous tissue because it conforms to the client's body and acts like a cushion. Consequently, it redistributes pressure over a greater area, reducing the compressive effect on skin and tissue. Foam also contains channels and cells filled with air that allow for the evaporation of moisture and the escape of heat.

Some foam mattresses are convoluted or made with a series of elevations and depressions, resembling an egg crate (see Chap. 18) or waffle. The density of the foam and the manner in which the foam is formed determine the degree of pressure reduction.

Egg-crate foam mattresses provide minimal pressure reduction and are recommended for comfort only. Thicker, waffle-shaped foam mattresses offer greater pressure reduction; nurses can use them to prevent skin breakdown.

Gel is an alternative substance used to fill cushions and mattresses. It differs from foam in that it suspends and supports the body part. Nurses place gel and foam cushions in wheelchairs to prevent the "hammock effect"—the posterior and lateral compression that occurs when sitting in a sling-like seat.

Static Air Mattress

A static air pressure mattress is filled with a fixed volume of air. It is similar in appearance to those used for recreational purposes. It suspends the client on a buoyant surface, distributing the pressure on the underlying tissue. If the mattress becomes underinflated, however, it loses its effectiveness as a pressure-relieving device. Because plastic is nonabsorbent, air mattresses permit less evaporation of moisture than foam. Also, sharp objects can damage the integrity of the mattress.

Alternating Air Mattress

An alternating air mattress (Fig. 23-16) is similar to a static one with one exception: every other channel inflates as the next one deflates. The process is then reversed. The wave-like redistribution of air cyclically relieves pressure over bony prominences. This repetitive process promotes blood flow and keeps the tissues supplied with oxygen. The tubing connecting the mattress to its motor-driven compressor must not become kinked. The noise may disturb some clients.

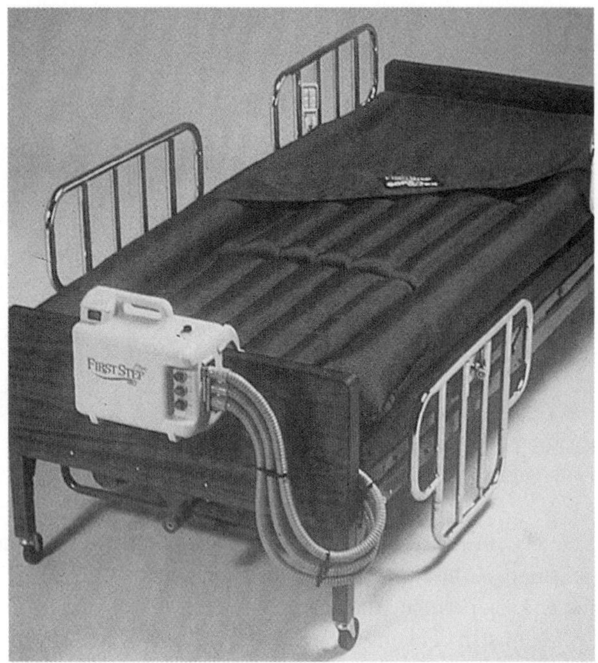

FIGURE 23-16 An alternating air mattress. (First Step Plus; Courtesy of KCI Therapeutic Services, San Antonio, TX.)

Water Mattress

A water mattress supports the body and equalizes the pressure per square inch over its surface. The pressure-relieving effect is maintained regardless of any shift in the client's position. Many claim that sleeping on a waterbed produces a feeling of tranquility, which may provide beneficial emotional effects. Water mattresses are heavy; therefore, the floor and the bed frame must be able to support the weight.

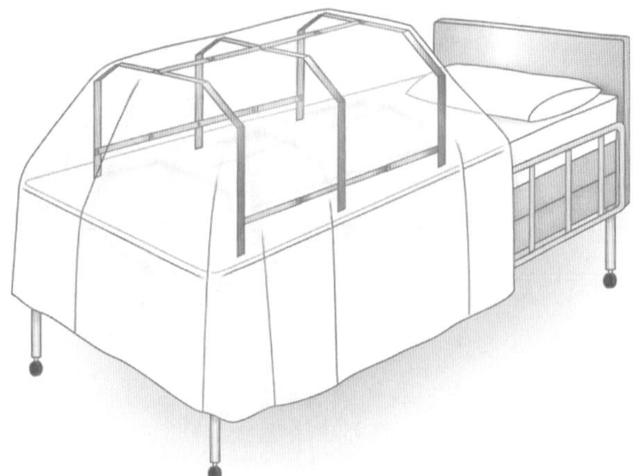

FIGURE 23-17 A bed cradle beneath the top sheet.

Puncturing leads to damage. Filling and emptying, although done infrequently, are time-consuming.

Cradle

A cradle is a metal frame secured to or placed on top of the mattress. It forms a shell over the client's lower legs to keep bed linen off the feet or legs (Fig. 23-17). A cradle is often used for clients with burns, painful joint disease, and fractures of the leg.

Specialty Beds

Specialty beds such as low–air-loss beds, air-fluidized beds, oscillating support beds, and circular beds offer more functions than standard hospital beds. Like mattress overlays, they are used to relieve pressure and to prevent other problems associated with inactivity and immobility (Table 23-3).

TABLE 23-3 Pressure-Relieving Devices

DEVICE	EXAMPLES	INDICATIONS FOR USE
Foam mattress or gel cushion	Egg crate Geo-Matt	Intact skin and minimal risk for breakdown Changes in position occur spontaneously or require minimal assistance
Static air, alternating air, or water mattress	TENDER Cloud Sof-Care Pulsair Lotus	At some risk for skin breakdown A superficial or single deep break in skin but pressure easily relieved Need for prolonged bed rest with immobilization
Oscillating support bed	Roto Rest Tilt and Turn Paragon 9000	At high risk for systemic effects of immobility, such as pneumonia and skin breakdown
Low–air-loss bed	KinAir FLEXICAIR Mediscus	Combination of the following: Impaired skin Continued existence of risk factors for further skin breakdown Alternative positions limited, less than adequate, or impossible Assistance required for frequent transfers from bed
Air-fluidized bed	Clinitron FluidAir	Combination of the following: Impaired skin Continued existence of risk factors for further skin breakdown Alternative positions limited, less than adequate, or impossible Seldom transferred from bed
Circular bed	CircOlectric	Current or high risk for skin breakdown because of multiple trauma, especially if it involves the head, neck, or spine Burns that require frequent dressing changes or topical applications

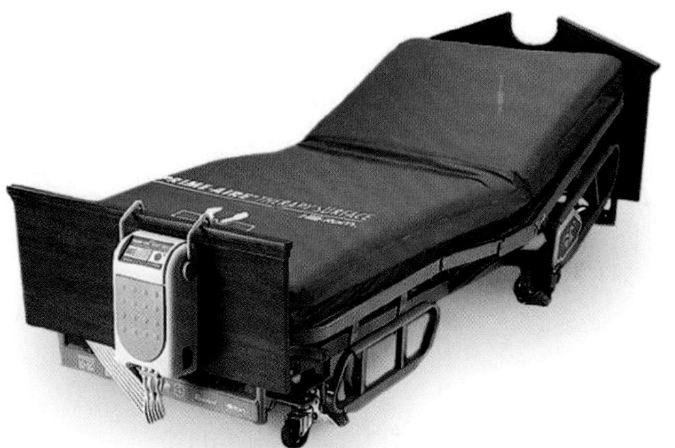

FIGURE 23-18 A low–air-loss bed. (Courtesy of Hill-Rom Company, Inc., Batesville, Indiana.)

Low–Air-Loss Bed

A low–air-loss bed (Fig. 23-18) contains inflated air sacs within the mattress. It maintains capillary pressure well below that which can interfere with blood flow. Regardless of changes in body position, the mattress selectively responds by redistributing the air to maintain low pressure to all skin areas.

Air-Fluidized Bed

An air-fluidized bed (Fig. 23-19) contains a collection of tiny beads within a mattress cover. The beads are blown upward on warm air. When suspended, the dry beads take on the characteristics of fluid, allowing the client to float on the lifted beads. Excretions and secretions drain away from the body and through the beads, thereby preventing skin irritation and maceration from moisture. The pressure-relieving effects of this type of bed have been shown to speed the healing of severely impaired tissue.

An air-fluidized bed is better used for a client who is likely to remain in bed for long periods. Fluid balance may become a problem because of the accelerated evaporation caused by the warm, blowing air. Puncturing or tearing the mattress is also a potential problem.

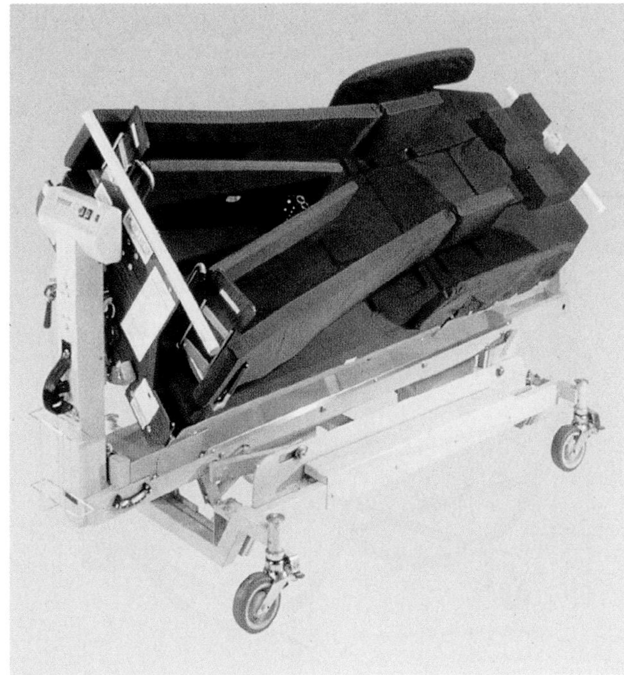

FIGURE 23-20 An oscillating bed. (Courtesy of Kinetic Concepts, Inc., San Antonio, TX.)

Oscillating Support Bed

An oscillating bed (Fig. 23-20) slowly and continuously rocks the client from side to side in a 124-degree arc. Oscillation relieves skin pressure and helps to mobilize respiratory secretions. Foam-covered supports applied to the head, arms, and legs prevent sliding and skin **shearing** (the force exerted against the surface and layers of the skin as tissues slide in opposite but parallel directions). Compartments within the bed are removed temporarily to facilitate assessment and care of the posterior body.

Circular Bed

A circular bed supports the client on a 6 or 7-ft anterior or posterior platform suspended across the diameter of the frame (Fig. 23-21). This type of bed allows the client to

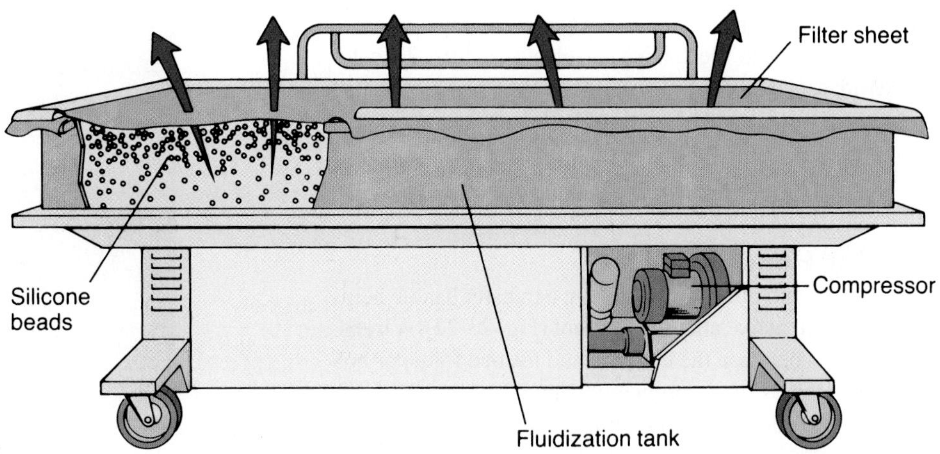

FIGURE 23-19 An air-fluidized bed.

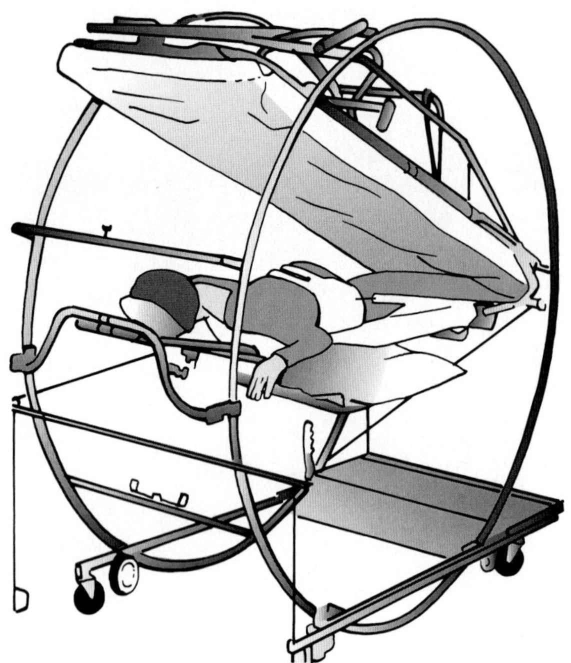

FIGURE 23-21 A circular bed.

remain passively immobilized during a position change. The bed has the capacity to rotate the client, who is sandwiched between the anterior and posterior frames, in a 180-degree arc. Turning permits access to the client for nursing care. Clients learn how to operate the bed to make minor adjustments in their position. This promotes a sense of control among otherwise dependent clients.

TRANSFERRING CLIENTS

Transfer (moving a client from place to place) refers to moving a client from the bed to a chair, toilet, or stretcher and back to bed again. The client assists in an active transfer. A transfer done with the help of one or more nursing personnel with an assistive device is a passive transfer. Transfer aids are assistive devices that help clients move laterally. Several devices are available to help transfer clients. Some examples of transfer aids are transfer handles, transfer belts, transfer boards, and mechanical or electrical lifts. Transfer devices are especially helpful for decreasing the potential for injury to caregivers and clients or for times when caring for clients who fear falling or lack confidence in the ability of personnel to transfer them safely and comfortably.

Transfer Handle

Some clients with disabilities find that a transfer handle helps them to remain active and independent (Fig. 23-22). A transfer handle fits between the mattress and the bed frame or box spring and serves as a combination grab bar and handrail to support the client's weight while exiting and returning to bed. A transfer handle is not considered a restrictive device

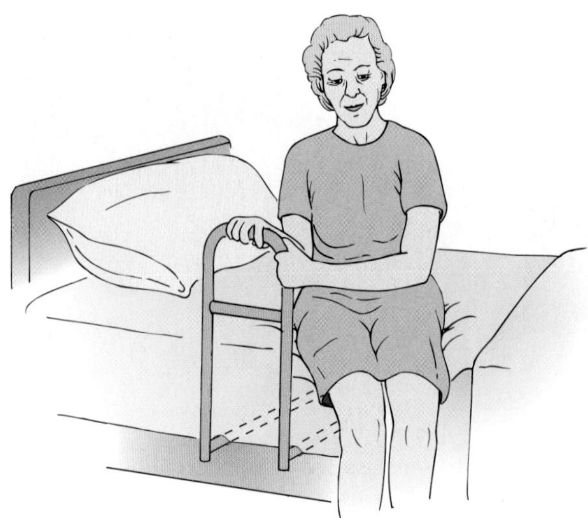

FIGURE 23-22 A transfer handle.

like side rails because the client is free to move around. It promotes activity and mobility for many who are physically challenged.

Transfer Belt

A transfer belt is a padded device secured around the client's waist. Its handles provide a means of gripping and supporting the client (Fig. 23-23). This device is designed for clients who can bear weight and help with the transfer but are unsteady. It also may be used as a walking belt to provide safety and security while assisting a client with ambulation (see Chap. 26).

Transfer Boards

A transfer board serves as a supportive bridge between two surfaces such as the bed and a wheelchair, the bed and a

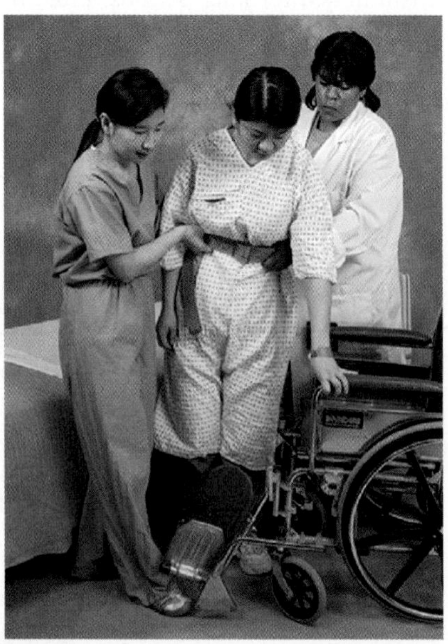

FIGURE 23-23 A belt is used to assist with transferring a client from the bed to a wheelchair and back to bed.

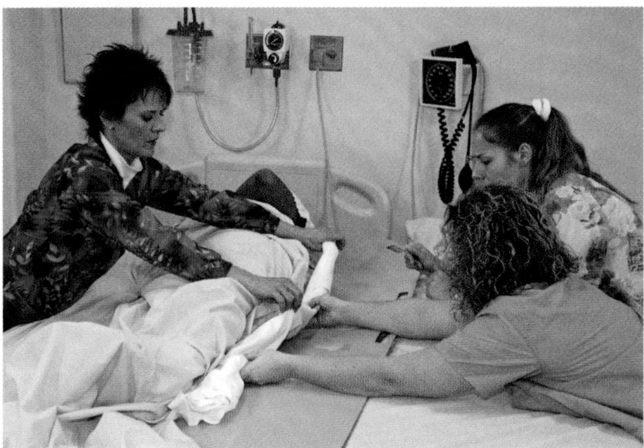

FIGURE 23-24 A transfer board is used to move a client from the bed to a stretcher.

stretcher, the wheelchair and a car seat, or the wheelchair and the toilet. Transfer boards come in a variety of widths and lengths. Some are curved to facilitate transferring around fixed armrests; others may have wheels on their underneath side. Transfer boards are positioned in such a way that the client's buttocks or body can slide across what would otherwise be an open space or a gap in height between two surfaces (Fig. 23-24). Some clients with strong arm and upper body muscles can use a transfer board independently. For clients who need assistance, the nurse uses a transfer belt in conjunction with a transfer board. Full-body transfer boards also are available for moving supine clients to a stretcher or an X-ray table. A low-friction roller sheet may be used in conjunction with a transfer board.

Mechanical Lift

A mechanical lift (Fig. 23-25) helps to move heavy clients or those with limited ability to assist from the bed to a chair, toilet, or tub, and back again. Both electric and hydraulic models are available with a lifting capacity of 350 to 600 lb. Using a mechanical lift enables a caregiver to raise

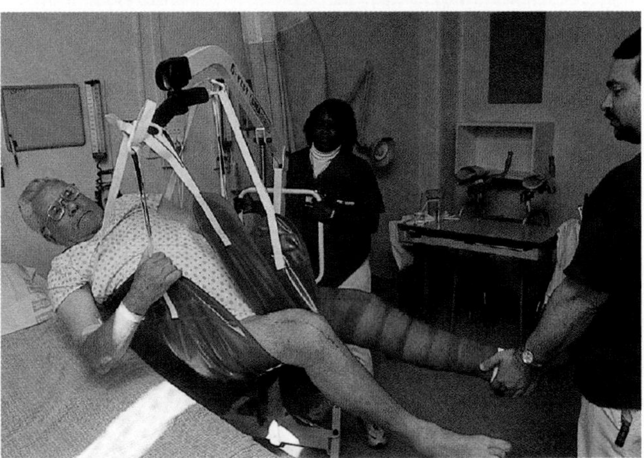

FIGURE 23-25 A hydraulic mechanical lift is used to raise and transfer an obese or helpless client to some other location and return the client to bed.

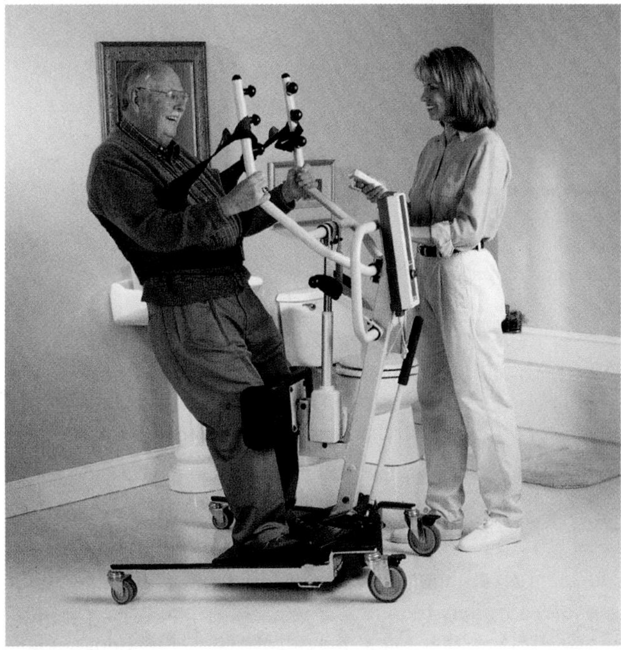

FIGURE 23-26 A standing lift supports a client who can bear some body weight. It also facilitates lowering the client to a sitting position on a chair or toilet.

and lower clients secured in a canvas sling and move them around on a wheeled frame. The wheels are locked when a stationary position is desired such as when lowering a client into place. Standing assist lifts are an alternative for use when clients have some ability to bear weight (Fig. 23-26).

It is best to use assistive devices when they are needed, observe the guidelines in Nursing Guidelines 23-3, and use the recommendations in Skill 23-2 when transferring clients.

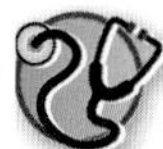

NURSING GUIDELINES 23-3

Assisting with Client Transfer

- Be realistic about how much you can safely lift. *Not exceeding one's capabilities demonstrates good judgment.*
- Always practice good body mechanics. *They reduce the potential for injury.*
- Put on braces and other supportive devices before getting a client out of bed. *Doing so maximizes time management.*
- Have the client wear shoes or nonskid slippers. *Appropriate footwear provides support and prevents foot injuries.*
- Plan to transfer clients across the shortest distance. *A short transfer reduces the potential for injury.*
- Make sure that the client's stronger leg, if there is one, is nearest the chair to which the client is transferring. *This action ensures safety.*
- Stand on the side of the bed to which the client will be moving. *This position helps the nurse assist the client.*
- Explain to the client what will be done, step by step, and solicit the client's help as much as possible. *These actions inform the client, encourage self-help, and reduce the workload.*

BOX 23-2 Levels of Functional Status

0 = Completely independent
1 = Requires the use of an assistive device
2 = Needs minimal help
3 = Needs assistance and/or some supervision
4 = Needs total supervision
5 = Needs total assistance or unable to assist

(Carpenito-Moyet, 2005)

Stop, Think, and Respond Box 23-3

List the various devices for transferring clients in a sequence from the one that requires the least work on the part of the nurse to the one that may require the most.

NURSING IMPLICATIONS

During the initial and subsequent client assessments, the nurse determines the client's level of dependence on nursing assistance. One scale for quantifying the client's status is shown in Box 23-2. The nurse selects positioning, transfer, and protective devices according to whether the client is independent or requires partial or total assistance.

Various nursing diagnoses may apply to inactive clients:

- Impaired Physical Mobility
- Risk for Injury
- Risk for Disuse Syndrome
- Risk for Perioperative Positioning Injury
- Impaired Transfer Ability
- Impaired Bed Mobility
- Risk for Impaired Skin Integrity

Nursing Care Plan 23-1 illustrates how nurses apply the steps in the nursing process when caring for a client with the nursing diagnosis of Risk for Disuse Syndrome. The NANDA-I taxonomy (2012, p. 222) describes this diagnostic category as a state in which a person is "at risk for deterioration of body systems as the result of prescribed or unavoidable musculoskeletal inactivity."

While providing nursing care, there may be opportunities to teach clients and their caregivers about techniques that promote activity or reduce the potential for complications from inactivity. See Client and Family Teaching 23-1.

Client and Family Teaching 23-1
Promoting Activity and Mobility

The nurse teaches the client and the family as follows:

- Balance periods of activity with periods of rest.
- Become aware of the dangers of inactivity.
- Allow adequate time for performing activities.
- Join a club that involves social activities.
- Develop hobbies or recreational interests.
- Become a volunteer at the hospital, your church, or a municipal group.
- Join a local group—a coffee club, a needlework group, football friends, or bingo or card players.
- Remove objects that might pose safety hazards, such as throw rugs or electrical cords. Make sure chair legs are not in the way. Promptly mop up any water spilled on the floor.
- Rent or purchase hospital equipment from a medical supply company.
- Investigate the loan of equipment for homebound terminal clients from national organizations such as the American Cancer Society.
- Ask about community services that encourage independent living, such as homemaker services, trained dogs, Meals on Wheels, social services, and church organizations.

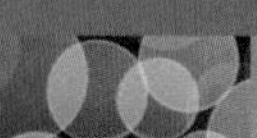

NURSING CARE PLAN 23-1 Risk for Disuse Syndrome

Assessment

- Assess the client's independent movement and activity status.
- Inspect the integrity of the skin.
- Inquire as to the client's bowel elimination pattern and characteristics of stool.
- Observe the client's depth of respirations and the ability to raise pulmonary secretions.
- Check skin color, capillary refill of nail beds, and urinary output for evidence of circulatory perfusion.
- Palpate distal peripheral pulses for rate and quality.
- Check the Homans' sign.
- Determine if there is a potential for infection of any type such as an indwelling urinary or venous catheter, artificial airway, wound, etc.
- Observe if the client has sufficient muscle strength and coordination to protect himself or herself from a potential injury.
- Assess if there is any impairment of vision, hearing, and tactile sensation.
- Note the client's mental status for signs of dementia, depression, or apathy.

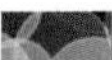

NURSING CARE PLAN 23-1 Risk for Disuse Syndrome (continued)

Nursing Diagnosis. **Risk for disuse syndrome** (A syndrome diagnosis contains its etiology in the diagnosis; consequently, when a syndrome diagnosis is made, it is identified in a one-part statement [Carpenito-Moyet, 2010, p. 20]).

Expected Outcome. The client will have no evidence of complications associated with disuse as evidenced by intact skin/tissue integrity; full range of joint motion; clear lung sounds; capillary refill in less than 3 seconds; strong peripheral pulses; negative Homans' sign; regular bowel movements of soft stool; urinary output greater than 1,500 mL/day throughout length of care.

Interventions	Rationales
Reposition the client every 2 hours around the clock.	Position changes relieve pressure and maintain sufficient capillary circulation to ensure cellular and tissue integrity.
Provide clean, dry, and wrinkle-free bedding at all times.	Clean dry linen prevents the maceration of skin from prolonged contact with moisture. Keeping the linen wrinkle-free prevents compromised circulation from increased pressure per square inch (psi) of skin.
Use and check incontinence pads on bed every 2 hr; change immediately when soiled.	Incontinence pads wick moisture away from the client and keep the bed linen dry. Changing soiled incontinence pads prevents skin maceration from contact with moisture and waste products of elimination.
Assist the client to the bedside commode every 4 hr when awake.	Transferring from bed to a commode promotes use of the musculoskeletal system, increases circulation and breathing, and relieves pressure on skin from lying positions in bed. Use of the commode promotes continence and dignity.
Use a foam mattress on the bed.	Foam acts like a layer of subcutaneous tissue and redistributes pressure over a greater area, reducing the potential for skin breakdown.
Use trochanter rolls for supine positioning.	Trochanter rolls prevent external rotation of the hips and legs. Maintaining a neutral position facilitates the potential for ambulation and independence.
Apply a footboard to the bed or foot splints to both legs.	These devices prevent foot drop and help to ensure the potential for normal ambulation.
Encourage active exercise with a bed trapeze and participation in activities of daily living such as assisting with bathing, grooming, oral hygiene, and eating.	Activity reduces the potential for complications associated with disuse.
Vary the daily routine when possible.	Variety in the routine stimulates the mind and cognitive processes.
Include the client in planning the daily routine.	Giving the client a locus of control maintains dignity and self-esteem.
Teach the family how to turn and position the client.	Involving the client's family provides a sense of personal satisfaction for being involved in the care of a loved one. Teaching helps to prepare them to assist the client when eventually discharged or transferred to another level of care.

Evaluation of Expected Outcomes

- The client's skin is pink, dry, and intact in all areas.
- The client has full range of motion in all joints.
- The client's lungs are clear to auscultation anteriorly, posteriorly, and laterally.
- The pedal pulses are present and strong bilaterally.
- The Homans' sign is negative bilaterally when the feet are dorsiflexed.
- The capillary refill in nail beds of great toes is 2 to 3 seconds.
- The client has a daily bowel movement without straining.
- The client's urine is clear yellow with a daily volume between 2,000 and 2,200 mL.
- No foot drop or external rotation of hips and legs is noted when footboard and trochanter rolls are in use.

CRITICAL THINKING EXERCISES

1. You observe a coworker using incorrect body mechanics while giving care to a client. How would you approach this coworker? What suggestions would you give?
2. List nursing activities that predispose one to work-related injuries. How can the nurse reduce the risk for injury during each?
3. What precautions would you advocate for repositioning or moving a **bariatric client**, one who is defined by the American Obesity Association (2005) as severely overweight with a body mass index (BMI) of 30 to 39.9 or morbidly obese with a BMI over 40?
4. What factors pose unique challenges in positioning and moving geriatric clients?

NCLEX-STYLE REVIEW QUESTIONS

1. Which client position is most correct when a nurse assists with a diagnostic examination involving the lower gastrointestinal tract, such as a sigmoidoscopy?
   1. Lithotomy position
   2. Sims' position
   3. Supine position
   4. Fowler's position
2. Which of the following body positions is best for the nurse to use to promote drainage from an abdominal wound?
   1. Lithotomy position
   2. Fowler's position
   3. Supine position
   4. Trendelenburg position
3. Before turning a postoperative client from a supine to a lateral position, which nursing instruction is most appropriate?
   1. "Hold your breath as you are turning."
   2. "Bend your knee as far as possible over the other."
   3. "Curl up in a ball before I help you turn."
   4. "Let me roll you as if you were a log."
4. What is the purpose for using a trochanter roll when positioning a client?
   1. Preventing hip adduction
   2. Preventing hip abduction
   3. Preventing hip flexion
   4. Preventing hip rotation
5. Which of the following is most helpful for facilitating a client's independent movement?
   1. A bed cradle
   2. A bed board
   3. An overbed trapeze
   4. Lower side rails

SKILL 23-1 Turning and Moving a Client

Suggested Action	Reason for Action
ASSESSMENT	
Assess for risk factors that may contribute to inactivity.	Indicates a need to reposition more frequently.
Determine the time of the last position change.	Ensures following the plan for care.
Assess the physical, mental, and emotional ability to assist in turning, positioning, or moving.	Determines if additional help or assistive devices are needed.
Inspect for drainage tubes and equipment.	Ensures that they will not be displaced or cause discomfort to the client.
PLANNING	
Explain the procedure to the client.	Increases cooperation and decreases anxiety.
Remove all pillows and current positioning devices, such as trochanter rolls.	Reduces interference during repositioning.
Raise the bed to elbow height, which is a suitable working height.	Prevents back strain by maintaining the center of gravity.
Secure two or three additional caregivers, positioning and moving devices (eg, roller sheets, repositioning sling, mechanical lift), or both as needed.	Ensures safety.
Close the door or draw the bedside curtain.	Demonstrates respect for privacy.
IMPLEMENTATION	
Turning the Client from Supine to Lateral or Prone Position	
Wash hands or perform an alcohol-based hand rub when appropriate (see Chap. 10).	Reduces the transmission of microorganisms.
Help or have the client slide to one side of the bed.	Provides room when repositioning.
Raise the side rail.	Ensures safety.
Flex the client's knee over the other with the arms across the chest.	Aids in turning and protects the client's arms.
Spread your feet, flex your knees, and place one foot behind the other.	Provides a broad base of support.
Place one hand on the client's shoulder and one on the hip.	Facilitates turning.
Roll the client toward the side rail (Fig. A).	Reduces effort.

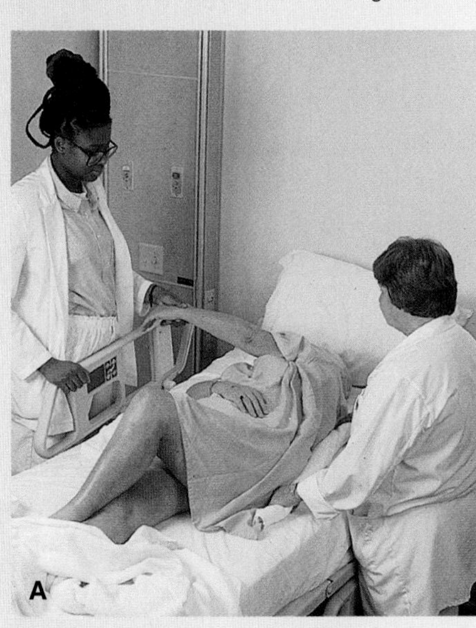

Directing the client to turn.

(continued)

Turning and Moving a Client (continued)

IMPLEMENTATION (CONTINUED)

Replace pillows behind the back, between the legs, and under the upper arm (Fig. B). — Aids in maintaining position and provides comfort.

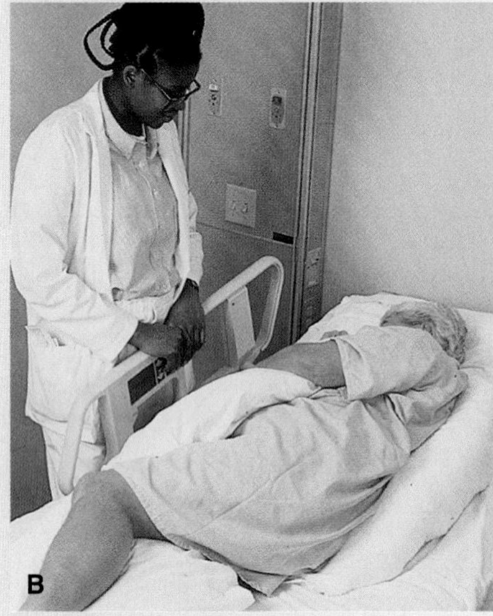

Supporting arms and legs with pillows.

Raise the side rails and lower the height of the bed. — Ensures safety.

Wash hands or perform an alcohol-based hand rub when appropriate (see Chap. 10). — Reduces the transmission of microorganisms.

For a Prone Position

Begin as described earlier for the lateral position. — Follows the same principles.

Have the client turn his or her head opposite to the direction for rolling and leave the arms extended at each side (Fig. C). — Prevents pressure on the face and arms during and after repositioning.

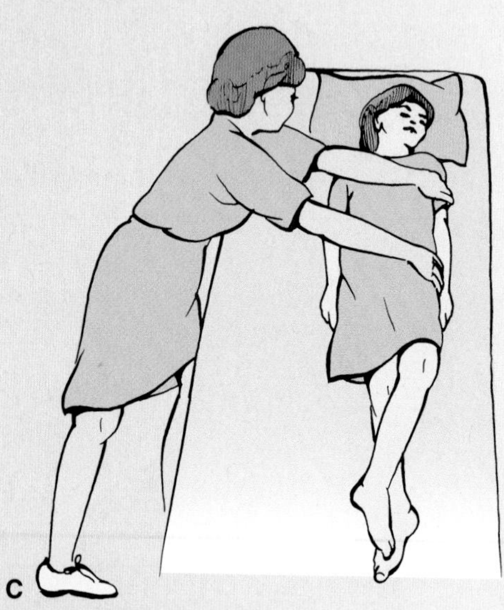

Preparing for prone positioning.

(continued)

Turning and Moving a Client (continued)

IMPLEMENTATION (CONTINUED)

Shift your hands from the posterior of the shoulder and hip to the anterior as the client rolls independently onto his or her abdomen (Fig. D).	Controls the speed with which the client is repositioned.

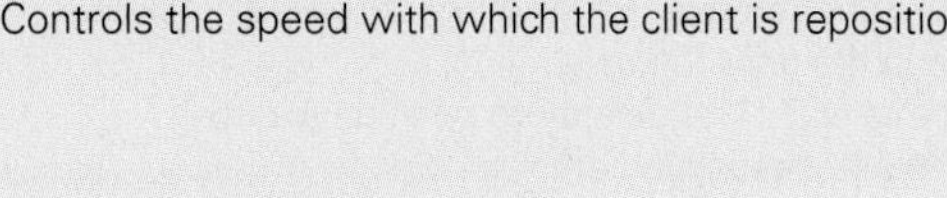

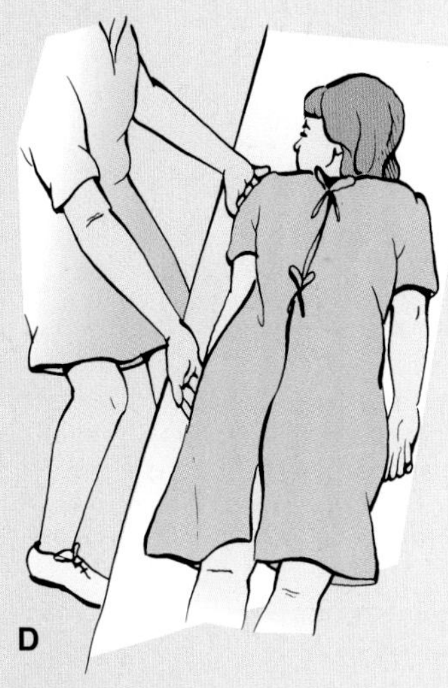

Bracing the client during turning.

Center the client in bed.	Prevents pressure on arms.
Arrange pillows.	Provides for comfort and support.
Raise the side rails and lower the height of the bed.	Ensures safety.
Wash hands or perform an alcohol-based hand rub when appropriate (see Chap. 10).	Reduces the transmission of microorganisms.

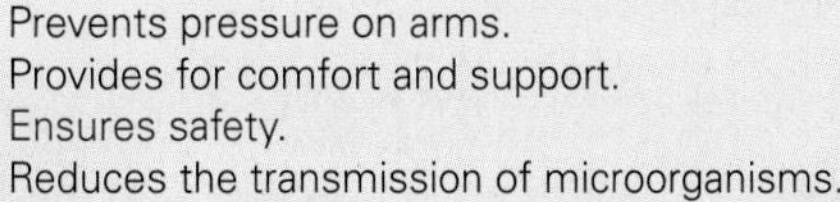

Moving the Mobile Client up in Bed (One-Nurse and Client Technique)

Wash hands or perform an alcohol-based hand rub when appropriate (see Chap. 10).	Reduces the transmission of microorganisms.
Remove the pillow from under the client's head.	Prevents strain on the neck and head during moving.
Place the pillow against the headboard.	Cushions the head from contact with the headboard.
Raise the bed to elbow height.	Reduces back strain.
Place a roller/slider sheet beneath the buttocks to facilitate movement if needed if the client is weak or unable to fully assist.	Promotes gliding and reduces friction.
Instruct the client to bend both knees and grasp a trapeze if one is available.	Aids in assisting by using the stronger muscles of the arms and legs.
Ask the client to push down with his or her feet, causing the legs to straighten (Fig. E). Repeat again if necessary.	Creates momentum to facilitate moving.

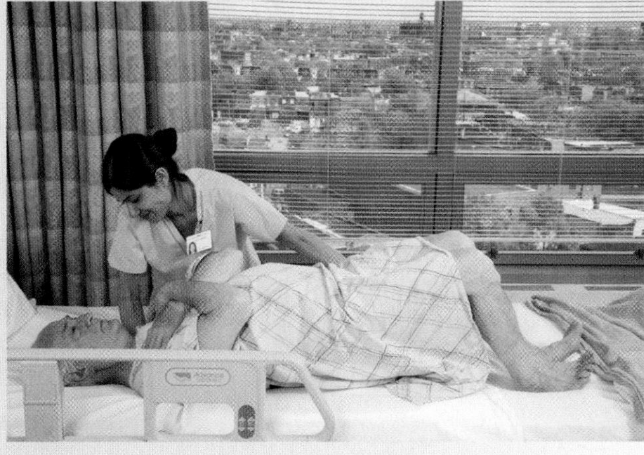

Moving up in bed.

(continued)

Turning and Moving a Client (continued)

IMPLEMENTATION (CONTINUED)

Action	Rationale
Rearrange pillows and remove the roller sheet unless it will be needed again in the near future.	Restores comfort.
Place the client in a slight Trendelenburg position if sliding downward is a persistent problem.	Gravity keeps the client from sliding downward.
Wash hands or perform an alcohol-based hand rub when appropriate (see Chap. 10).	Reduces the transmission of microorganisms.
Two-Nurse and Roller Sheet Technique	
Wash hands or perform an alcohol-based hand rub when appropriate (see Chap. 10).	Reduces the transmission of microorganisms.
Protect the headboard with a pillow.	Ensures client safety.
Raise the bed to elbow height.	Reduces back strain.
Place a roller/slider sheet beneath the client's shoulders and buttocks.	Facilitates gliding the client rather than lifting.
Stand facing each other on opposite sides of the bed between the client's hips and shoulders.	Aids in coordinating movement between nurses.
Roll the slider sheet to the sides of the client.	A palms-up grip provides more strength by keeping the elbows close to the body, thus reducing the workload.
Grasp the rolled sheet with the palms up and the knuckles in contact with the bed sheet.	A palms-up grip provides more strength by keeping the elbows close to the body, thus reducing the workload. Keeping the knuckles in contact with the bed sheet ensures a sliding, rather than a lifting, motion.
Bend hips and knees; spread feet.	Follows principles of good body mechanics and provides momentum to facilitate sliding.
Slide the client up on reaching a previously agreed signal (Fig. F), such as the count of three.	Promotes coordination of effort.

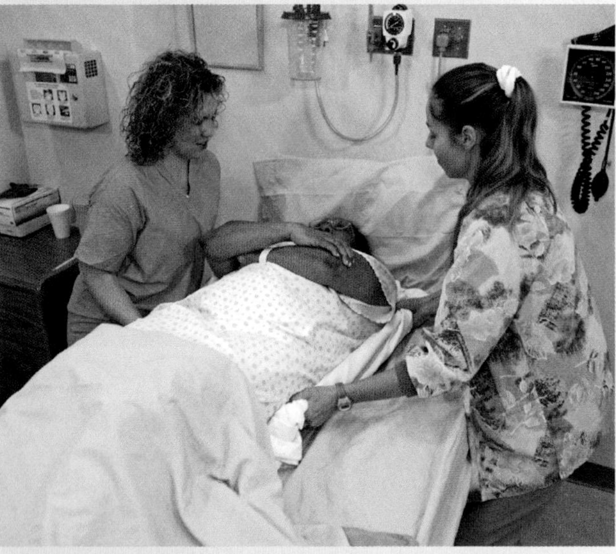

Moving the client up in bed with a rolled sheet and the assistance of two people.

Action	Rationale
Avoid shrugging the shoulders while moving the client.	Shrugging the shoulders indicates that the client is being lifted.
Rearrange pillows; remove the roller sheet unless it will be needed again in the near future.	Restores comfort.
Place the client in a slight Trendelenburg position if sliding downward is a persistent problem.	Gravity keeps the client from sliding downward.
Wash hands or use an alcohol-based hand rub when appropriate (see Chap. 10).	Reduces the transmission of microorganisms.

Evaluation

- Movement is achieved.
- Client is comfortable.
- Pressure is relieved.
- Joints and limbs are supported.

(continued)

Turning and Moving a Client (continued)

Document

- Frequency of turning and moving
- Positions used
- Use of positioning devices
- Assistance required
- Client's response

SAMPLE DOCUMENTATION

Date and Time Position changed q 2 h from supine to R and L lateral positions with assistance of client. Pillows used to support limbs and maintain positions. Foot board in place. No shortness of breath noted. No evidence of discomfort during repositioning. —— SIGNATURE/TITLE

SKILL 23-2 Transferring Clients

Suggested Action	Reason for Action
ASSESSMENT	
Check the Kardex, nursing care plan, and medical orders for activity level.	Complies with the plan for care.
Assess the client's strength and mobility, as well as his or her mental and emotional status.	Determines the need for additional personnel or a mechanical lifting device.
PLANNING	
Consult with the client on the preferred time for getting out of bed.	Helps client participate in decision making.
Locate a straight-backed chair, wheelchair, or stretcher to which the client will be transferred.	Facilitates efficient time management.
Arrange the chair or stretcher next to or close to the bed on the client's stronger side, if there is one.	Ensures safety.
Lock the wheels of the bed, wheelchair, or stretcher.	Prevents rolling and ensures safety.
Explain how the transfer will be accomplished.	Reduces anxiety and promotes cooperation.
From Bed to Chair	
Wash hands or perform an alcohol-based hand rub when appropriate (see Chap. 10).	Reduces the transmission of microorganisms.
Assist the client to a sitting position on the side of the bed.	Reduces dizziness; enables the client to stand.
Help the client don a bathrobe and nonskid slippers.	Ensures warmth, modesty, and safety.
Place the chair parallel to the bed on the client's stronger side; raise the footrests if using a wheelchair.	Provides for easy access.
Apply a transfer belt or other assistive device, if needed (Fig. A).	Reduces the risk for falling.

A

Applying a transfer belt.

(continued)

Transferring Clients (continued)

PLANNING (CONTINUED)

Grasp the transfer belt or reach under the client's arms.	Helps support the upper body.
Instruct the client to grasp your shoulders.	Gives the client leverage for rising.
Bend the hips and knees; brace the client's knees (Fig. B).	Stabilizes the client and follows principles of good body mechanics.

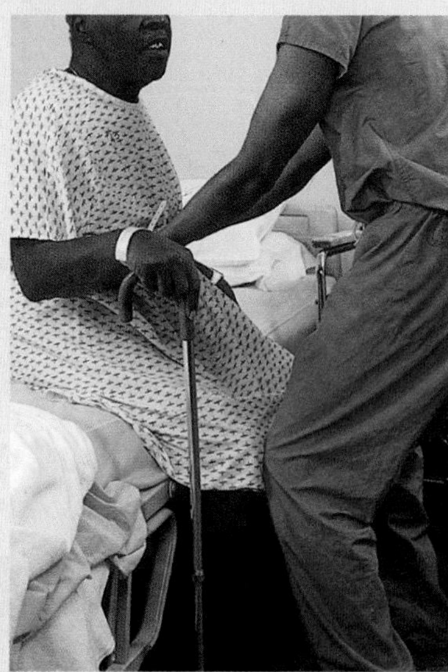

Bracing the client's knees.

Rock the client to a standing position at an agreed signal while encouraging the client to straighten his or her knees and hips.	Provides momentum and reduces the need to lift the client.
Pivot the client with his or her back toward the chair.	Positions the client for sitting.
Tell the client to step back until he or she feels the chair at the back of the legs.	Places the client in close proximity with the chair.
Instruct the client to grasp the arms of the chair while you stabilize his or her knees and lower the client into the chair (Fig. C).	Promotes safety.

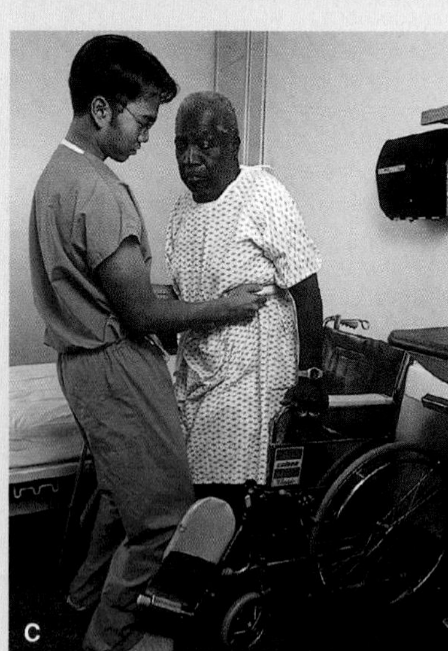

Backing into a wheelchair.

Support the feet on the footrests.	Facilitates good posture.
Using a Transfer Board	
Wash hands or perform an alcohol-based hand rub when appropriate (see Chap. 10).	Reduces the transmission of microorganisms.
Remove an arm from the wheelchair.	Reduces interference with transfer.
Lock the brakes on the bed and wheelchair.	Prevents rolling and ensures safety.
Slide the client to the edge of the bed.	Maintains shortest distance for transfer.

(continued)

Transferring Clients (continued)

PLANNING (CONTINUED)

Angle the transfer board from the client's buttocks and hips down toward the seat of the chair.	Places the board where there is maximum weight.
Position the transfer board beneath the client.	Supports upper body.
Support and brace the client's knee with your knees while maintaining proper body mechanics.	Prevents injury.
Slide the client down the transfer board into the seat of the chair at an agreed-on signal (Fig. D).	Reduces the need to lift the client.

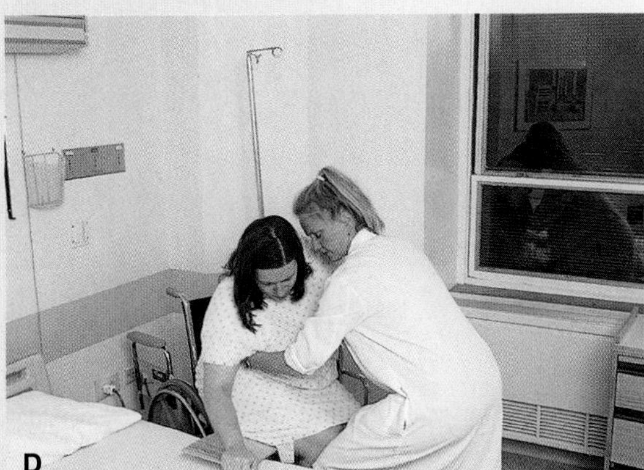

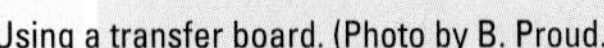

Using a transfer board. (Photo by B. Proud.)

Wash hands or perform an alcohol-based hand rub if appropriate (see Chap. 10).	Reduces the transmission of microorganisms.
Using a Mechanical Lift	
Wash hands or perform an alcohol-based hand rub if appropriate (see Chap. 10).	Reduces the transmission of microorganisms.
Raise the bed to a height that places the client near the nurse's center of gravity.	Reduces the risk for back injury.
Lock the brakes on the bed.	Prevents the bed from moving and causing injury.
Place the canvas sling under the client from the shoulders to midthigh (Fig. E).	Positions the sling where it will support the greatest mass of the client.

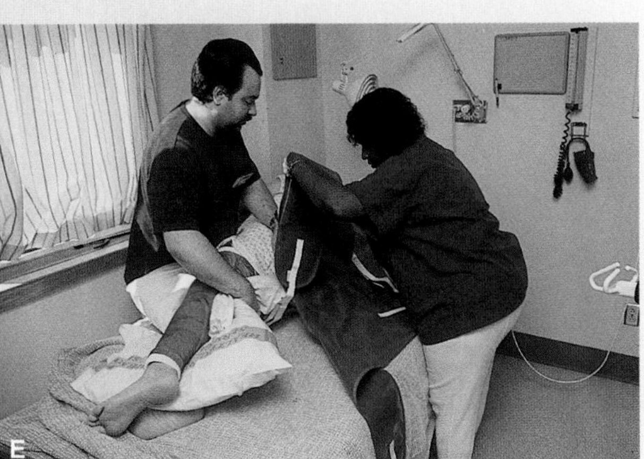

Applying the lift's sling.

Move the lift device on the same side of the bed as the chair or stretcher to which the client will be transferred.	Facilitates safety when the client and equipment are within close proximity.
Position the boom on the lift over the client's torso.	Enables the attachment of lifting chains to the canvas sling.
Lock the wheels on the lift.	Stabilizes the lift in place.

(continued)

Transferring Clients (continued)

PLANNING (CONTINUED)

Attach the hooks on the lifting chain or straps to the holes in the canvas sling (Fig. F). — Connects the lift to the client.

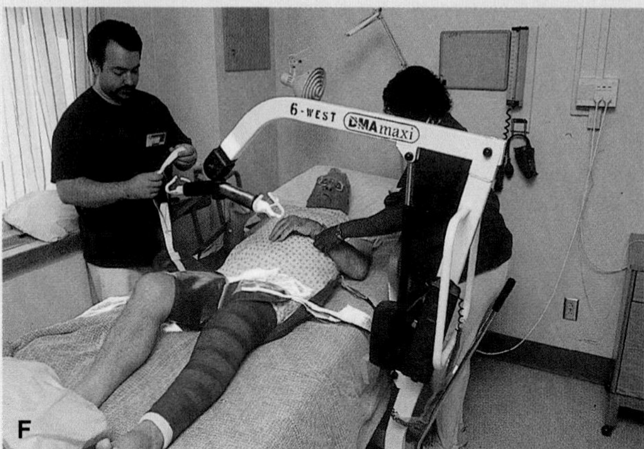

Positioning the lift and the client.

Position the client's arms across his or her chest. — Protects the client's arms and hands from being injured.

Pump the jack handle to elevate the client to about 6 inches above the mattress (Fig. G). — Aids in assessing whether the client is properly and safely within the sling.

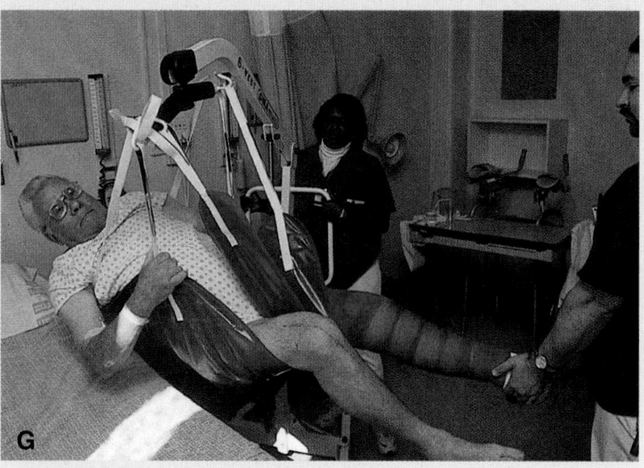

Raising the client.

Unlock the wheels on the lift and move the lifted client directly over the chair or stretcher. — Relocates the client to the desired location.

Relock the wheels of the lift. — Ensures the client's safety.

Release the jack handle slowly. — Lowers the client from the suspended position.

Remove the lifting chains, but leave the canvas sling in place beneath the client. — Facilitates returning the client to bed.

Wash hands or perform an alcohol-based hand rub if appropriate (see Chap. 10). — Reduces the transmission of microorganisms.

Evaluation

- Client is relocated.
- No injury occurs to client or personnel.

Document

- Method of transfer
- Response of client

SAMPLE DOCUMENTATION

Date and Time Transferred from bed to wheelchair by standing and pivoting with weight bearing on right leg. Transient pain rated at 1 on a scale of 0 to 10 experienced in left hip during transfer. Declined offer for pain medication. Up in chair approximately 1 hour ——— SIGNATURE/TITLE

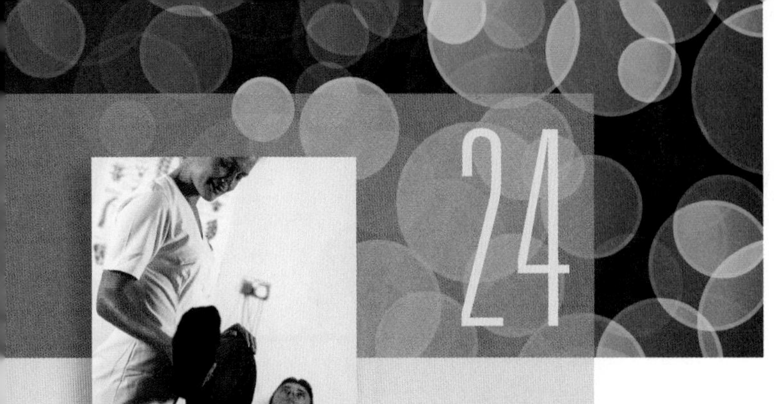

24 Therapeutic Exercise

Words To Know

active exercise
aerobic exercise
ambulatory electrocardiogram
ankylosis
body composition
cardiac ischemia
continuous passive motion machine
exercise
fitness
fitness exercise
isometric exercise
isotonic exercise
maximum heart rate
metabolic energy equivalent
passive exercise
range-of-motion exercises
recovery index
step test
stress electrocardiogram
submaximal fitness test
target heart rate
therapeutic exercise
walk-a-mile test

Learning Objectives

On completion of this chapter, the reader should be able to:

1. List at least five benefits of regular exercise.
2. Define fitness.
3. Identify seven factors that interfere with fitness.
4. Name at least two methods of fitness testing.
5. Describe how to calculate a person's target heart rate.
6. Define metabolic energy equivalent.
7. Differentiate fitness exercise from therapeutic exercise.
8. Differentiate isotonic exercise from isometric exercise.
9. Give at least one example of isotonic and isometric exercises.
10. Differentiate between active exercise and passive exercise.
11. Discuss how and why range-of-motion exercises are performed.
12. Provide at least two suggestions for helping older adults become or stay physically active.

Exercise (purposeful physical activity) is beneficial to people of all age groups (Box 24-1), and the health risks of a sedentary lifestyle are well documented. This chapter addresses techniques for improving health and maintaining or restoring muscle and joint function by promoting exercise. Because exercise must be individualized, nurses are responsible for assessing each person's fitness level before initiating an exercise program with a client.

FITNESS ASSESSMENT

Fitness means the capacity to exercise. Factors such as a sedentary lifestyle, health problems, compromised muscle and skeletal function, obesity, advanced age, smoking, and high blood pressure can impair a client's fitness and stamina. They could even result in injury during exercise. Therefore, before a client begins an exercise program, assessment of his or her fitness level is necessary. Some assessment techniques include measuring body composition, evaluating trends in vital signs, and performing fitness tests.

Body Composition

Body composition is the amount of body tissue that is lean versus the amount that is fat. Determining factors include anthropometric measurements such as height, weight, body-mass index, skin-fold thickness, and mid-arm muscle circumference (see Chap. 13). Inactivity without reduced food intake tends to promote obesity. Overweight or obese people are less fit than their leaner counterparts and need to proceed gradually when initiating an exercise program.

BOX 24-1 Benefits of Physical Exercise

- Improved cardiopulmonary function
- Reduced blood pressure
- Increased muscle tone and strength
- Greater physical endurance
- Increased lean mass and weight loss
- Reduced blood glucose level
- Decreased low-density blood lipids
- Improved physical appearance
- Increased bone density
- Regularity of bowel elimination
- Promotion of sleep
- Reduced tension and depression

Vital Signs

Vital signs—temperature, pulse rate, respiratory rate, and blood pressure—reflect a person's physical status (see Chap. 12). Elevated pulse rate, respiratory rate, and blood pressure while resting are signs that the person may have life-threatening cardiovascular symptoms during exercise. After a period of modified exercise, vital signs may decrease, thus reducing the potential for heart-related complications.

Fitness Tests

Fitness tests provide an objective measure of a person's current fitness level and his or her potential for safe exercise. They also help to establish safe parameters for the level and duration of exercise. Two methods of fitness testing are a stress electrocardiogram (ECG) and an ambulatory ECG. Another is a **submaximal fitness test**, which is an exercise test that does not stress a person to exhaustion. Examples of submaximal fitness tests include a step test and a walk-a-mile test. Because submaximal tests are less demanding, the validity of their results is less reliable than results obtained through ECG testing.

Stress Electrocardiogram

A **stress electrocadiogram** tests electrical conduction through the heart during maximal activity and is performed in an acute care facility or an outpatient clinic (Fig. 24-1). The client first walks slowly on a flat treadmill. As the test progresses, the speed and incline of the treadmill are increased. The examiner notes the client's heart rate and rhythm, blood pressure, breathing, and symptoms such as dizziness and chest pain. A pulse oximeter (see Chap. 21) is used to measure peripheral oxygenation. The examiner stops the test if the client develops an abnormal heart rhythm, **cardiac ischemia** (impaired blood flow to the heart), elevated blood pressure, or exhaustion.

Ambulatory Electrocardiogram

An **ambulatory electrocardiogram** is a continuous recording of heart rate and rhythm during normal activity. It requires the client to wear a device called a Holter monitor for 24 hours. This less taxing version of a stress ECG is used when the person has had prior cardiac-related symptoms, such as chest pain, or has major health risks that contraindicate a stress ECG.

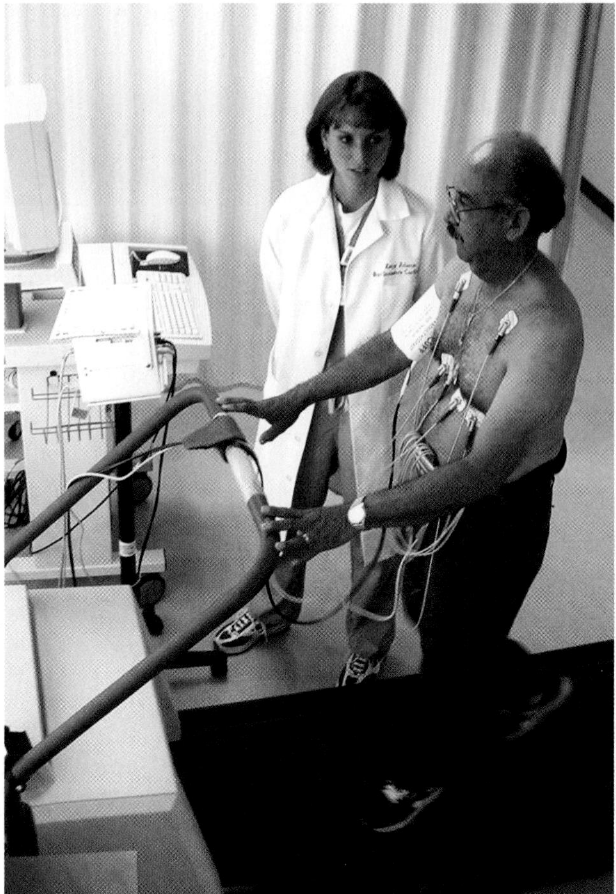

FIGURE 24-1 A stress electrocardiogram. (Image© Texas Heart Institute, www.texasheart.org.)

Ambulatory electrocardiography helps to assess the heart's response to normal activity rather than activity imposed during a stress ECG. It also helps to evaluate how a person is responding to cardiac rehabilitation and medical therapy.

The Holter monitor, which is connected to chest leads, is attached to a belt or shoulder strap or carried in a pocket (Fig. 24-2). During ambulatory electrocardiography, the client should not shower or swim; a sponge bath is permitted as long as the monitor does not get wet. The client also should avoid magnets, metal detectors, electric blankets, and high-voltage areas that may cause artifacts on the recordings that interfere with an accurate interpretation of the test results.

The client keeps a diary of the time and type of activities performed, when he or she took medications, and when he or she experienced symptoms, if any. After the test period, the client returns the monitor, and then a computer and the physician check the electrically recorded information. The physician compares the client's diary with the ECG. The assessment results help to determine whether oxygenation to the heart muscle was temporarily impaired during an activity or if an abnormal heart rhythm developed. Either finding indicates that exercise should begin at a very low intensity and for a short duration.

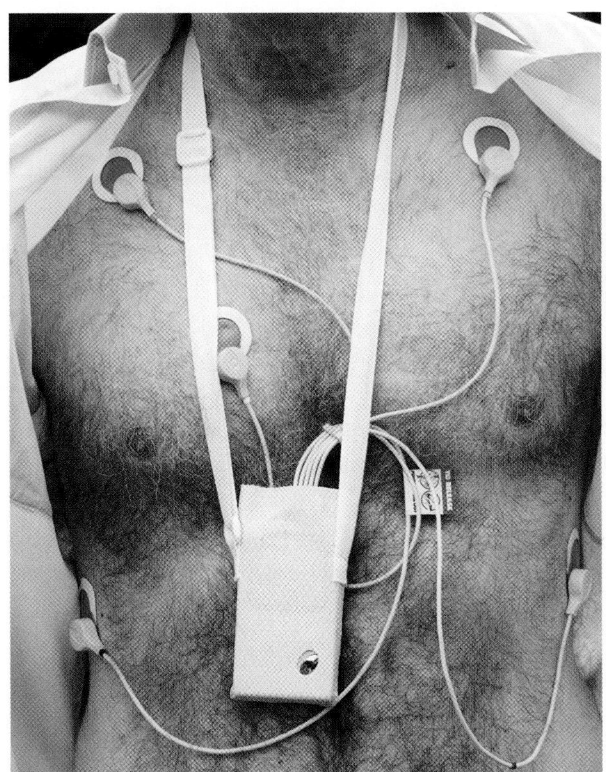

FIGURE 24-2 Ambulatory electrocardiography.

Step Test

A **step test** is a submaximal fitness test involving a timed stepping activity. Several variations include the Harvard Step Test, the Queens College Step Test, and the Chester Step Test. A person undergoing this type of fitness analysis will step up and down on a platform of a prescribed height (20 in. for men, 16 in. for women) for 3 to 5 minutes at a rate of at least 76 steps per minute. A step up or down is considered one step. The time is shortened when the client can no longer sustain the prescribed rate or develops discomfort. The examiner uses a metronome and a stopwatch to keep track of the rate and the time.

Examiners calculate the client's **recovery index** (a guide for determining a person's fitness level) by taking a 30-second pulse rate at 1, 2, and 3 minutes after the test and using the following formula:

$$\text{Recovery index} = \frac{(100 \times \text{test duration in seconds})}{2 \times \text{total of the 30-second pulse assessments}}$$

The examiner compares results with standardized fitness levels (Table 24-1). A fit person has a smaller decline in heart rate at each assessment. Another fitness indicator is how close the pulse rate at the end of recovery compares with the pretest pulse rate. The more similar the pretest and posttest pulse rates, the more fit is the person.

The step test must be used with caution. Personnel certified in cardiopulmonary resuscitation and use of an automatic cardiac defibrillator (see Chap. 37) should be available to assist if there is an adverse cardiac event.

TABLE 24-1 Cardiovascular Endurance Fitness Levels

SCORE	FITNESS CLASSIFICATION
≥90	Excellent
89–80	Good
79–65	Average
64–56	Below average
≤55	Poor

From *Fitness testing; Harvard step test.* Accessed April 27, 2010, from http://www.topendsports.com/testing/tests/step-harvard.htm.

Walk-a-Mile Test

The **walk-a-mile test**, devised by the American College of Sports Medicine (2009), measures the time it takes a person to walk 1 mile. The person is instructed to walk 1 mile on a flat surface as fast as possible. The examiner calculates the time from start to finish and interprets results using the guidelines in Table 24-2.

EXERCISE PRESCRIPTIONS

The prescription for an exercise program involves determining the person's target heart rate and the metabolic energy equivalents (METs) of particular activities based on the person's fitness level.

Target Heart Rate

Target heart rate means the goal for heart rate during exercise. It is determined by first calculating the person's **maximum heart rate** (the highest limit for heart rate during exercise). Maximum heart rate is calculated by subtracting a person's age from 220. Thus, a 20-year-old has a maximum heart rate of 200 beats per minute (bpm), whereas a 50 year old has a maximum heart rate of 170 bpm. The target heart rate for moderate intensity is 50% to 70% of the maximum heart rate (Centers for Disease Control and Prevention, 2010). Beginners should not exceed 50%, intermediates can exercise up to 70%, and competitive athletes may tolerate 70% to 85% of their maximum heart rate during vigorous intensive physical activity.

Stop, Think, and Respond Box 24-1

What is the maximum heart rate and minimum target heart rate for a person who is 25 years old and a competitive athlete who is 32 years old?

TABLE 24-2 Evaluation Criteria for the Walk-a-Mile Test

PERFORMANCE TIME FOR MEN (MIN)	PERFORMANCE TIME FOR WOMEN (min)	FITNESS LEVEL*
≥15:3	≥17:3	Poor
14:01–14:42	15:07–16:06	Average
12:54–14:00	14:12–15:06	Good
<12:54	<14:12	Excellent

*Based on adults age 40–49.

TABLE 24-3 Levels of Physical Activity

METABOLIC ENERGY EQUIVALENT (MET)	EXAMPLES OF ACTIVITIES
1	Sewing Watching television Dressing
1–2	Walking 1 mph on level ground Bowling
2–3	Golfing with a cart Mowing lawn with a power mower
3–4	Playing badminton (doubles) Raking leaves
4–5	Slow swimming Lifting 50 lb
5–6	Square dancing Shoveling snow
6–7	Water skiing Moving heavy furniture
7–8	Playing basketball Playing noncompetitive handball
8–9	Cross-country skiing Playing contact football
≥10	Running 6 mph or faster

Exercising at the target rate for 15 minutes (excluding the warm-up and cool-down periods) three or more times per week strengthens the heart muscle and promotes the use of fat reserves for energy. Exercising beyond the target heart rate reduces endurance by increasing fatigue.

Metabolic Energy Equivalent

Because fitness levels vary, exercises also are prescribed according to their **metabolic energy equivalent** (MET; the measure of energy and oxygen consumption during exercise). This is the prescribed amount that a person's cardiovascular system can safely support. Low-to-vigorous physical activities and their approximate METs are listed in Table 24-3.

TYPES OF EXERCISE

Exercise is performed to promote fitness or to achieve therapeutic outcomes. The two major types of exercise are fitness exercise and therapeutic exercise.

Fitness Exercise

Fitness exercise means physical activity performed by healthy adults. Fitness exercise develops and maintains cardiorespiratory function, muscular strength, and endurance (Fig. 24-3). The two categories of fitness exercise are isotonic and isometric.

Isotonic exercise is activity that involves movement and work. The prime example is **aerobic exercise**, which involves rhythmically moving all parts of the body at a moderate to slow speed without hindering the ability to breathe. In other words, the person can talk comfortably if the exercise is within his or her level of fitness. To promote cardiorespiratory conditioning and increase lean muscle mass, a person should perform isotonic exercise at his or her target heart rate.

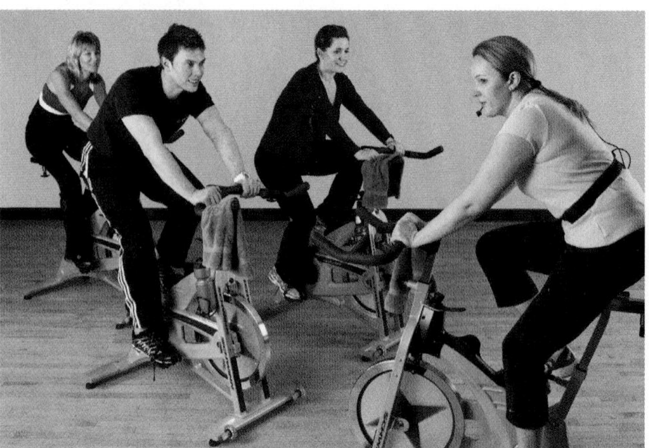

FIGURE 24-3 Stationary cycling.

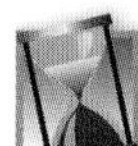

Gerontologic Considerations

- Older adults need to eliminate their intake of caffeinated and alcoholic beverages before and during physical activity to avoid depleting fluid volume. Water is the preferred drink for fluid replacement.
- Encourage families and caregivers of older adults with cognitive impairment to help older persons participate in physical activities such as walking and ball throwing. If the older person has difficulty with balance, exercises may be done while sitting or lying down. Active range-of-motion (ROM) exercises should be scheduled daily and may be divided into short sessions. If the older adult cannot participate actively in an exercise program, the caregivers can perform passive ROM exercises, at least daily, to prevent muscle atrophy and disuse syndrome.
- Many shopping malls permit, and even encourage, people to walk through the mall before stores open for business.
- Swimming or exercising in water puts less stress on joints and is beneficial for older adults.
- Many physically challenging sports, such as bowling, golfing, walking in marathons, and weight lifting, have competition categories for older adults.
- Precautions, such as wearing safe shoes with nonskid soles, are necessary to prevent falls when older adults exercise. Complications from falls contribute to morbidity and mortality among older people.

Isometric exercise consists of stationary exercises generally performed against a resistive force. Examples include body building, weight lifting, and less intense activities such as simply contracting and relaxing muscle groups while sitting or standing. Isometric exercises increase muscle mass and strength, and tone and define muscle groups. Although they improve blood circulation, they do *not* promote cardiorespiratory function. In fact, strenuous isometric exercises elevate blood pressure temporarily (see Client and Family Teaching 24-1).

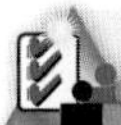

Client and Family Teaching 24-1
A Safe Exercise Program

The nurse teaches the client and the family as follows:

- Seek a pre-exercise fitness evaluation from a health care provider or a certified sports trainer.
- Determine the target heart rate according to fitness level.
- Determine the appropriate level of METs.
- Choose a form of exercise that seems pleasurable and involves as many muscle groups as possible.
- Plan at least 20-minute exercise periods at a convenient time 3–5 days each week (American College of Sports Medicine, 2009).
- Build up to 30 minutes or more of moderate-intensity physical activity on most (preferably all) days of the week (Thompson et al., 2003).
- Exercise with a partner for safety and motivation.
- Avoid exercising in extreme weather conditions (high humidity, smog).
- Dress in layers according to the temperature and weather conditions.
- Wear supportive shoes.
- Wear reflective clothing after dark.
- Walk or jog against traffic; cycle in the same direction as traffic.
- Eat complex carbohydrates (pasta, rice, cooked cereal) rather than fasting or eating simple sugars (cookies, chocolate, sweetened drinks) before exercising.
- Avoid drinking alcohol, which dilates the blood vessels, promotes heat loss, and interferes with good judgment.
- Warm up for 5 minutes by stretching muscle groups or doing light calisthenics.
- Measure the heart rate two or three times while exercising.
- Slow down if the heart rate exceeds the pre-established target.
- Try to sustain the target heart rate for at least 12 to 15 minutes.
- Never stop exercising abruptly.
- Cool down for at least 5 minutes in a manner similar to the warm-up.

Therapeutic Exercise

Therapeutic exercise is activity performed by people with health risks or those being treated for an existing health problem. Clients perform therapeutic exercise to prevent health-related complications or to restore lost functions (see Performing Leg Exercises in Chap. 27 and Strengthening Pelvic Floor Muscles in Chap. 30). Therapeutic exercise may be isotonic or isometric; isotonic exercises are performed actively or passively.

Active Exercise

Active exercise is therapeutic activity that the client performs independently after proper instruction. For example, clients who have undergone a mastectomy learn to exercise the arm on the surgical side by combing their hair, squeezing a soft ball, finger-climbing the vertical surface of a wall, and swinging a rope attached to a doorknob.

Active therapeutic exercise often is limited to a particular part of the body that is in a weakened condition. It is assumed that clients will use their unaffected muscle groups while performing activities of daily living such as bathing and dressing.

Passive Exercise

Passive exercise is therapeutic activity that the client performs with assistance and is provided when a client cannot move one or more parts of the body. For example, for clients who are comatose or paralyzed from a stroke or spinal injury, nurses perform exercises that maintain muscle tone and flexible joints. One form of frequently provided passive therapeutic exercise is ROM exercise. Another form is delivered with a continuous passive motion (CPM) machine.

Range-of-Motion Exercises

Range-of-motion exercises are therapeutic activities that move the joints. They are performed for the following reasons:

- To assess joint flexibility before initiating an exercise program
- To maintain joint mobility and flexibility in inactive clients
- To prevent **ankylosis** (the permanent loss of joint movement)
- To stretch joints before performing more strenuous activities
- To evaluate the client's response to a therapeutic exercise program

During ROM exercises, the client moves or is assisted to move joints in the positions that the joint normally permits (Table 24-4). Whenever possible, the client actively

TABLE 24-4 Joint Positions

POSITION	DESCRIPTION
Flexion	Bending so as to decrease the angle between two adjoining bones
Extension	Straightening so as to increase the angle between two adjoining bones up to 180 degrees
Hyperextension	Increasing the angle between two adjoining bones more than 180 degrees
Abduction	Moving away from the midline
Adduction	Moving toward the midline
Rotation	Turning from side to side as in an arc
External rotation	Turning outward, away from the midline of the body
Internal rotation	Turning inward, toward the midline of the body
Circumduction	Forming a circle
Pronation	Turning downward
Supination	Turning upward
Plantar flexion	Bending toward the sole of the foot
Dorsiflexion	Bending the foot toward the dorsum or anterior side
Inversion	Turning the sole of the foot toward the midline
Eversion	Turning the sole of the foot away from the midline

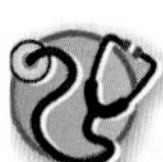

NURSING GUIDELINES 24-1

Performing Range-of-Motion Exercises

- Use good body mechanics (see Chap. 23). *Doing so conserves energy and avoids muscle strain and injury.*
- Remove pillows and other positioning devices. *Such items can interfere with the exercises.*
- Position the client to facilitate movement of the joint through all its usual positions. *This positioning makes it easier to perform a comprehensive exercise program.*
- Follow a systematic, repetitive pattern—such as beginning at the head and moving down. *A routine prevents overlooking a joint.*
- Perform similar movements with each extremity. *Doing so exercises the joints bilaterally.*
- Support the joint being exercised. *Support reduces discomfort.*
- Move each joint until there is resistance but not pain. *This method exercises each joint to its point of limitation.*
- Watch for nonverbal communication. *Nonverbal signs may indicate the client's response.*
- Avoid exercising a painful joint. *Doing so can contribute to injury.*
- Stop if spasticity develops, as manifested by a sudden, continuous muscle contraction. *Taking a break gives muscles time to relax and recover.*
- Apply gentle pressure to the muscle or move the spastic limb more slowly. *These actions relieve spasticity.*
- Expect the client's respiratory and heart rates to increase during exercise but to return to a resting rate later. *This is a normal cardiopulmonary response to activity.*
- Teach the family to perform ROM exercises. *A regular exercise program improves the potential for regaining function.*

exercises as many joints as possible while the nurse assists with those that are compromised (see Nursing Guidelines 24-1).

Nurses perform ROM exercises whenever they care for inactive clients (Skill 24-1).

Stop, Think, and Respond Box 24-2

Why would a nurse promote active ROM exercises in the upper body for a client who is paralyzed below the waist after a motor vehicle collision?

Continuous Passive Motion Machine

A **continuous passive motion machine** is an electrical device used as a supplement or substitute for manual ROM exercise (Fig. 24-4). A machine-assisted ROM sometimes

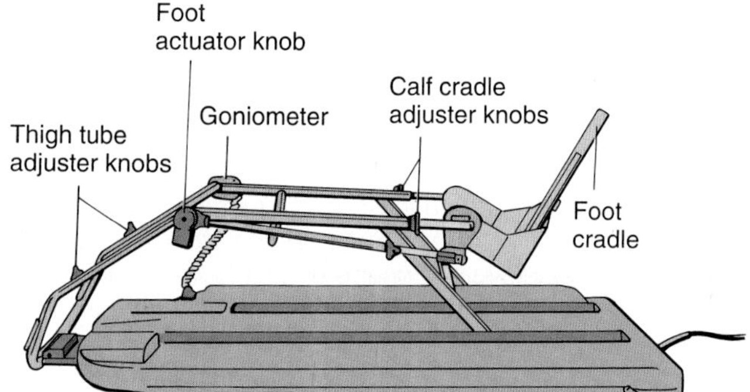

FIGURE 24-4 A continuous passive motion machine.

TABLE 24-5 Physical Activity Guidelines for Americans

GOAL	RECOMMENDATION	STRATEGIES	EXAMPLES
Increase aerobic physical activities	Do at least 2 1/2 hours of moderate level activities or 1 1/4 hours of vigorous activities per week	Build up time slowly Do at least 10 minutes at a time Combine moderate and vigorous activities	*Moderate* (can talk, but not sing during performance): Walking briskly Ballroom and line dancing Biking on level ground or with few hills
Increase muscle strengthening activities	Do at least 2 days/week	Include all the major muscle groups (legs, hips, back, chest, stomach, shoulders, and arms) Repeat 8–12 times for each muscle group per session	General gardening (raking, trimming shrubs) Sports where you catch and throw (baseball, softball, volleyball) Water aerobics *Vigorous* (can say a few words without stopping for a breath) Jogging Fast or aerobic dancing Biking faster than 10 mph Heavy gardening (digging, hoeing) Jumping rope Swimming fast or swimming laps Sports with a lot of running (basket-ball, soccer, hockey)

From US Department of Health and Human Services. (2008). *Be active your way: A fact sheet for adults.* Accessed April 28, 2010, from http://www.health.gov/paguidelines/factSheetAdults.aspx.

is preferred during the rehabilitation of clients who have experienced burns or have had knee or hip replacement surgery because the machine precisely controls the degree of joint movement and can increase it in specific increments throughout recovery.

In addition to restoring and increasing joint ROM, the movement created by the machine prevents the pooling of venous blood, thus decreasing the risk of blood clots. Also, it accelerates wound healing because the synovial fluid circulates around the joint.

Most machines produce 0 to 110 degrees of motion 2 to 10 times per minute. Initially, the nurse sets the machine at very low speeds and degrees of movement—it is common to begin with 5 or 10 degrees of flexion cycling twice a minute for at least six times a day. The nurse increases the settings as the client's tolerance builds. The nurse positions the client's extremity in the machine and programs the speed and the degree of desired joint flexion according to the physician's exercise prescription (Skill 24-2).

Stop, Think, and Respond Box 24-3

List the assessment findings that indicate a positive response to the use of a CPM machine.

NURSING IMPLICATIONS

Few people exercise sufficiently to promote optimal health. With this in mind, the Department of Health and Human Services has established Physical Activity Guidelines for Americans for improving the health of US citizens (Table 24-5). Nurses can set an example for others

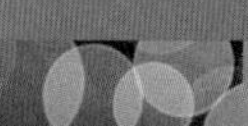

NURSING CARE PLAN 24-1 Unilateral Neglect

Assessment

- Observe the client's bilateral movement or unilateral lack of movement.
- Note whether the client uses both sides of the body in an integrated and coordinated manner.
- Determine whether the client omits, ignores, or favors activities or objects consistently on one side.
- Check the client's vision and sensation bilaterally.

Nursing Diagnosis. **Unilateral Neglect** related to a lack of awareness of objects in the left visual field secondary to stroke as manifested by a lack of attention to food on the left side of the plate and tray, an inability to see objects placed on the left side, combing only the right side of hair, no response to touch or pain stimuli on the left side, and an inability to differentiate between warm and cold on the left.

Expected Outcome. The client will identify his or her own body parts on the left side, attend to his or her care, and incorporate objects within his or her extrapersonal environment located to the client's left side by 4/21.

Interventions	Rationales
Approach the client always from the right side.	The client's perception and attention are limited to the unaffected side.
Place items for safety, such as the signal cord, and those for self-care, such as a glass of water, on the client's right side.	The neurologic deficit predisposes the client to ignore objects on the affected side.
Suggest that the client turn his or her head from side to side for a panoramic view of the environment.	Directing the client to scan the environment uses the visual areas in the unaffected structures of the brain.
Show the client three objects on the right side of the visual field each shift; then relocate objects to the left side and encourage the client to turn his or her head and identify where they are located.	Repetition in scanning both sides helps the client to develop awareness skills.
Have the client locate and touch the left arm and other body structures on the left side.	Attending to the affected side helps to retrain the client's brain to recognize and integrate parts of the self.
Add one self-care task at a time such as bathing the affected arm, inserting the arm into a gown or shirt, and grasping and exercising the affected hand with the unaffected hand as the client's awareness and competence develop.	Practice and repetition facilitate progress in reaching goals.

Evaluation of Expected Outcomes

- The nurse transfers the client to a room with a door on the right side of the client to facilitate awareness.
- The client locates and identifies one of three objects such as pen, watch, and banana after looking at them in the right visual field and then in the left.
- The client states "That's my arm and leg" when instructed to look to the left side of his or her body.
- The client touches and moves the affected left arm with the right arm.
- The client performs ROM exercises with assistance from the nurse for affected extremities.
- The client continues to practice bathing and exercise.

in the community by improving their own physical fitness and encouraging others to do so.

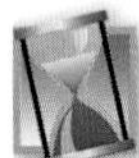

Gerontologic Considerations

■ Older adults, especially those who are disabled, need to balance periods of physical activity with periods of rest. Shortness of breath or an increased heart rate indicates that the level of activity is beyond the client's tolerance.

For people with medical disorders, nurses may identify one or more of the following nursing diagnoses that are treated with activity or an exercise regimen:

- Impaired Physical Mobility
- Risk for Disuse Syndrome
- Unilateral Neglect
- Risk for Delayed Surgical Recovery
- Activity Intolerance

Nursing Care Plan 24-1 illustrates how a nurse can incorporate exercise into the care of a client with a stroke using the nursing diagnosis of Unilateral Neglect. The NANDA-I taxonomy (2012, p. 259) defines this diagnosis as "inattention to one side (of the body) and overattention to the opposite side."

CRITICAL THINKING EXERCISES

1. List at least five excuses people give for not exercising and offer counterarguments for each.
2. A client with paralysis of the lower extremities is depressed and questions the purpose for performing passive ROM exercises on the lower body. Assuming paralysis is permanent and the client will never walk again, how would you respond?
3. What advantages would you offer to a friend who is physically inactive and could benefit from exercise?
4. What are some reasons the federal government sets goals and objectives for physical activity and fitness in its Healthy People campaigns?

NCLEX-STYLE REVIEW QUESTIONS

1. What will the nurse observe if a client performs isometric exercises of the quadriceps muscles correctly?
   1. The client moves the toes toward and away from the head.
   2. The client contracts and relaxes the muscles of the thigh.
   3. The client lifts the lower leg up and down from the bed.
   4. The client bends the knee and pulls the lower leg upward.

2. When the nursing team develops a plan of care for a client with a stroke, which area of nursing management is most important to the client's rehabilitation?
   1. Regulating bowel and bladder elimination
   2. Dealing with problems of disturbed body image
   3. Preventing contractures and joint deformities
   4. Facilitating positive outcomes from grieving

3. What nursing explanation best describes the primary purpose of a CPM machine?
   1. A CPM machine is used to strengthen leg muscles.
   2. A CPM machine is used to relieve foot swelling.
   3. A CPM machine is used to reduce surgical pain.
   4. A CPM machine is used to restore joint function.

4. What information is essential to document in relation to a client's progress in using a CPM machine? Select all that apply.
   1. Condition of the sutures around the incision
   2. Degree of joint flexion
   3. Amount of time the client used the machine
   4. Characteristics of drainage from the wound
   5. Number of cycles per minute
   6. Presence and quality of arterial pulses

5. When a client asks of what use a stress ECG will be, what is the most accurate answer the nurse can give?
   1. A stress ECG shows how the heart performs during exercise.
   2. A stress ECG helps determine the client's potential target heart rate.
   3. A stress ECG verifies how much exercise is needed to improve fitness.
   4. A stress ECG can predict whether the client will have a heart attack soon.

SKILL 24-1 Performing Range-of-Motion Exercises

Suggested Action	Reason for Action
ASSESSMENT	
Review the medical record and nursing plan for care.	Determines whether activity problems have been identified.
Assess the client's level of activity and joint mobility.	Indicates whether, and the extent to which, joints should be passively exercised.
Assess the client's understanding of the hazards of inactivity and purposes for exercise.	Determines the type and amount of health teaching needed.
PLANNING	
Explain the procedure for performing ROM exercises.	Reduces anxiety and promotes cooperation.
Consult with the client on when ROM exercises may be best performed.	Shows respect for independent decision making.
Suggest performing ROM exercises during a time that requires general activity, such as bathing.	Demonstrates efficient time management.
Perform ROM exercises at least twice a day.	Promotes recovery or maintains functional use.
Exercise each joint at least two to five times during each exercise period.	Increases exercise benefits.
IMPLEMENTATION	
Wash your hands or perform an alcohol-based hand rub (see Chap. 10).	Reduces the potential for transferring microorganisms.
Help the client to a sitting or lying position.	Promotes relaxation and access to the body.
Pull the privacy curtains.	Demonstrates respect for modesty.
Drape the client loosely or suggest loose-fitting underwear or shorts.	Avoids exposing the client.
Begin at the head.	Facilitates organization.
Support the client's neck and bring the chin toward the chest and then as far back in the opposite position as possible.	Flexes and hyperextends the neck (Fig. A).

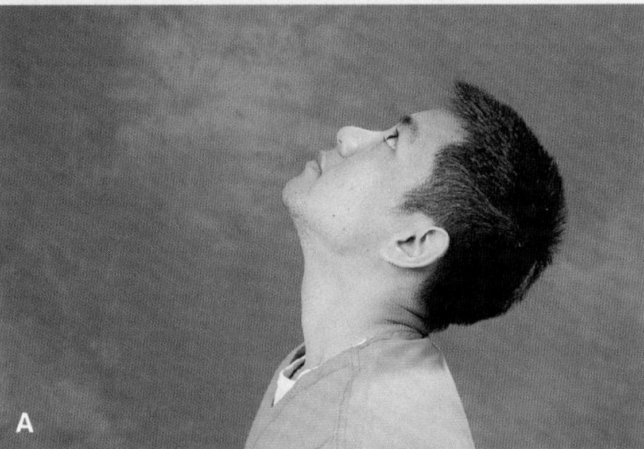

Neck hyperextension.

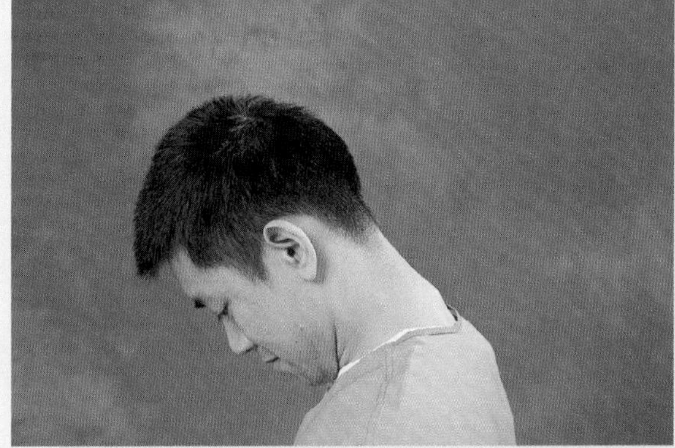

Neck flexion.

Suggested Action	Reason for Action
Place a hand on either side of the head and move the neck from side to side.	Rotates the neck (Fig. B).

B

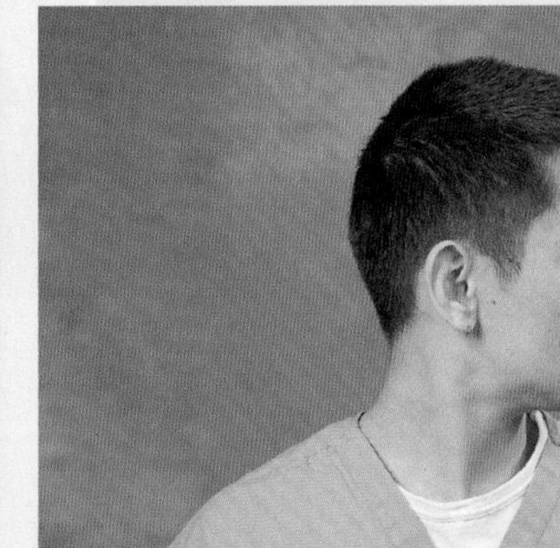

Neck rotation.

(continued)

Performing Range-of-Motion Exercises (continued)

IMPLEMENTATION (CONTINUED)

Turn the head in a circular fashion.

Puts the head and neck through circumduction (Fig. C).

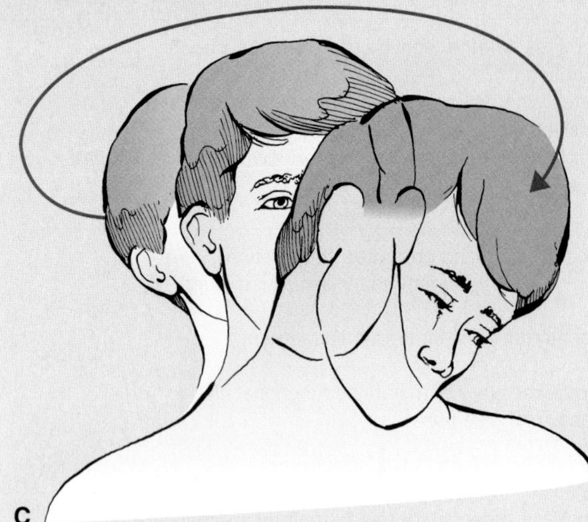

Circumduction of the neck.

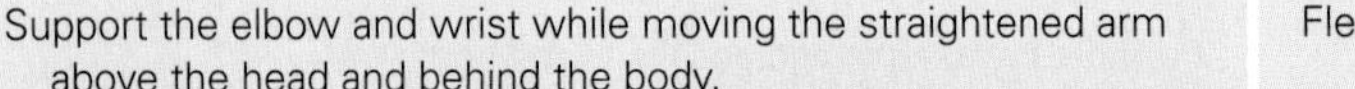

Support the elbow and wrist while moving the straightened arm above the head and behind the body.

Flexes, extends, then hyperextends the shoulder (Fig. D).

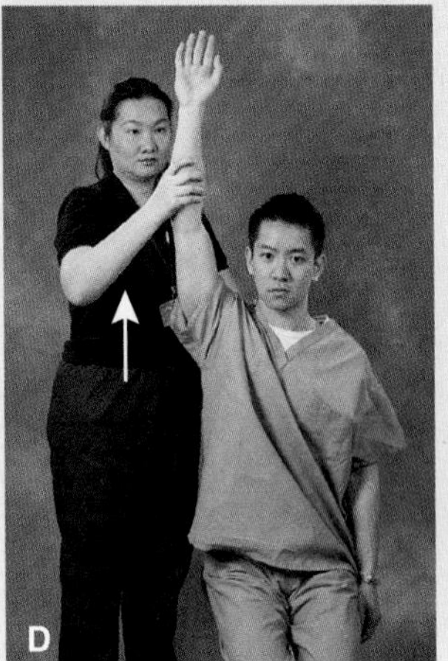

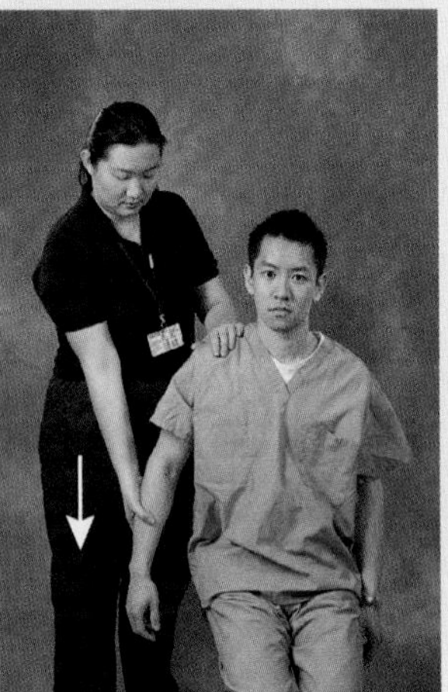

Flexion and extension of the shoulder.

Move the straightened arm away from the body and then toward the midline.

Abducts and adducts the shoulder (Fig. E).

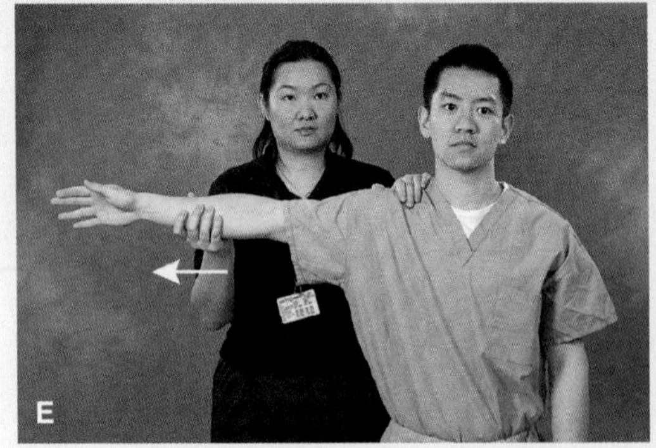

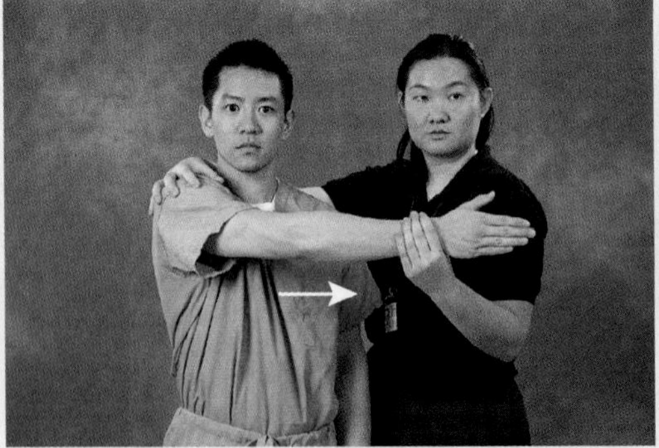

Abduction and adduction of the shoulder.

(continued)

Performing Range-of-Motion Exercises (continued)

IMPLEMENTATION (CONTINUED)

Bend the elbow and move the arm so that the palm is upward and then downward.

Produces internal and external rotation of the shoulder (Fig. F).

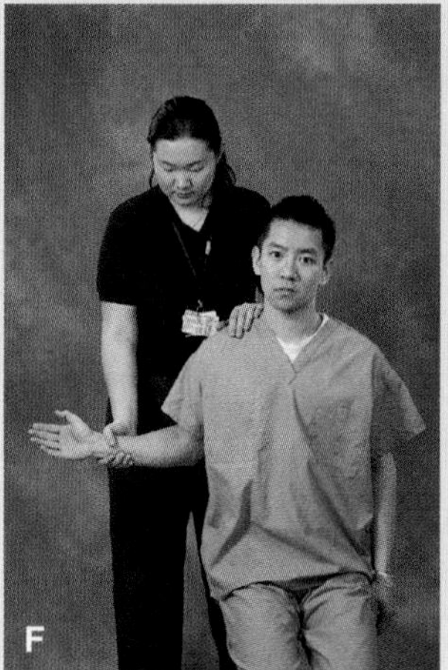

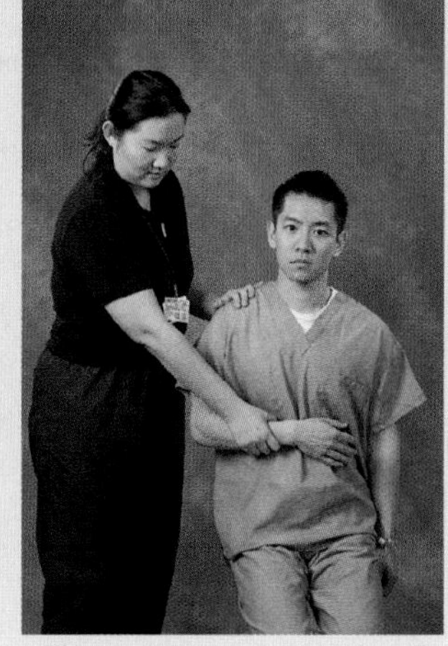

Internal and external rotation of the shoulder.

Move the arm in a full circle.

Circumducts the shoulder (Fig. G).

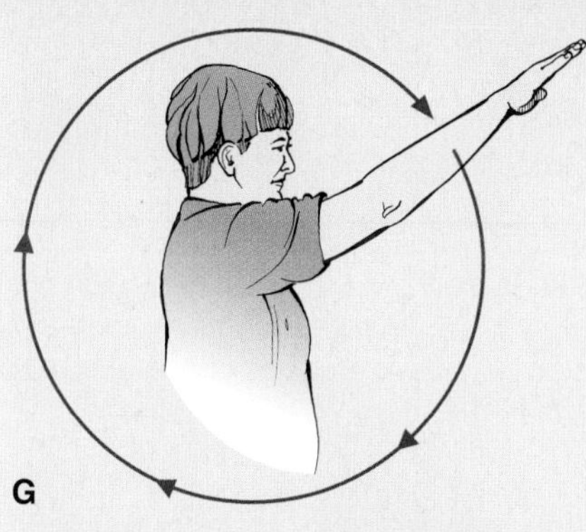

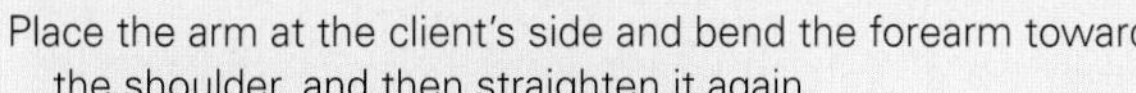

Circumduction of the shoulder.

Place the arm at the client's side and bend the forearm toward the shoulder, and then straighten it again.

Flexes and extends the elbow (Fig. H).

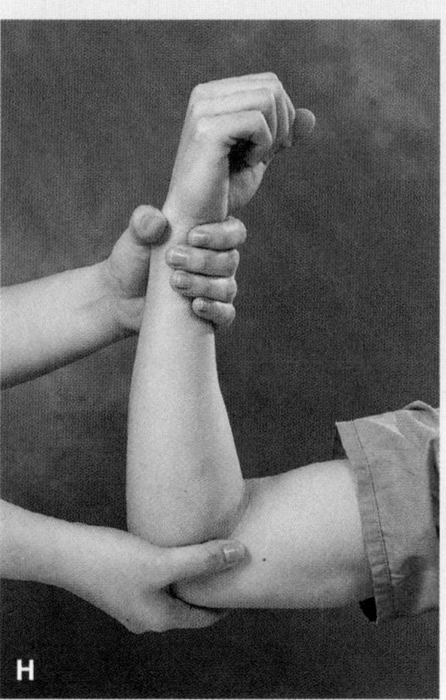

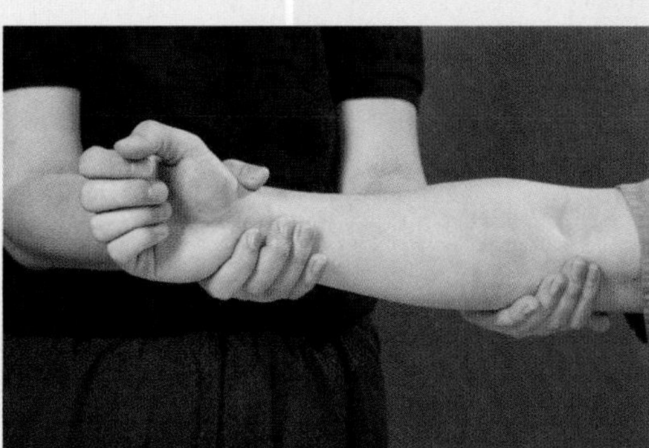

Flexion and extension of the elbow.

(continued)

Performing Range-of-Motion Exercises (continued)

IMPLEMENTATION (CONTINUED)

Bend the wrist forward and then backward.

Moves the wrist from flexion to extension and then hyperextension (Fig. I).

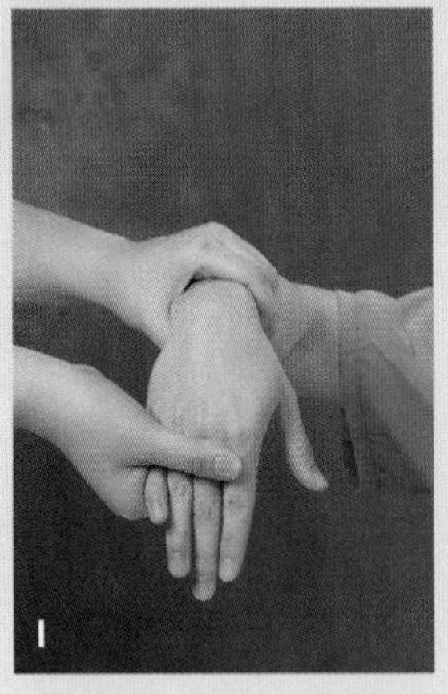

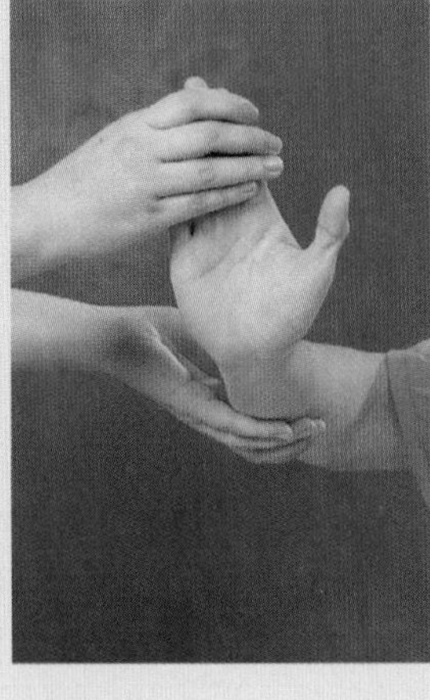

Flexion and extension of the wrist.

Twist the wrist to the right and then left.

Rotates the wrist joint (Fig. J).

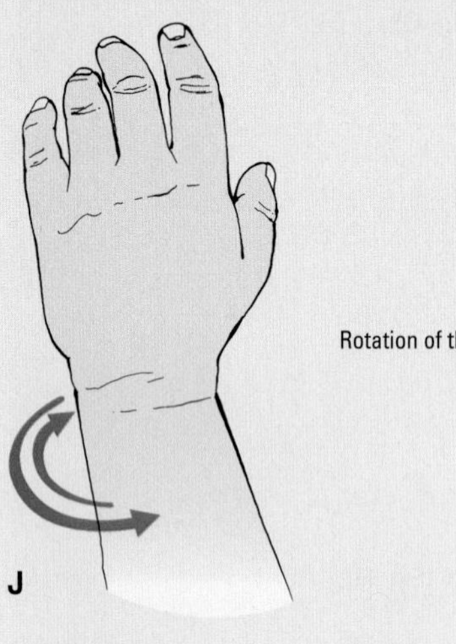

Rotation of the wrist.

Bend the thumb side of the hand way from the wrist and then in the opposite direction.

Provides adduction and then abduction of the wrist (Fig. K).

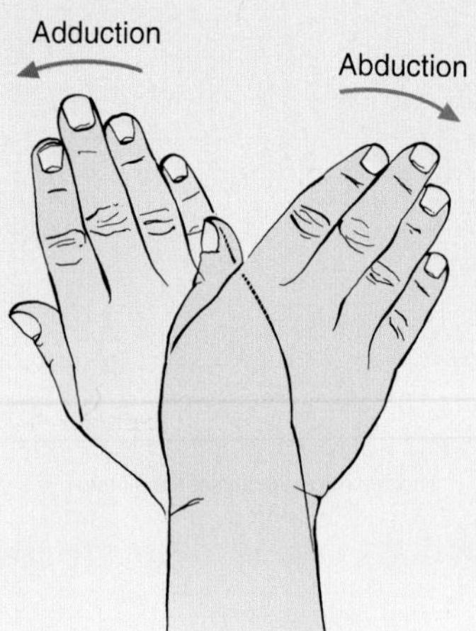

Abduction and adduction of the wrist.

(continued)

Performing Range-of-Motion Exercises (continued)

IMPLEMENTATION (CONTINUED)

Turn the palm downward and then upward. Pronates and supinates the wrist (Fig. L).

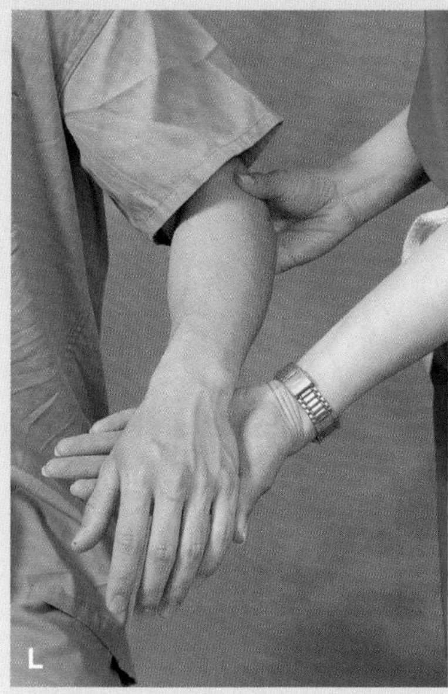

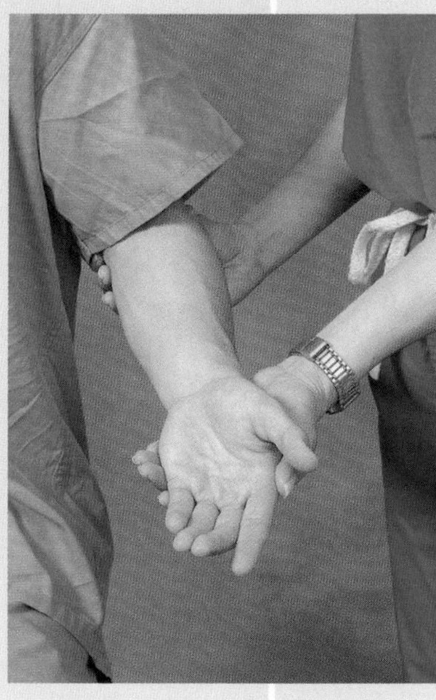

Pronation and supination of the wrist.

Open and close the fingers as though making a fist. Extends and flexes the fingers (Fig. M).

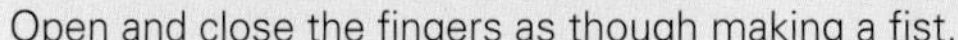

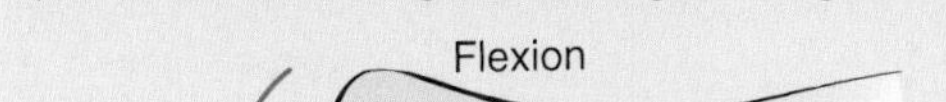

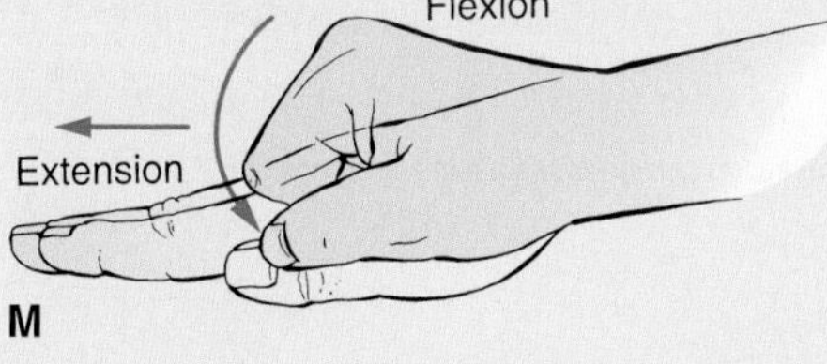

Flexion and extension of the fingers.

Bend the thumb toward the center of the palm and then back to its original position. Flexes and extends the thumb (Fig. N).

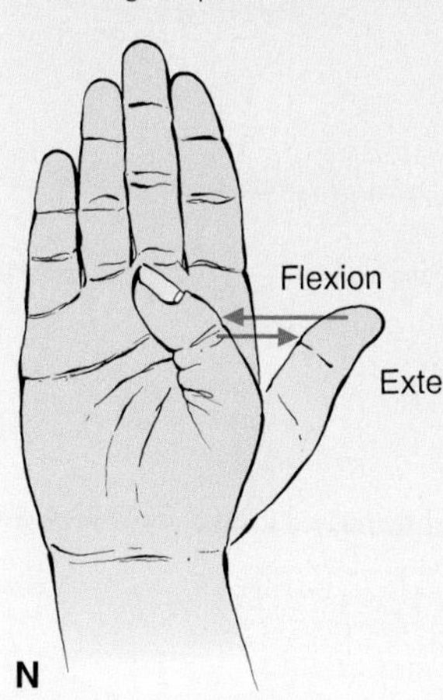

Flexion and extension of the thumb.

(continued)

Performing Range-of-Motion Exercises (continued)

IMPLEMENTATION (CONTINUED)

Spread the fingers and thumb as widely as possible and then bring them back together again.

Abducts and adducts the fingers and thumb (Fig. O).

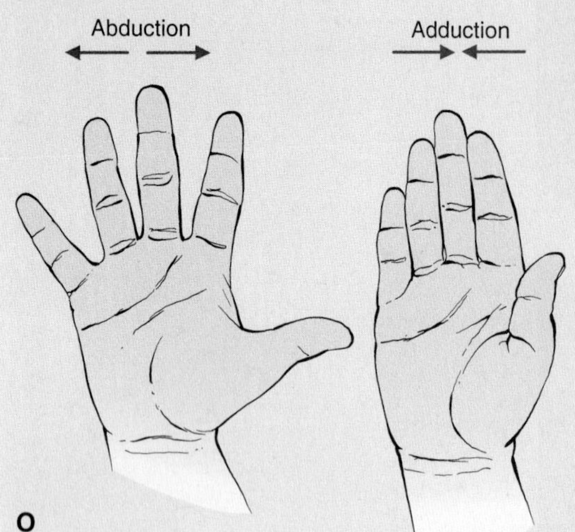

Abduction and adduction of the fingers and thumb.

Bring the straightened leg forward of and backward from the body in a standing position.

Flexes, extends, and hyperextends the hip (Fig. P).

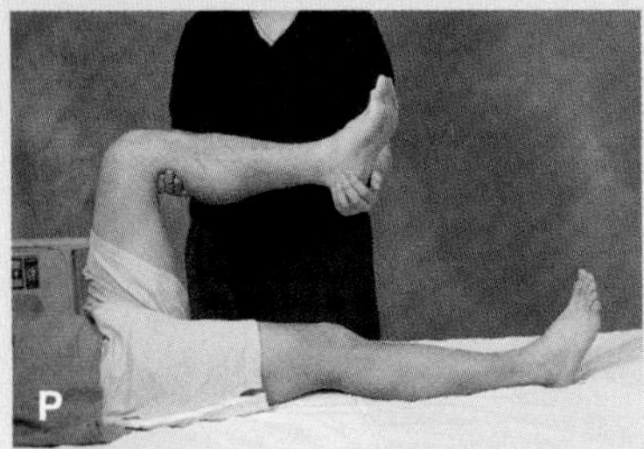

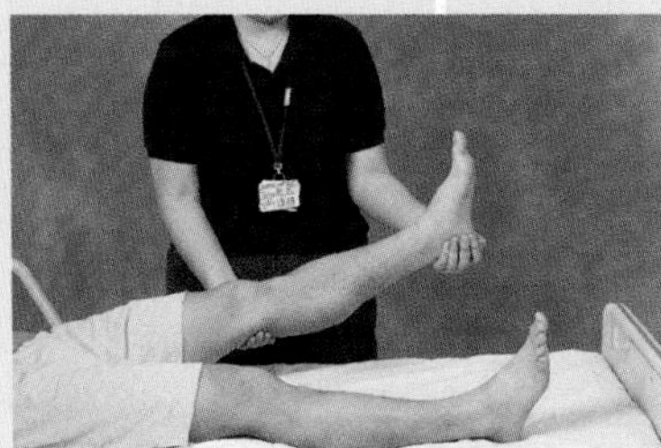

Flexion and extension of the hip in a lying position.

Move the straightened leg away from the body and back beyond the midline.

Abducts and then adducts the hip (Fig. Q).

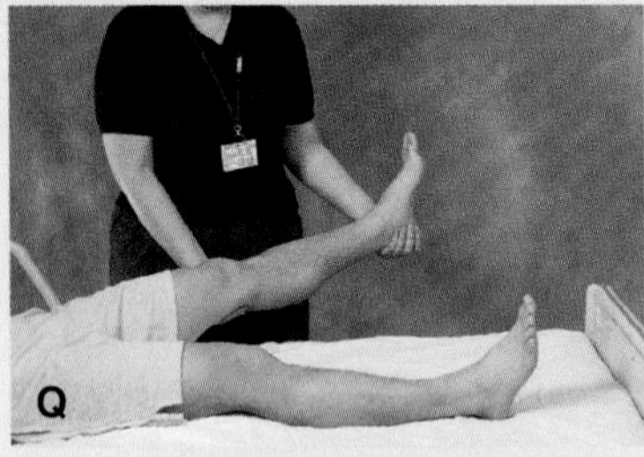

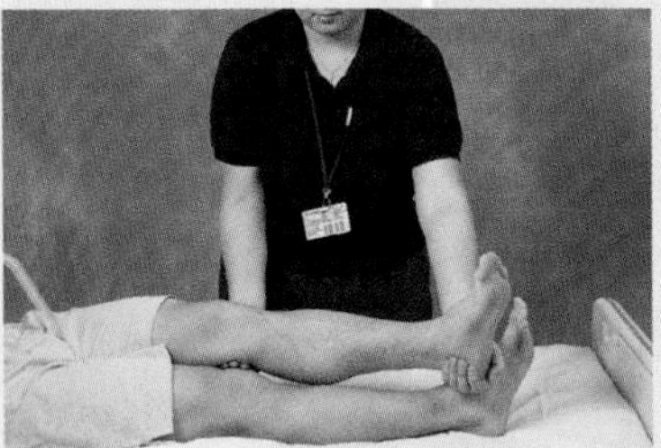

Abduction and adduction of the hip.

Turn the leg away from the other leg and then toward it.

Rotates the hip externally and then internally (Fig. R).

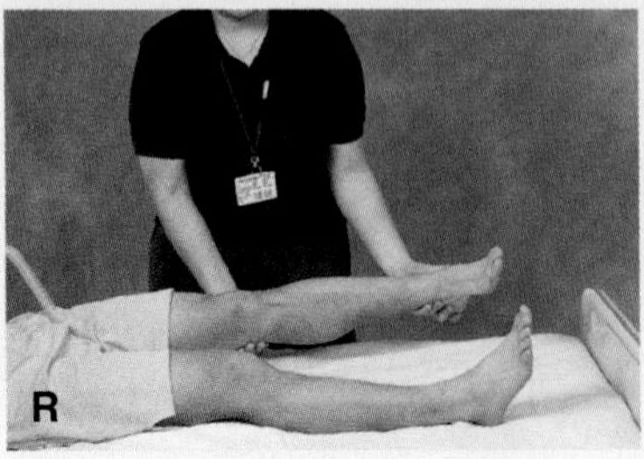

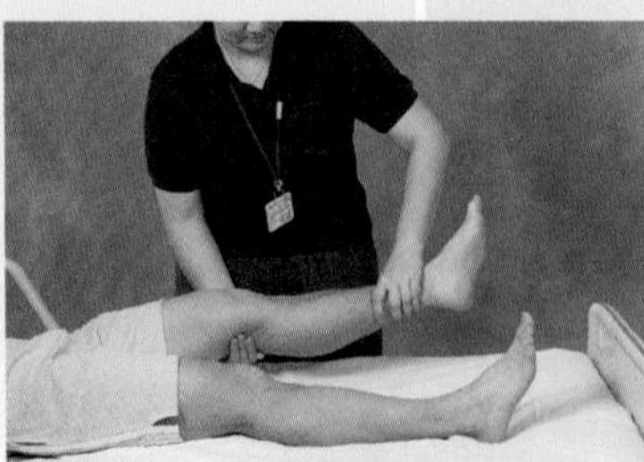

Internal and external rotation of the hip.

(continued)

Performing Range-of-Motion Exercises (continued)

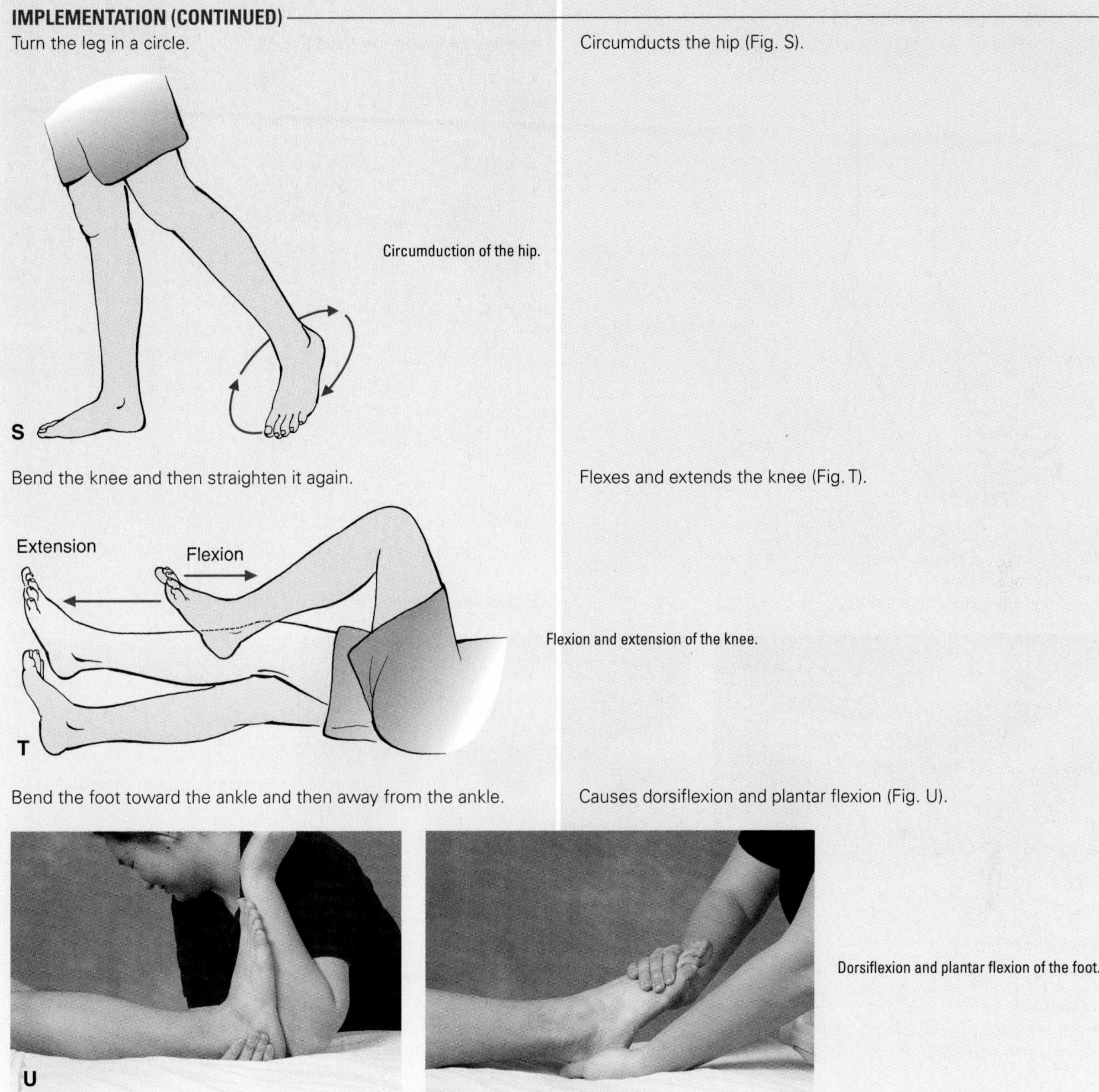

IMPLEMENTATION (CONTINUED)

Turn the leg in a circle. — Circumducts the hip (Fig. S).

Circumduction of the hip.

Bend the knee and then straighten it again. — Flexes and extends the knee (Fig. T).

Flexion and extension of the knee.

Bend the foot toward the ankle and then away from the ankle. — Causes dorsiflexion and plantar flexion (Fig. U).

Dorsiflexion and plantar flexion of the foot.

(continued)

Performing Range-of-Motion Exercises (continued)

IMPLEMENTATION (CONTINUED)

Bend the sole of the foot toward the midline and then away from midline.

Inverts and everts the ankle (Fig. V).

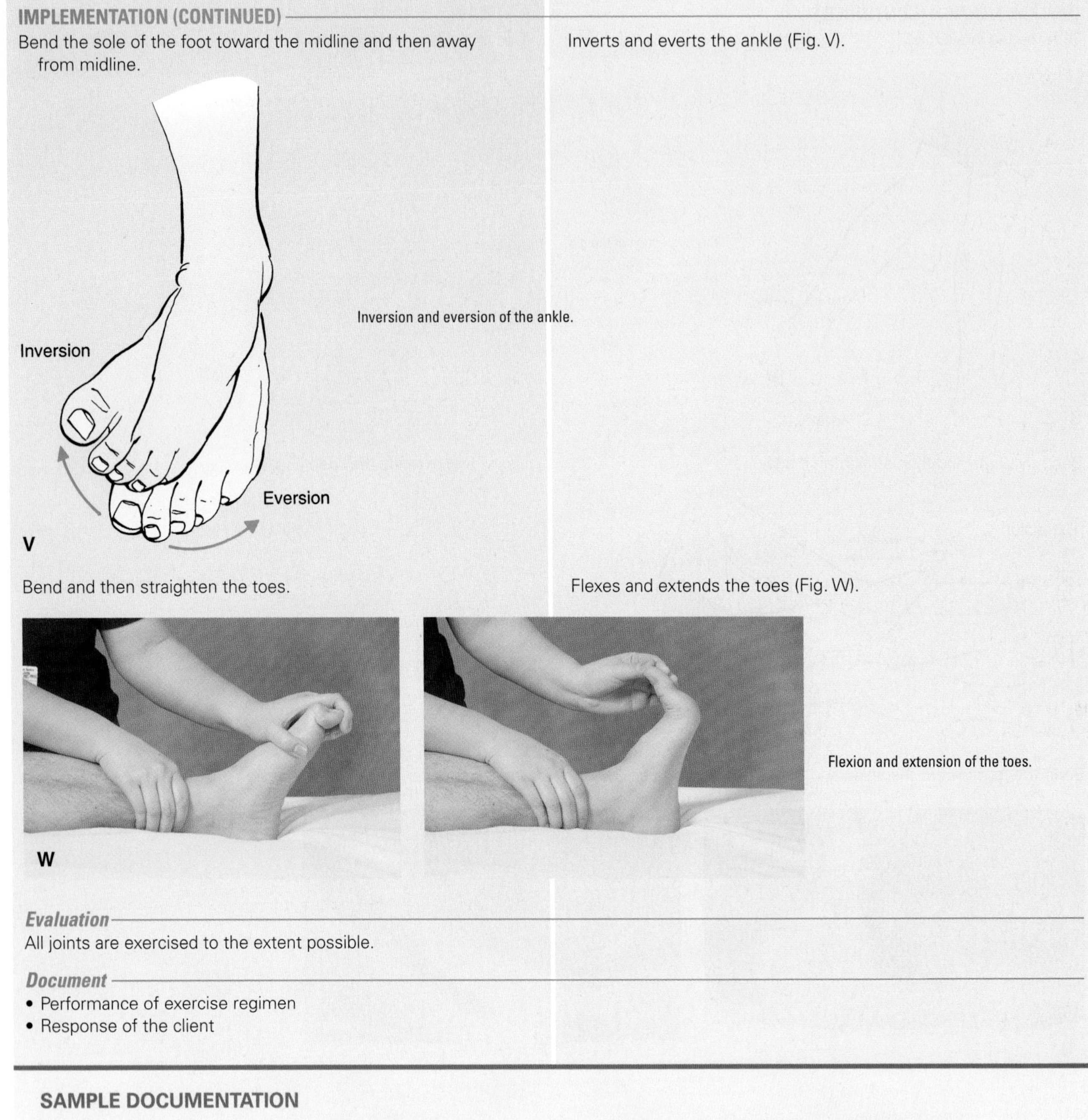

Inversion and eversion of the ankle.

Bend and then straighten the toes.

Flexes and extends the toes (Fig. W).

Flexion and extension of the toes.

Evaluation

All joints are exercised to the extent possible.

Document

- Performance of exercise regimen
- Response of the client

SAMPLE DOCUMENTATION

Date and Time Assisted to perform ROM exercises during bath. Actively moves all joints on the right side of the body. Joints on the left side passively exercised through full ranges. No resistance or pain experienced. ——————————SIGNATURE/TITLE

SKILL 24-2 Using a Continuous Passive Motion Machine

Suggested Action	Reason for Action
ASSESSMENT	
Review the medical record and nursing care plan for the amount of joint flexion, cycles per minute, frequency, and duration of exercise.	Determines the exercise prescription for the client.
Explore how much the client understands about CPM, especially if this is the first time it is being used.	Determines the level and type of health teaching to provide.
Assess the quality of peripheral pulses, capillary refill, edema, temperature, sensation, and mobility of the affected extremity.	Provides a baseline of data for future comparisons.
Compare assessment findings with the unaffected extremity.	Provides comparative data.
Determine the client's need for pain-relieving medication before use of the CPM machine.	Controls pain before it intensifies with exercise.
PLANNING	
Develop a schedule with the client for using the machine.	Involves the client in decision making.
Instruct the client on techniques for muscle relaxation and pain control such as deep breathing, listening to tapes, watching television, or applying an ice bag.	Empowers the client with techniques for controlling pain.
Obtain the CPM machine and secure a length of sheepskin or soft flannel cloth to the horizontal bars to form a cradle (sling) for the calf.	Prepares the machine for supporting the leg.
Wash hands or perform an alcohol-based hand rub (see Chap. 10).	Reduces the transmission of microorganisms.
Don gloves and empty any wound drainage containers; change or reinforce the dressing (see Chap. 28).	Prevents leakage during exercise, when drainage is likely to increase.
IMPLEMENTATION	
Explain the purpose, application, and use of the CPM machine.	Reduces anxiety and promotes cooperation.
Position the client flat or slightly elevate the head of the bed.	Promotes comfort during exercise.
Place the CPM machine on the bed and position the client's foot so that it rests against the foot cradle (Fig. A).	Prepares the client for exercise.

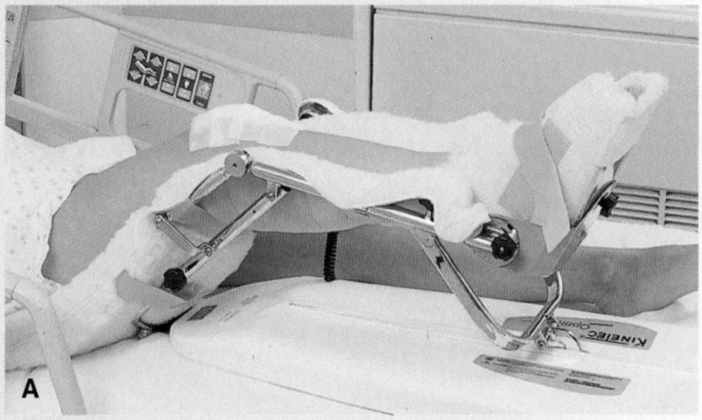

A

Range of motion of the knee with a continuous passive motion machine. (Photo by B. Proud.)

Suggested Action	Reason for Action
Check that the knee joint corresponds to the foot actuator knob and *goniometer,* a device for measuring ROM.	Positions the knee correctly.
Use Velcro or canvas straps to secure the leg within the fabric cradle of the machine.	Supports and stabilizes the leg.
Adjust the machine to a lower than prescribed rate and degree of flexion.	Provides gradual progression to prescribed parameters.
Turn on the machine and observe the client's response.	Indicates the client's level of tolerance.
Readjust the alignment of the leg or position of the machine for optimal comfort.	Demonstrates concern for the client's well-being.
Increase the degree of flexion and cycles per minute gradually until the prescribed levels are reached.	Facilitates adaptation.
Turn off the machine with the leg in an extended position at the end of the prescribed period of exercise.	Facilitates lifting the leg from the machine.
Release the straps and support the joints beneath the knee and ankle while lifting the leg.	Reduces discomfort.
Remove the machine from the bed; encourage active ROM exercises and isometric exercises.	Potentiates effects from CPM.

(continued)

Using a Continuous Passive Motion Machine (continued)

Evaluation

CPM applied and used according to exercise prescription.

Document

- Assessment data
- Use of machine
- Current amount of flexion, cycles per minute, and duration
- Tolerance of exercise

SAMPLE DOCUMENTATION

Date and Time Knee incision is dry and intact. Toes on both feet are warm with capillary refill <3 seconds. Pedal pulses present and strong bilaterally. CPM machine used for 15 minutes with ROM at 30-degree knee flexion for 5 cycles per minute. Discomfort increased from a level 4 before exercise to level 7 during exercise. Pain at a level of 5 after 15 minutes of rest following exercise. ———————— SIGNATURE/TITLE

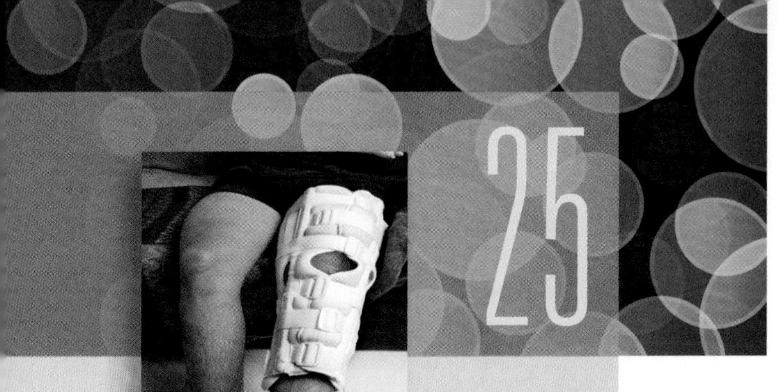

Mechanical Immobilization

Words To Know

bivalved cast
body cast
braces
cast
cervical collar
compartment syndrome
cylinder cast
external fixator
functional braces
immobilizers
inflatable splints
manual traction
molded splints
orthoses
petals
pin site
prophylactic braces
rehabilitative braces
skeletal traction
skin traction
sling
spica cast
splint
traction
traction splints
window

Learning Objectives

On completion of this chapter, the reader should be able to:

1. List at least three purposes of mechanical immobilization.
2. Name four types of splints.
3. Discuss why slings and braces are used.
4. Explain the purpose of a cast.
5. Name three types of casts.
6. Describe at least five nursing actions that are appropriate when caring for clients with casts.
7. Discuss how casts are removed.
8. Explain what traction implies.
9. List three types of traction.
10. Name seven principles that apply to maintaining effective traction.
11. Describe the purpose of an external fixator.
12. Identify the rationale for performing pin site care.

Some clients are inactive and physically immobile as a result of an overall debilitating condition. For others, impaired mobility results from trauma or its treatment. Such is the case for clients with **orthoses**, which are orthopedic devices that support or align a body part and prevent or correct deformities. Examples of orthoses include splints, immobilizers, and braces. Other clients have limited mobility when the use of slings, casts, traction, and external fixators is necessary. Caring for clients who are mechanically immobilized with orthopedic devices requires specialized nursing skills described in this chapter.

PURPOSES OF MECHANICAL IMMOBILIZATION

Most clients who require mechanical immobilization have suffered trauma to the musculoskeletal system. Such injuries are painful and heal less rapidly than injuries to the skin or soft tissue. They require a period of inactivity to allow new cells to restore integrity to the damaged structures.

Mechanical immobilization of a body part accomplishes the following:

- Relieves pain and muscle spasm
- Supports and aligns skeletal injuries
- Restricts movement while injuries heal
- Maintains a functional position until healing is complete

- Allows activity while restricting movement of an injured area
- Prevents further structural damage and deformity

MECHANICAL IMMOBILIZING DEVICES

The use of various immobilizing devices can achieve therapeutic benefits. Examples of such devices include splints, slings, braces, casts, and traction.

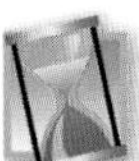

Gerontologic Considerations

- As adults live longer, many are dealing with the pain and loss of function associated with arthritis. Treatment options involve rehabilitation with various types of mechanical devices in the home or rehabilitation setting.
- Some fractures in older adults, particularly of the upper extremities, are treated nonsurgically with immobilization. Occupational and physical therapists are helpful in assisting older adults to regain function and range of motion following any period of immobilization to prevent a decrease or a permanent loss of function.
- Because of diminished tactile sensation, older adults may be unaware of skin pressure from a splint, cast, traction, or other mechanical device. Assess the skin of an older person daily for redness or other signs of pressure (a reddened area that does not resolve in 30 minutes of pressure relief). If the older person cannot change positions, the caregiver is responsible for ensuring that pressure is relieved at least every 2 hours.

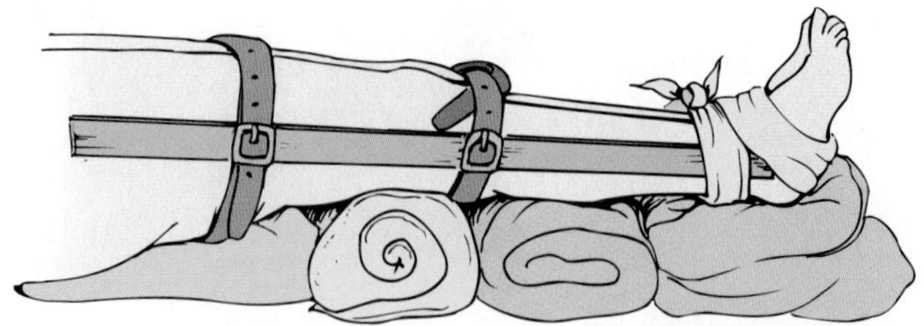

FIGURE 25-1 Emergency first-aid splinting immobilizes the injured leg to the uninjured leg with a make shift splint, such as a board, broom handle, or golf club. Neckties, belts, or scarves keep the splint in place.

Splints

Some conditions are treated with a **splint**, which is a device that immobilizes and protects an injured body part. Splints are used before or instead of casts or traction.

Emergency Splints

Splints often are applied as a first-aid measure for suspected sprains or fractures (Fig. 25-1) (see Nursing Guidelines 25-1).

Commercial Splints

Commercial splints are more effective than improvised splints. They are available in various designs depending on the injury. Examples include inflatable splints, traction splints, immobilizers, molded splints, and cervical collars. Inflatable and traction splints are intended for short-term use; they usually are applied just after the injury and are removed shortly after a more thorough assessment of the injury. Immobilizers and molded splints are used for longer periods.

Inflatable Splints

Inflatable splints, also called "pneumatic splints," are immobilizing devices that become rigid when filled with

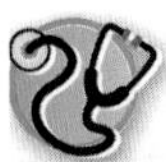

NURSING GUIDELINES 25-1

Applying an Emergency Splint

- Avoid changing the position of the injured part even if it appears grossly deformed. *Keeping the injured part in place prevents additional injuries.*
- Leave a high-top shoe or a ski boot in place if the injury involves an ankle. *The shoe or boot limits movement and reduces pain and swelling.*
- Cover any open wounds with clean material. *Such a covering absorbs blood and prevents dirt and additional pathogens from entering.*
- Select a rigid splinting material such as a flat board, broom handle, or rolled-up newspaper. *Rigid material provides support while restricting movement.*
- Pad bony prominences with soft material. *Padding reduces pressure and prevents friction on the skin.*
- Apply the splinting device so that it spans the injured area from the joint above to the joint below the injury. *Such placement immobilizes the injured tissue.*
- Use an uninjured area of the body adjacent to the injured part as a splint, if no other sturdy material is available. *The uninjured part can serve as a substitute for an external splint.*
- Use wide tape or wide strips of fabric to confine the injured part to the splint. *Securing the body part prevents displacement and reduces the risk for compromising circulation.*
- Loosen the splint or the material used to attach it if the fingers or toes are pale, blue, or cold. *Loosening the splint facilitates circulation.*
- Elevate the immobilized part, if possible, so that the lowest point is higher than the heart. *Elevation reduces swelling and enhances venous return to the heart.*
- Keep the client warm and safe. *Shock is a risk.*
- Seek assistance in transporting the client to a health care agency. *The client requires more sophisticated treatment.*

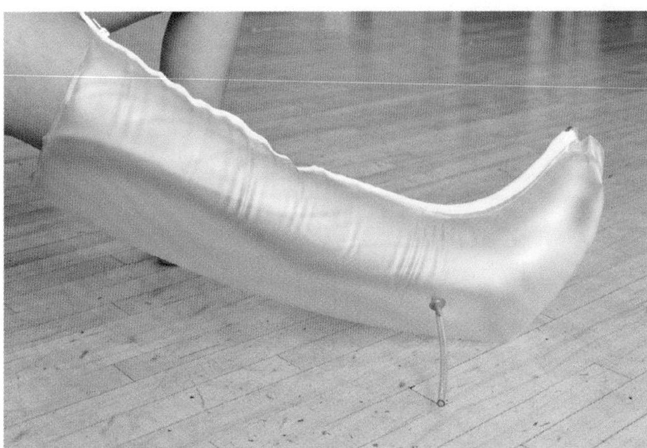

FIGURE 25-2 An inflatable splint.

air (Fig. 25-2). In addition to limiting motion, they control bleeding and swelling. The injured body part is inserted into the deflated splint. When air is infused, the splint molds to the contour of the injured part, preventing movement. The splint is filled with air to the point at which it can be indented 0.5 in. (1.3 cm) with the fingertips. The injury should be examined and treated within 30 to 45 minutes after application of the splint; otherwise, circulation may be affected.

Traction Splints

Traction splints are metal devices that immobilize and pull on contracted muscles. They are not as easy to apply as inflatable splints. One example is a *Thomas splint*, which requires special training for its application to prevent additional injuries (Fig. 25-3).

Immobilizers

Immobilizers are commercial splints made from cloth and foam and held in place by adjustable hook and loop tape (such as Velcro) straps (Fig. 25-4). As the name implies, immobilizers limit motion in the area of a painful but healing injury such as the neck and the knee. They are removed for brief periods during hygiene and dressing.

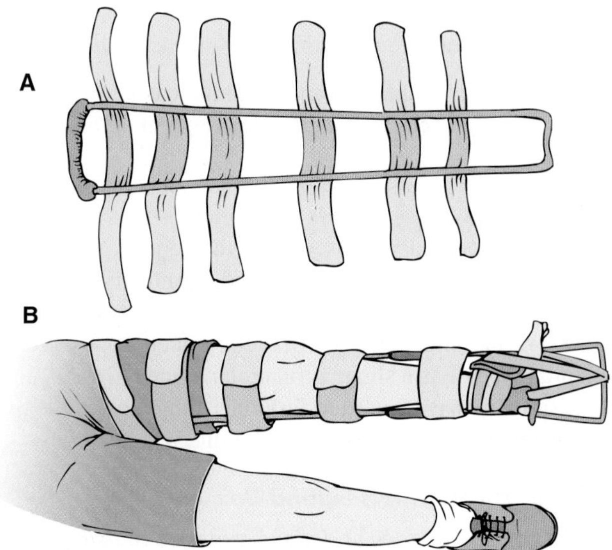

FIGURE 25-3 **A.** A Thomas splint. **B.** A Thomas splint applied to the lower extremity.

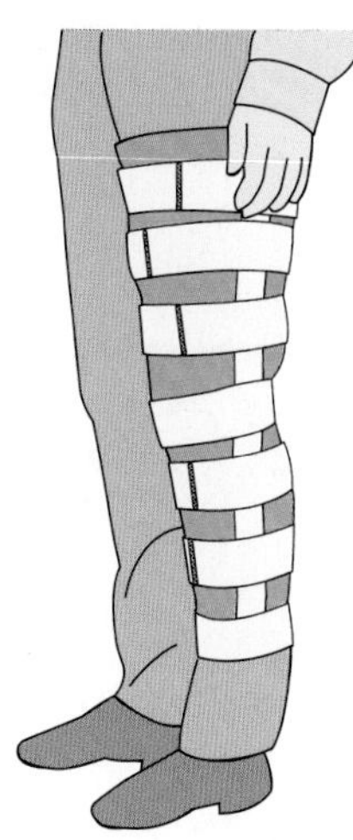

FIGURE 25-4 A leg immobilizer.

Molded Splints

Molded splints are orthotic devices made of rigid materials and are used for chronic injuries or diseases. They may be appropriate for clients with repetitive motion disorders such as carpal tunnel syndrome. They provide prolonged support and limit movement to prevent further injury and pain (Fig. 25-5). They maintain the body part in a functional position to prevent contractures and muscle atrophy during immobility.

Cervical Collars

A **cervical collar** is a foam or rigid splint placed around the neck. It is used to treat athletic neck injuries and other trauma that results in a neck sprain or strain (Fig. 25-6). Neck strain is sometimes referred to as *whiplash* or a *whiplash injury.* The incidence of whiplash injuries has decreased primarily for two reasons: improved athletic protective equipment and use of shoulder harnesses and neck supports in automobiles.

When a neck injury—which is generally more painful the day after trauma—is mild or moderate, a foam collar,

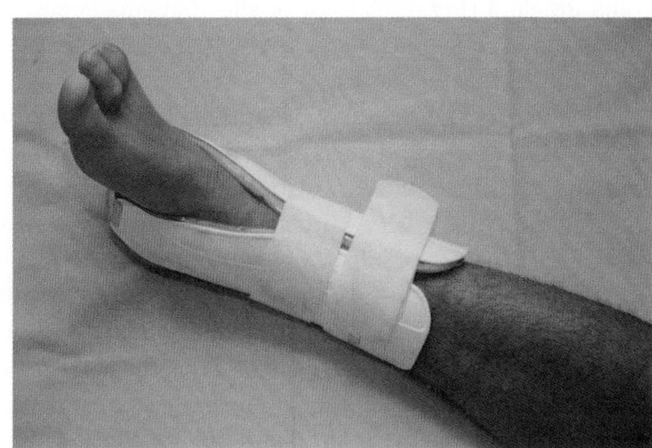

FIGURE 25-5 A molded splint.

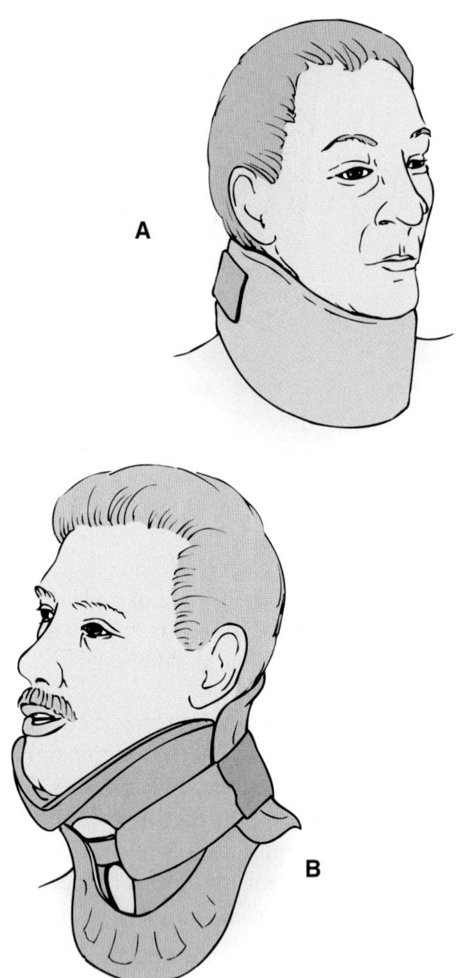

FIGURE 25-6 **A.** A foam cervical collar. **B.** A rigid cervical collar.

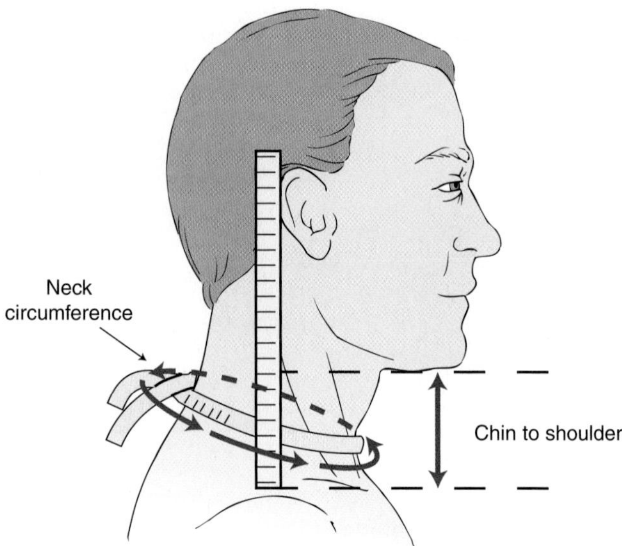

FIGURE 25-7 Vertical and circumferential measurements for cervical collar size.

covered with stockinette (a stretchable cotton fabric), is used. When the client wears it, it reminds him or her to limit neck and head movements. For more serious injuries, a rigid splint made from polyurethane is used to control neck motion and support the head, reducing its load-bearing force on the cervical spine.

To determine the proper collar size, the nurse measures the neck circumference and the distance between the shoulder and the chin (Fig. 25-7). He or she compares measurements with the size guide suggested by the collar manufacturer. For example, a person with a neck size of 15 to 20 in. and a shoulder-to-chin height of 3 in. probably would require a regular adult size. Adult sizes also come in short, tall, and extra tall. Pediatric collars are also available.

When applying a cervical collar, the head is placed in a neutral position (see Chap. 23). The front of the collar is positioned well beneath the chin and slid upward until the chin is well supported. The opening of the collar is centered at the back of the neck. Straps made of Velcro or other materials are used to secure the collar in the desired position. When applied appropriately, the client can breathe and swallow effortlessly while wearing the collar.

Clients wear cervical collars almost continuously, even while sleeping, for 10 days to 2 weeks. They remove them to do gentle range-of-motion neck exercises (see Chap. 24). The sooner a client performs exercise (within his or her pain tolerance), the faster revascularization and recovery occur. Prolonged dependence on the collar for comfort can lead to permanent stiffness in the neck.

During recovery, the nurse assesses the client's neuromuscular status by having the client perform movements that correlate with muscular functions controlled by cervical spine and peripheral nerve roots. If neuromuscular function is intact, the client can do the following:

- Elevate both shoulders
- Flex and extend the elbows and the wrists
- Generate a strong hand grip
- Spread the fingers
- Touch the thumb to the little finger on each hand

The nurse documents and communicates to the physician any difference in strength or movement on one side or the other.

Slings

A **sling** is a cloth device used to elevate, cradle, and support parts of the body. Slings are applied commonly to the arm (Fig. 25-8), leg, or pelvis after immobilization and examination of the injury. Many ambulatory clients use the commercial type of arm sling; a triangular piece of muslin cloth occasionally may be used to fashion a sling. To be effective, slings require proper application (Skill 25-1).

Stop, Think, and Respond Box 25-1

List the advantages and disadvantages of using a commercially made canvas sling and a triangular cloth sling.

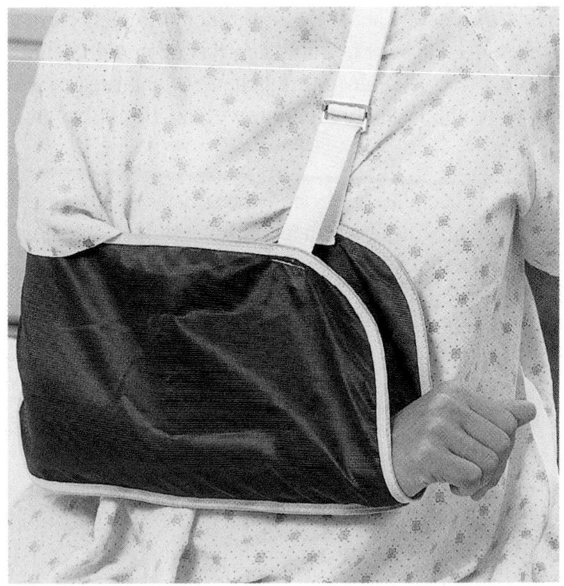

FIGURE 25-8 A commercial sling used for arm suspension. (Photo by B. Proud.)

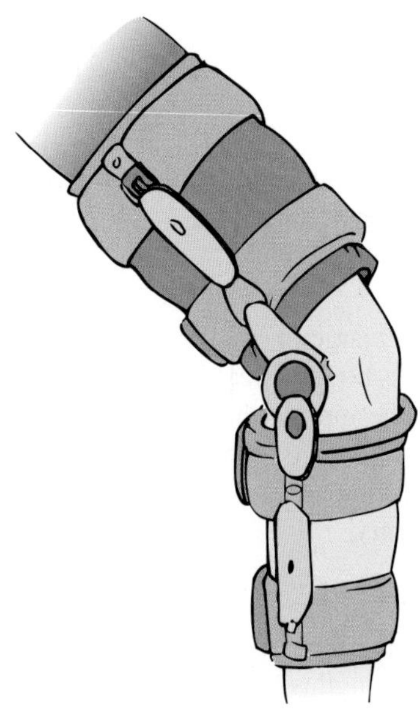

FIGURE 25-9 A rehabilitative brace that ensures appropriate control of knee motion following an operative procedure.

Braces

Braces are custom-made or custom-fitted devices designed to support weakened structures. The three categories of braces are (1) **prophylactic braces** (those used to prevent or reduce the severity of a joint injury), (2) **rehabilitative braces** (those that allow protected motion of an injured joint that has been treated operatively; Fig. 25-9), and (3) **functional braces** (those that provide stability for an unstable joint).

Because clients generally wear braces during active periods, braces are made of sturdy materials such as metal or leather. Leg braces may be incorporated into a shoe. Some back braces are made of cloth with metal staves, or strips, sewn within the fabric of the brace. An improperly applied or ill-fitting brace can cause discomfort, deformity, and skin ulcerations from friction or prolonged pressure.

Casts

A **cast** is a rigid mold placed around an injured body part after it has been restored to correct the anatomic alignment. The purpose of the cast is to immobilize the injured structure. Casts usually are applied to fractured (broken) bones. They are formed using either wetted rolls of plaster of Paris or premoistened rolls of fiberglass (Table 25-1).

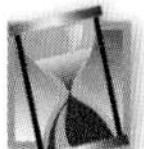

Gerontologic Considerations

- Hip fractures are common in older adults, especially postmenopausal women not treated for osteoporosis. The fracture may result from weakness of the bone and lead to a fall, or a fall may cause the fracture of a weakened bone.
- With aging, bones become brittle and weak, resulting in longer healing time for fractures.

Types of Casts

There are basically three types of casts: cylinder, body, and spica. Cylinder and body casts may be bivalved.

TABLE 25-1 Cast Materials

SUBSTANCE	ADVANTAGES	DISADVANTAGES
Plaster of Paris	Inexpensive Easy to apply Low incidence of allergic reactions	Takes 24–48 hours to dry; large casts may take up to 72 hours to dry Weight bearing must be delayed until thoroughly dried Heavy Prone to cracking or crumbling, especially at the edges Softens when wet
Fiberglass	Lightweight Porous Dries in 5–15 minutes Allows immediate weight bearing Durable Unaffected by water	Expensive Not recommended for severe injuries or those accompanied by excessive swelling Macerates skin if padding becomes wet Cast edges may be sharp and may cause skin abrasions

Cylinder Cast

A **cylinder cast** encircles an arm or leg and leaves the toes or fingers exposed. The cast extends from the joints above and below the affected bone. This prevents movement in the injured area, thereby maintaining correct alignment during healing. As healing progresses, the cast may be trimmed or shortened.

Body Cast

A **body cast** is a larger form of a cylinder cast and encircles the trunk of the body instead of an extremity. It generally extends from the nipple line to the hips. For some clients with spinal problems, the body cast extends from the back of the head and chin areas to the hips, with modifications for exposing the arms.

Bivalved Cast

The physician may create a **bivalved cast** (one that is cut into two pieces lengthwise) from either a body or a cylinder cast. Creating a front and a back for a body cast facilitates bathing and skin care. A bivalved cast on an extremity (Fig. 25-10) is created when:

- Swelling compresses tissue and interferes with circulation
- The client is being weaned from the cast
- A sharper X-ray image is needed
- Painful joints need to be immobilized temporarily for a client with arthritis

Creating a front and a back for a body cast facilitates bathing and skin care. If the physician approves, half of the shell is removed temporarily for hygiene while the other half remains in place. The process is repeated when caring for the opposite body area. Once care has been completed, the removed piece is replaced and the two halves are held in place by wrapping them together with an elastic bandage.

Spica Cast

A **spica cast** encircles one or both the arms or legs and the chest or trunk. It may have an abduction bar to help maintain the position of the repaired injury. When applied to the upper body, the cast is referred to as a *shoulder spica*; one applied to the lower extremities is called a *hip spica* (Fig. 25-11). Spica casts, especially those on the lower extremities, are heavy, hot, and frustrating because they severely restrict movement and activity.

When applied to a lower extremity, the cast is trimmed in the anal and genital areas to allow for the elimination of urine and stool. Clients with a hip spica cannot sit during elimination, so the nurse protects the cast from soiling using plastic wrap and positions the client on a small bedpan known as a fracture pan (see Chap 30).

Cast Application

Cast application generally requires more than one person. The nurse prepares the client, assembles the cast supplies, and helps the physician during the cast application (Skill 25-2). A light-cured fiberglass cast requires exposure to ultraviolet light to harden.

Basic Cast Care

Some clients need extended care after surgery that has included the application of a cast. The nurse is responsible for caring for the cast and making appropriate assessments

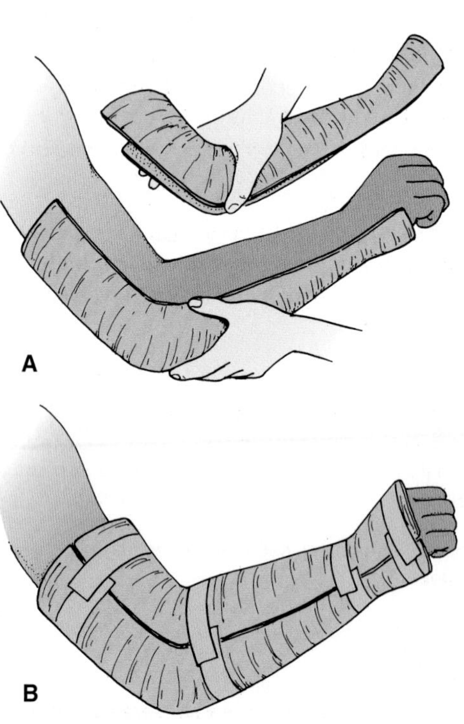

FIGURE 25-10 **A.** A bivalved cast. **B.** The two halves are rejoined.

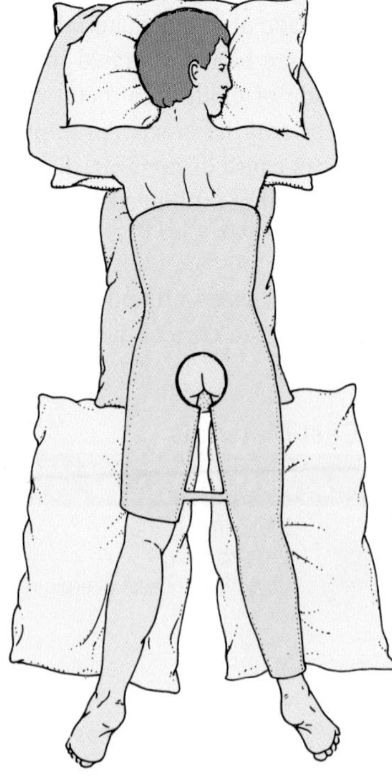

FIGURE 25-11 Hip spica cast. (Timby, B.K., & Smith, N. [2010]. *Introductory medical-surgical nursing* [10th ed., p. 970]. Philadelphia: Lippincott Williams & Wilkins.)

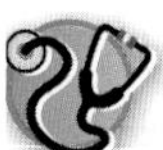

NURSING GUIDELINES 25-2

Making and Applying Petals

- Cut multiple strips of adhesive tape approximately 2 in. wide by 2 to 3 in. in length or use precut ovals from moleskin. *The width of the tape is optional depending on the circumference of the cast that needs to be covered. Each petal must be of sufficient length for placement of an end both inside and outside the cast edges.*
- Round the end of each adhesive strip like a flower petal or trim to create chevrons that resemble arrows; moleskin may already be shaped in an oval. *Modifying the ends of the tape reduces the potential for wrinkles.*
- Tuck one end of the tape or moleskin inside the cast edge, taking care to avoid wrinkles. *Wrinkles can cause friction on the skin and may lead to abrasions.*
- Overlap the strips of tape or moleskin around the rough cast edge (see Fig. 25-12). *Overlapping ensures that there are no gaps that expose a rough area that will continue to irritate the skin.*
- Continue to monitor the skin for signs of impairment. *If petals do not relieve skin irritation, the physician may need to smooth the edge with additional strips of plaster.*

to prevent complications (Skill 25-3). See Nursing Guidelines 25-2 and Figure 25-12 for instructions on making and applying **petals**, strips of adhesive tape or moleskin for the purpose of reducing skin irritation from the rough edges of a cast.

Stop, Think, and Respond Box 25-2

Discuss the discharge teaching for a client who has had a cast applied.

Cast Removal

In most cases, casts are removed when they need to be changed and reapplied, or when the injury has healed sufficiently that the cast is no longer necessary. A cast is removed prematurely if complications develop.

Most casts are removed with an electric cast cutter, an instrument that looks like a circular saw (Fig. 25-13). The cast cutter is noisy and may frighten clients. There is a natural expectation that an instrument sharp enough to cut a cast is sharp enough to cut skin and tissue. Proper use of an electric cast cutter, however, leaves the skin intact.

When the cast is removed, the unexercised muscle is usually smaller and weaker. The joints may have a limited range of motion. The skin usually appears pale and waxy and may contain scales or patches of dead skin. The skin is washed as usual with soapy warm water, but the semi-attached areas of skin are left in place; they are not forcibly removed. Applying lotion to the skin adds moisture and tends to prevent the rough skin edges from catching on clothing. Eventually, the dead skin fragments will slough free.

Traction

Traction is a pulling effect exerted on a part of the skeletal system. It is a treatment measure for musculoskeletal trauma and disorders. Traction is used to accomplish the following:

- Reduce muscle spasms
- Realign bones
- Relieve pain
- Prevent deformities

The pull of the traction generally is offset by the counterpull from the client's own body weight. Except for traction exerted with the hands, application of traction involves the use of weights connected to the client through a system of ropes, pulleys, slings, and other equipment.

Types of Traction

The three basic types of traction are manual, skin, and skeletal. The categories reflect the manner in which traction is applied.

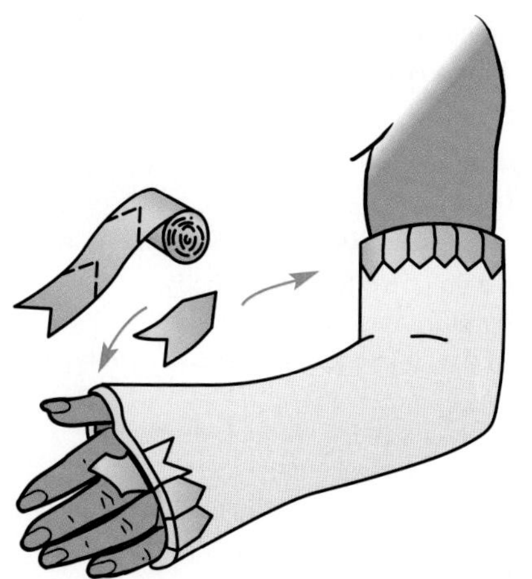

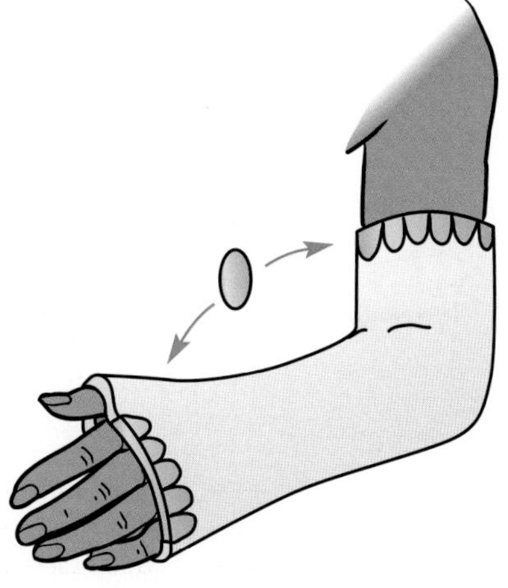

FIGURE 25-12 Petals are overlapped and applied around the edge circumference of a cast.

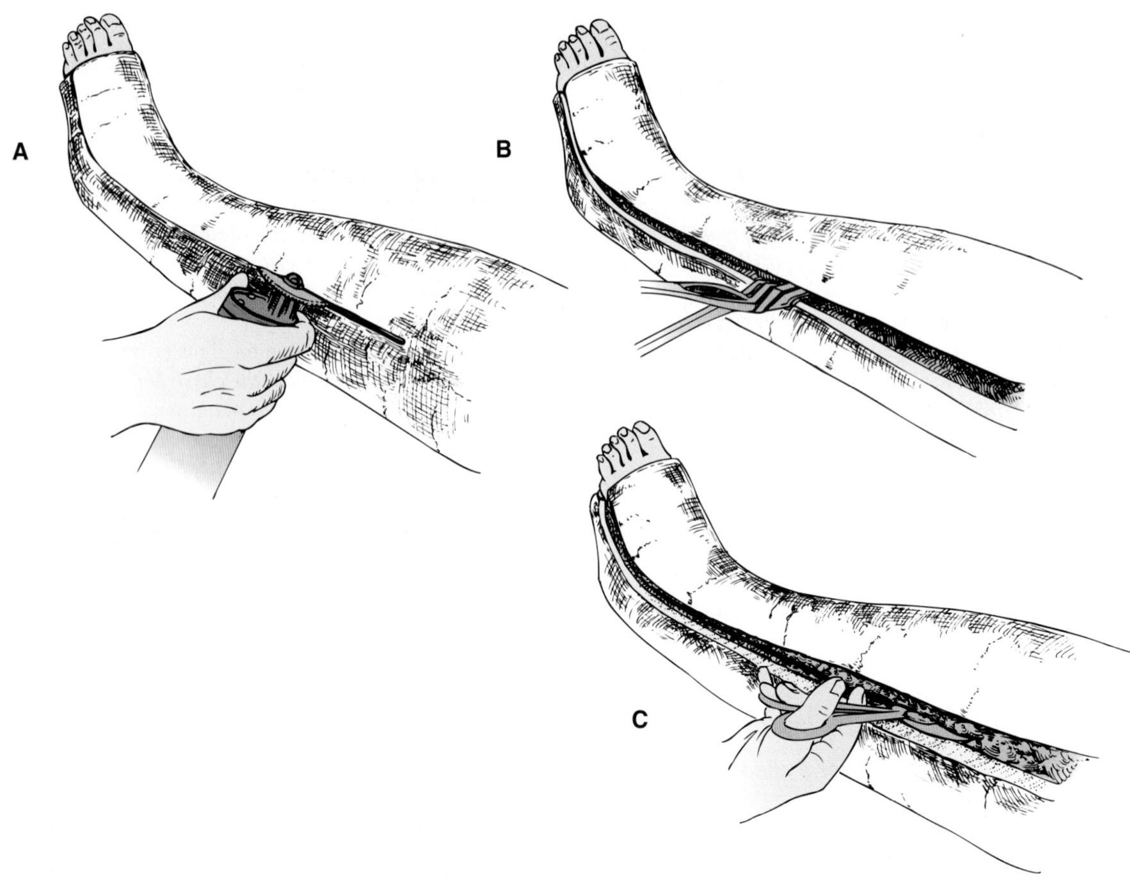

FIGURE 25-13 A cast removal. **A.** The cast is bivalved with an electric cast cutter. **B.** The cast is split. **C.** The padding is manually cut.

Manual Traction

Manual traction means pulling on the body using a person's hands and muscular strength (Fig. 25-14). It most often is used briefly to realign a broken bone. It is also used to replace a dislocated bone into its original position within a joint.

Skin Traction

Skin traction means a pulling effect on the skeletal system by applying devices to the skin, such as a pelvic belt and a cervical halter (Fig. 25-15). Other names for commonly applied forms of skin traction are Buck's traction and Russell's traction (Fig. 25-16).

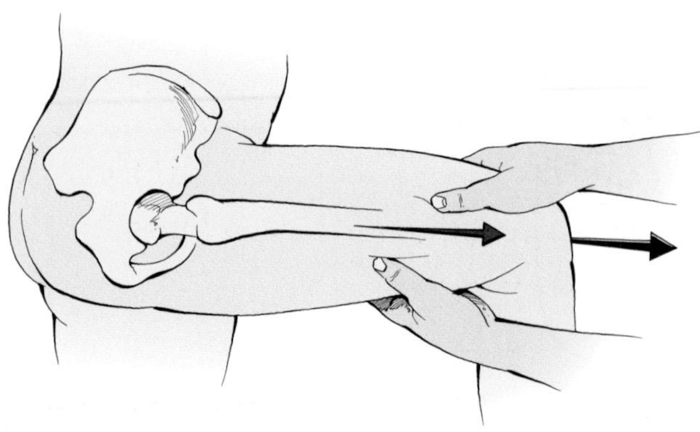

FIGURE 25-14 Manual traction.

Skeletal Traction

Skeletal traction means pull exerted directly on the skeletal system by attaching wires, pins, or tongs into or through a bone (Fig. 25-17). Skeletal traction is applied continuously for an extended period.

Traction Care

Regardless of the type of traction used, its effectiveness depends on the application of certain principles during the client's care (see Box 25-1 and Skill 23-4).

External Fixators

An **external fixator** is a metal device inserted into and through one or more broken bones to stabilize fragments during

BOX 25-1 Principles for Maintaining Effective Traction

- Traction must produce a pulling effect on the body.
- Countertraction (counterpull) must be maintained.
- The pull of traction and the counterpull must be in exactly opposite directions.
- Splints and slings must be suspended without interference.
- Ropes must move freely through each pulley.
- The prescribed amount of weight must be applied.
- The weights must hang free.

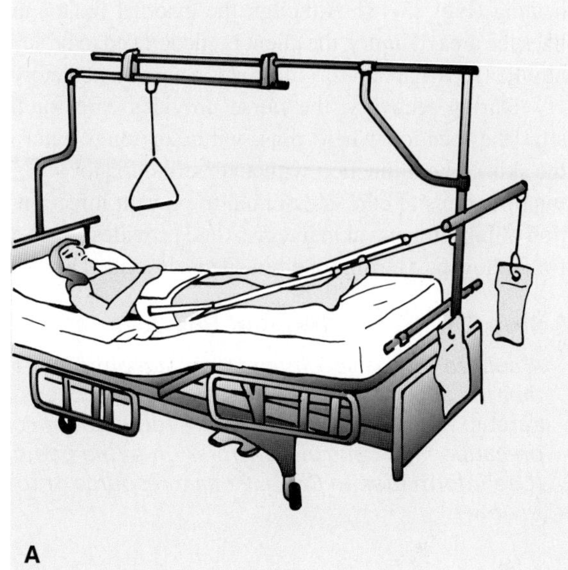

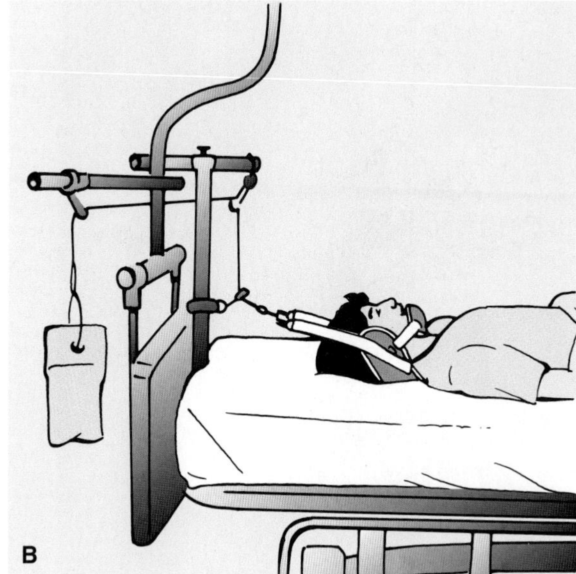

FIGURE 25-15 **A.** A pelvic belt. **B.** A cervical halter.

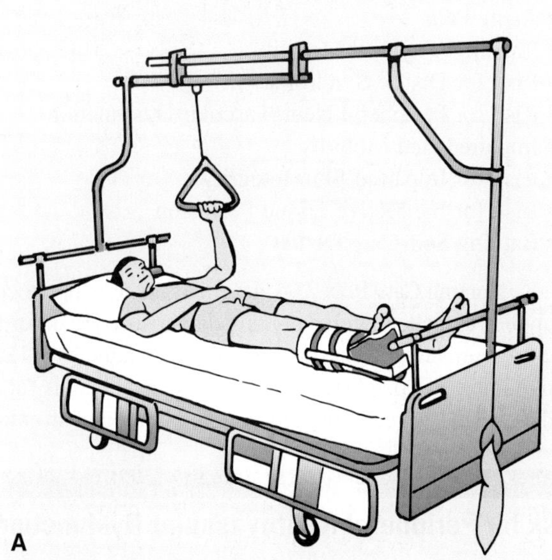

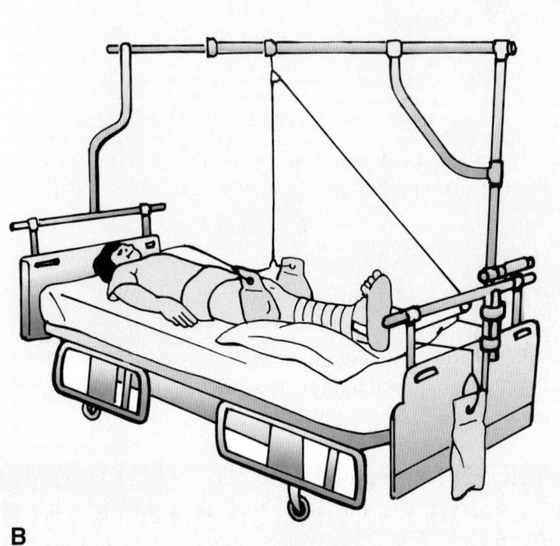

FIGURE 25-16 **A.** Buck's traction. **B.** Russell's traction.

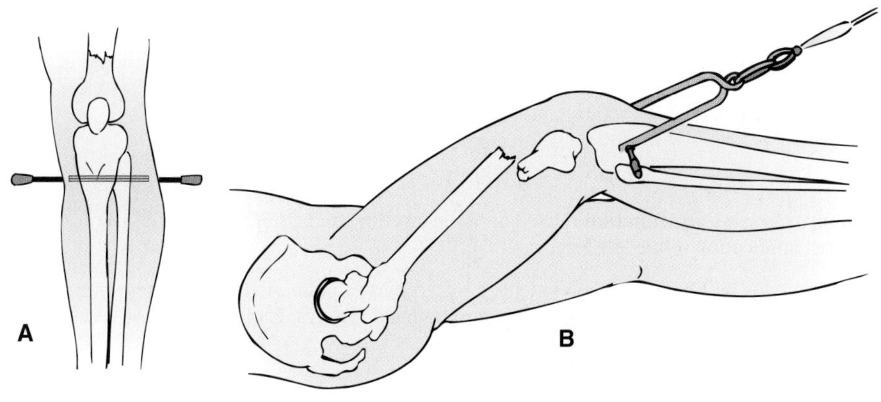

FIGURE 25-17 The application of skeletal traction. **A.** A pin transects the bone. **B.** Traction is applied.

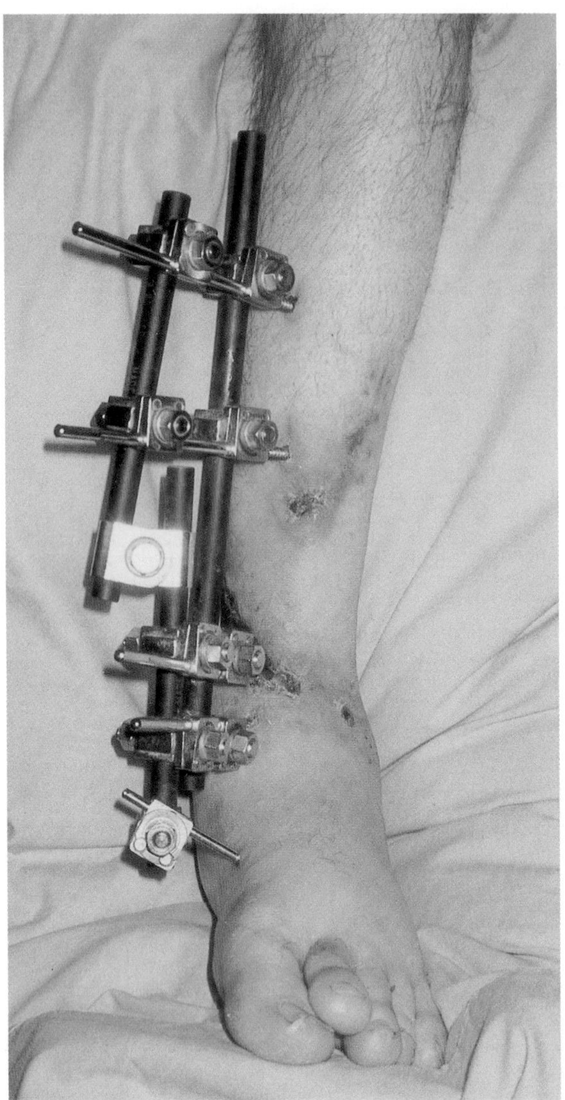
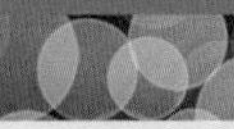

FIGURE 25-18 An external fixator. Metal rods exert traction between two sets of skeletal pins.

healing (Fig. 25-18). Although the external fixator immobilizes the area of injury, the client is encouraged to be active and mobile (see Chap. 26 for information about ambulatory aids).

During recovery, the nurse provides care for the **pin site** (the location where pins, wires, or tongs enter or exit the skin). In conjunction with an external fixator and skeletal traction, pin site care is essential to prevent infection. Insertion of pins impairs skin integrity and provides a port of entry for pathogens. Caring for a pin site is described in Skill 25-5.

Stop, Think, and Respond Box 25-1

A culture from a specimen taken at a pin site reveals that the pin site is infected with Staphylococcus aureus. *What nursing actions are required for contact precautions to control transmission of the pathogen? (Use information in Chap. 22 as a resource or to review.)*

NURSING IMPLICATIONS

Clients with immobilizing devices such as casts and traction may have one or more of the following nursing diagnoses:

- Acute Pain
- Impaired Physical Mobility
- Risk for Disuse Syndrome
- Risk for Peripheral Neurovascular Dysfunction
- Impaired Bed Mobility
- Risk for Impaired Skin Integrity
- Risk for Ineffective Tissue Perfusion
- Bathing Self-Care Deficit

Nursing Care Plan 25-1 describes the nursing process as it applies to a client with a nursing diagnosis of Risk for Peripheral Neurovascular Dysfunction, defined in the NANDA-I taxonomy (2012, p. 434) as a state in which a client is "at risk for disruption in circulation, sensation, or motion of an extremity."

NURSING CARE PLAN 25-1 Risk for Peripheral Neurovascular Dysfunction

Assessment

- Monitor peripheral circulation:
  - Check for the presence and quality of peripheral pulses in affected and unaffected extremities.
  - Feel the temperature of exposed toes or fingers and compare findings with the opposite extremity.
  - Compress the nailbeds and determine the time for the color to return following blanching.
  - Observe for swelling in the affected extremity in comparison to the unaffected extremity.
  - Look at the skin color and compare differences in the extremities.
- Assess the client's neurologic status in both extremities:
  - Ask the client to move the toes or fingers in the extremities.
  - Touch the client's extremities with objects that are sharp, dull, warm, or cold to determine whether the client can differentiate the stimuli without actually seeing the source of stimulation.
  - Quantify the client's level of pain, its location, characteristics, and whether it decreases or increases with usual pain-relieving measures.

Nursing Diagnosis. **Risk for Peripheral Neurovascular Dysfunction** related to tissue swelling and compression of blood vessels and nerves secondary to injury and recent cast application to the left leg.

Expected Outcome. The client's neurovascular status will be normal as evidenced by a report of pain relief from present rate of 9 to ≤7. Pedal pulses will be equally strong. Movement and sensation will be equal in both extremities. Capillary refill will be ≤3 seconds bilaterally within 3 hours today (8/20).

(continued)

NURSING CARE PLAN 25-1 Risk for Peripheral Neurovascular Dysfunction (continued)

Interventions	Rationales
Elevate the casted left leg so that toes are higher than the client's heart.	Use of gravity facilitates the venous return of blood from distal areas to the heart.
Have client exercise toes of left foot in cast every 15 minutes while awake.	Contraction of skeletal muscles compresses capillaries and veins, which propels venous blood toward the heart.
Apply an ice bag on the cast over the area of injury; empty and refill ice bag every 20 minutes.	Application of cold causes blood vessels to constrict and reduces tissue swelling.
Monitor circulatory status, sensation including tactile and pain, and mobility of toes in affected extremity every 30 minutes.	Lack of improvement or escalation of signs suggesting neurovascular impairment indicate a medical emergency.
Report worsening of symptoms to the charge nurse and physician immediately.	Failure to report and implement additional interventions can cause the client to permanently lose function in the limb or require surgical amputation.

Evaluation of Expected Outcomes

- The pedal pulse is diminished in extremity in cast; pulse is strong and regular in unaffected foot despite the elevation of casted leg on three pillows. The client performs active exercises with toes every 15 minutes. Ice bag is applied to cast over lateral ankle.
- Client rates pain at 10 after receiving Demerol 75 mg intramuscularly.
- The nurse notifies the doctor, who gives orders to obtain a cast cutter for bivalving cast.
- Capillary refill is 2 seconds in toes on both feet. Pedal pulses are palpable and equal bilaterally. The client moves and detects sensation equally bilaterally and rates pain at 5 after cast is bivalved.
- Affected leg remains elevated with ice bag applied. Client does exercises as directed.

CRITICAL THINKING EXERCISES

1. Although slings are applied most often to support injured extremities, discuss possible reasons for applying a sling on an arm paralyzed by a stroke.
2. Discuss the differences and similarities between caring for clients with casts and caring for clients in traction.
3. Discuss ways to provide diversions for clients with a cast or in traction who are confined to bed while their injuries heal.
4. A nursing assistant reports that a client with a cast is experiencing pain that is being rated at higher and higher levels since the cast was applied this morning. What actions should the nurse take? What complication could be the cause of the client's discomfort?

NCLEX-STYLE REVIEW QUESTIONS

1. As the physician wraps the arm of a client with rolls of wet plaster, what is the most appropriate method the nurse should use for supporting the wet cast?
   1. Support the wet cast on a soft mattress.
   2. Support the wet cast on a firm surface.
   3. Support the wet cast with the tips of the fingers.
   4. Support the wet cast with the palms of the hands.
2. Which one of the following is accurate when a nurse describes the advantage of fiberglass casts?
   1. Fiberglass casts are generally less expensive.
   2. Fiberglass casts are generally more lightweight.
   3. Fiberglass casts are generally more flexible.
   4. Fiberglass casts are generally less restrictive.
3. Which of the following techniques is best for assessing circulation in the casted extremity of a client with a long leg plaster cast?
   1. Ask the client whether the cast feels exceptionally heavy.
   2. Feel the cast to determine whether it is unusually cold.
   3. Depress the nail bed and time the return of color.
   4. See whether there is room to insert a finger within the cast.
4. Which finding is most suggestive that a client in skeletal traction has an infection at the pin site?
   1. There is serous drainage at the pin site.
   2. There is bloody drainage at the pin site.
   3. There is mucoid drainage at the pin site.
   4. There is purulent drainage at the pin site.
5. While providing nursing care for a client in Buck's skin traction, which of the following indicates a need for immediate action?
   1. The traction weights are hanging above the floor.
   2. The leg is in line with the pull of the traction.
   3. The client's foot is touching the end of the bed.
   4. The rope is in the groove of the traction pulley.

SKILL 25-1 Applying an Arm Sling

Suggested Action	Reason for Action
ASSESSMENT	
Check the medical orders.	Integrates nursing activities with medical treatment.
Assess the skin color and temperature, capillary refill time, and amount of edema; verify the presence of peripheral pulses in the injured arm (don gloves if there is a potential for contact with blood or nonintact skin).	Provides baseline objective data for future comparisons.
Ask the client to describe how the fingers and arm feel and to rate any pain on a scale of 0–10.	Provides baseline subjective data for future comparisons.
Determine whether the client had required an arm sling in the past.	Indicates the level and type of health teaching needed.
PLANNING	
Explain the purpose for the sling.	Adds to the client's understanding.
Obtain a canvas or triangular sling, depending on what is available or prescribed for use.	Complies with medical practice.
IMPLEMENTATION	
Wash your hands or perform an alcohol-based hand rub (see Chap. 10).	Reduces the potential for transferring microorganisms.
Position forearm across the client's chest with the thumb pointing upward.	Flexes the elbow.
Avoid more than 90 degrees of flexion, especially if the elbow has been injured.	Facilitates circulation.
Canvas Sling	
Slip the flexed arm into the canvas sling so that the elbow fits flush with the corner of the sling (Fig. A).	Encloses the forearm and wrist.

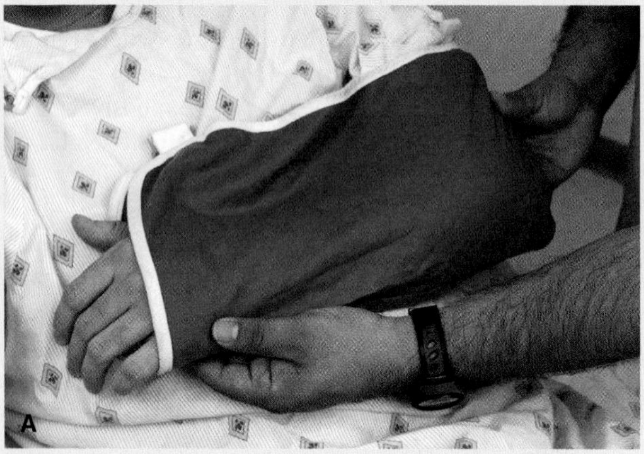

A

Positioning a commercial arm sling.

Suggested Action	Reason for Action
Bring the strap around the opposing shoulder and fasten it to the sling (Fig. B).	Provides the means for support.

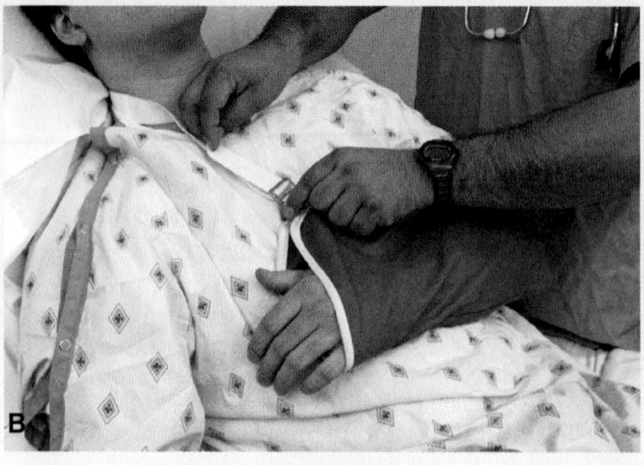

B

Placing the strap around the neck.

(continued)

Applying an Arm Sling (continued)

IMPLEMENTATION (CONTINUED)

Pad and tighten the strap sufficiently (Fig. C). — Reduces friction and pressure to preserve skin integrity.

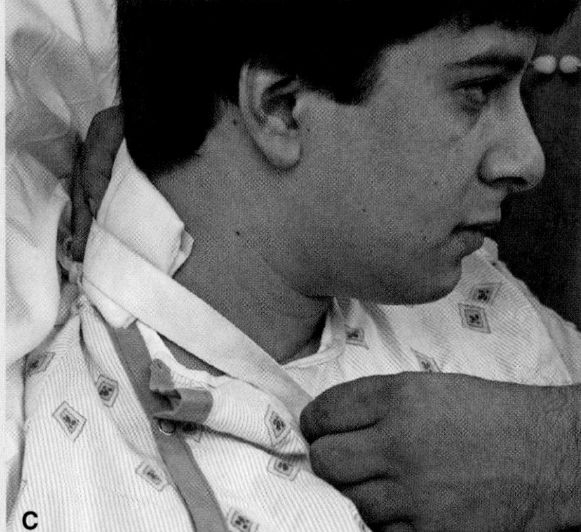

Placing padding between the strap and neck.

Keep the elbow flexed and the wrist elevated (Fig. D). — Promotes circulation.

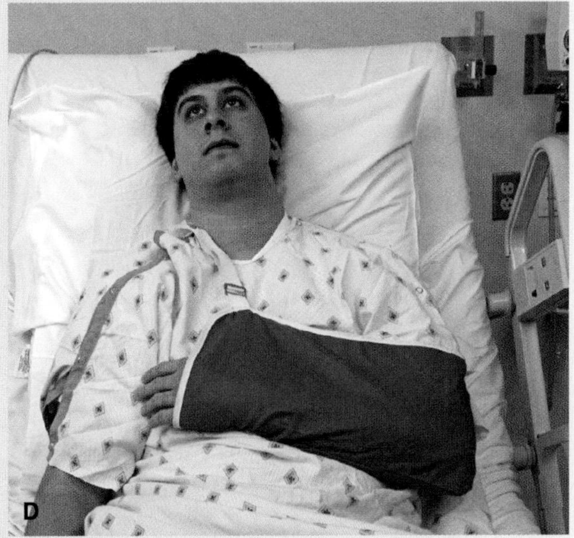

The sling in place.

Triangular Sling

Place the longer side of the sling from the shoulder opposite the injured arm to the waist. — Positions the sling where length is needed.

(continued)

Applying an Arm Sling (continued)

IMPLEMENTATION (CONTINUED)

Position the apex or point of the triangle under the elbow (Fig. E). — Facilitates making a hammock for the arm.

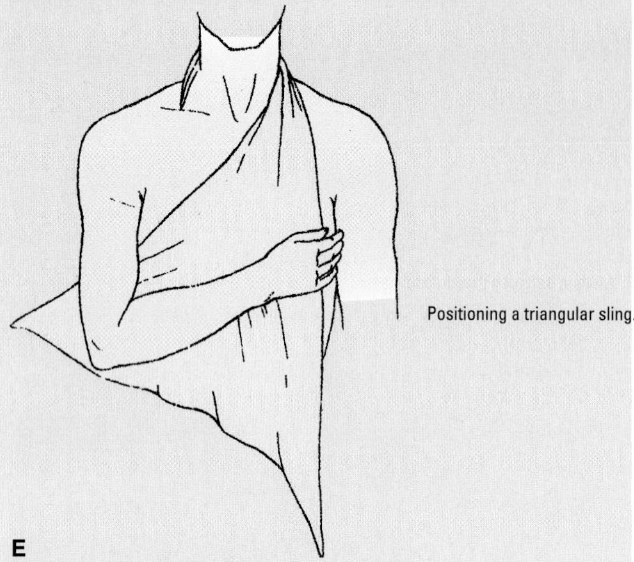

Positioning a triangular sling.

E

Bring the point at the waist up to join the point at the neck and tie them. — Encloses the injured arm.

Position the knot to the side of the neck. — Avoids pressure on the vertebrae.

Fold in and secure excess fabric at the elbow; a safety pin may be necessary (Fig. F). — Keeps the elbow enclosed.

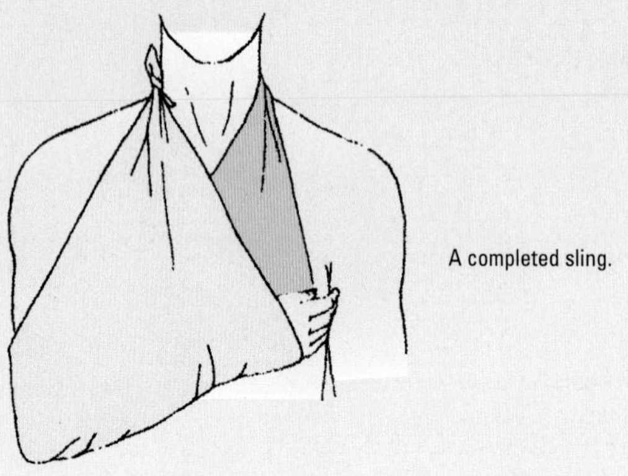

A completed sling.

F

Inspect the condition of the skin at the neck and the circulation, mobility, and sensation of the fingers at least once per shift. — Provides comparative data.

Pad the skin at the neck with soft gauze or towel material if the skin becomes irritated. — Reduces pressure and friction.

Tell the client to report any changes in sensation, especially pain with limited movement or pressure. — Indicates developing complications.

(continued)

Applying an Arm Sling (continued)

Evaluation

- Forearm is supported.
- Wrist is elevated.
- Pain and swelling are reduced.
- Circulation, mobility, and sensation are maintained.

Document

- Baseline and comparative assessment data
- Type of sling applied or used
- To whom significant abnormal assessments were reported
- Outcomes of the verbal report

SAMPLE DOCUMENTATION

Date and Time **Fingers on R. hand are pale, cool, and swollen. Capillary refill is sluggish, taking 4 seconds for color to return. Can move all fingers. Can discriminate sharp and dull stimuli. No tingling identified. Pain rated at 8 on a scale of 0–10. All above data reported to Dr. Stuckey. Orders received for pain medication and canvas sling. Demerol 75 mg given IM in vastus lateralis. Sling applied. ——————— SIGNATURE/TITLE**

SKILL 25-2 Assisting with a Cast Application

Suggested Action	Reason for Action
ASSESSMENT	
Check the medical orders.	Integrates nursing activities with the medical treatment.
Assess the appearance of the skin that the cast will cover; also check circulation, mobility, and sensation.	Provides a baseline of data for future comparisons.
Ask the client to describe the location, type, and intensity of any pain.	Determines whether the client needs analgesic medication.
Determine what the client understands about the application of a cast.	Indicates the type of health teaching needed.
Check with the physician as to whether a plaster of Paris or fiberglass cast will be applied.	Facilitates assembling appropriate supplies.
PLANNING	
Obtain a signature on a treatment consent form, if required.	Ensures legal protection.
Administer pain medication, if prescribed.	Relieves discomfort.
Remove the client's clothing that may not stretch over the cast once it is applied.	Avoids having to cut and destroy clothing.
Provide a gown or drape.	Preserves dignity and protects clothing.
Assemble materials, which may include a stockinette, felt padding, cotton batting, rolls of cast material, gloves, and apron.	Facilitates organization and efficient time management.
Anticipate that if the cast is being applied to a lower extremity, the client will need crutches and instructions on their use (see Chap. 26).	Shows awareness of discharge planning.
Have an arm sling available if applying the cast to an upper extremity.	Shows awareness of discharge planning.
IMPLEMENTATION	
Explain how the cast will be applied. If using plaster of Paris, be sure to tell the client that it will feel warm as it dries.	Reduces anxiety and promotes cooperation.
Wash your hands or perform an alcohol-based hand rub (see Chap. 10).	Reduces the potential for transferring microorganisms.
Wash the client's skin with soap and water and dry well.	Removes dirt, body oil, and some microorganisms.

(continued)

Assisting With a Cast Application (continued)

IMPLEMENTATION (CONTINUED)

Cover the skin with a stockinette and protective padding as directed (Fig. A).

Protects the skin from direct contact with the cast material and provides a fabric cushion that protects the skin.

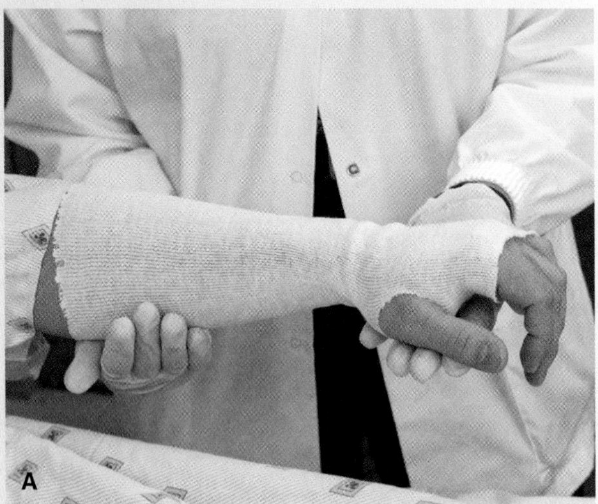

A stockinette in place.

If applying a plaster cast, open rolls and strips of plaster gauze material. Dip them, one at a time, briefly in water and wring out the excess moisture.

Prepares the cast material for application.

If using fiberglass material, open the foil packets one at a time.

Reduces the risk of rapidly drying and becoming unfit for use.

Support the extremity while the physician wraps the cast material around the arm or leg (Fig. B).

Facilitates going around the injured area; ensures proper alignment because fiberglass is harder to mold.

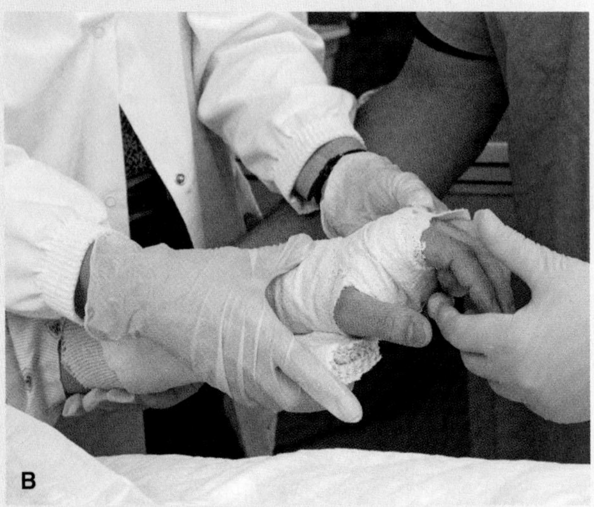

Casting material being applied.

For a fiberglass cast, hold the extremity in this position until the cast is dry (approximately 15 minutes).

(continued)

Assisting With a Cast Application (continued)

IMPLEMENTATION (CONTINUED)

Help to fold back the edges of the stockinette at each end of the cast just before the final layer of cast material is applied (Fig. C). — Forms a smooth, soft edge at the margins of the cast, which may protect the skin from becoming irritated.

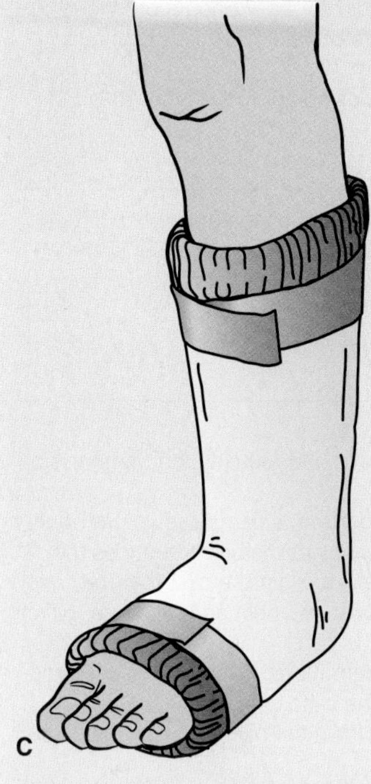

C

The folded stockinette beneath the cast protects the skin from the sharp edges of the cast.

Elevate the cast on pillows or other support. — Helps to reduce swelling and pain.

If a plaster cast was applied, use a special sink with a plaster trap to dispose of the water in which plaster rolls were soaked. — Prevents clogging of plumbing.

Provide verbal and written instructions on cast care. — Facilitates independence and safe self-care.

Evaluation

- Skin has been cleaned and protected.
- Cast has been applied and is drying or dried.
- Circulation and sensation are within acceptable parameters.
- Client can repeat discharge instructions.

Document

- Assessment data
- Type of cast
- Cast material
- Name of physician who applied the cast
- Discharge instructions

SAMPLE DOCUMENTATION

Date and Time Wrist appears swollen but skin is warm, dry, and intact. Capillary refill <3 seconds. X-ray department reports a fracture of the wrist. Dr. Roberts notified. Dr. Roberts applied cylinder fiberglass cast from middle of hand to above elbow. Assessment findings remain unchanged after cast application. Casted arm supported in a canvas sling. Standard instructions for cast care provided (see copy attached). Instructed to call Dr. Roberts if pain or swelling increases and make an office appointment in 2 weeks.

SIGNATURE/TITLE

SKILL 25-3 Providing Basic Care of a Client With a Cast

Suggested Action	Reason for Action
ASSESSMENT	
Determine the type of cast, the body location, and when the cast was initially applied.	Plaster casts do not completely dry for 24–72 hours or longer depending on the size and type of cast; fiberglass casts dry within 30 minutes.
Check whether there is a trapeze on the client's bed.	A trapeze helps a client change position or move up or down in bed.
PLANNING	
Plan to check the condition of the cast, the neurovascular status, and the condition of the skin on the limb enclosed by the cast every 30 minutes initially and twice per shift once it has dried.	A plaster cast is vulnerable to changing shape until it has dried; neurovascular complications are more likely to occur in the early hours after the initial cast application; and the risk for impaired skin integrity and infection is ongoing.
Explain the purpose and methods for assessment to the client.	Adds to the client's understanding.
IMPLEMENTATION	
Place the bed at a comfortable height.	Prevents back strain.
Wash your hands or perform an alcohol-based hand rub (see Chap. 10).	Removes transient microorganisms and reduces the transmission of pathogens.
Observe and feel the condition of the cast on the anterior as well as posterior surfaces. Position a fresh plaster cast on pillows without plastic covers.	A dry cast is white, shiny, and odorless; a damp cast is gray, dull, and musty-smelling. The buoyancy of the pillow reduces the direct force of the hard mattress against the cast that may alter its shape. Plastic covered pillows trap heat and moisture, which retards drying.
Use the palms of the hands, not the fingers, to move or reposition the cast before it is thoroughly dry.	Use of the fingers can cause indentations, which can cause pressure sores to develop under the cast.
Leave a freshly applied plaster cast uncovered until it is dry; turn the client periodically to expose all the surfaces of the cast to air.	Aids in the evaporation of water from the plaster which is necessary for drying the cast.
Avoid using the abduction bar in a hip spica cast when turning a client.	Pulling on the abduction bar is likely to break it free from its attachment to the cast.
Observe the color, temperature, and size of the fingers or toes on the extremity with the cast; compare with those on the opposite extremity.	Digits that are pink, warm, and of a similar size bilaterally suggest that there is an adequate distal blood supply.
Assess capillary refill in exposed fingers or toes (Fig. A); compare with the uncasted digits.	Color should reappear in 2–3 seconds as the capillaries refill following blanching; checking the opposite nailbeds provides comparative data.

A

Assessing capillary refill. (Photo by B. Proud.)

Suggested Action	Reason for Action
Elevate an extremity that appears swollen.	Elevation promotes the return of venous blood to the heart that may be trapped distally by a swelling extremity.
Circle areas where blood has seeped through the cast; note the time on the cast. Recircle any expanding blood seepage and identify the time.	Identification helps in evaluating the significance of blood loss.

(continued)

Providing Basic Care of a Client With a Cast (continued)

IMPLEMENTATION (CONTINUED)

Apply ice packs to the cast at the level of injury or where surgery has been performed if swelling is evident (Fig. B).

Cold is conducted through the skin causing vasoconstriction, which helps to control swelling and bleeding.

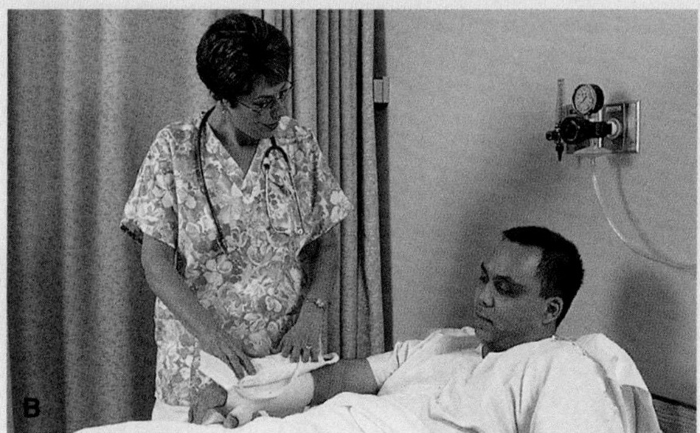

Applying an ice pack. (Photo by B. Proud.)

Monitor the mobility of the fingers or toes (Fig. C).

The ability to move the fingers or toes upon request reflects intact neuromuscular status.

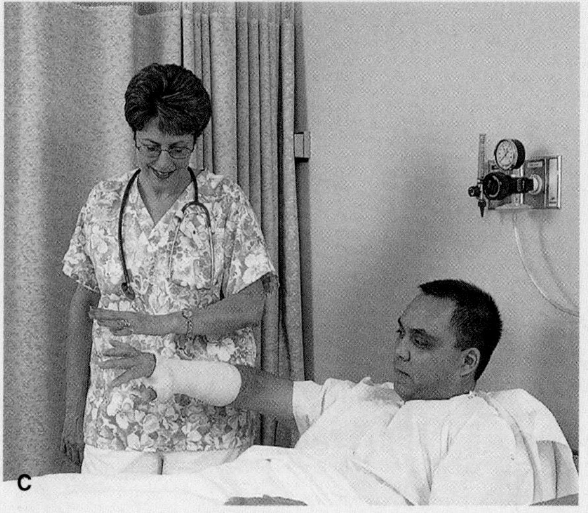

Checking mobility. (Photo by B. Proud.)

Assess sensation in exposed fingers or toes (Fig. D).

The ability to feel sensation indicates intact neurologic status.

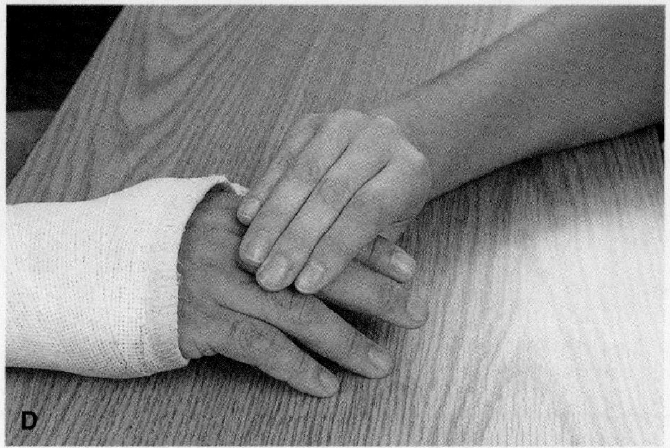

Assessing sensation in exposed fingers. (Photo by B. Proud.)

Assess the presence and quality of pain in the area covered by the cast, especially if it is unrelieved by elevation, cold applications, and analgesic medication.

Unrelieved pain of increasing intensity suggests a complication known as **compartment syndrome**, which is caused by pressure due to swelling within the inelastic fascia that surrounds muscles.

Report pain that escalates and does not respond to pain relieving measures.

The pressure from compartment syndrome, if unrelieved, disrupts circulation and damages nerves, which may cause permanent disability.

(continued)

Providing Basic Care of a Client With a Cast (continued)

IMPLEMENTATION (CONTINUED)

Be aware of any foul odor or purulent drainage coming from within the cast. — A foul odor and purulent drainage suggests a possible infection.

Encourage the client to exercise fingers or toes frequently. — Exercise helps to increase circulation, decrease swelling, and prevent stiffness.

Swab remnants of plaster from the skin with a damp cloth; remove fiberglass resin from the skin with alcohol or acetone. — Water moistens plaster, allowing it to be removed; alcohol and acetone are chemical solvents.

Avoid getting a cast wet. If it becomes wet, dry the area using a blow dryer on a cool setting. — Water softens plaster and may saturate the padding next to the skin of both plaster and fiberglass casts. Prolonged dampness weakens plaster; damp padding can macerate the skin integrity.

Ensure that the edges of the cast are smooth and padded (Fig. E). — Padding reduces the risk for skin irritation and breakdown.

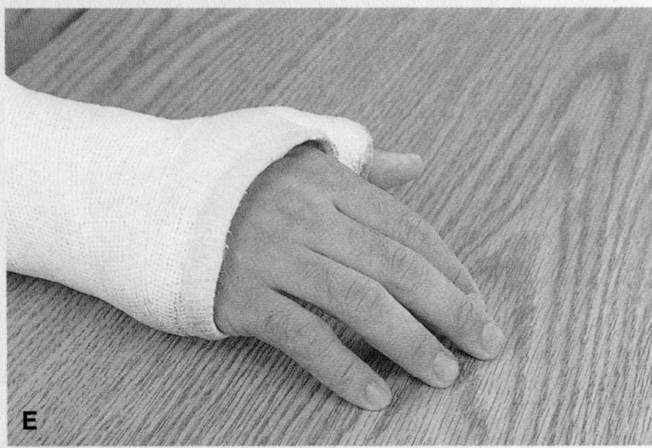

Soft cast edges minimizes the risk for skin impairment. (Photo by B. Proud.)

Rough edges can be reinforced with petals made of tape or moleskin (Nursing Guidelines 25-2).

Caution clients not to insert objects (eg, straws, combs, utensils) within the cast. — Foreign objects can impair the skin by causing abrasions or prolonged pressure if retained within the cast.

Report itching, which may be treated with oral medication or by blowing cool air from a hair dryer down the cast. — Antipruritic medications relieve itching, but may cause drowsiness. Cool blown air is not harmful nor does it cause side effects.

Advise clients not to paint a fiberglass cast, but friends may write or draw on either type of cast. — Painting fiberglass interferes with its porosity.

Replace a **window**, a small square cut from a cast for the purpose of inspecting the skin or incision beneath a cast, by taping it back in place. — Replacing a window prevents the skin from bulging into the open space, causing impaired skin and circulation in the area.

Ambulate clients as soon as possible or have them exercise in bed. — Movement prevents complications from immobility.

Evaluation

- The cast is dry without any evidence of dents or cracks.
- The skin is warm and pink without evidence of swelling.
- Pain is absent or reduced using pain-relieving measures.
- The client is able to move fingers or toes and has normal sensory perception.
- The exposed skin at the cast edges is intact.
- There is no evidence of purulent drainage.

Document

- Date, time, and results of assessments
- Measures used to relieve swelling or itching, if any occurred
- Level of pain, pain relieving techniques, and outcome following their use
- Skin care that is provided
- To whom abnormal findings were communicated, the content of the reported information, and the response of the caregiver receiving the information

SAMPLE DOCUMENTATION

Date and Time Long leg cast on left leg is dry and shiny, and elevated on two pillows. No evidence of dents or cracks in cast. Toes are pink, warm, and similar in size to those on the right. Capillary refill of toes on left is 2 seconds. Can move all toes and perceives being touched. Rates pain at a level 3 and refuses any pain relieving measures. ——— SIGNATURE/TITLE

SKILL 25-4 Caring for Clients in Traction

Suggested Action	Reason for Action
ASSESSMENT	
Check the medical orders to determine the type of traction and amount of weight that has been prescribed.	Integrates nursing activities with medical treatment.
Note whether there is a trapeze attached to the overbed frame.	Facilitates mobility and self-care.
Inspect the mechanical equipment used to apply traction.	Inspection determines the status of the equipment.
Check whether traction ropes move freely through the pulleys.	Fraying or knots in the traction ropes may interfere with the pull of traction.
Determine whether the weights are hanging free of the bed or floor.	Unobstructed and unsupported weights ensure the effectiveness of traction.
Observe the client's body position.	Effective traction occurs when the body part is positioned in an opposite line with the pull of the traction equipment.
Wash your hands or perform an alcohol-based hand rub (see Chap. 10).	Removes transient microorganisms and reduces the transmission of pathogens.
Inspect the skin and pin sites.	Pressure from traction equipment, immobility, and tissue compromised by skeletal pins predispose a client to impaired skin integrity and the risk of infection.
Assess the client's circulation and sensation in the area to which traction has been applied.	Neurovascular complications can occur when a part of the body is immobilized.
Determine the client's last date of bowel elimination.	Immobility and having to use a bedpan predisposes the client to constipation and fecal impaction.
Note the frequency, volume, and color of urine.	Certain traction positions interfere with the complete emptying of the bladder; urinary stasis predisposes the client to stone formation and bladder infection.
Auscultate the client's lungs.	Immobilized clients tend to breathe shallowly, creating a risk for pneumonia.
Review the trend in the client's temperature.	An elevation in body temperature is suggestive of infection.
Assess the client's level of pain or discomfort.	Pain is the fifth vital sign.
Observe the client's emotional state.	Prolonged confinement, immobilization, and decreased sensory stimulation place the client at risk for boredom, depression, and loneliness.
PLANNING	
Explain the purpose of the traction and the care that will follow.	Adds to the client's understanding.
IMPLEMENTATION	
Keep the traction applied continuously unless there are medical orders to the contrary.	Continuous traction fosters the achievement of desired outcomes.
Raise the height of the bed to ensure that the weights hang above the floor.	Weights provide the musculoskeletal pull in traction.
Limit the client's positions to those indicated in the medical orders or standards for care.	Positions that alter the pull and counterpull of traction interfere with therapy.
Provide for the client's hygiene and oral needs.	Clients are encouraged to perform as much self-care as possible.
Bathe the back of clients who must remain in a supine or other back-lying position by depressing the mattress enough to insert a hand.	Facilitates skin care and hygiene.
Remove and apply bottom bed linen from the foot of the bed rather than turning the client from side to side.	Maintains body alignment.
Avoid tucking top sheets, blankets, or bedspread beneath the mattress.	Bedding tucked under the mattress interferes with the pull of traction equipment.
Do not use a pillow if the client's head or neck is in traction unless medical orders indicate otherwise.	Using a pillow could disturb the line of pull and counterpull.
Use pressure-relieving devices (see Chaps. 23 and 28) and a regimen of frequent conscientious skin care if the client is confined to bed for a prolonged time.	Prevents impaired skin integrity.
Insert padding within slings if they tend to wrinkle.	Helps to cushion and distribute pressure, prevents interference with circulation, and reduces the risk for skin breakdown.
Cleanse the skin around a skeletal pin insertion using an antimicrobial agent (See Skill 25-5).	Reduces the risk of infection.
Cover the tips of protruding metal pins or other sharp traction devices with corks or other protective material.	Prevents accidental injury.
Use a small bedpan, called a "fracture pan," if elevating the hips alters the line of pull.	Ensures alignment and maintains the effectiveness of traction.

(continued)

Caring for Clients in Traction (continued)

Suggested Action	Reason for Action
IMPLEMENTATION (CONTINUED)	
Encourage isometric, isotonic, and active range-of-motion exercises.	Maintains the tone, strength, and flexibility of the musculoskeletal system.
Provide diversional activities as often as possible.	Relieves boredom and sensory deprivation.

Evaluation

- The type of traction and amount of traction weight correlates with the medical orders.
- The weights hang freely above the floor.
- There are no knots in the traction rope close to the pulleys.
- The traction ropes are unfrayed and move freely through the pulleys.
- The client lies in the center of the bed in proper alignment with the pull of the traction.
- There is a trapeze within reach of the client.
- Physical assessment data are normal.
- Hygiene is accomplished on a regular basis.

Document

- Date and time of care
- Type of traction and location of application
- Amount of weight currently applied
- Results of physical assessment
- To whom abnormal findings were reported and changes recommended as a result of the report

SAMPLE DOCUMENTATION

Date and Time Buck's skin traction applied to left leg with 5 lbs. of weight attached. Ropes move freely through pulleys and weights are hanging freely off the floor. Client in supine position with left leg aligned with pull of traction. Peripheral pulses are present and strong in both extremities; capillary refill is less than 2–3 seconds in toes on the left, the toes on the left are warm and move when instructed to do so, sensation in left foot is normal. Skin remains intact and free of redness. Eliminating stool and urine regularly. Lung sounds are clear upon auscultation. Pain rated at 2 which is within a tolerable range. Mood is appropriate for situation. ——— SIGNATURE/TITLE

SKILL 25-5 Providing Pin Site Care

Suggested Action	Reason for Action
ASSESSMENT	
Check the medical orders or standards for care regarding the frequency of pin site care and the preferred cleansing agent.	Demonstrates collaboration with the medical treatment.
Review the medical record for trends in the client's temperature, white blood cell count, reports of pain, and frequency for treating pain.	Uses data that reflect indications of infection.
Inspect the area around the pin insertion site for redness, swelling, increased tenderness, and drainage.	Provides data for current and future comparisons.
Examine the pin for signs of bending or shifting.	Identifies potential problems with maintaining traction and desired position.
PLANNING	
Explain the purpose and technique for pin site care to the client.	Adds to the client's understanding.
Assemble gloves, the prescribed cleansing agent (usually hydrogen peroxide or povidone iodine), and sterile cotton-tipped applicators. Sometimes presaturated swabs are used.	Contributes to organization and efficient time management.
Place the bed at a comfortable height.	Prevents back strain.
IMPLEMENTATION	
Wash your hands or perform an alcohol-based hand rub (see Chap. 10).	Removes transient microorganisms and reduces the transmission of pathogens.
Don gloves; clean gloves can be used to hold the stick end of the applicator.	Prevents skin contact with blood or body fluid.

(continued)

Providing Pin Site Care (continued)

IMPLEMENTATION (CONTINUED)

Action	Rationale
Open the package containing cotton-tipped applicators without touching the applicator tips.	Avoids contaminating the point of contact between the applicator tip and the client's skin.
Pour enough cleansing agent to saturate the dry applicators while holding them over a basin or wastebasket.	Prepares applicators for use while maintaining the sterility of the applicator tip.
Cleanse the skin at the pin site moving outward in a circular manner (Fig. A).	Prevents moving microorganisms toward the area of open skin.

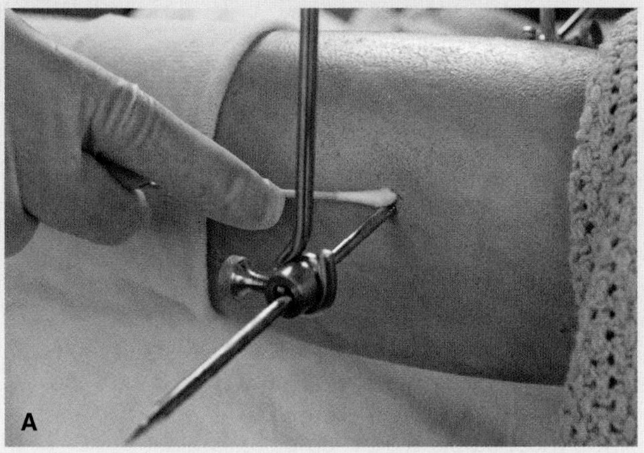

Providing pin site care.

Action	Rationale
Gently remove crusted secretions.	Removes debris that supports the growth of microorganisms.
Use a separate applicator for each pin site or if the site needs more than one circular swipe for additional cleansing.	Prevents reintroducing microorganisms into cleaned areas.
Avoid applying ointment to pin sites unless prescribed.	Reduces retained moisture at the site and occludes drainage, both of which increase the risk for microbial growth.
Check with the physician or infection-control policy about obtaining a wound culture if *purulent drainage* (that which contains pus) is present.	Aids in determining the identity of pathogenic microorganisms and the need to institute infection-control measures, such as contact precautions (see Chap. 22).
Teach the client to not touch the pin sites.	Prevents introducing transient and resident microorganisms into the wound.
Discard soiled supplies in an enclosed, lined container; remove gloves; and wash hands or perform an alcohol-based hand rub.	Demonstrates the principles of medical asepsis (see Chap. 10).

Evaluation

- The skin and tissue around the pin site are free of redness, swelling, or pain.
- There is no evidence of purulent drainage.
- The client's temperature and white blood cell count are within normal ranges.

Document

- Date, time, and location of pin site care
- Type of cleansing agent
- Appearance of the pin site and the client's subjective remarks regarding the presence of tenderness or pain
- Collection of a wound specimen for a culture test, if ordered, and time of its delivery to the laboratory
- To whom abnormal findings were communicated, the content of the reported information, and the response of the caregiver receiving the information

SAMPLE DOCUMENTATION

Date and Time **Pin sites on medial and lateral sides of left thigh cleansed with povidone–iodine. Sites appear dry and without evidence of inflammation. No complaints of pain or discomfort. ———— SIGNATURE/TITLE**

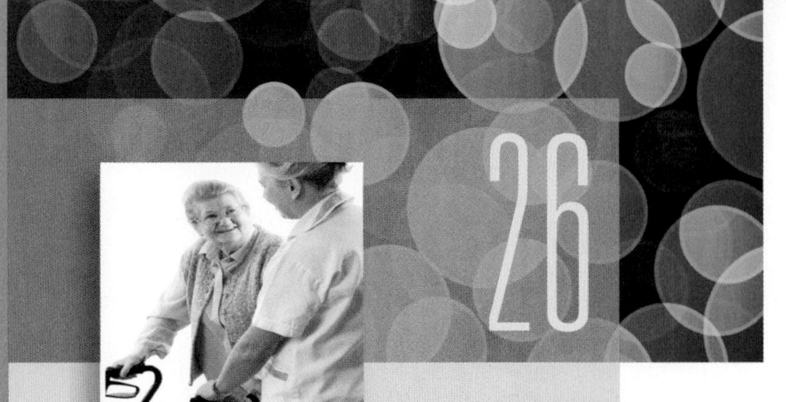

Ambulatory Aids

Words To Know

axillary crutches
cane
crutches
crutch palsy
dangling
forearm crutches
gluteal setting
parallel bars
platform crutches
prosthetic limb
prosthetist
quadriceps setting
strength
tilt table
tone
walker
walking belt

Learning Objectives

On completion of this chapter, the reader should be able to:

1. Name four activities that prepare clients for ambulation.
2. Give two examples of isometric exercises that tone and strengthen lower extremities.
3. Identify one technique for building upper arm strength.
4. Explain the reason for dangling clients or using a tilt table.
5. Name two devices used to assist clients with ambulation.
6. Give three examples of ambulatory aids.
7. Identify the most stable type of ambulatory aid.
8. Describe three characteristics of appropriately fitted crutches.
9. Name four types of crutch-walking gaits.
10. Explain the purpose of a temporary prosthetic limb.
11. Discuss two criteria that must be met before constructing a permanent prosthetic limb.
12. Name four components of above-the-knee and below-the-knee prosthetic limbs.
13. Describe how a prosthetic limb is applied.
14. Discuss age-related changes that affect the gait and ambulation of older adults.

Clients with disorders of or injuries to the musculoskeletal system and those who are weak or unsteady because of age-related or neurologic problems may have difficulty walking. This chapter provides information on nursing activities and devices used to promote or enhance mobility.

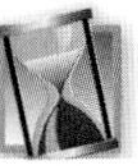

Gerontologic Considerations

■ Maintaining independence is important to the older person. Mobility facilitates staying active and independent.

■ An older adult's self-perception is often linked to their functional ability. Functional ability involves both mobility and making adaptations to compensate for changes occurring with aging or disease processes. Older people may need encouragement and support to integrate adaptations for mobility to maintain their activities of daily living.

■ An elevated toilet seat and grab bars may be needed to improve an older adult's ability to transfer and to maintain independence.

PREPARING FOR AMBULATION

Debilitated clients (those who are frail or weak from prolonged inactivity) require physical conditioning before they can ambulate again. Some techniques for increasing muscular strength and the ability to bear weight include performing isometric exercises with the lower limbs, performing isotonic exercises with the upper arms, dangling at the bedside, and using a device called a tilt table.

Isometric Exercises

Isometric exercises (see Chap. 24) are used to promote muscle tone and strength. **Tone** means the ability of muscles to respond when stimulated; **strength** means the power to perform. Both tone and strength are inherent in maintaining mobility. Frequent contraction of muscle fibers retains or improves muscle tone and strength. Active people maintain these two qualities through everyday activities, but inactive people and those who have been immobilized in casts or traction may require focused periods of exercise to reestablish their previous ability to walk.

Quadriceps setting and gluteal setting exercises are two types of isometric exercises that promote tone and strength in weight-bearing muscles. Both types are easily performed in bed or in a chair. They are initiated long before the anticipated time when ambulation will start. Most clients can perform these exercises independently once they have been instructed (see Client and Family Teaching 26-1).

Quadriceps Setting

Quadriceps setting is an isometric exercise in which the client alternately tenses and relaxes the quadriceps muscles. This type of exercise is sometimes referred to as quad setting. The quadriceps muscles (rectus femoris, vastus intermedius, vastus medialis, and vastus lateralis) cover the front and side of the thigh. Together they aid in extending the leg. Exercising the quadriceps muscles, therefore, enables clients to stand and support their body weight.

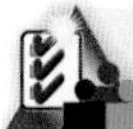

Client and Family Teaching 26-1
Quadriceps and Gluteal Setting Exercises

The nurse teaches the client and the family as follows:

- Tighten (contract) the quadriceps muscles by flattening the backs of the knees into the mattress. If that is not possible, place a rolled towel under the knee or heel before attempting to tighten the quadriceps muscles.
- Check to see that the kneecaps move upward. This is an indication that the client is performing the exercise correctly.
- Hold the contracted position for a count of five.
- Relax and repeat two or three times each hour.
- Tighten (contract) the gluteal muscles by pinching the cheeks of the buttocks together.
- Hold the contracted position for a count of five.
- Relax and repeat two or three times each hour.

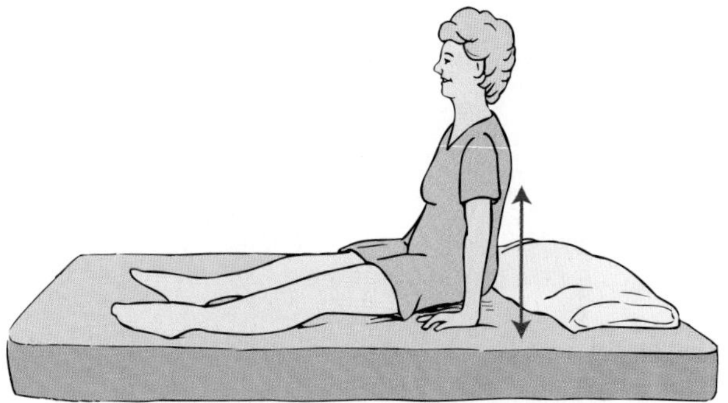

FIGURE 26-1 Modified hand push-ups are performed by extending the elbows and flexing the wrists to lift the buttocks slightly off the mattress.

Gluteal Setting

Gluteal setting is the contraction and relaxation of the gluteal muscles (gluteus maximus, gluteus medius, and gluteus minimus) to improve their strength and tone. As a group, the muscles in the buttocks aid in extending, abducting, and rotating the leg—functions that are essential to walking.

Upper Arm Strengthening

Clients who will use a walker, cane, or crutches need upper arm strength. An exercise regimen to strengthen the upper arms typically includes flexion and extension of the arms and wrists, raising and lowering weights with the hands, squeezing a ball or spring grip, and performing modified hand push-ups in bed (Fig. 26-1).

Clients perform modified push-ups (exercises in which clients support their upper body on the arms) several ways, depending on age and condition. While sitting in bed, a client may lift the hips off the bed by pushing down on the mattress with the hands. If the mattress is soft, the nurse places a block or books on the bed under the client's hands. If a sturdy armchair is available, the client can raise his or her body from the seat while pushing on the armrests.

If the client can lie on the abdomen, he or she performs push-ups in the following sequence:

1. Flex the elbows.
2. Place the hands, palms down, at approximately shoulder level.
3. Straighten the elbows to lift the head and chest off the bed.

For effectiveness, clients must perform push-ups three or four times a day.

Dangling

Dangling (sitting on the edge of the bed; Fig. 26-2) helps to normalize blood pressure, which may drop when the client rises from a reclining position (see the section on postural hypotension in Chap. 12; see Nursing Guidelines 26-1).

Using a Tilt Table

A **tilt table** is a device that raises the client from a supine to a standing position (Fig. 26-3). It helps clients adjust to being

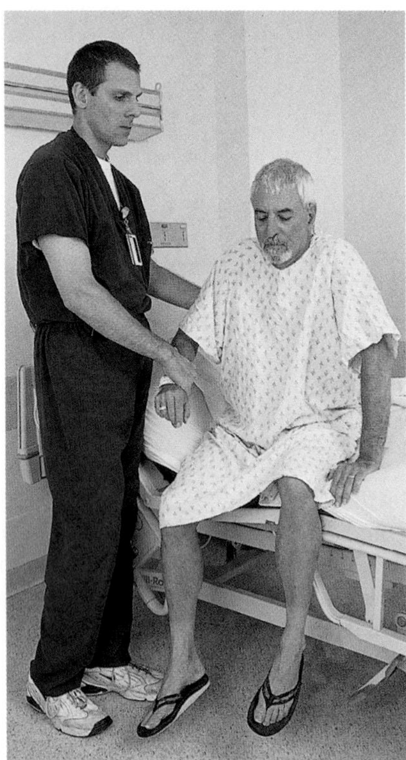

FIGURE 26-2 Dangling. (Copyright B. Proud.)

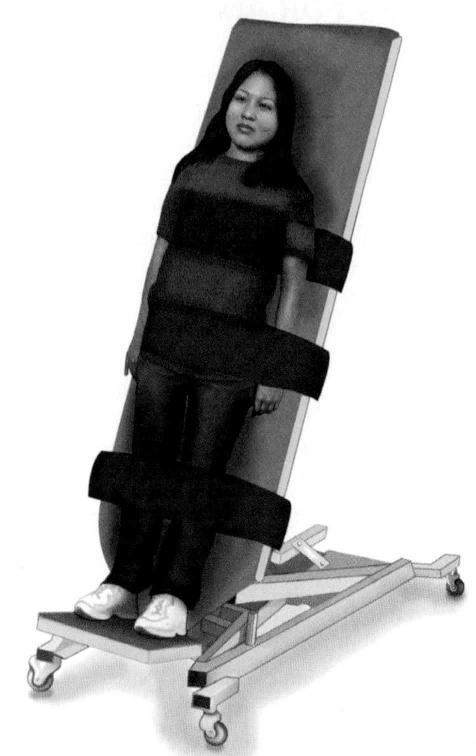

FIGURE 26-3 A tilt table.

upright and bearing weight on their feet. Although the tilt table is usually located in the physical therapy department, nurses often prepare the client for this type of preambulation therapy and communicate with the therapists about the client's response.

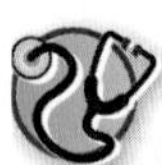

NURSING GUIDELINES 26-1

Assisting Clients to Dangle

- Perform dangling before ambulating whenever a client has been inactive for an extended period. *Performing dangling before ambulating demonstrates concern for the client's safety.*
- Place the client in a Fowler's position for a few minutes. *This position maintains safety should the client become dizzy or faint.*
- Lower the height of the bed. *With a lowered bed, the client can use the floor for support.*
- Provide a footstool if the client's feet do not reach the floor. *A footstool is an alternative for supporting the feet.*
- Fold back the top linen. *Linen can interfere with movement.*
- Provide the client with a robe and slippers. *Doing so maintains warmth and shows respect for the client's modesty.*
- Help the client pivot a quarter of a turn to swing the legs over the side and sit on the edge of the bed. *This position helps the client adjust to the sitting position.*
- Stay with the client until he or she no longer feels dizzy or light-headed. *The nurse can provide immediate assistance.*

Just before using a tilt table, the nurse applies elastic stockings (see the section on antiembolism stockings in Chap. 27). These stockings help to compress vein walls, thus preventing the pooling of blood in the extremities, which may trigger fainting.

After being transferred from the bed or stretcher to the horizontal tilt table, the client is strapped securely to prevent a fall. The feet are positioned against the foot rest. The entire table is then tilted in increments of 15 to 30 degrees until the client is in a vertical position. If symptoms such as dizziness and hypotension develop, the table is lowered or returned to the horizontal position.

ASSISTIVE DEVICES

Some clients still need assistance to ambulate independently even after performing strengthening exercises. Two devices used to provide support and assistance with walking are parallel bars and a walking belt, which is also known as a gait belt.

Clients use **parallel bars** (a double row of stationary bars) as handrails to gain practice in ambulating. Sometimes a tilt table is positioned just in front of the parallel bars so that the client can progress from being upright to actually walking again (Fig. 26-4).

A **walking belt** is applied around the client's waist. If the client loses balance, the nurse can support him or her and prevent injuries. When assisting a client to ambulate, the nurse

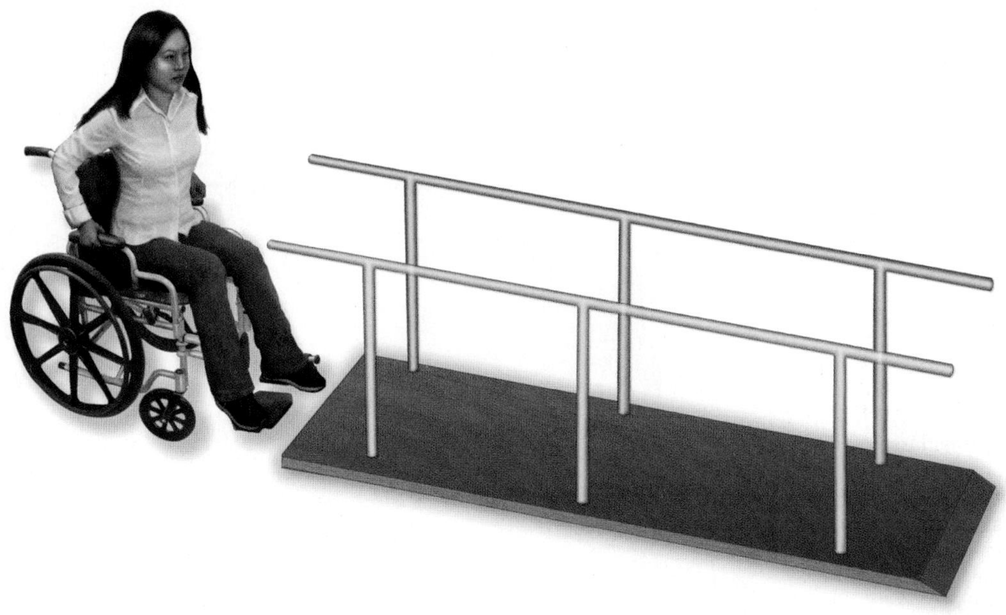

FIGURE 26-4 Parallel bars.

walks alongside the client, holding the walking belt or the client's own belt and supporting the client's arm (Fig. 26-5).

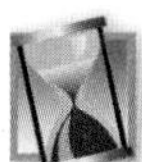

Gerontologic Considerations

- A walking or gait belt can be used to assist an older person with transferring, even if the client is not ambulatory. The older client balances on the stronger extremity while being supported with the gait belt. The client should never be forced to walk if unable.

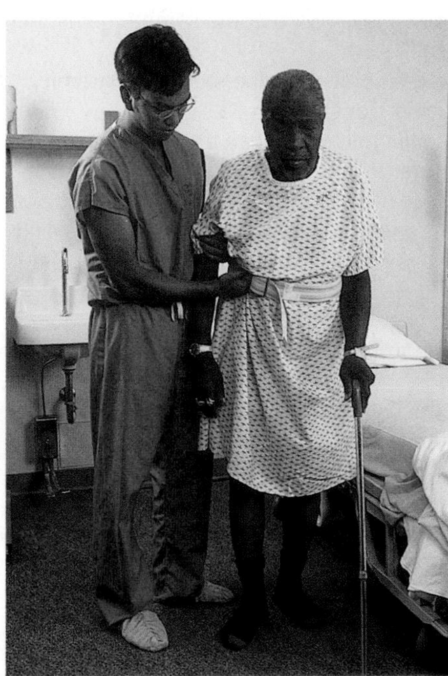

FIGURE 26-5 Using a walking belt.

While ambulating, the nurse observes the client for pallor, weakness, or dizziness. If fainting seems likely, the nurse supports the client by sliding an arm under the axilla and placing a foot to the side, forming a wide base of support. With the client's weight braced, the nurse balances the client on a hip until help arrives or slides the client down the length of the nurse's leg to the floor (Fig. 26-6).

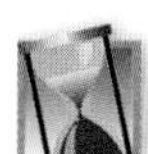

Gerontologic Considerations

- Limited or unsteady mobility may be a problem for some older adults as a result of age-related postural changes. It may lead to the development of a swaying or shuffling gait. As a person ages, he or she may develop flexion of the spine, which can alter the center of gravity and may result in an increase in falls.
- If a client appears to have an unusual gait, assess the feet for corns, calluses, bunions, and ingrown or very long toenails. If any of these conditions are found, a podiatry referral may be indicated. Vascular changes may lead to numbness and a decreased sensory ability to perceive contact with the ground, which can also change a person's gait.

AMBULATORY AIDS

Three aids are used to help with ambulation: canes, walkers, and crutches.

Canes

A client who has weakness on one side of the body uses a **cane**, which is a handheld ambulation device made of wood or aluminum. Aluminum canes are more common. Canes have rubber tips to reduce the potential for slipping.

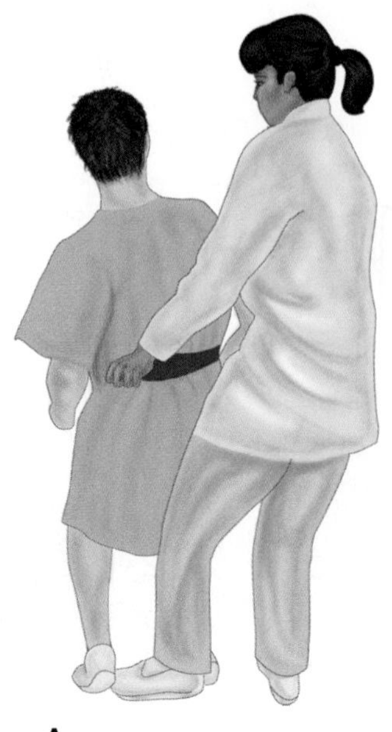

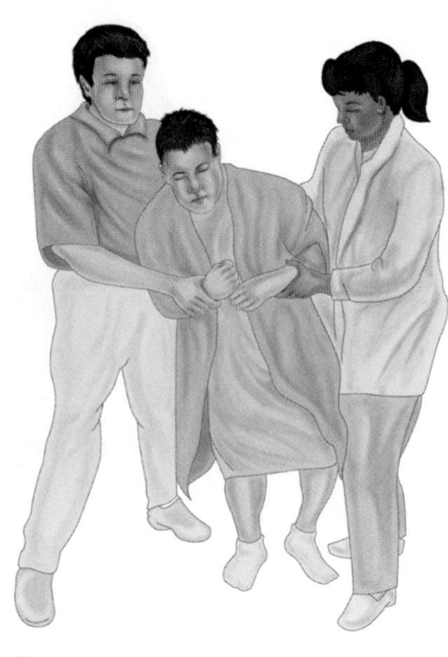

FIGURE 26-6 A. One nurse guides a client to the floor. **B.** A client is lowered to the floor with two nurses. (From Taylor, C., Lillis, C., LeMone, P., et al. [2008]. *Fundamentals of nursing* [6th ed. p. 1304]. Philadelphia: Lippincott Williams & Wilkins.)

Clients may use different types of canes depending on their physical deficits. For clients who need minimal support, a cane with a half-circle handle is appropriate. A T-handle cane has a handgrip with a slightly bent shaft, offering the user more stability. A quad cane has four supports at the base and provides even more stability than the other types. (Fig. 26-7).

A cane must be the right height for the client. The cane's handle should be parallel with the client's hip, providing an elbow flexion of approximately 30 degrees. Removing a portion of the lower end can shorten wooden canes. Depressing metal buttons in the telescoping shaft can shorten or lengthen aluminum canes (see Client and Family Teaching 26-2).

When clients are beginning to use a cane, the nurse assists by applying a walking belt and standing toward the back of the client's stronger side.

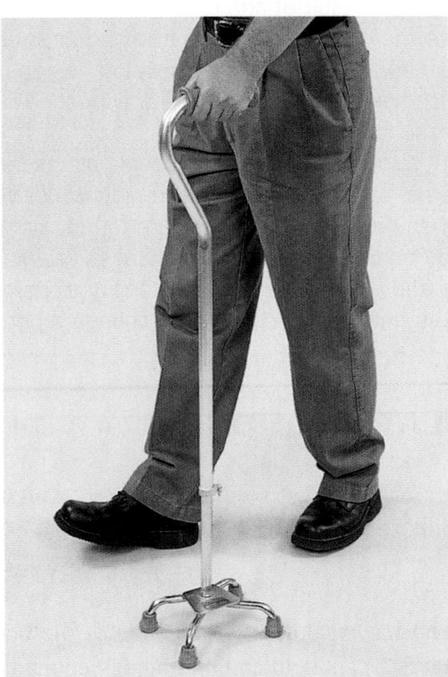

FIGURE 26-7 A quad cane. Note that the handle is parallel to the client's hip. (Photo by B. Proud.)

Client and Family Teaching 26-2
Using a Cane

The nurse teaches the client and the family as follows:

- Place the cane on the stronger side of the body.
- Stand upright with the cane 4 to 6 in. (10–15 cm) to the side of the toes.
- Move the cane forward at the same time as the weaker extremity.
- Take the next step with the stronger extremity.
- When using stairs:
  - Use a stair rail rather than the cane when going up or down stairs, if possible.
  - Take each step up with the stronger leg followed by the weaker one. Reverse the pattern for descending the stairs.
  - If there is no stair rail, advance the cane just before rising or descending with the weaker leg.
- When sitting:
  - Back up to the chair until the seat is against the back of the legs.
  - Rest the cane close by.
  - Grip the arm rests with both hands.
  - Sit down.
- When getting up from a chair:
  - Grip the arm rests while holding the cane in the stronger hand.
  - Advance the stronger leg.
  - Lean forward.
  - Push with both arms against the arm rests.
  - Stand until balanced and any symptoms of dizziness pass.

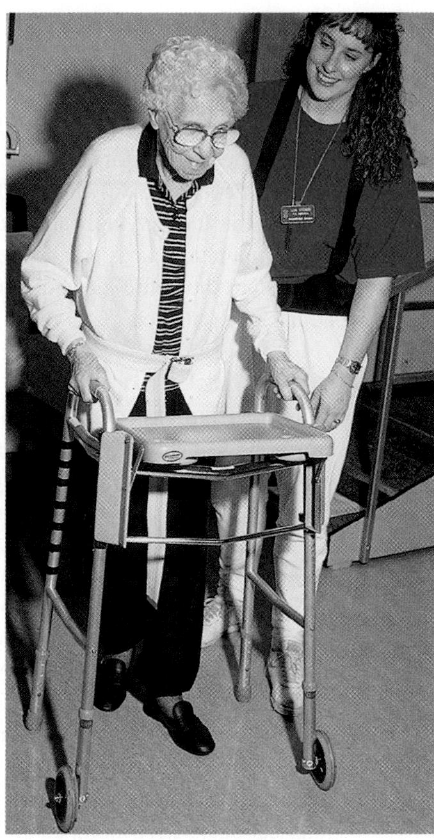

FIGURE 26-8 Using a walker with wheels.

Walkers

Clients who require considerable support and assistance with balance use a **walker**, the most stable form of ambulatory aid. Examples of clients who commonly use walkers are those beginning to ambulate after prolonged bed rest or after hip surgery.

Standard walkers are constructed of curved aluminum bars that form a three-sided enclosure with four legs for support. Some have front wheels (Fig. 26-8) or a seat. Other adaptations are made for clients who have compromised use of one or both arms or those who must use stairs. The height of a walker as well as a cane is adjustable.

Nurses instruct clients who use a walker to:

- Stand within the walker
- Hold on to the walker at the padded handgrips
- Pick up the walker and advance it 6 to 8 in. (15 to 20 cm)
- Take a step forward
- Support the body weight on the handgrips when moving the weaker leg (for clients with partial or non–weight-bearing on one leg)

When the client with a walker wants to sit down, the technique is similar to that with a cane, with one exception. When the legs are at the front of the chair seat, the client grips an arm rest with one arm while placing the other hand on the walker and using the stronger leg for support. The client releases the grip on the walker while using the free hand to grasp the opposite arm rest and lowers himself or herself into the chair. To rise, the client moves to the edge of the chair and repositions the walker. After pushing up on the arm rests with both arms until the body weight is centered, the client uses one hand, then the other to grasp the walker.

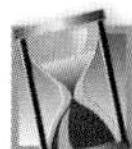

Gerontologic Considerations

- Older adults sometimes use a "step-stop" pattern when using an ambulatory aid; that is, they take one step, then stop, and repeat again. If that is the case, encourage a smooth, progressive cadence.
- Some older adults develop the habit of picking up and carrying a walker rather than having it make contact with the floor. In these situations, the person may benefit from another type of walker such as a walker with wheels or a three-wheeled walker. A physical therapist can assess the situation and recommend an appropriate walker.
- Rubber tips and handgrips on ambulatory aids should be kept clean and replaced when they are worn. Worn or dirty tips and handgrips contribute to falls and unsafe mobility.
- Before discharging an older person who will be using a mobility device, advise the family to make the home safer by removing scatter rugs and ensuring that lighting is adequate and that no electric cords are in passageways. Furniture may have to be rearranged and railings or grab bars may need to be added to bathrooms and outside entrances.
- A ramp with a hand rail helps older adults to enter and leave their residence more conveniently and safely when they are using an ambulatory aid.

Crutches

Crutches, an ambulatory aid generally used in pairs, are constructed of wood or aluminum. Because the use of crutches requires a great deal of upper arm strength and balance, older adults or weak clients do not commonly use them.

The three basic types of crutches are axillary, forearm, and platform (Fig. 26-9). The most familiar type is **axillary crutches** (the standard type of crutches) that have a bar that fits beneath the axilla. Clients who need brief, temporary assistance with ambulation are likely to use axillary crutches. Lofstrand and Canadian crutches are examples of **forearm crutches**; they have an arm cuff but no axillary bar. Forearm crutches generally are used by experienced clients who need permanent assistance with walking. **Platform crutches** (crutches that support the forearm) are used by clients who cannot bear weight with their hands and wrists. Many clients with arthritis use them. Sometimes a client uses one axillary crutch and one platform crutch—for example, when one arm is broken.

Once the type of ambulatory aid is medically prescribed, the client is measured (Skill 26-1).

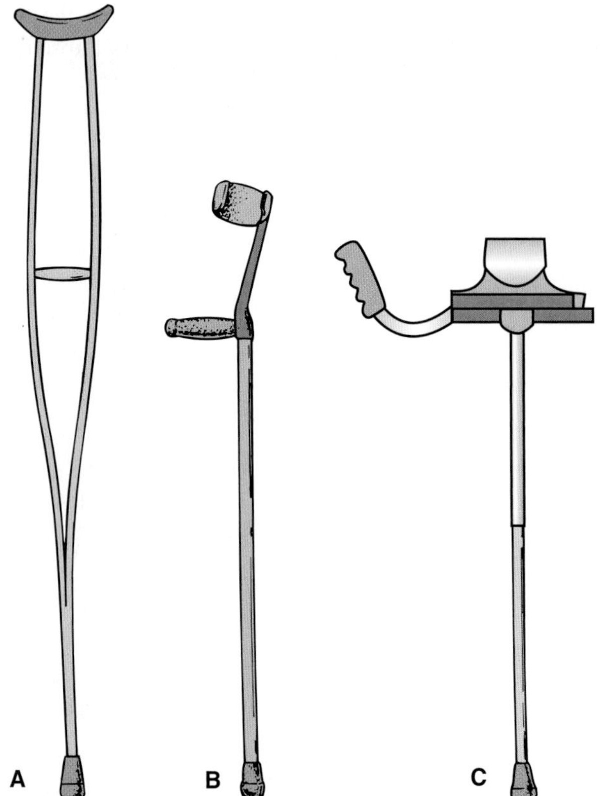

FIGURE 26-9 Three types of crutches: axillary (A), forearm (B), and platform (C).

Crutch-Walking Gaits

The term *gait* refers to one's manner of walking. A crutch-walking gait is the walking pattern used when ambulating with crutches; clients use some of the same gaits with walkers or canes.

The four types of crutch-walking gaits are the four-point gait, the three-point gait (non–weight-bearing or partial weight-bearing), the two-point gait, and the swing-through gait (Table 26-1). The word *point* refers to the sum of the crutches and legs used when performing the gait. Nurses are responsible for assisting clients who are learning to walk with crutches (Skill 26-2).

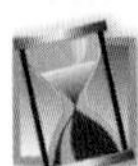

Gerontologic Considerations

- Older adults who have difficulty going up and down stairs may consider rearranging their homes so all necessary furnishings are on one level. A bedside commode decreases the number of trips up and down stairs if the bathroom is not on the same level as the bedroom or living area.

Stop, Think, and Respond Box 26-1

What negative consequences can occur when a client uses ambulatory aids?

PROSTHETIC LIMBS

Some clients with leg amputations ambulate using a **prosthetic limb** (a substitute for an arm or leg) without the assistance of crutches or other ambulatory aids. The design of a prosthetic limb varies depending on whether the lower extremity is amputated at the foot (Syme's amputation), is a below-the-knee (BK) amputation, or is an above-the-knee (AK) amputation, or whether the entire leg and a portion of the hip (hemipelvectomy) are removed.

Temporary Prosthetic Limb

In many cases, clients return from surgery with an *immediate postoperative prosthesis* (IPOP), which is a temporary artificial limb. It consists of a walking pylon, a lightweight tube, attached to a shell made of plaster or plastic on the stump, and a rigid foot (Fig. 26-10). A belt with garters keeps the temporary prosthesis in place. The belt is loosened while the client is in bed and is tightened during ambulation. Some IPOPs are attached to the residual limb with a pneumatic air bag or with a clamshell design, which permits removal when the client is not ambulating. An IPOP facilitates early ambulation and promotes an intact body image immediately after surgery. It also helps to control stump swelling.

The nurse is responsible for ensuring that the incision heals and that no complications, such as joint contractures or infection, develop. Complications delay rehabilitation. Contractures interfere with limb and prosthetic alignment, which ultimately affects the client's ability to walk.

Permanent Prosthetic Components

Construction of a permanent prosthesis is delayed for several weeks or months until the wound heals and the stump size is

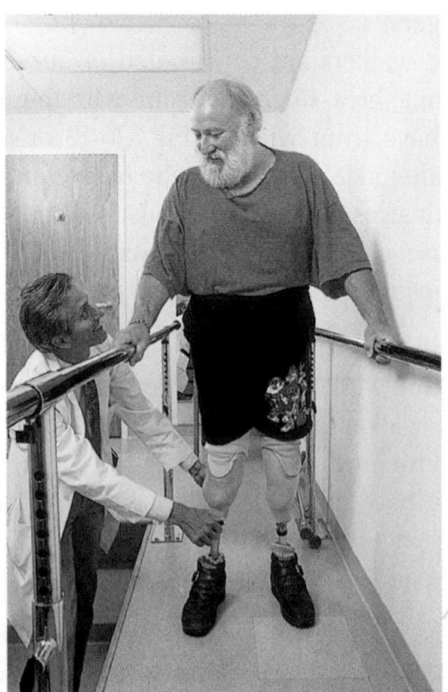

FIGURE 26-10 Many amputees receive prostheses soon after surgery and begin learning to use them with the support of the rehabilitation team.

TABLE 26-1 Crutch-Walking Gaits

GAIT	INDICATIONS FOR USE	GAIT PATTERN	ILLUSTRATION
Four-point	Bilateral weakness or disability such as arthritis or cerebral palsy	One crutch, opposite foot, other crutch, remaining foot	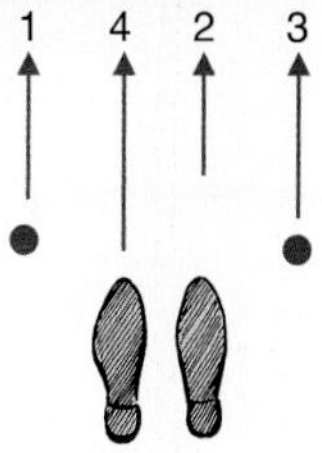 1 4 2 3
Two-point	Same as for four-point, but clients have more strength, coordination, and balance	One crutch and opposite foot moved in unison, followed by the remaining pair	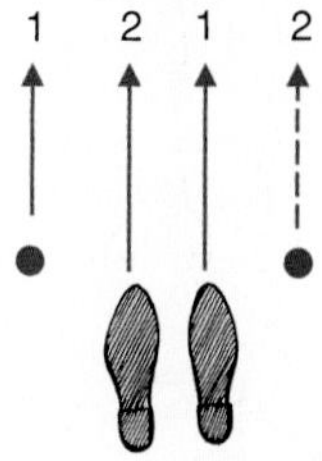 1 2 1 2
Three-point non–weight-bearing	One amputated, injured, or disabled extremity (fractured leg or severe ankle sprain)	Both crutches move forward followed by the weight-bearing leg	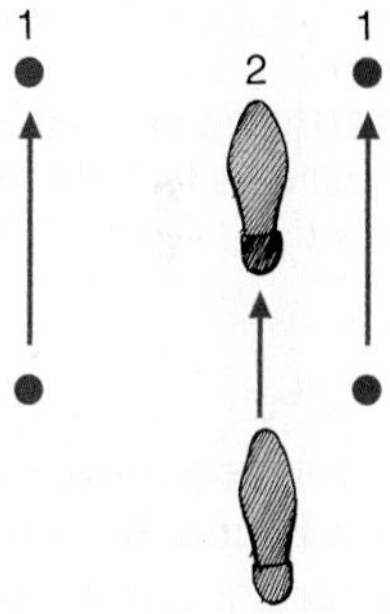 1 2 1
Three-point partial weight-bearing	Amputee learning to use prosthesis, minor injury to one leg, or previous injury showing signs of healing	Both crutches are advanced with the weaker leg; the stronger leg is placed parallel to the weaker leg	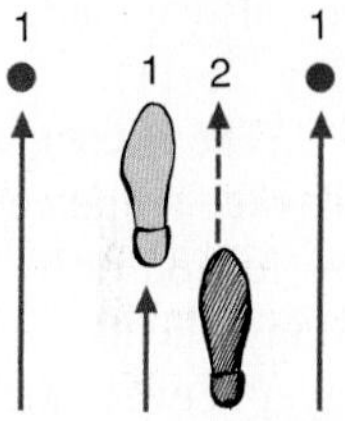 1 1 2 1
Swing-through	Injury or disorder affecting one or both legs, such as a paralyzed client with leg braces or an amputee before being fitted with a prosthesis	Both crutches are moved forward; one or both legs are advanced beyond the crutches	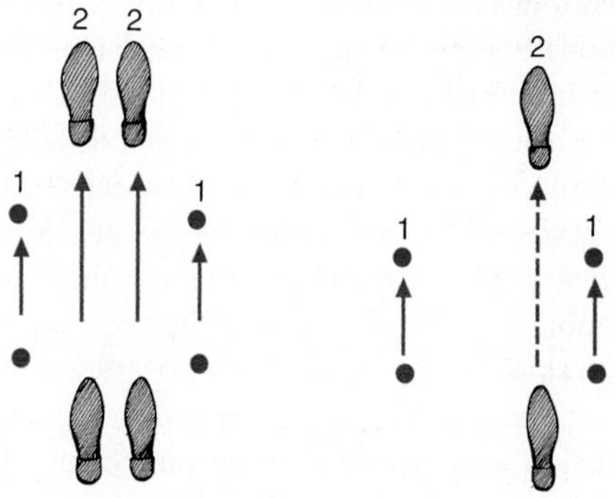 2 2 1 1; 2 1 1

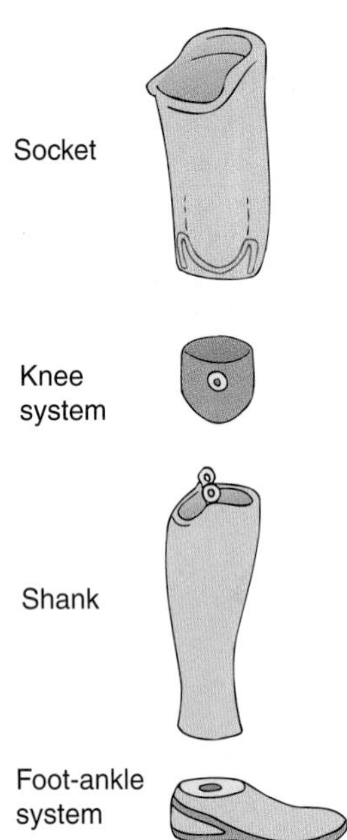

FIGURE 26-11 Components of a permanent prosthetic limb; a prosthesis for a BK amputation does not contain a knee system or a thigh socket.

relatively stable. The permanent prosthesis is custom-made to conform to the stump and to meet the client's needs.

Permanent prostheses for BK amputees include a socket, a shank, and an ankle/foot system. AK prostheses also include a knee system to replace the knee joint (Fig. 26-11).

The socket, a molded cone, holds the stump and enables the amputee to move the prosthesis. It is held in place by suction or by a leather belt, also referred to as a sling. Many clients wear one or more socks over the stump as a layer between the skin and the socket. Stump socks, made of wool or cotton, come in a variety of thicknesses to accommodate slight changes in stump size. Tube socks are not an appropriate substitute. Despite the expense, stump socks must be replaced whenever holes develop or they become worn; a darned stump sock can cause skin breakdown as a result of friction within the socket. Some amputees also wear a nylon sheath beneath the stump sock to wick perspiration from the skin toward the sock and reduce friction on the skin.

For AK amputees, the prosthetic knee system allows flexion and extension to accommodate sitting and a more natural gait while walking. The knee system connects the socket to the shank of the prosthesis.

The shank usually is shaped like a natural lower leg. It transfers the body weight to the walking surface. The shank is painted to resemble the client's skin color.

There are two basic types of ankle/foot systems: those that have one or more moving artificial joints (articulated systems) and those that do not. Although articulated systems allow more motion, the nonarticulated type has a cushion in the heel that permits compression during walking. The client wears a sock and shoe on the prosthetic foot. The client can vary his or her shoes, but all should be of similar height to ensure alignment of the prosthesis and a near-normal gait pattern.

Client Care

Nurses are responsible for managing the care of the stump and ensuring maintenance of the prosthesis (Skill 26-3).

Ambulation With a Lower Limb Prosthesis

Ambulation with a lower limb prosthesis requires strength and endurance. The more natural joints that are preserved, the more natural the gait appears, and the more easily it is performed. To ensure as normal a gait as possible, clients learn to stand erect and look ahead when walking. They keep the feet close together and take each step without hiking the hip unnaturally to swing the artificial limb forward. If using a cane, the client holds it in the hand opposite the prosthetic limb. When going up or down stairs, curbs, or hills, the client moves the unaffected leg first, followed by the one with the prosthesis.

Amputees who wish to participate in strenuous activities such as snow skiing can use a sturdier modified prosthesis.

Stop, Think, and Respond Box 26-2

Give some reasons why amputees may abandon rehabilitation and the use of a prosthesis; discuss how clients can overcome these impediments.

NURSING IMPLICATIONS

Many nursing diagnoses are possible for clients who need to use an ambulatory aid. Applicable nursing diagnoses include the following:

- Impaired Physical Mobility
- Risk for Disuse Syndrome
- Unilateral Neglect
- Risk for Trauma
- Risk for Peripheral Neurovascular Dysfunction
- Risk for Activity Intolerance

Nursing Care Plan 26-1 demonstrates how the nurse would devise a care plan for a client with the nursing diagnosis of Impaired Physical Mobility, defined in the NANDA-I taxonomy (2012, p. 224) as a "limitation in independent, purposeful physical movement of the body or of one or more extremities." This diagnosis can be used for clients who are completely independent; those who require help from another person for assistance, supervision, or teaching; those who require help from another person for assistance and a device; or those who are totally dependent.

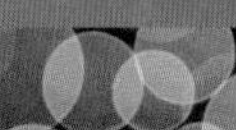

NURSING CARE PLAN 26-1 Impaired Physical Mobility

Assessment

- Assess motor strength and range of motion in both lower extremities.
- Observe the client's ability to turn himself or herself, rise from a lying or sitting position, and move from one location to another.
- Watch the client walk, noting whether the client has a stable or unstable gait.
- Ask whether the client uses any type of ambulatory assistive device like crutches, cane, or walker.
- Inspect the client's lower extremities to determine whether the client wears a lower limb prosthesis or a mechanical brace.
- Review the client's health history for disorders that affect or impair mobility such as a previous stroke, joint disease like arthritis, or neurologic deficits that affect balance and coordination such as Parkinson's disease.
- Gather information about the client's current use of prescription and nonprescription medications and research possible actions or side effects that can cause sedation, dizziness, and physical instability.

Nursing Diagnosis. **Impaired Physical Mobility** related to restricted positioning, limited weight bearing, pain, and fear of ambulating as manifested by hip replacement surgery 3 days earlier, joint position of operative hip limited to extension, slight flexion, and continuous abduction, partial weight bearing on operative leg with three-point gait following physical therapy instruction, and statement, "My hip hurts and I feel so scared about walking."

Expected Outcome. The client will ambulate 6 ft with the assistance of a walker following physical therapy on 2/10.

Interventions	Rationales
Instruct and supervise the client to dorsiflex, plantar flex, and perform quad-setting exercises of both lower extremities every hour while awake.	Active exercise and range of motion promote joint flexibility and muscle tone.
Maintain abduction wedge between legs to keep knees apart at all times while in bed.	Maintaining abduction prevents the hip prosthesis from becoming displaced until healing is complete.
Keep flat with slight elevation (30–45 degrees) of head.	Preventing hip flexion helps to maintain the placement of the hip prosthesis until healing is complete.
Encourage the use of a patient-controlled analgesia (PCA) pump at frequent intervals to control pain.	Relieving pain facilitates the client's comfort and cooperation in performing rehabilitative exercise and mobility.
Transfer from the bed to a standing position at the bedside, following these directions: • Slide affected left leg to edge of bed; remove abduction wedge. • Have client use trapeze or elbows and hands to slide buttocks and legs perpendicular to bed. Remind client to avoid leaning forward and praise efforts at moving. • Lower unaffected right foot to floor and help with lowering affected left foot, keeping knees apart. • Dangle at bedside for approximately 5 minutes. • Apply walking safety belt around waist. • Brace feet and pull forward on belt. • Stand at bedside, putting only partial weight on left leg. • Reverse actions for returning the client to bed.	Preventing hip flexion helps to maintain the placement of the hip prosthesis until healing is complete.

Evaluation of Expected Outcomes

- Client maintains postoperative positions as ordered by physician.
- Abduction wedge is in place while client is in bed.
- Client performs active isotonic and isometric (quad-setting) exercises.
- Use of PCA pump reduces pain to a level that facilitates exercise.
- Client can transfer from bed and stand at bedside following the procedure outlined in the written plan of care.
- Client alternates full weight bearing on right leg with partial weight bearing on left leg in preparation for ambulation in the physical therapy department.

CRITICAL THINKING EXERCISES

1. Compare the differences in using two types of ambulatory aids, such as crutches and a walker.
2. Discuss stereotypes of people who use ambulatory aids.
3. What are some advantages of implementing an exercise regimen to promote early ambulation?
4. What rationales could the nurse offer a client for providing an IPOP on an amputated limb?

NCLEX-STYLE REVIEW QUESTIONS

1. What is the best evidence that a client using a walker is performing a three-point partial weight-bearing gait correctly?
   1. The client advances the walker and the operative leg while putting most of the weight on the hand grips of the walker.
   2. The client advances the walker and the operative leg while putting most of the weight on the back legs of the walker.
   3. The client advances the walker and the operative leg while putting most of the weight on the toes of the operative leg.
   4. The client advances the walker and the operative leg while putting most of the weight on the heel of the unoperative leg.
2. When the nurse observes a client with arthritis using a cane, which finding indicates that the client needs more instruction about its use?
   1. The client's cane tip is covered with a rubber cap.
   2. The client wears athletic shoes with nonskid soles.
   3. The client uses the cane on the painful side.
   4. The client holds the head up and looks straight ahead.
3. After a client undergoes a total hip replacement, which position of the operative hip is essential for the nurse to maintain?
   1. Adduction
   2. Abduction
   3. Flexion
   4. Rotation
4. Which activity is best to plan immediately after surgery for strengthening the muscles of a client before ambulating with crutches?
   1. Standing at the side of the bed
   2. Balancing between parallel bars
   3. Lifting with the overbed trapeze
   4. Transferring from bed to a chair
5. Which of the following observations is most indicative that the crutches a client is using need further adjustment?
   1. The client stands straight without bending forward.
   2. The elbows are slightly flexed when standing in place.
   3. The top bars of the crutches fit snugly into the axillae.
   4. The wrists are hyperextended when grasping the handgrips.

SKILL 26-1 Measuring for Crutches, Canes, and Walkers

Suggested Action	Reason for Action
ASSESSMENT	
Check the medical orders.	Collaborates nursing activities with the medical treatment.
Determine the type of ambulatory aid the client will use.	Indicates the type of measurements needed.
Check agency policy about personnel responsible for measuring and dispensing ambulatory aids.	Complies with agency procedures; clients in health care agencies sometimes are referred to personnel in the physical therapy department.
Determine the strength of the client's arm and leg muscles.	Indicates the client's potential for weight bearing; weakness suggests a need to measure the client in bed or for further collaboration with the physician concerning muscle strengthening.
PLANNING	
Obtain a long tape measure.	Facilitates measuring clients with a range of heights.
Wash your hands or perform an alcohol-based hand rub (see Chap. 10).	Reduces the transmission of microorganisms.
Assist the client with donning socks and walking shoes, if the client can stand for the measurement.	Aids in more accurate measurement that accommodates added height of the heel.
IMPLEMENTATION	
Axillary Crutches	
Assist the client who can support his or her body weight to a standing position at the bedside with supportive shoes.	Positions the client in a posture for the actual use of crutches.
Measure from the anterior skinfold of the axilla to approximately 4–8 in. (10–20 cm) diagonally from the foot (Fig A).	Approximates the length required for appropriate use.

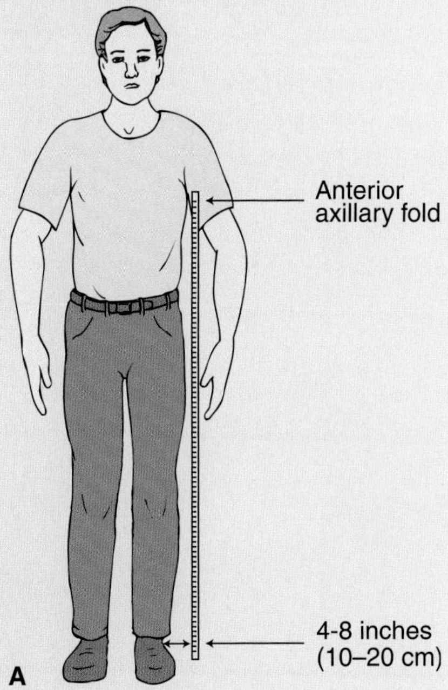

Measuring for crutches in a standing position.

(continued)

Measuring for Crutches, Canes, and Walkers (continued)

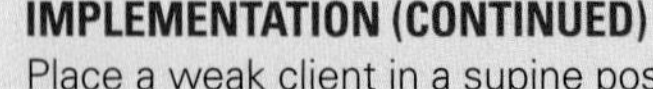

IMPLEMENTATION (CONTINUED)

Action	Rationale
Place a weak client in a supine position.	Simulates the client's height in a standing position.
Measure the distance from the anterior skinfold of the axilla to heel and add 2 in. (5 cm) or subtract 16 in. (40 cm) from the client's height (Fig. B).	Accommodates for the added height of the heel.

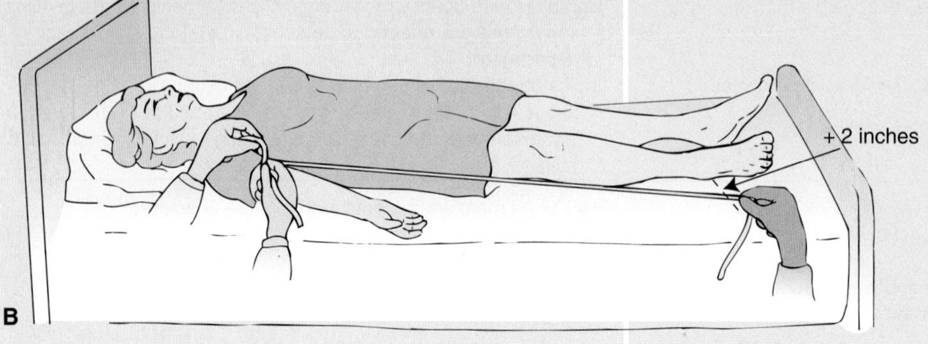

Measuring for crutches in a supine position.

Action	Rationale
Adjust the handgrips so there is 30 degrees of elbow flexion and 15 degrees of wrist hyperextension when client grasps the handgrips standing upright (Fig. C).	Ensures the potential for extending the elbow and supporting body weight.

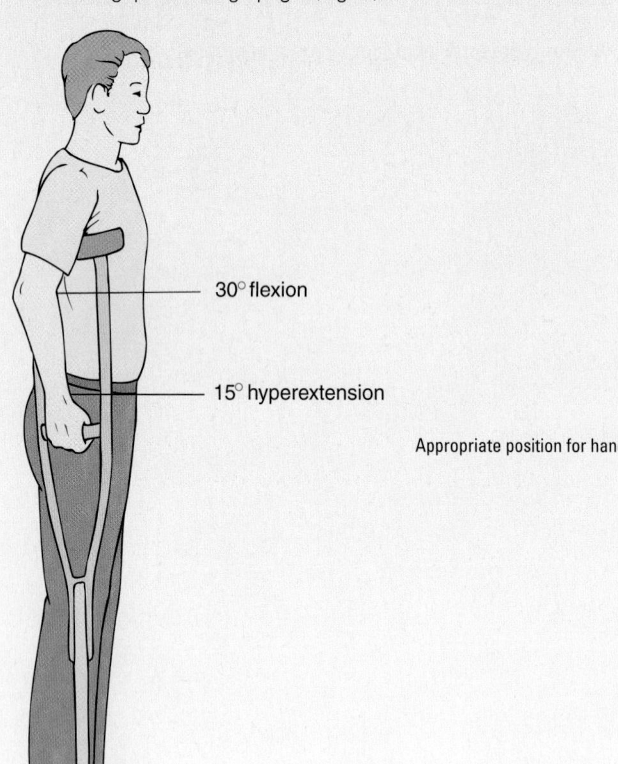

Appropriate position for handgrips.

(continued)

Measuring for Crutches, Canes, and Walkers (continued)

IMPLEMENTATION (CONTINUED)

Lengthen or shorten axillary crutches by removing wing nuts and replacing metal screws in the appropriate hole in the stem of the crutch. Adjust handgrips in the same way (Fig. D).

Customizes the length of the crutches according to the client's height.

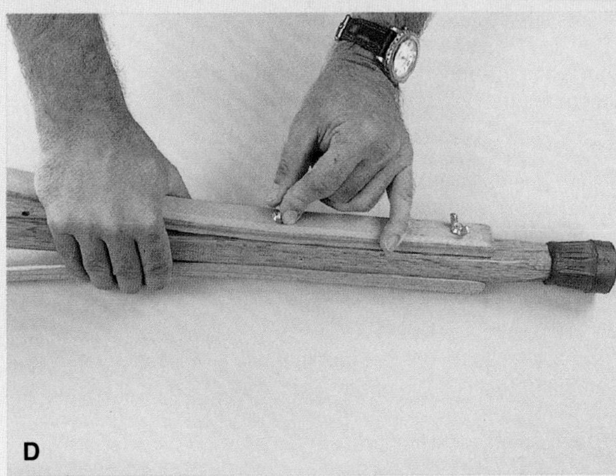

Adjusting length of an axillary crutch. (Photo by B. Proud.)

Forearm Crutches

Stand the client in shoes with the elbows flexed so the crease of the wrist is at the hip.

Simulates the appropriate posture when using forearm crutches.

Measure the forearm from 3 in. below the elbow, then add the distance between the wrist and floor (Fig. E).

Adjusts total length to accommodate for elbow and wrist flexion.

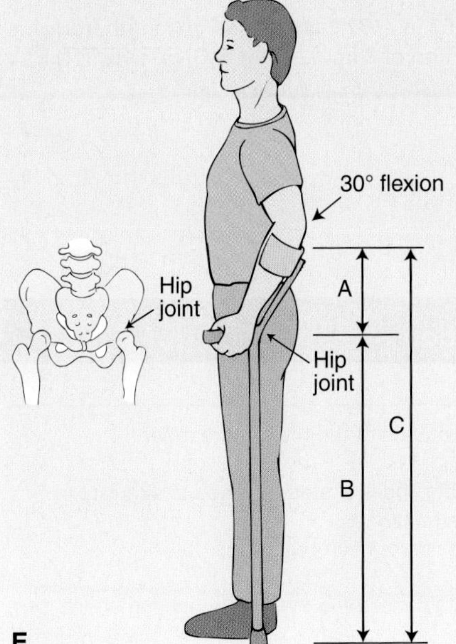

Measuring forearm crutches. Total length C = sum of A (3 in. below elbow to wrist) + B (wrist to floor).

Adjust the length of the forearm crutches by telescoping them up or down.

Customizes the final fit.

(continued)

Measuring for Crutches, Canes, and Walkers (continued)

Suggested Action	Reason for Action
IMPLEMENTATION (CONTINUED)	
Canes	
Have the client stand erect in shoes that he or she wears most often for ambulating.	Incorporates the height of the client's shoes.
Instruct the client to avoid leaning forward or elevating the shoulders.	Ensures an accurate measurement.
Measure from the wrist to the floor.	Determines the appropriate length of the cane.
Adjust the length of cane to provide 30 degrees of elbow flexion with the hand on the grip.	Customizes the final height of the cane.
Walkers	
Have the client stand while wearing supportive shoes.	Accommodates for the added height of shoes.
Measure from the mid-buttocks to the floor.	Facilitates the approximate height of the walker.
Adjust the legs of the walker to provide approximately 30 degrees of elbow flexion.	Customizes the final fit of the walker.

Evaluation

- The client stands upright with the shoulders relaxed.
- With axillary crutches, there is space for two fingers between the axilla and axillary bar to prevent **crutch palsy** (a weakened forearm, wrist, and hand muscles from nerve impairment secondary to pressure on the brachial plexus of nerves in the axilla) from incorrectly fitted crutches or poor posture.
- There is 30 degrees of elbow flexion and slight hyperextension of the wrist when standing in place.

Document

- Type of ambulatory aid
- Measurements for ambulatory aid
- Method for measuring client

SAMPLE DOCUMENTATION

Date and Time Measured for axillary crutches. Approximate length of crutches is 53 in. (132.5 cm) based on length from axillary fold to heel (51 in.) while in a supine position and the addition of 2 in. ——— SIGNATURE/TITLE

SKILL 26-2 Assisting with Crutch-Walking

Suggested Action	Reason for Action
ASSESSMENT	
Review the medical orders for the type of activity and crutch-walking gait.	Reflects the implementation of the medical treatment.
Read any previous nursing documentation regarding the client's efforts at crutch-walking.	Provides evaluative data and indicates the need to simulate or modify nursing interventions.
Wash hands or perform an alcohol-based hand rub (see Chap. 10).	Reduces the transmission of microorganisms.
Observe the condition of the client's axillae and palms.	Provides objective data concerning the weight-bearing effects on the upper body.
Ask the client whether there is any muscle or joint pain or tingling or numbness in the fingers.	Provides subjective data concerning the effects of crutch-walking and possible nerve irritation.
Inspect the conditions of the axillary pads and rubber crutch tips.	Demonstrates concern for safety.
PLANNING	
Consult with the client about the preferred time for ambulation.	Shows respect for individual decision making.
Assist the client to don clothes or a robe and supportive shoes or slippers with nonskid soles.	Demonstrates concern for modesty and safety.
Apply a walking belt if the client is weak or inexperienced in the use of crutches.	Demonstrates concern for safety.
Clear a pathway where the client will ambulate.	Demonstrates concern for safety.
Review the technique for performing the prescribed crutch-walking gait.	Reinforces prior learning.

(continued)

Assisting with Crutch-Walking (continued)

IMPLEMENTATION

Help the client to a standing position. — Prepares the client for ambulation.

Offer the crutches and observe that they are placed 4–8 in. (10–20 cm) to the side of the feet (Fig. A). — Forms a triangle for good balance.

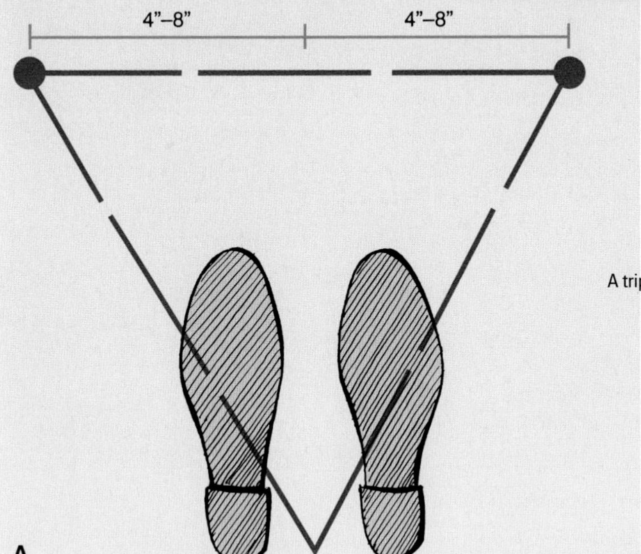

A tripod of support.

Remind the client to stand straight with the shoulders relaxed. — Reduces muscle strain.

Position yourself to the side and slightly behind the client on the weaker side (Fig. B). — Facilitates assistance without causing interference.

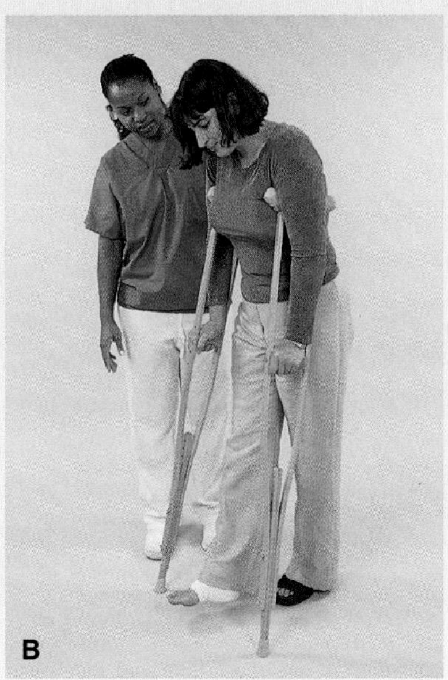

Positioning for assistance. (Photo by B. Proud.)

Take hold of the walking belt. — Helps steady or support the client.

Instruct the client to advance the crutches, lean forward, put some weight on the handgrips, and move one or both feet, depending on the prescribed gait. — Promotes walking.

Remind the client to slow down if there is evidence of fatigue or intolerance to the activity. — Demonstrates concern for the client's well-being.

(continued)

Assisting with Crutch-Walking (continued)

IMPLEMENTATION (CONTINUED)

For Sitting

Action	Rationale
Recommend backing up to the seat of the chair.	Promotes a position for sitting.
Have the client place both crutches in the hand on the same side as the weaker leg (Fig. C).	Frees the opposite hand.

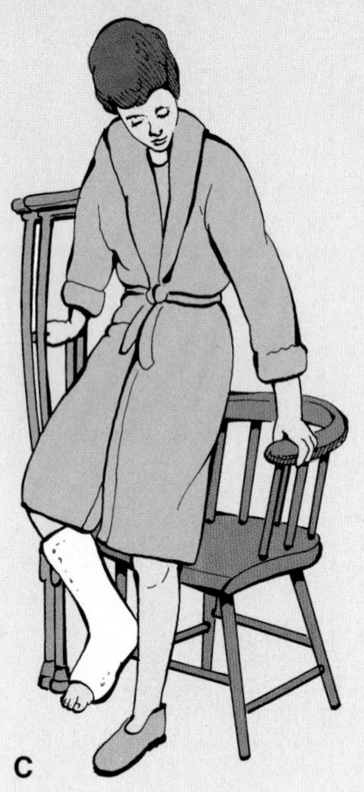

C Sitting down.

Action	Rationale
While using the handgrips on the crutches for support, have the client grasp one armrest with the free hand.	Reduces the potential for falling.
When balanced, tell the client to lower himself or herself into the seat of the chair.	Facilitates sitting.
To get up, help the client to the edge of the chair.	Facilitates using the stronger muscles of the thighs.
Instruct the client to hold the crutches upright on the weaker side, balancing the crutches with one hand.	Positions crutches for support.
Tell the client to position the weaker leg forward of the body and the stronger leg toward the base of the chair.	Helps to distribute weight over the stronger leg.
Tell the client to push on the handgrips and armrest, lean forward, and press down with the stronger leg.	Raises the client from the chair.

To Climb Stairs

Action	Rationale
Have the client use a handrail on the stronger side of the body, if possible.	Balances needed support.
Have the client transfer both crutches to the hand opposite the handrail.	Frees one hand for grasping the handrail for support.

(continued)

Assisting with Crutch-Walking (continued)

IMPLEMENTATION (CONTINUED)

Tell the client to push down on the handrail and step up with the good leg (Fig. D).	Uses the stronger muscles for bearing weight.

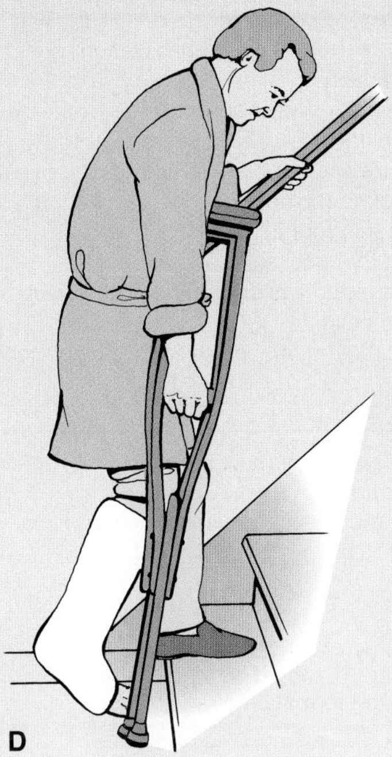

D Climbing stairs.

Follow by raising the weaker leg.	Brings both legs to the same stair.
Remind the client that when going down the stairs, the weaker leg is advanced first with the support of the crutches or handrail; then the stronger leg is moved.	Enables a safe descent.

Evaluation

- Crutches fit appropriately.
- Client performs crutch-walking gait correctly.
- No fatigue or other symptoms develop.
- Client remains free of injury.

Document

- Distance ambulated
- Gait used
- Response of the client

SAMPLE DOCUMENTATION

Date and Time Ambulated length of hospital corridor (approximately 100 ft) using crutches and a three-point non–weight-bearing gait. No breathlessness noted. States upper arms "ache" and attributes discomfort to "muscle strain" from previous day's ambulation efforts. Refuses medication for muscle discomfort.
________________ SIGNATURE/TITLE

SKILL 26-3 Applying a Leg Prosthesis

Suggested Action	Reason for Action
ASSESSMENT	
Wash hands or perform an alcohol-based hand rub (see Chap. 10).	Reduces the transmission of microorganisms.
Inspect the stump for evidence of bleeding, wound drainage, skin abrasions, blisters, and edema.	Detects complications that delay healing and rehabilitation or that interfere with ambulation.
Weigh the client at regular intervals.	Helps to detect fluctuations in weight that alter the size of the stump and the fit of the prosthesis.
Observe the ease or difficulty of inserting the stump within the socket.	Indicates changes in stump size and the need to add or decrease the numbers or thickness of stump socks.
Examine the joint connections in the prosthetic limb.	Determines whether lubrication or prosthetic maintenance is necessary; concerns about the mechanical features of the prosthesis or its fit are referred to a **prosthetist** (a person who constructs prostheses) immediately.
Inspect the shoe on the prosthetic limb for signs of wear or moisture.	Establishes whether heels or the entire shoe need to be replaced or dried.
PLANNING	
Cleanse the skin on the stump each evening, not in the morning.	Allows sufficient time for the skin to be moisture-free.
Rinse the soap from the stump and dry it well.	Avoids skin impairment and irritation.
Encourage the client to lie supine or prone periodically during the day.	Promotes venous circulation, reduces stump edema, and avoids joint contractures.
Instruct the client to avoid crossing the legs or keeping the natural knee flexed for a prolonged period.	Prevents circulatory problems.
Wash the socket each evening with water and mild soap.	Removes soil and perspiration.
Dry the socket well before application.	Prevents skin breakdown.
Use a small brush to clean the valve on a prosthesis with a suction socket.	Removes dust and facilitates the formation of a vacuum.
Keep a supply of clean stump socks to facilitate a daily change and a nylon sheath if one is used.	Promotes cleanliness and comfort.
Store clean wool stump socks for several days before use.	Allows the restoration of wool fiber resiliency.
Wash a nylon sheath in soapy lukewarm water, rinse well, and stretch it lengthwise before air drying; never remove water by twisting the sheath.	Maintains shape and integrity.
Advise the client with a new prosthesis to wear it for short periods initially and then increase the wearing time each day.	Prevents overexertion and impaired skin integrity.
IMPLEMENTATION	
Cover the prosthetic foot with the stocking and shoe of choice.	Coordinates apparel and helps to conceal the appearance of the prosthetic limb.
Apply the nylon sheath, if used, and the appropriate number or ply of stump socks.	Promotes comfort and the fit of the stump within the prosthesis.
Place a nylon stocking over the stump sock, allowing a long portion of the toe to extend from the base of the stump (Fig. A).	Helps to slide the stump within the socket.

A nylon stocking covers the stump sock.

A

(continued)

Applying a Leg Prosthesis (continued)

IMPLEMENTATION (CONTINUED)

Stand and position the prosthetic limb next to the residual limb.	Facilitates application.
Pull the toe of the nylon stocking through the valve at the base of the socket (Fig. B).	Locates the stump well within the lower area of the socket.

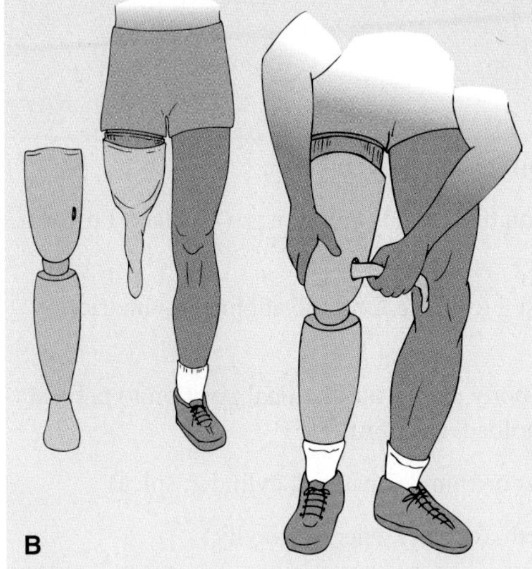

B

The nylon is pulled through the valve hole on the socket of the prosthesis.

Pump the stump up and down as the nylon stocking is completely removed.	Expels air and creates a vacuum that keeps the prosthesis attached to the stump.
Replace the plug within the valve opening.	Ensures the retention of vacuum suction.
Fasten all slings if other than a suction-socket type of prosthesis is used.	Secures the prosthesis to the stump.

Evaluation

- Stump size is unchanged.
- Skin is intact.
- Circulation is adequate based on similar skin color in the stump and the remaining limb.
- Joints above the amputation have full range of motion.
- Prosthesis is mechanically sound.
- Client ambulates without discomfort or injury.

Document

- Care and condition of the stump
- Care of stump socks
- Care and condition of the prosthesis
- Level of client performance in stump care and application of the prosthesis
- Client's performance in ambulation

SAMPLE DOCUMENTATION

Date and Time Stump washed and dried by client. No evidence of skin breakdown. Soiled stump socks exchanged with spouse for supply of clean socks. Inside of prosthetic socket cleaned and dried. Client observed while independently donning prosthesis. Procedure completed accurately and appropriately. Ambulated for approximately 15 min. without loss of balance or other difficulties. ———— SIGNATURE/TITLE

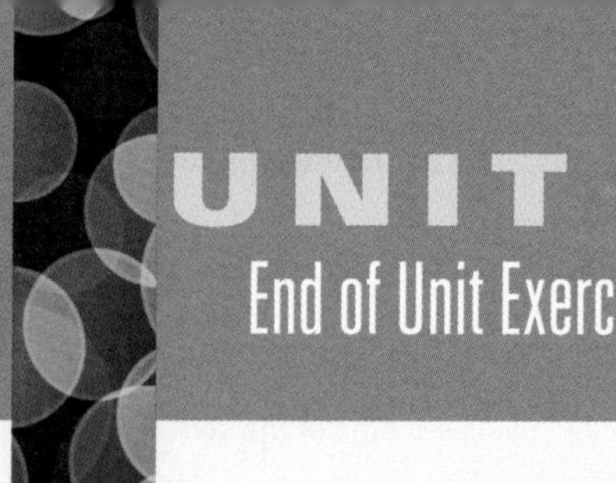

UNIT 6

End of Unit Exercises for Chapters 23, 24, 25, and 26

Section I: Reviewing What You've Learned

Activity A: *Fill in the blanks by choosing the correct word from the options given in parentheses.*

1. ________________ crutches are used by clients who cannot bear weight on their hands and wrists. (Axillary, Forearm, Platform)
2. ________________ exercises are stationary movements performed against a resistive force. (Dangling, Isometric, Isotonic)
3. A(n) ________________ splint is made of rigid materials that maintain a body part in a functional position to prevent contractures and muscle atrophy during periods of immobility. (inflatable, molded, traction)
4. A ________________ cast encircles one or both arms or legs and the chest or trunk. (bivalved, cylinder, spica)
5. The force of ________________ pulls objects toward the center of the earth. (density, energy, gravity)
6. Permanent shortening of muscles that resist stretching is called a ________________. (contraction, contracture, fracture)
7. The capacity to which a person can exercise is called ________________. (fitness, power, strength)
8. The range-of-motion exercise that involves spreading the fingers and thumb as widely as possible is called ________________. (abduction, adduction, flexion)

Activity B: *Mark each statement as either T (True) or F (False). Correct any false statements.*

1. T____F____ The ability of the muscles to respond to stimulation is referred to as strength.
2. T____F____ The gluteal muscles in the buttocks aid in extending, abducting, and rotating the leg.
3. T____F____ Braces are custom-made or custom-fitted devices designed to support weakened structures.
4. T____F____ A bivalved cast is cut in two pieces lengthwise from either a body or a cylinder cast.
5. T____F____ Skin shearing is the force exerted against the surface and layers of the skin as tissues slide in opposite but parallel directions.
6. T____F____ A trapeze is a rectangular piece of metal hung by a chain over the foot of the bed.
7. T____F____ Target heart rate means the goal for heart rate during exercise.

Activity C: *Write the correct term for each description below.*

1. Amputation of the foot ________________
2. Metal device inserted into and through one or more broken bones to stabilize fragments during healing ________________
3. Large cylinder cast that encircles the trunk, rather than an extremity ________________
4. Pulling effect directly exerted on a bone by attaching wires, pins, or tongs into or through it ________________
5. Field of engineering science devoted to promoting comfort, performance, and health in the workplace ________________

Activity D: *1. Match the types of mechanical immobilizing devices in Column A with their uses in Column B.*

Column A	Column B
1. ________ Inflatable splint	A. Prevents or reduces the severity of a joint injury
2. ________ Prophylactic brace	B. Prevents movement to maintain alignment during healing
3. ________ Manual traction	C. Controls bleeding and swelling
4. ________ Cylinder cast	D. Realigns a broken bone briefly by pulling on the body using muscular strength

2. Match the common body positions in Column A with their descriptions in Column B.

Column A	Column B
1. ________ Supine position	A. Semi-prone with the right knee drawn toward the chest
2. ________ Lateral position	B. Semi-sitting
3. ________ Prone position	C. Side lying with the hip and knee of the top leg in flexion
4. ________ Sims' position	D. Back lying
5. ________ Fowler's position	E. Abdomen lying
6. ________ Lateral oblique position	F. Side-lying

Activity E: *1. Differentiate between casts made from plaster of Paris and from fiberglass in the categories identified below.*

	Plaster of Paris	Fiberglass
Application		
Cost		
Durability		
Weight		
Weight bearing		
Effect of water		

2. Differentiate between active exercise and passive exercise in the categories listed below.

	Active Exercise	Passive Exercise
Definition		
Uses		
Examples		

Activity F: *Consider the following figure.*

1.

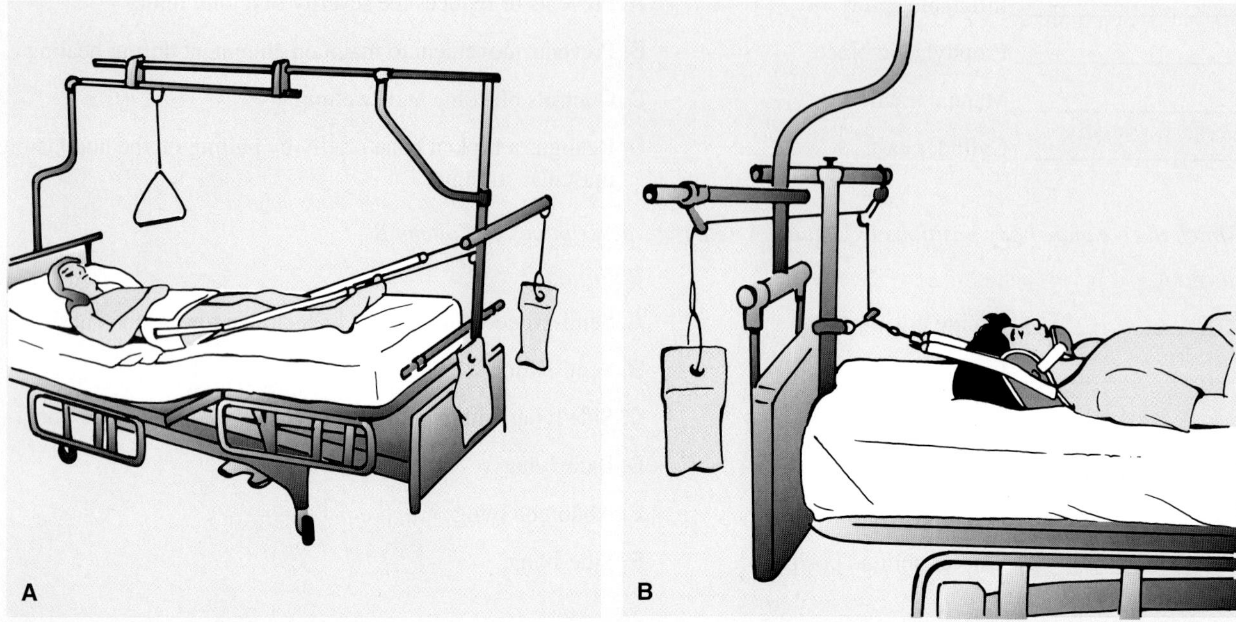

a. Identify the devices shown in the figure.

b. What are they used for?

Activity G: *A trochanter is the bony protrusion at the head of the femur near the hip. Trochanter rolls prevent the legs from turning outward. Write in the boxes provided below the correct sequence for using trochanter rolls.*

1. Roll the sheet around the blanket so that the end of each roll is underneath.
2. Fold a sheet lengthwise in half or in thirds and place it under the client's hips.
3. Secure the rolls next to each hip and thigh.
4. Permit the leg to rest against the trochanter roll.
5. Place a rolled-up bath blanket under each end of the sheet that extends on either side of the client.

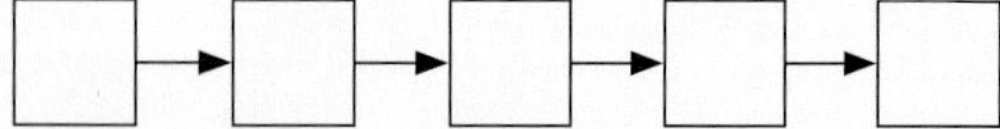

Activity H: *Answer the following questions.*

1. What is the purpose of a tilt table?

2. What are the functions of mechanical immobilization of a body part?

3. What is a cast? When is it used?

4. What are common nursing diagnoses applicable to a client with an immobilizing device?

5. How can one maintain a good standing posture?

6. What methods are used to prevent foot drop?

7. What are seven factors that may compromise a client's fitness and stamina?

Section II: Applying Your Knowledge

Activity I: *Give rationales for the following questions.*

1. Why should the nurse encourage a client who is being fitted with a prosthetic limb to lie supine or prone periodically during the day?

2. Why are bedridden older adults prone to developing problems from skin pressure?

3. Why is it important for the nurse to provide meticulous care to a pin site?

4. Why is the Fowler's position helpful for clients with dyspnea?

5. Why is a continuous passive motion machine used for the rehabilitation of clients who have undergone hip replacement surgery?

Activity J: *Answer the following questions focusing on nursing roles and responsibilities.*

1. A nurse is caring for a client recovering from hip surgery who is learning to ambulate with a walker.
   a. What instructions should the nurse give to the client regarding the use of the walker?

   b. How should the nurse teach this client the techniques of sitting down and rising from a chair?

2. A nurse is caring for a client who has a whiplash injury.
   a. How should the nurse determine the size of the cervical collar for this client?

   b. How should the nurse assess the client's neuromuscular function during recovery?

3. A nurse is preparing to transfer an elderly client from a bed to a chair. What general guidelines should the nurse follow when assisting with this client transfer?

4. A nurse is caring for an obese client with cardiovascular symptoms. The physician has ordered a balanced diet and an exercise program aimed at weight reduction for the client.

a. What methods can the nurse use to assess the client's fitness level?

b. How is the client's target heart rate calculated, and how does the client's fitness influence the prescription of a metabolic energy equivalent?

5. A nurse is caring for elderly clients at an extended care facility who can maintain some regular activity and exercise.

a. How can the nurse help to ensure that fluid intake is appropriate for these clients?

b. How can the nurse help these clients stay physically active?

6. The nurse is caring for a client who will need to use crutches.

a. How can the nurse ensure that the client will be strong enough to use crutches?

b. What kind of push-ups should the nurse teach a client who is still bedfast?

Activity K: *Consider the following questions. Discuss them with your instructor or peers.*

1. A nurse is caring for a 32-year-old client who is to be fitted with a prosthetic limb following a below-the-knee amputation of his right leg. The client is struggling to accept his condition.

a. What actions can the nurse take to ensure that the prosthetic limb is comfortable for the client?
b. How can the nurse help the client begin accepting the amputation and the need for the prosthetic limb?

2. A nurse is caring for a 64-year-old client with a fractured leg in a cast following a fall. The client is taking prescribed analgesics for pain. She has not been eating well, and her mobility is restricted.

a. What actions can the nurse take regarding the client's nutritional intake and use of analgesics?
b. What are major concerns when caring for elderly clients with casts?

3. A nurse is providing care for a client with paraplegia who requires assistance with activities of daily living.

a. How can the nurse help to prevent disuse syndrome?
b. What positioning devices might be considered for this client?

4. A nurse is working with a client who has lost movement on one side of his body following a cerebrovascular accident. What interventions can the nurse perform to maintain or restore functional use when caring for this client?

Section III: Getting Ready for NCLEX

Activity L: *Answer the following questions.*

1. A nurse is teaching a client with a fractured right leg how to climb stairs with a pair of crutches. Which of the following should the nurse tell the client?
   a. Step up by raising the right leg.
   b. Use the handrail if it is on the right side.
   c. Grasp both crutches at the handpiece in the right hand.
   d. Follow the right leg with the left leg.
2. A nurse is measuring an elderly client for a cane following an ankle sprain. Which of the following actions by the nurse is correct?
   a. Instruct the client to lean forward.
   b. Have the client stand barefoot with a support.
   c. Ensure 40 degrees of elbow flexion with the hand on the grip.
   d. Measure from the client's wrist to the floor.
3. What guidelines should the nurse follow when applying an emergency splint to a client? Select all that apply.
   a. Cover any open wounds with clean material.
   b. Swab the skin using alcohol or acetone.
   c. Select rigid material to provide support.
   d. Use wide tape to confine the injured part to the splint.
   e. Encourage the client to exercise fingers and toes frequently.
4. A nurse is caring for a client with a fractured wrist in a cylinder cast. Which of the following actions should the nurse perform to obtain information about the client's neuromuscular function? Select all that apply.
   a. Monitor the mobility of the fingers.
   b. Assess for sensation in the exposed fingers.
   c. Elevate the cast on pillows or another support.
   d. Apply an ice pack at the level of injury.
   e. Depress nail beds and time the color return.
5. The nurse is caring for a client with impaired mobility who is to be moved to another unit of the health care facility. What principles of body mechanics should the nurse follow to avoid self-injury when transferring the client to a wheelchair? Select all that apply.
   a. Stretch the muscles as far as possible.
   b. Keep feet apart for a broad base of support.
   c. Rest between periods of exertion.
   d. Keep the knees bent.
   e. Avoid contracting the abdominal muscles.

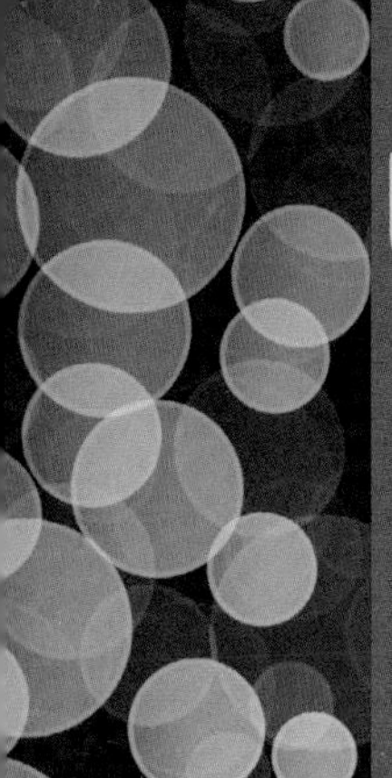

UNIT 7
The Surgical Client

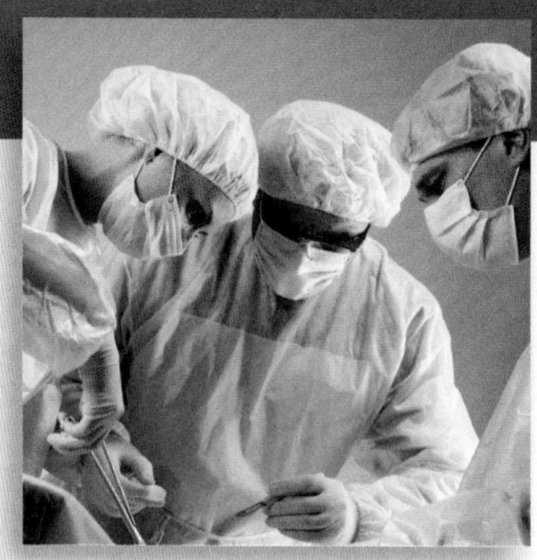

27 Perioperative Care

Words To Know

anesthesiologist
anesthetist
antiembolism stockings
atelectasis
autologous transfusion
conscious sedation
depilatory agent
directed donors
discharge instructions
emancipated minor
emboli
forced coughing
informed consent
inpatient surgery
intraoperative period
microabrasions
outpatient surgery
perioperative care
plume
pneumatic compression device
pneumonia
postanesthesia care unit
postoperative care
postoperative period
preoperative checklist
preoperative period
receiving room
reversal drugs
substituted judgment
surgical waiting area
thrombophlebitis
thrombus

Learning Objectives

On completion of this chapter, the reader should be able to:

1. Define perioperative care.
2. Identify the three phases of perioperative care.
3. Differentiate inpatient from outpatient surgery.
4. List at least four advantages of laser surgery.
5. Discuss two methods for donating blood before surgery.
6. Identify four major activities that nurses perform for all clients immediately before surgery.
7. Name three topics to address in preoperative teaching.
8. Explain the purpose of antiembolism stockings.
9. Name two recommended methods for removing hair when preparing the skin for surgery.
10. List at least five items that are verified on the preoperative checklist.
11. Name three areas of the surgical department used during the intraoperative period.
12. Describe the focus of nursing care during the immediate postoperative period.
13. Give four examples of common postoperative complications.
14. Discuss the purpose of a pneumatic compression device.
15. Describe at least two items of information included in discharge instructions for postsurgical clients.
16. Discuss at least two ways in which the surgical care of older adults differs from that of other age groups.

Perioperative care (care that clients receive before, during, and after surgery) is unique. The current trend is to facilitate as short a perioperative period as possible. This trend is driven by efforts to control health care costs by facilitating the client's recovery in the comfort and support of his or her home environment. This chapter discusses the general responsibilities nurses assume when caring for clients during the preoperative, intraoperative, and postoperative periods of perioperative care.

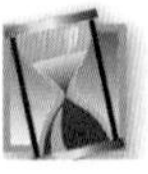

Gerontologic Considerations

■ Chronic health concerns may be present in older adults and may increase the complexity of both the preoperative, intraoperative, and postoperative periods.

TABLE 27-1 Types of Surgery According to Their Urgency

TYPE	DESCRIPTION	EXAMPLE
Optional	Surgery is performed at the client's request.	Surgery for cosmetic purposes
Elective	Surgery is planned at the client's convenience. Failure to have the surgery does not result in catastrophe.	Surgery for the removal of a superficial cyst
Required	Surgery is necessary and should be done relatively promptly.	Surgery for the removal of a cataract
Urgent	Surgery is required promptly, within 1 or 2 days if at all possible.	Surgery for the removal of a malignant tumor
Emergency	Surgery is required immediately for survival.	Surgery to relieve an intestinal perforation

PREOPERATIVE PERIOD

The **preoperative period** starts when clients, or their families in an emergency, learn that surgery is necessary and ends when clients are transported to the operating room. This period can be short or long; one major factor affecting its length is the urgency with which the surgery must be performed (Table 27-1).

Inpatient Surgery

Surgery is performed for various reasons (Table 27-2). **Inpatient surgery** is the term used for procedures performed on a client who is admitted to the hospital, expected to remain at least overnight, and in need of nursing care for more than 1 day after surgery. All except the sickest of clients usually are admitted the morning of the scheduled surgery.

Many people who have inpatient surgery undergo prior laboratory and diagnostic tests. Some have met with an **anesthesiologist** (a physician who administers chemical agents that temporarily eliminate sensation and pain; Table 27-3) or an **anesthetist** (a nurse specialist who administers anesthesia under the direction of a physician). Most clients will have received preoperative instructions from either the surgeon's office nurse or a hospital nurse.

Outpatient Surgery

Outpatient surgery, also called ambulatory surgery and same-day surgery, is the term used for operative procedures performed on clients who return home the same day. It generally is reserved for clients in an optimal state of health whose recovery is expected to be uneventful. Advantages and disadvantages of outpatient surgery are listed in Table 27-4.

Outpatient surgical units are located in either a hospital or a separate building that the hospital owns. Others are free-standing, privately owned facilities not affiliated with a hospital. The client remains in the outpatient surgical suite for a brief time and is discharged by midafternoon or early evening when (1) the client is awake and alert, (2) vital signs are stable, (3) pain and nausea are controlled, (4) oral fluids are retained, (5) the client voids a sufficient quantity of urine, and (6) the client has received discharge instructions. If a complication develops, the client is transferred and admitted to a hospital unit.

Outpatient procedures have increased dramatically as a result of advances in techniques such as those using endoscopes, an instrument for performing internal procedures in lieu of those requiring an incision (see Chap. 14), and lasers; methods of anesthesia; prospective reimbursement; managed care; and changes in Medicare and Medicaid provisions (Smeltzer & Bare, 2009).

Laser Surgery

The acronym LASER stands for **l**ight **a**mplification by the **s**timulated **e**mission of **r**adiation. Lasers convert a solid, gas, or liquid into light. When focused, the energy from the light is converted to heat, causing the vaporization of tissue and

TABLE 27-2 Reasons for Surgery

TYPE OF SURGERY	PURPOSE	EXAMPLES
Diagnostic	Removal and study of tissue to make a diagnosis	Breast biopsy Biopsy of skin lesion
Exploratory	More extensive means to diagnose a problem; usually involves exploration of a body cavity or use of scopes inserted through small incisions	Exploration of abdomen for unexplained pain Exploratory laparoscopy
Curative	Removal or replacement of defective tissue to restore function	Cholecystectomy Total hip replacement
Palliative	Relief of symptoms or enhancement of function without cure	Resection of a tumor to relieve pressure and pain
Cosmetic	Correction of defects, improvement of appearance, or change to a physical feature	Rhinoplasty Cleft lip repair Mammoplasty

TABLE 27-3 Types of Anesthesia

TYPE	DESCRIPTION
General Anesthesia	Eliminates all sensation and consciousness or memory of the event
Inhalants	Includes gas or volatile liquids
Injectables	Are given intravenously
Regional Anesthesia	Blocks sensation in an area, but consciousness is unaffected
Spinal (includes epidural)	Eliminates sensation in lower extremities, lower abdomen, and pelvis
Local	Blocks sensation in a circumscribed area of skin and subcutaneous tissue
Topical	Inhibits sensation where directly applied in epithelial tissues such as skin and mucous membranes

coagulation of blood vessels. Examples include the carbon dioxide laser, the argon laser, the ruby laser, and the yttrium–aluminum–garnet (YAG) laser.

Laser surgery is used as an alternative to many previously conventional surgical techniques such as reattaching the retina, removing skin tattoos, and revascularizing ischemic heart muscle (instead of coronary artery bypass graft surgery). Laser surgery offers the following advantages:

- Cost effectiveness
- Reduced need for general anesthesia
- Smaller incisions
- Minimal blood loss
- Reduced swelling
- Less pain
- Decreased incidence of wound infections
- Reduced scarring
- Less time recuperating

TABLE 27-4 Advantages and Disadvantages of Outpatient Surgery

ADVANTAGES	DISADVANTAGES
Lowers the surgical costs because of the reduced use of hospital services	Reduces the time for establishing a nurse–client relationship
Reduces the time spent away from home, school, or place of employment	Requires intensive preoperative teaching in a short amount of time
Interferes less with the client's usual daily routine	Reduces the opportunity for reinforcement of teaching and for answering questions
Provides the potential for more rest and sleep before and after surgery	Allows for fewer delays in assessing and preparing a client once he or she arrives for surgery
Allows more opportunity for family contact and support	Requires that care of the client after discharge be carried out by unskilled people

Laser technology requires unique safety precautions such as eye, fire, heat, and vapor protection. Depending on the type of laser used, everyone—including the client—wears goggles. In some cases, prescription glasses with side shields are sufficient, but contact lenses are not allowed.

Because lasers produce heat, fire, and electrical discharge, safety is paramount. Volatile substances such as alcohol and acetone are not used around lasers because of their flammability. Surgical instruments are coated black to avoid absorbing scattered light that causes them to heat up. Sometimes even the client's teeth are covered with plastic or a rubber mouth guard to shield metal dental fillings. For the same reason, no jewelry is allowed.

When a laser is used, it releases a **plume** (a substance composed of vaporized tissue, carbon dioxide, and water) that may contain intact cells. Plumes are accompanied by smoke, an offensive odor, and (for some) burning and itching eyes. The latter effects are not hazardous and usually can be reduced with the use of smoke evacuators. The greater concern involves the consequences of inhaling plumes. Airborne cells in the inhaled plume may contain viruses, possibly including HIV. Although no cases of HIV transmission through lasers have been documented, high-efficiency respirator masks (see Chap. 22) are better than conventional surgical masks for reducing the risk for infection transmission.

Informed Consent

Regardless of whether surgery is performed conventionally, endoscopically, or with a laser, clients commonly are fearful and anxious. They often have many questions and preconceived ideas about what surgery involves. Health care providers may answer some of these questions. Nevertheless, the physician is responsible for providing information that meets the criteria for **informed consent** (permission a client gives after an explanation of the risks, benefits, and alternatives; see Chap. 14). A signed form, witnessed by a nurse, is evidence that consent has been obtained (Fig. 27-1).

If an adult client is confused, unconscious, or mentally incompetent, the client's spouse, nearest blood relative, or someone with a durable power of attorney for the client's health care must sign the consent form. If an adult client is under the influence of a mind-altering drug such as a narcotic or is alcohol intoxicated, obtaining consent must be delayed until the drug has been metabolized. In a life-threatening emergency, a court may waive the need to obtain a written or verbal consent from a client who requires immediate surgery on the basis of **substituted judgment**; that is, the court believes that if the client had the capacity to consent, he or she would have done so. Refer to Chapter 14 for the elements that constitute informed consent.

If the client is younger than 18 years, a parent or legal guardian must sign the consent form. In an emergency, health care personnel make every effort to obtain consent by telephone, telegram, or fax. Adolescents younger than 18 years, living independently, and supporting themselves are regarded as **emancipated minors** and may sign their own consent forms.

THREE RIVERS AREA HOSPITAL
THREE RIVERS, MICHIGAN 49093

AUTHORIZATION FOR MEDICAL
AND/OR
SURGICAL TREATMENT

Date July 18 2010 Time 2:30 a.m. / p.m. (p.m. circled)

I, the undersigned, a patient in Three Rivers Area Hospital, hereby authorize Dr. Robert Morrison, M.D. (and whomever he may designate as his assistant) to administer such treatment as is necessary, and to perform the following operation Exploratory Laparotomy and Appendectomy.

(Name of operation and/or procedure)

and such additional operations or procedures as are considered therapeutically necessary on the basis of findings during the course of said operation, with the following exception, None.

I also consent to the administration of such anesthetics as are necessary, with the exception of None.

(None, spinal anesthesia, or other)

I hereby certify that I have read and fully understand the above AUTHORIZATION FOR MEDICAL and/or SURGICAL TREATMENT, the reasons why the above named surgery is considered necessary, its advantages and possible complications, if any, as well as possible alternative modes of treatments, which were explained to me by Dr. Morrison.

I also certify that no guarantee or assurance has been made as to the results that may be obtained.

Gary Holmes
(Patient or nearest relative)

Judi Ebbert, RN
(Witness)

(Relationship)

I hereby certify that I have explained to Gary Holmes (a patient at Three Rivers Area Hospital), the reasons why the above named surgery is considered necessary, its advantages and possible complications, if any, as well as possible alternative modes of treatment.

Robert Morrison, M.D.
(Surgeon signature)

7-18-10
(Date)

FIGURE 27-1 A surgical consent form.

Each nurse must be familiar with agency policies and state laws regarding surgical consent forms. Clients must sign the consent form before receiving any preoperative sedatives. When the client or designated person has signed the permit, an adult witness also signs it to indicate that the client or designee signed voluntarily. This witness usually is a member of the health care team or an employee in the admissions department. The nurse is responsible for ensuring that all necessary parties have signed the consent form and that it is in the client's chart before the client goes to the operating room.

Preoperative Blood Donation

The low risk for acquiring HIV from a blood transfusion sometimes is discussed during the preoperative period. Although publicly donated blood is tested for several pathogens including HIV and hepatitis B, the potential, although slight, for acquiring a blood-borne disease still exists. Therefore, some clients undergoing surgery donate their own blood preoperatively. Predonated blood is held on reserve in the event that the client needs a blood transfusion during or after surgery. Receiving one's own blood is called an **autologous transfusion** (self-donated blood). Autologous transfusions also are prepared by salvaging blood lost during or immediately after surgery. The salvaged blood is suctioned, cleaned, and filtered from drainage collection devices.

Clients who do not meet the time or health requirements for self-donation may select **directed donors** (blood donors chosen from among the client's relatives and friends). The client's siblings should not donate blood for the client. Doing so would rule them out as future organ or tissue donors for the client because antigens in the transfused blood would sensitize the recipient, increasing the risk for organ or tissue rejection. Also, a male sexual partner of a woman in her reproductive years should not be a directed donor to avoid possible antibody reactions against a fetus in any future pregnancy.

Most authorities believe that receiving blood from directed donors is no safer than receiving blood from public donors. Although predonation of blood is available in the United States, the criteria for autologous and directed donors (Table 27-5) vary among regions and hospitals. Because directed donors must meet the same requirements as public donors, if the intended recipient does not use the blood, it is released into the public pool and can be given to someone else.

Immediate Preoperative Care

Although some presurgical activities take place weeks in advance, others cannot be performed until just before surgery. During the immediate preoperative period—the few hours before the procedure—several major tasks must be completed: conducting a nursing assessment, providing preoperative teaching, performing methods of physical preparation, administering medications, assisting with psychosocial preparation, and completing the surgical checklist.

Nursing Assessment

Nurses share with physicians the responsibility for assessing preoperative clients. The assessment varies depending on the urgency of the surgery and if the client is admitted the same day of surgery or earlier. Although assessment of the surgical client is always necessary, the particular circumstances dictate the extent of the process. There may not be time to perform a detailed assessment.

When surgery is not an emergency, the nurse performs a thorough history and physical examination. He or she assesses the client's understanding of the surgical procedure, postoperative expectations, and ability to participate in recovery. The nurse also considers cultural needs, specifically as they relate to beliefs about surgery, personal privacy, and presence of family members during the preoperative and postoperative phases. The nurse may question the client regarding strong culturally influenced feelings about disposal of body parts and blood transfusions.

On admission, the nurse reviews preoperative instructions, such as diet and fluid restrictions, bowel and skin preparations, and the withholding or self-administration of medications, to ensure that the client has followed them. If the client has not carried out a specific portion of the instructions, the nurse immediately notifies the surgeon.

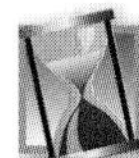

Gerontologic Considerations

- The older person should be educated about taking usual medications before surgical procedures and about resuming usual or new medications after surgery.

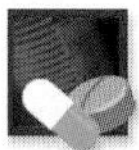

Pharmacologic Considerations

- Many adults are on anticoagulation therapy—including self-therapy with low-dose aspirin—and may need to have this addressed as a preoperative consideration. Evaluate the person's use of aspirin and medications containing salicylates. Ibuprofen (Advil) and naproxen (Aleve) may also increase the risk for gastrointestinal (GI) side effects such as bleeding. Assessment of alternative therapies, such as herbs (eg, ginkgo, ginseng), is necessary because these therapies may increase the risk for bleeding postoperatively.

The nurse identifies the client's potential risks for complications during or after the surgery. Certain surgical

TABLE 27-5 Criteria for Autologous and Directed Blood Donation

AUTOLOGOUS DONATION	DIRECTED DONATION
To bank one's own blood, the donor must:	**To be a directed donor, the person must:**
Have a physician's recommendation	Be at least 17 years of age
Have a hematocrit within a safe range	Meet all the criteria of a public donor
Be free of infection at the time of donation	Have the same blood type as the potential recipient or one that is compatible
Meet the blood collection center's minimum weight requirement	Not have received a blood transfusion within the last 6 months
Donate 40 to 3 days before the anticipated date of use	Donate 20 to 3 days before the anticipated use
Donate no more frequently than every 3–5 days; once per week is preferred	Be free from blood-borne pathogens and high-risk behaviors
Assume responsibility for costs above the usual processing fees even if blood is not used	
Be advised that his or her blood will be discarded if unused	

risk factors increase the likelihood of perioperative complications:

- Extremes of age
- Dehydration
- Malnutrition
- Obesity
- Smoking
- Diabetes
- Cardiopulmonary disease
- Drug and alcohol abuse
- Bleeding tendencies
- Low hemoglobin and red cells
- Pregnancy

Some problems, such as an unexplained elevation in temperature, abnormal laboratory data, current infectious disease, or significant deviations in vital signs, are causes for postponing or canceling the surgery (Table 27-6).

Preoperative Teaching

Preoperative teaching varies with the type of surgery and the length of hospitalization. Preoperatively, clients are alert and free from pain or in less pain at this time, which facilitates their participation. Knowledge of what to expect on the part of clients and family can enhance recovery from surgery.

The following are examples of information to include in preoperative teaching:

- Preoperative medications—when they are given and their effects
- Postoperative pain control
- Explanation and description of the postanesthesia recovery room or postsurgical protocol
- Discussion of the frequency of assessing vital signs and the use of monitoring equipment

The nurse also explains and demonstrates how to perform deep breathing, coughing, and leg exercises.

Deep Breathing

Deep breathing, a form of controlled ventilation that opens and fills small air passages in the lungs (see Chap. 21), is especially advantageous for clients who receive general anesthesia or who breathe shallowly after surgery because of pain. Deep breathing reduces the postoperative risk for

TABLE 27-6 Surgical Risk Factors and Potential Complications

VARIABLE	POTENTIAL COMPLICATION
Age	
Very young—Immaturity of organ systems and regulatory mechanisms	Respiratory obstruction, fluid overload, dehydration, hypothermia, and infection
Elderly—Multiple organ degeneration and slowed regulatory mechanisms	Decreased metabolism and excretion of anesthetics and pain medications, fluid overload, renal failure, formation of blood clots, delayed wound healing, infection, confusion, and respiratory complications
Nutritional Status	
Malnourished—Low weight and nutrient deficiencies	Fluid and electrolyte imbalances, cardiac dysrhythmias, delayed wound healing, and wound infections
Obese—Stressed cardiovascular system, decreased circulation, and decreased pulmonary function	Atelectasis, pneumonia, blood clots, delayed wound healing, wound infection, delayed metabolism, and excretion of anesthetics and pain medication
Substance Abuse	
Alcohol, tobacco, sedatives—Altered respiratory function, nutritional status, or liver function	Atelectasis, pneumonia, altered effectiveness of anesthetics and pain medications, drug interactions, and drug withdrawal
Medical Problems	
Immune—Allergies and immunosuppression secondary to corticosteroid therapy, transplants, chemotherapy, or diseases such as AIDS	Adverse reactions to medications, blood transfusions, or latex; infection
Respiratory—Acute and chronic respiratory problems and history of tobacco use	Atelectasis, bronchopneumonia, and respiratory failure
Cardiovascular—Hypertension, coronary artery disease, and peripheral vascular disease	Hypotension, hypertension, fluid overload, congestive heart failure, shock, dysrhythmias, myocardial infarction, stroke, and blood clots
Hepatic—Liver dysfunction	Delayed drug metabolism leading to drug toxicity, disrupted clotting mechanisms leading to excessive bleeding or hemorrhage, confusion, and increased risk for infection
Renal—Kidney disease, chronic renal insufficiency, and renal failure	Fluid and electrolyte imbalances, congestive heart failure, dysrhythmias, delayed excretion of drugs leading to drug toxicity
Endocrine—Diabetes	Hypoglycemia, hyperglycemia, hypokalemia, infection, and delayed wound healing

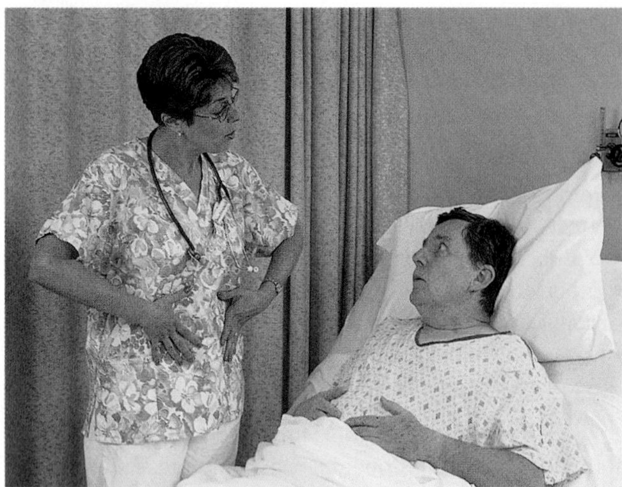

FIGURE 27-2 Teaching deep breathing. (Photo by B. Proud.)

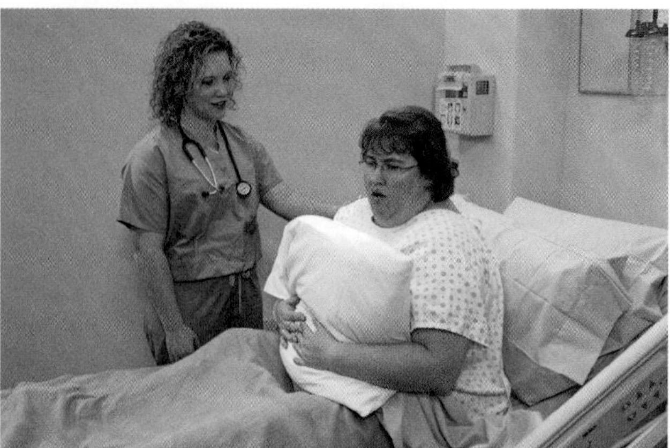

FIGURE 27-3 Teaching the client to splint the incision and to cough. (Photo by Ken Kasper.)

respiratory complications such as **atelectasis** (airless, collapsed lung areas) and **pneumonia** (lung infection), both of which can lead to hypoxemia.

The nurse practices deep breathing with clients before they undergo surgery (Fig. 27-2). Deep breathing involves inhaling deeply using the abdominal muscles, holding the breath for several seconds, and exhaling slowly. Pursing the lips may extend the period of exhalation. Incentive spirometers (see Chap. 21) also are used to promote deep breathing.

Coughing

Thickened respiratory secretions often accompany impaired ventilation. Coughing is a natural method for clearing secretions from the airways. Deep breathing alone is sometimes sufficient to produce a natural cough. **Forced coughing** (coughing that is purposely produced) may not be necessary for all postoperative clients. Forced coughing is most appropriate for clients who have diminished or moist lung sounds or who raise thick sputum. Nevertheless, all clients need to be prepared for the possibility of having to perform this technique and should receive instructions about it (see Client and Family Teaching 27-1).

Coughing is painful for clients with abdominal or chest incisions. Administering pain medication approximately 30 minutes before coughing or splinting the incision during coughing can reduce discomfort. Methods of splinting include pressing on the incision with both hands, pressing on a pillow placed over the incision, or wrapping a bath blanket around the client (Fig. 27-3).

Leg Exercises

Leg exercises help to promote circulation and reduce the risk for forming a **thrombus** (a stationary blood clot) in the veins. Blood clots form when venous circulation is sluggish and when the fluid component of blood is reduced. Surgical clients are predisposed to both. Surgical clients have reduced circulatory volume because of the preoperative restriction of food and fluids and blood loss during surgery. Also, blood tends to pool in the lower extremities because of the stationary position during surgery and the clients' reluctance to move afterward. With the use of leg exercises, efforts to reduce circulatory complications begin as soon as the client recovers from anesthesia (see Client and Family Teaching 27-2 and Fig. 27-4).

Client and Family Teaching 27-1
Performing Forced Coughing

The nurse teaches the client and the family as follows:

- Sit upright.
- Take a slow, deep breath through the nose.
- Make the lower abdomen rise as much as possible.
- Lean slightly forward.
- Exhale slowly through the mouth.
- Pull the abdomen inward.
- Repeat, but this time cough three times in a row while exhaling.

Client and Family Teaching 27-2
Performing Leg Exercises

The nurse teaches the client and the family as follows:

- Sit with the head slightly raised.
- Bend one knee. Raise and hold the leg above the mattress for a few seconds (see Fig. 27-4).
- Straighten the raised leg.
- Lower the leg back to the bed gradually.
- Do the same with the other leg.
- Rest both legs on the bed.
- Point the toes toward the mattress and then toward the head.
- Move both feet in clockwise and then counterclockwise circles.
- Repeat the exercises five times at least every 2 hours while awake.

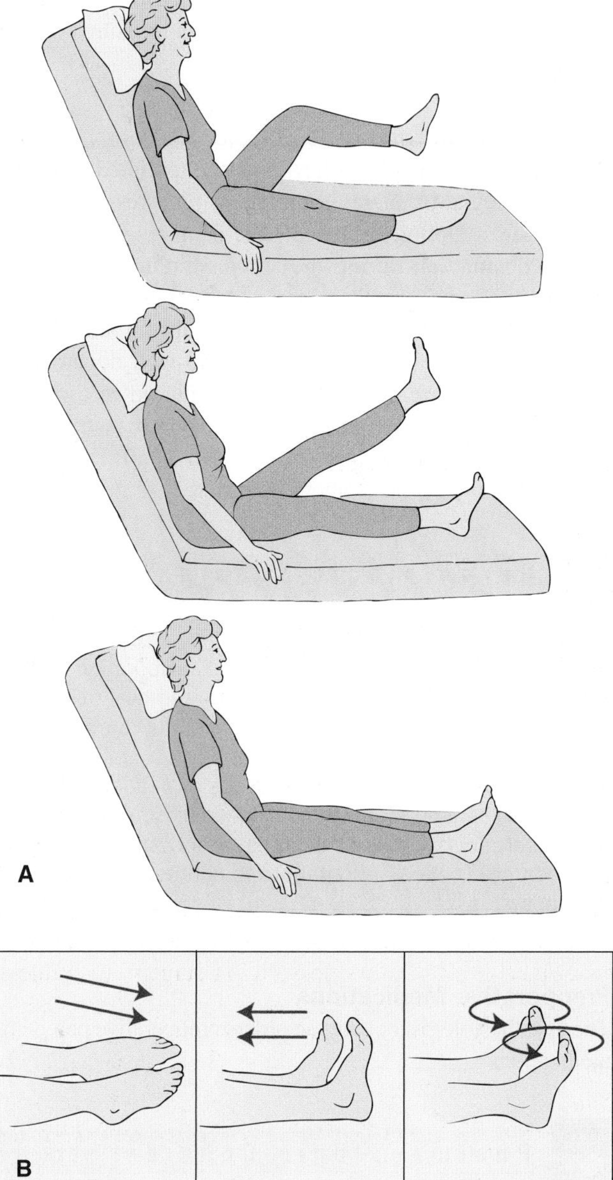

FIGURE 27-4 Components of leg exercises. **A.** Exercising the lower legs. **B.** Exercising the feet.

Antiembolism stockings are knee-high or thigh-high elastic stockings. They are sometimes called thromboembolic disorder (TED) hose. Antiembolism stockings help to prevent thrombi and **emboli** (mobile blood clots) by compressing superficial veins and capillaries, redirecting more blood to larger and deeper veins, where it flows more effectively toward the heart. Intermittent pneumatic compression devices (discussed later in this chapter) are used for the same purpose but are applied postoperatively.

Antiembolism stockings must fit the client properly and must be applied correctly (Skill 27-1). Stockings that become dirty are laundered, during which a second pair is used. If washed by hand, the stockings are laid flat to dry to prevent loss of their elasticity.

Stop, Think, and Respond Box 27-1

Discuss reasons why surgical clients are not as active and mobile as nonsurgical clients.

Physical Preparation

Depending on the time of admission to the hospital or surgical facility, the nurse may perform some physical preparation that includes skin preparation, attention to elimination, restriction of food and fluids, care of valuables, donning of surgical attire, and disposition of prostheses.

Skin Preparation

Skin preparation involves cleansing the skin and, in some cases, hair removal because skin and hair are reservoirs for microorganisms (Skill 27-2). The goal is to decrease transient and resident bacteria without compromising skin integrity. Reducing bacteria helps to prevent postoperative wound infections.

For planned surgery, the client may be asked to bathe or shower twice at home with chlorhexidine gluconate for a minimum of 2 minutes contact time; dry with a fresh, clean dry towel; and don clean clothing afterwards (AORN, 2008). Hair usually is not removed before surgery unless it is likely to interfere with the incision. Shaving causes **microabrasions** (tiny cuts that provide an entrance for microorganisms). For this reason, institutions are switching from razors to electric or battery-operated clippers for hair removal. **Depilatory agents**, chemicals that remove hair, are another alternative, but their use is associated with skin irritation and allergic reactions. Some authorities believe that simply washing the skin and hair is sufficient to prevent infections. (Joanna Briggs Institute, 2007; Pfiedler Enterprises, 2009).

Stop, Think, and Respond Box 27-2

Correlate the potential for transmitting an infection using a razor for presurgical skin preparation with the chain of infection discussed in Chapter 10.

Elimination

The nurse may need to insert an indwelling urinary catheter (see Chap. 30) preoperatively for some surgeries, particularly of the lower abdomen. A distended bladder increases the risks for bladder trauma and difficulty in performing the procedure. The catheter keeps the bladder empty during surgery. If a catheter is not inserted, the nurse instructs the client to urinate immediately before receiving preoperative medication.

Enemas or a laxative may be ordered to clean the lower bowel (see Chap. 31) if the client is having abdominal or pelvic surgery. A clean bowel allows for improved visualization of the surgical site and prevents trauma to the intestines or accidental contamination of the abdominal cavity with feces. A cleansing enema or laxative is prescribed the evening before surgery and may be repeated the morning of surgery.

If bowel surgery is scheduled, antibiotics may be prescribed to destroy intestinal microorganisms.

Food and Fluids

The physician gives specific instructions about how long to restrict food and fluids preoperatively. Fasting from food and water from midnight onward before surgery is common, but the basis for the practice is now questionable. Fasting is used to reduce the potential for aspirating (inhaling) stomach contents while a client is anesthetized. However, aspiration is uncommon today with standard practices used by those administering general anesthesia. Consequently, the American Society of Anesthesiology (1999) recommends that healthy preoperative clients can consume clear liquids 2 hours before elective surgery, have a light breakfast 6 hours before a surgical procedure, and eat a heavier meal 6 to 8 hours beforehand (deAguilar-Nascimento & Dock-Nascimento, 2010). Despite these newer recommendations, old practices persist. The nurse, therefore, encourages clients to maintain good nutrition and hydration before the restricted time to promote nutrients, such as protein and ascorbic acid (vitamin C), which are needed for healing.

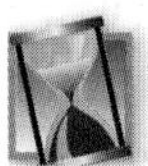

Gerontologic Considerations

- The period of fluid restriction before surgery may be shortened for older adults to reduce their risk for dehydration and hypotension. Vital signs, weight, and sternal skin turgor should be assessed before fluid restriction to serve as a baseline for comparison.

Valuables

The nurse instructs the client preoperatively to leave valuables at home. If the client forgets or does not follow this instruction, he or she must entrust valuables to a family member. Otherwise, health care agency personnel itemize them, place them in an envelope, and lock them in a designated area. The client signs a receipt, and the nurse notes the items' whereabouts in the client's medical record.

If the client is reluctant to remove a wedding band, the nurse may slip a ribbon of gauze under the ring and then loop the gauze around the finger and wrist or apply adhesive tape around a plain wedding band. The client also removes eyeglasses and contact lenses, which the nurse places in a safe location or gives to a family member.

Surgical Attire

Usually, clients wear a hospital gown and surgical cap to the operating room. The physician may order thigh-high or knee-high antiembolism stockings or order the client's legs wrapped in elastic roller bandages (see Chap. 28) before surgery to prevent venous stasis.

Hair ornaments are removed to avoid injury with equipment used to administer oxygen and inhalant anesthetics. Makeup and nail polish are omitted to facilitate assessing oxygenation. If a client has acrylic nails, one usually is removed to attach a pulse oximeter, which measures oxygen saturation (see Chap. 21).

Dentures and Prostheses

Depending on agency policy and the preference of the anesthesiologist or surgeon, the client removes full or partial dentures. Doing so prevents the dentures from causing airway obstruction during the administration of a general anesthetic. Some anesthesiologists prefer that well-fitting dentures remain in place to preserve facial contours, but that information must be communicated and well documented. When dentures are removed, they are placed in a denture container and stored at the client's bedside or with the client's belongings. Other prostheses, such as artificial limbs, also are removed unless otherwise ordered.

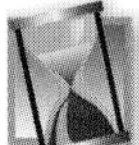

Gerontologic Considerations

- Older adults also are likely to be self-conscious when dentures are removed before surgery. Collaboration with operating room personnel regarding the removal of dentures, eyeglasses, and hearing aids is helpful to ensure their use as much or as long as possible.
- Older adults who rely on eyeglasses or hearing aids may experience sensory deprivation if these aids are removed before surgery or other procedures. Removal may interfere with communication or contribute to confusion and altered mental status.

Preoperative Medications

The anesthesiologist or surgeon orders preoperative parenteral medications.

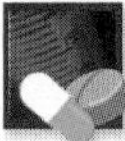

Pharmacologic Considerations

Common preoperative medications include one or more of the following:

- *Anticholinergics*, such as glycopyrrolate (Robinul), decrease respiratory secretions, dry mucous membranes, and prevent vagal nerve stimulation during endotracheal intubation.
- *Antianxiety* drugs, such as lorazepam (Ativan), reduce preoperative anxiety, cause slight sedation, slow motor activity, and promote the induction of anesthesia.
- *Histamine-2 receptor antagonists*, such as cimetidine (Tagamet), decrease gastric acidity and volume.
- *Narcotics*, such as morphine sulfate, sedate the client and decrease the amount of anesthesia.
- *Sedatives*, such as midazolam (Versed), promote sleep or conscious sedation and decrease anxiety.
- *Antibiotics*, such as kanamycin (Kantrex), destroy enteric microorganisms.

Before administering preoperative medications, the nurse uses at least two methods to verify the identity of the client. An example would be checking the client's identification bracelet and asking the client to state his or her name and date of birth (see Chaps. 19, 32, and 34). The nurse asks about drug allergies, obtains vital signs, asks the client to void, and ensures that the surgical consent form has been signed.

Psychosocial Preparation

Preparing the client emotionally and spiritually is as important as doing so physically. Psychosocial preparation should begin as soon as the client is aware that surgery is necessary. Anxiety and fear, if extreme, can affect a client's condition during and after surgery. Anxious clients have a poor response to surgery and are prone to complications (Heisler, 2009). Many clients are fearful because they know little or nothing about what will happen before, during, and after surgery. Careful listening and explaining by the nurse about what will happen and what to expect can help to allay some of these fears and anxieties. The nurse also must assess methods the client uses for coping. Religious faith is a source of strength for many clients; therefore, nurses facilitate contact with a client's clergyperson or the hospital chaplain, if requested.

Preoperative Checklist

A **preoperative checklist** (Fig. 27-5) is a form that identifies the status of essential presurgical activities and is completed before surgery. The nurse verifies the following:

- The history and physical examination have been documented.
- The name of the procedure on the surgical consent form matches that scheduled in the operating room.
- The surgical consent form has been signed and witnessed.
- All laboratory and diagnostic test results, such as a fasting blood sugar or electrocardiogram (ECG), have been returned and reported if abnormal.
- Allergies have been identified.
- The client is wearing an identification bracelet and allergy bracelet, if any exist.
- The client has had nothing by mouth (NPO, *nil per os*) since midnight or the number of hours prescribed.
- Skin preparation has been completed.
- Vital signs have been assessed and recorded.
- Nail polish, glasses, contact lenses, and hairpins have been removed.

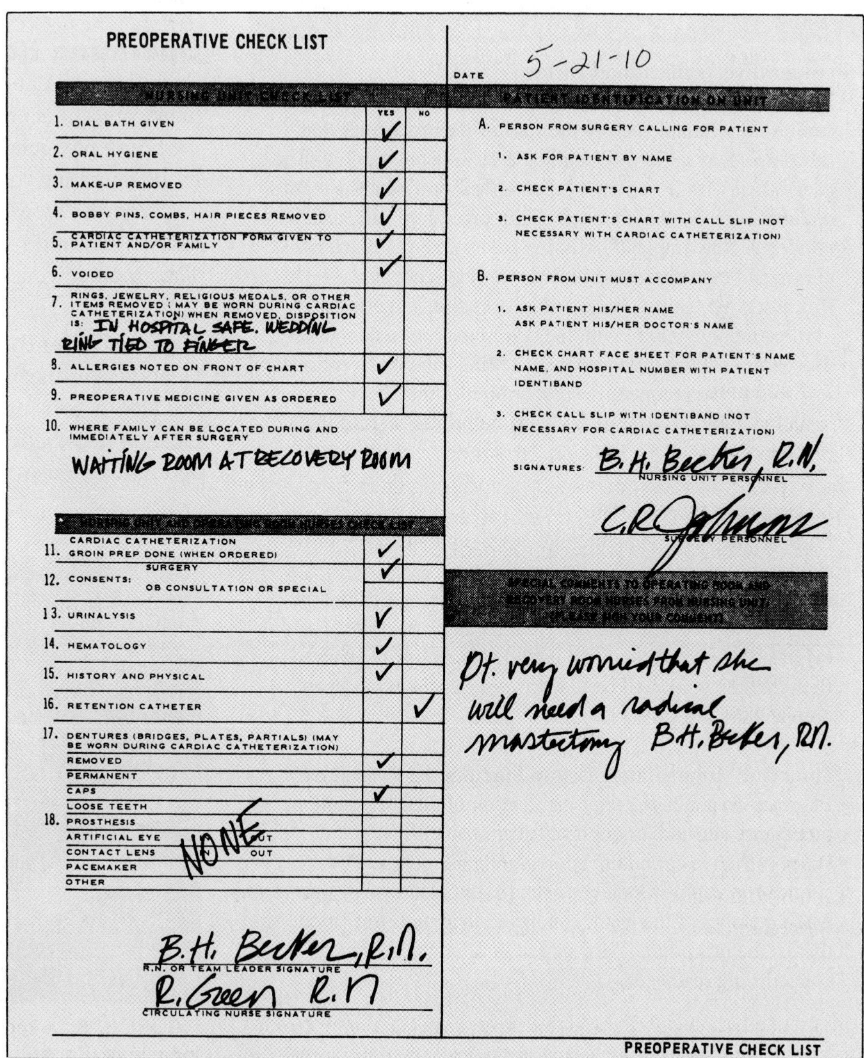

PREOPERATIVE CHECK LIST

DATE 5-21-10

NURSING UNIT CHECK LIST

	YES	NO
1. DIAL BATH GIVEN	✓	
2. ORAL HYGIENE	✓	
3. MAKE-UP REMOVED	✓	
4. BOBBY PINS, COMBS, HAIR PIECES REMOVED	✓	
5. CARDIAC CATHETERIZATION FORM GIVEN TO PATIENT AND/OR FAMILY	✓	
6. VOIDED	✓	
7. RINGS, JEWELRY, RELIGIOUS MEDALS, OR OTHER ITEMS REMOVED (MAY BE WORN DURING CARDIAC CATHETERIZATION) WHEN REMOVED, DISPOSITION IS: IN HOSPITAL SAFE. WEDDING RING TIED TO FINGER		
8. ALLERGIES NOTED ON FRONT OF CHART	✓	
9. PREOPERATIVE MEDICINE GIVEN AS ORDERED	✓	

10. WHERE FAMILY CAN BE LOCATED DURING AND IMMEDIATELY AFTER SURGERY

WAITING ROOM AT RECOVERY ROOM

NURSING UNIT AND OPERATING ROOM NURSES CHECK LIST

	YES	NO
11. CARDIAC CATHETERIZATION GROIN PREP DONE (WHEN ORDERED)	✓	
12. CONSENTS: SURGERY	✓	
OB CONSULTATION OR SPECIAL		
13. URINALYSIS	✓	
14. HEMATOLOGY	✓	
15. HISTORY AND PHYSICAL	✓	
16. RETENTION CATHETER		✓
17. DENTURES (BRIDGES, PLATES, PARTIALS) (MAY BE WORN DURING CARDIAC CATHETERIZATION)		
REMOVED	✓	
PERMANENT		
CAPS	✓	
LOOSE TEETH		
18. PROSTHESIS		
ARTIFICIAL EYE IN OUT		
CONTACT LENS IN OUT		
PACEMAKER		
OTHER		

NONE

B.H. Becker, R.N.
R.N. OR TEAM LEADER SIGNATURE

R. Green R.N.
CIRCULATING NURSE SIGNATURE

PATIENT IDENTIFICATION ON UNIT

A. PERSON FROM SURGERY CALLING FOR PATIENT

1. ASK FOR PATIENT BY NAME
2. CHECK PATIENT'S CHART
3. CHECK PATIENT'S CHART WITH CALL SLIP (NOT NECESSARY WITH CARDIAC CATHETERIZATION)

B. PERSON FROM UNIT MUST ACCOMPANY

1. ASK PATIENT HIS/HER NAME
   ASK PATIENT HIS/HER DOCTOR'S NAME
2. CHECK CHART FACE SHEET FOR PATIENT'S NAME NAME, AND HOSPITAL NUMBER WITH PATIENT IDENTIBAND
3. CHECK CALL SLIP WITH IDENTIBAND (NOT NECESSARY FOR CARDIAC CATHETERIZATION)

SIGNATURES: B.H. Becker, R.N.
NURSING UNIT PERSONNEL

C.R. Johnson
SURGERY PERSONNEL

SPECIAL COMMENTS TO OPERATING ROOM AND RECOVERY ROOM NURSES FROM NURSING UNIT (PLEASE SIGN YOUR COMMENT)

Pt. very worried that she will need a radical mastectomy B.H. Becker, RN.

PREOPERATIVE CHECK LIST

FIGURE 27-5 Preoperative checklist.

- Jewelry has been removed or the wedding ring has been secured.
- Dentures have been removed or left in place if requested by the person administering inhalant anesthesia.
- The client is wearing only a hospital gown and hair cover.
- The client has urinated.
- Location of intravenous (IV) site, type of IV solution, and rate of infusion are identified.
- The prescribed preoperative medication has been given.

The nurse is responsible for completing and signing the checklist. Operating room personnel review it when they arrive to transport the client. Surgery may be delayed if the checklist is incomplete.

Emphasis has increased relative to ensuring that the right client has the proper procedure on the correct side (if that applies). See Box 27-1 for the universal protocol developed by The Joint Commission (2010) to prevent errors in these categories.

BOX 27-1 Universal Protocol for Preventing Wrong Site, Wrong Procedure, Wrong Person Surgery

Preoperative Verification Process

- Purpose: To ensure that all of the relevant documents and studies are available before the start of the procedure; that they have been reviewed; and that they are consistent with each other, with the client's expectations, and with the team's understanding of the intended client, procedure, site, and, as applicable, any implants. Missing information or discrepancies must be addressed before starting the procedure.
- Process: An ongoing process of information gathering and verification, beginning with the determination to do the procedure, continuing through all settings and interventions involved in the preoperative preparation of the client, up to and including the "time out" just before the start of the procedure.

Marking the Operative Site

- Purpose: To identify unambiguously the intended site of incision or insertion.
- Process: For procedures involving right/left distinction, multiple structures (such as fingers and toes), or multiple levels (as in spinal procedures), the intended site must be marked such that the mark will be visible after the client has been prepped and draped.

"Time Out" Immediately Before Starting the Procedure

- Purpose: To conduct a final verification of the correct client, procedure, site and, as applicable, implants.
- Process: Active communication among all members of the surgical/procedure team, consistently initiated by a designated member of the team, conducted in a "fail-safe" mode; that is, the procedure is not started until any questions or concerns are resolved.

Adapted from The Joint Commission (2010). Accessed May 26, 2010, from http://www.jointcommission.org/patientsafety/universalprotocol.

INTRAOPERATIVE PERIOD

The **intraoperative period** (the time during which the client undergoes surgery) takes place in the operating suite. It involves transportation to a receiving room then to the operating room where anesthesia is administered and the procedure is performed. The family is directed to a surgical waiting area during this time.

Receiving Room

The **receiving room** (Fig. 27-6) is a place in the surgery department where clients are observed until the operating room and surgical team are ready. In some hospitals, preoperative medication is administered when clients reach the receiving room rather than before leaving the nursing unit. This practice coordinates the client's sedation more closely with the actual time of surgery.

Skin preparation may be delayed until this time as well. There is a direct relationship between the time the skin preparation is performed and the rate of microbial proliferation (Centers for Disease Control and Prevention, 2008; Odom-Forren, 2006).

Operating Room

Eventually, clients are taken to the operating room, where their care and safety are in the hands of a team of experts including physicians and nurses. Anesthesia is administered in the operating room.

Various types of anesthesia cause partial or complete loss of sensation with or without a loss of consciousness. They include general, regional, and local anesthesia.

General Anesthesia

General anesthesia acts on the central nervous system to produce a loss of sensation, reflexes, and consciousness. General anesthetics commonly are administered via inhaled and intravenous routes.

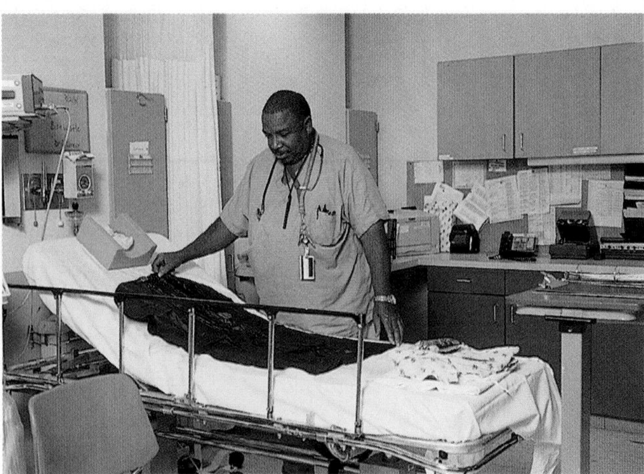

FIGURE 27-6 A receiving room being prepared for an incoming client. (Photo by B. Proud.)

Throughout the duration of and recovery from anesthesia, the client is monitored closely for effective breathing and oxygenation; effective circulatory status, including blood pressure (BP) and pulse within normal ranges; effective temperature regulation; and adequate fluid balance. During weaning from the anesthetic at the end of surgery, the client's consciousness will be elevated sufficiently for him or her to follow commands and breathe independently. The recovery period can be brief or long. Many effects of general anesthesia take some time for the client to eliminate completely. Usually, clients do not remember much about the initial recovery period.

Regional Anesthesia

Regional anesthesia interferes with the conduction of sensory and motor nerve impulses to a specific area of the body. The client experiences loss of sensation and decreased mobility to the specific anesthetized area. He or she does not lose consciousness. Depending on the surgery, the client may receive a sedative to promote relaxation and comfort during the procedure. Types of regional anesthesia include local and spinal anesthesia and epidural and peripheral nerve blocks.

The major advantage of regional anesthesia is the decreased risk for respiratory, cardiac, and GI complications. Team members must monitor the client for signs of allergic reactions, changes in vital signs, and toxic reactions. In addition, they must protect the anesthetized area if sensation is absent because the client is at risk for injury.

Conscious Sedation

Conscious sedation refers to a state in which clients are sedated, a state of relaxation and emotional comfort, but are not unconscious. They are free of pain, fear, and anxiety and can tolerate unpleasant diagnostic and short therapeutic surgical procedures, such as endoscopies or bone marrow aspiration, while maintaining independent cardiorespiratory function. They can respond verbally and physically.

The intravenous route is used to administer medications that create conscious sedation. If other routes are used, the client must have venous access for the treatment of possible adverse effects such as hypoxemia and central nervous system depression. The responsibility for ensuring client safety and comfort during sedation rests with the nurse directly involved in the client's care. Although numerous types of equipment for monitoring clients are available, no equipment replaces a nurse's careful observations. Clients are discharged shortly after the procedure in which conscious sedation is used.

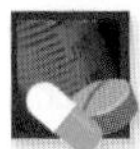

Pharmacologic Considerations

- **Reversal drugs,** medications that counteract the effects of those used for conscious sedation, must be readily available in case the client becomes overly sedated. Two examples of reversal drugs are naloxone (Narcan), which is the antagonist for opiates like morphine, and flumazenil (Romazicon), which reverses antianxiety drugs like midazolam (Versed).

Surgical Waiting Area

The **surgical waiting area** is the room where family and friends await information about the client. It is staffed by volunteers who provide comfort, support, and news about how the client's surgery is progressing. Many agencies provide food and beverages, public telephones, television, and magazines in this area. Often, the surgeon comes to the waiting area immediately after the procedure to contact the family. The family and surgeon generally go to a private room where the surgeon discusses the client's status and the procedure so as to ensure confidentiality.

POSTOPERATIVE PERIOD

The **postoperative period** begins after the operative procedure is completed and the client is transported to an area to recover from the anesthesia and ends when the client is discharged. The **postanesthesia care unit** (PACU), also known as the *postanesthesia reacting* (PAR) room or the *recovery room*, is the area in the surgical department where clients are intensively monitored (Fig. 27-7). Nurses in the PACU ensure the safe recovery of surgical clients from anesthesia.

Immediate Postoperative Care

The focus of **postoperative care** (nursing care after surgery) is different during the immediate postoperative period than it is later, when clients are more stable. The immediate postoperative period refers to the first 24 hours after surgery. During this time, nurses monitor the client for complications as he or she recovers from anesthesia and is sufficiently stable to be transferred to a nursing unit for continued assessment.

Initial Postoperative Assessments

The circulating surgical nurse or anesthesiologist reports pertinent information regarding the surgery and the client's

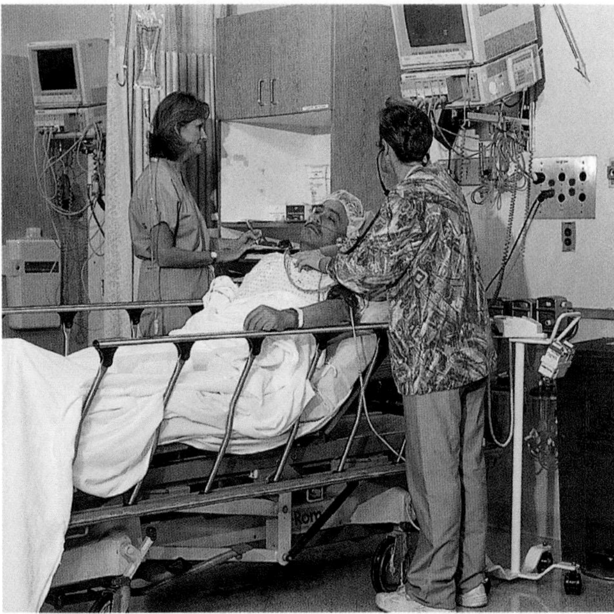

FIGURE 27-7 A postanesthesia care unit. (Photo by B. Proud.)

condition to the nurse in the PACU. Once the care of the client is transitioned to the recovery room nurse, the PACU nurse's major responsibilities are to ensure a patent airway; help to maintain adequate circulation; prevent or assist with the management of shock; maintain proper positions and function of drains, tubes, and intravenous infusions; and detect evidence of any complications. The nurse systematically checks the following:

- Level of consciousness
- Vital signs
- Effectiveness of respirations
- Presence or need for supplemental oxygen
- Condition of the wound and dressing
- Location of drains and drainage characteristics
- Location, type, and rate of intravenous fluid
- Level of pain and need for analgesia
- Presence of a urinary catheter and urine volume

Continuing Postoperative Care

Once the client is stable, the client is readied for transport to the general surgical unit where the client's room is prepared and assessments will continue to prevent, detect, or minimize complications.

Preparing the Room

The next stage of care begins with getting the client's bed and the environment ready.

The nurses fold the top bed linen toward the foot or side of the bed. They place the bed in a high position to facilitate transferring the client from the stretcher. Often, they keep additional blankets ready for use because some clients feel cold after being quiet and inactive.

Additionally, nurses assemble bedside supplies and equipment that facilitate caring for the client. Potentially useful items include oxygen equipment (see Chap. 21), a pole or electronic infusion device for continuing the administration of intravenous fluids (see Chap. 16), an emesis basin if the client vomits, paper tissues, and a device for collecting and measuring urine (see Chap. 30). Suction canisters may be necessary for clients who have gastric tubes (see Chap. 29).

Monitoring for Complications

Postoperative clients are at risk for many complications (Table 27-7), some of which are more likely to develop soon after surgery. Frequently focused assessments of the client and equipment facilitate a safe postoperative recovery (see Nursing Guidelines 27-1).

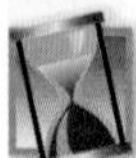

Gerontologic Considerations

- The cardiac status of older adults is monitored carefully after surgery because they may not be able to tolerate or eliminate intravenous fluids given at standard rates. Similarly, rates of intravenous fluids may need to be adjusted for older adults, especially if their renal or cardiac status is compromised.

Providing Food and Oral Fluids

After surgery, the client needs to resume eating. Food and oral fluids are withheld until surgical clients are awake, are free of nausea and vomiting, and bowel sounds are active. Postoperative clients usually progress from a clear liquid diet to a surgical soft diet unless complications develop. Nurses monitor fluid intake and output to ensure that clients are adequately hydrated.

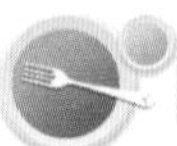

Nutrition Notes

- The postsurgical diet order may be "Progress from clear liquids to a regular diet as tolerated." A quick progression to self-selected regular food by the second postsurgical meal is safe for most clients, even those who have had major GI surgery, and may even hasten recovery.

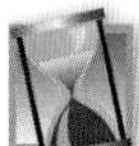

Gerontologic Considerations

- If an indwelling catheter is inserted before surgery, it is best to remove it as soon as possible after surgery to prevent urinary tract infections. Prompt attention to the client's bladder schedule is indicated to ensure adequate voiding amounts and timing, especially if a bedpan will be required during a period of ambulatory restrictions.

Promoting Venous Circulation

Surgical clients ambulate with assistance as soon as possible to reduce the potential for pulmonary and vascular complications. After some surgical procedures, however, antiembolism stockings, leg exercises, ambulation, and elevation of the lower extremities may not be enough to reduce swelling of the lower extremities and the potential for thrombus formation.

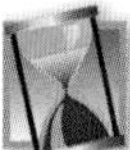

Gerontologic Considerations

- Muscle atrophy occurs in older adults who have been on bed rest even for 1 or 2 days. Range of motion and muscle tone can be maintained through routine active or passive range-of-motion exercises.

For clients who have the potential for impaired circulation in one or both extremities, a **pneumatic compression device** a machine that promotes the circulation of venous blood and relocation of excess fluid into the lymphatic vessels) may be medically prescribed. Various companies make pneumatic compression devices, but they all consist of an extremity sleeve with tubes that connect to an electrical air pump (Fig. 27-8). The device compresses the sleeved extremity either intermittently or sequentially from distal to proximal areas. Most devices cycle on for a few seconds and then cycle off for a longer period. Depending on the manufacturer,

TABLE 27-7 Postoperative Complications

COMPLICATION	DESCRIPTION	TREATMENT
Airway occlusion	Obstruction of throat	Tilt the head and lift the chin Insert an artificial airway
Hemorrhage	Severe, rapid blood loss	Control bleeding Administer intravenous fluid Replace blood
Shock	Inadequate blood flow	Place the client in a modified Trendelenburg position A modified Trendelenburg position. Replace fluids Administer oxygen Give emergency drugs
Pulmonary embolus	Obstruction of circulation through the lung as a result of a wedged blood clot that began as a thrombus	Give oxygen Administer anticoagulant drugs
Hypoxemia	Inadequate oxygenation of blood	Give oxygen
Adynamic ileus	Lack of bowel motility	Treat the cause Give nothing by mouth Insert a nasogastric tube and connect to suction Administer intravenous fluid
Urinary retention	Inability to void	Insert a catheter
Wound infection	Proliferation of pathogens at or beneath the incision	Cleanse with antimicrobial agents Open and drain incision Administer antibiotics
Dehiscence	Separation of incision	Reinforce wound edges Apply a binder
Evisceration	Protrusion of abdominal organs through separated wound	Cover with wet dressing Reapproximate wound

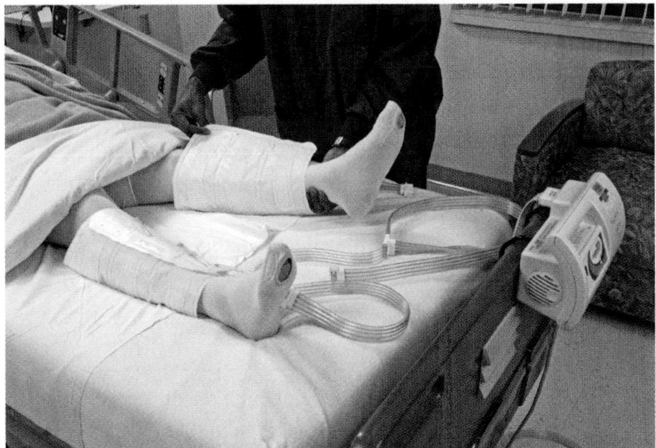

FIGURE 27-8 A pneumatic compression device.

pumps may cycle one to four times per minute. The nurse is responsible for applying this device (Skill 27-3).

Other measures to prevent thrombi include drinking plenty of fluids, avoiding long periods of sitting, keeping the legs uncrossed (especially at the knees), ambulating, and changing position frequently.

Stop, Think, and Respond Box 27-3

Compare the use of TED hose with a pneumatic compression device; list advantages and disadvantages for each.

Performing Wound Management

Nurses assess the condition of the wound and the characteristics of drainage at least once in each shift. Dressings are reinforced or changed if they become loose or saturated.

Eventually, sutures or staples are removed (see Chap. 28). Most hospitalized clients are discharged within 3 to 5 days of surgery or sooner to continue their recuperation at home.

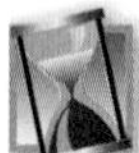

Gerontologic Considerations

■ Wound healing in older adults may occur more slowly because of age-related skin changes and impaired circulation and oxygenation. Poor hydration and nutrition further interfere with wound healing. A registered dietitian can recommend nutritional interventions such as protein, zinc, and vitamin C to improve wound healing.

■ If older adults develop postoperative infections, the manifestations are likely to be subtle or delayed. Older adults are likely to have a lower "normal" temperature. Therefore, it is imperative to document the client's usual baseline temperature so that deviations can be assessed. A change in mental status may be an early indicator of infection.

Providing Discharge Instructions

The nurse provides **discharge instructions** (directions for managing self-care and medical follow-up) before the client leaves. Common areas to address when discharging clients who have undergone surgery include the following:

- How to care for the incision site
- Signs of complications to report
- What drugs to use to relieve pain
- How to self-administer prescribed drugs
- When presurgical activity can be resumed
- If and how much weight can be lifted
- Which foods to consume or avoid
- When and where to return for a medical appointment

The nurse gives information verbally and in written form.

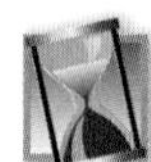

Gerontologic Considerations

■ A thorough assessment of an older client's support system must be done well before discharge. It should include the ability of the support system to provide assistance once the client is discharged. Support people should be included in discharge teaching, with plenty of time to provide any return demonstration of learning regarding the needs of the older adult. Additionally, the home's environment should be assessed before discharge for safety issues (eg, use of scatter rugs, lighting, rails, grab bars).

■ If the older person cannot manage his or her postoperative care independently or with the assistance of supportive family or friends, options relative to extended or skilled

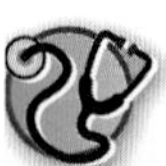

NURSING GUIDELINES 27-1

Providing Postoperative Care

- Obtain a summary report from a PACU nurse. *This report provides current assessment data concerning the client's progress.*
- Check the postoperative medical orders on the chart. *The medical orders provide instructions for individualized care.*
- Assist PACU personnel to transfer the client to bed. *The client should be observed continuously at this time.*
- Observe the client's respiratory pattern and auscultate the lungs. *Maintaining breathing is a priority for care.*
- Check oxygen saturation using a pulse oximeter if the client seems hypoxic (see Chap. 21). *An oximeter indicates the quality of internal respiration.*
- Administer oxygen if the oxygen saturation is less than 90% or if prescribed by the physician. *Oxygen administration increases oxygen available for binding with hemoglobin and for becoming dissolved in the plasma.*
- Note the client's level of consciousness and response to stimulation. *Findings indicate the client's neurologic status.*
- Orient the client and instruct him or her to take several deep breaths, as taught preoperatively. *Deep breathing improves ventilation and gas exchange.*
- Check vital signs. *Findings provide data for assessing the client's current general condition.*
- Repeat vital sign assessments at least every 15 minutes until they are stable; then follow agency policy and retake them every hour to every 4 hours depending on the client's condition or medical orders. *Repeat assessment of vital signs provides comparative data.*
- Check the incisional area and the dressing for drainage. *Findings provide data concerning the status of the wound and blood loss.*
- Inspect all tubes, insertion sites, and connections. *For optimal outcomes, the equipment must function properly.*
- Check the type of intravenous fluid, rate of administration, and volume that remains. *Findings provide data regarding fluid therapy.*
- Monitor urination; report failure to void within 8 hours of surgery. *Failure to void indicates urinary retention.*
- Auscultate bowel sounds. *Findings provide data concerning bowel motility.*
- Assess the client's level of pain, its location, and characteristics. *Pain indicates the need for analgesia.*
- Administer analgesic drugs according to prescribed medical orders, if doing so is safe. *Analgesic drugs relieve pain.*
- Remind the client to perform leg exercises or apply antiembolism stockings. *Leg exercises and antiembolism stockings promote circulation.*
- Use a side-lying position if the client is lethargic or unresponsive. *This position prevents airway obstruction by the tongue and aspiration of emesis if vomiting occurs.*
- Raise the side rails unless providing direct care. *Keeping the side rails up ensures safety.*
- Fasten the signal device within the client's reach. *The signal device is a way for the client to communicate and obtain assistance.*

nursing care should be explored and discussed. Options for skilled nursing or rehabilitation services may be available for home settings.

NURSING IMPLICATIONS

Surgical clients offer unique nursing care problems. Applicable nursing diagnoses include the following:

- Deficient Knowledge
- Fear
- Acute Pain
- Impaired Skin Integrity
- Risk for Infection
- Risk for Deficient Fluid Volume
- Ineffective Breathing Pattern
- Ineffective Airway Clearance
- Risk for Impaired Gas Exchange
- Disturbed Body Image
- Risk for Self-Health Management

Nursing Care Plan 27-1 shows how the nurse can use the nursing process to identify and resolve a diagnosis of disturbed body image, defined in the NANDA-I taxonomy (2012, p. 291) as "confusion in (the) mental picture of one's physical self." This diagnosis is especially pertinent to clients who have had their appearance altered as a result of surgery.

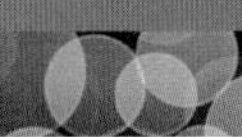

NURSING CARE PLAN 27-1 Disturbed Body Image

Assessment

- Observe the client's reaction to his or her body changes.
- Note if the client refuses to touch or look at the body part that has been altered.
- Scrutinize the client's involvement, or lack of it, in learning techniques for self-care or rehabilitation.
- Observe if the client seeks others to manage care for which he or she is capable.
- Watch the quality and quantity of the client's social interactions or avoidance of others.
- Listen for self-depreciating remarks or hostility toward others.

Nursing Diagnosis. **Disturbed Body Image** related to fear of rejection based on altered elimination secondary to a colectomy with ileostomy as evidenced by asking that room freshener be sprayed frequently, applying perfume heavily, positioning herself more than 5′ from visitors, and stating, "I hate myself for agreeing to this operation. This 'thing' fills up, it bulges, and it smells. No one will ever want to come near me again."

Expected Outcome. The client will demonstrate acceptance and less self-consciousness about changed body image by interacting with a visitor within 3 feet by 10/9.

Interventions	Rationales
Spend at least 15 minutes with the client midmorning, midafternoon, and early evening without performing direct care.	Social interaction not associated with performing a task communicates interest and acceptance of the client as a worthwhile person.
During interaction, sit within 3′ of the client.	Sitting closely provides evidence that closeness is not a problem.
Acknowledge verbally that the ostomy and resulting change in elimination are difficult to accept.	Verbalizing what the client is implying nonverbally and actively demonstrating shows empathy.
Offer to contact another person with an ostomy through the United Ostomy Association.	Interacting with another person who is coping well with a similar change can help the client to share feelings and acquire a different perspective from an objective role model.
Offer a referral to an enterostomal nurse therapist.	An enterostomal nurse therapist has knowledge and skills for managing problems experienced by clients with ostomies, such as odor control and other wound and skin impairments.
During ostomy teaching sessions and care of the stoma, avoid facial expressions that may communicate disgust or repulsion.	Nonverbal behavior is more accurate than verbal expressions during communication.
Use terminology such as "your stoma," and avoid any depersonalized or slang names for the changed body part.	Using inappropriate terms trivializes the significance of the issue with which the client is coping.

Evaluation of Expected Outcomes

- Client moved away to provide more distance during close interaction.
- Client looked at stoma while skin care and changing of appliance were demonstrated.
- Client read booklet provided by the United Ostomy Association.
- Client agreed to meet with the enterostomal therapist.

CRITICAL THINKING EXERCISES

1. The following data is reviewed by a nurse preparing a client for surgery: The client is 60 years old; weighs 205 lb; has a history of chronic pulmonary disease; quit smoking 10 years ago, vital signs are BP 140/88, temperature is 101.8°F, pulse is 92, and respiratory rate is 28 breaths per minute. Which finding is most important to report to the surgeon?

2. A client reports having taken only one shower with chlorhexidine gluconate rather than two the night before surgery. What actions could the nurse take?

3. A nurse assesses a postoperative client and obtains the following data: BP 102/64, pulse rate 90, respirations 32 and shallow, responds when shaken, and experiences nausea. What finding is most serious at this time, and what nursing actions are appropriate?

4. A preoperative client who is Native American wants you to attach a dream catcher, a circular object with a woven web, to the IV pole. What is an appropriate way to respond to the client's request?

NCLEX-STYLE REVIEW QUESTIONS

1. Assuming a client is admitted the evening before surgery, when is it best for the nurse to perform preoperative skin antisepsis and hair removal, if the latter is necessary, on a client who is scheduled for a procedure at 1300?
1. The night before surgery
2. After the morning shower
3. Before transport to the receiving area
4. When in the operating room

2. From whom is it most appropriate to obtain consent to perform surgery on an adolescent with a fractured tibia?
1. The client
2. The client's physician
3. The client's minister
4. The client's parent

3. If a client who will undergo surgery is wearing a ring, which action is most correct?
1. Put the ring in the bedside stand.
2. Leave the ring on the client's finger.
3. Give the ring to the security guard.
4. Lock the ring with his valuables.

4. What is the most important nursing action after giving a preoperative medication containing a narcotic?
1. Raise the side rails.
2. Help the client to the toilet.
3. Provide oral hygiene.
4. Teach leg exercises.

5. When the nurse assesses a client postoperatively, which assessment is most indicative of shock?
1. Bounding pulse
2. Slow respirations
3. Low blood pressure
4. High body temperature

SKILL 27-1 Applying Antiembolism Stockings

Suggested Action	Reason for Action
ASSESSMENT	
Review the medical orders and the nursing plan for care.	Directs client care.
Wash your hands or perform an alcohol-based hand rub (see Chap. 10).	Reduces the transmission of microorganisms.
Check the *Homans' sign* by dorsiflexing the foot and noting if the client experiences pain in the calf. Report a positive finding.	Indicates the possibility of **thrombophlebitis** (inflammation of a vein as a result of a thrombus).
Measure the client's leg from the flat of the heel to the bend of the knee or to midthigh.	Determines the length needed for knee-high or thigh-high stockings.
Measure the calf or thigh circumference.	Determines the size needed.
Assess the client's understanding of the purpose and use of elastic stockings.	Determines the type and amount of health teaching needed.
Check the fit of stockings that the client is currently wearing.	Identifies the potential complications from tight, loose, or wrinkled stockings.
PLANNING	
Obtain the correct size of stockings before surgery or as soon as possible after they are ordered.	Facilitates early preventive treatment.
Plan to remove the stockings for 20 minutes once in each shift or at least twice a day and then reapply them.	Allows for assessment and hygiene.
Elevate the legs for at least 15 minutes before applying the stockings if the client has been sitting or standing for some time.	Promotes venous circulation and avoids trapping venous blood in the lower extremities.
IMPLEMENTATION	
Wash and dry the feet.	Removes dirt, skin oil, and some microorganisms.
Apply corn starch or talcum powder if desired.	Reduces friction when applying the stockings.
Avoid massaging the legs.	Prevents dislodging a thrombus if one is present.
Turn the stockings inside out (Fig. A).	Facilitates threading the stockings over the foot and leg.

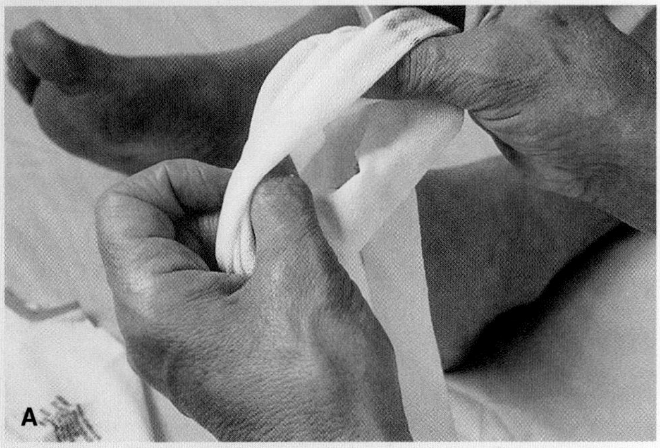

A

Turning the stocking inside out and tucking the heel inside. (Photo by B. Proud.)

(continued)

Applying Antiembolism Stockings (continued)

IMPLEMENTATION (CONTINUED)

Insert the toes and pull the stocking upward a few inches until it covers the foot (Fig. B).

Reduces bunching and bulkiness.

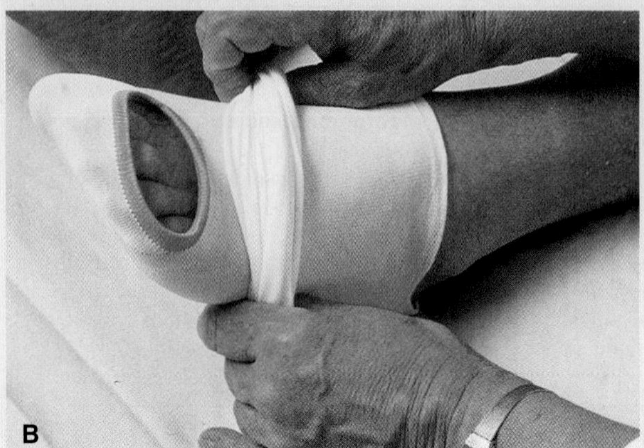

Easing the foot section over the toe and heel. (Photo by B. Proud.)

Gather the remaining length of the stocking and pull it upward a few inches at a time (Fig. C).

Eases application and avoids forming wrinkles.

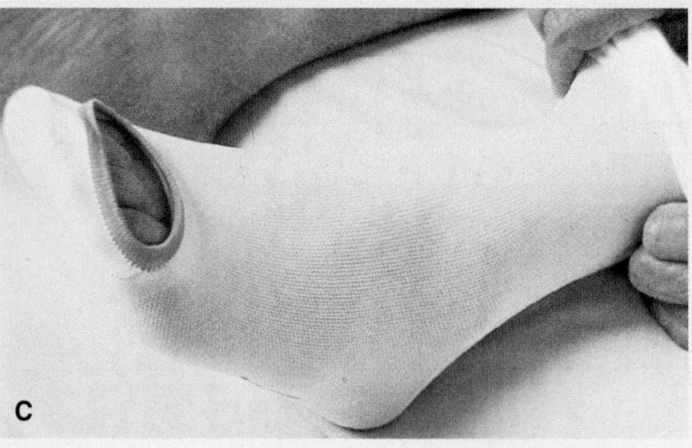

Pulling the stocking upward over the rest of the leg. (Photo by B. Proud.)

Evaluation

- Skin remains intact and circulation is adequate.
- No calf pain on dorsiflexion of the foot.
- Stockings are removed and reapplied at least b.i.d.

Document

- Assessment findings
- Removal and reapplication of elastic stockings
- To whom abnormal assessment findings have been reported and the outcome of the communication

SAMPLE DOCUMENTATION

Date and Time Toes are warm. Blood returns to nail beds within 3 seconds of compression. Skin over legs is smooth and intact. Homans' sign is negative. TED hose applied after bathing. ——————— SIGNATURE/TITLE

SKILL 27-2 Performing Presurgical Skin Preparation

Suggested Action	Reason for Action
ASSESSMENT	
Determine that the client has followed instructions regarding showering and avoiding shaving the surgical site before coming to the facility.	Washing and rinsing with an antiseptic removes microorganisms from the skin; shaving the surgical area hours or the day before surgery significantly increases the risk for a surgical site infection.
Consult the preoperative medical orders to determine if it is necessary to remove hair in the area of the potential surgical incision.	Studies indicate that surgical site infections are reduced by omitting hair removal or only removing hair without a razor at or around the incision site if it will interfere with the procedure.
Wash your hands or perform an alcohol-based hand rub (see Chap. 10).	Reduces the transmission of microorganisms.
Assess the condition of the skin, looking especially for skin lesions.	Indicates areas that may bleed if irritated or provide a reservoir of microorganisms.
Explore how much the client understands about the purpose and extent of skin preparation.	Helps to identify the extent and level of health teaching needed.
PLANNING	
Arrange to perform the skin preparation before the client is transported for surgery.	Reduces the time during which microorganisms will recolonize the skin.
Explain the procedure.	Reduces anxiety and promotes cooperation.
Provide an opportunity for the client to don a hospital gown.	Protects personal clothing and provides access for care.
Obtain electric or battery-operated clippers or depilatory agent, if ordered, a towel, a bath blanket, and gloves.	Provides essential supplies.
Braid scalp hair or use a nonflammable gel to keep hair out of the way prior to surgical procedures in which an incision will be made in the scalp.	Leaving scalp hair in place has not been shown to increase the incidence of surgical site infections and promotes a client's self-esteem postoperatively.
IMPLEMENTATION	
Wash your hands or perform an alcohol-based hand rub (see Chap. 10) and don clean gloves.	Reduces the transmission of microorganisms.
Provide privacy.	Shows respect for dignity.
Position the client so the area to be prepared is accessible.	Facilitates performing the procedure.
Drape the client with a bath blanket.	Maintains dignity as well as warmth.
Protect the bed with towels or a disposable pad.	Contains the dispersal of loose hair.
Use a single-use hair clippers or clippers with a reusable head that can be disinfected to remove hair from the designated area.	Prevents transmission of microorganisms to other clients.
Follow the manufacturer's directions regarding skin testing in a small area if a depilatory is used.	Determines if hypersensitivity or skin irritation develops.
Keep a depilatory away from the client's eyes and genitalia.	Reduces the potential for skin and tissue irritation.
Deposit or dispose of items used for skin antisepsis and hair removal in appropriate containers.	Confines sources of infectious disease transmission, and restores comfort and orderliness.
Remove the reusable head from a non disposable hair clipper and follow the agency's policy for disinfection.	Reduces the transmission of microorganisms.
Remove gloves and wash hands.	Reduces the transmission of microorganisms.
Return reusable clippers to their designated location and recharge the battery.	Ensures that reusable hair clippers are in working condition for future use.

Evaluation

- Skin has been prepared according to policy and medical orders
- Skin remains essentially intact

Document

- Assessment findings
- Technique for preoperative skin antisepsis (ie, bathing, showers, hair removed with clippers, depilatory, or not removed)
- Area prepared

SAMPLE DOCUMENTATION

Date and Time Client reports taking two showers with chlorhexidine gluconate the evening before surgery. No hair removed from the potential site of the incision. Skin is intact. No evidence of lesions or body piercings. ——— SIGNATURE/TITLE

SKILL 27-3 Applying a Pneumatic Compression Device

Suggested Action	Reason for Action
ASSESSMENT	
Review the medical orders and the nursing plan for care.	Directs client care.
Determine whether the device will be applied to one or both extremities.	Gives direction for gathering assessment data and applying the device.
Wash your hands or perform an alcohol-based hand rub (see Chap. 10).	Reduces the potential for the transmission of microorganisms.
Assess the circulation of the toes and integrity of the skin.	Provides a baseline of data for future comparison.
Check the Homans' sign (see Skill 27-1) and report if it is positive.	Indicates a possible thrombophlebitis; if positive, it is a contraindication for use of a pneumatic compression device.
Measure the calf circumference and assess for pitting edema in extremities.	Provides a baseline of data for future comparisons.
Palpate the pedal pulses.	Validates arterial blood flow to the foot if present and strong.
Assess the client's understanding of the purpose and use of a pneumatic compression device.	Determines the type and amount of health teaching needed.
PLANNING	
Obtain the extremity sleeves, electric air pump, and accompanying air tubes.	Facilitates expeditious implementation of the medical order.
Assist the client with any elimination needs.	Avoids having to disconnect the equipment shortly after the device is applied.
Arrange supplies the client may need within his or her reach, including the signal device.	Promotes independence yet ensures that the client can call for assistance.
Help the client to a position of comfort such as a supine or low Fowler's position.	Fosters rest and relaxation.
IMPLEMENTATION	
Wrap the extremity sleeve snugly around the extremity (Fig. A).	Positions the sleeve where compression is desired.

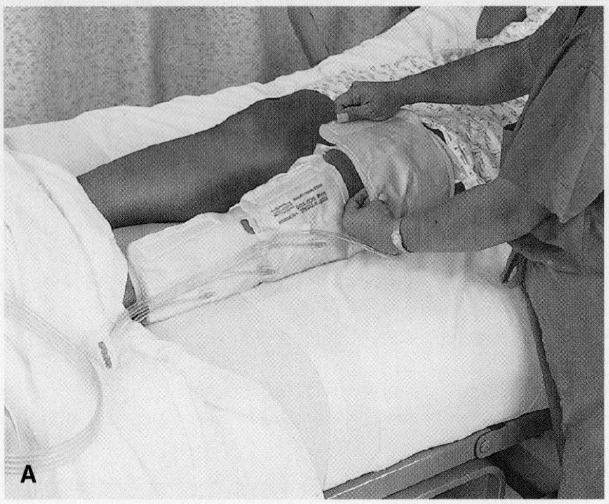

A

Applying the extremity sleeve. (Photo by B. Proud.)

Suggested Action	Reason for Action
Secure the sleeve once it encircles the leg; most are secured with Velcro.	Ensures that the sleeve will remain in the applied position.
Secure the air pump to the bottom of the bed or a stable surface.	Protects the device from damage and prevents injury to staff or visitors.

(continued)

Applying a Pneumatic Compression Device (continued)

IMPLEMENTATION (CONTINUED)

Action	Rationale
Attach the air tubes to the ports that extend from the sleeve and to the adapter within the air pump (Fig. B).	Provides a channel through which air is delivered to the extremity sleeve.

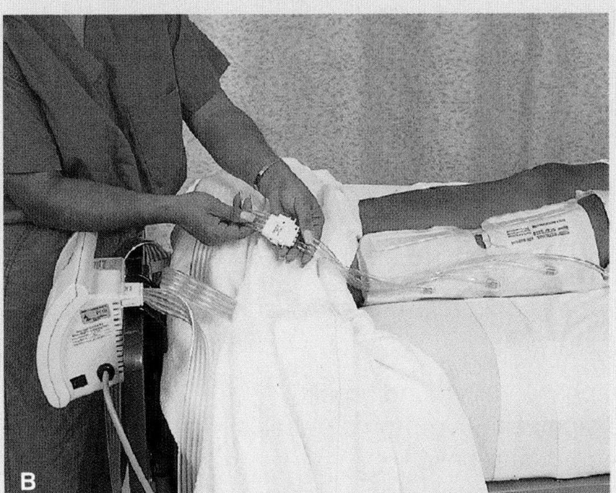

Attaching air tubes so that the arrows align. (Photo by B. Proud.)

Action	Rationale
Check that the air tubes are unkinked and not compressed under the client or the wheels of the bed.	Ensures the unobstructed delivery of air.
Plug the air pump into an electrical outlet.	Delivers power to the air pump motor.
Set the pressure on the air pump to the amount prescribed (most medical orders range from 35 to 55 mm Hg, with a common average of 40 mm Hg).	Provides intermittent compression at an appropriate pressure to promote venous circulation.
Turn the power switch on and observe that the function lights illuminate during compression and turn off between compressions.	Indicates that the machine is operational.
Assess the client's circulatory status and comfort every 2–4 hours throughout the therapeutic treatment, which is continuous for some clients.	Focuses assessment on signs that indicate adverse effects.
Remove the extremity sleeve before ambulation or other out-of-bed activities.	Allows freedom of movement from the tether of the air tubes and pump.
Discontinue the compressions if serious impairment of circulation and sensation, tingling, numbness, or leg pain occurs.	Helps to avoid serious complications.
Remove the extremity sleeve and assess calf size and circulation to distal areas of the extremity at least once per day.	Provides comparative data with which to evaluate the therapeutic response.
Apply elastic stockings and reinforce the need to perform leg exercises every hour when the machine is not in use.	Promotes venous circulation.
Place equipment in a safe area where it is available for the next use.	Demonstrates regard for safety and efficient time management.

Evaluation

- Calf size is reduced or does not increase in diameter.
- Homans' sign is negative.
- Skin in lower extremity is intact, warm, and is the appropriate color for ethnicity.
- Capillary refill is less than 2–3 seconds.
- Pedal pulses are present and strong.

Document

- Assessment findings before and after application
- Extremity to which device was applied
- Setting and duration of application
- To whom abnormal assessment findings have been reported and the outcome of the communication

SAMPLE DOCUMENTATION

Date and Time Right calf measures 18 in. (45 cm). Left calf is 20 in. (50 cm). Toes are warm. Blood returns to nail beds within 3 seconds of compression. Skin over legs is pink, warm, and intact. Homans' sign is negative bilaterally. Pneumatic compression device applied to calves of both legs and set at a pressure of 40 mm Hg.
________________ SIGNATURE/TITLE

Date and Time Pneumatic compression device removed after 2 hours of use to facilitate bathing and reapplied at 40 mm Hg.
________________ SIGNATURE/TITLE

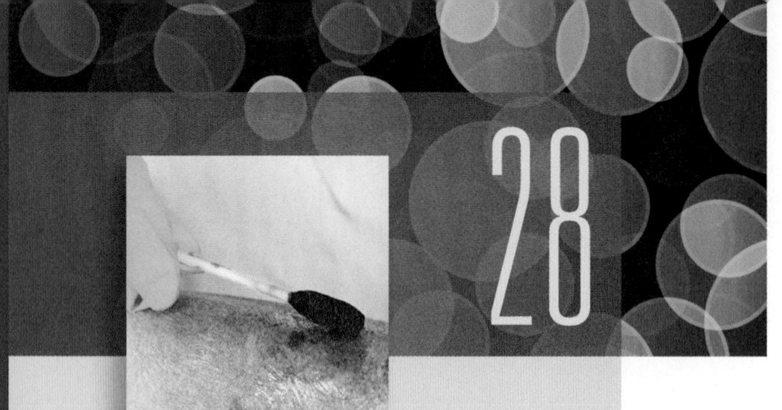

28 Wound Care

Words To Know

aquathermia pad
bandage
binder
capillary action
closed wound
collagen
compresses
debridement
dehiscence
douche
drains
dressing
evisceration
first-intention healing
granulation tissue
hydrotherapy
inflammation
irrigation
leukocytes
leukocytosis
macrophages
Montgomery straps
necrotic tissue
open wound
pack
phagocytosis
pressure ulcer
proliferation
purulent drainage
regeneration
remodeling
resolution
scar formation
second-intention healing
sepsis
serous drainage
shearing force
sitz bath
skin tear
slough
soak
staples
sutures
therapeutic baths
third-intention healing
trauma
undermining
wound

Learning Objectives

On completion of this chapter, the reader should be able to:

1. Define the term wound.
2. Name three phases of wound repair.
3. Identify five signs and symptoms classically associated with the inflammatory response.
4. Discuss the purpose of phagocytosis, including the two types of cells involved.
5. Name three ways in which the integrity of a wound is restored.
6. Explain first-, second-, and third-intention healing.
7. Name two types of wounds.
8. State at least three purposes for using a dressing.
9. Explain the rationale for keeping wounds moist.
10. Describe two types of drains, including the purpose of each.
11. Name the two major methods for securing surgical wounds together until they heal.
12. Explain three reasons for using a bandage or binder.
13. Discuss the purpose for using one type of binder.
14. Give examples of four methods used to remove nonliving tissue from a wound.
15. List three commonly irrigated structures.
16. State two uses each for applying heat and for applying cold.
17. Identify at least four methods for applying heat and cold.
18. List at least five risk factors for developing pressure ulcers.
19. Discuss three techniques for preventing pressure ulcers.

Body tissues have a remarkable ability to recover when injured. This chapter discusses several types of tissue injury, including those caused by surgical incisions and prolonged pressure. It also addresses nursing interventions to support the healing process and actions to prevent tissue injury.

WOUNDS

A **wound** (damaged skin or soft tissue) results from **trauma** (a general term referring to injury). Examples of tissue trauma include cuts, blows, poor circulation, strong chemicals, and excessive heat or cold. Such trauma produces two basic types of wounds: open and closed (Table 28-1).

An **open wound** is one in which the surface of the skin or mucous membrane is no longer intact. It may be caused accidentally or intentionally, as when a surgeon incises the tissue. In a **closed wound**, there is no opening in the skin or mucous membrane. Closed wounds occur more often from blunt trauma or pressure.

TABLE 28-1 Types of Wounds

WOUND TYPES	DESCRIPTION
Open Wounds	
Incision	A clean separation of skin and tissue with smooth, even edges
Laceration	A separation of skin and tissue in which the edges are torn and irregular
Abrasion	A wound in which the surface layers of skin are scraped away
Avulsion	Stripping away of large areas of skin and underlying tissue, leaving cartilage and bone exposed
Ulceration	A shallow crater in which the skin or the mucous membrane is missing
Puncture	An opening of skin, underlying tissue, or mucous membrane caused by a narrow, sharp, pointed object
Closed Wounds	
Contusion	Injury to soft tissue underlying the skin from the force of contact with a hard object, sometimes called a bruise

WOUND REPAIR

Regardless of the type of wound, the body immediately attempts to repair the injury and heal the wound. The process of wound repair proceeds in three sequential phases: inflammation, proliferation, and remodeling.

Inflammation

Inflammation, the physiologic process immediately after tissue injury, lasts approximately 2 to 5 days. Its purposes are to (1) limit the local damage, (2) remove injured cells and debris, and (3) prepare the wound for healing. Inflammation progresses through several stages (Fig. 28-1).

During the first stage, local changes occur. Immediately following an injury, blood vessels constrict to control blood loss and confine the damage. Shortly thereafter, the blood vessels dilate to deliver platelets that form a loose clot. The membranes of the damaged cells become more permeable, causing the release of plasma and chemical substances that transmit a sensation of discomfort. The local response produces the characteristic signs and symptoms of inflammation: *swelling*, *redness*, *warmth*, *pain*, and *decreased function*.

A second wave of defense follows the local changes when **leukocytes** and **macrophages** (types of white blood cells) migrate to the site of injury, and the body produces more and more white blood cells to take their place. **Leukocytosis** (an increased production of white blood cells) is confirmed and monitored by counting the number and type of white blood cells in a sample of the client's blood. The laboratory test is called a white blood cell count and differential count. Increased production of white blood cells, particularly neutrophils and monocytes, suggests an inflammatory and, in some cases, infectious process.

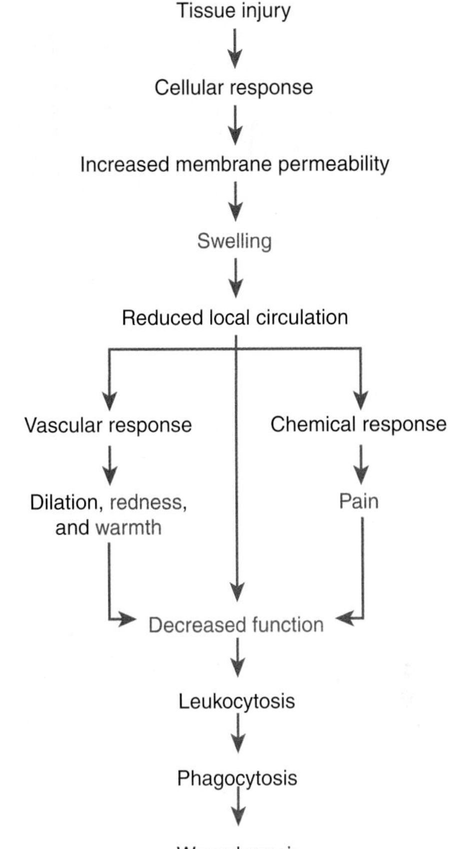

FIGURE 28-1 The inflammatory response. The words in red are the five classic signs and symptoms of inflammation.

Neutrophils and monocytes, specific kinds of white blood cells, are primarily responsible for **phagocytosis**, which is a process by which these cells consume pathogens, coagulated blood, and cellular debris. Collectively, neutrophils and monocytes clean the injured area and prepare the site for wound healing.

Proliferation

Proliferation (a period during which new cells fill and seal a wound) occurs from 2 days to 3 weeks after the inflammatory phase. It is characterized by the appearance of **granulation tissue** (a combination of new blood vessels, fibroblasts, and epithelial cells), which is bright pink to red because of the extensive projections of capillaries in the area.

Granulation tissue grows from the wound margin toward the center. It is fragile and easily disrupted by physical or chemical means. As more and more fibroblasts produce **collagen** (a tough and inelastic protein substance), the adhesive strength of the wound increases. Toward the end of the proliferative phase, the new blood vessels degenerate, causing the previously pink color to regress.

Generally, the integrity of skin and damaged tissue is restored by (1) **resolution** (a process by which damaged cells recover and reestablish their normal function), (2) **regeneration** (cell duplication), or (3) **scar formation** (replacement of damaged cells with fibrous scar tissue). Fibrous scar tissue

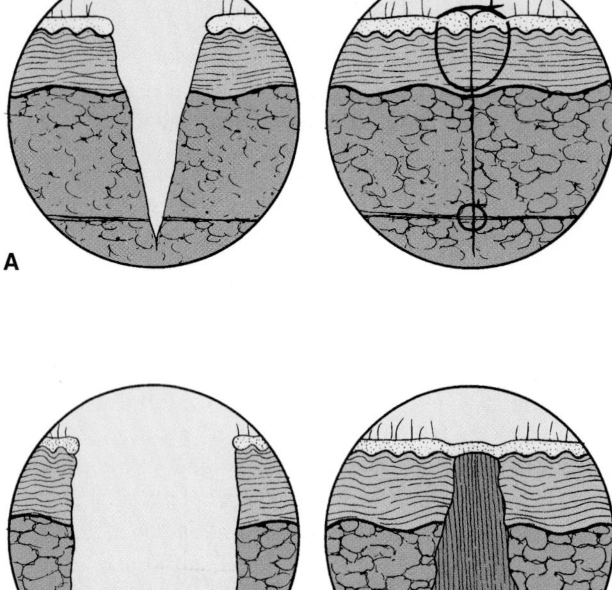

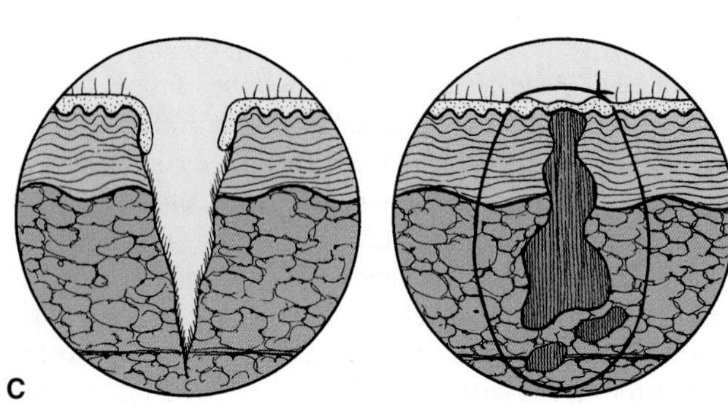

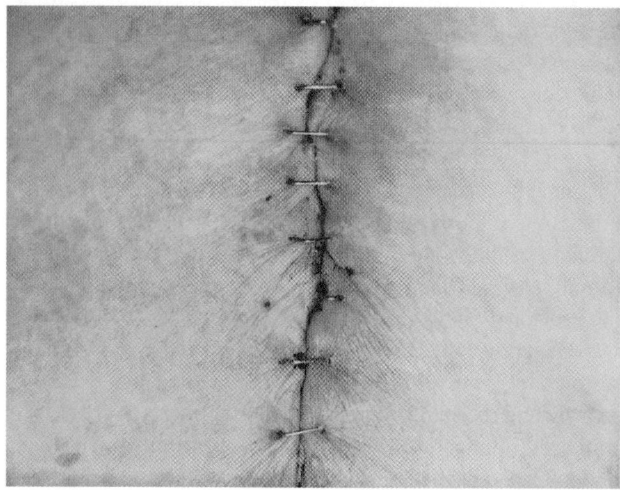

FIGURE 28-2 A. First-intention healing. **B.** Second-intention healing. **C.** Third-intention healing.

FIGURE 28-3 Example of a first-intention wound healing.

acts as a nonfunctioning patch. The extent of scar tissue that forms depends on the magnitude of tissue damage and the manner of wound healing (discussed later in this chapter).

Remodeling

Remodeling (a period during which the wound undergoes changes and maturation) follows the proliferative phase and may last 6 months to 2 years (Porth & Matfin, 2008). During this time, the wound contracts, and the scar shrinks.

WOUND HEALING

Several factors affect wound healing:

- Type of wound injury
- Expanse or depth of wound
- Quality of circulation
- Amount of wound debris
- Presence of infection
- Status of the client's health

The speed of wound repair and the extent of scar tissue that forms depend on whether the wound heals by first, second, or third intention (Fig. 28-2).

First-intention healing, also called healing by primary intention, is a reparative process in which the wound edges are directly next to each other. Because the space between the wound is so narrow, only a small amount of scar tissue forms. Most surgical wounds that are closely approximated heal by first intention (Fig. 28-3).

In **second-intention healing**, the wound edges are widely separated, leading to a more time-consuming and complex reparative process. Because the margins of the wound are not in direct contact, the granulation tissue needs additional time to extend across the expanse of the wound. Generally, a conspicuous scar results. Healing by second intention is prolonged when the wound contains body fluid or other wound debris. Wound care must be performed cautiously to avoid disrupting the granulation tissue and retarding the healing process.

With **third-intention healing**, the wound edges are intentionally left widely separated and are later brought together with some type of closure material. This reparative process results in a broad, deep scar. Generally, wounds that heal by third intention are deep and are likely to contain extensive drainage and tissue debris. To speed up healing, they may contain drainage devices or be packed with absorbent gauze.

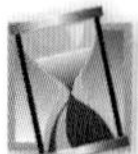

Gerontologic Considerations

- Wound healing is delayed in older adults. Regeneration of healthy skin takes twice as long for an 80-year-old client as it does for a 30-year-old client.
- Age-related changes that affect wound healing include diminished collagen and blood supply and decreased quality of elastin. Long-term exposure to ultraviolet rays from the sun compounds these age-related changes.

■ Factors such as depression, poor appetite, cognitive impairments, and physical or economic barriers that interfere with adequate nutrition in older adults may impair wound healing. These factors may be addressed by enlisting the assistance of registered dietitians, who can suggest appropriate nutritional interventions, and by making referrals to community resources such as home-delivered meals or homemaker/home health aide services.

Nutrition Notes

■ Wounds may require increased amounts of protein depending on their severity and the client's nutritional status. For instance, pressure ulcers may increase protein requirement by 50% to 100% depending on the stage and number of ulcers, whereas minor surgery may have no impact on nutrient needs. Adequate calories must be provided so that protein is not used for energy but for tissue healing. Often, high-protein beverages are given to boost protein intake; they are easy to consume and may be less filling than solid food.
■ Vitamin C and zinc play important roles in tissue repair and may be given as supplements to facilitate healing.

WOUND-HEALING COMPLICATIONS

The key to wound healing is adequate blood flow to the injured tissue. Factors that may interfere include compromised circulation, infection, and purulent, bloody, or serous fluid accumulation that prevent skin and tissue approximation. In addition, excessive tension or pulling on wound edges contributes to wound disruption and delays healing. One or several of these factors may be secondary to poor nutrition, impaired inflammatory or immune responses related to drugs like corticosteroids, and obesity (see discussion on surgical risks in Chap. 27).

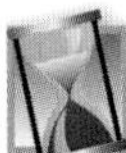

Gerontologic Considerations

■ Diminished immune response from reduced T-lymphocyte cells predisposes older adults to wound infections.
■ Signs of inflammation may be subtle in older adults (see Chap. 22).
■ Diabetes or other conditions that may interfere with circulation increase the older adult's susceptibility to delayed wound healing and wound infections.

The nurse assesses the wound to determine whether it is intact or shows evidence of unusual swelling, redness, warmth, drainage, and increasing discomfort. When assessing the wound it is important to look for **undermining**, erosion of tissue from underneath intact skin at the wound edge; **slough**, which is dead tissue on the wound surface that is moist, stringy, yellow, tan, gray, or green; and **necrotic tissue**, which is dry, brown or black devitalized tissue (Fig. 28-4). The latter two must be removed to facilitate wound healing (see the later discussion on debridement).

Two potentially serious surgical wound complications include **dehiscence** (the separation of wound edges) and **evisceration** (wound separation with the protrusion of organs) (Fig. 28-5). These complications are most likely within 7 to 10 days after surgery. They may be caused by insufficient dietary intake of protein and sources of vitamin C; premature removal of sutures or staples; unusual strain on the incision from severe coughing, sneezing, vomiting, dry heaves, or hiccupping; weak tissue or muscular support secondary to obesity; distention of the abdomen from accumulated intestinal gas; or compromised tissue integrity from previous surgical procedures in the same area.

The client may describe that something has "given way." Pinkish drainage may appear suddenly on the dressing. If wound disruption is suspected, the nurse positions the client to put the least strain on the operated area. If evisceration occurs, the nurse places sterile dressings moistened with normal

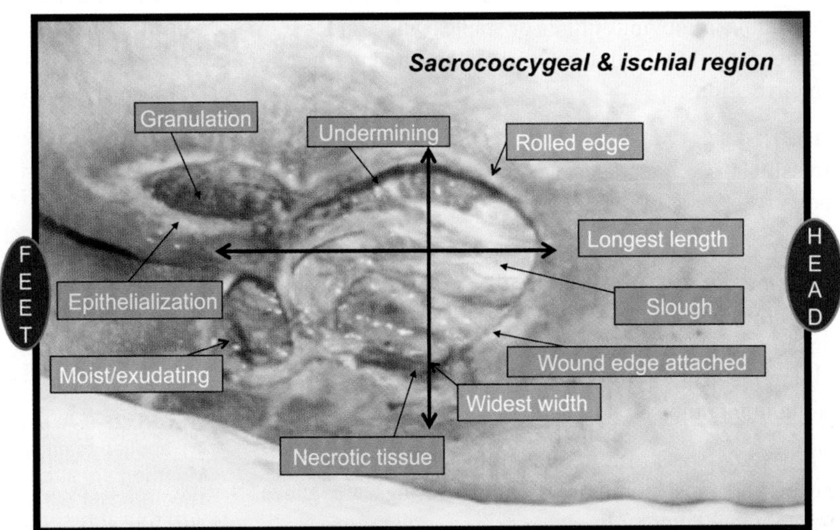

FIGURE 28-4 Components in wound assessment.

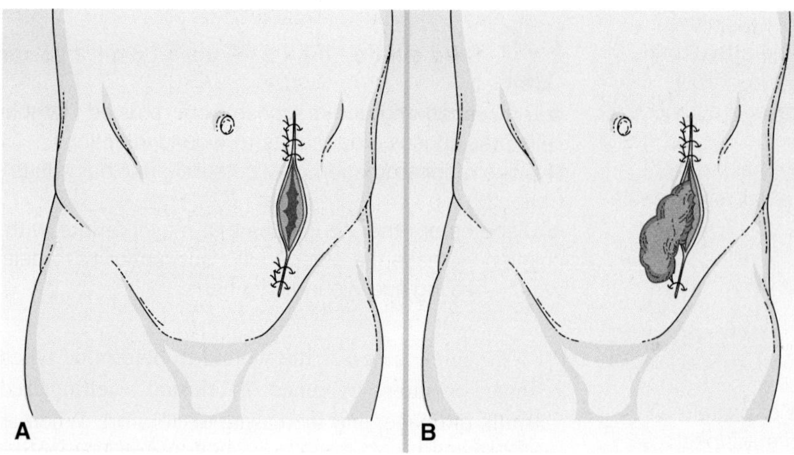

FIGURE 28-5 A. Wound dehiscence. **B.** Wound evisceration.

saline over the protruding organs and tissues. For any wound disruption, the nurse notifies the physician immediately. The nurse must be alert for signs and symptoms of impaired blood flow such as swelling, localized pallor or mottled appearance, and coolness of the tissue in the area around the wound.

Stop, Think, and Respond Box 28-1

Discuss the signs and symptoms a person would exhibit if a wound were infected.

WOUND MANAGEMENT

Wound management involves techniques that promote wound healing. Surgical wounds result from incising tissue with a laser (see Chap. 27) or an instrument called a scalpel. The primary goal of surgical or open wound management is to reapproximate the tissue to restore its integrity.

A **pressure ulcer** is a wound caused by prolonged capillary compression that is sufficient to impair circulation to the skin and underlying tissue. The primary goal in managing pressure ulcers is prevention. Once a pressure ulcer forms, however, the nurse implements measures to reduce its size and to restore skin and tissue integrity.

Wound management involves changing dressings, caring for drains, removing sutures or staples when directed by the surgeon, applying bandages and binders, and performing wound irrigations.

Dressings

A **dressing** (the cover over a wound) serves one or more purposes:

- Keeping the wound clean
- Absorbing drainage
- Controlling bleeding
- Protecting the wound from further injury
- Holding medication in place
- Maintaining a moist environment

Types and sizes of dressings differ depending on their purpose. The most common wound coverings are gauze, transparent, and hydrocolloid dressings.

Gauze Dressings

Gauze dressings are made of woven cloth fibers. Their highly absorbent nature makes them ideal for covering fresh wounds that are likely to bleed or wounds that exude drainage. Unfortunately, gauze dressings obscure the wound and interfere with wound assessment. Unless an ointment is used on the wound or the gauze is lubricated with an ointment such as petroleum, granulation tissue may adhere to the gauze fibers and disrupt the wound when removed.

Gauze dressings usually are secured with tape. If gauze dressings need frequent changing, **Montgomery straps** (strips of tape with eyelets) may be used (Fig. 28-6). Another method may be necessary if the client is allergic to tape (see the discussion on bandages and binders later in this chapter).

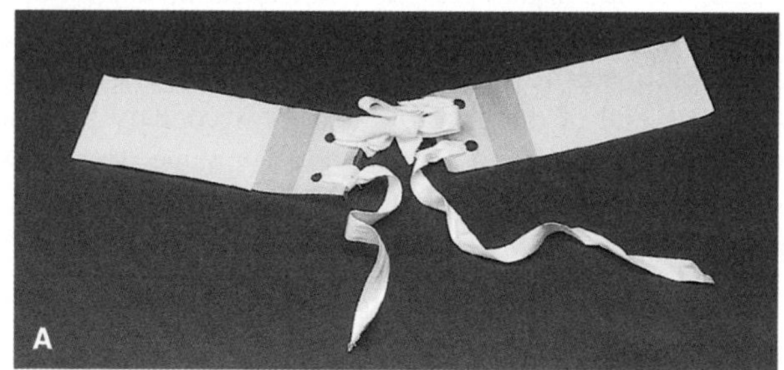

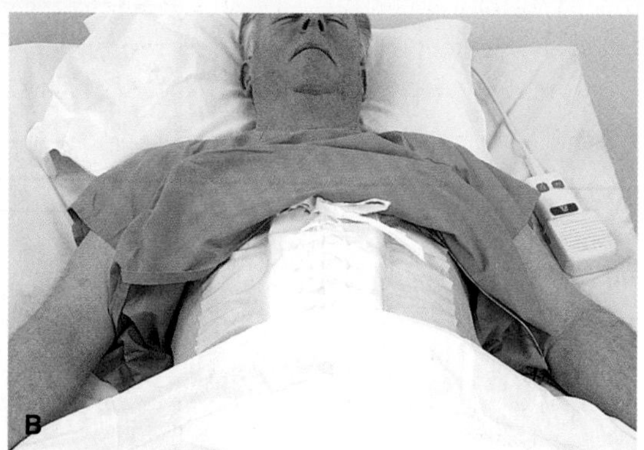

FIGURE 28-6 A. The adhesive outer edge of Montgomery straps are applied to either side of a wound. **B.** The inner edges of Montgomery straps are tied to hold a dressing over a wound. They prevent skin breakdown and wound disruption from repeated tape removal when checking or changing a dressing.

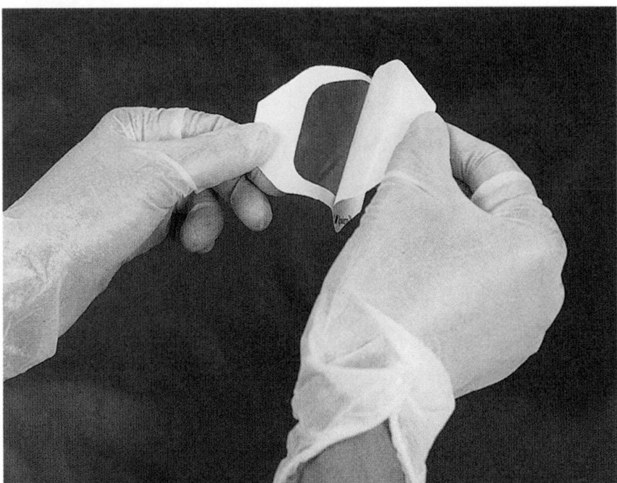

FIGURE 28-7 A transparent dressing. (Photo by B. Proud.)

Transparent Dressings

Transparent dressings, such as Op-Site, are clear wound coverings. One of their chief advantages is that they allow the nurse to assess a wound without removing the dressing. In addition, they are less bulky than gauze dressings and do not require tape because they consist of a single sheet of adhesive material (Fig. 28-7). They commonly are used to cover peripheral and central intravenous insertion sites. Transparent dressings are not absorbent; therefore, if wound drainage accumulates, they tend to loosen. Once a dressing is no longer intact, many of its original purposes are defeated.

Hydrocolloid Dressings

Hydrocolloid dressings, such as DuoDerm, are self-adhesive, opaque, air- and water-occlusive wound coverings (Fig. 28-8). They keep wounds moist. Moist wounds heal more quickly because new cells grow more rapidly in a wet environment. If the hydrocolloid dressing remains intact, it can be left in place for up to 1 week. Its occlusive nature also repels other body substances such as urine or stool. For proper use, a hydrocolloid dressing must be sized generously, allowing at least a 1-in. margin of healthy skin around the wound.

Dressing Changes

Health care professionals change dressings when a wound requires assessment or care and when the dressing becomes loose or saturated with drainage. In some cases, the physician may choose to assume total responsibility for changing the dressing—at least for the initial dressing change. Nurses, however, commonly *reinforce* dressings (apply additional absorbent layers), when dressings become moist. Reinforcing a dressing prevents wicking microorganisms toward the wound (see Chap. 10).

Because most surgical wounds are covered with gauze dressings, this example is used when describing the technique for changing a dressing in Skill 28-1. When using dressings made of materials other than gauze, nurses can modify the technique by following the manufacturer's directions.

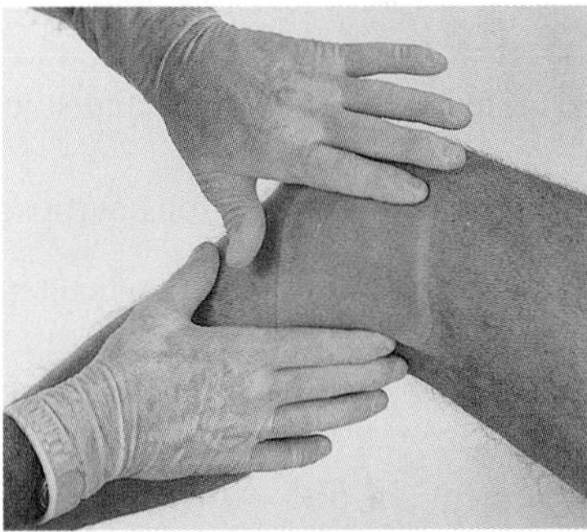

FIGURE 28-8 A hydrocolloid dressing absorbs drainage into its matrix.

Drains

Drains are tubes that provide a means for removing blood and drainage from a wound. They promote wound healing by removing fluid and cellular debris. Although some drains are placed directly within a wound, the current trend is to insert them so that they exit from a separate location beside the wound. This approach keeps the wound margins approximated and avoids a direct entry site for pathogens. The physician may choose to use an open or closed drain.

Open Drains

Open drains are flat, flexible tubes that provide a pathway for drainage toward the dressing. Draining occurs passively by gravity and **capillary action** (the movement of a liquid at the point of contact with a solid, which in this case is the gauze dressing). Sometimes, a safety pin or long clip is attached to the drain as it extends from the wound. This prevents the drain from slipping within the tissue. As the drainage decreases, the physician may instruct the nurse to shorten the drain, enabling healing to take place from inside toward the outside of the wound. To shorten a drain, the nurse pulls it from the wound for the specified length. He or she then repositions the safety pin or clip near the wound to prevent the drain from sliding back internally within the wound (Fig. 28-9).

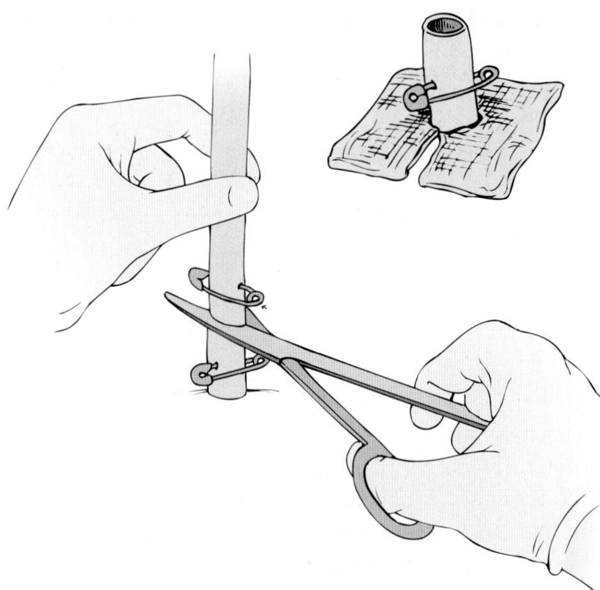

FIGURE 28-9 An open drain is pulled from the wound, and the excess portion is cut. A drain sponge is placed around the drain, and the wound is covered with a gauze dressing.

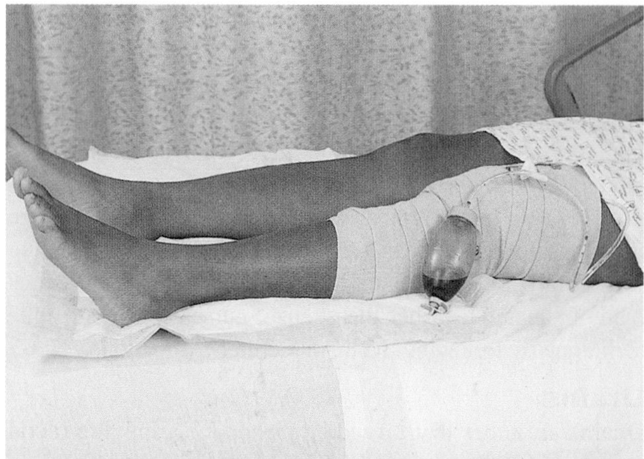

FIGURE 28-10 A Jackson-Pratt (closed) drain. (Photo by B. Proud.)

Closed Drains

Closed drains are tubes that terminate in a receptacle. Some examples of closed drainage systems are the Hemovac and the Jackson-Pratt drain (Fig. 28-10). Closed drains are more efficient than open drains because they pull fluid by creating a vacuum or negative pressure. This is done by opening the vent on the receptacle, compressing the drainage collection chamber, then capping the vent (Fig. 28-11).

When caring for a wound with a drain, the nurse cleans the insertion site in a circular manner from the center outward. After cleansing, he or she places a precut drain sponge or gauze, which is open to its center, around the base of the drain. An open drain may require additional layers of gauze because the drainage does not collect in a receptacle.

Sutures and Staples

Sutures, knotted ties that hold an incision together, generally are constructed from silk or synthetic materials such as nylon. **Staples** (wide metal clips) perform a similar function. Staples do not encircle a wound like sutures; instead, they form a bridge that holds the two wound margins together. Staples are advantageous because they do not compress the tissue if the wound swells.

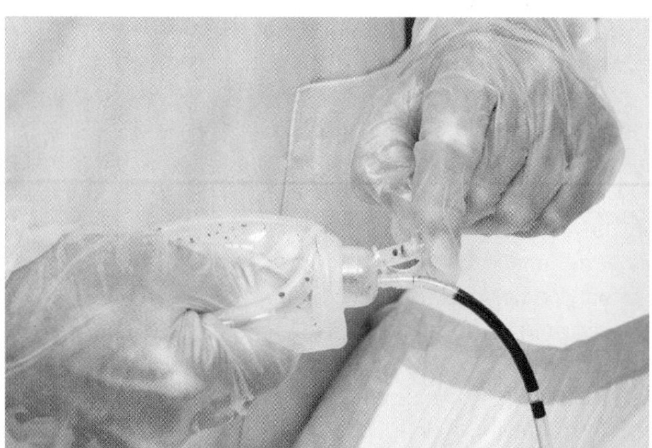

FIGURE 28-11 Compressing the bulb on a Jackson-Pratt drain and capping the vent reestablishes negative pressure that allows the collection of wound drainage.

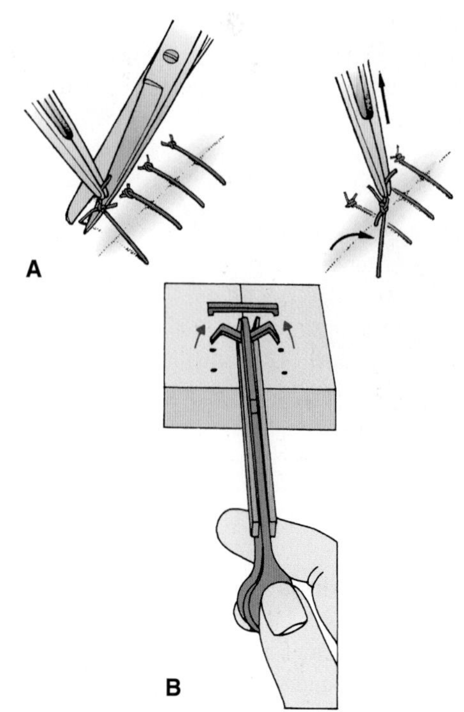

FIGURE 28-12 **A.** A technique for suture removal. **B.** A technique for staple removal.

Sutures and staples are left in place until the wound has healed sufficiently to prevent reopening. Depending on the location of the incision, this may be a few days to as long as 2 weeks.

The physician may direct the nurse to remove sutures and staples (Fig. 28-12), sometimes half on one day and the other half on another day. Adhesive *Steri-Strips*, also known as *butterflies* because of their winged appearance, can hold a weak incision together temporarily. Sometimes Steri-Strips are used instead of sutures or staples to close superficial lacerations.

Bandages and Binders

A **bandage** is a strip or roll of cloth wrapped around a body part. One example is an Ace bandage. A **binder** is a type of cloth cover generally applied to a particular body part such as the abdomen or breast. Bandages and binders are made from gauze, muslin, elastic rolls, and stockinette (see Chap. 25).

Bandages and binders serve various purposes:

- Holding dressings in place, especially when tape cannot be used or if the dressing is extremely large
- Supporting the area around a wound or injury to reduce pain
- Limiting movement in the wound area to promote healing

Roller Bandage Application

Most bandages are prepared in rolls of varying widths. The nurse holds the end in one hand while passing the roll around the part being bandaged.

Nurses follow several principles when applying a roller bandage:

- Elevate and support the limb.
- Wrap from a distal to proximal direction.
- Avoid gaps between each turn of the bandage.
- Exert equal, but not excessive, tension with each turn.
- Keep the bandage free of wrinkles.
- Secure the end of the roller bandage with metal clips.
- Check the color and sensation of exposed fingers or toes often.
- Remove the bandage for hygiene and replace at least twice a day.

Six basic techniques are used to wrap a roller bandage (Fig. 28-13): circular turn, spiral turn, spiral-reverse turn, figure-of-eight turn, spica turn, and recurrent turn.

A *circular turn* is used to anchor and secure a bandage where it starts and ends. It simply involves holding the free end of the rolled material in one hand and wrapping it around the area, bringing it back to the starting point.

A *spiral turn* partly overlaps a previous turn. The amount of overlapping varies from one-half to three-fourths of the width of the bandage. Spiral turns are used when wrapping cylindrical parts of the body such as the arms and legs.

A *spiral-reverse turn* is a modification of a spiral turn. The roll is reversed or turned downward halfway through the turn.

A *figure-of-eight turn* is best when bandaging a joint such as the elbow or knee. This pattern is made by making oblique turns that alternately ascend and descend, simulating the number eight.

A *spica turn* is a variation of the figure-of-eight pattern. It differs in that the wrap includes a portion of the trunk or chest (see spica cast, Chap. 25).

A *recurrent turn* is made by passing the roll back and forth over the tip of a body part. Once several recurrent turns are made, the bandage is anchored by completing the application with another basic turn such as the figure-of-eight turn. A recurrent turn is especially beneficial when wrapping the stump of an amputated limb or the head.

Binder Application

Binders are not used as commonly as bandages; more convenient commercial devices have largely replaced binders. For example, brassieres frequently are used instead of breast binders. Sometimes, after rectal or vaginal surgery, nurses apply a T-binder, which, as the name implies, looks like the letter T (Fig. 28-14). T-binders are used to secure a dressing to the anus or perineum or within the groin. To apply a T-binder, the nurse fastens the crossbar of the T around the waist. Then, he or she passes the single or double tails between the client's legs and pins the tails to the belt. Adhesive sanitary napkins worn inside underwear briefs are an alternative to a T-binder for stabilizing absorbent materials.

Debridement

Most wounds heal rapidly with conventional care. Nevertheless, some wounds require **debridement** (the removal of dead tissue) to promote healing. Four methods of debridement are sharp, enzymatic, autolytic, and mechanical.

Sharp Debridement

Sharp debridement is the removal of necrotic nonliving tissue from the healthy areas of a wound with sterile scissors, forceps, or other instruments (Fig. 28-15). This method is preferred if the wound is infected because it helps the wound to heal quickly and well. The procedure is done at the bedside or in the operating room if the wound is extensive. Sharp debridement is painful, and the wound may bleed afterward.

Enzymatic Debridement

Enzymatic debridement involves the use of topically applied chemical substances that break down and liquefy wound debris. A dressing is used to keep the enzyme in contact with the wound and to help absorb the drainage. This form of debridement is appropriate for uninfected wounds or for clients who cannot tolerate sharp debridement.

Autolytic Debridement

Autolytic debridement, or self-dissolution, is a painless, natural physiologic process that allows the body's enzymes to soften, liquefy, and release devitalized tissue. It is used when a wound is small and free of infection. The main disadvantage in autolysis is the prolonged time it takes to achieve desired results. To accelerate autolysis, an occlusive or semi-occlusive dressing keeps the wound moist. Because removal of tissue debris is slow, the nurse monitors the client closely for signs of wound infection.

Mechanical Debridement

Mechanical debridement involves the physical removal of debris from a deep wound. One technique is the application of wet-to-dry dressings. The wound is packed with moist gauze, which is removed approximately 4 to 6 hours later when the gauze is dry. Dead tissue adheres to the meshwork of the gauze and is removed when the dressing is changed. Recently, the use of wet-to-dry dressings for debridement has come under questioning. Some disadvantages include: (1) impeded healing from local tissue cooling, (2) disruption of angiogenesis (formation of new blood vessels), and (3) increased risk for infection from frequent dressing changes (Moses, 2009). It has also been described as being nonselective, traumatic, painful, costly, and time-consuming. An alternative to wet-to-dry dressings is to use a calcium alginate dressing such as Algiderm, which consists of absorbent, nonadherent, biodegradable, nonwoven fibers derived from

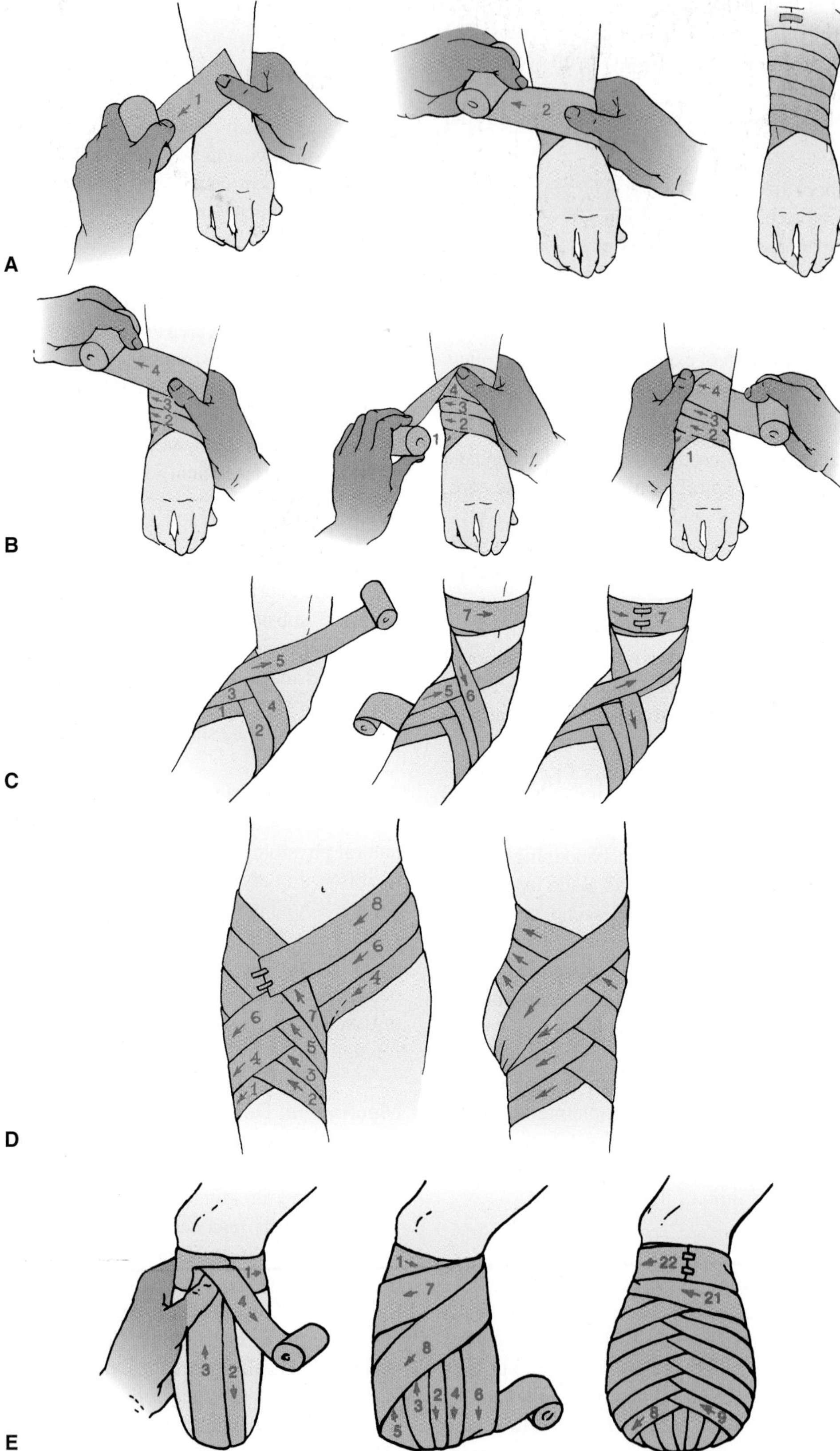

FIGURE 28-13 A. A circular and spiral turn. **B.** A spiral-reverse turn. **C.** A figure-of-eight turn. **D.** A spica turn. **E.** A recurrent turn.

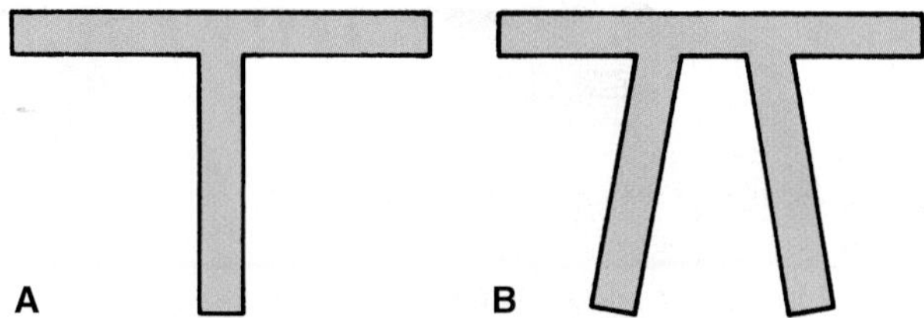

FIGURE 28-14 **A.** A single T-binder. **B.** A double T-binder.

seaweed and other chemicals. Its contents form a gel when in contact with wound drainage, thus facilitating debridement when it is removed. Calcium alginate dressings are supplied in sheets, pads, and ribbons depending on the wound requirements.

Another approach to the mechanical removal of wound debris is **hydrotherapy** (the therapeutic use of water), in which the body part with the wound is submerged in a whirlpool tank. The agitation of the water, which contains an antiseptic, softens the dead tissue. Loose debris that remains attached is removed afterward by sharp debridement.

A third method for mechanically removing wound debris is **irrigation** (a technique for flushing debris). An irrigation is used when caring for a wound and also when cleaning an area of the body such as the eyes, ears, and vagina.

Stop, Think, and Respond Box 28-2

List an advantage and disadvantage of methods used for wound debridement.

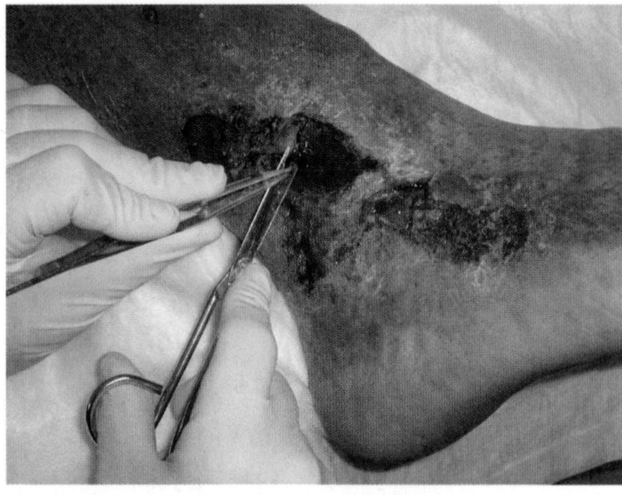

FIGURE 28-15 A sharp debridement at the bedside.

Wound Irrigation. Wound irrigation (Skill 28-2) generally is carried out just before applying a new dressing. This technique is best used when granulation tissue has formed. Surface debris should be removed gently without disturbing the healthy proliferating cells.

Eye Irrigation. An eye irrigation flushes a toxic chemical from one or both eyes or displaces dried mucus or other drainage that accumulates from inflamed or infected eye structures (see Nursing Guidelines 28-1 and Fig. 28-16).

Ear Irrigation. An ear irrigation removes debris from the ear. An ear irrigation is contraindicated if the tympanic

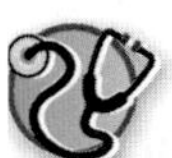

NURSING GUIDELINES 28-1

Eye Irrigation

- Assemble supplies: a bulb syringe, an irrigating solution, gauze squares, gloves and other standard precaution apparel, absorbent pads, and at least one towel. *Assembling equipment ahead of time ensures organization and efficient time management.*
- Warm the solution to approximately body temperature by placing the container in warm water except when administering emergency first aid. *A warm solution is more comfortable for the client.*
- Position the client with the head tilted slightly toward the side. *This position facilitates drainage.*
- Place absorbent material in the area of the shoulder. *Use of absorbent material prevents saturating the client's gown and bed linen.*
- Give the client an emesis basin to hold beneath the cheek. *The basin can be used to collect the irrigating solution.*
- Wash hands or use an alcohol-based hand rub and don gloves. *Hand hygiene and glove use reduce the transmission of microorganisms.*
- Open and prepare supplies. *This enables the nurse to perform the irrigation efficiently.*
- Wipe a moistened gauze square from the nasal corner of the eye toward the temple; use additional gauze squares, one at a time, as needed. *This removes gross debris.*
- Separate the eyelids widely with the fingers of one hand. *This action widens the exposed surface area.*
- Direct the solution onto the conjunctiva, holding the syringe or irrigating device about 1 in. (2.5 cm) above the eye (see Fig. 28-16). *Holding the syringe away from the eye prevents injury to the cornea.*
- Instruct the client to blink periodically. *Blinking distributes solution under the eyelid and around the eye.*
- Continue irrigating until the debris is removed. *This accomplishes the desired result.*
- Dry the client's face and replace a wet gown or linen. *These actions promote client comfort.*
- Dispose of soiled materials and gloves; wash hands. *These measures reduce the transmission of microorganisms.*
- Record assessment data, the specifics of the procedure, and the outcome. *Documentation records performance of the nursing intervention and the client's response.*

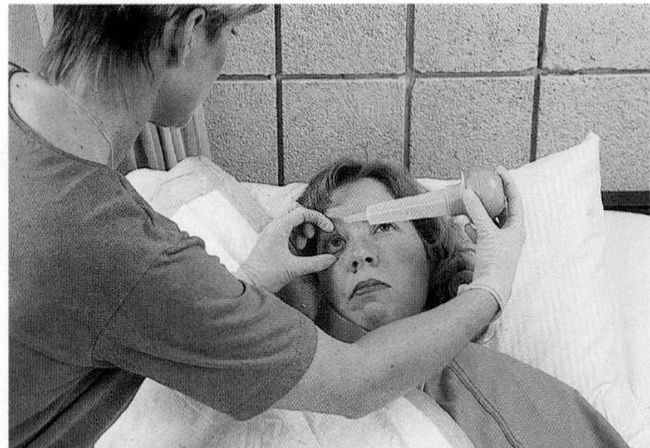

FIGURE 28-16 Eye irrigation. (Photo by B. Proud.)

membrane (eardrum) is perforated. Performing a gross inspection of the ear is important if a foreign body is suspected because a bean, pea, or other dehydrated substance can swell if the ear is irrigated, causing it to become even more tightly fixed. Solid objects may require removal with an instrument.

If an ear irrigation is not contraindicated, it is performed much like an eye irrigation except that the nurse directs the solution toward the roof of the auditory canal (Fig. 28-17). Also, the nurse takes care to avoid occluding the ear canal with the tip of the syringe because the pressure of the trapped solution could rupture the eardrum. After the irrigation, the nurse places a cotton ball loosely within the ear to absorb drainage but not to obstruct its flow.

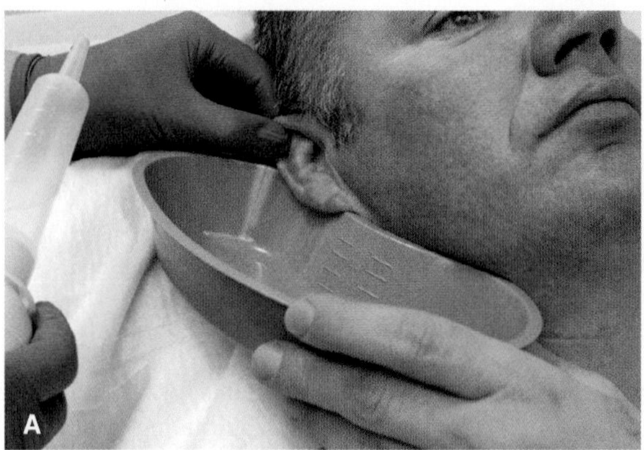

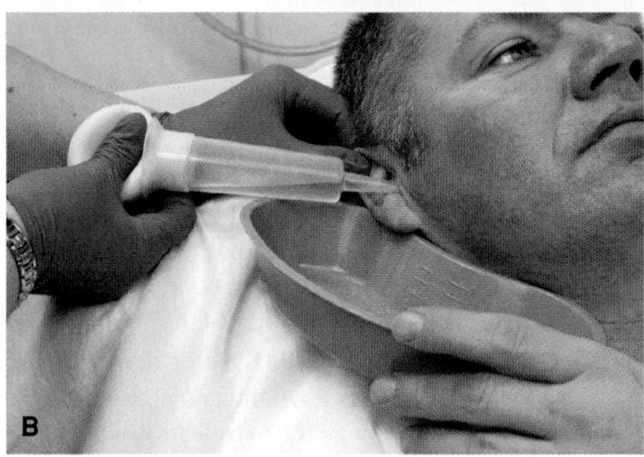

FIGURE 28-17 (**A.** and **B.**) Ear irrigation.

Vaginal Irrigation. A vaginal irrigation, also known as a **douche** (a procedure for cleansing the vaginal canal), is sometimes necessary to treat an infection (see Client and Family Teaching 28-1).

Heat and Cold Applications

Heat and cold have various therapeutic uses (Box 28-1), and each can be used in several ways. Examples include an ice bag, collar, chemical pack, compress, and aquathermia pad. Heat is also applied with soaks, moist packs, and therapeutic baths.

The terms *hot* and *cold* are subject to wide interpretation. Table 28-2 correlates common terms with temperature ranges. Because exposing the skin to extremes of temperature can result in injuries, the nurse assesses the temperature of the application and frequently monitors the condition of the skin. Direct contact between the skin and the heating or cooling device is avoided. Hot and cold applications are used cautiously in children younger than 2 years, older adults, clients with diabetes, and clients who are comatose or neurologically impaired.

Client and Family Teaching 28-1 Douching

The nurse teaches the client or the family as follows:

- Do not douche routinely because douching removes microbes, called *Döderlein bacilli,* that help prevent vaginal infections.
- Do not douche 24–48 hours before a Pap test (see Chap. 14). Douching may wash away diagnostic cells.
- Consult a physician about symptoms such as itching, burning, or drainage rather than attempting self-diagnosis.
- Find out from the physician if sexual partners also need to be treated with medications to avoid reinfection.
- Buy douching equipment from a drugstore; prefilled disposable containers are available.
- Warm the solution to a comfortable temperature (no more than 110°F [43.3°C]).
- Clamp the tubing (on reusable equipment) and fill the reservoir bag.
- Undress and lie down in the bathtub.
- Suspend the douche bag (if used) about 18–24 in. (45–60 cm) above the hips.
- Insert the lubricated tip of the nozzle or the prefilled container downward and backward within the vagina about the distance of a tampon.
- Unclamp the tubing and rotate the nozzle as the fluid is instilled.
- Contract the perineal muscles as though trying to stop urinating and then relax the muscles. Repeat the exercise four or five times while douching.
- Sit up to facilitate drainage or shower afterward.
- Use a sanitary napkin or perineal pad to absorb residual drainage.

BOX 28-1 Common Uses for Heat and Cold Applications

USES FOR HEAT	USES FOR COLD
• Provides warmth	• Reduces fevers
• Promotes circulation	• Prevents swelling
• Speeds healing	• Controls bleeding
• Relieves muscle spasm	• Relieves pain
• Reduces pain	• Numbs sensation

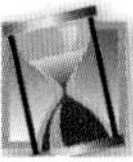

Gerontologic Considerations

■ The risk for thermal skin injury is increased in older adults with impaired tactile sensation or sensory nerve damage because of circulatory or neurological disorders. Older adults who have problems with the ability to sense temperatures need to take special precautions such as using a thermometer to ensure that applications involving heat are less than 100°F (38°C) to avoid burns or injury.

Ice Bag and Ice Collar

Ice bags and ice collars are containers for holding crushed ice or small ice cubes (Fig. 28-18). Ice collars usually are applied after tonsil removal. Ice bags are applied to any small injury in the process of swelling. Although ice bags are available commercially, they can also be improvised. A rubber or plastic glove, a plastic bag with a zipper closure, or a bag of small frozen vegetables, such as peas, can be used. Client instruction minimizes the risk for injury (see Client and Family Teaching 28-2).

Chemical Packs

Commercial cold packs are struck or crushed to activate the chemicals inside, causing them to become cool. Most first-aid kits generally include this type of cold pack. Commercial cold packs can be used only once. Gel packs, designed for cold or hot application, are reusable. They are stored in the freezer until needed or heated in a microwave.

Compresses

Compresses (moist, warm, or cool cloths) are applied to the skin. Before applying the compress, the nurse soaks it in tap water or a medicated solution at the appropriate temperature and then wrings out excess moisture. To maintain the moisture and temperature, a piece of plastic or plastic wrap is used to cover the compress, and the area is secured in a towel. As the compress material cools or warms outside the range of the intended temperature, the nurse removes it and reapplies it if necessary.

TABLE 28-2 Temperature Ranges for Applications of Heat and Cold

LEVEL OF HEAT OR COLD	TEMPERATURE RANGE
Very hot	40.5°–46.1°C (105°–115°F)
Hot	36.6°–40.5°C (98°–105°F)
Warm and neutral	33.8°–36.6°C (93°–98°F)
Tepid	26.6°–33.8°C (80°–93°F)
Cool	18.3°–26.6°C (65°–80°F)
Cold	10°–18.3°C (50°–65°F)
Very cold	Below 10°C (below 50°F)

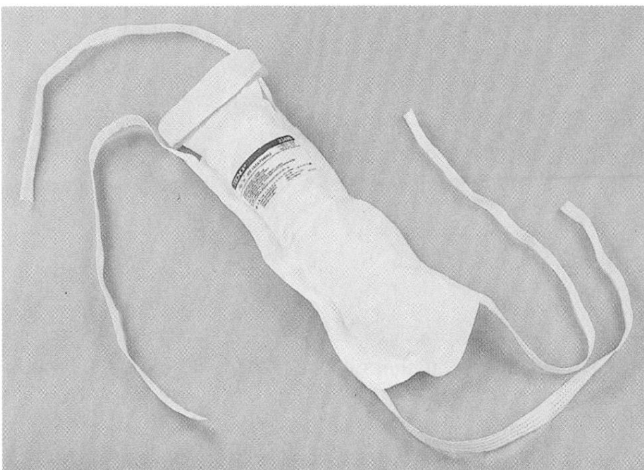

FIGURE 28-18 An ice bag filled with crushed ice.

If the skin is not intact, as in the case of a draining wound, nurses wear gloves when applying a compress. They use aseptic surgical technique when applying compresses to an open wound.

Aquathermia Pad

An **aquathermia pad** (an electrical heating or cooling device) is sometimes called a K-pad. It resembles a mat but contains hollow channels through which heated or cooled distilled water circulates (Fig. 28-19). An aquathermia pad is used alone or as a cover over a compress. A thermostat is used to keep the temperature of the water at a specified setting. As with other forms of hot and cold therapeutic devices, the nurse assesses the skin frequently and removes the device periodically.

Before placing the client on the aquathermia pad or wrapping it around a body part, the nurse covers the pad to help prevent thermal skin damage. A roller bandage may help hold the pad in place. The nurse positions the electrical unit slightly higher than the client to promote gravity circulation of the fluid.

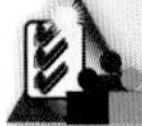

Client and Family Teaching 28-2 Using an Ice Bag

The nurse teaches the client or the family as follows:

- Test the ice bag for leaks.
- Fill it one-half to two-thirds full of crushed ice or small cubes so it can be molded easily to the injured area.
- Eliminate as much air from the bag as possible.
- Pour water over the ice to provide slight melting. This tends to smooth the sharp edges from frozen ice crystals.
- Cover the ice bag with a layer of cloth before placing it on the body.
- Leave the ice bag in place no more than 20–30 minutes. Allow the skin and tissue to recover for at least 30 minutes before reapplying.
- If the skin becomes mottled or numb, remove the ice bag—it is too cold.

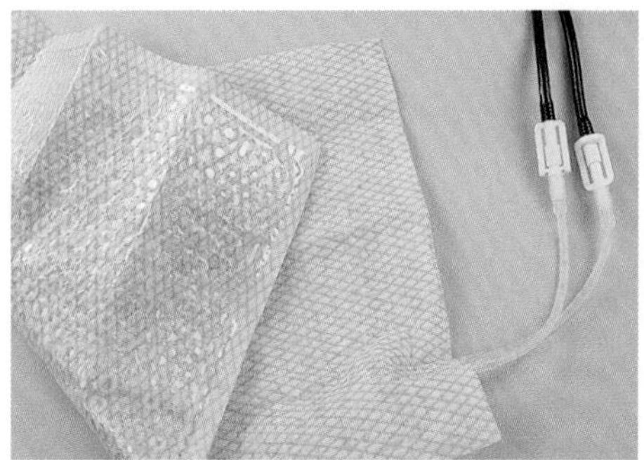

FIGURE 28-19 An aquathermia pad (K-pad). (Photo by B. Proud.)

Larger styles are used to warm clients who are hypothermic or to cool those with heat stroke. Because these clients have dangerously altered body temperatures, the nurse must monitor vital signs continuously.

Soaks and Moist Packs

A **soak** is a technique in which a body part is submerged in fluid to provide warmth or to apply a medicated solution. A **pack** (a commercial device for applying moist heat) also can be used. Moist heat is more comforting and therapeutic than dry heat.

A soak usually lasts 15 to 20 minutes. The nurse keeps the temperature of the fluid as constant as possible, which requires frequent emptying and refilling of the basin. The newly added water should not be too hot; overly hot water causes discomfort or tissue damage.

Packs differ from soaks in two major ways: the duration of the application is usually longer, and the initial application of heat is generally more intense. Packs usually are applied at temperatures as warm as the client can tolerate. Because of the potential for causing burns, a pack never is used on a client who is unresponsive or paralyzed and cannot perceive temperatures. The nurse must make frequent assessments and remove the pack if there is any likelihood of a thermal injury.

Therapeutic Baths

Therapeutic baths (those performed for other than hygiene purposes) help reduce a high fever or apply medicated substances to the skin to treat skin disorders or discomfort. Examples are baths to which sodium bicarbonate (baking soda), cornstarch, or oatmeal paste are added.

The most common type of therapeutic bath is a **sitz bath** (a soak of the perianal area). Sitz baths reduce swelling and inflammation and promote healing of wounds after a *hemorrhoidectomy* (the surgical removal of engorged veins inside and outside the anal sphincter) or an *episiotomy* (an incision that facilitates vaginal birth). Some health care agencies have special tubs for administering sitz baths, but most provide clients with disposable equipment (Skill 28-3).

Stop, Think, and Respond Box 28-3

What assessment findings suggest that a sitz bath is providing a therapeutic effect?

PRESSURE ULCERS

Pressure ulcers or sores, also referred to as *decubitus ulcers*, most often appear over bony prominences of the sacrum, hips, and heels. They also can develop in other locations such as the elbows, shoulder blades, the back of the head, and places where pressure is unrelieved because of infrequent movement (Fig. 28-20). The tissue in these areas is particularly vulnerable because body fat, which acts as a pressure-absorbing cushion, is minimal. Consequently, the tissue is compressed between the bony mass and a rigid surface such as a chair seat or a bed mattress. If the compression reduces the pressure in local capillaries to less than 32 mm Hg for 1 to 2 hours without intermittent relief, the cells die from a lack of oxygen and nutrients.

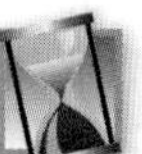

Gerontologic Considerations

- Age-related changes (ie, a thinning dermal layer of skin, decreased subcutaneous tissue) result in increased susceptibility to pressure ulcers and shear-type injuries in older adults. Because of the decreased blood supply to the skin, an older adult may need position changes every 60 to 90 minutes, rather than every 120 minutes. Take special care when moving older adults to avoid friction on the skin.
- Absorbent undergarments may contribute to skin breakdown because they may not allow for air circulation. Urine or feces next to the skin will cause damage and possible skin breakdown. Therefore, any incontinent older adult must be checked every 60 to 90 minutes to prevent skin damage. If urinary incontinence interferes significantly with wound healing, an indwelling catheter (see Chap. 30) may be necessary. It should be removed as soon as feasible, however, and efforts must be made to restore continence.
- Older adults with diminished mobility require aggressive skin care to prevent pressure ulcers. The elbows, heels, coccyx, shoulder blades, and hips are especially vulnerable, as are the creases above the ears if oxygen tubing is in use. Special precautions include heel and elbow protectors, pressure-relief pads, and mattresses, and a strict routine of changing the client's position at least every 2 hours or more frequently if the person's skin becomes reddened in a shorter period. Assessment of at-risk pressure point areas should be done before the 2-hour period.

Stages of Pressure Ulcers

Pressure ulcers are grouped into four stages according to the extent of tissue injury (Fig. 28-21). Care and healing depend on the stage of injury. Without aggressive nursing care, early stage pressure ulcers can easily progress to much more serious ones.

Stage I is characterized by intact but reddened skin. The hallmark of cellular damage is skin that remains red and fails to resume its normal color when pressure is relieved.

A stage II pressure ulcer is red and accompanied by blistering or a **skin tear** (a shallow break in the skin) without slough. Impairment of the skin may lead to colonization and infection of the wound.

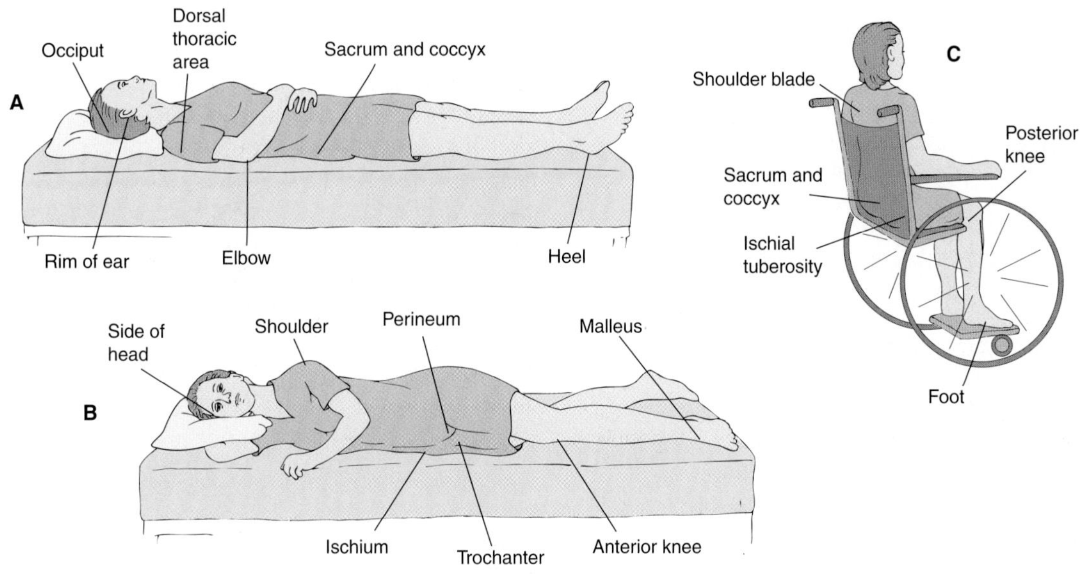

FIGURE 28-20 Locations where pressure ulcers commonly form. **A.** The supine position. **B.** A side-lying position. **C.** The sitting position.

A stage III pressure ulcer has a shallow skin crater that extends to the subcutaneous tissue. It may be accompanied by **serous drainage** (leaking plasma), undermining, slough, or **purulent drainage** (white or greenish fluid) caused by a wound infection. The area is relatively painless despite the severity of the ulcer.

Stage IV pressure ulcers are life-threatening. The tissue is deeply ulcerated, exposing muscle and bone (Fig. 28-22). Slough and necrotic tissue may be evident. The dead or infected tissue may produce a foul odor. If an infection is present, it easily spreads throughout the body, causing **sepsis** (a potentially fatal systemic infection).

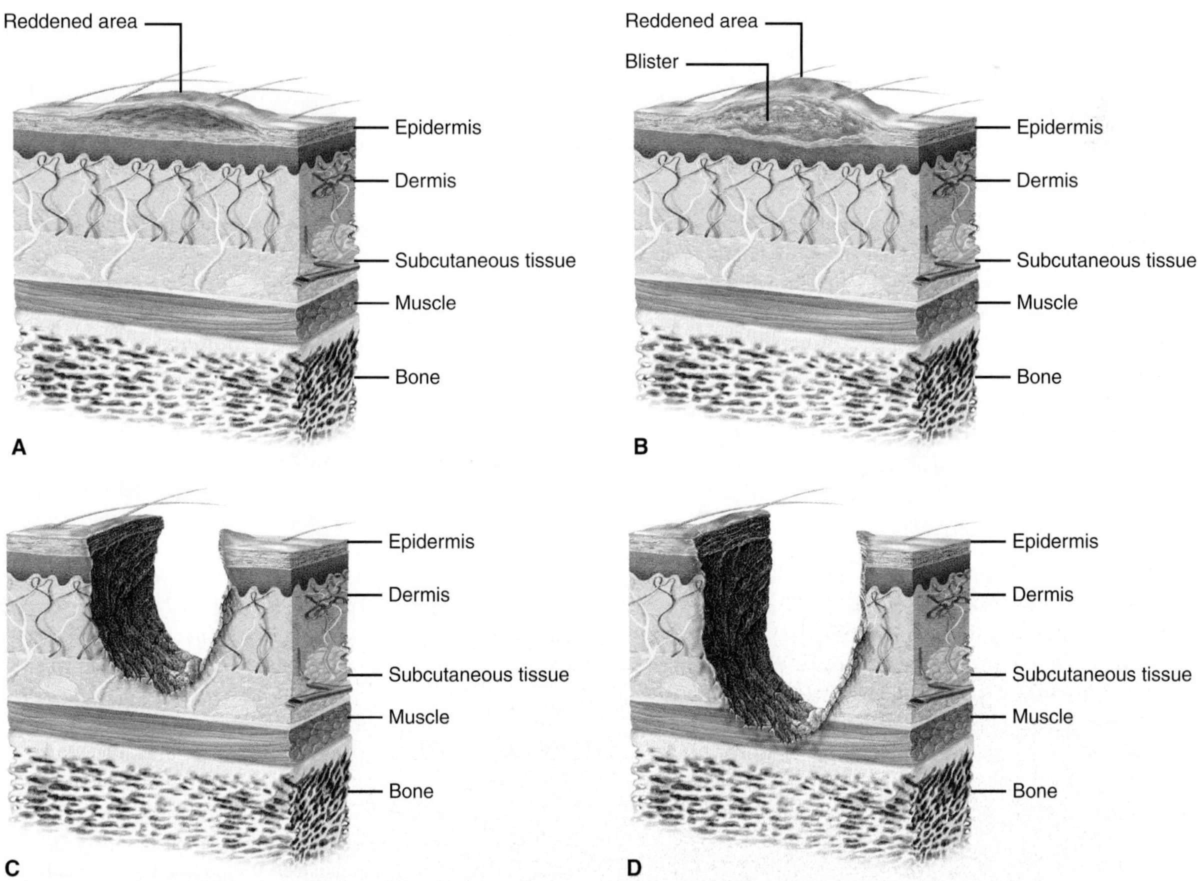

FIGURE 28-21 Pressure sore stages. **A.** Stage I. **B.** Stage II. **C.** Stage III. **D.** Stage IV.

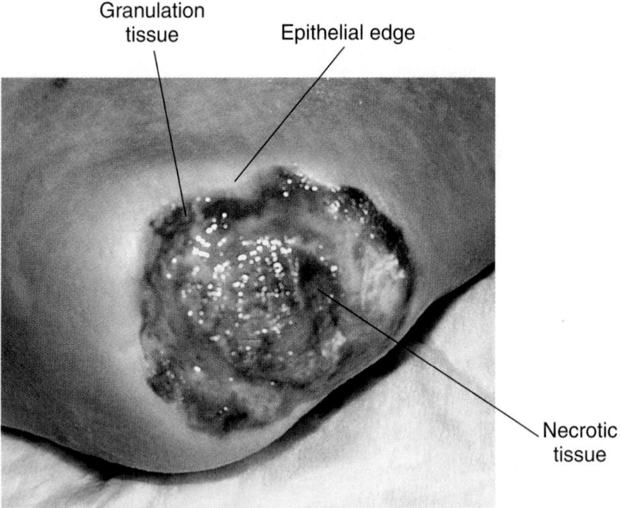

FIGURE 28-22 Example of stage IV pressure sore.

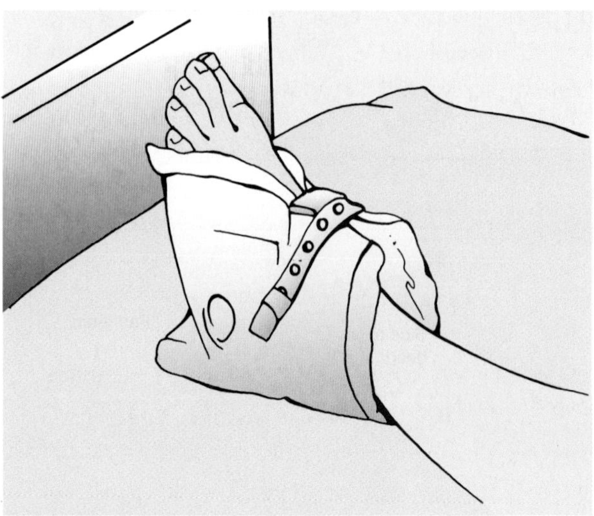

FIGURE 28-23 Heel and ankle protection.

Prevention of Pressure Ulcers

The first step in prevention is to identify clients with risk factors for pressure ulcers (Box 28-2). The second step is to implement measures that reduce conditions under which pressure ulcers are likely to form (see Nursing Guidelines 28-2 and Fig. 28-23).

BOX 28-2 Risk Factors for Developing Pressure Ulcers

- Inactivity
- Immobility
- Malnutrition
- Emaciation
- Diaphoresis
- Incontinence
- Vascular disease
- Localized edema
- Dehydration
- Sedation

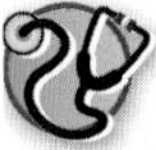

NURSING GUIDELINES 28-2

Preventing Pressure Ulcers

- Change the bedridden client's position frequently. Remind a client who is sitting in a chair to stand and move hourly or at least to shift his or her weight every 15 minutes while sitting. *Changing positions relieves pressure and restores circulation.*
- Lift rather than drag the client during repositioning. *Dragging causes friction, which abrades the skin and damages underlying blood vessels.*
- Avoid using plastic-covered pillows when positioning clients. *Plastic prevents evaporation of perspiration because it is nonporous. It also raises skin temperature, further contributing to the growth of microorganisms.*
- Use positioning devices such as pillows to keep two parts of the body from direct contact with each other. *Such devices absorb perspiration, reduce localized heat, and avoid the compression of tissue between two body parts.*
- Use the lateral oblique position (see Chap. 23) rather than the conventional lateral position for side lying. *The lateral oblique position more effectively reduces the potential for pressure on vulnerable bony prominences.*
- Massage bony prominences only if the skin blanches with pressure relief. *Massage improves circulation to normal tissue but causes further damage to areas where pressure ulcers—even those that are stage I—are already established.*
- Keep the skin clean and dry especially when clients cannot control their bladder or bowel function. *Cleansing removes substances that chemically injure the skin.*
- Use a moisturizing skin cleanser rather than soap, if possible. *A nonsoap cleanser maintains skin hydration and avoids altering the skin's natural acidity, which protects it from bacterial colonization.*
- Rinse and dry the skin well. *Cleansing then drying removes chemical residues and surface moisture.*
- Use pressure-relieving devices such as special beds or mattresses (see Chap. 23). *These special devices maintain capillary blood flow by reducing pressure.*
- Pad body areas such as the heels, ankles, and elbows, which are vulnerable to friction and pressure (see Fig. 28-23). *Padding prevents friction and adds a cushioning layer over the bony prominence.*
- Use seat cushions such as a commercial gel-filled pad when clients sit for extended periods. *These cushions distribute pressure over a wider area, relieving direct pressure on the coccyx.*
- Keep the head of the bed elevated no more than 30 degrees. *Sliding down in bed can produce a* ***shearing force*** *(the effect that moves layers of tissue in opposite directions).*
- Provide a balanced diet and adequate fluid intake. *Adequate nutrition maintains and restores cells and keeps tissues hydrated.*

NURSING IMPLICATIONS

Clients with a surgical wound, pressure ulcer, or other type of tissue injury are likely to have one or more of the following nursing diagnoses:

- Acute Pain
- Impaired Skin Integrity
- Ineffective Peripheral Tissue Perfusion
- Impaired Tissue Integrity
- Risk for Infection

Nursing Care Plan 28-1 shows how nurses use the nursing process to care for a client with Impaired Tissue Integrity, defined in the 2012 NANDA-I taxonomy (p. 443) as "damage to mucous membrane, corneal, integumentary, or subcutaneous tissue."

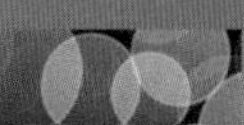

NURSING CARE PLAN 28-1 Impaired Tissue Integrity

Assessment

- Inspect the skin especially over bony prominences.
- Look for skin redness that does not blanch with relief of pressure, evidence of skin tears, or ulceration.
- Observe the client's ability to move and reposition himself or herself independently.
- Assess the status of the client's hydration and nutrition.
- Determine if the client is incontinent or feverish or has other contributing factors to skin and tissue breakdown such as conditions accompanied by edema, those that require the application of devices such as a cast or traction, or treatments that increase the potential for impairment of the integument such as radiation cancer therapy.

Nursing Diagnosis. **Impaired Tissue Integrity** related to unrelieved pressure secondary to immobility from a spinal cord injury at the C7 (7th cervical vertebrae) level 2 years ago as manifested by stage III pressure ulcer over the coccyx and a stage I ulcer over the bilateral heels and elbows.

Expected Outcome. The tissue integrity in the area of the coccygeal pressure sore will be restored as evidenced by the development of granulation tissue around the circumference of the wound by 8/30 and closure by 10/1. The elbows and heels will blanch with pressure relief by 8/18.

Interventions	Rationales
Reposition the client every 2 hours until an air-fluidized bed can be obtained.	Frequent repositioning maintains capillary pressure above 32 mm Hg to facilitate the oxygenation of tissue.
Avoid the supine and Fowler's positions as much as possible.	These positions increase the potential for shear forces and pressure over bony prominences on posterior body areas such as the coccyx, shoulders, and heels.
After bathing, spray heels and elbows with Bard Barrier Film.	Skin products, such as Bard Barrier Film, form a clear, breathable film that is impervious to liquids and potential irritants and protects against skin abrasion and friction.
Until the results of wound culture are obtained, care for the open coccygeal wound as follows: • Mix the antimicrobial solution with water and cleanse the wound. • Rinse with normal saline. • Pack the wound loosely with a continuous strip of gauze moistened with normal saline. • Cover with an abdominal pad. • Repeat above routine every 4 hours as the packing becomes dry.	An antimicrobial reduces the transient and resident microorganisms that can increase the extent and severity of the pressure sore and delay healing. Packing the wound with moist gauze is a form of mechanical debridement that removes devitalized tissue and promotes granulation of the wound.
If wound culture is negative for pathogens: • Eliminate wet-to-dry dressing. • Clean, dry, and cover wound with transparent dressing (Op-Site) and leave in place for 5 days. • If drainage collects, pierce Op-Site and aspirate fluid from underneath. Seal the opened area with a small reinforcement of Op-Site over the punctured area.	A transparent dressing creates a moist environment that accelerates the healing process. Accumulation of fluid beneath the dressing increases the potential for loosening the wound cover. The aspiration of fluid through the dressing reduces fluid volume. Sealing the puncture area restores the occlusive nature of the dressing without the need to replace it.
Measure the open pressure sore every 3 days (8/18, 8/21, etc.) during the day shift.	Regular assessment of the wound helps to determine the need to continue or revise the plan for wound care.

Evaluation of Expected Outcomes

- Pressure ulcer in area of coccyx measures 2 × 3 × 1/2 in. on 8/18 with 1/16 in. of granulation tissue around the circumference of the wound.
- Heels and elbows no longer appear red.

CRITICAL THINKING EXERCISES

1. What nursing assessments would be evident to suggest that a wound is healing?

2. A nurse notes that the gauze dressing that covers a wound comes loose repeatedly. What measures could a nurse take?

3. Describe the wound care appropriate for a client with a stage I pressure ulcer, one with an abdominal incision, and one with a peripheral intravenous infusion site.

4. A 75-year-old client is admitted from a nursing home to have surgery to repair a fractured hip. Discuss the factors that may threaten this client's wound healing.

NCLEX-STYLE REVIEW QUESTIONS

1. Which of the following body positions will promote wound drainage from an abdominal incision with an open drain?
1. Lithotomy
2. Fowler's
3. Recumbent
4. Trendelenburg

2. When the nurse changes a client's dressing, which nursing action is correct?
1. The nurse removes the soiled dressing with sterile gloves.
2. The nurse frees the tape by pulling it away from the incision.
3. The nurse encloses the soiled dressing within a latex glove.
4. The nurse cleans the wound in circles toward the incision.

3. When a nurse empties the drainage in a Jackson-Pratt reservoir, which nursing action is essential for reestablishing the negative pressure within this drainage device?
1. The nurse compresses the bulb reservoir and closes the vent.
2. The nurse opens the vent, allowing the bulb to fill with air.
3. The nurse fills the bulb reservoir with sterile normal saline.
4. The nurse secures the bulb reservoir to the skin near the wound.

4. Which one of the following explanations is best when a client asks why the nurse is applying wet-to-dry dressings over a skin ulcer?
1. "These dressings help to prevent wound infections."
2. "These dressings help to remove dead cells and debris."
3. "These dressings help to absorb blood and drainage."
4. "These dressings help to protect the skin from injury."

5. Which of the following is the best evidence that a Stage III pressure ulcer is healing?
1. The size becomes smaller and there is more drainage.
2. The size becomes smaller and there is less discomfort.
3. The size becomes smaller and the edges appear pink.
4. The size becomes smaller with a gap under the wound margin.

SKILL 28-1 Changing a Gauze Dressing

Suggested Action	Reason for Action
ASSESSMENT	
Inspect the current dressing for drainage, integrity, and type of dressing supplies used.	Provides assessments indicating a need to change the dressing and supplies that may be needed.
Check the medical orders for a directive to change the dressing.	Shows collaboration with the prescribed medical treatment.
Determine if the client has allergies to tape or antimicrobial wound agents.	Helps to determine the dressing supplies to use.
Assess the client's level of pain and its characteristics.	Determines if analgesia will be beneficial before changing the dressing.
PLANNING	
Explain the need and technique for changing the dressing.	Relieves anxiety and promotes cooperation.
Consult the client on a preferred time for the dressing change if there is no immediate need for it.	Empowers the client to participate in decision making.
Give pain medication, if needed, 15–30 minutes before the dressing change.	Allows time for medication absorption and effectiveness.
Gather the necessary supplies, which are likely to include a paper bag for the soiled dressing, clean and sterile gloves, individually packaged gauze dressings, tape, and, in some cases, an antimicrobial agent such as povidone-iodine swabs for wound cleansing.	Facilitates organization and efficient time management.
IMPLEMENTATION	
Wash your hands or use an alcohol-based hand rub (see Chap. 10).	Reduces the transmission of microorganisms.
Pull the privacy curtain.	Shows respect for the client's dignity.
Position the client to allow access to the dressing.	Facilitates comfort and dexterity.
Drape the client to expose the area of the wound.	Ensures modesty but facilitates care.
Loosen the tape securing the dressing; pull the tape toward the wound (Fig. A).	Facilitates removal without separating the healing wound.

A

Loosen the tape. (Photo by B. Proud.)

(continued)

Changing a Gauze Dressing (continued)

IMPLEMENTATION (CONTINUED)

Don at least one glove and lift the dressing from the wound (Fig. B).
Provides a barrier against contact with blood and body substances.

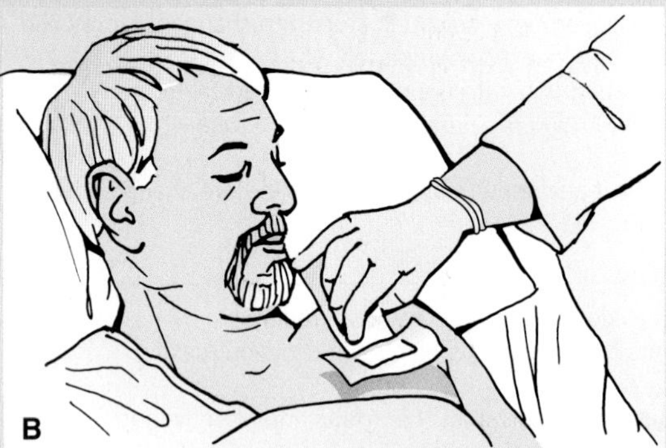

B Remove the dressing.

Moisten the gauze with sterile normal saline if it adheres to the wound.
Prevents the disrupting of granulation tissue.

Discard the soiled dressing in a paper bag or other receptacle along with the glove(s) (Fig. C).
Confines the sources of pathogens.

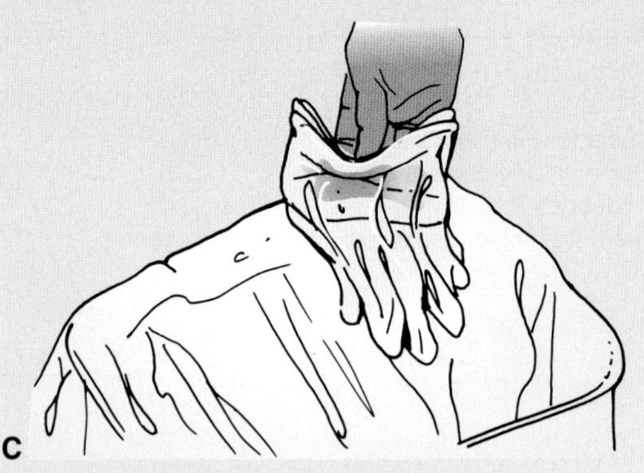

C Dispose of the dressing.

Wash your hands again or repeat the alcohol-based hand rub.
Removes transient microorganisms.

Tear several long strips of tape and fold the ends over, forming tabs (Fig D).
Facilitates handling tape later when wearing gloves and eases tape removal during the next dressing change.

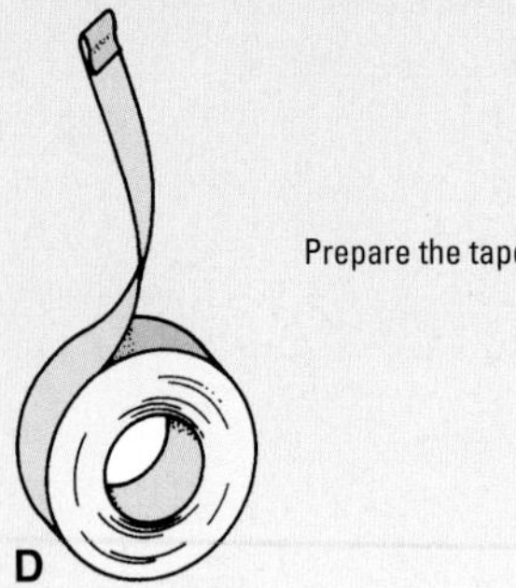

D Prepare the tape.

(continued)

Changing a Gauze Dressing (continued)

IMPLEMENTATION (CONTINUED)

Open sterile supplies using the inside wrapper of one of the gauze dressings as a sterile field, if needed.	Ensures an aseptic technique.
Don sterile gloves.	Ensures sterility.
Inspect the wound.	Provides data for description and comparison.
Cleanse the wound with the antimicrobial agent.	Removes drainage and microorganisms.
Use a technique that prevents transferring microorganisms back to a cleaned area (Fig. E).	Supports principles of medical asepsis.

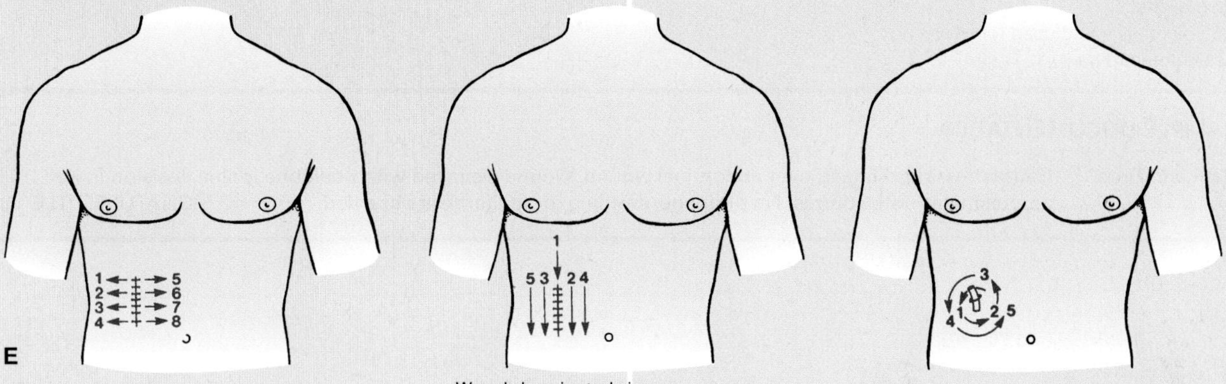

Wound cleansing techniques.

Use a single swab or a small gauze square for each stroke.	Prevents transferring microorganisms to clean areas.
Allow the antimicrobial agent to dry.	Ensures that the tape will stay secured when applied.
Cover the wound with the gauze dressing (Fig. F).	Protects the wound.

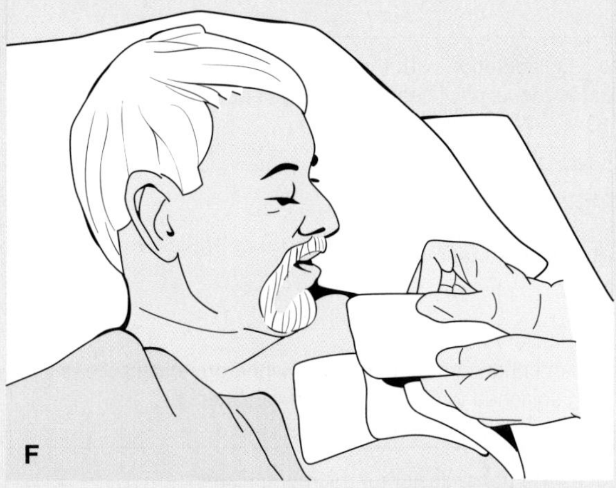

Apply the dressing.

Secure the dressing with tape in the opposite direction of the incision or across a joint. Place a strip of tape at each end of the dressing and in the middle if needed (Fig. G).	Prevents loosening with activity; holds the dressing in place without exposing the wound or incision.

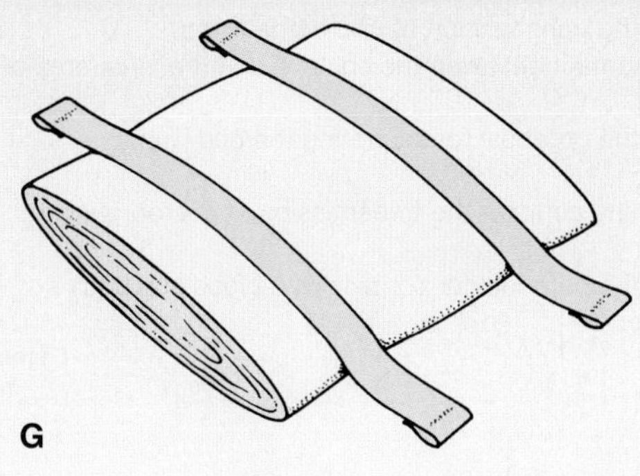

Position the tape.

(continued)

Changing a Gauze Dressing (continued)

IMPLEMENTATION (CONTINUED)	
Remove and discard gloves.	Confines the sources of microorganisms.
Rewash hands or repeat the alcohol-based hand rub.	Removes transient microorganisms.
Evaluation	
• Dressing covers the entire wound. • Dressing is secure, dry, and intact.	
Document	
• Type of dressing • Antimicrobial agent used for cleansing • Assessment data	

SAMPLE DOCUMENTATION

Date and Time Gauze dressing changed over abdominal wound. Wound cleansed with povidone iodine. Incision is well approximated with sutures. No drainage, swelling, or tenderness observed. ——— SIGNATURE/TITLE

SKILL 28-2 Irrigating a Wound

Suggested Action	Reason for Action
ASSESSMENT	
Check the medical orders for a directive to irrigate the wound.	Shows collaboration with the prescribed medical treatment.
Determine how much the client understands about the procedure.	Indicates the level of health teaching needed.
PLANNING	
Plan to irrigate the wound at the same time that the dressing requires changing.	Makes efficient use of time.
Gather the equipment required, which is likely to include a container of solution, a basin, a bulb or asepto syringe, gloves, and absorbent material including a towel to dry the skin.	Facilitates organization.
Bring supplies for changing the dressing.	Makes efficient use of time.
Consider additional items for standard precautions such as goggles or face shield and cover apron or gown.	Follows infection control guidelines when there is a potential for being splashed with blood or body substances.
IMPLEMENTATION	
Wash your hands or use an alcohol-based hand rub (see Chap. 10).	Reduces the transmission of microorganisms.
Pull the privacy curtain.	Shows respect for the client's dignity.
Drape the client to expose the area of the wound.	Ensures modesty but facilitates care.
Follow directions in Skill 28-1 for removing the dressing.	Provides access to the wound.
Wash your hands or repeat the alcohol-based hand rub.	Reduces the transmission of microorganisms.
Position the client to facilitate filling the wound cavity with solution.	Ensures contact between the solution and the inner area of the wound.
Pad the bed with absorbent material and place an emesis basin adjacent to and below the wound.	Reduces the potential for saturating the bed linens
Open and prepare supplies following the principles of surgical asepsis.	Confines and controls the transmission of microorganisms.
Don gloves and other standard precautions apparel.	Reduces the potential for contact with blood and body substances.

(continued)

Irrigating a Wound (continued)

IMPLEMENTATION (CONTINUED)

Fill the syringe with solution and instill it into the wound without touching the wound directly (Fig. A).
Dilutes and loosens debris.

A

Instill the irrigant.

Hold the emesis basin close to the client's body to catch the solution as it drains from the wound (Fig. B).
Collects and contains the irrigating solution.

B

Position the client to drain the irrigant.

Repeat the process until the draining solution seems clear.
Indicates the evacuation of debris.

Tilt the client toward the basin.
Drains the remaining solution from the wound.

Dry the skin.
Facilitates applying a dressing.

Dispose of the drained solution, soiled equipment, and linens.
Reduces the potential for transmitting microorganisms.

Remove gloves, wash hands, and prepare to change the dressing.
Provides for the absorption of residual solution and coverage of the wound.

Evaluation

- Irrigation solution shows evidence of debris removal.
- Wound shows evidence of healing.

Document

- Assessment data
- Type and amount of solution
- Outcome of procedure

SAMPLE DOCUMENTATION

Date and Time Dressing removed. Moderate purulent drainage on soiled dressing. Wound is separated 3 inches. Approximately 300 mL of sterile NSS instilled within wound. Drained solution is cloudy with particles of debris.
———————————————— SIGNATURE/TITLE

SKILL 28-3 Providing a Sitz Bath

Suggested Action	Reason for Action
ASSESSMENT	
Check the medical orders for a directive to administer a sitz bath.	Shows collaboration with the prescribed medical treatment.
Determine how much the client understands about the procedure.	Indicates the level of health teaching needed.
Assess the condition of the rectal or perineal wound and the client's level of pain.	Provides baseline data for future comparisons; indicates if pain medication is needed.
PLANNING	
Explain the procedure.	Relieves anxiety and promotes cooperation.
Ask if the client prefers the sitz bath before or after routine hygiene.	Involves the client in the decision-making process.
Obtain disposable equipment unless specially installed tubs are available.	Facilitates organization and efficient time management.
Assemble other supplies such as a bath blanket and towels.	Prepares for maintaining warmth and provides a means for drying the skin.
Inspect and clean the bathroom area or the tub room.	Supports principles of medical asepsis.
Place the basin inside the rim of the raised toilet seat (Fig. A).	Allows for submerging the rectum and the perineum.

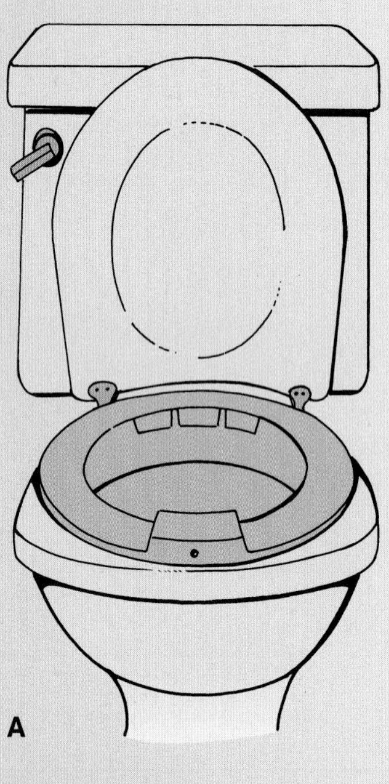

A — Position the sitz bath basin.

Suggested Action	Reason for Action
IMPLEMENTATION	
Wash your hands or use an alcohol-based hand rub (see Chap. 10).	Reduces the transmission of microorganisms.
Help the client don a robe and slippers.	Maintains warmth, safety, and comfort.
Help the client to ambulate to the location where the sitz bath will be administered.	Demonstrates concern for safety.
Shut the door to the bathroom or tub room.	Provides privacy.
Clamp the tubing attached to the water bag.	Prevents a loss of fluid.

(continued)

Providing a Sitz Bath (continued)

IMPLEMENTATION (CONTINUED)

Fill the container with warm water, no hotter than 110°F (43.3°C) (Fig. B). — Provides comfort without the danger of burning the skin.

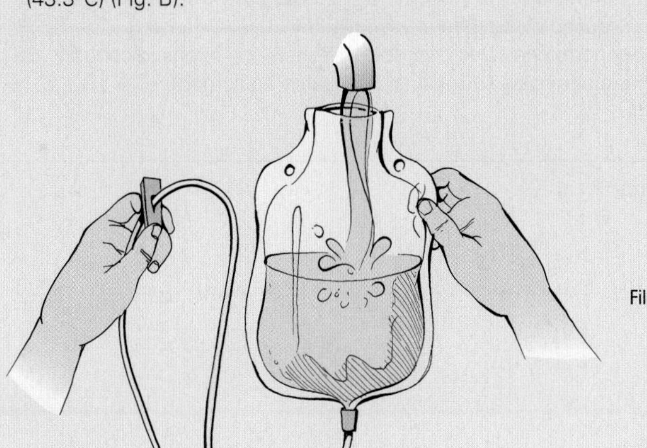

Fill the solution container.

Hang the bag above the toilet seat (Fig. C). — Facilitates gravity flow.

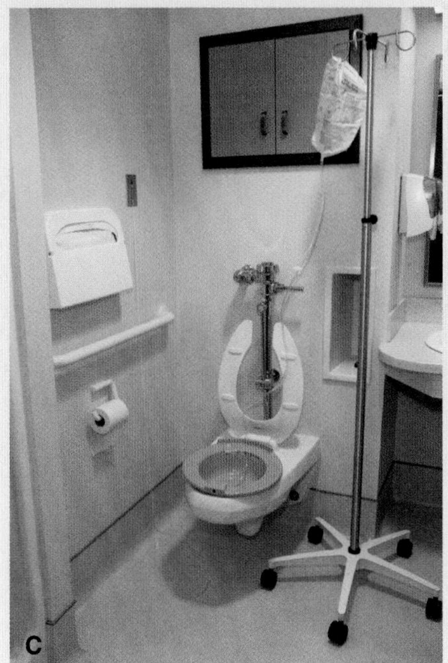

Hang the bag and insert the tubing into the basin.

Insert the tubing from the bag into the front of the basin. — Provides a means for filling the basin.

Help the client to sit on the basin and unclamp the tubing. — Facilitates filling the basin.

Cover the client's shoulders with a bath blanket if the client feels chilled. — Promotes comfort.

Instruct the client on how to signal for assistance. — Ensures safety.

Leave the client alone, but recheck frequently to add more warm water to the reservoir bag. — Provides a sustained application of warm water.

(continued)

Providing a Sitz Bath (continued)

IMPLEMENTATION (CONTINUED)

Help the client pat the skin dry after soaking for 20–30 minutes.	Restores comfort.
Assist the client back to bed.	Ensures safety in case the client feels dizzy from hypotension caused by peripheral vasodilation.
Don gloves and clean the disposable equipment and bath area.	Supports principles of medical asepsis and infection control.
Replace the sitz bath equipment in the client's bedside cabinet or leave it in the client's private bathroom.	Reduces costs by reusing disposable equipment.

Evaluation

- A sitz bath is administered according to the agency's policy or standards of care.
- Safety is maintained.
- The client reports that symptoms are relieved.

Document

- Procedure
- Response of the client
- Assessment data

SAMPLE DOCUMENTATION

Date and Time Sitz bath provided over 30 minutes. Client states, "I always feel so good after this treatment." Perineum is slightly swollen. Margins of episiotomy are approximated. Continues to have moderate bloody vaginal drainage. ——— SIGNATURE/TITLE

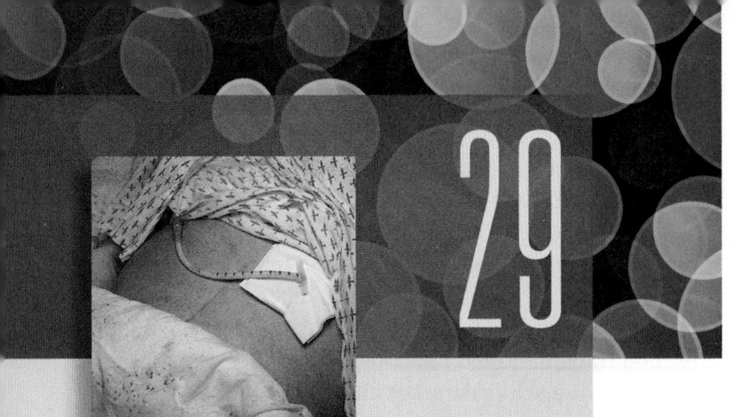

29 Gastrointestinal Intubation

Words To Know

bolus feeding
continuous feeding
cyclic feeding
decompression
dumping syndrome
enteral nutrition
gastric reflux
gastric residual
gastrostomy tube (G-tube)
gavage
intermittent feeding
intestinal decompression
intubation
jejunostomy tube (J-tube)
lavage
lumen
nasogastric intubation
nasogastric tube
nasointestinal intubation
nasointestinal tubes
NEX measurement
orogastric intubation
orogastric tube
ostomy
percutaneous endoscopic gastrostomy (PEG) tube
percutaneous endoscopic jejunostomy (PEJ) tube
stylet
sump tubes
tamponade
transabdominal tubes

Learning Objectives

On completion of this chapter, the reader should be able to:

1. Define intubation and list reasons for gastrointestinal intubation.
2. Identify four general types of gastrointestinal tubes.
3. Name at least four assessments that are necessary before inserting a tube nasally.
4. Explain the purpose of and how to obtain a NEX measurement.
5. Describe three techniques for checking distal placement in the stomach.
6. Discuss three ways that nasointestinal feeding tubes or their insertion differ from their gastric counterparts.
7. Name four schedules for administering tube feedings.
8. Explain the purpose of assessing gastric residual.
9. Name five nursing activities involved in managing the care of clients who are being tube-fed.
10. Name two nursing responsibilities for assisting with the insertion of a tungsten-weighted intestinal decompression tube.

Clients, especially those undergoing abdominal or gastrointestinal (GI) surgery, may require some type of tube placed within their stomach or intestine. The use of a gastric or intestinal tube reduces or eliminates problems associated with surgery or conditions affecting the GI tract, such as impaired peristalsis, vomiting, or gas accumulation. Tubes also can be used to nourish clients who cannot eat. This chapter discusses the multiple uses for gastric and intestinal tubes and the nursing guidelines and skills for managing related client care.

INTUBATION

Intubation generally means the placement of a tube into a body structure; in this chapter, it refers specifically to insertion of a tube into the stomach or intestine by way of the mouth or nose. **Orogastric intubation** (the insertion of a tube through the mouth into the stomach), **nasogastric intubation** (the insertion of a tube through the nose into the stomach; Fig. 29-1), and **nasointestinal intubation** (the insertion of a tube through the nose to the intestine) are performed to remove gas or fluids or to administer liquid nourishment.

A tube also may be inserted within an **ostomy** (a surgically created opening). A prefix identifies the anatomic site of the ostomy; for instance, a *gastrostomy* is an artificial opening into the stomach.

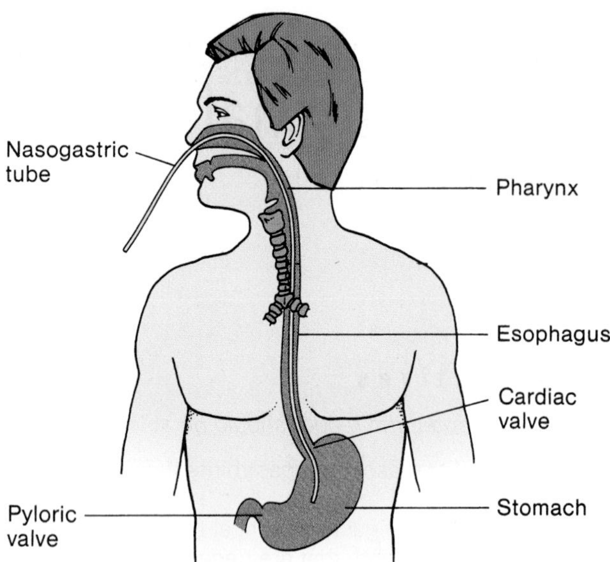

FIGURE 29-1 The nasogastric intubation pathway.

Gastric or intestinal tubes are used for a variety of reasons, including the following:

- Performing a **gavage** (providing nourishment)
- Administering oral medications that the client cannot swallow
- Obtaining a sample of secretions for diagnostic testing
- Performing a **lavage** (removing substances from the stomach, typically poisons)
- Promoting **decompression** (removing gas and liquid contents from the stomach or bowel)
- Controlling gastric bleeding, a process called compression or **tamponade** (pressure)

TYPES OF TUBES

Although all gastric and intestinal tubes have a proximal and distal end, their size, construction, and composition vary according to their use (Table 29-1). The outside diameter of most tubes is measured using the French scale, indicated by a number followed by the letter F. Each number on the French scale equals approximately 0.33 mm. The larger the number, the larger the diameter of the tube.

Tubes can be identified according to the location of their insertion (mouth, nose, or abdomen) or the location of their distal end (stomach [gastric] or intestinal).

Orogastric Tubes

An **orogastric tube** (a tube inserted through the mouth into the stomach), such as an Ewald tube, is used in an emergency to remove toxic substances that have been ingested. The diameter of the tube is large enough to remove pill fragments and stomach debris. Because of its size, the tube is introduced through the mouth rather than the nose.

Nasogastric Tubes

A **nasogastric tube** (a tube placed through the nose and advanced to the stomach) is smaller in diameter than an orogastric tube but larger and shorter than a nasointestinal tube. Some nasogastric tubes have more than one **lumen** (channel) within the tube.

A Levin tube is a commonly used, single-lumen gastric tube with multiple uses, one of which is decompression. Gastric **sump tubes** (double-lumen tubes) are used almost exclusively to remove fluid and gas from the stomach (Fig. 29-2). The second lumen serves as a vent. The use of sump tubes decreases the possibility that the stomach wall will adhere to and obstruct the drainage openings when suction is applied.

Because nasogastric tubes remain in place for several days or more, many clients complain of nose and throat discomfort. If the tube's diameter is too large or pressure from the tube is prolonged, tissue irritation or breakdown may occur. Furthermore, gastric tubes tend to dilate the esophageal sphincter also known as the cardiac valve, a circular muscle between the esophagus and stomach. The stretched

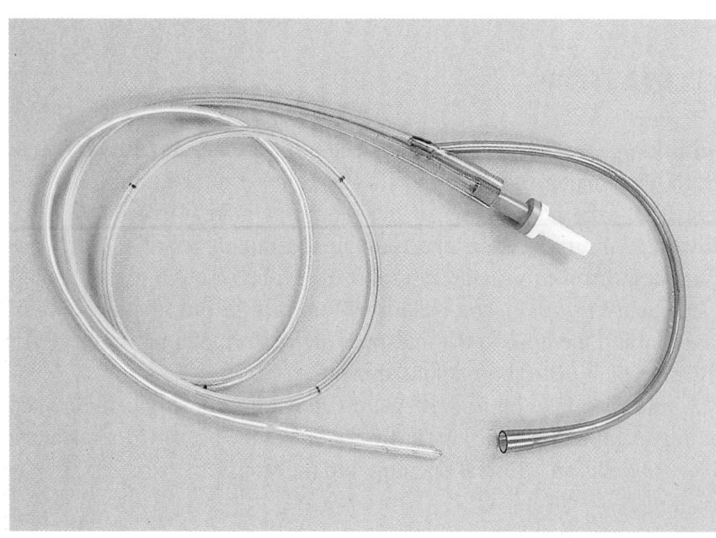

FIGURE 29-2 Vented nasogastric (Salem sump) tube with a one-way valve. (Photo by B. Proud.)

TABLE 29-1 Types of Gastrointestinal Tubes

TUBE	PURPOSE	CHARACTERISTICS
Orogastric		
Ewald	Lavage	• Large diameter: 36–40 F • Single lumen • Multiple distal openings for drainage
Nasogastric		
Levin	Lavage Gavage Decompression Diagnostics	• Usual adult size 14–18 F • Single lumen • 42–50 in. (107–127 cm) long • Multiple drain openings
Salem sump	Decompression	• Same diameter as Levin • Double lumen • Pigtail vent • 48 in. (122 cm) long • Marked at increments to indicate depth of insertion • Radiopaque
Sengstaken–Blakemore	Compression Drainage	• Usual diameter: 20 F • 36 in. (90 cm) long • Triple lumen; two lead to balloons in the esophagus and stomach and the third is for removing gastric drainage; a fourth lumen may be used to remove pharyngeal secretions
Nasointestinal		
Keofeed	Gavage	• Small diameter: 8 F • 36 in. (90 cm) long • Polyurethane or silicone • Weighted tip • Extremely flexible and may require the use of a stylet during insertion • Radiopaque • Bonded lubricant that becomes activated with moisture
Maxter	Intestinal decompression	• Usual size: 18 F • 100 in. (250 cm) long • Double lumen • Tungsten-weighted tip • Graduated marks every 10 in. (25 cm)
Transabdominal		
Gastrostomy	Gavage; may be used for decompression while the client is fed through a jejunostomy tube	• Sizes 12–24 F for adults • Rubber or silicone • May have additional side ports for balloon inflation to maintain placement • May be capped or plugged between feedings • Radiopaque
Jejunostomy	Gavage	• Sizes 5–14 F for adults • Silicone or polyurethane • Radiopaque

opening may contribute to **gastric reflux** (the reverse flow of gastric contents), especially when the tube is used to administer liquid formula. If gastric reflux occurs, the liquid could enter the airway and interfere with respiratory function.

Nasointestinal Tubes

Nasointestinal tubes (tubes inserted through the nose for distal placement below the stomach) are longer than their gastric counterparts. The added length permits them to be placed in the small bowel. They are used to provide nourishment (feeding tubes) or to remove gas and liquid contents from the small intestine (decompression tubes).

Feeding Tubes

Nasointestinal tubes used for nutrition, such as a Keofeed tube, are usually small in diameter and made of a flexible substance such as polyurethane or silicone. Their narrow width and soft composition allow them to remain in the same nostril for 4 weeks or longer. In addition, they reduce the potential for gastric reflux because they deliver liquid nutrition beyond the stomach.

Narrow tubes are not problem free. They tend to curl during insertion because they are so flexible. Therefore, some are supplied with a **stylet** (metal guidewire) that helps straighten and support them during insertion. Almost all

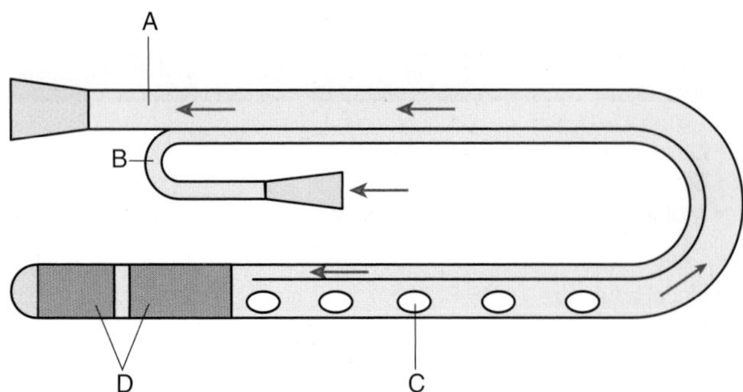

FIGURE 29-3 An intestinal decompression tube, (**A**) including the suction lumen, (**B**) the vent lumen, (**C**) openings for suction, (**D**) and the radiopaque tungsten tip.

have a weighted tip that helps them descend past the stomach. Checking the placement of the distal end is more difficult; these tubes also become obstructed more easily.

Despite the problems associated with maintenance, small-diameter tubes are preferred for their comfort. They are ideal for providing a continuous infusion of nourishment.

Intestinal Decompression Tubes

Although surgery is often the most common intervention when a client has a partial or complete bowel obstruction, **intestinal decompression** (the removal of gas and intestinal contents) also may be used. A tube used for intestinal decompression has a double lumen and a weighted tip (Fig. 29-3). One lumen is used to suction the intestinal contents; the other acts as a vent to reduce suction-induced trauma to intestinal tissue. The weighted tip and peristalsis, if present, propel the tube beyond the stomach and into the intestine. The progress of the radiopaque tip through the GI tract is monitored by X-ray.

At one time, intestinal tubes, such as the Cantor and Miller-Abbott tubes, were weighted with mercury. Because of mercury's hazards to both the client and the environment, however, mercury-weighted tubes are not used today. Instead, intestinal tubes, like the Maxter tube (see Table 29-1), are now weighted with tungsten.

Transabdominal Tubes

Transabdominal tubes (tubes placed through the abdominal wall) provide access to various parts of the GI tract. Two examples are a **gastrostomy tube** or G-tube (a transabdominal tube located within the stomach) and a **jejunostomy tube** or J-tube (a transabdominal tube that leads to the jejunum of the small intestine).

A G-tube is placed surgically or with the use of an endoscope. A surgically inserted G-tube resembles a long rubber catheter sutured to the abdomen. A **percutaneous endoscopic gastrostomy (PEG) tube** (a transabdominal tube inserted under endoscopic guidance) is anchored with internal and external crossbars called bumpers (Fig. 29-4A).

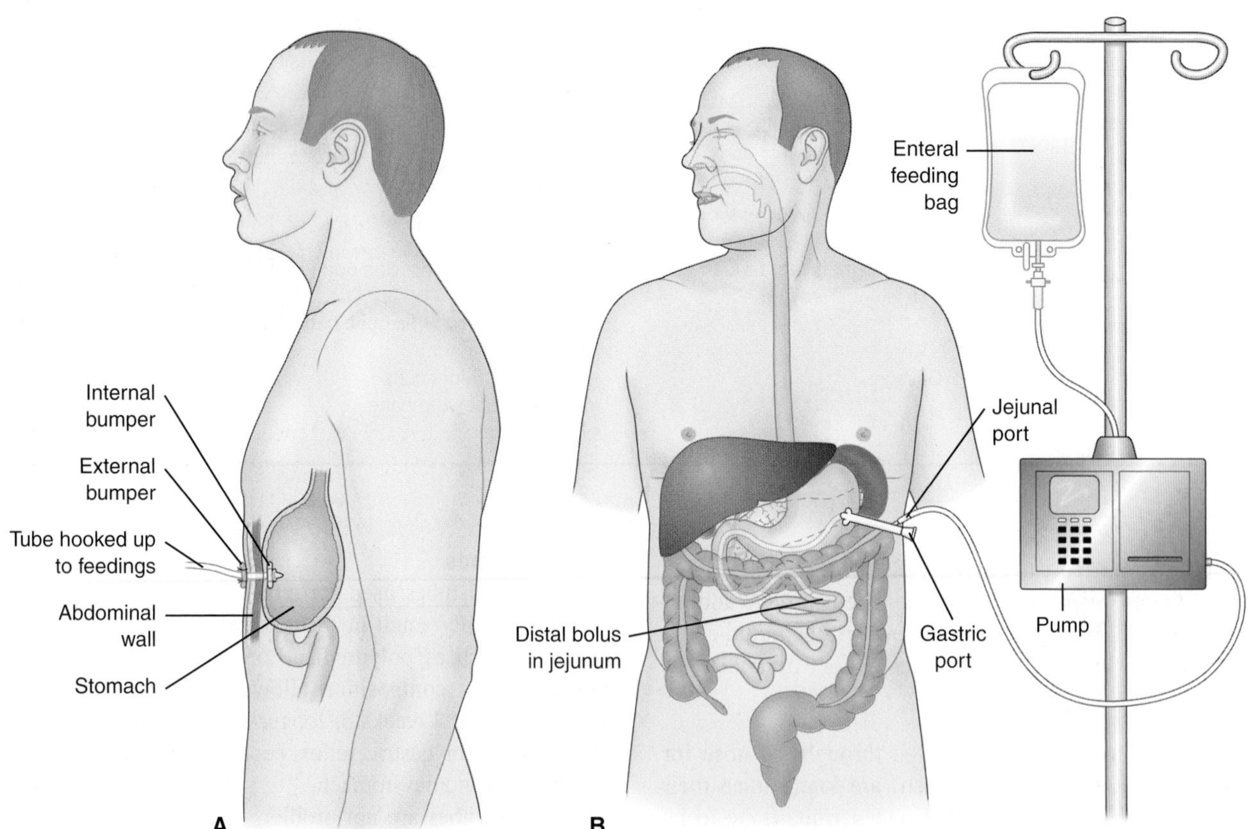

FIGURE 29-4 Transabdominal tubes. **A.** A percutaneous endoscopic gastrostomy (PEG) tube. **B.** A percutaneous endoscopic jejunostomy (PEJ) tube. (Courtesy of IVAC Corporation, San Diego, CA.)

A **percutaneous endoscopic jejunostomy (PEJ) tube** (a tube that is passed through a PEG tube into the jejunum) is small in diameter so that it can be inserted through the larger PEG tube (see Fig. 29-4B).

Transabdominal tubes are used instead of nasogastric or nasointestinal tubes when clients require an alternative to oral feeding for more than 1 month.

NASOGASTRIC TUBE MANAGEMENT

Usually, nurses insert nasogastric tubes. Additional nursing responsibilities include keeping the tube patent (or unobstructed), implementing the prescribed use, and removing the tube when it has accomplished its therapeutic purpose.

Insertion

Inserting a nasogastric tube involves preparing the client, conducting preintubation assessments, and placing the tube.

Client Preparation

Most clients are anxious about having to swallow a tube. Suggesting that the diameter of the tube is smaller than most pieces of food may foster a positive outcome. Explaining the procedure and giving instructions on how the client can assist while the tube is being passed may further reduce anxiety. One of the most important ways to support clients is to provide them with some means of control. The nurse can establish with the client a signal, such as the client raising a hand, to indicate the need for a pause during the tube's passage.

Preintubation Assessment

Before insertion, the nurse conducts a focused assessment that includes the client's:

- Level of consciousness
- Weight
- Bowel sounds
- Abdominal distention
- Integrity of nasal and oral mucosa
- Ability to swallow, cough, and gag
- Any nausea and vomiting

Assessment findings serve as a baseline for future comparisons and may suggest a need to modify the procedure or the equipment used. One main goal of the assessment is to determine which nostril is best to use when inserting the tube and the length to which the tube will be inserted.

Nasal Inspection

After the client clears nasal debris by blowing into a paper tissue, the nurse inspects each nostril for size, shape, and patency. The client should exhale while each nostril in turn is occluded. The presence of nasal polyps (small growths of tissue), a deviated septum (nasal cartilage deflected from the midline of the nose), or a narrow nasal passage excludes a nostril for tube insertion.

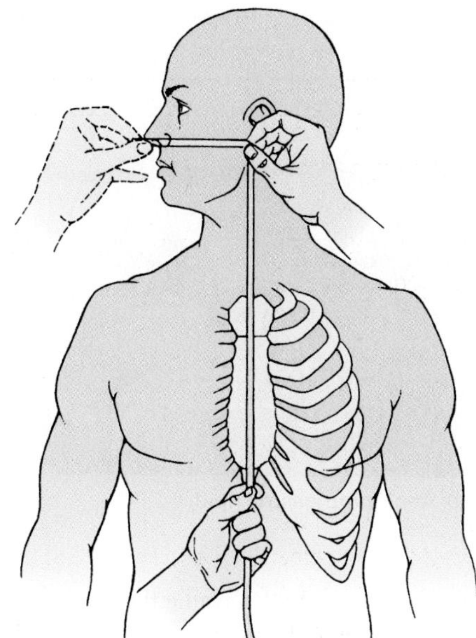

FIGURE 29-5 Obtaining the NEX measurement.

Tube Measurement. Some tubes are already marked to indicate the approximate length at which the distal tip will be located within the stomach. These markings, however, may not correlate exactly with the client's anatomy. Therefore, before inserting a tube, the nurse obtains the client's **NEX measurement** (length from Nose to Earlobe to the Xiphoid process [tip of the sternum]; Fig. 29-5) and marks the tube appropriately.

The first mark on the tube is made at the measured distance from the nose to the earlobe. It indicates the distance to the nasal pharynx–a location that places the tip at the back of the throat but above where the gag reflex is stimulated. A second mark is made at the point where the tube reaches the xiphoid process, indicating the depth required to reach the stomach.

Tube Placement

When inserting a nasogastric tube, the nurse's primary concerns are to cause as little discomfort as possible, to preserve the integrity of the nasal tissue, and to locate the tube within the stomach, not in the respiratory passages.

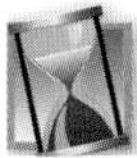

Gerontologic Considerations

- An age-related reduction in the number of laryngeal nerve endings contributes to diminished efficiency of the gag reflex. Other conditions that depress the gag reflex include neurologic disorders such as dementia and strokes and the repeated insertion and removal of dentures.

Once the tube is at its final mark, the nurse must verify the location within the stomach. The physical assessment

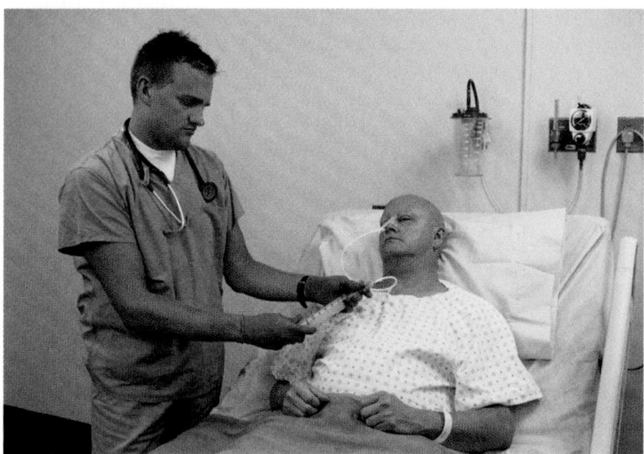

FIGURE 29-6 Aspirating gastric fluid.

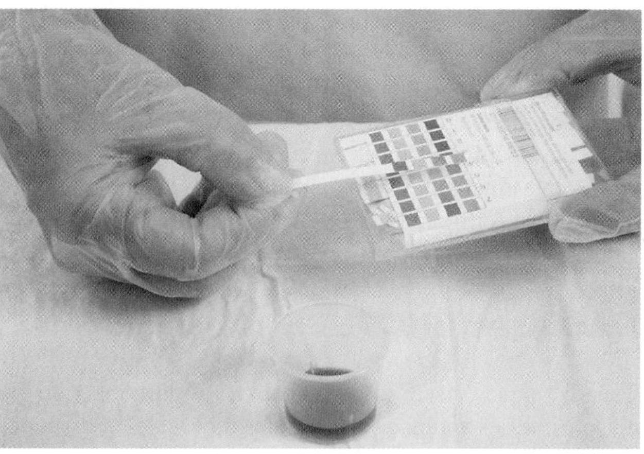

FIGURE 29-7 Checking the pH.

methods that nurses use to determine the distal location of a nasogastric tube are as follows:

- Aspirating fluid: If aspirated fluid appears clear, brownish-yellow, or green, the nurse can presume that its source is the stomach (Fig. 29-6).
- Auscultating the abdomen: The nurse instills 10 mL or more of air while listening with a stethoscope over the abdomen. If a swooshing sound is heard, the nurse can infer that the cause was air entering the stomach. Belching often indicates that the tip is still in the esophagus.
- Testing the pH of aspirated liquid: The first two techniques provide only presumptive signs that the tube is in the stomach; testing pH confirms acidic gastric contents. Other than obtaining an abdominal X-ray, the pH test is the most accurate technique for checking tube placement (see Nursing Guidelines 29-1 and Fig. 29-7).

Once the nurse has confirmed stomach placement (using two methods is best), he or she secures the tube to avoid upward or downward migration (Fig. 29-8). The tube is then ready to use for its intended purpose. The steps to follow when inserting a nasogastric tube are outlined in Skill 29-1.

Stop, Think, and Respond Box 29-1

Discuss the consequences of inserting a nasogastric tube into the respiratory passages.

Use and Maintenance

Nasogastric tubes are connected to suction for gastric decompression or are used for tube feeding.

Gastric Decompression

Suction is either continuous or intermittent. Continuous suctioning with an unvented tube can cause the tube to adhere to the stomach mucosa, resulting in localized irritation and interfering with drainage. Using a vented tube or intermittent suction prevents or minimizes these effects.

The tube is connected to a wall outlet or portable suction machine (Fig. 29-9). The suction setting is prescribed by the physician or indicated in the agency's standards for care. Usually low pressure (40 to 60 mm Hg) is used.

The tube is clamped or plugged during ambulation or after instilling medications (see Chap. 32).

Promoting Patency

Even with intermittent suctioning, the tube may become obstructed. Giving ice chips or occasional sips of water to

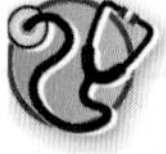

NURSING GUIDELINES 29-1

Assessing the pH of Aspirated Fluid

- Wash hands or perform an alcohol-based hand rub (see Chap. 10). *Hand hygiene reduces the transmission of microorganisms.*
- Don gloves. *They provide a physical barrier between the nurse's hands and body fluids.*
- Aspirate a small volume of fluid from the tube with a clean syringe. *Doing so ensures valid test results.*
- Drop a sample of gastric fluid onto an indicator strip. *This step initiates a chemical reaction on contact and saturation.*
- Compare the color on the test strip with the color guide on the container of reagent strips (see Fig. 29-7). *The color of the test strip changes according to the hydrogen ion concentration of the liquid. Stomach fluid usually has a pH of 1 to 3—very acid on the pH scale. If the pH is 5 or 6, the client may be receiving medications to decrease gastric acidity or the fluid may be from the duodenum. A pH of 7 or greater indicates that the tube is in the respiratory tract.*

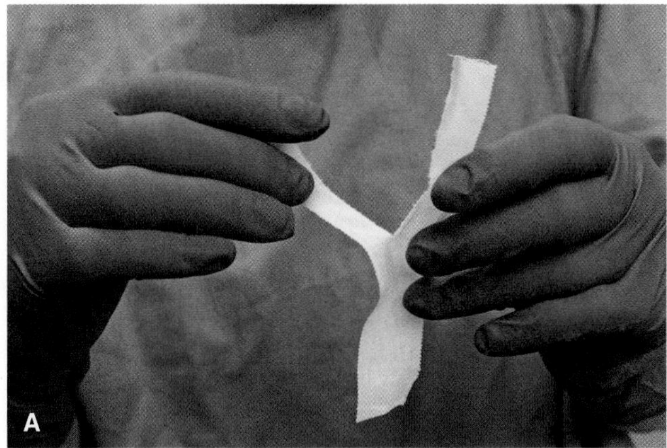

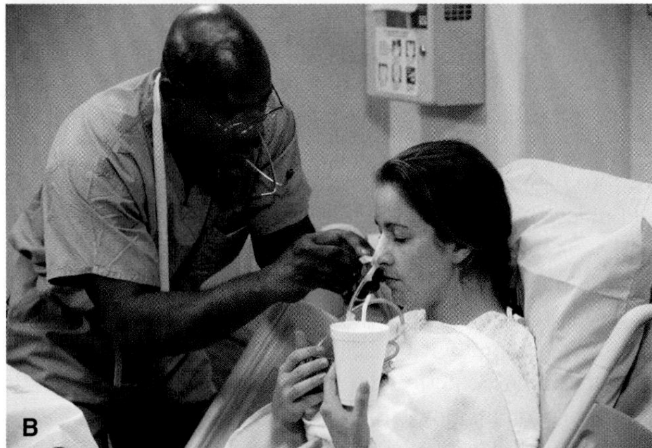

FIGURE 29-8 A. One end of a piece of tape is split, forming two narrower strips, and the opposite end is left intact. B. The wider intact end of the tape is applied to the nose, and the narrower strips are wound around the tube in opposite directions to secure the nasogastric tube.

a client who is otherwise NPO (receives nothing by mouth) promotes tube patency. The fluid helps dilute the gastric secretions. Both must be given sparingly, however, because water is hypotonic and draws electrolytes into the gastric fluid. Because the diluted fluid is ultimately removed, giving the client liberal amounts of water can deplete serum electrolytes (see Chap. 16).

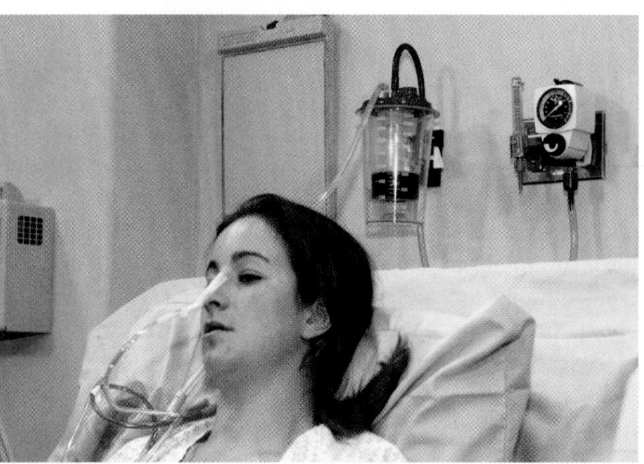

FIGURE 29-9 Suction removes liquids and gas from the stomach.

Restoring Patency

The nurse assesses tube patency frequently by monitoring the volume and characteristics of drainage and observing for signs and symptoms suggesting an obstruction (nausea, vomiting, and abdominal distention). Inspection of the equipment helps to identify possible causes for the assessment findings (Table 29-2). Once the cause is identified, a variety of simple nursing interventions can resolve it. Sometimes the nasogastric tube must be irrigated to maintain or restore patency (Skill 29-2). The nurse must obtain a medical order before attempting an irrigation.

Stop, Think, and Respond Box 29-2

Explain the reason for using an isotonic saline solution, rather than a hypotonic or hypertonic solution, to irrigate a nasogastric tube.

Enteral Nutrition

Enteral nutrition (nourishment provided through the stomach or small intestine rather than by the oral route) is delivered by instilling formula through a tube. Although a nasogastric tube can be used, it is more likely that liquid formula will be administered through a nasointestinal or transabdominal tube. Both are discussed later in this chapter.

TABLE 29-2 Troubleshooting a Poorly Draining Nasogastric Tube

POSSIBLE CAUSES	SOLUTIONS
The drainage holes are adhering to the gastric mucosal wall.	Turn the suction off momentarily. Change the client's position.
The tube is displaced above the esophageal sphincter.	If the measured mark is not at the tip of the nose, remove the tape, advance the tube, check placement, and resecure.
The portable suction machine is disconnected or turned off.	Replace the plug into the electrical outlet or turn on power.
The drainage container is filled beyond capacity.	Empty and record the amount of drainage in the suction container.
The vent is acting as a siphon.	Instill a bolus of air into the vent to restore patency.
The vent is capped or plugged.	Remove the cap and restore the port to atmospheric pressure.
The tubing is kinked or disconnected.	Straighten tubing or reconnect to the suction machine.
The suction is inadequate.	Check that the pressure is 40–60 mm Hg.
The cover on the suction container is loose.	Resecure the lid to the container.
A solid particle or thick mucus obstructs the lumen.	Increase suction pressure momentarily. Obtain and implement a medical order for an irrigation.

Removal

Nurses remove a nasogastric tube (Skill 29-3) when the client's condition improves, when the tube becomes hopelessly obstructed, or according to the agency's standards for maintaining the integrity of the nasal mucosa. Unobstructed larger diameter tubes usually are removed and changed at least every 2 to 4 weeks for adults. Small-diameter, flexible tubes are removed and changed every 4 weeks to 3 months, depending on the agency's policy. Tubes used for pediatric clients are changed more frequently because the tissue is more fragile and there is a greater potential for infection.

Before permanent removal, some physicians prescribe a trial period during which the tube is clamped and the client is allowed to consume oral fluids. Remaining asymptomatic (ie, no nausea, vomiting, or gastric distention) is a good indication that the client no longer requires intubation. If symptoms develop, the tube is already in place and can be easily reconnected to suction. This practice avoids subjecting the client to the discomfort associated with tube replacement.

Stop, Think, and Respond Box 29-3

If the client who has just had a nasogastric tube removed wants something to eat, what nursing actions are appropriate?

NASOINTESTINAL TUBE MANAGEMENT

Nurses also insert nasointestinal tubes used for enteral feeding.

Insertion

The techniques for client preparation, positioning, and advancement of nasointestinal tubes are similar to those for nasogastric tubes. Some modifications are necessary, however, because nasointestinal tubes are constructed differently.

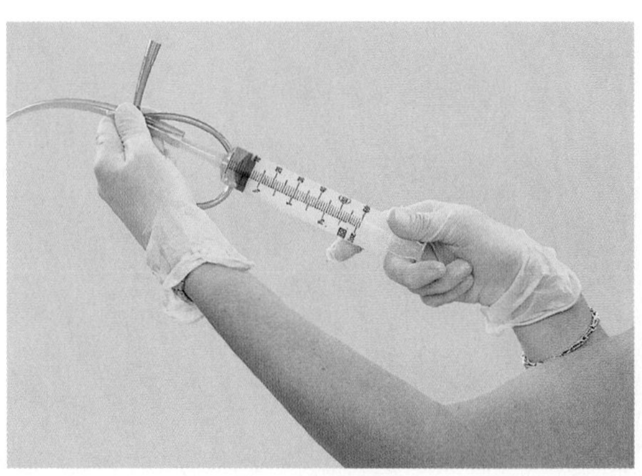

FIGURE 29-10 Aspirating to assess the pH. (Photo by B. Proud.)

To estimate the length of tube required for an intestinal placement, the nurse determines the NEX measurement and adds 9 in. (23 cm). He or she also marks the additional measurement on the tubing (see Nursing Guidelines 29-2 and Figs. 29-10 and 29-11).

New technologies that promise to promote safety and efficacy in nasoenteric tube placement are becoming available. A computer system that uses electromagnetic technology to direct and locate a feeding tube has also been developed. It consists of an electronically modified feeding tube and a receiver that is placed externally over the mid abdomen. A computer then converts the signal into a graphic display. This helps to identify misplacement immediately, and subsequent use eliminates the need for repeated

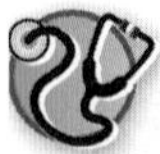

NURSING GUIDELINES 29-2

Inserting a Nasointestinal Feeding Tube

- Wash hands or perform an alcohol-based hand rub (see Chap. 10). *Hand hygiene reduces the transmission of microorganisms.*
- Don gloves. *Gloves provide a physical barrier between the nurse's hands and body fluids.*
- Follow the manufacturer's suggestions for activating the lubricant bonded to the tube. Two common techniques are to instill water through the tube and to immerse the tip in water. *Activation of the lubricant transforms the dry bond to a gelatinous consistency.*
- Secure the stylet within the tube. *This measure stiffens the tube and facilitates insertion.*
- Insert the tube to the second mark. *Doing so places the tube in the presumed area of the stomach.*
- Aspirate fluid using a 50-mL syringe (see Fig. 29-10) and test the fluid pH. *The results provide data for determining gastric placement.*
- Loop the tubing and tape it temporarily to the cheek, if the test for placement suggests that the tip is in the stomach. *Looping provides slack so the tube can descend into the small intestine.*
- Ambulate or position the client on his or her right side for at least 1 hour or the time specified in the agency's policy. *This duration allows the tube to move by gravity through the pyloric valve.*
- Secure the tube at the nose when the third measured mark is at the nasal tip. *This prevents the tube from migrating further than the desired distance.*
- Verify placement by X-ray, especially in unconscious clients or those with a depressed gag reflex. An *X-ray confirms the distal location.*
- Remove the stylet using gentle traction (see Fig. 29-11) or follow the manufacturer's suggestions. *Opening of the lumen allows for the instillation of water and liquid nourishment.*
- Store the stylet in a clean wrapper at the client's bedside. *This measure avoids charging the client for a new tube should the current one need to be removed and reintroduced.*
- Never reinsert the stylet while the tube is in the client. *Reinsertion might cause trauma to the client and damage to the tube.*
- Measure and record the length of tubing extending from the nose. *Documentation provides data for reassessing distal placement.*

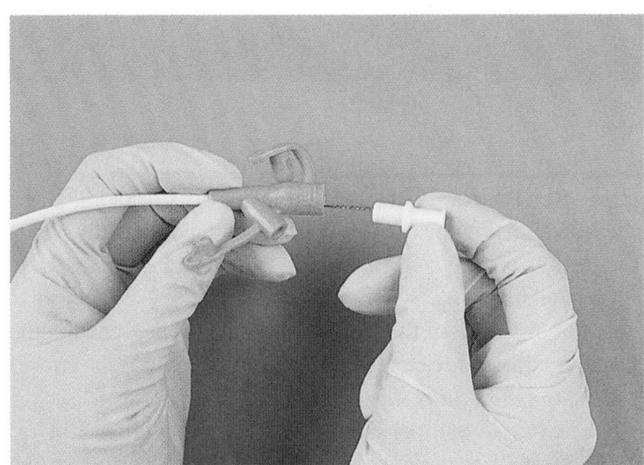

FIGURE 29-11 Removing a stylet. (Photo by B. Proud.)

radiographic verification of its location (Mathus-Vliegen et al., 2010; Young et al., 2005).

Checking Tube Placement

Initial tube placement is traditionally verified with an X-ray and eventually may be identified in real time using an electromagnetic system once the technology becomes more widely used. Other techniques for determining placement of small-diameter nasogastric feeding tubes are less reliable. Checking the placement by auscultating air may be inconclusive because the air that escapes from the distal tip is less pronounced as a result of the small diameter of the tube. Also, aspiration of stomach contents from small-diameter tubes is not always possible because the negative pressure causes the tube to collapse. Nonetheless, once the feeding tube is inserted and secured to avoid slipping, its continued safe location requires frequent checking. Repeated X-rays to reassess tube placement are expensive, impractical, and potentially harmful. Currently, nurses verify the tube's distal placement throughout its use by modifying the aspiration technique after the initial X-ray. The modification involves using a large-volume (50-mL) rather than a small-volume (3- to 5-mL) syringe to obtain a sample of fluid. The larger syringe creates less negative pressure during aspiration and, therefore, provides enough fluid to test the pH. The placement of weighted-tip feeding tubes also has been confirmed using bedside ultrasonography (Duggan et al., 2008; Vigneau et al., 2005). In a small research sample of adults, the technique proved to be 97% accurate in determining distal tube location.

TRANSABDOMINAL TUBE MANAGEMENT

The physician inserts transabdominal tubes, such as G- and J-tubes, but the nurse is responsible for assessing and caring for them and their insertion sites. Conscientious care is necessary because G-tubes may leak (Box 29-1) and cause skin breakdown (see Nursing Guidelines 29-3 and Fig. 29-12).

BOX 29-1 Causes of Gastrostomy Leaks

- Disconnection between the feeding delivery tube and G-tube
- Clamped G-tube while tube feeding is infusing
- Mismatch between the size of the G-tube and stoma
- Increased abdominal pressure from formula accumulation, retching, sneezing, and coughing
- Underinflation of the balloon beneath the skin
- Less than optimal stoma or stomal location

TUBE FEEDINGS

Providing nutrition by the oral route is always best. However, if oral feedings are impossible or jeopardize the client's safety, nourishment is provided enterally or parenterally (see section on "Total Parenteral Nutrition," Chap. 16). Tube feedings are used when clients have an intact stomach or intestinal function but are unconscious, have undergone extensive mouth surgery, have difficulty swallowing, or have esophageal or gastric disorders. Skill 29-4 describes the technique for administering tube feedings.

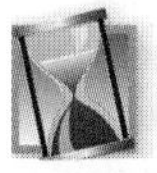

Gerontologic Considerations

■ Long-term use of tube feedings in older adults with dementia or other chronic declining conditions involves many ethical considerations. Refusal to eat (intentional starvation) may be seen as a possible means of suicide in the older person or as a symptom of depression. Caregivers must carefully assess an individual client's decision to refuse food or desire to have a feeding tube removed. Older people who are institutionalized have more limited decision-making power in these cases than the person living at home may have. Nurses should follow the 2001 American Nurses Association position statement regarding advance directives related to a client's wish to avoid artificial nutrition and hydration. Nurses, especially those working in home care and long-term care settings, need up-to-date knowledge about ethical and legal issues related to the use of tube feedings (see Chap. 3).

Benefits and Risks

Tube feedings are delivered through a nasogastric, nasointestinal, or transabdominal tube. Each has its advantages and disadvantages (Table 29-3).

Instilling nutritional formulas into the stomach uses the body's natural reservoir for food. It also reduces the potential for enteritis (inflammation of the intestine) because the chemicals in the stomach tend to destroy microorganisms. Gastric feedings increase the potential for gastric reflux, however, because of their volume and temporary retention within the stomach.

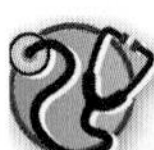

NURSING GUIDELINES 29-3

Managing a Gastrostomy

- Wash hands or perform an alcohol-based hand rub (see Chap. 10). *Hand hygiene reduces the transmission of microorganisms.*
- Don gloves. *They provide a physical barrier between the nurse's hands and body fluids.*
- Assess and replace the gauze dressing over a new gastrostomy if it becomes moist; slight bleeding or a clear serous drainage from the wound is normal for a few weeks after the procedure. *These measures reduce the conditions that support the growth of microorganisms and maceration of the skin.*
- Remove and discontinue the dressing after the first 24 hours unless the physician orders otherwise. *This facilitates assessment.*
- Inspect the skin around the tube daily. *Regular monitoring provides assessment data about the status of wound repair.*
- Make sure that the sutures holding a surgically placed tube are intact. *Checking prevents tube migration.*
- Report any redness or tissue maceration. *These findings indicate early skin impairment.*
- Apply a skin barrier ointment such as zinc oxide, karaya gum wafer, hydrocolloid dressing, or ostomy pouch if the skin appears irritated (see section on "Ostomy Care," Chap. 31). *Such barriers protect the skin and promote healing.*
- Press down on the skin at the base of the tube (see Fig. 29-12A). If the client has a PEG tube, compress the arms of the external bumper together and lift them about 1 in. (2.5 cm) (see Fig. 29-12B). *These steps aid in assessing for drainage, which normally disappears by the end of the first week.*
- Clean the skin with half-strength hydrogen peroxide or 0.9% saline. After 1 week, using soap and water is sufficient. Dry the skin well using air or a blow dryer on a cool or low heat setting. *Appropriate cleaning removes secretions and reduces microorganisms.*
- Rotate the direction of the external bumper 90 degrees or other external retaining device at least once a day. *Doing so relieves pressure and maintains skin integrity.*
- Slide the external bumper down so it is flush with the skin. *Sliding restabilizes the tube.*
- Avoid placing any type of dressing material under the arms of the external bumper. *This helps to avoid creating pressure on the internal bumper and damaging the tissue.*
- Replace the water in the balloon weekly using a Luer-tip (not Luer-lok) syringe. *This keeps the balloon fully inflated and prevents tube migration.*
- Tape the G-tube to the abdomen or secure it with an abdominal binder or commercial tube stabilizer. *Appropriately securing the tube maintains its position.*
- Make sure the tube is not kinked and the skin is not stretched. *These assessments ensure tube patency and skin integrity.*
- Insert a Foley catheter (see Chap. 30), if the client is not sensitive to latex, 2–5 in. (5–10 cm) within the opening, and inflate the balloon if the tube comes out. *Doing so maintains temporary access to the stomach and, if done within 3 hours of accidental extubation, prevents the site from closing.*
- Use the G-tube in a manner similar to how a nasogastric tube is used for administering feedings. *The tube facilitates nourishment.*

Although the placement of tubes within the intestine reduces the risk for gastric reflux, it does not eliminate that risk. Additional problems are associated with intestinal tube feedings. For example, an intestinally placed tube may lead to **dumping syndrome** (a cluster of symptoms from the rapid deposition of calorie-dense nourishment into the small intestine). The symptoms, which include weakness, dizziness, sweating, and nausea, are caused by fluid shifts from the circulating blood to the intestine and a low blood glucose level related to a surge of insulin. Diarrhea also may result when administering hypertonic formula solutions.

Formula Considerations

In addition to the type of tube and the access site, the type of formula also is individualized based on the client's nutritional needs (Table 29-4). Factors include the client's weight,

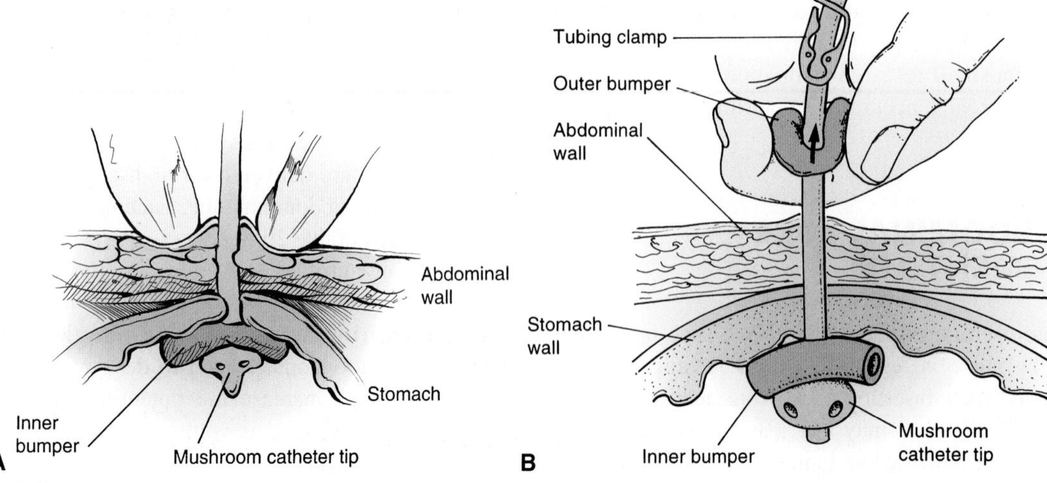

FIGURE 29-12 Inspection. **A.** Inspecting for drainage. **B.** Inspecting the skin.

TABLE 29-3 Comparison of Feeding Tubes

TUBE	ADVANTAGES	DISADVANTAGES
Nasogastric	Low incidence of obstruction Accommodates crushed medications Facilitates bolus or intermittent feedings Easy to check distal placement and gastric residual	Can damage nasal and pharyngeal mucosa from pressure or friction Dilates esophageal sphincter, potentiating gastric reflux Potential for aspiration Requires frequent replacement to ensure the integrity of nasal tissue
Nasointestinal	Easy to insert Comfortable Only slight dilation of esophageal sphincter Reduced danger for aspiration Can remain in place for 4 weeks or longer	Requires X-ray to verify placement Becomes obstructed easily Best used for continuous feeding
Gastrostomy	No nasal tube Easily concealed Accommodates long-term use Infrequent tube replacement Client can be taught self-care	Must wait 24 hours to use after initial placement May leak and cause skin breakdown Increased incidence of infection Requires skin care at tube site Can migrate or become dislodged if tube is not secured Gastric overfill and aspiration possible
Jejunostomy	Same as gastrostomy Reduced potential for reflux and aspiration	Same as gastrostomy

nutritional status, concurrent medical conditions, and the projected length of therapy. The feeding schedule also affects the choice of formula: calories may need to be concentrated if the client is being fed several times a day rather than continuously. Most formulas provide 0.5 to 2.0 kcal/mL.

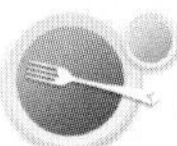

Nutrition Notes

- Specialty formulas are available with altered nutritional profiles for specific disease states, such as for clients with diabetes, renal failure, hepatic failure, respiratory insufficiency, and wound healing. Pediatric formulas are also available.
- Products like Boost, Carnation Breakfast, and Ensure are primarily intended as oral supplements, not for tube feedings.

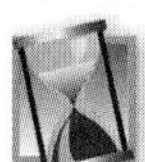

Gerontologic Considerations

- Tube-feeding formulas may vary based on the older client's condition (ie, malabsorption syndromes, glucose intolerance). Several lactose-free tube-feeding formulas on the market today may be beneficial to older clients who experience malabsorption syndromes.
- Clients with or who are at risk for pressure sores benefit from formulas fortified with additional zinc, protein, and other nutrients.
- In home and long-term care settings, registered dietitians may be helpful in the ongoing assessment of tube feedings.

Tube-Feeding Schedules

Tube feedings may be administered on bolus, intermittent, cyclic, or continuous schedules.

TABLE 29-4 Tube-Feeding Formulas

TYPE	EXAMPLES	DESCRIPTION
Standard, isotonic	Osmolite Isocal Nutren 1.0	Routine formulas for clients with normal digestion and absorption; do not alter water distribution. Provide approximately 1.0 cal/mL
High calorie	Comply Nutren 1.5 Nutren 2.0 Deliver 2.0	Provide up to double the amount of calories of standard formulas for clients who require a fluid restriction or have high calorie needs.
High protein	Promote Isocal HN Ultracal HN plus	Provide up to double the amount of protein of standard formulas.
Fiber containing	Jevity Compleat Ultracal	Provide fiber to normalize bowel function in clients with diarrhea or constipation.
Partially hydrolyzed	Criticare HN Optimental Vivonex T.E.N.	Provide nutrients in simple form that require little or no digestion for clients with impaired digestion or absorption.

Bolus Feedings

A **bolus feeding** (the instillation of liquid nourishment in less than 30 minutes four to six times a day) usually involves 250 to 400 mL of formula per administration. This schedule is the least desirable because it distends the stomach rapidly, causing gastric discomfort and an increased risk for reflux. Bolus feedings may be used because they mimic, to some extent, the natural filling and emptying of the stomach. Some clients experience discomfort from the rapid delivery of this quantity of fluid. Clients who are unconscious or who have delayed gastric emptying are at greater risk for regurgitation, vomiting, and aspiration with this method of administration.

Intermittent Feedings

An **intermittent feeding** (the gradual instillation of liquid nourishment four to six times a day) is administered over 30 to 60 minutes, the time most people spend eating a meal. The usual volume is 250 to 400 mL per administration. Intermittent feedings generally are given by gravity drip from a suspended container or with a feeding pump. Gradual filling of the stomach at a slower rate reduces the bloated feeling that can accompany bolus feedings. The container and feeding tube that holds the formula requires thorough flushing after each feeding to reduce the growth of microorganisms. Tube-feeding administration sets are replaced every 24 hours regardless of the feeding schedule.

Cyclic Feedings

A **cyclic feeding** (the continuous instillation of liquid nourishment for 8 to 12 hours) is followed by a 16- to 12-hour pause. This routine often is used to wean clients from tube feedings while continuing to maintain adequate nutrition. The tube feeding is given during the late evening and hours of sleep. During the day, clients eat some food orally. As oral intake increases, the volume and duration of the tube feeding gradually decreases.

Continuous Feedings

A **continuous feeding** (the instillation of liquid nutrition without interruption) is administered at a rate of approximately 1.5 mL/minute. A feeding pump is used to regulate the instillation. Because only a small amount of fluid is instilled at any one time, the formula does not need to be held in the reservoir of the stomach; it can be delivered directly into the small intestine. Instilling small amounts of fluid beyond the stomach reduces the risk of vomiting and aspiration. Continuous feeding creates some inconvenience, though, because the pump must go wherever the client goes.

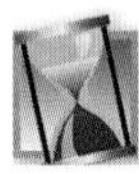

Gerontologic Considerations

- Older adults tend to tolerate small, continuous feedings.

Client Assessment

The following daily assessments are standard for almost every client who receives tube feedings: weight, fluid intake and output, bowel sounds, lung sounds, temperature, condition of the nasal and oral mucous membranes, breathing pattern, gastric complaints, status of abdominal distention, vomiting, bowel elimination patterns, and skin condition at the site of a transabdominal tube. Once tube feedings have been initiated, it is also necessary to routinely assess the client's **gastric residual** (the volume of liquid within the stomach). The nurse measures the gastric residual to determine whether the rate or volume of feeding exceeds the client's physiologic capacity. Overfilling the stomach can cause gastric reflux, regurgitation, vomiting, aspiration, and pneumonia. As a rule of thumb, the gastric residual should be no more than 100 mL or no more than 20% of the previous hour's tube-feeding volume. If the gastric residual is high, the feeding is stopped and the gastric residual is rechecked every 30 minutes until it is within a safe volume for resuming the feeding (see Nursing Guidelines 29-4).

Stop, Think, and Respond Box 29-4

If a client's nutritional needs are met entirely with tube feedings, what effects might that have on the person physically, emotionally, and socially?

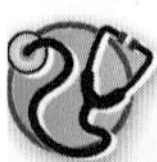

NURSING GUIDELINES 29-4

Checking the Gastric Residual

- Wash hands or perform an alcohol-based hand rub (see Chap. 10). *Hand hygiene reduces the transmission of microorganisms.*
- Don gloves. *Gloves provide a physical barrier between the nurse's hands and body fluids.*
- Stop the infusion of the tube-feeding formula. *This measure facilitates assessment.*
- Aspirate fluid from the feeding tube using a 50-mL syringe. *Doing so allows for the collection of a large volume of fluid.*
- Continue aspirating until no more fluid is obtained. *This ensures an accurate assessment.*
- Measure the aspirated fluid and record the amount. *Documentation provides objective data for evaluation.*
- Reinstill the aspirated fluid. *This measure returns partially digested nutrients and electrolytes to the client.*
- Postpone tube feeding and report residual amounts that exceed agency guidelines or those established by the physician. *Doing so reduces the risk of aspiration.*
- Check gastric residual again in 30 minutes. *This duration allows time for part of the stomach contents to empty into the small intestine.*
- Provide or resume tube feeding if the gastric residual is within an acceptable range. *Doing so prevents overfeeding.*

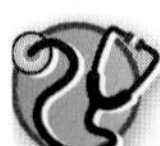

NURSING GUIDELINES 29-5

Clearing an Obstructed Feeding Tube

- Select a syringe with a capacity of at least 50 mL. *This capacity reduces negative pressure during aspiration, which could lead to the collapse of the tube walls.*
- Wash hands or perform an alcohol-based hand rub (see Chap. 10). *Hand hygiene reduces the transmission of microorganisms.*
- Don gloves. *They provide a physical barrier between the nurse's hands and potential contact with body fluids.*
- Aspirate as much as possible from the feeding tube. *Aspiration clears the path above the obstructing debris.*
- Instill 5 mL of the selected solution. *Instillation allows for direct contact between the irrigating solution and debris.*
- Clamp the tube and wait 15 minutes. *This duration gives the substance in the solution time to physically affect the obstructing debris.*
- Aspirate or flush the tube with water. *Repeat if necessary. Use of negative pressure or positive pressure restores patency.*

Nursing Management

Caring for clients with feeding tubes generally involves maintaining tube patency, clearing any obstructions, providing adequate hydration, dealing with common formula-related problems, and preparing clients for home care.

Maintaining Tube Patency

Feeding tubes, especially those smaller than 12 F, are prone to obstruction. Common causes are using formulas with large-molecule nutrients, refeeding partially digested gastric residual, administering formula at a rate less than 50 mL/hour, and instilling crushed or hydrophilic (water-absorbing) medications into the tube. To maintain patency, it is best to flush feeding tubes with 30 to 60 mL of water immediately before and after administering a feeding or medications, every 4 hours if the client is being continuously fed, and after refeeding the gastric residual.

Although tap water is effective as a flush solution, cranberry juice and carbonated beverages may be used. Formula tends to curdle when it comes in contact with cranberry juice, which detracts from the efficacy of this approach.

Clearing an Obstruction

If an obstruction occurs, the nurse consults the physician. Occasionally, it is possible to clear the tube with a solution of meat tenderizer or pancreatic enzyme, but both methods require written medical orders (see Nursing Guidelines 29-5).

When an obstruction cannot be cleared, the tube is removed and another is inserted rather than compromising nutrition by the delay.

Providing Adequate Hydration

Although tube feedings are approximately 80% water, clients usually require additional hydration. Adults require 30 mL of water per kilogram of body weight, or 1 mL/kcal, on a daily basis (Dudek, 2009).

To determine whether or not a client's hydration needs are being met, the nurse identifies the amount of water on the label of commercial formula. He or she can then add this amount to the total volume of flush solution and compare it with the recommended amount. If there is a significant deficit, the nurse revises the plan of care to increase either the volume or, preferably, the frequency of flushing the tube. If the fluid volume is excessive, the nurse monitors the client's urine output and lung sounds to determine whether or not the client can excrete comparable amounts (see Chap. 16).

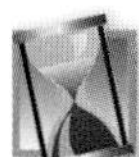

Gerontologic Considerations

- Most tube-feeding formulas are highly concentrated; therefore, the hydration status of the older client must be closely monitored.

Dealing With Miscellaneous Problems

Clients who require enteral feeding experience several common or potential problems. Many are associated with tube-feeding formulas or the mechanical effects of the tubes themselves (Table 29-5). Nurses report problems promptly and make necessary adjustments to the plan of care.

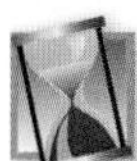

Gerontologic Considerations

- Older adults are at increased risk for fluid and electrolyte disturbances and, as a result, may develop hyperglycemia (elevated blood glucose levels) when tube feedings are administered.
- If an older client is receiving tube feedings with full-strength formula concentrations, it is important to check capillary blood glucose levels every 4 hours for a 48-hour period until the client's results are within a normal range.
- Monitor older adults for agitation or confusion, which may cause them to pull out feeding tubes inadvertently. Also, a change in mental status is an early indicator of a fluid or electrolyte imbalance.

Preparing for Home Care

Because of shortened lengths of stay in hospitals, some clients who continue to need tube feedings are discharged to care for themselves at home. Before demonstrating the procedure, the nurse provides a written instruction sheet that includes the following:

- Places to obtain equipment and formula
- The amount and schedule for each feeding and flush, using household measurements

TABLE 29-5 Common Tube-Feeding Problems

PROBLEM	COMMON CAUSES	SOLUTIONS
Diarrhea	Highly concentrated formula Rapid administration	Dilute initial tube feeding to one-quarter to one-half strength. Start at 25 mL/hr and increase rate by 25 mL q12hr. Hang no more than 4 hours' worth of formula.
	Bacterial contamination	Wash hands. Change formula bag and tubing q24hr. Refrigerate unused formula.
	Lactose intolerance	Consult with the physician on using a milk-free formula.
	Inadequate protein content	Raise serum albumin levels with total parenteral nutrition solutions containing supplemental protein, or administer albumin intravenously.
	Medication side effects	Consult with the physician about adjusting drug therapy or administering an antidiarrheal.
Nausea and vomiting	Rapid feeding	Instill bolus and intermittent feedings by gravity.
	Overfeeding	Delay feeding until gastric residual is <100 mL or <20% of hourly volume.
	Air in stomach	Maintain sitting position for at least 30 minutes after feeding. Consult with the physician about ordering medication that facilitates gastric emptying. Administer continuous feedings. Instill feedings within the small intestine. Keep tubing filled with formula or water.
	Medication side effects	Consult with the physician about adjusting drug therapy or administering drugs to control symptoms.
Aspiration	Incorrect tube placement	Check placement before instilling liquids.
	Vomiting	Keep head elevated at least 30 degrees during feedings and for 30 minutes afterward. Keep cuffed tracheostomy and endotracheal tubes inflated. Refer to measures for controlling vomiting.
Constipation	Lack of fiber	Change formula.
	Dehydration	Increase supplemental water. Consult with the physician on giving a laxative, enema, or suppository.
Elevated blood glucose level	Calorie-concentrated formula	Instill diluted formula and gradually increase concentration. Administer insulin according to medical orders.
Weight loss	Inadequate calories	Increase calories in formula. Increase rate or frequency of feedings.
Elevated electrolytes	Dehydration	Increase supplemental water.
Dry oral and nasal mucous membranes	Mouth breathing Dried nasal mucus	Provide frequent oral and nasal hygiene.
Middle ear inflammation	Narrowing or obstruction of eustachian tube from presence of tube in pharynx	Turn from side to side q2hr. Insert a small-diameter feeding tube.
Sore throat	Pressure and irritation from tube	Use a small-diameter feeding tube.
Plugged feeding tube	Instilling crushed or powdered medications through the tube	Use liquid medications. Dilute crushed drugs.
	Formula coagulation from drug-food interactions	Flush the tubing liberally after drug administration. Flush tubing with water before and after drug administration. Follow agency policy for alternative flush solutions such as carbonated beverages or solutions of meat tenderizer.
	Kinked tube	Maintain neck in neutral position or change position frequently.
	Large molecules in formula	Dilute formula. Flush tubing at least q4hr. Use a larger diameter feeding tube.
Dumping syndrome	Rapid and large instillation of highly concentrated formula into the intestine	Administer small, continuous volume. Adjust glucose content of formula.

- Guidelines for delaying a feeding
- Special instructions for skin, nose, or stomal care, including frequency and types of products to use
- Problems to report such as weight loss, reduced urination, weakness, diarrhea, nausea and vomiting, and breathing difficulties
- Names and phone numbers of people to call if questions arise
- Date, time, and place for continued medical follow-up

Depending on the client's self-confidence and competence in self-administering tube feedings, health care providers often make a referral to a home health agency for post-discharge nursing support.

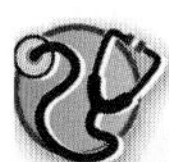

NURSING GUIDELINES 29-6

Inserting an Intestinal Decompression Tube

- Assemble all the necessary equipment as for any nasally inserted tube. *Doing so ensures organization and efficient time management.*
- Follow the techniques in Skill 29-1 for inserting a nasogastric tube. *The same principles are involved during the initial insertion.*
- Thread excess tubing through a sling of folded gauze taped to the forehead (see Fig. 29-13) once gastric placement is confirmed. *The sling supports the tube as it advances.*
- Ambulate the client, if possible. *Ambulation helps the tube to move through the pyloric valve into the small intestine.*
- When the radiograph indicates that the intestinal tube has advanced beyond the stomach, position the client on the right side for 2 hours, then on the back in a Fowler's position for 2 hours, then on the left side for 2 hours. *Gravity and positioning promote movement through intestinal curves.*
- Follow agency policy or physician's instructions for manually advancing the tube several inches each hour. *This advancement supplements the natural peristaltic advancement.*
- Observe the graduated marks on the tube. *They provide a means for monitoring the tube's progression and approximate anatomic location.*
- Request an X-ray confirmation when the tube has reached the prescribed distance. *An X-ray provides objective evidence of the terminal location of the distal tip.*
- Secure the tube to the nose once its distal location has been confirmed. *This measure stabilizes the tube and prevents further migration.*
- Coil the excess tubing and attach it to the client's pajamas or gown. *Coiling and attachment prevent accidental extubation.*
- Connect the proximal end to a wall or a portable suction source. *This measure produces negative pressure to pull substances from the intestine.*

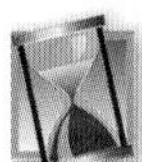

Gerontologic Considerations

■ When teaching older adults or older caregivers how to manage a G-tube or administer tube feedings at home, allow more time for processing information and include several practice sessions. A referral for skilled nursing care, which may be covered by Medicare/Medicaid or private health insurance plans, may be appropriate for ongoing teaching and assessments for clients being discharged with tube feedings.

■ For older adults living on a fixed income, dietitians can suggest ways to prepare less costly, home-blended formulas that meet the client's nutritional needs.

INTESTINAL DECOMPRESSION

Most nasogastric, nasointestinal, and transabdominal tubes are used for enteral feeding or gastric decompression. Sometimes, however, clients require intestinal decompression, which is performed with a tungsten-weighted tube (see Table 29-1). Intestinal decompression sometimes makes it possible to avoid surgery.

Tube Insertion

A nasointestinal decompression tube is inserted in the same manner as a nasogastric tube. The nurse then promotes and monitors its passage into the intestine. In the presence of peristalsis, the weight of the tungsten propels the tip of the tube beyond the stomach. Openings through the distal end provide channels through which the intestinal contents are suctioned. An intestinal decompression tube generally remains in place until the intestinal lumen is patent or until surgical treatment is instituted (see Nursing Guidelines 29-6).

Removal

Once the intestinal decompression tube has served its purpose, the nurse begins the process of removing it. An intestinal decompression tube is removed slowly because removal is in a reverse direction through the curves of the intestine and the valves of the lower and upper ends of the stomach.

First, the tube is disconnected from the suction source. Next, the tape that secures the tube to the face is removed and the tube is withdrawn 6 to 10 in. (15 to 25 cm) at 10-minute intervals. When the last 18 in. (45 cm) remains, the tube is pulled gently from the nose. Afterward, nasal and oral hygiene measures are provided. The tube cannot be removed nasally if the distal end descends below the ileocecal valve between the small and large intestine. Instead, the proximal end is cut and the tube is gradually removed manually or by peristalsis when it descends through the anus.

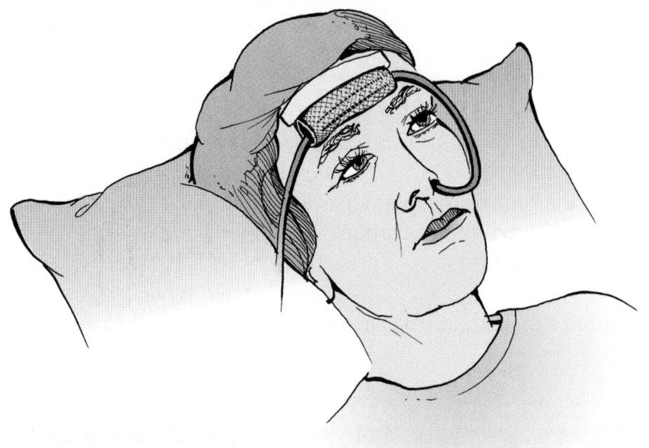

FIGURE 29-13 Fashioning a gauze sling.

NURSING IMPLICATIONS

Depending on data collected during client care, the nurse may identify one or more of the following nursing diagnoses:

- Imbalanced Nutrition: Less Than Body Requirements
- Feeding Self-Care Deficit
- Impaired Swallowing
- Risk for Aspiration
- Impaired Oral Mucous Membrane
- Diarrhea
- Constipation

Nursing Care Plan 29-1 is a model for managing the care of a client with a large gastric residual with a nursing diagnosis of Risk for Aspiration, defined by NANDA-I (2012, p. 422) as "at risk for entry of gastrointestinal secretions, oropharyngeal secretions, solids or fluids into tracheobronchial passages."

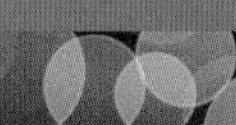

NURSING CARE PLAN 29-1 Risk for Aspiration

Assessment

- Note client's level of consciousness and prescribed drug therapy that may cause sedation.
- Check for a cough and gag reflex.
- Determine the client's ability to swallow effectively or review the results of a swallow study ordered by the physician.
- Measure the gastric residual if the client is receiving tube feedings.
- Auscultate bowel sounds.
- Palpate the abdomen and measure abdominal girth for evidence of distention.
- Ask an alert client about feeling full, nauseous, or vomiting.
- Check if any medical orders restrict the positioning of a client in a Fowler's position.

Nursing Diagnosis. **Risk for Aspiration** related to slow gastric emptying as manifested by the measurement of the gastric residual of 150 mL from a 16 F nasogastric tube 4 hours after previous bolus feeding of 400 mL, unresponsiveness except for eye opening and pulling away from painful stimuli following head trauma in a motor vehicle collision, and mechanical ventilation with an endotracheal tube that has been placed orally.

Expected Outcome. The client's risk for aspiration will be reduced as evidenced by a gastric residual of less than 100 mL within 1 hour of feeding.

Interventions	Rationales
Keep cuff of endotracheal tube inflated at the prescribed pressure.	An inflated cuff acts as a barrier that prevents stomach contents from entering the airway.
Maintain head elevation at no less than 30 degrees at all times.	Elevating the upper body promotes the deposition of the tube-feeding formula within the stomach and movement toward the small intestine.
Monitor bowel sounds; report if absent or fewer than five per minute.	Active bowel sounds suggest that peristalsis is sufficient to facilitate gastric emptying and intestinal absorption and the elimination of liquid nourishment.
Check the placement of the distal end of the gastric tube before administering any liquid substance.	Checking the distal placement provides evidence that the end of the tube is located within the stomach rather than the esophagus, airway, or small intestine.
Measure gastric residual before all tube feedings.	This standard of care helps to determine the client's response to liquid nourishment via a gastric tube.
Refeed gastric residual and follow with a 30 mL tap water flush.	Gastric residual contains partially digested nutrients that should not be discarded; flushing the tube following refeeding helps to prevent obstruction within the tube and provides additional water intake.
Postpone tube feeding for 30 minutes if the gastric residual measures 100 mL or more or 20% above the hourly rate for infusion.	Distention of the stomach with additional formula predisposes the client to regurgitation and the potential for aspiration.
Report the gastric residual volume to the physician if it remains above the maximum volume after delaying feeding for 30 minutes.	Sharing the assessment findings with the physician facilitates collaboration in modifying the plan of care by changing the type, volume, or frequency of the tube feeding, or administering a medication that promotes gastric emptying.
Maintain the suction machine at the bedside.	Having equipment for performing oral–pharyngeal suctioning ensures a rapid response for clearing the upper gastrointestinal tract and airway following episodes in which the client vomits.

Evaluation of Expected Outcomes

- Gastric residual measures 50 mL.
- Bowel sounds are present and active in all quadrants.
- The endotracheal tube cuff remains inflated.
- Head is elevated 30 degrees.
- Tube feeding is infusing at 100 mL/hr with the feeding pump rather than with bolus feeding following a change in medical order.

CRITICAL THINKING EXERCISES

1. What nutritional suggestions could a nurse make for a client who has a chronic disease that impairs the ability to swallow food?
2. When a client experiences persistent gagging during attempts to insert a nasogastric tube, what actions can the nurse take?
3. Describe the similarities and differences between inserting a tube for gastric decompression and one for intestinal decompression.
4. What questions would be important to ask if a client receiving tube feedings at home calls to report the onset of diarrhea?

NCLEX-STYLE REVIEW QUESTIONS

1. What is the most correct nursing action to determine the length for inserting a nasogastric sump tube?
   1. Place the distal tip of the tube at the client's nose and measure the distance from there to the jaw, then midway to the sternum.
   2. Place the distal tip of the tube at the client's nose and measure the distance from there to the mouth, then between the nipples.
   3. Place the distal tip of the tube at the client's nose and measure the distance from there to the mid-sternum, then to the umbilicus.
   4. Place the distal tip of the tube at the client's nose and measure the distance from there to the ear, then to the xiphoid process.
2. When a practical nurse assists with the insertion of a single lumen nasogastric tube, which of the following instructions is correct when the tube is in the client's oropharynx?
   1. Breathe deeply as the tube is advanced.
   2. Hold your head in a sniffing position.
   3. Press your chin to your upper chest.
   4. Avoid coughing until the tube is down.
3. What is the most appropriate technique for determining whether the distal end of a tube for gastric decompression is in the stomach?
   1. Request a portable X-ray of the stomach.
   2. Check the pH of aspirated fluid.
   3. Instill 100 mL of tap water into the tube.
   4. Feel for air at the tube's proximal end.
4. Immediately after insertion of a transabdominal G-tube, which finding should the nurse consider normal when assessing the gastrostomy site?
   1. Milky-appearing drainage
   2. Serosanguineous drainage
   3. Green-tinged drainage
   4. Bright bloody drainage
5. When a client with a nasogastric tube for gastric decompression indicates that he or she is very thirsty, which nursing intervention is most appropriate to add to the plan of care?
   1. Offer fluids at least every 2 hours.
   2. Provide crushed ice in sparse amounts.
   3. Increase oral liquids on the dietary tray.
   4. Refill the water carafe twice each shift.

SKILL 29-1 Inserting a Nasogastric Tube

Suggested Action	Reason for Action
ASSESSMENT	
Check that a medical order has been written.	Ensures that care is within the legal scope of practice.
Determine the reason for the nasogastric tube.	Facilitates the evaluation of outcomes.
Identify the client.	Ensures that the procedure will be performed on the correct client.
Assess how much the client understands about the procedure.	Indicates the need for and the level of health teaching.
Inspect the nose after the client blows into a paper tissue (Fig. A).	Provides data that will determine which naris to use.

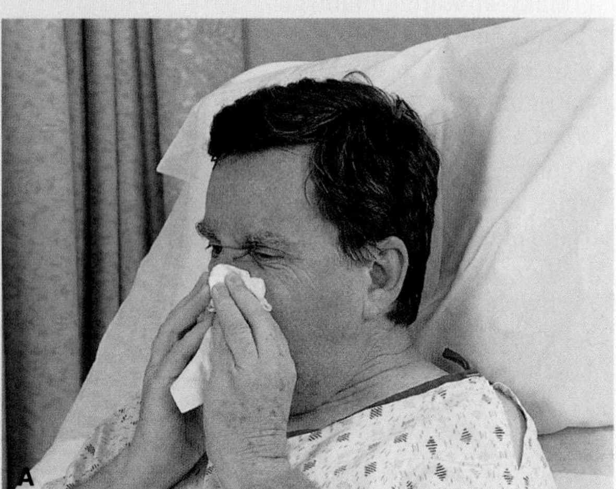

Clearing the nose. (Photo by B. Proud.)

Suggested Action	Reason for Action
Unwrap and uncoil the tube.	Straightens the tube and releases bends from product packaging.
Obtain the NEX measurements (Fig. B).	Determines length for insertion.

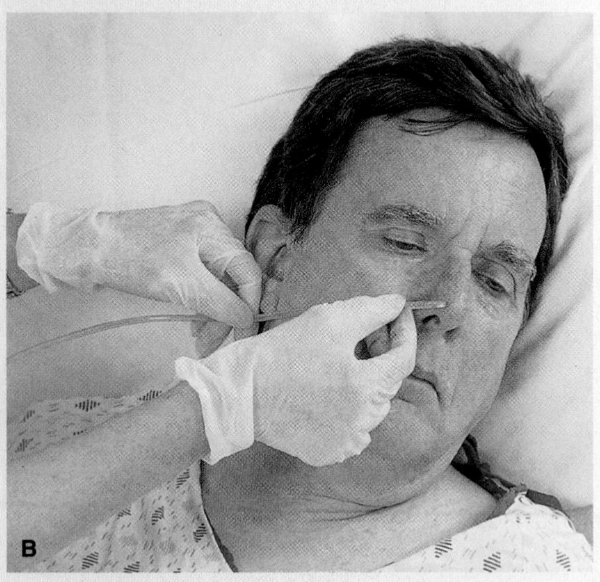

Measuring the tube. (Photo by B. Proud.)

(continued)

Inserting a Nasogastric Tube (continued)

ASSESSMENT (CONTINUED)

Action	Rationale
Mark the tube at the NE (nose-to-ear) and EX (ear-to-xiphoid) measurements (Fig. C).	Provides a guide during insertion.

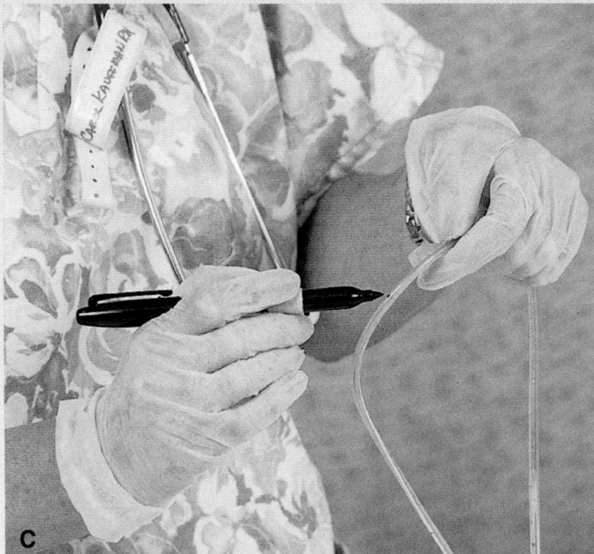

Marking the tube. (Photo by B. Proud.)

PLANNING

Action	Rationale
If a plastic tube feels rigid, place it in or flush it with warm water.	Promotes flexibility.
Assemble the following equipment, in addition to the tube: water, straw, towel, lubricant, tissues, tape, emesis basin, flashlight, stethoscope, clean gloves, and 50-mL syringe.	Contributes to organization and efficient time management.
Place a suction machine at the bedside if the client is unresponsive or has difficulty swallowing.	Provides a method for clearing the client's airway of vomitus.
Remove dentures.	Avoids choking should they become loose or displaced.
Establish a hand signal for pausing.	Relieves anxiety by providing the client with some locus for control.

IMPLEMENTATION

Action	Rationale
Wash your hands or perform an alcohol-based hand rub (see Chap. 10).	Reduces the transmission of microorganisms.
Pull the privacy curtain.	Demonstrates respect for the client's dignity.
Assist the client to sit in semi-Fowler's or high-Fowler's position and hyperextend the neck as if in a sniffing position.	Ensures the visualization of the nasal passageway to facilitate inserting the tube.
Protect the client, bedclothing, and linen with a towel.	Avoids linen changes.
Don gloves.	Reduces the transmission of microorganisms.
Lubricate the tube with water-soluble gel over 6–8 in. (15–20 cm) at the distal tip.	Reduces friction and tissue trauma.

(continued)

Inserting a Nasogastric Tube (continued)

IMPLEMENTATION (CONTINUED)

Action	Rationale
Insert the tube into the nostril while pointing the tip backward and downward (Fig. D).	Follows the normal contour of the nasal passage.

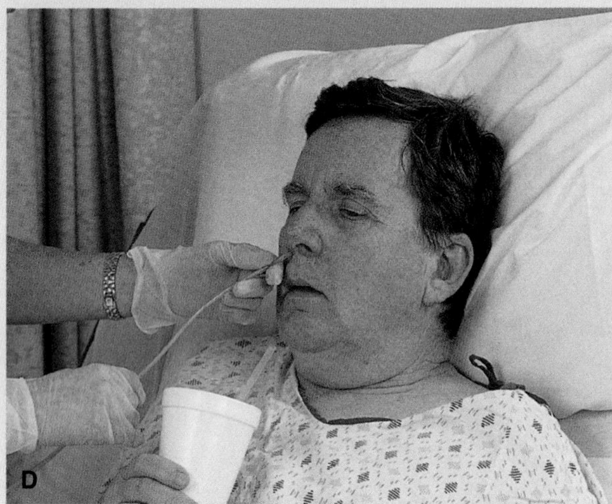

Preparing to insert the tube. (Photo by B. Proud.)

Action	Rationale
Do not force the tube. Relubricate or rotate it if there is resistance.	Prevents trauma.
Stop when the first mark on the tube is at the tip of the nose.	Places the tip above the area where the gag reflex may be stimulated.
Use a flashlight to inspect the back of the throat.	Confirms that the tube has been maneuvered around the nasal curve.
Instruct the client to lower his or her chin to the chest and swallow sips of water.	Narrows the trachea and opens the esophagus; helps to advance the tube.
Advance the tube 3–5 in. (7.5–12.5 cm) each time the client swallows.	Coordinates insertion; reduces the potential for gagging or vomiting.
Pause if the client gives the preestablished signal.	Demonstrates respect and cooperation.
Discontinue the procedure and raise the tube to the first mark if there are signs of distress such as gasping, coughing, a bluish skin color, or the inability to speak or hum.	Indicates that the tube is possibly in the airway.
Assess placement, preferably using two different methods when the second mark is reached (Fig. E).	Provides data on distal placement.

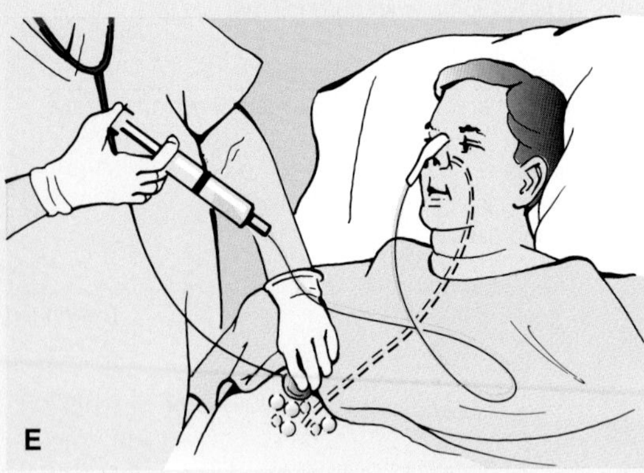

Assessing the placement.

(continued)

Inserting a Nasogastric Tube (continued)

IMPLEMENTATION (CONTINUED)

Withdraw the tube to the first mark and reattempt insertion if the assessment findings are inconclusive, or consult with the physician about obtaining an X-ray.	Ensures safety.
Proceed to secure the tube if the data indicate the tube is in the stomach (Fig. F).	Prevents tube migration.

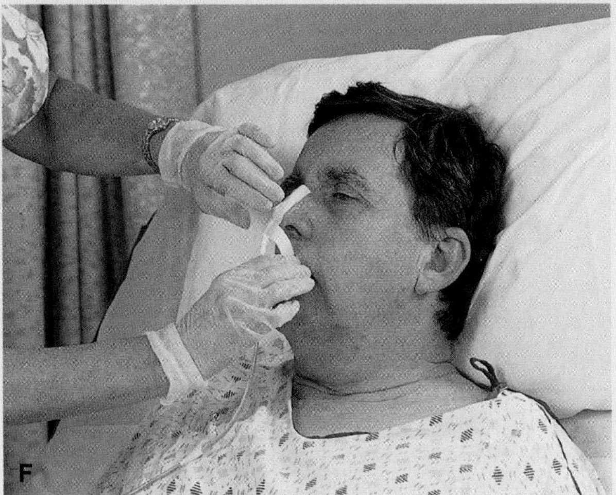

Securing the tube. (Photo by B. Proud.)

Connect the tube to suction or clamp it while awaiting further orders.	Promotes gastric decompression or potential use.
Remove gloves and wash your hands or use an alcohol-based hand rub.	Reduces the transmission of microorganisms.
Position the client with a minimum head elevation of 30 degrees.	Prevents gastric reflux.
Remove equipment from the bedside.	Restores orderliness and supports the principles of medical asepsis.
Measure and record the volume of drainage at least every 8 hours.	Provides data for evaluating fluid balance.

Evaluation

- Distal placement within the stomach is confirmed.
- Client exhibits no evidence of respiratory distress.
- Client can speak or hum.
- Lung sounds are present and clear bilaterally.
- No bleeding or pain is noted in the area of nasal mucosa.

Document

- Type of tube
- Outcomes of the procedure
- Method for determining placement and outcome of assessment
- Description of drainage
- Type and amount of suction, if the tube is used for decompression

SAMPLE DOCUMENTATION

Date and Time A 16 F Salem sump tube inserted without difficulty. Placement verified by noting the sound of air while auscultating over the stomach and by aspirating gastric secretions, which are yellowish-green and reveal a pH of 3 when tested. Salem sump tube secured to nose and connected to low, intermittent wall suction. Positioned with the head of bed elevated 30 degrees. —————— SIGNATURE/TITLE

SKILL 29-2 Irrigating a Nasogastric Tube

Suggested Action	Reason for Action
ASSESSMENT	
Monitor the client's symptoms, the volume and rate of drainage, and evidence of abdominal distention.	Provides data for future comparisons.
Check that a medical order has been written, if that is the agency's policy.	Complies with the legal scope of the nursing practice.
Identify the client.	Ensures that the procedure will be performed on the correct client.
Assess how much the client understands about the procedure.	Provides an opportunity for client teaching.
PLANNING	
Assemble the following equipment: Asepto or irrigating syringe, irrigating fluid (isotonic saline solution), container, clean towel or pad, clean gloves, and cover or plug for end of tube.	Contributes to organization and efficient time management.
Turn off the suction.	Facilitates implementation.
IMPLEMENTATION	
Pull the privacy curtain.	Demonstrates respect for the client's dignity.
Wash your hands or perform an alcohol-based hand rub (see Chap. 10).	Reduces the transmission of microorganisms.
Place a clean pad or towel beneath where the tube will be separated.	Avoids changing bed linens and protects the client from soiling.
Don clean gloves.	Complies with standard precautions.
Disconnect the nasogastric tube from the suction tubing and apply cover or insert plug into suction tubing.	Keeps the connection area clean.
Check the distal placement of the tube.	Ensures safety.
Fill irrigating syringe with 30–60 mL of normal saline solution.	Provides an adequate quantity of isotonic solution to clear tubing.
Insert the tip of the syringe within the proximal end of the tube and allow the solution to flow in by gravity or apply gentle pressure (Fig. A).	Dilutes and mobilizes debris.

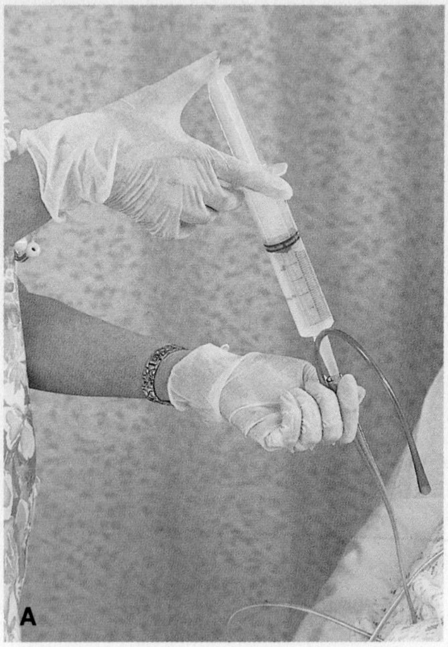

A

Instilling the irrigation solution. (Photo by B. Proud.)

(continued)

Irrigating a Nasogastric Tube (continued)

IMPLEMENTATION (CONTINUED)

Aspirate after the fluid has been instilled.	Removes substances that may impair future drainage.
Reconnect the tube to the source of suction.	Resumes therapeutic management.
Observe the characteristics of the aspirated solution; measure and discard.	Provides data for evaluating the effectiveness of the procedure.
Monitor for the flow of drainage through the suction tubing (Fig. B).	Provides evidence that patency is being maintained.

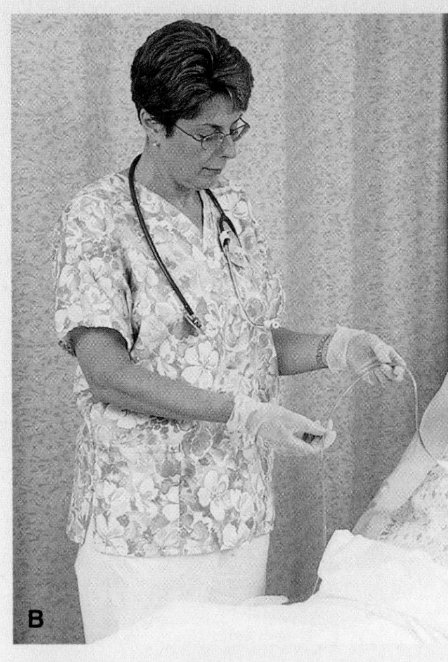

Monitoring drainage. (Photo by B. Proud.)

Remove gloves and perform hand hygiene.	Reduces the transmission of microorganisms.
Record the volume of instilled and drained fluid on the bedside intake and output sheet.	Provides accurate data for determining fluid balance.

Evaluation

- Drainage is restored.
- Nausea and vomiting are relieved.
- Abdominal distention is reduced.

Document

- Volume and type of fluid instilled
- Appearance and volume of returned drainage
- Response of client

SAMPLE DOCUMENTATION

Date and Time Salem sump tube irrigated with 60 mL of normal saline. Solution instilled with slight pressure. A 100 mL of solution returned with several large mucus particles. Reconnected to low, intermittent suction. Gastric tube draining well at the present time. Abdomen is soft. No vomiting. —————————— SIGNATURE/TITLE

SKILL 29-3 Removing a Nasogastric Tube

Suggested Action	Reason for Action
ASSESSMENT	
Assess bowel sounds, the condition of the mouth and nasal mucosa, the level of consciousness, and gag reflex.	Provides data for future comparisons and may affect how the procedure is performed.
Check that a medical order has been written.	Complies with the legal scope of nursing practice.
Identify the client.	Ensures that the procedure will be performed on the correct client.
Assess how much the client understands the procedure.	Provides an opportunity for client teaching.
PLANNING	
Assemble the following equipment: towel, emesis basin, cotton-tipped applicator sticks, oral hygiene equipment, and clean gloves.	Contributes to organization and efficient time management.
IMPLEMENTATION	
Pull the privacy curtain.	Demonstrates respect for dignity.
Wash your hands or perform an alcohol-based hand rub (see Chap. 10).	Reduces the transmission of microorganisms.
Place the client in a sitting position, if alert, or in a lateral position if not.	Prevents aspiration of stomach contents.
Cover the chest with a clean towel and place the emesis basin and tissues within easy reach.	Prepares for possible vomiting and protects the client from soiling.
Remove the tape securing the tube to the client's nose.	Facilitates pulling the tube from the stomach.
Don clean gloves.	Complies with standard precautions.
Turn off the suction and separate the tube.	Prepares for removal.
Instill a bolus of air into the lumen that drains gastric secretions.	Prevents residual fluid from leaking as the tube is withdrawn.
Clamp, plug, or pinch the tube (Fig. A).	Prevents fluid from leaking as the tube is withdrawn.

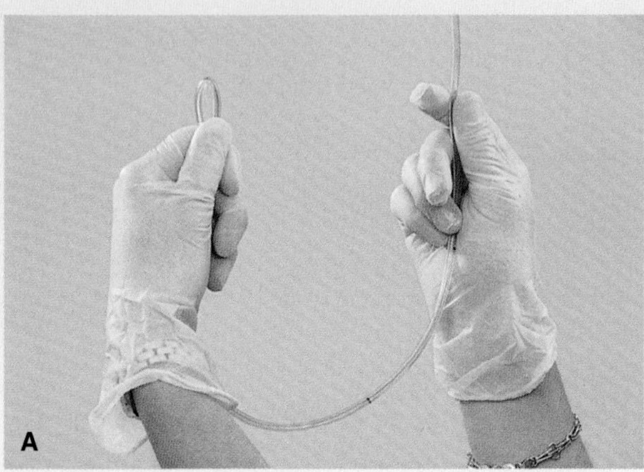

Occluding the tube. (Photo by B. Proud.)

Suggested Action	Reason for Action
Instruct the client to take a deep breath and hold it just before removing the nasogastric tube.	Reduces the risk for aspirating gastric fluid.
Remove the tube from the client's nose gently and slowly.	Lessens the potential for trauma.

(continued)

Removing a Nasogastric Tube (continued)

IMPLEMENTATION (CONTINUED)

Action	Rationale
Enclose the tube within the towel or glove and discard the tube in a covered container (Fig. B).	Provides a transmission barrier against microorganisms.

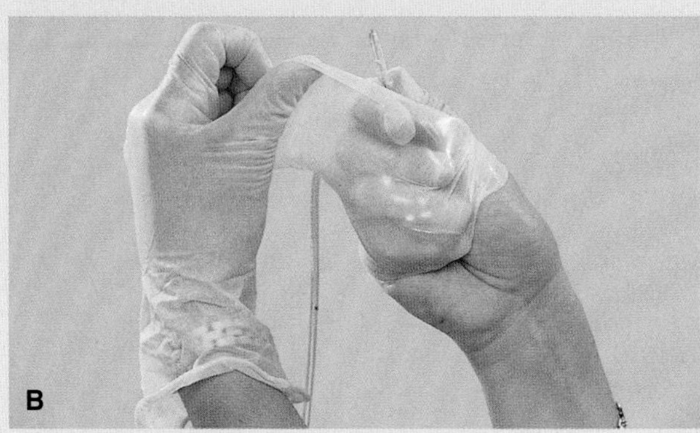

Enclosing the tube. (Photo by B. Proud.)

Action	Rationale
Empty, measure, and record the drainage in the suction container.	Provides data for evaluating the client's fluid status.
Remove gloves and perform hand hygiene.	Reduces the transmission of microorganisms.
Offer an opportunity for oral hygiene.	Removes disagreeable tastes from the client's mouth.
Encourage the client to clear the nose of mucus and debris with paper tissues or cotton-tipped applicators.	Promotes the integrity of nasal tissue.
Discard disposable equipment; rinse and return portable suction equipment.	Preserves cleanliness and orderliness in the client's unit; demonstrates accountability for equipment.

Evaluation

- The tube is removed.
- The client resumes eating and taking fluids.
- The client experiences no nausea or vomiting.
- The airway remains clear.
- The nasal mucosa is moist and intact.

Document

- Type of tube removed
- Response of client
- Appearance and volume of drainage
- Appearance of nose and nasopharynx

SAMPLE DOCUMENTATION

Date and Time Salem sump tube removed. Brief period of retching during removal. Total of 75 mL clear green drainage emptied from suction container. Oral care provided. L. naris swabbed with applicator lubricated with petroleum jelly. Mucosa is red but intact. —————————— SIGNATURE/TITLE

SKILL 29-4 Administering Tube Feedings

Suggested Action	Reason for Action
Bolus Feeding	
ASSESSMENT	
Check the medical order for the type of nourishment, volume, and schedule to follow.	Complies with the legal scope of nursing practice.
Check the date and identifying information on the container of tube-feeding formula.	Ensures accurate administration and avoids using outdated formula.
Wash your hands or perform an alcohol-based hand rub (see Chap. 10).	Reduces the transmission of microorganisms.
Identify the client.	Ensures that the procedure will be performed on the correct client.
Distinguish the tubing for gastric or intestinal feeding from the tubing to instill intravenous solutions.	Prevents administering nutritional formula into the vascular system.
Assess bowel sounds.	Provides data indicating the safety for instilling liquids through the tube.
Measure gastric residual if a 12 F or larger tube is in place (Fig. A).	Determines if the stomach has the capacity to manage the next instillation of formula; aspiration of fluid may be impossible with small-lumen tubes.

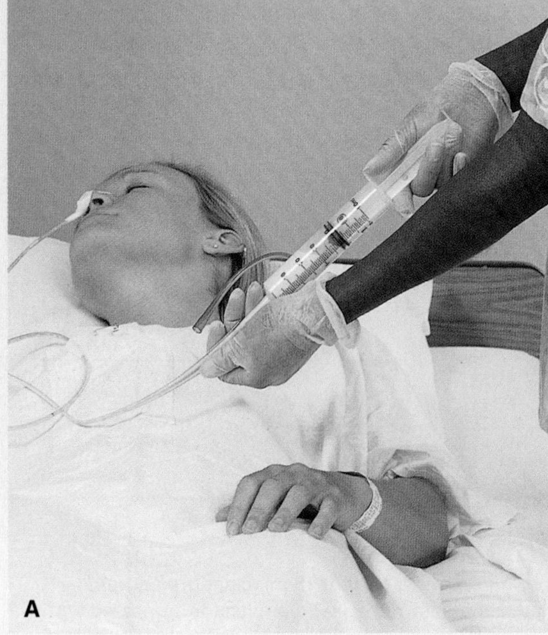

Measuring gastric residual. (Photo by B. Proud.)

Suggested Action	Reason for Action
Measure capillary blood glucose or glucose in the urine.	Provides data indicating response to caloric intake.
Assess how much the client understands the procedure.	Provides an opportunity for client teaching.

(continued)

Administering Tube Feedings (continued)

PLANNING	
Replace any unused formula every 24 hours.	Reduces the potential for bacterial growth.
Wait and recheck gastric residual in 30 minutes if it exceeds 100 mL.	Avoids overfilling the stomach.
Assemble the following equipment: Asepto syringe, formula, tap water.	Contributes to organization and efficient time management.
Warm refrigerated nourishment to room temperature in a basin of warm water.	Prevents chilling and abdominal cramping.
IMPLEMENTATION	
Perform hand hygiene.	Reduces the transmission of microorganisms.
Place the client in a 30- to 90-degree sitting position.	Prevents regurgitation.
Refeed gastric residual by gravity flow.	Returns predigested nutrients without excessive pressure.
Pinch the tube just before all the residual has instilled (Fig. B).	Prevents air from entering the tube.

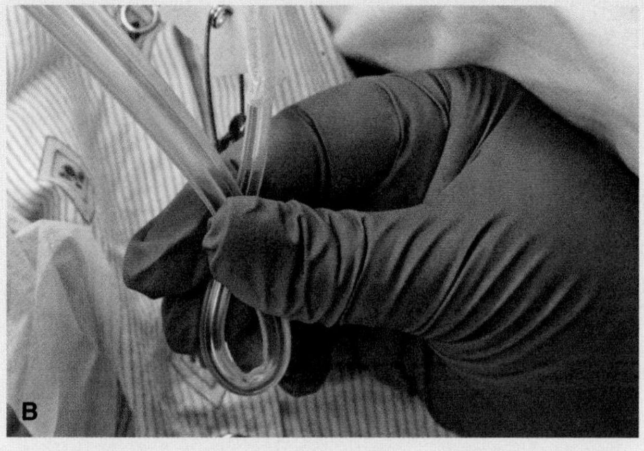

Pinch the tubing before it becomes empty.

Add fresh formula to the syringe and adjust the height to allow a slow but gradual instillation (Fig. C).	Provides nourishment.

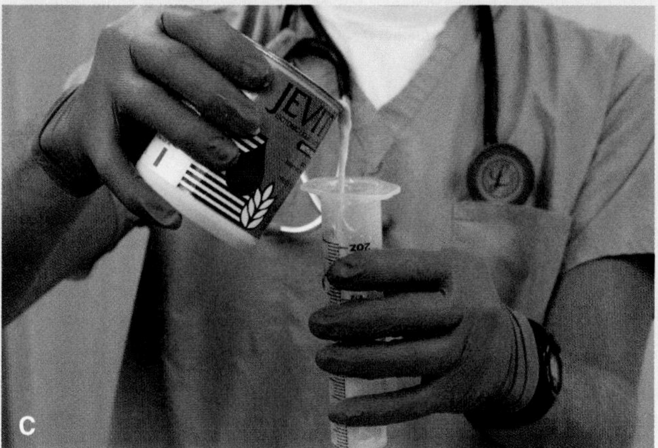

Administering a bolus feeding.

Continue filling the syringe before it becomes empty.	Prevents air from entering the tube.

(continued)

Administering Tube Feedings (continued)

IMPLEMENTATION (CONTINUED)

If a gastrostomy tube is being used, tilt the barrel of the syringe during the feeding (Fig. D).

Permits air displacement from the stomach.

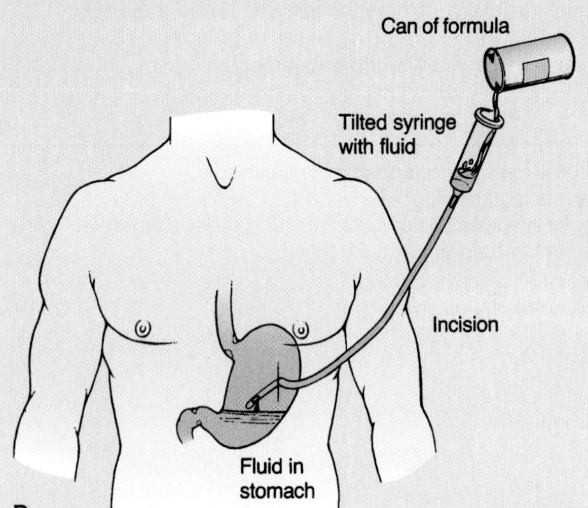

Bolus feeding through a gastrostomy tube (G-tube).

Flush the tubing with at least 30–60 mL of water after each feeding, or follow the agency's policy for suggested amounts (Fig. E).

Ensures that all nourishment has entered the stomach; prevents fermentation and coagulation of formula in the tube; provides water for fluid balance.

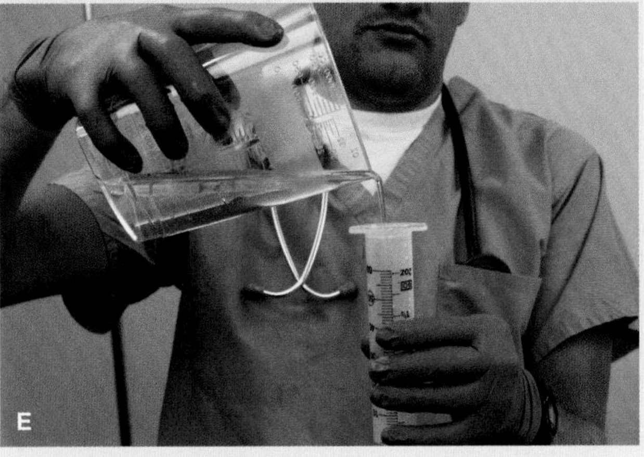

Instilling water to flush the tubing.

Plug or clamp the tube as the water leaves the syringe.

Prevents air from entering the tubing; maintains patency.

Keep the head of the bed elevated for at least 30–60 minutes after a feeding.

Prevents gastric reflux.

Wash and dry the feeding equipment. Return items to the bedside.

Supports principles of medical asepsis.

Record the volume of formula and water administered on the bedside intake and output record.

Provides accurate data for assessing fluid balance and caloric value of nourishment.

Provide oral hygiene at least twice daily.

Removes microorganisms and promotes comfort and hygiene of the client.

(continued)

Administering Tube Feedings (continued)

Intermittent Feeding

ASSESSMENT

Follow the previous sequence for assessment.	Principles remain the same.

PLANNING

In addition to those activities listed for bolus feeding, replace unused formula, feeding containers, and tubing every 24 hours.	Reduces the potential for bacterial growth.

IMPLEMENTATION

Fill the feeding container with room-temperature formula.	Prevents administration of cold formula, which can cause cramping; room-temperature formula will be instilled before supporting bacterial growth.
Gradually open the clamp on the tubing.	Purges air from the tube.
Connect the tubing to the nasogastric or nasoenteral tube.	Provides access to formula.
Open the clamp and regulate the drip rate according to the physician's order or the agency's policy.	Supports safe administration of liquid nourishment.
Check at 10-minute intervals (Fig. F).	Ensures early identification of infusion problems.

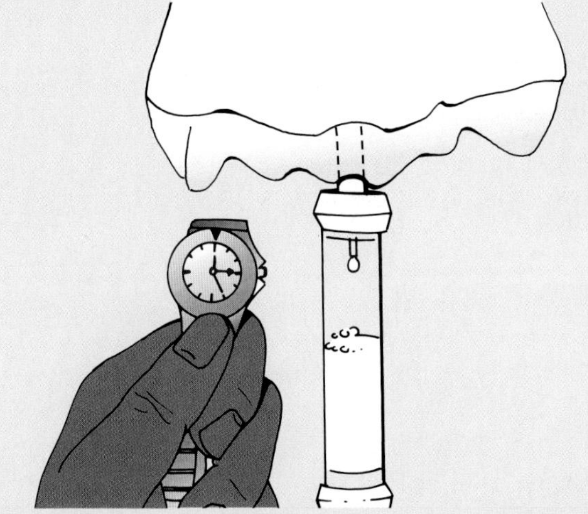

Checking the rate of flow.

Flush the tubing with water after the formula has infused (Fig. G).	Clears the tubing of formula, prevents obstruction, and provides water for fluid balance.

G

Flushing the tubing following feeding.

Pinch the feeding tube just as the last volume of water is administered.	Prevents air from entering the tube.
Clamp or plug the feeding tube.	Prevents leaking.
Record the volume of formula and water instilled.	Provides accurate data for assessing fluid balance and caloric value of nourishment.
Follow recommendations for postprocedural care as described with a bolus feeding.	Principles for care remain the same.

(continued)

Administering Tube Feedings (continued)

Continuous Feeding

ASSESSMENT

In addition to previously described assessments, check the gastric residual every 4 hours.

Principles remain the same. This method ensures a routine pattern for assessment to accommodate the schedule of continuous feedings and prevents inadvertent overfeeding.

PLANNING

In addition to previously described planning activities, obtain equipment for regulating continuous infusion (eg, tube-feeding pump).

Aids in an accurate administration and sounds an alarm if the infusion is interrupted.

Replace unused formula, feeding containers, and tubing every 24 hours.

Reduces the potential for bacterial growth.

Attach a time tape to a feeding container.

Facilitates periodic assessment.

IMPLEMENTATION

Flush the new feeding container with water.

Reduces surface tension within the tube and enhances the passage of large protein molecules.

Fill the feeding container with no more than 4 hours' worth of refrigerated formula. *Exception:* Commercially prepared, sterilized containers of formula, or formula that is kept iced while infusing may hang for longer periods.

Prevents growth of bacteria; body heat will warm cold formula when infused at a slow rate.

Purge the tubing of air.

Prevents distention of the stomach or intestine.

Thread the tubing within the feeding pump according to the manufacturer's directions (Fig. H).

Ensures the correct mechanical operation of equipment and accurate administration to the client.

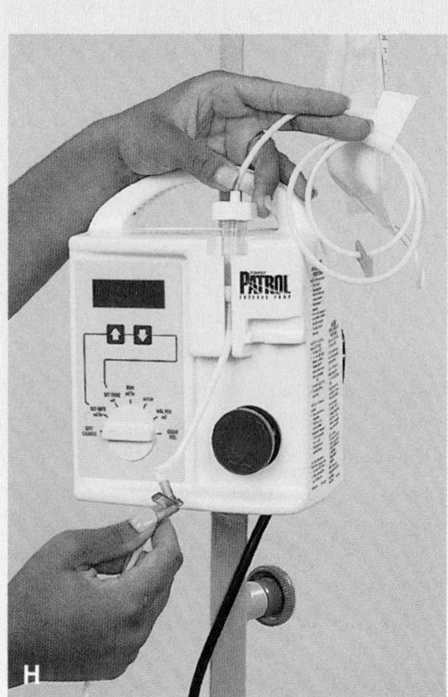

Preparing the pump. (Photo by B. Proud.)

(continued)

Administering Tube Feedings (continued)

IMPLEMENTATION (CONTINUED)

Connect the tubing from the feeding pump to the client's feeding tube (Fig. I).

Provides access to formula.

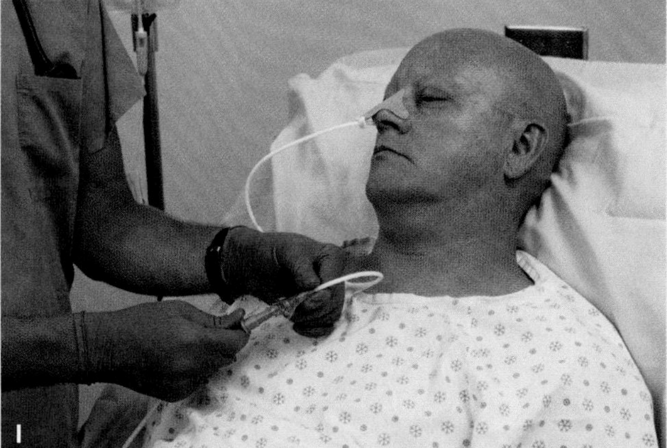

Connecting the feeding tube to the pump.

Set the prescribed rate on the feeding pump (Fig. J).

Complies with the medical order.

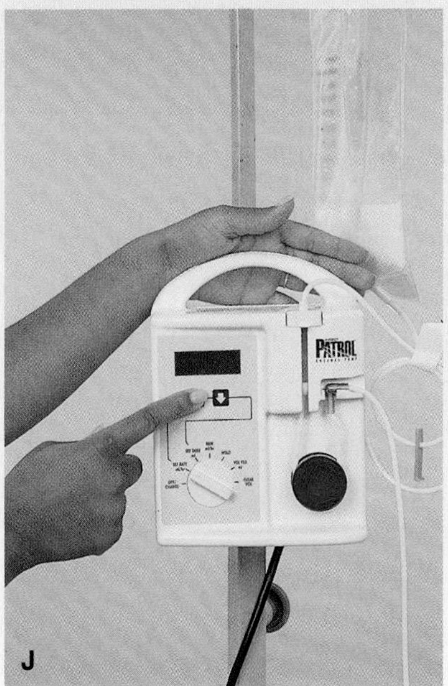

Programming the pump. (Photo by B. Proud.)

(continued)

Administering Tube Feedings (continued)

IMPLEMENTATION (CONTINUED)

Open the clamp on the feeding tube and start the pump (Fig. K). — Initiates infusion.

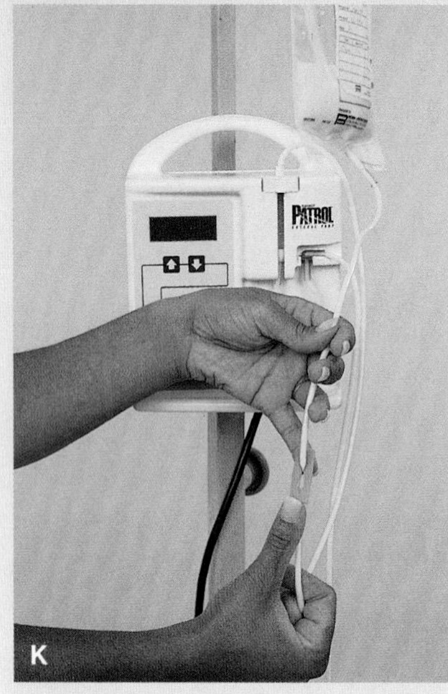

Releasing the clamp. (Photo by B. Proud.)

Keep the client's head elevated at all times. — Prevents reflux and aspiration.

Flush the tubing with 30–60 mL of water or more every 4 hours after checking and refeeding gastric residual and after administering medications. — Promotes patency and contributes to the client's fluid balance.

Record the instilled volume of formula and water. — Provides accurate data for assessing fluid balance and caloric value of nourishment.

Follow recommendations for postprocedural care as described with a bolus feeding. — Principles for care remain the same.

Evaluation

- The client receives a prescribed volume of formula according to an established feeding schedule.
- The client's weight remains stable or the client reaches the target weight.
- The lungs remain clear.
- Bowel elimination is within normal parameters for client.
- The client has a daily fluid intake between 2,000 and 3,000 mL unless intake is otherwise restricted.

Document

- Volume of gastric residual and actions taken, if excessive
- Type and volume of formula
- Rate of infusion, if continuous
- Volume of water used for flushes
- Response of client; if symptomatic, describe actions taken and results

SAMPLE DOCUMENTATION

Date and Time A 50 mL of gastric residual. Residual reinstilled and tube flushed with 60 mL of tap water. A 480 mL of Enrich with Fiber placed in tube-feeding bag. Formula infusing at 120 mL/hr. No diarrhea or gastric complaints at this time. ———————— SIGNATURE/TITLE

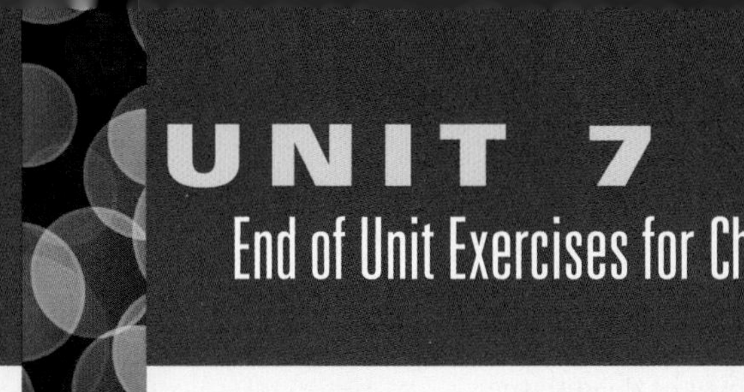

UNIT 7
End of Unit Exercises for Chapters 27, 28, and 29

Section I: Reviewing What You've Learned

Activity A: *Fill in the blanks by choosing the correct word from the options given in parentheses.*

1. A stationary blood clot in the veins is called a/an __________________. (embolus, thrombophlebitis, thrombus)
2. Surgery that removes or replaces defective tissue to restore function is called __________________. (curative, exploratory, palliative)
3. __________________ is confirmed and monitored by counting the number and type of white blood cells in a sample of the client's blood. (Leukocytosis, Phagocytosis, Pinocytosis)
4. __________________ dressings are self-adhesive, opaque, air- and water-occlusive wound coverings. (Gauze, Hydrocolloid, Transparent)
5. The use of gastrointestinal tubes to provide nourishment is called __________________ feeding. (bolus, gavage, lavage)
6. __________________ tubes are inserted through the nose for distal placement below the stomach. (Nasogastric, Nasointestinal, Orogastric)

Activity B: *Mark each statement as either T (True) or F (False). Correct any false statements.*

1. T____F____ The care that clients receive before, during, and after surgery is called perioperative care.
2. T____F____ A wound is damaged skin or soft tissue that results from trauma.
3. T____F____ Inflammation, the immediate physiologic response to tissue injury, lasts about 10 days.
4. T____F____ Gastric reflux is the reverse flow of gastric contents.
5. T____F____ Enteral nutrition is nourishment provided by the oral route.

Activity C: *Write the correct term for each description below.*

1. A physician who administers chemical agents that temporarily eliminate sensation and pain __________________
2. Blood donors chosen from among the client's relatives and friends __________________
3. The period from 2 days to 3 weeks after the inflammatory phase during which new cells fill and seal a wound __________________
4. A process by which damaged cells recover and reestablish their normal function __________________
5. The procedure of cleansing the vaginal canal to treat an infection __________________
6. Measuring the length from the nose to the earlobe to the xiphoid process __________________

Activity D: *1. Match the terms related to wounds and wound care in Column A with their explanations in Column B.*

Column A	Column B
1. ________ Collagen	A. Removal of dead tissue
2. ________ Remodeling	B. Tough and inelastic protein
3. ________ Dehiscence	C. Movement of a liquid at the point of contact with a solid
4. ________ Debridement	D. Separation of wound edges
5. ________ Capillary action	E. The period during which the wound undergoes changes and maturation

2. Match the terms related to tube feeding in Column A with their explanations in Column B.

Column A	Column B
1. ________ Intermittent feeding	A. Instillation of liquid nutrition without interruption at a rate of approximately 1.5 mL/min
2. ________ Continuous feeding	B. Instillation of liquid nourishment for 8 to 12 hours followed by a pause of 12 to 16 hours
3. ________ Cyclic feeding	C. Instillation of liquid nourishment four to six times a day

Activity E: *1. Differentiate between open drains and closed drains based on the categories given below.*

	Open Drains	Closed Drains
Definition		
Method of drainage		
Wound care		

Activity F: *Consider the following figure.*

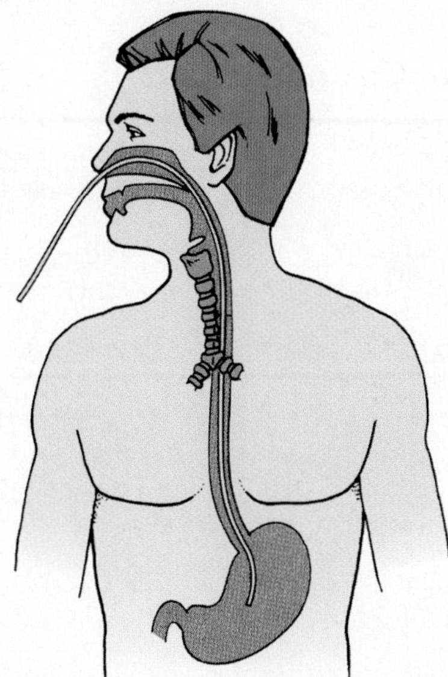

1. Label and identify what is shown in the figure.
2. What could be the adverse effects of this procedure?

Activity G: *Coughing is the natural method of clearing secretions from the airways. Write in the boxes provided below the correct sequence of performing forced coughing.*

1. Take a slow deep breath through the nose.
2. Exhale slowly through the mouth.
3. Sit upright.
4. Lean slightly forward.
5. Pull the abdomen inward.
6. Make the lower abdomen rise to the maximum.

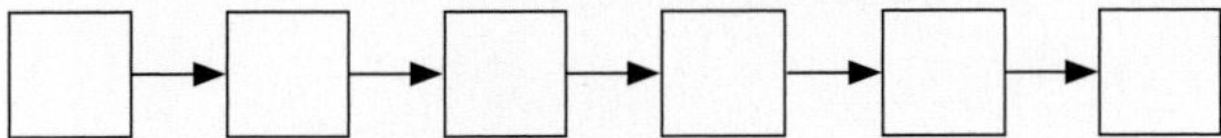

Activity H: *Answer the following questions.*

1. What is a pneumatic compression device?
2. What are the three methods for preparing the skin for surgery?
3. What are the three types of wound healing?

4. What are the causes of gastrostomy leaks?

5. What are the uses of gastric or intestinal tubes?

Section II: Applying Your Knowledge

Activity I: *Give rationales for the following questions.*

1. Why are volatile substances such as alcohol and acetone avoided around lasers?

2. Why do surgical clients have a reduced circulatory volume?

3. Why are transparent dressings less bulky than gauze dressings?

4. Why it is important to keep wounds moist?

5. Why are mercury-weighted tubes not used anymore?

6. Why should water be given sparingly to clients who are using a tube for gastric decompression?

Activity J: *Answer the following questions focusing on nursing roles and responsibilities.*

1. A nurse is caring for a client who is to undergo surgery the following day. What potential risks factors increase the likelihood of perioperative complications?

2. A nurse in a health care facility is caring for a middle-aged client scheduled for an incisional cholecystectomy.
   a. What general preoperative information should the nurse provide for this client?

   b. What preoperative physical preparations is the nurse likely to perform for the client?

3. A nurse is to perform an ear irrigation on a client.
   a. What process will the nurse follow?

   b. What post-irrigation technique should the nurse implement?

4. What six basic techniques should the nurse follow to wrap a roller bandage?

5. A nurse at an extended-care facility is caring for a client receiving tube feedings. The client has asked for self-care at home even if tube feeding is required.
   a. What written instructions should the nurse provide when preparing the client for home care?

   b. What are some nursing diagnoses that might be appropriate for this client?

6. What are common nursing guidelines for clients with intestinal decompression tubes?

Activity K: *Consider the following questions. Discuss them with your instructor or peers.*

1. A nurse is caring for a client who has received preoperative spinal anesthesia.
   a. What postoperative nursing care will be appropriate for this client?
   b. How does client care differ for general anesthesia versus regional anesthesia?
2. An elderly client at an extended care facility is experiencing chronic lower back pain.
   a. What measures can the nurse take to provide pain relief?
   b. What actions should the nurse perform to help prevent pressure ulcers resulting from restricted mobility in this client?

3. A client has been brought to the health care facility in a semiconscious state following a suicide attempt by drug overdose.
   a. What immediate care should the nurse provide for this client?
   b. What assistance should the nurse provide during a lavage procedure for this client?

Section III: Getting Ready for NCLEX

Activity L: *Answer the following questions.*

1. The physician has ordered a cold application for a client with a bruised and painful ankle. Which of the following explanations will the nurse give to the client regarding the benefit of cold applications?
   a. Speeds healing
   b. Relieves muscle spasm
   c. Promotes circulation
   d. Numbs sensation
2. How can the nurse clear a small-diameter orogastric feeding tube that is obstructed? Select all that apply.
   a. Aspirate as much as possible from the tube.
   b. Instill 5 mL of an enzymatic solution.
   c. Reinstill the aspirated fluid.
   d. Measure the aspirated fluid and record.
   e. Clamp the tube and wait for 15 minutes.
3. A physician has ordered tube feedings for a hospitalized client. Which of the following could contribute to the development of diarrhea in a tube-fed client? Select all that apply.
   a. Highly concentrated formula
   b. Rapid administration
   c. Bacterial contamination
   d. Incorrect tube placement
   e. Inadequate calories
4. A nurse is providing preoperative information to a client scheduled to undergo surgery. Which of the following explanations will the nurse give to the client regarding the benefits of deep breathing?
   a. Reduces postoperative risk for respiratory complications
   b. Helps clear secretions from the airways
   c. Eases postoperative pain and discomfort
   d. Decreases the risk for circulatory complications
5. An elderly client is scheduled to undergo surgery. Which of the following assessments should a nurse perform before fluid restriction? Select all that apply.
   a. Fluid intake and output
   b. Vital signs
   c. Level of consciousness
   d. Weight
   e. Skin turgor
6. A nurse is caring for an elderly client receiving tube feedings. Which of the following signs should the nurse closely monitor to identify hyperglycemia?
   a. Malabsorption syndrome
   b. Hydration status
   c. Change in skin turgor
   d. Elevated body temperature

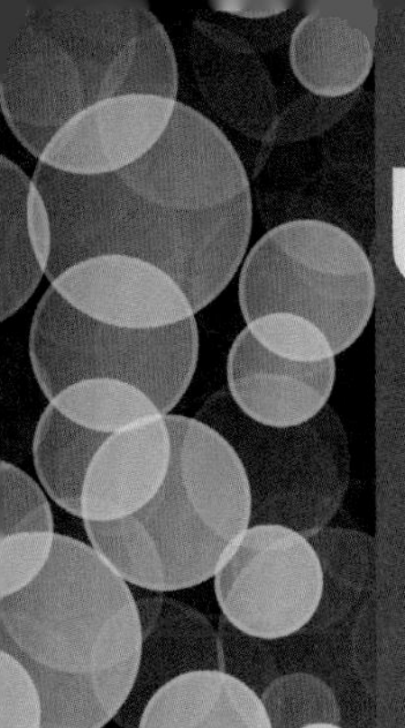

UNIT 8
Promoting Elimination

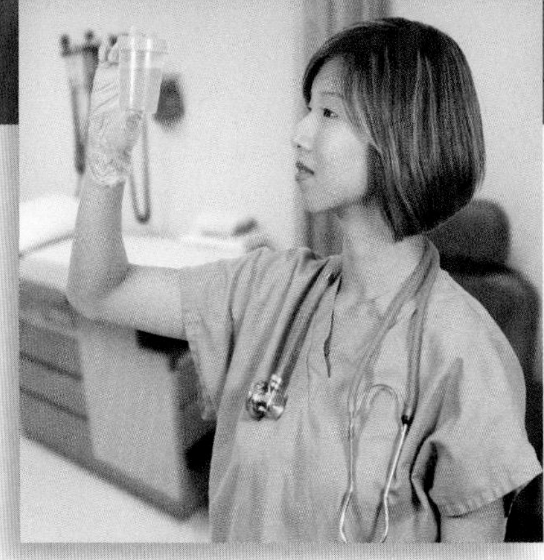

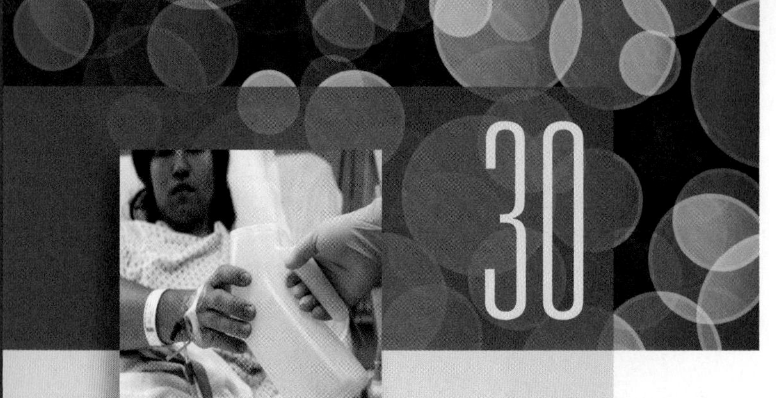

Urinary Elimination

Words To Know

anuria
bedpan
catheter care
catheter irrigation
catheterization
clean-catch specimen
closed drainage system
commode
continence training
continuous irrigation
Credé's maneuver
cutaneous triggering
dysuria
external catheter
fenestrated drape
frequency
incontinence
Kegel exercises
nocturia
oliguria
peristomal skin
polyuria
residual urine
retention catheter
stasis
straight catheter
24-hour specimen
urgency
urinal
urinary diversion
urinary elimination
urinary retention
urine
urostomy
voided specimen
voiding reflex

Learning Objectives

On completion of this chapter, the reader should be able to:

1. Identify the collective functions of the urinary system.
2. Describe the physical characteristics of urine and factors that affect urination.
3. Name four types of urine specimens that nurses commonly collect.
4. Identify three alternative devices for urinary elimination.
5. Define continence training.
6. Name three types of urinary catheters.
7. Describe two principles that apply to using a closed drainage system.
8. Explain why catheter care is important in the nursing management of clients with retention catheters.
9. Discuss the purpose for irrigating a catheter and methods for performing this skill.
10. Define urinary diversion.
11. Discuss factors that contribute to impaired skin integrity in clients with a urostomy.

This chapter reviews the process of urinary elimination and describes the nursing skills for assessing and maintaining urinary elimination.

OVERVIEW OF URINARY ELIMINATION

The urinary system (Fig. 30-1) consists of the kidneys, ureters, bladder, and urethra. These major components, along with some accessory structures such as the ring-shaped muscles called the internal and external sphincters, work together to produce **urine** (fluid within the bladder), collect it, and excrete it from the body.

Urinary elimination (the process of releasing excess fluid and metabolic wastes), or urination, occurs when urine is excreted. Under normal conditions, the average person eliminates approximately 1,500 to 3,000 mL of urine each day. The consequences of impaired urinary elimination can be life-threatening.

Urination takes place several times each day. The need to urinate becomes apparent when the bladder distends with approximately 150 to 300 mL of urine. The distention with urine causes increased fluid pressure, stimulating stretch receptors in the bladder wall and creating a desire to empty it of urine.

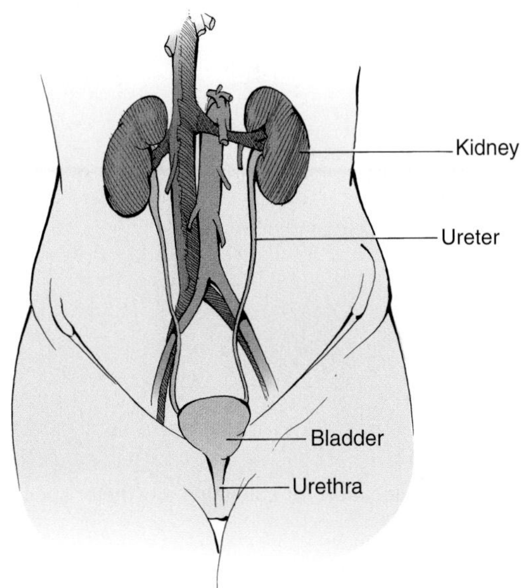

FIGURE 30-1 The major structures of the urinary system.

CHARACTERISTICS OF URINE

The physical characteristics of urine include its volume, color, clarity, and odor. Variations in what is considered normal are wide (Table 30-1).

FACTORS AFFECTING URINARY ELIMINATION

Patterns of urinary elimination depend on physiologic, emotional, and social factors. Examples include (1) the degree of neuromuscular development and the integrity of the spinal cord; (2) the volume of fluid intake and the amount of fluid losses, including those from other sources; (3) the amount and type of food consumed; and (4) the person's circadian rhythm, habits, opportunities for urination, and anxiety.

General measures to promote urination include providing privacy, assuming a natural position for urination (sitting for women, standing for men), maintaining an adequate fluid intake, and using stimuli such as running water from a tap to initiate voiding.

Urine Specimen Collection

Health care professionals collect urine specimens, or samples of urine, to identify microscopic or chemical constituents. Common urine specimens that nurses collect include voided specimens, clean-catch specimens, catheter specimens, and 24-hour specimens.

Voided Specimens

A **voided specimen** is a sample of fresh urine collected in a clean container. The first voided specimen of the day is preferred because it is most likely to contain substantial urinary components that have accumulated during the night. Nevertheless, the specimen can be voided and collected at any time it is needed.

The sample of urine is transferred into a specimen container and delivered to the laboratory for testing and analysis. If the specimen cannot be examined in less than 1 hour after collection, it is labeled and refrigerated.

Clean-Catch Specimens

A **clean-catch specimen** is a voided sample of urine considered sterile and is sometimes called a midstream specimen because of the way it is collected. To avoid contaminating the voided sample with microorganisms or substances other than those in the urine, the external structures through which urine passes (the urinary meatus, which is the opening to the urethra, and the surrounding tissues) are cleansed. The urine is collected after the initial stream has been released.

Clean-catch specimens are preferred to randomly voided specimens. This method of collection is also preferable when a urine specimen is needed during a woman's menstrual period. As soon as the specimen is collected, it

TABLE 30-1 Characteristics of Urine

CHARACTERISTIC	NORMAL	ABNORMAL	COMMON CAUSES OF VARIATIONS
Volume	500–3,000 mL/day 1,200 mL/day average	<400 mL/day	Low fluid intake Excess fluid loss Kidney dysfunction
		>3,000 mL/day	High fluid intake Diuretic medication Endocrine diseases
Color	Light yellow	Dark amber Brown Reddish-brown Orange, green, blue	Dehydration Liver/gallbladder disease Blood Water-soluble dyes
Clarity	Transparent	Cloudy	Infection Stasis
Odor	Faintly aromatic	Foul Strong Pungent	Infection Dehydration Certain foods

Client and Family Teaching 30-1
Collecting a Clean-Catch Specimen

The nurse teaches the female client as follows:

- Wash your hands.
- Remove the lid from the specimen container.
- Rest the lid upside down on its outer surface, taking care not to touch the inside areas.
- Sit on the toilet and spread your legs.
- Separate your labia with your fingers.
- Cleanse each side of the urinary meatus with a separate antiseptic swab, wiping from front to back toward the vagina.
- Use the final clean, moistened swab to wipe directly down the center of the separated tissue.
- Begin to urinate.
- After releasing a small amount of urine into the toilet, catch a sample of urine in the specimen container.
- Take care not to touch the mouth of the specimen container to your skin.
- Place the specimen container nearby on a flat surface.
- Release your fingers and continue voiding normally.
- Wash your hands.
- Cover the specimen container with the lid.

The male client should follow the same steps as above but should perform the following cleansing routine:

- Retract your foreskin, if you are uncircumcised, or cleanse in a circular direction around the tip of the penis toward its base using a premoistened antiseptic swab.
- Repeat with another swab.
- Continue retracting the foreskin while initiating the first release of urine and until you have collected the midstream specimen.

is labeled and taken to the laboratory. A clean-catch urine specimen is refrigerated if the analysis will be delayed more than 1 hour.

Research suggests that collecting a specimen in midstream after the use of soap, tap water, and nonsterile gauze for perineal cleansing provides results as reliable as those in which an antiseptic solution is used (Unlu et al., 2007). Nurses should follow their agency's policy.

When a clean-catch specimen is needed, nurses can instruct clients who are capable of performing the procedure on the collection technique (see Client and Family Teaching 30-1).

Catheter Specimens

A urine specimen can be collected under sterile conditions using a catheter, but this is usually done when clients are catheterized for other reasons such as to control incontinence in an unconscious client. For clients who are already catheterized, the nurse can aspirate a sample through the lumen of a latex catheter or from a self-sealing port that has been cleansed with an alcohol pad (Fig. 30-2).

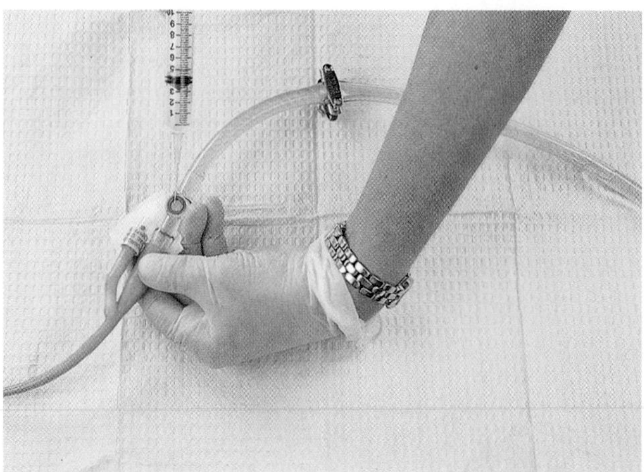

FIGURE 30-2 The location for collecting a catheter specimen. (Photo by B. Proud.)

24-Hour Specimens

The nurse collects, labels, and delivers a **24-hour specimen** (a collection of all urine produced in a full 24-hour period) to the laboratory for analysis. Because the contents in urine decompose over time, the nurse places the collected urine in a container with a chemical preservative or puts the container in a basin of ice or in a refrigerator.

To establish the 24-hour collection period accurately, the nurse instructs the client to urinate just before starting the test and then discards that urine. All urine voided thereafter becomes part of the collected specimen. Exactly 24 hours later, the nurse asks the client to void one last time to complete the test collection. The final urination and all collected voidings from the preceding 24 hours represent the total specimen, which the nurse labels and takes to the laboratory.

Abnormal Urine Characteristics

Laboratory analysis is a valuable diagnostic tool for identifying abnormal characteristics of urine. Specific terms describe particular abnormal characteristics of urine and urination. Many terms use the suffix *-uria,* which refers to urine or urination. For example:

- Hematuria: urine containing blood
- Pyuria: urine containing pus
- Proteinuria: urine containing plasma proteins
- Albuminuria: urine containing albumin, a plasma protein
- Glycosuria: urine containing glucose
- Ketonuria: urine containing ketones

ABNORMAL URINARY ELIMINATION PATTERNS

Assessment findings may indicate abnormal urinary elimination patterns. Some common problems include anuria, oliguria, polyuria, nocturia, dysuria, and incontinence.

Anuria

Anuria means the absence of urine or a volume of 100 mL or less in 24 hours. It indicates that the kidneys are not forming sufficient urine. In this case, the term "urinary suppression" is used. In urinary suppression, the bladder is empty; therefore, the client feels no urge to urinate. This distinguishes anuria from **urinary retention**, in which the client produces urine but does not release it from the bladder. A sign of urinary retention is a progressively distending bladder.

Oliguria

Oliguria, urine output less than 400 mL/24 hours, indicates the inadequate elimination of urine. Sometimes oliguria is a sign that the bladder is being only partially emptied during voidings. **Residual urine**, or more than 50 mL of urine that remains in the bladder after voiding, can support the growth of microorganisms, leading to infection. Also, when there is urinary **stasis** (a lack of movement), dissolved substances such as calcium can precipitate, leading to urinary stones.

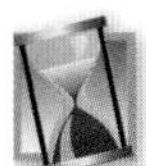

Gerontologic Considerations

■ Older adults are more likely to have chronic residual urine (excessive urine in the bladder after urinating), which increases the risk for urinary tract infections. They may benefit from learning double-voiding in which the person voids then waits a few more minutes to allow any residual urine to be voided.

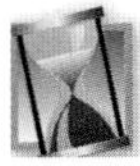

Gerontologic Considerations

■ The prevention of urinary tract infections is best accomplished by prompt attention to perineal hygiene. Women should always clean from the urinary area back toward the rectal area to prevent organisms from the stool entering the bladder. In addition, thorough hand washing by the client and caregiver is necessary.

Polyuria

Polyuria means greater than normal urinary elimination and may accompany minor dietary variations. For example, consuming higher than normal amounts of fluids, especially those with mild diuretic effects (eg, coffee and tea), or taking certain medications actually can increase urination. Ordinarily, urine output is nearly equal to fluid intake. When the cause of polyuria is not apparent, excessive urination may be the result of a disorder. Common disorders associated with polyuria include *diabetes mellitus*, an endocrine disorder caused by insufficient insulin or insulin resistance, and *diabetes insipidus*, an endocrine disease caused by insufficient antidiuretic hormone.

Nocturia

Nocturia (nighttime urination) is unusual because the rate of urine production is normally reduced at night. Consequently, nocturia suggests an underlying medical problem. In aging men, an enlarging prostate gland, which encircles the urethra, interferes with complete bladder emptying. As a result, there is a need to urinate more frequently, including during the usual hours of sleep.

Dysuria

Dysuria is the difficult or uncomfortable voiding and a common symptom of trauma to the urethra or a bladder infection. **Frequency** (the need to urinate often) and **urgency** (a strong feeling that urine must be eliminated quickly) often accompany dysuria.

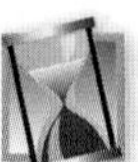

Gerontologic Considerations

■ Older adults are likely to experience urinary urgency and frequency because of normal physiologic changes such as diminished bladder capacity and degenerative changes in the cerebral cortex. Subsequently, when they perceive the urge to void, they need to access a bathroom as soon as possible.

Incontinence

Incontinence means the inability to control either urinary or bowel elimination and is abnormal after a person is toilet trained. The term *urinary incontinence* should not be used indiscriminately: anyone may be incontinent if his or her need for assistance goes unnoticed. Once the bladder becomes extremely distended, spontaneous urination may be more of a personnel problem than a client problem. (The client may not be incontinent if staff members are attentive to his or her need to urinate.)

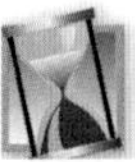

Gerontologic Considerations

■ Age-related changes, such as a diminished bladder capacity and a relaxation of the pelvic floor muscle tone, increase the risk for incontinence.

■ Fluid restriction may be used in an attempt to control urination, but it may actually contribute to incontinence by causing concentrated urine and eliminating the normal perception of a full bladder.

■ Older adults should be taught that odors may remain in clothing because of ammonia from urine leakage. Adding vinegar or using odor-controlling detergents may be useful when laundering soiled clothing.

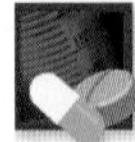

Pharmacologic Considerations

■ Diuretic therapy commonly can increase the risk for urinary incontinence especially among older adults with

mobility problems. Planning for access to a toilet within 30 to 120 minutes following medication administration should be included in client education regarding diuretic therapy.
■ A diuretic should be administered in the morning to avoid disturbing a client's sleep by the need to urinate.

ASSISTING CLIENTS WITH URINARY ELIMINATION

Stable clients who can ambulate are assisted to the bathroom to use the toilet. Clients who are weak or cannot walk to the bathroom may need a commode. Clients confined to the bed use a urinal or bedpan.

Commode

A **commode** (a chair with an opening in the seat under which a receptacle is placed) is located beside or near the bed (Fig. 30-3). It is used for eliminating urine or stool. Immediately afterward, the waste container is removed, emptied, cleaned, and replaced.

Urinal

A **urinal** is a cylindrical container for collecting urine. It is more easily used by males. When given to the client, the urinal should be empty; otherwise, the bed linen may become wet and soiled. If the client needs help placing the urinal:

- Pull the privacy curtain
- Don gloves
- Ask the client to spread his legs
- Hold the urinal by its handle
- Direct the urinal at an angle between the client's legs so that the bottom rests on the bed (Fig. 30-4)
- Lift the penis and place it well within the urinal

After use, the nurse promptly empties the urinal. He or she measures and records the volume of urine if the client's intake and output are being monitored (see Chap. 16). The nurse washes his or her hands and always offers the client an opportunity to wash his hands after voiding.

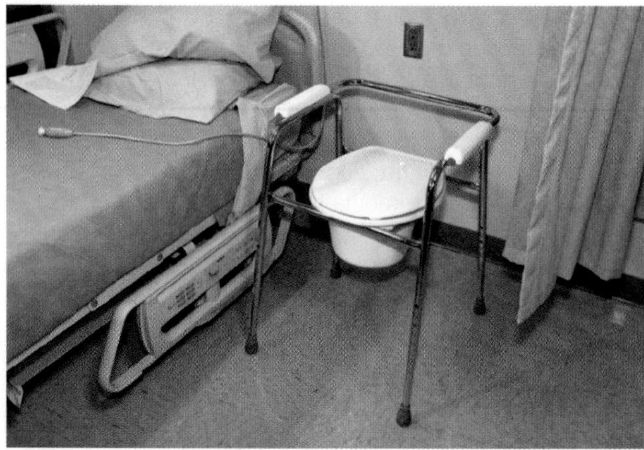

FIGURE 30-3 A bedside commode.

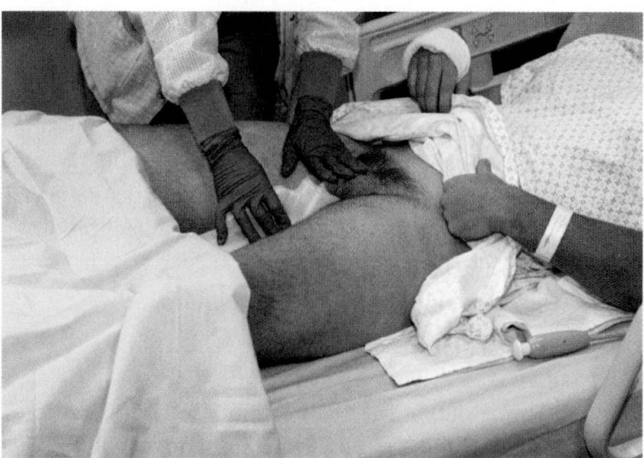

FIGURE 30-4 Placement of a urinal.

Using a Bedpan

A **bedpan** (a seatlike container for elimination) is used to collect urine or stool. Most bedpans are made of plastic and are several inches deep. A *fracture pan*, a modified version of a conventional bedpan, is flat on the sitting end rather than rounded (Fig. 30-5). Clients with musculoskeletal disorders who cannot elevate their hips and sit on a bedpan in the usual manner use a fracture pan. When a client confined to bed feels the need to eliminate, the nurse places a bedpan under the buttocks (Skill 30-1).

Stop, Think, and Respond Box 30-1

Describe measures that may reduce a client's concerns when he or she requires a bedpan.

MANAGING INCONTINENCE

Urinary incontinence, depending on its type, may be permanent or temporary. The six types of urinary incontinence are stress, urge, reflex, functional, total, and overflow (Table 30-2).

The management of incontinence is complex because there are so many variations. Treatment is further complicated when clients have more than one type of incontinence; for example, stress incontinence often accompanies urge incontinence.

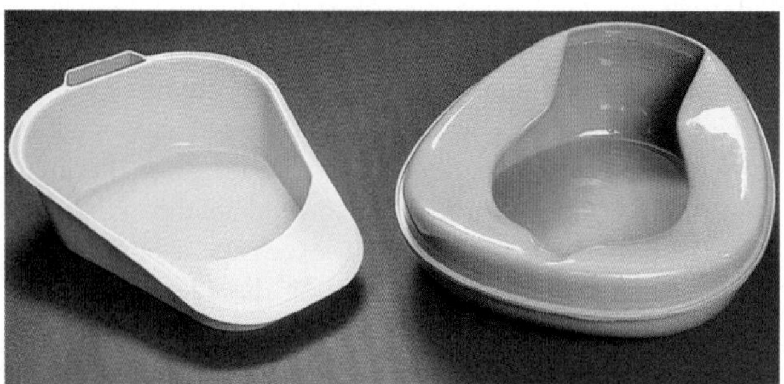

FIGURE 30-5 Two types of bedpans: a fracture pan (*left*) and a conventional bedpan (*right*). (Photo by B. Proud.)

TABLE 30-2 Types of Incontinence

TYPE	DESCRIPTION	EXAMPLE	COMMON CAUSES	NURSING APPROACH
Stress	The loss of small amounts of urine when intra-abdominal pressure rises	Dribbling is associated with sneezing, coughing, lifting, laughing, or rising from a bed or chair	Loss of perineal and sphincter muscle tone secondary to childbirth, menopausal atrophy, prolapsed uterus, or obesity	Pelvic floor muscle strengthening Weight reduction
Urge	Need to void perceived frequently, with short-lived ability to sustain control of the flow	Voiding commences when there is a delay in accessing a restroom	Bladder irritation secondary to infection; loss of bladder tone from recent continuous drainage with an indwelling catheter	Restriction of fluid intake of at least 2,000 mL/day Omit bladder irritants, such as caffeine or alcohol Administration of diuretics in the morning
Reflex	Spontaneous loss of urine when the bladder is stretched with urine, but without prior perception of a need to void	The person automatically releases urine and cannot control it	Damage to motor and sensory tracts in the lower spinal cord secondary to trauma, a tumor, or other neurologic conditions	Cutaneous triggering Straight intermittent catheterization
Functional	Control over urination lost because of inaccessibility of a toilet or a compromised ability to use one	Voiding occurs while attempting to overcome barriers such as doorways, transferring from a wheelchair, manipulating clothing, acquiring assistance, or making needs known	Impaired mobility, impaired cognition, physical restraints, inability to communicate	Clothing modification Access to a toilet, commode, or urinal Assistance to a toilet according to a preplanned schedule
Total	Loss of urine without any identifiable pattern or warning	The person passes urine without any ability or effort to control	Altered consciousness secondary to a head injury, loss of sphincter tone secondary to prostatectomy, anatomic leak through a urethral/vaginal fistula	Absorbent undergarments External catheter Indwelling catheter
Overflow	Urine leakage because the bladder is not completely emptied; bladder distended with retained urine	The person voids small amounts frequently, or urine leaks around a catheter	Overstretched bladder or weakened muscle tone secondary to obstruction of the urethra by debris within a catheter, an enlarged prostate, distended bowel, or postoperative bladder spasms	Hydration Adequate bowel elimination Patency of catheter Credé's maneuver

Some forms of incontinence respond to simple measures such as modifying clothing to make elimination easier. Other forms improve only with a more regimented approach like continence training. Inserting a retention catheter is the least desirable approach to managing incontinence because it is the leading cause of urinary tract infections in hospitals and nursing homes (Centers for Disease Control and Prevention, 2009; National Institute of Diabetes and Digestive and Kidney Diseases, 2005).

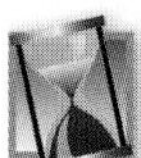

Gerontologic Considerations

■ Loss of control over urination often threatens an older adult's independence and self-esteem. It also may cause an older adult to restrict activities, possibly contributing to depression. Teaching older adults to structure activities with planned toileting breaks every 60 to 90 minutes results in less urine in the bladder and thus diminishes urge incontinence.

■ Older adults who experience difficulty controlling urine need an evaluation of contributing factors, which may be treated to reverse the diminished control of urination. Such causes may include constipation, urinary tract infection, and medication side effects.

■ Older adults need encouragement to discuss urinary incontinence with a knowledgeable, nonjudgmental health care provider. If they understand that urinary incontinence is a condition that frequently responds to medication or behavioral retraining, they are more likely to seek professional help.

■ Many resources are available to assist older adults in evaluating and treating incontinence. For example, some health care facilities offer special incontinence clinics and physical therapy departments to teach pelvic muscle exercises. In addition, biofeedback has been used to strengthen bladder control. The National Association for Continence

(800-252-3337; http://www.nafc.org) is an excellent source of information for products, resources, and continence programs. Nurses can encourage older adults to take advantage of these kinds of resources rather than accepting incontinence as an inevitable condition that compromises their quality of life.

■ When efforts to restore continence are unsuccessful, nurses can encourage older adults to verbalize their feelings and identify interventions helpful in maintaining dignity, ultimately enabling older adults to participate in meaningful activities.

Continence training to restore the control of urination involves teaching the client to refrain from urinating until an appropriate time and place. This process sometimes is referred to as *bladder retraining*, but this term is inaccurate because the various techniques used involve mechanisms other than those unique to the bladder.

Continence training primarily benefits clients with the cognitive ability and desire to participate in a rehabilitation program. This includes clients with lower body paralysis who wish to facilitate urination without the use of urinary drainage devices such as catheters. Clients who are not candidates for continence training require alternative methods such as absorbent undergarments.

Continence training is often a slow process that requires the combined effort and dedication of the nursing team, client, and family (see Nursing Guidelines 30-1 and Fig. 30-6).

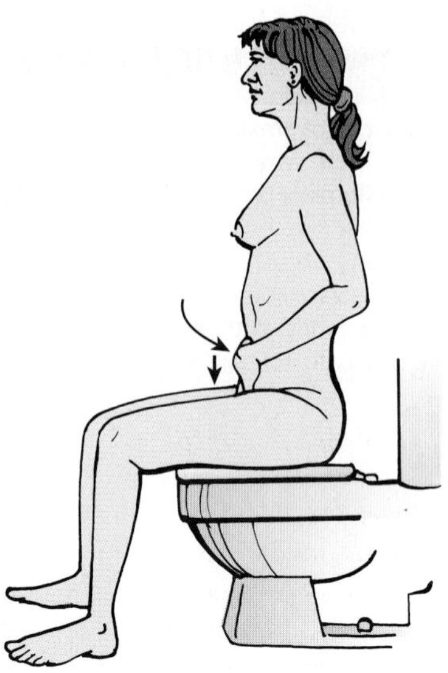

FIGURE 30-6 Credé's maneuver.

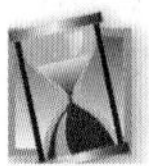

Gerontologic Considerations

■ Routine toileting schedules must be offered every 90 to 120 minutes to clients who have problems with incontinence.

■ Absorbent products are likely to interfere with the person's independence in toileting and may lead to skin breakdown. Incontinence products are never used primarily for staff convenience in institutional settings. In addition, an older person should never be reprimanded for an episode of incontinence.

■ When efforts to restore continence are unsuccessful, nurses can encourage older adults to verbalize their feelings and identify interventions helpful in maintaining dignity, ultimately enabling older adults to participate in meaningful activities.

CATHETERIZATION

Catheterization (the act of applying or inserting a hollow tube), in this case, refers to using a device inside the bladder, or externally about the urinary meatus. A urinary catheter is used for various reasons:

- Keeping incontinent clients dry (catheterization is a last resort that is used only when all other continence measures have been exhausted)
- Relieving bladder distention when clients cannot void
- Assessing fluid balance accurately
- Keeping the bladder from becoming distended during procedures such as surgery
- Measuring the residual urine
- Obtaining sterile urine specimens
- Instilling medication within the bladder

Types of Catheters

The three common types of catheters are external, straight, and retention. Most catheters are made of latex. For clients who are sensitive or allergic to latex, latex-free catheters such as those made of silicone are used.

External Catheters

An **external catheter** (a urine-collecting device applied to the skin) is not inserted within the bladder; instead, it surrounds the urinary meatus. Examples of external catheters are a condom catheter (Fig. 30-7) and a urinary bag (U-bag). External catheters are more effective for male clients.

Condom catheters are helpful for clients receiving care at home because they are easy to apply. A condom catheter has a flexible sheath that is unrolled over the penis. The narrow

BOX 30-1 Technique for Performing Kegel Exercises

- Tighten the internal muscles used to prevent urination or interrupt urination once it has begun.
- Keep the muscles contracted for at least 10 seconds.
- Relax the muscles for the same period.
- Repeat the pattern of contraction and relaxation 10 to 25 times.
- Perform the exercise regimen three or four times a day for 2 weeks to 1 month.

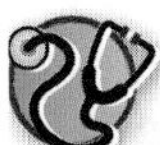

NURSING GUIDELINES 30-1

Providing Continence Training

- Compile a log of the client's urinary elimination patterns. *The data help to reveal the client's type of incontinence.*
- Set realistic, specific, short-term goals with the client. *Short-term goals prevent self-defeating consequences and promote client control.*
- Discourage strict limitation of liquid intake. *Intake maintains fluid balance and ensures adequate urine volume.*
- Plan a trial schedule for voiding that correlates with the times when the client is usually incontinent or experiences bladder distention. *This schedule reduces the potential for accidental voiding or sustained urinary retention.*
- In the absence of any identifiable pattern, plan to assist the client with voiding every 2 hours during the day and every 4 hours at night. *This duration provides time for urine to form.*
- Communicate the plan to nursing personnel, the client, and the family. *Collaboration promotes continuity of care and dedication to reaching goals.*
- Assist the client to a toilet or commode; position the client on a bedpan or place a urinal just before the scheduled time for trial voiding. *These measures prepare the client for releasing urine.*
- Simulate the sound of urination such as by running water from the faucet. *Doing so simulates relaxation of the sphincter muscles, allowing the release of urine.*
- Suggest performing **Credé's maneuver** (the act of bending forward and applying hand pressure over the bladder; see Fig. 30-6). *Credé's maneuver increases abdominal pressure to overcome the resistance of the internal sphincter muscle.*
- Instruct paralyzed clients to identify any sensation that precedes voiding such as a chill, muscular spasm, restlessness, or spontaneous penile erection. *These cues can help the client anticipate urination.*
- Suggest that paralyzed clients with reflex incontinence use **cutaneous triggering** (lightly massaging or tapping the skin above the pubic area). *Cutaneous triggering initiates urination in clients who have retained a **voiding reflex** (the spontaneous relaxation of the urinary sphincter in response to physical stimulation).*
- Teach clients with stress incontinence to perform **Kegel exercises** (isometric exercises to improve the ability to retain urine within the bladder; see Box 30-1). *Kegel exercises strengthen and tone the pubococcygeal and levator ani muscles used voluntarily to hold back urine and intestinal gas or stool.*
- Assist clients with urge incontinence to walk slowly and concentrate on holding their urine when nearing the toilet. *These measures reverse previous mental conditioning in which the urge to urinate becomes stronger and more overpowering close to the toilet.*

end is connected to tubing that serves as a channel for draining urine. The drainage tube may be attached to a leg bag (Fig. 30-8) or connected to a larger urine-collection device.

Three potential problems accompany the use of condom catheters. First, the sheath may be applied too tightly, restricting blood flow to the skin and tissues of the penis. Second, moisture tends to accumulate beneath the sheath, leading to skin breakdown. Third, condom catheters frequently leak. Applying the catheter correctly and managing care appropriately can prevent these problems (Skill 30-2).

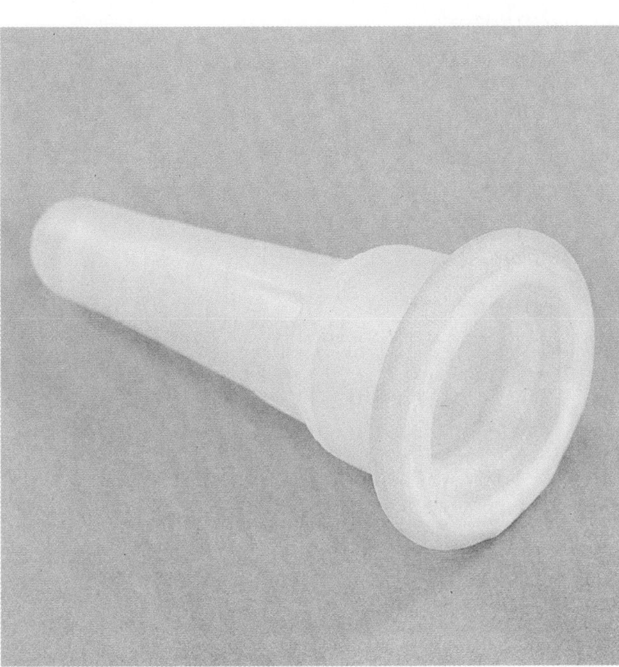

FIGURE 30-7 A condom catheter is an example of an external urine collection device. (Photo by B. Proud.)

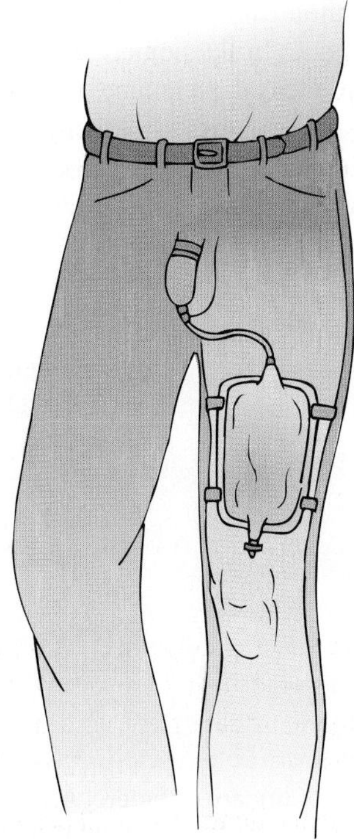

FIGURE 30-8 A leg bag collects urine from a catheter but is concealed under clothing.

Stop, Think, and Respond Box 30-2

Discuss assessments that indicate common problems associated with the use of a condom catheter and nursing measures that can reduce or eliminate negative outcomes.

A U-bag is more often used to collect urine specimens from infants. It is attached by adhesive backing to the skin surrounding the genitals. Urine collects in the self-contained bag. Once enough urine is collected, the bag is removed.

Straight Catheters

A **straight catheter** is a urine drainage tube inserted but not left in place. It drains urine temporarily or provides a sterile urine specimen (Fig. 30-9).

Retention Catheters

A **retention catheter**, also called an indwelling catheter, is left in place for a period of time (see Fig. 30-9). The most common type is a Foley catheter.

Unlike straight catheters, retention catheters are secured with a balloon that is inflated once the distal tip is within the bladder. Both straight and retention catheters are available in various diameters, sized according to the French (F) scale (see Chap. 29). For adults, sizes 14, 16, and 18 F are commonly used.

Inserting a Catheter

The techniques for inserting straight and retention catheters are similar, although the steps for inflating the retention balloon do not apply to a straight catheter. When inserting a straight or a retention catheter in a health agency, the nurse uses sterile technique. In the home, nurses and clients who self-catheterize use clean technique because most clients have adapted to the organisms in their own environment. Because of anatomic differences, techniques for insertion differ in men and women and are described in Skills 30-3 and 30-4.

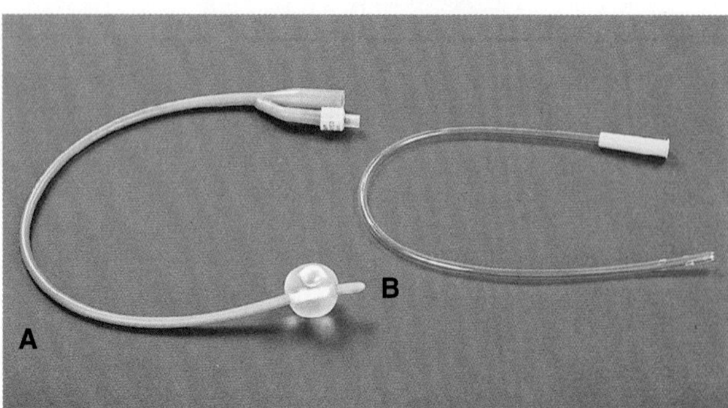

FIGURE 30-9 Types of urinary catheters. **A.** A retention (Foley) catheter with balloon. **B.** A straight catheter. (Photo by B. Proud.)

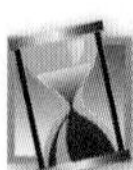

Gerontologic Considerations

■ Enlargement of the prostate, a common problem among older men, can totally obstruct urinary outflow and make catheterization difficult or impossible. Insertion of a urinary catheter should never be forced. Sometimes a catheter is inserted into the bladder through the abdominal wall when it cannot be inserted into a narrowed urethra.

Stop, Think, and Respond Box 30-3

Discuss factors that predispose a female with a Foley catheter to develop a urinary tract infection.

Connecting a Closed Drainage System

A **closed drainage system** (a device used to collect urine from a catheter) consists of a calibrated bag, which can be opened at the bottom; tubing of sufficient length to accommodate for turning and positioning clients; and a hanger from which to suspend the bag from the bed (Fig. 30-10). The nurse coils excess tubing on the bed but keeps the section from the bed to the collection bag vertical. Dependent loops in the tubing interfere with gravity flow. The nurse also takes care to avoid compressing the tubing, which can obstruct drainage. Placing the tubing over the client's thigh is acceptable.

The nurse always positions the drainage system lower than the bladder to avoid a backflow of urine. When

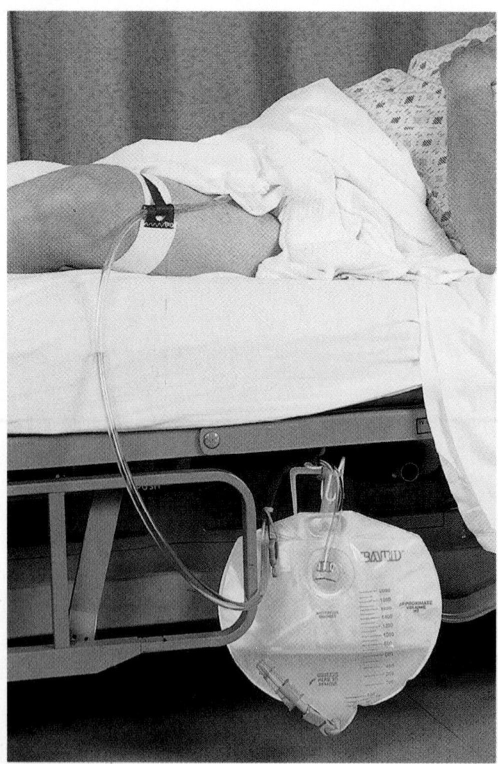

FIGURE 30-10 A closed urine drainage system. (Photo by B. Proud.)

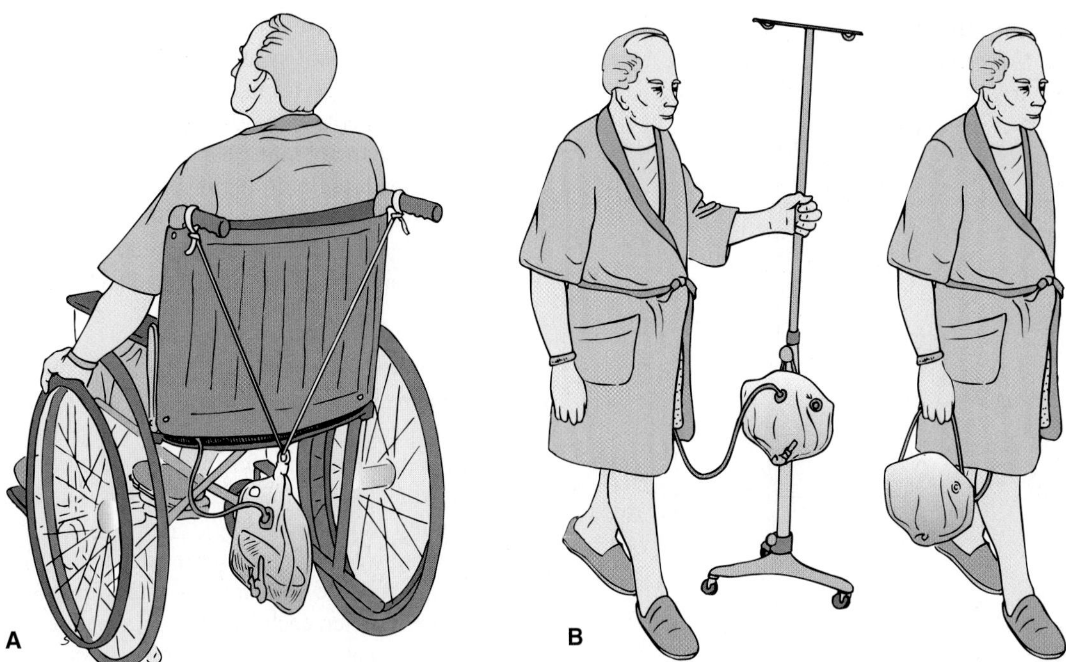

FIGURE 30-11 Techniques for suspending a drainage system below the bladder. A. A wheelchair patient. B. An ambulating patient with and without an IV pole.

transporting the client in a wheelchair, the nurse suspends the drainage bag from the chair below the level of the bladder. When the client is ambulating, the nurse secures the drainage bag to the lower part of an IV pole or allows the client to carry the bag by hand (Fig. 30-11).

To reduce the potential for the drainage system becoming a reservoir of pathogens, the entire drainage system is replaced whenever the catheter is changed and at least every 2 weeks in clients with a urinary tract infection.

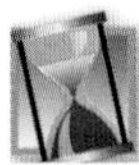

Gerontologic Considerations

■ Indwelling catheters should be avoided if at all possible because older people have increased susceptibility to urinary tract infections. Bladder training is much more desirable. If indwelling catheters are necessary, meticulous daily care is required. The tubing should never be placed higher than the bladder to prevent any backflow of urine into the bladder.

Stop, Think, and Respond Box 30-4

Discuss possible explanations for why urine may not flow from a catheter.

Providing Catheter Care

A retention catheter keeps the meatus slightly dilated, providing pathogens with a direct pathway to the bladder where an infection could develop. Bacteria also tend to adhere to the matrix of catheters forming a slimy substance known as biofilm, which supports bacterial growth and subsequent antibiotic resistance (Lu, 2008; Falkinham, 2007).

Catheter care (hygiene measures used to keep the meatus and adjacent area of the catheter clean) helps to deter the growth and spread of colonizing pathogens. Nursing Guidelines 30-2 describes the technique for providing catheter care. Nurses must follow agency policy for using antiseptic and antimicrobial agents because the use of these substances is not a standard recommendation by the Centers for Disease Control and Prevention (2009).

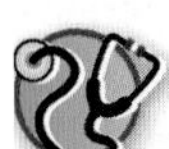

NURSING GUIDELINES 30-2

Providing Catheter Care

- Plan to cleanse the meatus and a nearby section of the catheter at least once a day. *Regular cleansing reduces colonizing microorganisms.*
- Gather clean gloves, soap, water, washcloth, towel, and a disposable pad. *Organization facilitates efficient time management.*
- Wash your hands or perform an alcohol-based hand rub (see Chap. 10). *Hand hygiene reduces the potential for transmitting microorganisms.*
- Place a disposable pad beneath the hips of a female and beneath the penis of a male. *The pad protects the bed linen from becoming wet or soiled.*
- Don clean gloves and wash the meatus, the catheter where it meets the meatus, the genitalia, and the perineum (in that order) with warm, soapy water. *Rinse and dry. Routine hygiene removes gross secretions and transient microorganisms while following the principles of asepsis.*
- Remove soiled materials and gloves, and repeat hand hygiene measures. *These steps remove colonizing microorganisms.*

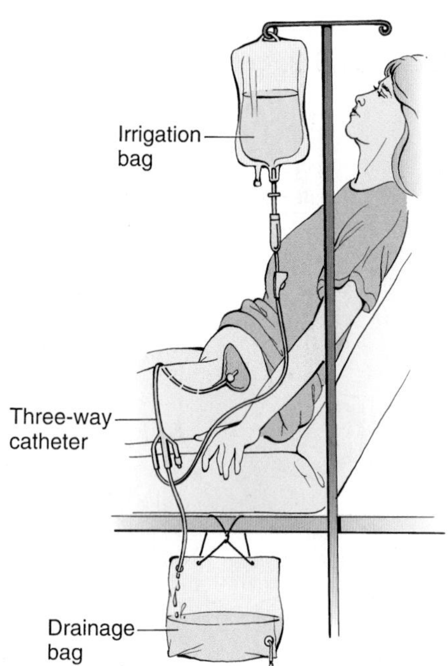

FIGURE 30-12 Bladder irrigation using a three-way catheter.

Catheter Irrigation

Catheter irrigation (flushing the lumen of a catheter) is a technique for restoring or maintaining catheter patency. A catheter that drains well, however, does not need irrigating. A generous oral fluid intake is usually sufficient to produce dilute urine, which thus keeps small shreds of mucus or tissue debris from obstructing the catheter. Occasionally, however, the catheter may need to be irrigated, such as after a surgical procedure that results in bloody urine.

Depending on the type of indwelling catheter, nurses irrigate continuously through a three-way catheter or periodically using an open system or a closed system (Skill 30-5).

Using an Open System

An open system is one in which the retention catheter is separated from the drainage tubing to insert the tip of an irrigating syringe. Opening the system creates the potential for infection because it provides an opportunity for pathogens to enter the exposed connection. Consequently, it is the least desirable of the three methods.

Using a Closed System

A closed system is irrigated without separating the catheter from the drainage tubing. To do so, the catheter or drainage tubing must have a self-sealing port. After cleansing the port with an alcohol swab, the nurse pierces the port with an 18- or 19-gauge, 1.5 in. needle (see Chap. 34). He or she attaches the needle to a 30- to 60-mL syringe containing a sterile irrigation solution. The nurse pinches or clamps the tubing beneath the port and instills the solution. He or she releases the tubing for drainage. The nurse records the volume of irrigant as fluid intake or subtracts it from the urine output to maintain an accurate intake and output record.

Continuous Irrigation

A **continuous irrigation** (the ongoing instillation of solution) instills irrigating solution into a catheter by gravity over a period of days (Fig. 30-12). Continuous irrigations keep a catheter patent after prostate or other urologic surgery in which blood clots and tissue debris collect within the bladder and catheter.

A three-way catheter is necessary to provide a continuous irrigation. The catheter has three lumens or channels within the catheter, each leading to a separate port. One port connects the catheter to the drainage system; another provides a means for inflating the balloon in the catheter; and the third instills the irrigating solution (Fig. 30-13). The steps involved in providing a continuous irrigation are as follows:

- Hang the sterile irrigating solution from an intravenous pole.
- Purge the air from the tubing.
- Connect the tubing to the catheter port for irrigation (Fig. 30-14).
- Regulate the rate of instillation according to the medical order.
- Monitor the appearance of the urine and volume of urinary drainage.

Stop, Think, and Respond Box 30-5

Discuss what actions might be appropriate if irrigating a catheter is unsuccessful in promoting catheter patency.

Indwelling Catheter Removal

A catheter is removed when it needs to be replaced or when its use is discontinued. The best time to remove a catheter is in the morning when there is more opportunity to address any urination difficulties without depriving a client of sleep (see Nursing Guidelines 30-3).

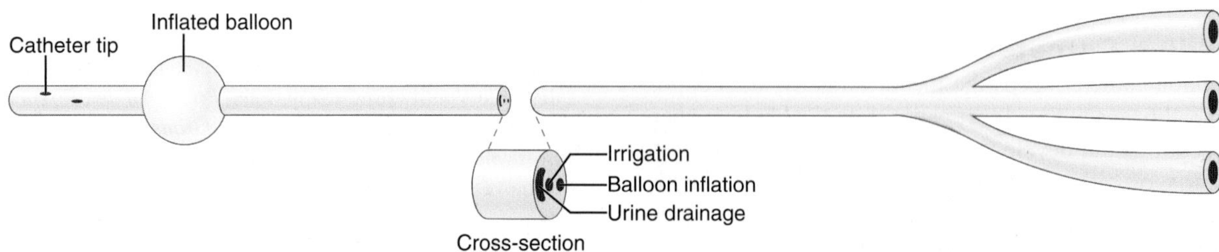

FIGURE 30-13 Components of a three-way catheter.

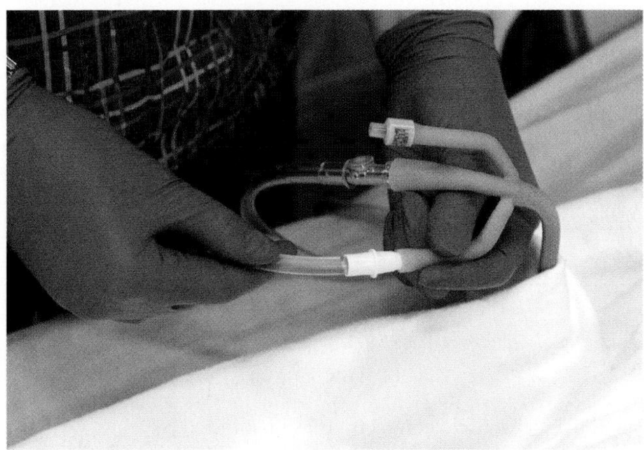

FIGURE 30-14 Attaching irrigation tubing to a port on a three-way catheter.

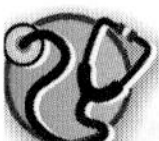

NURSING GUIDELINES 30-3

Removing a Foley Catheter

- Wash your hands or perform an alcohol-based hand rub (see Chap. 10) and don clean gloves. *These measures follow standard precautions.*
- Empty the balloon by aspirating the fluid with a syringe. *This step ensures that all the fluid has been withdrawn.*
- Gently pull the catheter near the point where it exits from the meatus. *Doing so facilitates withdrawal.*
- Inspect the catheter and discard if it appears to be intact. *This ensures safety.*
- Clean the urinary meatus. *This promotes comfort and hygiene.*
- Monitor the client's voiding especially for the next 8 to 10 hours; measure the volume of each voiding. *Findings determine whether or not elimination is normal as well as characteristics of the urine.*

URINARY DIVERSIONS

In a **urinary diversion**, one or both ureters are surgically implanted elsewhere. This procedure is done for various life-threatening conditions. The ureters may be brought to and through the skin of the abdomen (Fig. 30-15) or implanted within the bowel (called an ileal conduit). A **urostomy** (a urinary diversion that discharges urine from an opening on the abdomen) is the focus of this discussion.

Care for an ostomy, a surgically created opening, is discussed in more detail in Chapter 31 because those formed for bowel elimination are more common. Chapter 31 also provides a detailed description of an ostomy appliance, the device used for collecting stool or urine, and the manner in which it is applied and removed from the skin.

Caring for a urostomy and changing a urinary appliance are more challenging than the care of intestinal stomas. Urine drains continuously from a urostomy, increasing the risk for skin breakdown. In addition, because moisture and the weight of the collected urine tend to loosen the appliance from the skin, a urinary appliance may need to be changed more frequently. When changing the appliance, it may help to place a tampon within the stoma to absorb urine temporarily while the skin is cleansed and prepared for another appliance.

It is often difficult to maintain the integrity of the **peristomal skin** (the skin around the stoma) because of the frequent appliance changes and the ammonia in urine. Skin barrier products are used, and sometimes an antibiotic or steroid ointment is applied.

NURSING IMPLICATIONS

Clients with urinary elimination problems may have one or more of the following nursing diagnoses:

- Toileting Self-Care Deficit
- Impaired Urinary Elimination
- Risk for Infection
- Stress Urinary Incontinence
- Urge Urinary Incontinence
- Reflex Urinary Incontinence
- Functional Urinary Incontinence
- Situational Low Self-Esteem
- Risk for Impaired Skin Integrity

Nursing Care Plan 30-1 is developed for a client with Urge Urinary Incontinence, defined by NANDA-I (2012, p. 198) as "the involuntary passage of urine occurring soon after a strong sense of urgency to void."

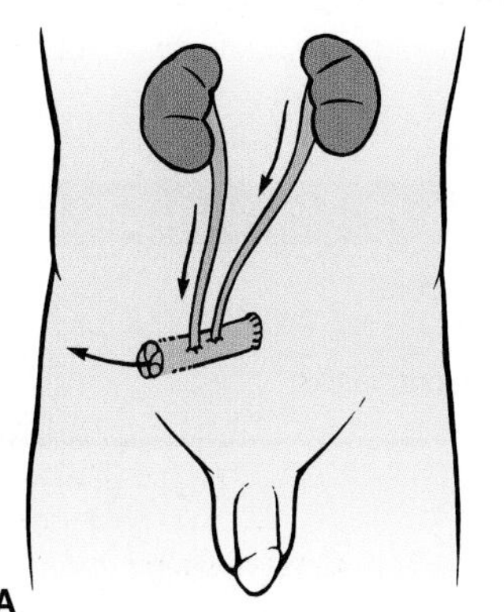

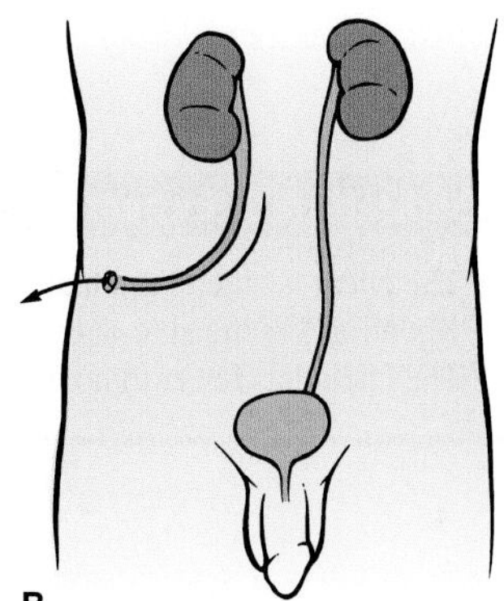

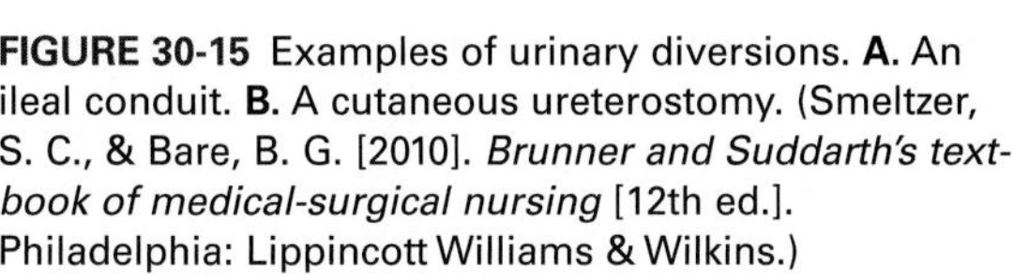

FIGURE 30-15 Examples of urinary diversions. **A.** An ileal conduit. **B.** A cutaneous ureterostomy. (Smeltzer, S. C., & Bare, B. G. [2010]. *Brunner and Suddarth's textbook of medical-surgical nursing* [12th ed.]. Philadelphia: Lippincott Williams & Wilkins.)

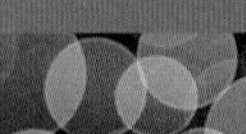

NURSING CARE PLAN 30-1 Urge Urinary Incontinence

Assessment

- Inquire about the number of voidings per day; voiding more than eight times in 24 hours or waking up two or more times at night to urinate, or urinating soon after the bladder has been emptied suggests a pattern of urgency or what has also been referred to as an overactive bladder.
- Identify the interim the client can wait to postpone urination following the sensation of a need to empty the bladder, commonly referred to as warning time (Carpenito-Moyet, 2006).
- Ask the client if the need to urinate is less easily controlled as the person gets nearer to the location of a toilet.
- Determine if the client experiences accidental loss of urine when there is an almost unstoppable need to urinate.

Nursing Diagnosis. **Urge Urinary Incontinence** related to uninhibited bladder muscle contractions as manifested by 14 to 18 voidings per day including awakening three times at night to urinate; daily episodes of urinary incontinence with impaired ability to delay urge to void.

Expected Outcome. The client will report a decrease in the number of daily voidings to <8 per day; absence or limited occasions of nocturia; ability to delay urination by 15 minutes or more when urination seems imminent; and absence of urinary incontinence within 6 to 8 weeks of implementing therapeutic interventions, for example, by 9/15.

Interventions	Rationales
Keep a record of the frequency of voidings and the length of time between the warning sign for voiding and actual voiding for 3 days beginning 8/1 through 8/3.	Documenting the client's unique pattern of urination facilitates appropriate nursing interventions.
Alert all nursing team members to respond as soon as possible to the client's signal for assistance.	Responding promptly reduces episodes of incontinence and demonstrates a united effort to help the client achieve control of urination.
Instruct the client to restrain urination as long as possible after the warning sign is perceived.	Efforts to delay urination help to reverse an established habit of over-responding to an urgent need to void.
Suggest that the client uses a technique such as breathing deeply, singing a song, or talking about family to delay voiding.	Focusing thoughts on something other than urination may provide sufficient distraction to extend the interval between the warning sign and actual voiding.
Encourage the client to eliminate the intake of beverages that contain caffeine or alcohol.	Caffeine promotes urination; alcohol inhibits the antidiuretic hormone, which prevents the reabsorption of water in the nephrons and leads to an increased formation of urine.
Ensure an oral fluid intake of at least 1,500–2,000 mL/day.	An adequate fluid intake reduces the potential for urinary infection or renal stone formation.
Assist the client to the toilet for the purpose of urination at a frequency that corresponds with the client's preconditioning pattern of urination (ie, approximately q1 1/2h), and extend the time by 15 minutes until there is an interval of 2 hours between voidings.	Increasing the length of time between voidings reduces chronic low-volume voiding, improves bladder muscle tone, and increases bladder capacity, which potentiates achieving continence.
Continue to extend the intervals between voiding until the client is voiding no more frequently than q4h in a 24-hour period.	Reconditioning the control of urination is facilitated by repetition and gradually extending the efforts to control voiding.
Praise the client every time a short-term goal of delaying or controlling urination is achieved.	Positive reinforcement helps to motivate the client to continue efforts to control incontinence.
Share the client's progress with the physician.	Medical interventions such as prescribing a medication that blocks acetylcholine (anticholinergic agent) may help to inhibit bladder muscle contractions and promote contraction of the urinary sphincter.

Evaluation of Expected Outcomes

- The client is able to gradually delay urination.
- Nocturia is reduced to once per night.
- The client has fewer to no episodes of incontinence.

CRITICAL THINKING EXERCISES

1. During a nursing assessment, a female client reports periodic dribbling of urine. What additional information is important to obtain?
2. An older adult client confides that she would like to participate in activities outside her home, but she is worried that others will notice her problem with urinary incontinence. What response might help this client? What suggestions could you offer?
3. A resident in a nursing home who has had a retention catheter for the last 6 months says, "I'd do anything if I didn't have to have this catheter." What suggestions would be appropriate at this time?
4. The physician orders the removal of a urinary retention catheter. What actions should the nurse take?

NCLEX-STYLE REVIEW QUESTIONS

1. What is the most important nursing assessment before beginning continence retraining?
   1. Recording the times when the client is incontinent
   2. Checking the results of a routine urinalysis
   3. Palpating the extent of bladder distention
   4. Observing the characteristics of the client's urine
2. During continence retraining, what is the best nursing response when a client wants to restrict fluid intake to remain dry for longer periods?
   1. Encourage the practice because it shows evidence of client cooperation.
   2. Encourage the practice because it leads to accomplishing the goal.
   3. Discourage the practice because it contributes to constipation.
   4. Discourage the practice because it predisposes to fluid imbalance.
3. When applying an external condom catheter, which nursing action is correct?
   1. Lubricate the penis before applying the catheter.
   2. Measure the length and circumference of the penis.
   3. Leave space between the penis and bottom of the catheter.
   4. Retract the foreskin and roll the catheter over the penis.
4. After inserting an indwelling retention catheter into a male client, which of the following describes an appropriate technique for stabilizing the catheter to avoid a penoscrotal fistula?
   1. Tape the catheter to the abdomen.
   2. Pass the catheter under the client's leg.
   3. Fasten the drainage tube to the bed with a safety pin.
   4. Insert the catheter into the tubing of a collecting bag.
5. When the nurse instructs a female client on the technique for collecting a clean-catch midstream urine specimen for routine urinalysis, which statement is correct?
   1. Cleanse the urethral area using several circular motions.
   2. Void into the plastic liner that is under the toilet seat.
   3. After voiding a small amount, collect a sample of urine.
   4. Mix the antimicrobial solution with the collected urine specimen.

SKILL 30-1 Placing and Removing a Bedpan

Suggested Action	Reason for Action
ASSESSMENT	
Ask the client if he or she feels the need to void.	Anticipates elimination needs.
Palpate the lower abdomen for signs of bladder distention.	Indicates bladder fullness.
Determine if a fracture pan is necessary or if there are any restrictions in turning or lifting.	Prevents injury.
PLANNING	
Gather needed supplies such as clean gloves, bedpan, toilet tissue, and a disposable pad.	Promotes organization and efficient time management.
Warm the bedpan by running warm water over it especially if it is made of metal.	Demonstrates concern for the client's comfort.
IMPLEMENTATION	
Wash your hands or perform an alcohol-based hand rub (see Chap. 10); don clean gloves.	Reduces the transmission of microorganisms.
Place the adjustable bed in high position.	Promotes use of good body mechanics.
Close the door and pull the privacy curtains.	Demonstrates concern for the client's right to privacy and dignity.
Raise the top linen enough to determine the location of the client's hips and buttocks.	Prevents unnecessary exposure.
Instruct the client to bend the knees and press down with the feet.	Helps to elevate the hips.
Place a disposable pad over the bottom sheets, if necessary.	Protects bed linen from becoming wet and soiled.
Slip the bedpan beneath the client's buttocks (Fig. A).	Ensures proper placement.

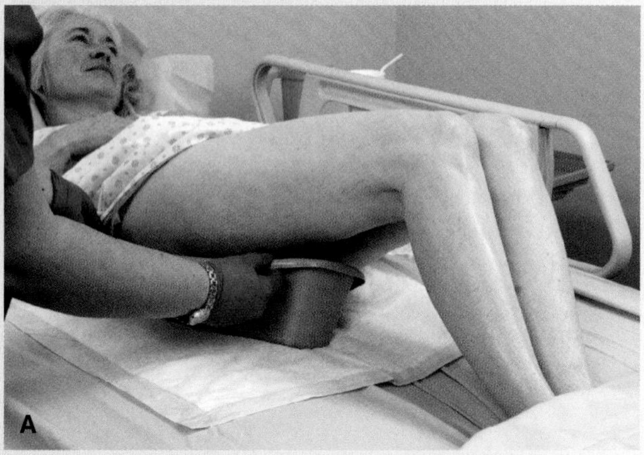

A

Placing a bedpan.

Suggested Action	Reason for Action
Or roll the client to the side and position the bedpan (Fig. B).	Reduces work effort and the potential for a work-related injury; aids in placement if client cannot lift buttocks.

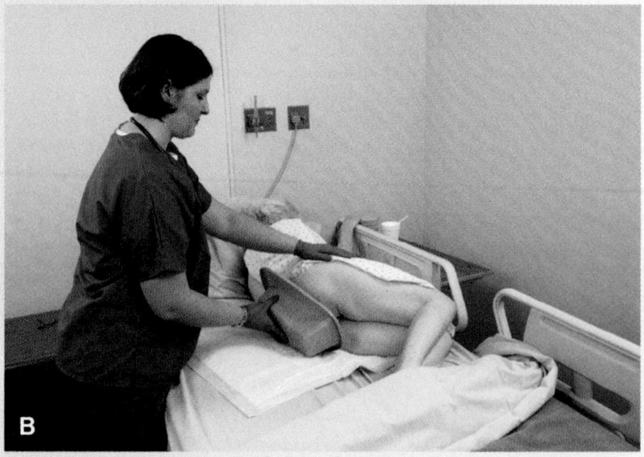

B

Placing a bedpan from a side-lying position.

(continued)

Placing and Removing a Bedpan (continued)

Suggested Action	Reason for Action
IMPLEMENTATION (CONTINUED)	
Raise the head of the bed (Fig. C).	Simulates the natural position for elimination.

C

The position for elimination.

Suggested Action	Reason for Action
Ensure that toilet tissue is within the client's reach.	Provides supplies for hygiene.
Identify the location of the signal device and leave the client, if doing so is safe.	Respects privacy yet provides a mechanism for communicating a need for assistance.
Return and remove the bedpan.	Prevents discomfort.
Assist with removing residue of urine from the skin, if necessary.	Prevents offensive odors and skin irritation.
Wrap the gloved hand with toilet tissue and wipe from the meatus of a female toward the anal area.	Supports the principles of medical asepsis.
Place soiled tissue in the bedpan unless it requires measuring.	Contains soiled tissue until the time of disposal.
Help the client to a comfortable position.	Ensures the client's well-being.
Provide supplies for hand hygiene.	Removes residue of urine and colonizing microorganisms.
Measure the volume of urine if the client's intake and output are being monitored.	Ensures accurate data collection.
Save a sample of urine if it appears abnormal in any way.	Facilitates laboratory examination or further assessment.
Empty the urine into a toilet and flush.	Facilitates disposal.
Clean the bedpan and replace it in a place that is separate from clean supplies.	Supports the principles of asepsis.
Remove gloves and repeat hand hygiene.	Removes colonizing microorganisms.

Evaluation

- Bedpan is positioned without injury.
- Urine is eliminated.
- Hygiene measures are performed.

Document

- Volume of urine eliminated (for monitoring intake and output)
- Appearance and other characteristics of the urine

SAMPLE DOCUMENTATION

Date and Time Assisted to use the bedpan. Voided 300 mL of clear, amber urine without difficulty. — SIGNATURE/TITLE

SKILL 30-2 Applying a Condom Catheter

Suggested Action	Reason for Action
ASSESSMENT	
Wash your hands or perform an alcohol-based hand rub (see Chap. 10).	Reduces the potential for transmitting microorganisms.
Assess the penis for swelling or skin breakdown.	Provides data for future comparison or a basis for using some other method for urine collection.
Determine the client's understanding about the application and use of an external catheter.	Provides an opportunity for health teaching.

(continued)

Applying a Condom Catheter (continued)

ASSESSMENT (CONTINUED)

Action	Rationale
Verify the client's willingness to use a condom catheter.	Respects the client's right to participate in making decisions.
Check the medical record to determine if the client has a latex allergy.	Maintains client safety and prevents possible allergic reaction.

PLANNING

Action	Rationale
Gather supplies such as soap, water, a towel, a condom catheter, drainage tubing, a collection device, and clean gloves. Some devices come packaged with an adhesive strip or Velcro for securing the catheter.	Promotes organization and efficient time management.
Provide privacy.	Demonstrates respect for the client's dignity.
Place the client in a supine position and cover him with a bath blanket.	Facilitates the application of the catheter and maintains privacy.

IMPLEMENTATION

Action	Rationale
Wash your hands or perform an alcohol-based hand rub (see Chap. 10) and don clean gloves.	Reduces the transmission of microorganisms and follows standard precautions.
Wash and dry the penis well.	Promotes skin integrity.
Wind the adhesive strip in an upward spiral around the penis (Fig. A).	Reduces the potential for restricting blood flow.

A

Applying the adhesive strip in a spiral.

Action	Rationale
Ensure that the wider end of the condom catheter is rolled to the narrower tip (Fig. B).	Facilitates application to the penis.

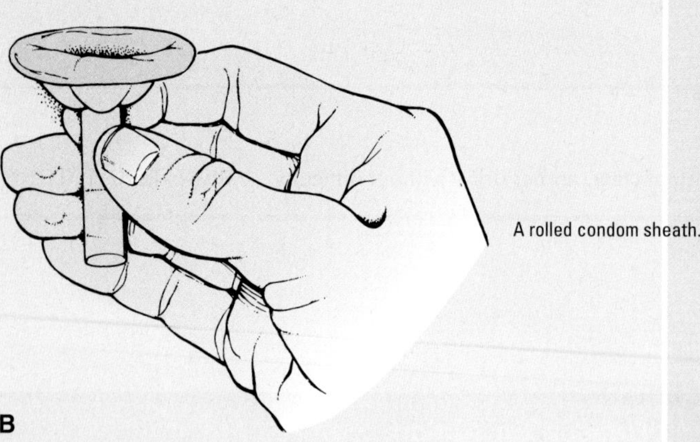

B

A rolled condom sheath.

(continued)

Applying a Condom Catheter (continued)

IMPLEMENTATION (CONTINUED)

Action	Rationale
Hold approximately 1–2 in. (2.5–5 cm) of the lower sheath below the tip of the penis and unroll the sheath upward (Fig. C).	Leaves space below the urethra to prevent the irritation of the meatus.

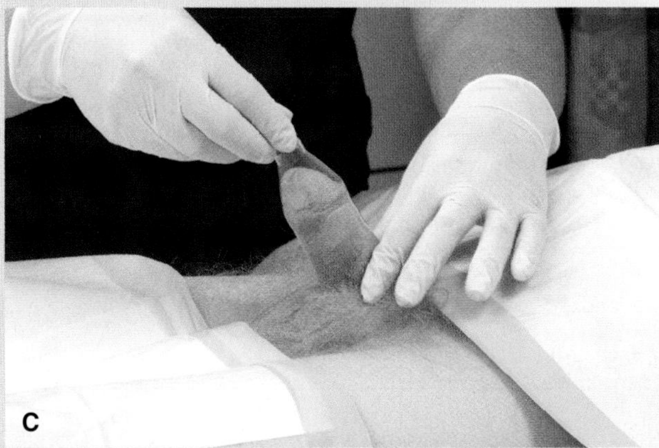

Unrolling the condom catheter sheath over the penis.

Action	Rationale
Secure the upper end of the unrolled sheath to the skin firmly with a second strip of adhesive or a Velcro strap but not so tight as to interfere with circulation (Fig. D).	Ensures that the catheter will remain in place.

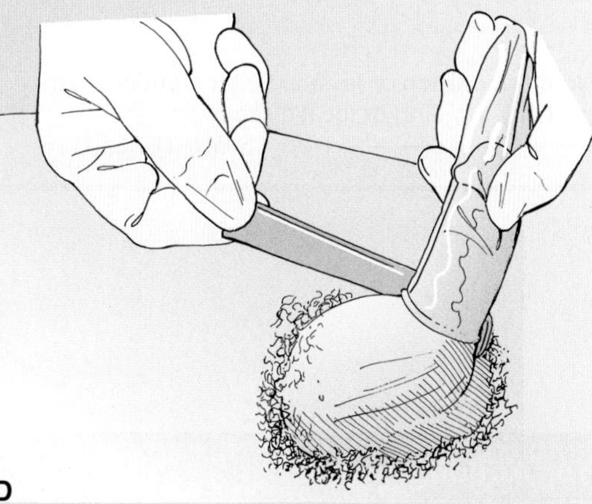

Securing a condom catheter.

Action	Rationale
Connect the drainage tip to a drainage collection device (Fig. E).	Allows for urine drainage and collection.

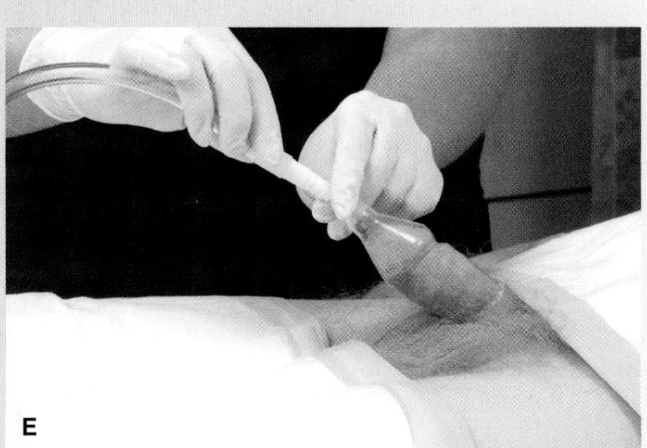

Connecting the condom catheter to a drainage collection system.

(continued)

Applying a Condom Catheter (continued)

IMPLEMENTATION (CONTINUED)

Suggested Action	Reason for Action
Keep the penis in a downward position.	Promotes urinary drainage.
Assess the penis at least every 2 hours.	Ensures prompt attention to signs of impaired circulation.
Check that the catheter has not become twisted.	Maintains catheter patency.
Empty the leg bag, if one is used, as it becomes partially filled with urine.	Ensures that the catheter will not be pulled from the penis by the weight of the collected urine.
Remove and change the catheter daily or more often if it becomes loose or tight.	Maintains skin integrity.
Substitute a waterproof garment during periods of nonuse.	Provides a mechanism for absorbing urine.
Wash the catheter and collection bag with mild soap and water and rinse with a 1:7 solution of vinegar and water.	Extends the use of the equipment and reduces offensive odors.

Evaluation

- Catheter remains attached to the penis.
- Penis exhibits no evidence of skin breakdown, swelling, or impaired circulation.
- Linen and clothing remain dry.

Document

- Preapplication assessment data
- Hygiene measures performed
- Time of catheter application
- Content of teaching
- Postapplication assessment data

SAMPLE DOCUMENTATION

Date and Time Penis washed with soap and water. Penile skin is intact. No discoloration or lesions noted. Condom catheter applied and connected to a leg bag. Instructed to report any swelling or local discomfort.
———————————————— SIGNATURE/TITLE

SKILL 30-3 Inserting a Foley Catheter in a Female

ASSESSMENT

Suggested Action	Reason for Action
Check the client's record to verify that a medical order has been written.	Demonstrates the legal scope of nursing; catheterization is not an independent measure.
Inspect the medical record to determine if the client has a latex allergy.	Determines if it is safe to use a latex catheter or if a latex-free type is needed.
Determine the type of catheter that has been prescribed.	Ensures the selection of an appropriate catheter.
Review the client's record for documentation of genitourinary problems.	Provides data by which to modify the procedure or equipment.
Assess the client's age, size, and mobility.	Influences the size of the catheter and the need for additional assistance.
Assess the time of the last voiding.	Indicates how full the bladder may be.
Determine how much the client understands about catheterization.	Provides an opportunity for health teaching.

(continued)

Inserting a Foley Catheter in a Female (continued)

ASSESSMENT (CONTINUED)

Familiarize yourself with the anatomic landmarks (Fig. A). — Facilitates insertion in the appropriate location.

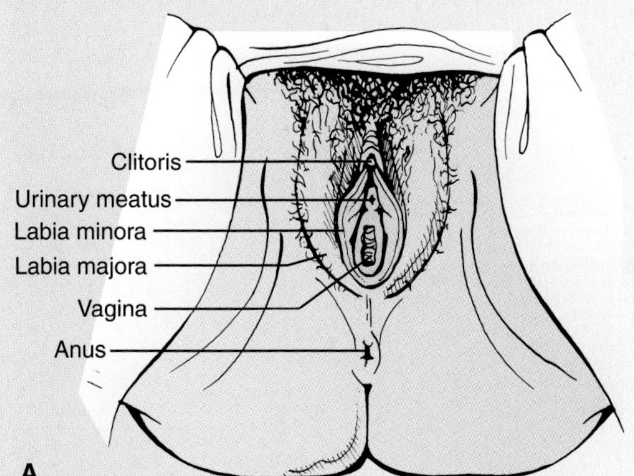

Female anatomical landmarks.

PLANNING

Gather supplies, which include a catheterization kit, a bath blanket, and additional light, if necessary. — Promotes organization and efficient time management.

IMPLEMENTATION

Close the door and pull the privacy curtain. — Demonstrates concern for the client's dignity.

Raise the bed to a high position. — Prevents back strain.

Wash your hands or perform an alcohol-based hand rub (see Chap. 10). — Reduces the potential for transmitting microorganisms.

Cover the client with a bath blanket and pull the top linen to the bottom of the bed. — Avoids unnecessary exposure.

Position an additional light at the bottom of the bed or ask an assistant to hold a flashlight. — Ensures good visualization.

Use the corners of the bath blanket to cover each leg. — Provides warmth and maintains modesty.

Place the client in a dorsal recumbent position with the feet about 2 feet apart (Fig. B). — Provides access to the female urinary system.

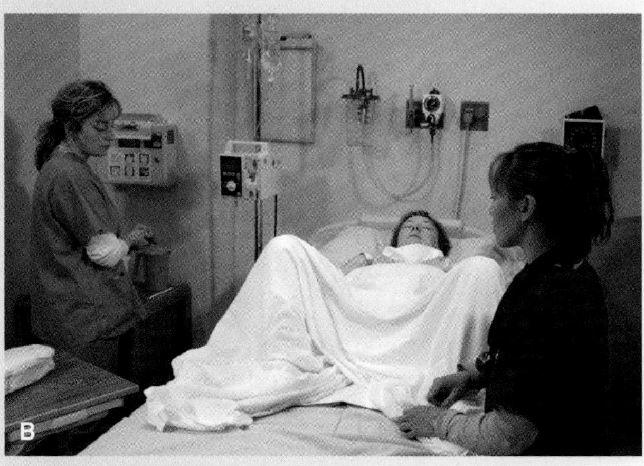

A client draped and placed in a dorsal recumbent position.

Use a lateral or Sims' position for clients who have difficulty maintaining a dorsal recumbent position. — Provides access to the female urinary system, but neither is the preferred position.

If the client is soiled, don gloves, wash the client, remove gloves, and perform hand hygiene measures again. — Supports the principles of asepsis.

Remove the wrapper from the catheterization kit and position it nearby. — Provides a receptacle for collecting soiled supplies.

(continued)

Inserting a Foley Catheter in a Female (continued)

IMPLEMENTATION (CONTINUED)

Unwrap the sterile cover to maintain the sterility of the supplies inside (see Chap. 10) (Fig. C).

Prevents contamination and the potential for infection.

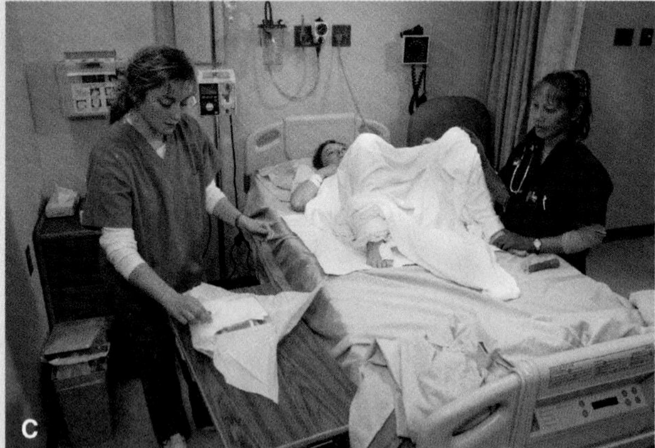

Opening the sterile catheter tray.

Remove and don the packaged sterile gloves (see Chap. 10).

Facilitates handling the remaining equipment without transferring microorganisms.

Remove the sterile towel from the kit and place it beneath the client's hips (Fig. D).

Provides a sterile field.

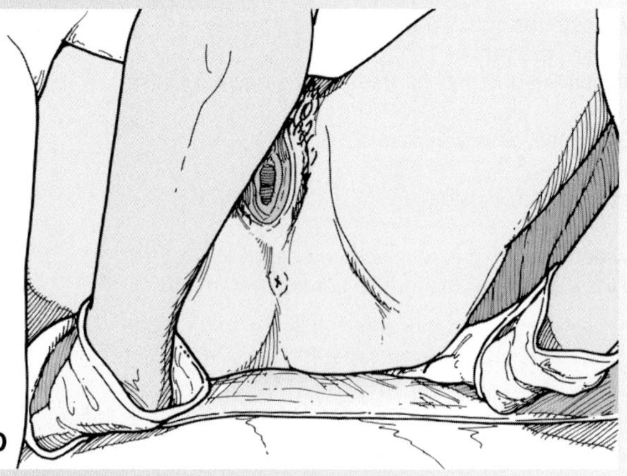

Placing a sterile towel.

Place a **fenestrated drape** (one with an open circle in its center) over the perineum (Fig. E).

Provides a sterile field.

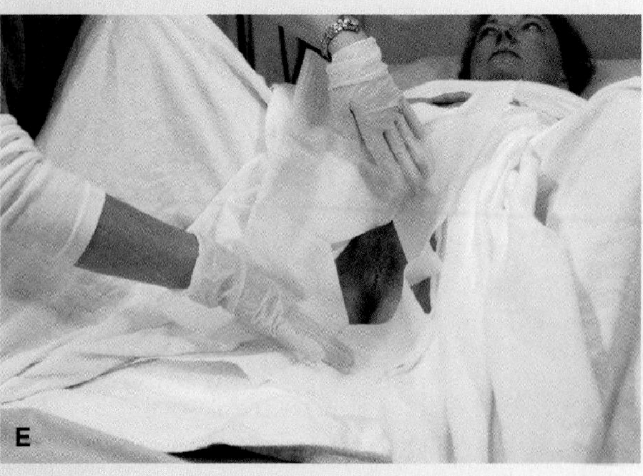

Placing a fenestrated drape over the perineum.

(continued)

Inserting a Foley Catheter in a Female (continued)

IMPLEMENTATION (CONTINUED)

Action	Rationale
Open and pour the packet of antiseptic solution (Betadine) over the cotton balls.	Prepares the sterile supplies before contaminating one of two hands later in the procedure.
Test the balloon on the catheter by instilling fluid from the prefilled syringe; then aspirate the fluid back within the syringe (Fig. F).	Determines if the balloon is intact or defective.

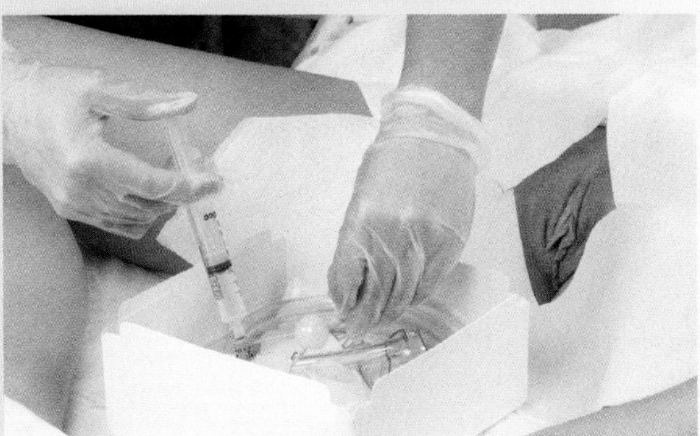

Testing the balloon.

Action	Rationale
Spread lubricant on the tip of the catheter (Fig. G).	Facilitates insertion.

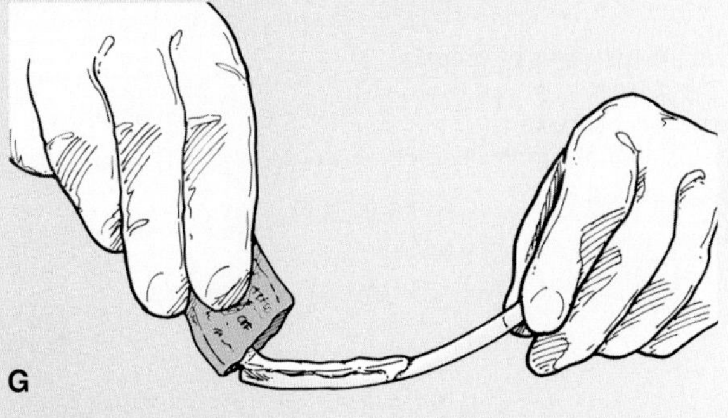

Lubricating the catheter.

Action	Rationale
Place the catheterization tray on top of the sterile towel between the client's legs.	Promotes access to supplies and reduces the potential for contamination.
Pick up a moistened cotton ball with the sterile forceps and wipe one side of the labia majora from an anterior to posterior direction.	Cleanses outer skin before cleansing deeper areas of tissue.
Discard the soiled cotton ball in the outer wrapper of the catheterization kit; repeat cleansing the other side of the labia majora.	Completes the bilateral cleansing.
Separate the labia majora and minora with the thumb and fingers of the nondominant hand, exposing the urinary meatus (Fig. H).	Facilitates the visualization of anatomic landmarks and prevents contaminating the catheter during insertion.

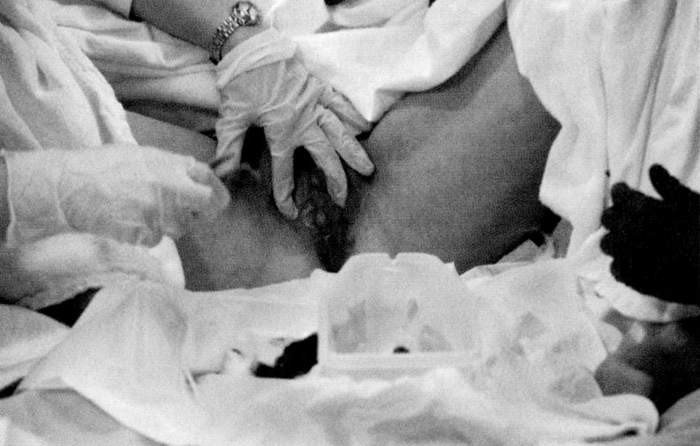

Separating the labia.

(continued)

Inserting a Foley Catheter in a Female (continued)

IMPLEMENTATION (CONTINUED)

Consider the hand separating the labia to be contaminated.	Avoids transferring microorganisms to sterile equipment and supplies.
Clean each side of the labia minora with a separate cotton ball while continuing to retract the tissue with the nondominant hand.	Removes colonizing microorganisms.
Use the last cotton ball to wipe centrally, starting above the meatus down toward the vagina (Fig. I).	Completes the cleaning of external structures.

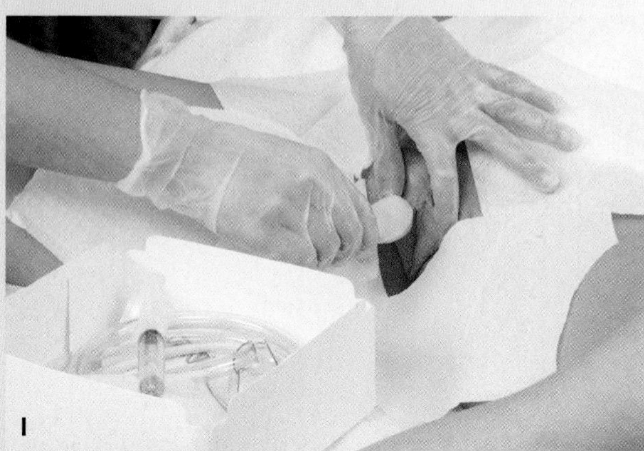

Wiping from above the meatus downward.

Discard the forceps with the last cotton ball into the wrapper for contaminated supplies.	Follows the principles of asepsis.
Keep the clean tissue separated.	Prevents recontamination.
Pick up the catheter, holding it approximately 3–4 in. (7.5–10 cm) from its tip (Fig. J).	Facilitates control during insertion.

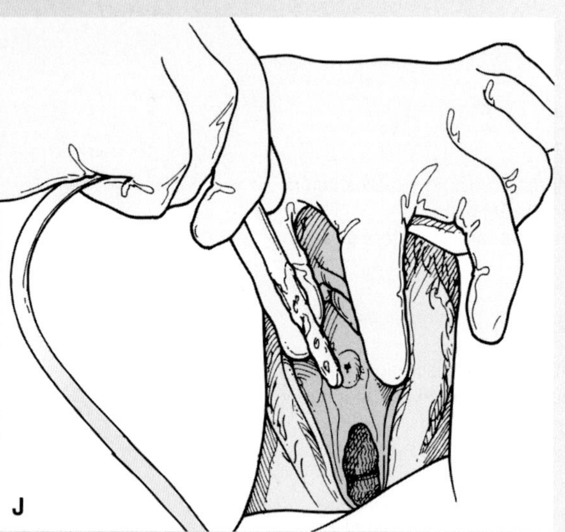

Preparing to insert the catheter.

Insert the tip of the catheter into the meatus approximately 2–3 in. (5–7.5 cm) or until urine begins to flow.	Locates the tip beyond the length of the female urethra, which is approximately 1.5–2.5 in. (4–6.5 cm).
Recheck anatomic landmarks if there is no evidence of urine; remove an incorrectly placed catheter and repeat, using another sterile catheter.	Indicates one of two possibilities: either the bladder is empty or the catheter has been placed within the vagina by mistake; ensures sterility of equipment.
Advance the catheter another 0.5–1 in. (1.3–2.5 cm) after urine begins to flow.	Ensures that the catheter is well within the bladder, where the balloon can be safely inflated.
Direct the end of the catheter so that it drains into the equipment tray or specimen container.	Avoids wetting the linens.
Hold the catheter in place with the fingers and thumb that were separating the labia.	Stabilizes the catheter externally.

(continued)

Inserting a Foley Catheter in a Female (continued)

IMPLEMENTATION (CONTINUED)

Pick up the prefilled syringe with the sterile, dominant hand, insert it into the opening to the balloon, and instill the fluid (Fig. K). — Stabilizes the catheter internally.

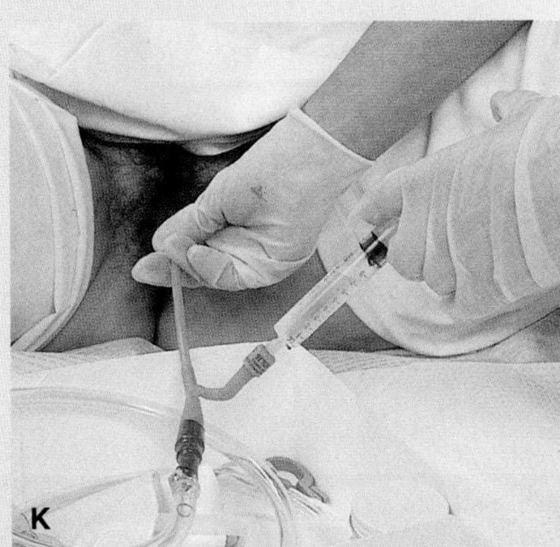

K Inflating the balloon.

Withdraw the fluid from the balloon if the client describes feeling pain or discomfort, advance the catheter a little more, and try again. — Prevents internal injury.

Tug gently on the catheter after the balloon has been filled. — Tests whether or not the catheter is well anchored within the bladder.

Connect the catheter to a urine collection bag. — Provides a means of assessing the urine and its volume.

Wipe the meatus and labia of any residual lubricant. — Demonstrates concern for the client's comfort.

Secure the catheter to the leg with tape or other commercial device (Fig. L). — Prevents pulling on the balloon within the catheter.

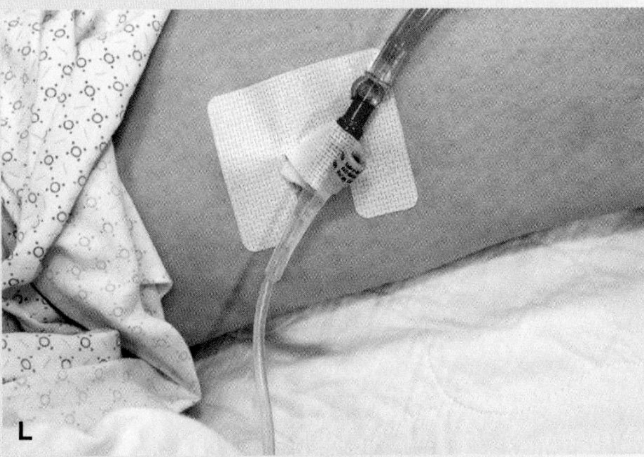

L Securing the catheter to the thigh.

Hang the collection bag below the level of the bladder; coil excess tubing on the mattress. — Ensures gravity drainage.

Discard the catheterization tray and wrapper with soiled supplies. — Follows the principles of asepsis.

Remove your gloves and perform hand hygiene. — Removes colonizing microorganisms.

Remove the drape, restore the top sheets, make the client comfortable, and lower the bed. — Restores comfort and safety.

Evaluation

- The catheter is inserted under aseptic conditions.
- The urine is draining from the catheter.
- The client exhibits no evidence of discomfort during or after the insertion.

(continued)

Inserting a Foley Catheter in a Female (continued)

Document
- Preassessment data
- Size and type of catheter
- Amount and appearance of urine
- Client's response

SAMPLE DOCUMENTATION

Date and Time Unable to void in past 8 hours. Bladder feels distended. Dr. Peter notified. 16 F Foley catheter inserted per order and connected to gravity drainage. 550 mL of urine drained from bladder at this time. Urine appears light amber. No discomfort reported. ———————— SIGNATURE/TITLE

SKILL 30-4 Inserting a Foley Catheter in a Male

Suggested Action	Reason for Action
ASSESSMENT	
Check the client's record to verify that a medical order has been written.	Demonstrates the legal scope of nursing; catheterization is not an independent measure.
Inspect the medical record to determine if the client has a latex allergy.	Determines if it is safe to use a latex catheter or if a latex-free type is needed.
Determine the type of catheter that has been prescribed.	Ensures the selection of the appropriate catheter.
Review the client's record for documentation of genitourinary problems.	Provides data by which to modify the procedure or equipment.
Assess the client's age, size, and mobility.	Influences the size of the catheter and need for additional assistance.
Assess the time of the last voiding.	Indicates the potential fullness of the bladder.
Determine how much the client understands about catheterization.	Provides an opportunity for health teaching.
Familiarize yourself with the anatomic landmarks (Fig. A).	Facilitates insertion.

Male anatomical landmarks. **A.** Circumcised. **B.** Uncircumcised.

Suggested Action	Reason for Action
PLANNING	
Gather supplies, which include a catheterization kit, a bath blanket, and additional light.	Promotes organization and efficient time management.
IMPLEMENTATION	
Close the door and pull the privacy curtain.	Demonstrates concern for the client's dignity.
Raise the bed to a high position.	Prevents back strain.
Perform handwashing or an alcohol-based hand rub (see Chap. 10).	Reduces the potential for transmitting microorganisms.
Place the client in a supine position.	Provides access to the male urinary system.

(continued)

Inserting a Foley Catheter in a Male (continued)

IMPLEMENTATION (CONTINUED)

Cover the client's upper body with a bath blanket and lower the top linen to expose just the penis.	Provides minimal exposure.
Position an additional light at the bottom of the bed or ask an assistant to hold a flashlight.	Ensures good visualization.
If the client is soiled, don gloves, wash the client, remove gloves, and repeat hand hygiene measures.	Supports the principles of asepsis.
Remove the wrapper from the catheterization kit and position it nearby.	Provides a receptacle for collecting soiled supplies.
Unwrap the sterile inner cover so as to maintain the sterility of the supplies inside (see Chap. 10).	Prevents contamination and the potential for infection.
Remove and don the packaged sterile gloves (see Chap. 10).	Facilitates handling the remaining equipment without transferring microorganisms.
Place the fenestrated drape over the client's penis without touching the upper surface of the drape (Fig. B).	Provides a sterile field.

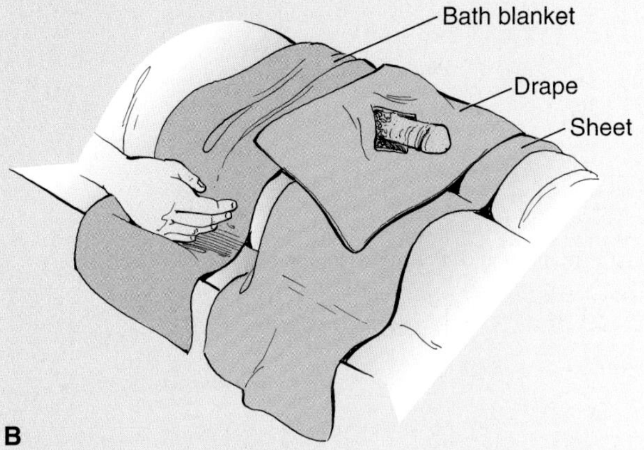

Placing a fenestrated drape.

Open and pour the packet of antiseptic solution (Betadine) over the cotton balls.	Prepares sterile supplies before contaminating one of two hands later in the procedure.
Test the balloon on the catheter by instilling fluid from the prefilled syringe; then aspirate the fluid back within the syringe.	Determines whether the balloon is intact or defective.
Place the catheterization tray between the client's thighs.	Promotes ease of access to supplies and reduces the potential for contamination.
Lift the penis at its base with the nondominant hand; retract the foreskin if the client is uncircumcised.	Promotes visualization and support during catheter insertion.
Consider the gloved hand holding the penis to be contaminated.	Avoids transferring microorganisms to sterile equipment and supplies.
Pick up a moistened cotton ball with the sterile forceps and wipe the penis in a circular manner from the meatus toward the base; repeat using a different cotton ball each time (Fig. C).	Moves microorganisms away from the meatus.

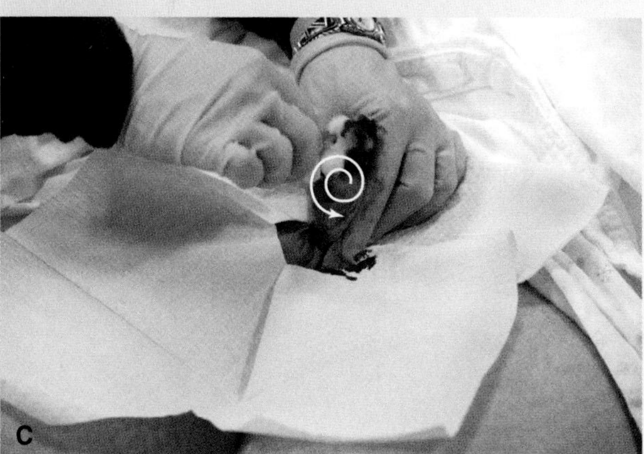

Cleaning the penis.

(continued)

Inserting a Foley Catheter in a Male (continued)

IMPLEMENTATION (CONTINUED)

Discard the forceps with the last cotton ball into the wrapper for contaminated supplies. — Follows the principles of asepsis.

Apply gentle traction to the penis by pulling it straight up with the nondominant gloved hand. — Straightens the urethra.

Instill the contents of a prefilled syringe containing lubricant directly through the meatus into the urethra (Fig. D). — Avoids trauma to the urethra caused by insufficient lubrication; this technique replaces the traditional practice of lubricating the outer surface of the catheter, which resulted in its accumulation at the meatus only (Gerard & Sueppel, 1997).

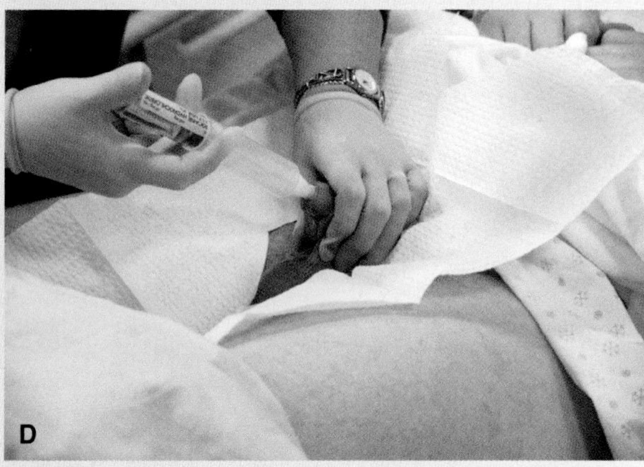

Instilling lubricant.

Insert, but never force the catheter; rather, rotate the catheter, apply more traction to the penis, encourage the client to breathe deeply, or angle the penis toward the toes (Fig. E). — Adjusts for passing the catheter beyond the prostate gland.

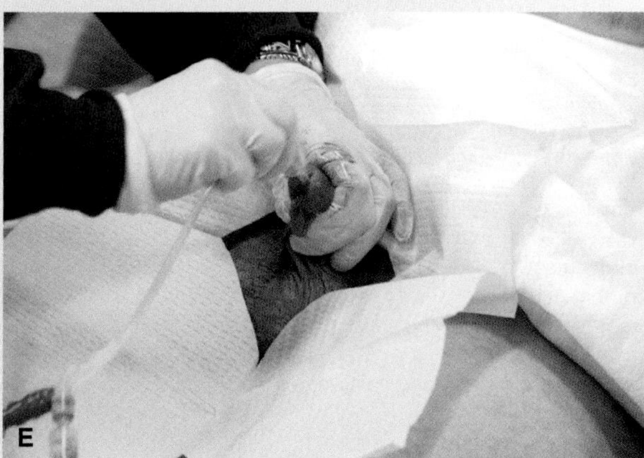

Catheter insertion.

Continue insertion until only the inflation and drainage ports are exposed and urine flows. — Locates the tip beyond the length of the male urethra.

Pick up the prefilled syringe with the sterile, dominant hand, insert it into the opening to the balloon, and instill the fluid (Fig. F). — Stabilizes the catheter internally.

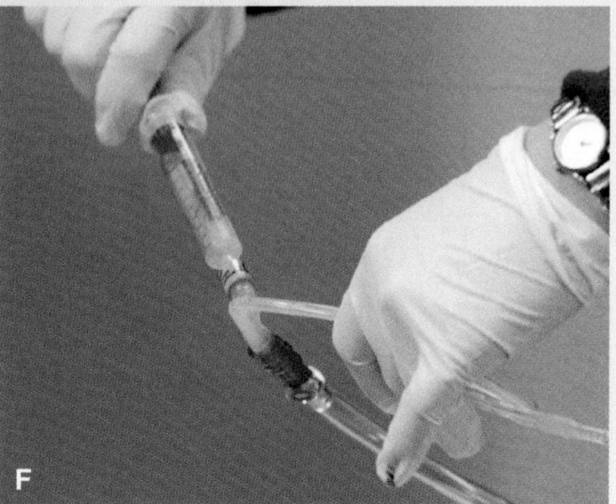

Inflating the balloon.

(continued)

Inserting a Foley Catheter in a Male (continued)

IMPLEMENTATION (CONTINUED)

Withdraw the fluid from the balloon if the client describes feeling pain or discomfort, advance the catheter a little more, and try again.	Prevents internal injury.
Tug gently on the catheter after the balloon has been filled.	Tests whether or not the catheter is well anchored within the bladder.
Connect the catheter to a urine collection bag.	Provides a means of assessing the urine and its volume.
Wipe the meatus and penis of any residual lubricant.	Demonstrates concern for the client's comfort.
Secure the catheter to the leg or abdomen with tape or other commercial device (Fig. G).	Prevents pulling on the balloon within the catheter.

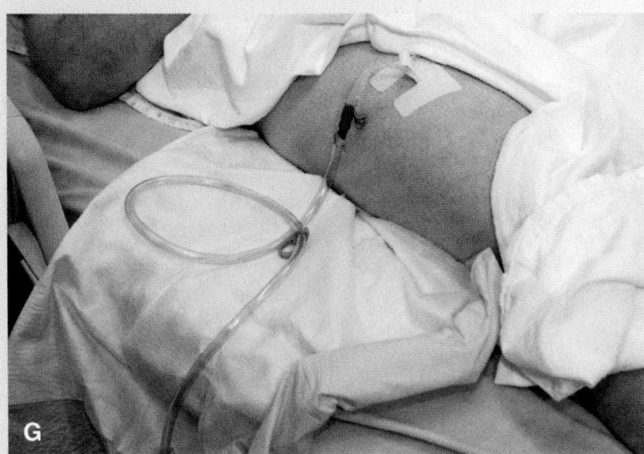

Securing a catheter.

Hang the collection bag below the level of the bladder; coil excess tubing on the mattress.	Ensures gravity drainage.
Discard the catheterization tray and wrapper with soiled supplies.	Follows the principles of asepsis.
Remove your gloves and repeat hand hygiene measures.	Removes colonizing microorganisms.
Remove the drape, restore the top sheets, make the client comfortable, and lower the bed.	Restores comfort and safety.

Evaluation

- The catheter is inserted under aseptic conditions.
- The urine is draining from the catheter.
- The client demonstrates no evidence of discomfort during or after insertion.

Document

- Preassessment data
- Size and type of catheter
- Amount and appearance of urine
- Client's response

SAMPLE DOCUMENTATION

Date and Time 16 F Foley catheter inserted before surgery according to preoperative orders. 350 mL of urine obtained before connecting the catheter to gravity drainage. Urine appears light yellow and clear. ———————————— SIGNATURE/TITLE

SKILL 30-5 Irrigating a Foley Catheter

Suggested Action	Reason for Action
ASSESSMENT	
Check the client's record to verify that a medical order has been written.	Demonstrates the legal scope of nursing; a catheter irrigation is not an independent measure.
Verify the type of irrigating solution prescribed, or follow the standard for practice, which usually advises using sterile normal saline solution.	Complies with medical the directives or standards for care.
Assess the urine characteristics.	Provides a baseline for assessing the outcome of the procedure.
Determine how much the client understands about a catheter irrigation.	Provides an opportunity for health teaching.
Locate the port on the drainage tube through which fluid can be instilled (Fig. A).	Ensures a safe procedure and maintains the integrity of the catheter.

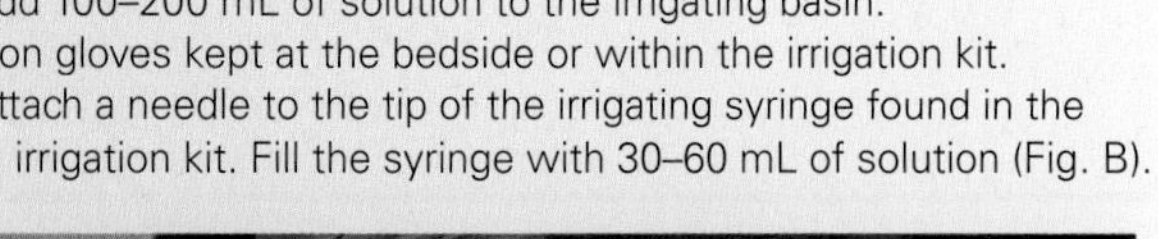

A Identifying the self-sealing irrigation port.

Suggested Action	Reason for Action
PLANNING	
Gather needed equipment and supplies: an irrigation kit, a flask of sterile irrigating solution, a 30- to 60-mL syringe, and alcohol swabs.	Promotes organization and efficient time management.
IMPLEMENTATION	
Wash hands or perform an alcohol-based hand rub (see Chap. 10).	Follows the principles of asepsis and standards of practice.
Raise the height of the bed.	Reduces back strain.
Pull the privacy curtain.	Demonstrates concern for the client's dignity.
Add 100–200 mL of solution to the irrigating basin.	Avoids contaminating and wasting all the solution in the flask.
Don gloves kept at the bedside or within the irrigation kit.	Complies with standard precautions.
Attach a needle to the tip of the irrigating syringe found in the irrigation kit. Fill the syringe with 30–60 mL of solution (Fig. B).	Provides a means for penetrating the self-sealing port.

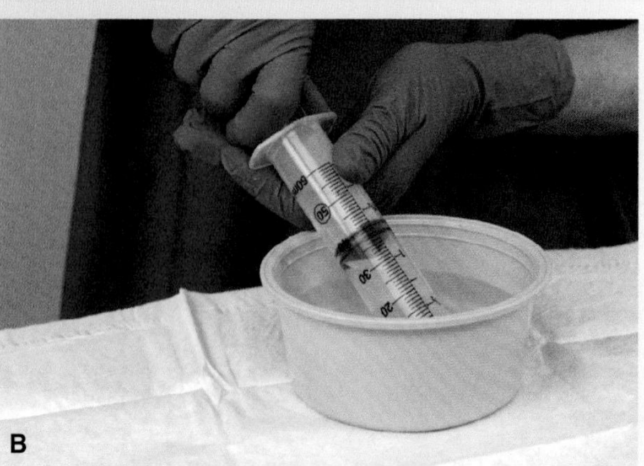

B Filling the syringe with solution.

(continued)

Irrigating a Foley Catheter (continued)

IMPLEMENTATION (CONTINUED)

Clean the port on the catheter with an alcohol swab (Fig. C).

Removes gross debris and colonizing microorganisms.

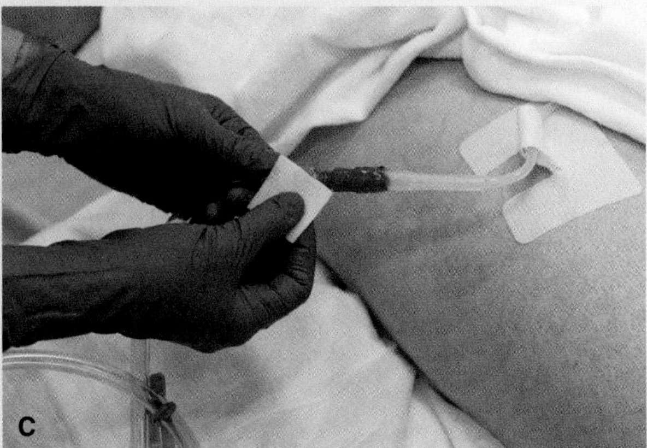

Cleaning the irrigation port.

Clamp or kink the tubing below the port through which the irrigating solution will be instilled (Fig. D).

Ensures that the solution will move forward into the catheter and not into the drainage system.

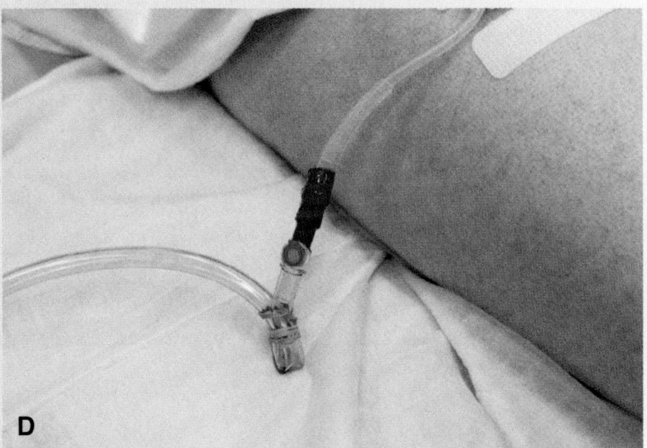

Clamping the drainage tubing.

While holding the catheter with one hand, insert the syringe into the port (Fig. E).

Maintains sterility.

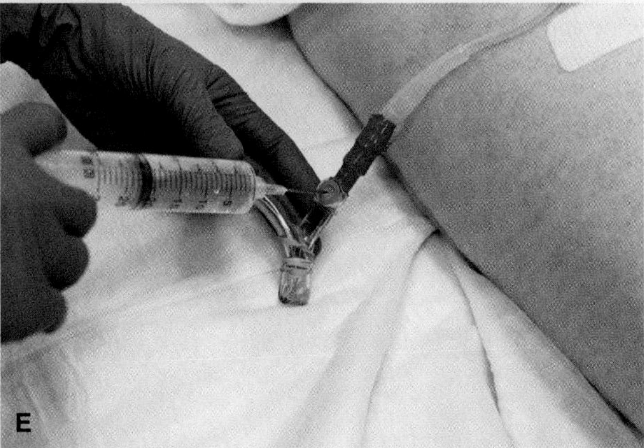

Instilling the irrigation solution.

Gently instill the solution.

Clears the catheter of debris and dilutes particles within the catheter.

Remove the syringe.

Prevents leaking.

(continued)

Irrigating a Foley Catheter (continued)

IMPLEMENTATION (CONTINUED)

Release the clamp from the drainage tubing and observe the flow of urine through the tubing (Fig. F).	Facilitates gravity drainage.

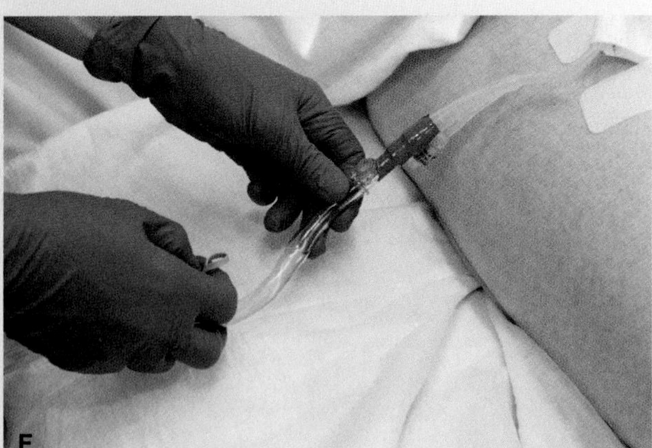

Draining the irrigation solution.

Repeat the instillation and drainage if the urine appears to contain appreciable debris.	Promotes patency.
Record the volume of instilled solution as fluid intake.	Maintains accurate assessment data.
Discard or protect the sterility of the irrigating equipment, which may be reused for the next 24 hours as long as it is not contaminated.	Complies with the principles of infection control.

Evaluation

- The prescribed amount and type of solution are instilled.
- The principles of asepsis have been maintained.
- The urine continues to drain well through the catheter.
- The client reports no discomfort.

Document

- Preassessment data
- Volume and type of solution
- Volume and appearance of drainage

SAMPLE DOCUMENTATION

Date and Time Urine appears amber with some evidence of white particles. 60 mL of sterile normal saline solution instilled into catheter. 120 mL drainage returned. Urine appears to have less sediment. Catheter remains patent. ——— SIGNATURE/TITLE

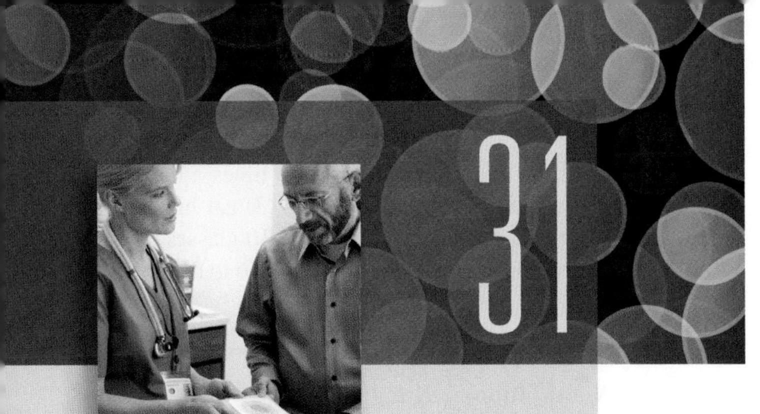

31

Bowel Elimination

Words To Know

anal sphincters
appliance
colostomy
constipation
continent ostomy
defecation
diarrhea
enema
enterostomal therapist
excoriation
fecal impaction
fecal incontinence
feces
flatulence
flatus
gastrocolic reflex
ileostomy
ostomy
peristalsis
retention enema
stoma
suppository
Valsalva maneuver

Learning Objectives

On completion of this chapter, the reader should be able to:

1. Describe the process of defecation.
2. Name two components of a bowel elimination assessment.
3. List five common alterations in bowel elimination.
4. Name four types of constipation.
5. Identify measures within the scope of nursing practice for treating constipation.
6. Identify two interventions that promote bowel elimination when it does not occur naturally.
7. Name two categories of enema administration.
8. List at least three common solutions used in a cleansing enema.
9. Explain the purpose of an oil retention enema.
10. Name four nursing activities involved in ostomy care.

This chapter briefly reviews the process of intestinal elimination and discusses measures to help promote it. It also describes nursing skills that may assist clients who have alterations in bowel elimination.

DEFECATION

Defecation (bowel elimination) is the act of expelling **feces** (stool) from the body. To do so, all structures of the gastrointestinal tract, especially the components of the large intestine (also referred to as the *bowel* or *colon*), must function in a coordinated manner (Fig. 31-1). In the large intestine, a remarkable volume of water is removed from the remnants of digestion, causing the bowel's contents to become a consolidated mass of residue before being eliminated.

Peristalsis means the rhythmic contractions of intestinal smooth muscle that facilitate defecation. Peristalsis moves fiber, water, and nutritional wastes along the ascending, transverse, descending, and sigmoid colon toward the rectum. Peristalsis becomes even more active during eating; this increased peristaltic activity is called the **gastrocolic reflex**.

The gastrocolic reflex usually precedes defecation. Its accelerated wavelike movements, sometimes perceived as slight abdominal cramping, propel stool forward, packing it within the rectum. As the rectum distends, the person feels the urge to defecate. Stool is eventually released when the **anal sphincters** (ring-shaped bands of muscles) relax. Performing the **Valsalva maneuver** (closing the glottis and contracting the pelvic and abdominal muscles to increase abdominal pressure)

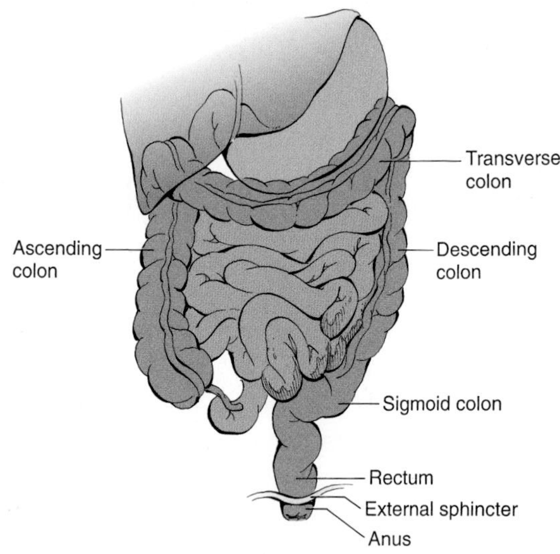

FIGURE 31-1 The large intestine.

facilitates this process. Several dietary, physical, social, and emotional factors can influence the bowel's mechanical function (Table 31-1).

ASSESSMENT OF BOWEL ELIMINATION

A comprehensive assessment of bowel elimination involves collecting data about the client's elimination patterns (bowel habits) and the actual characteristics of the feces.

Elimination Patterns

Because various elimination patterns can be normal, it is essential to determine the client's usual patterns, including the frequency of elimination, the effort required to expel stool, and what elimination aids, if any, he or she uses. Health education regarding bowel elimination includes the following points: (1) adults should identify their own patterns of bowel regularity, which can range from 3 times a day to 3 times a week; (2) include daily exercise, (3) eat high-fiber foods on a regular basis, and (4) drink 8 to 10 glasses of liquid a day (unless contraindicated), and respond to the urge to defecate as soon as possible.

TABLE 31-1 Common Factors Affecting Bowel Elimination

FACTOR	EFFECT
Types of food consumed	Influence color, odor, volume, and consistency of stool, and fecal velocity
Fluid intake	Influences moisture content of stool
Drugs	Slow or speed motility
Emotions	Alter bowel motility
Neuromuscular function	Affects the ability to control rectal muscles
Abdominal muscle tone	Affects the ability to increase intra-abdominal pressure (Valsalva maneuver)
Opportunity for defecation	Inhibits or facilitates elimination

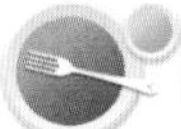

Nutrition Notes

- Foods that are high in fiber include apples and pears with skin, nuts, bran, whole wheat products, oatmeal, brown rice, beans, lentils, and raw carrots.
- Adults may be receptive to eating bran cereal or adding bran to casseroles or muffins as a means to increase fiber intake.

Stool Characteristics

Health care providers can obtain objective data about stool characteristics by inspecting the stool or asking the client to describe its appearance. Information that is particularly diagnostic includes stool color, odor, consistency, shape, and unusual components (Table 31-2). The incidence of colorectal cancer increases with age. One early sign is a change in bowel elimination patterns and stool characteristics. Therefore, advise older adults to have regular endoscopic bowel examinations after 50 years of age. Any change in bowel elimination that does not respond to simple dietary or lifestyle changes requires further investigation.

Whenever stool appears abnormal, a sample is saved in a covered container for the physician's inspection. In some instances, nurses may independently perform screening tests on stool samples, such as those that determine the presence of blood (see Nursing Guidelines 31-1). Nurses then report the results, which can be falsely positive, to the physician, who may order more specific laboratory or diagnostic tests.

TABLE 31-2 Characteristics of Stool

CHARACTERISTIC	NORMAL	ABNORMAL
Color	Brown	Black Clay colored (tan) Yellow Green
Odor	Aromatic	Foul
Consistency	Soft, formed	Soft, bulky Hard, dry Watery Paste like
Shape	Round, full	Unformed Flat Pencil-shaped Stone like
Components	Undigested fiber	Worms Blood Pus Mucus

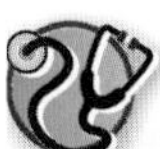

NURSING GUIDELINES 31-1

Testing Stool for Occult Blood

- Collect stool within a toilet liner or bedpan. *Use of such devices prevents mixing stool with water or urine.*
- Don gloves and use an applicator stick to collect the specimen. *These measures reduce the transmission of microorganisms.*
- Take a sample from the center area of the stool. *A sample from here provides more diagnostic value because it is not superficially tainted with blood from local tissue.*
- Apply a thin smear of stool onto the test area supplied with the screening kit. *Correct use of the kit ensures thorough contact with the chemical reagent.*
- Cover the entire test space. *Doing so ensures more accurate findings.*
- Place two drops of the chemical reagent onto the test space. *This step promotes a chemical reaction.*
- Wait for 60 seconds. *This duration is the time needed for chemical interaction with the stool.*
- Observe for a blue color. *This finding indicates that blood is present.*

By analyzing assessment findings, nurses may help physicians to diagnose a medical problem or use the conclusions to identify alterations within the scope of nursing management.

COMMON ALTERATIONS IN BOWEL ELIMINATION

Clients often have temporary or chronic problems with bowel elimination and intestinal function such as constipation, fecal impaction, flatulence, diarrhea, and fecal incontinence. If these conditions are a component of a serious disorder, nurses and physicians collaborate to address them. Nurses may treat alterations within the scope of nursing practice independently.

Constipation

Constipation is an elimination problem characterized by dry, hard stool that is difficult to pass. Various accompanying signs and symptoms include the following:

- Complaints of abdominal fullness or bloating
- Abdominal distention
- Complaints of rectal fullness or pressure
- Pain on defecation
- Decreased frequency of bowel movements
- Inability to pass stool
- Changes in stool characteristics such as oozing, liquid stool or hard, small stool

The infrequent elimination of stool does not necessarily indicate that a person is constipated. Some people may be constipated even though they have a daily bowel movement, whereas others who defecate irregularly may have normal bowel function.

The incidence of constipation tends to be high among those whose dietary habits lack adequate fiber (such as not eating sufficient raw fruits and vegetables, whole grains, seeds, and nuts). Dietary fiber, which includes undigested cellulose, is important because it attracts water within the bowel, resulting in bulkier stool that is more quickly and easily eliminated.

Some researchers speculate that a shortened transit time—the time between when a person eats food and eliminates stool—protects against serious medical disorders. They argue that the longer the stool is retained, the more contact with and absorption of toxic substances takes place that may contribute to the development of colorectal cancer (Johnson, Barret, Gishan, et al., 2006; Talley, Lasch, & Baum, 2008).

Constipation is classified into one of four distinct types (primary, secondary, iatrogenic, and pseudoconstipation), according to the underlying cause.

Primary Constipation

Primary or simple constipation is well within the treatment domain of nurses. It results from lifestyle factors such as inactivity, inadequate intake of fiber, insufficient fluid intake, or ignoring the urge to defecate.

Secondary Constipation

Secondary constipation is a consequence of a pathologic disorder such as a partial bowel obstruction. It usually resolves when the primary cause is treated.

Iatrogenic Constipation

Iatrogenic constipation occurs as a consequence of other medical treatments. For example, prolonged use of narcotic analgesia tends to cause constipation. These and other drugs slow peristalsis, delaying transit time. The longer the stool remains in the colon, the drier it becomes, making it more difficult to pass.

Pseudoconstipation

Pseudoconstipation, also referred to as Perceived Constipation by NANDA International (NANDA-I, 2012), is a term used when clients believe themselves to be constipated even though they are not. Pseudoconstipation may occur in people who are extremely concerned about having a daily bowel movement. In their zeal for regularity, they often overuse or abuse laxatives, suppositories, and enemas. Such self-treatment may ultimately cause rather than treat constipation.

Chronic purging eventually weakens bowel tone; consequently, bowel elimination is less likely unless it is artificially stimulated.

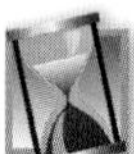

Gerontologic Considerations

- Age-related changes, such as a loss of elasticity in the intestinal walls and slower motility throughout the gastrointestinal tract, predispose older adults to constipation. Such changes alone, however, do not cause constipation. Other factors, such as adverse medication effects, diminished physical activity, and reliance on commercially prepared meals that are easy to heat and eat, but which are low in fiber, fresh fruits, and vegetables, contribute to the development of constipation.
- Older adults are likely to implement various home remedies such as drinking prune juice or hot water in the morning to promote bowel elimination. The consideration of benefits, potential risks, or lack of effect on an older person's usual health practices allows for collaboration regarding the efficacy of continuing the health care behavior with the older adult.
- Older adults may be open to increasing dietary fiber which is a healthier alternative to using laxatives to maintain bowel elimination.
- Older adults may be taught to incorporate a natural laxative into their diet. The "Power Pudding" recipe consists of 1 cup wheat bran, 1 cup applesauce, and 1 cup prune juice all mixed thoroughly and refrigerated. The older person can begin with 1 tbsp per day and increase the amount by small increments daily until an ease of bowel movement is achieved and no disagreeable symptoms occur (Touhy & Jett, 2010).

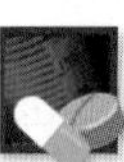

Pharmacologic Considerations

- Some adults may become very bowel conscious and overuse laxatives or have a sustained laxative abuse. They can develop healthier bowel elimination habits through use of bulk-forming products containing psyllium or polycarbophil, which are more effective and less irritating than other types of laxatives. Examples of these agents include Metamucil (Procter & Gamble, Cincinnati, OH) and FiberCon (Lederle Laboratories, Pearl River, NY).
- Adults who use mineral oil to prevent or relieve constipation need to be informed that its prolonged use interferes with the absorption of fat-soluble vitamins (A, D, E, and K).

Fecal Impaction

Fecal impaction occurs when a large, hardened mass of stool interferes with defecation, making it impossible for the client to pass feces voluntarily. Fecal impactions result from unrelieved constipation, retained barium from an intestinal X-ray, dehydration, and weakness of abdominal muscles.

Clients with a fecal impaction usually report a frequent desire to defecate but an inability to do so. Rectal pain may result from unsuccessful efforts to evacuate the lower bowel. Some clients with an impaction pass liquid stool, which may be misinterpreted as diarrhea. Forceful muscular contractions of peristalsis in higher bowel areas, where the stool is still fluid, cause the liquid stool. These contractions send the liquid around the margins of the impacted stool, but this passage of liquid stool does not relieve the initial condition.

To determine whether or not a fecal impaction is present, it may be necessary to insert a lubricated, gloved finger into the rectum. If the rectum is filled with a mass of stool, the nurse implements measures for its removal. Sometimes nurses administer enemas, first oil retention, and then cleansing. These therapeutic measures are discussed later in this chapter. Another intervention is to remove the stool digitally (see Nursing Guidelines 31-2 and Fig. 31-2).

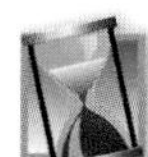

Gerontologic Considerations

- Older adults may have benign lesions such as hemorrhoids or polyps in their lower bowel, which may interfere with the passage of stool. If the digital removal of an impaction is required, gentle manipulation within the rectum should be used to prevent bleeding and tissue trauma.

Flatulence

Flatulence or **flatus** (an excessive accumulation of intestinal gas) results from swallowing air while eating or from sluggish peristalsis. Another cause is the gas that forms as a by-product of bacterial fermentation in the bowel. Vegetables such as cabbage, cucumbers, and onions are commonly known for producing gas. Beans are other gas formers. Eating beans creates intestinal gas because humans lack an enzyme to completely digest its particular form of complex carbohydrate.

Regardless of its cause, flatus may be expelled rectally, thus reducing intestinal accumulation and distention. Sometimes, however, this is not sufficient to eliminate the cramping pain or other symptoms. When clients are extremely uncomfortable and ambulating does not eliminate flatus, the nurse may insert a rectal tube to help the gas escape (Skill 31-1).

Stop, Think, and Respond Box 31-1

Discuss measures to include in a teaching plan that would help clients reduce or eliminate intestinal gas.

Diarrhea

Diarrhea is the urgent passage of watery stool and commonly is accompanied by abdominal cramping. Simple diarrhea usually begins suddenly and lasts for a short period. Other associated signs and symptoms include nausea and vomiting and blood or mucus in the stools.

Usually, diarrhea is a means of eliminating an irritating substance such as tainted food or intestinal pathogens.

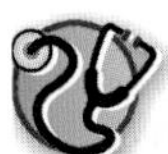

NURSING GUIDELINES 31-2

Removing a Fecal Impaction

- Wash your hands or perform an alcohol-based hand rub (see Chap. 10). *Hand hygiene reduces the transmission of microorganisms.*
- Don clean examination gloves. *Doing so complies with standard precautions by providing a barrier between the hands and a substance that contains body fluid.*
- Provide privacy. *Privacy demonstrates respect for the client's dignity.*
- Place the client in a Sims' position (see Chap. 14). *This position facilitates access to the rectum.*
- Cover the client with a drape and place a disposable pad under the client's hips. *Use of these materials prevents soiling.*
- Place a bedpan conveniently on the bed. *The bedpan acts as a container for removed stool.*
- Lubricate the forefinger of your dominant gloved hand. *Lubrication eases insertion within the rectum.*
- Insert your lubricated finger within the rectum to the level of the hardened mass. *Insertion to this level facilitates digital manipulation of the stool.*
- Move your finger about slowly and carefully to break up the mass of stool. *Movement facilitates removal or voluntary passage.*
- Withdraw segments of the stool (see Fig. 31-2) and deposit them in the bedpan. *Removal reduces the internal mass of stool.*
- Provide periods of rest but continue until the mass has been removed or sufficiently reduced. *Doing so restores patency to the lower bowel.*
- Clean the client's rectal area; dispose of the stool and soiled gloves; repeat hand hygiene measures. *These measures support the principles of medical asepsis.*

Diarrhea may also result from emotional stress, dietary indiscretions, laxative abuse, or bowel disorders.

Resting the bowel temporarily may relieve simple diarrhea. This means the person drinks clear liquids but avoids solid foods for 12 to 24 hours. Resumed eating begins with bland foods and those low in residue such as bananas, applesauce, and cottage cheese. If diarrhea is not relieved within 24 hours, it is best to consult a physician.

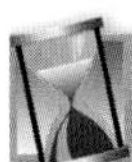

Gerontologic Considerations

■ Diarrhea can easily lead to dehydration and electrolyte imbalances (especially hypokalemia) in older adults, who tend to have less body fluid reserve than younger people.

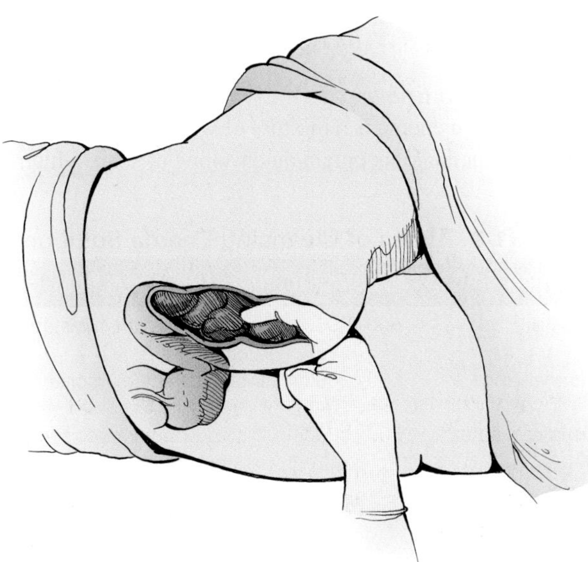

FIGURE 31-2 Removing impacted stool.

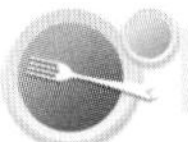

Nutrition Notes

■ Probiotics are beneficial bacteria present in some commercial products like yogurt that contain live cultures. These bacteria survive digestion and colonize within the bowel, making bowel contents more acidic. The lowered intestinal pH creates a hostile environment for unhealthy bacteria. Eating products containing probiotics is believed to regulate and improve elimination, thus reducing symptoms of diarrhea, constipation, intestinal gas, and bloating.

Fecal Incontinence

Fecal incontinence is the inability to control the elimination of stool. It does not necessarily imply that stool is loose or watery, although that may be the case. In some instances, bowel function is normal, but incontinence results from neurologic changes that impair muscle activity, sensation, or thought processes. Even a fecal impaction may be an underlying cause of incontinence. Incontinence also may occur when a person cannot reach a toilet in time to eliminate, such as after taking a harsh laxative.

Chronic fecal incontinence can be devastating socially and emotionally. Clients who cope with chronic fecal incontinence and their families require much support and understanding. They may benefit from teaching that the nurse offers (see Client and Family Teaching 31-1).

MEASURES TO PROMOTE BOWEL ELIMINATION

Nurses commonly use two interventions—inserting suppositories and administering enemas—to promote elimination when it does not occur naturally or when the bowel must

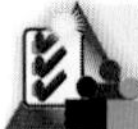

Client and Family Teaching 31-1 Managing Fecal Incontinence

The nurse teaches the client and the family as follows:

- Eat regularly and nutritiously.
- Monitor the pattern of incontinence to determine whether it occurs at a similar time each day.
- Sit on the toilet or bedside commode before the time elimination tends to occur.
- Consult the physician about inserting a suppository or administering an enema every 2 to 3 days to establish a pattern for bowel elimination.
- Use moisture-proof undergarments and absorbent pads to protect clothing and bed linen.
- Teach caregivers to do the following:
  - Do not imply, verbally or nonverbally, that the client is to blame for the incontinence or that cleaning him or her is disgusting.
  - Avoid anything that connotes diapering, to preserve the client's dignity and self-esteem.

be cleansed for other purposes, such as in preparation for surgery and endoscopic or X-ray examinations.

Inserting a Rectal Suppository

A **suppository** (an oval or cone-shaped mass that melts at body temperature) is inserted into a body cavity such as the rectum. The most common reason for inserting a suppository is to deliver a drug that will promote the expulsion of feces. Other medications, such as drugs to control vomiting and reduce fever, also are available in suppository form.

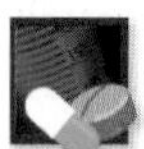

Pharmacologic Considerations

- Medications released from the suppository can have local or systemic effects. Depending on the drug, local effects may include softening and lubricating dry stool, irritating the wall of the rectum and anal canal to stimulate smooth muscle contraction, and liberating carbon dioxide, thus increasing rectal distention and the urge to defecate.

Drugs administered in suppository form are chosen when clients have difficulty retaining or absorbing oral medications because of chronic vomiting or an impaired ability to swallow, or it is undesirable to delay defecation while waiting for an oral medication to act. Administering a suppository is a form of medication administration (Skill 31-2). For additional principles, refer to Chapters 32 and 33.

▸ *Stop, Think, and Respond Box 31-2*

Discuss appropriate actions if a mass of stool is felt when inserting a suppository.

Administering an Enema

An **enema** introduces a solution into the rectum (Skill 31-3). Nurses give enemas to:

- Cleanse the lower bowel (most common reason)
- Soften feces
- Expel flatus
- Soothe irritated mucous membranes
- Outline the colon during diagnostic X-rays
- Treat worm and parasite infestations

Cleansing Enemas

Cleansing enemas use different types of solution to remove feces from the rectum (Table 31-3). Defecation usually occurs within 5 to 15 minutes after administration.

Large-volume cleansing enemas may create discomfort because they distend the lower bowel. Nurses must administer them cautiously to clients with intestinal disorders such as colitis (inflammation of the colon) because large-volume enemas may rupture the bowel or cause other secondary complications. In many health agencies and in the home, commercially prepared disposable administration sets have become the method of choice for cleansing the bowel. Their smaller volume makes them less fatiguing and distressing than large-volume enemas, and they can be easily self-administered.

Tap Water and Normal Saline Enemas

Tap water and normal saline solutions are preferred for their nonirritating effects, especially for clients with rectal diseases or those being prepared for rectal examinations. Tap water and normal saline appear to have about the same degree of effectiveness for cleansing the bowel.

Because tap water is hypotonic, the fluid can be absorbed through the bowel. Consequently, if several enemas are administered in succession, fluid and electrolyte imbalances may occur (see Chap. 16). Therefore, to ensure client safety, if stool continues to be expelled after the administration of three enemas, the nurse consults the physician before administering more.

Soap Solution Enemas

A soap solution enema is a mixture of water and soap. Many disposable enema kits contain an envelope of soap, which is

TABLE 31-3 Types of Cleansing Enema Solutions

SOLUTION	AMOUNT (ml)	MECHANISM OF ACTION
Tap water	500–1,000	Distends rectum, moistens stool
Normal saline	500–1,000	Distends rectum, moistens stool
Soap and water	500–1,000	Distends rectum, moistens stool, irritates local tissue
Hypertonic saline	120	Irritates local tissue and draws water into the bowel
Mineral, olive, or cottonseed oil	120–180	Lubricates and softens stool

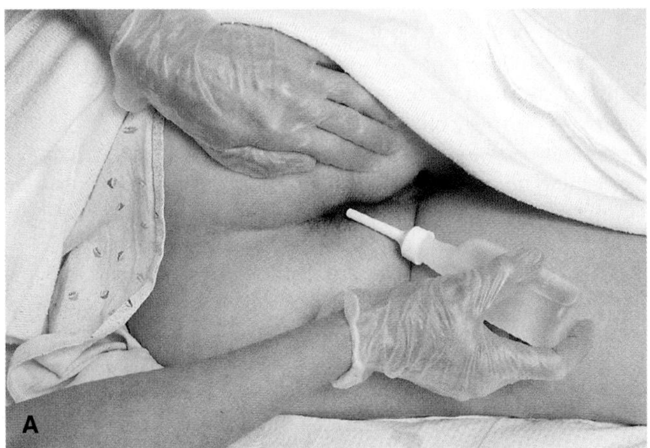

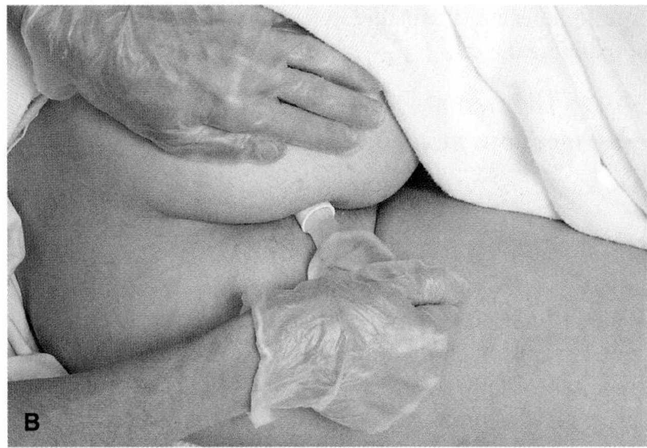

FIGURE 31-3 **A.** The enema tip is inserted fully within the rectum. **B.** The chamber that contains fluid is compressed to instill the solution.

mixed with up to 1 quart (1,000 mL) of water. If these soap packets are not available, a comparable mixture is 1 mL of mild liquid soap per 200 mL of solution, or a ratio of 1:200. Therefore, 5 mL of soap is added to prepare a volume of 1,000 mL.

Soap causes chemical irritation of the mucous membranes. Adding too much soap or using strong soap can potentiate the irritating effect.

Hypertonic Saline Enemas

A hypertonic saline (sodium phosphate) enema draws fluid from body tissues into the bowel. This increases the fluid volume in the intestine beyond what was originally instilled. The concentrated solution also acts as a local irritant on the mucous membranes.

Hypertonic enema solutions are available in commercially prepared, disposable containers holding approximately 4 oz (120 mL) of solution (Fig. 31-3). The container, which has a lubricated tip, substitutes for enema equipment and tubing (see Nursing Guidelines 31-3).

Retention Enemas

A **retention enema** uses a solution held within the large intestine for a specified period, usually at least 30 minutes. Some retention enemas are not expelled at all. One type of retention enema is called an oil retention enema because the fluid instilled is mineral, cottonseed, or olive oil. Oils lubricate and soften the stool, so it can be expelled more easily.

The oil may come in a prefilled container similar to those that contain hypertonic saline. If disposable equipment is not available, the nurse lubricates and inserts a 14- to 22-F tube in the rectum. A small funnel or large syringe is attached to the tube, and the nurse instills approximately 100 to 200 mL of warmed oil slowly to avoid stimulating an

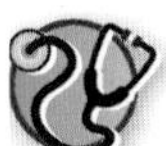

NURSING GUIDELINES 31-3

Administering a Hypertonic Enema Solution

- Warm the container of solution (if it is cold) by placing it in a basin or sink of warm water. *Warmth promotes comfort.*
- Assist the client to a Sims' position or use a knee–chest position (see Chap. 14). *These positions promote gravity distribution of the solution.*
- Wash hands or use an alcohol-based hand rub (see Chap. 10) and don gloves. *Hand hygiene reduces transmission of microorganisms; gloves provide a barrier from contact with a substance that contains body fluid.*
- Remove the cover from the lubricated tip. *This step facilitates administration.*
- Cover the tip with additional lubricant. *Lubricant eases insertion.*
- Invert the container. *Inversion causes air in the container to rise toward the upper end.*
- Insert the full length of the tip within the rectum. *This positioning places the tip at a level that promotes effectiveness.*
- Apply gentle, steady pressure on the solution container for 1 to 2 minutes or until the solution has been completely administered. *This method instills a steady stream of solution.*
- Compress the container as the solution instills. *Compression provides positive pressure rather than gravity to instill fluid.*
- Encourage the client to retain the solution for 5 to 15 minutes. *This duration promotes effectiveness.*
- Clean the client and position for comfort. *These measures demonstrate concern for the client's well-being.*
- Discard the container, remove gloves, and perform hand hygiene measures. *Doing so follows the principles of medical asepsis.*

urge to defecate. Premature defecation defeats the purpose of retaining the oil.

Stop, Think, and Respond Box 31-3

List measures for preventing constipation.

OSTOMY CARE

A client with an **ostomy** (a surgically created opening to the bowel or other structure; see Chap. 30) requires additional care for promoting bowel elimination. Two examples of intestinal ostomies are an **ileostomy** (a surgically created opening to the ileum) and a **colostomy** (a surgically created opening to a portion of the colon; Fig. 31-4). Materials enter and exit through a **stoma** (the entrance to the opening).

Most persons with an ostomy, also called ostomates, wear an **appliance** (a bag or collection device over the stoma) to collect stool. Depending on the type and location of the ostomy, client care may involve providing peristomal care, applying an appliance, draining a continent ileostomy, and, for clients with a colostomy, administering irrigations through the stoma.

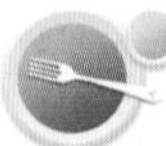

Nutrition Notes

- Because large amounts of fluid, sodium, and potassium are normally absorbed in the colon, the risk of fluid and electrolyte imbalances increases as the length of the remaining colon decreases. Clients with ileostomies are at higher risk of nutritional problems than are clients with colostomies in which some of the colon is retained.
- Clients with ileostomies are encouraged to consume 8 to 10 glasses of fluid daily to maintain a normal urine output and to minimize the risk of renal calculi. Assure clients that excess fluid is excreted through the kidneys, not the stoma. A liberal salt intake may be needed to replenish losses.
- Ileostomies are placed before the terminal ileum where vitamin B12 is absorbed. Nasal sprays or parenteral injections of vitamin B12 are necessary to prevent vitamin B12 deficiency anemia.

Providing Peristomal Care

Preventing skin breakdown is a major challenge in ostomy care. Enzymes in the stool can quickly cause **excoriation** (chemical injury of the skin). Washing the stoma and the surrounding skin with mild soap and water, and patting it dry

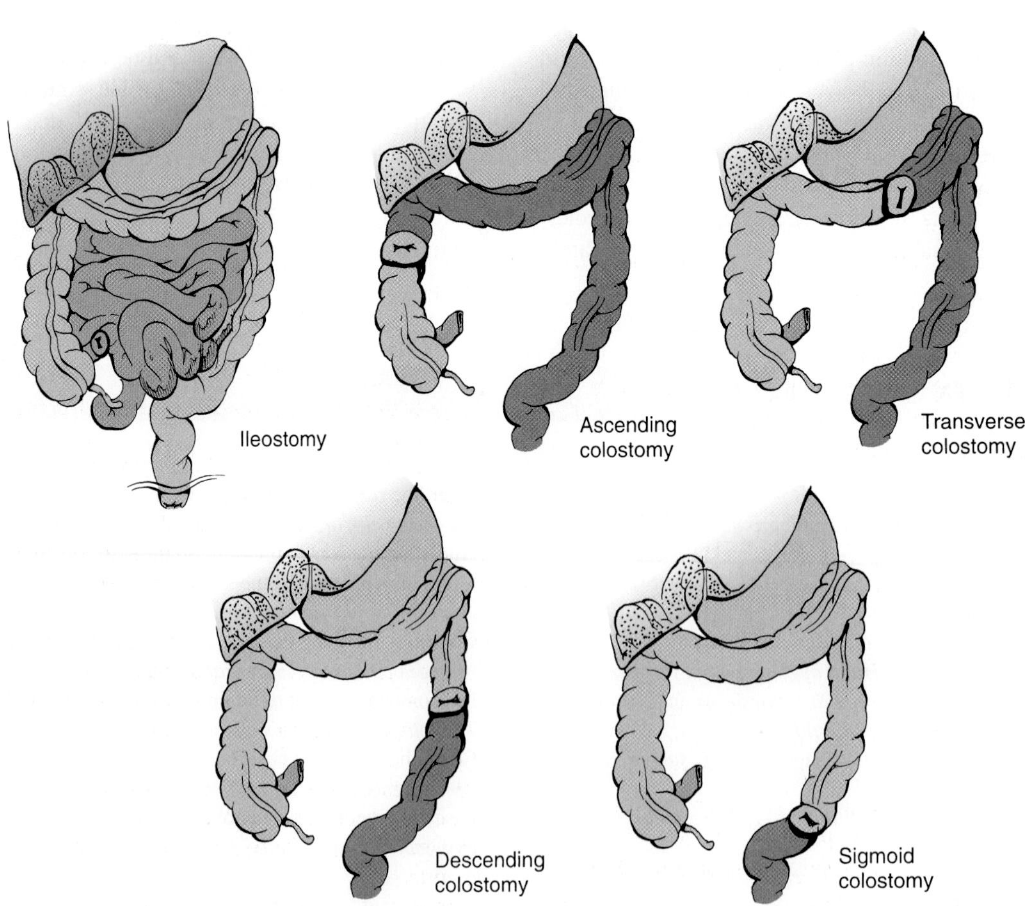

FIGURE 31-4 The locations of intestinal ostomies.

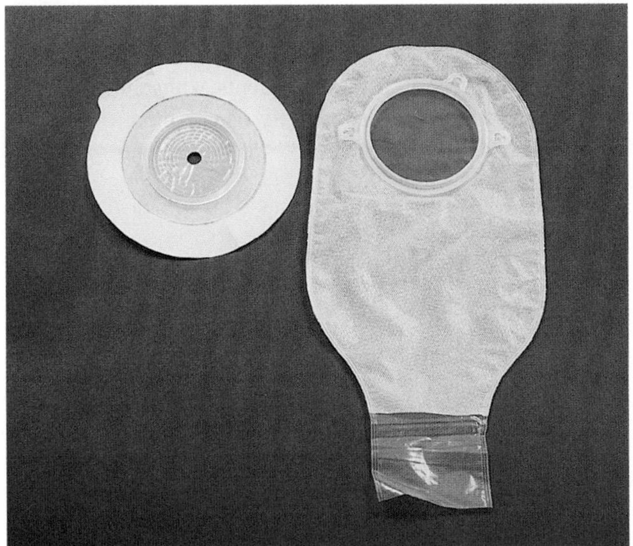

FIGURE 31-5 An ostomy appliance: a faceplate and pouch. (Photo by B. Proud.)

can preserve skin integrity. Another way to protect the skin is to apply barrier substances such as *karaya*, a plant substance that becomes gelatinous when moistened, and commercial skin preparations around the stoma. An **enterostomal therapist**, a nurse certified in caring for ostomies and related skin problems, may be consulted regarding skin and stomal care.

Applying an Ostomy Appliance

Various appliances are available, but all consist of a pouch for collecting stool and a faceplate, or disk, that attaches to the abdomen. The stoma protrudes through an opening in the center of the appliance (Fig. 31-5). The pouch fastens into position when pressed over the circular support on the faceplate. Some clients prefer a type that is also fastened to an elastic belt worn around the waist. The belt helps to support the weight of the fecal material and prevents the faceplate from being pulled away from the abdomen. The client empties the pouch by releasing the clamp at the bottom.

The faceplate usually remains in place for 3 to 5 days unless it becomes loose or causes skin discomfort. Pouches are emptied and rinsed or detached and replaced periodically. The client empties the pouch when it is one-third to one-half full; otherwise, it may become too heavy and pull the faceplate from the skin. Although design of the equipment varies, almost all types of appliances are changed similarly (Skill 31-4).

Draining a Continent Ileostomy

A **continent ostomy** (a surgically created opening that controls the drainage of liquid stool or urine by siphoning it from an internal reservoir) also is referred to as a *Kock pouch*, after the surgeon who developed the technique (Fig. 31-6). This type of ostomy requires no appliance; however, the client must drain the accumulating liquid stool or urine approximately every 4 to 6 hours. The client can use a gravity drainage system at night (see Client and Family Teaching 31-2).

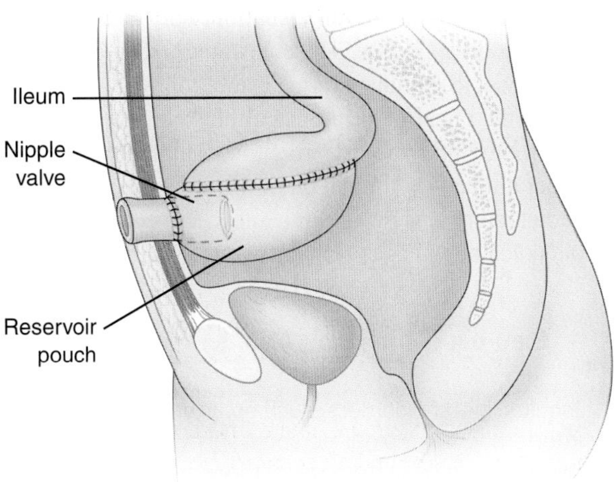

FIGURE 31-6 A continent ileostomy.

Irrigating a Colostomy

Clients with a colostomy whose stool is more solid sometimes require the instillation of fluid to promote elimination. Colostomy irrigation involves instilling the solution through the stoma into the colon, a process similar to administering an enema (Skill 31-5).

The purpose of the irrigation is to remove formed stool and, in some cases, to regulate the timing of bowel movements.

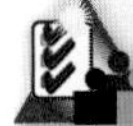

Client and Family Teaching 31-2
Draining a Continent Ileostomy

The nurse teaches the client and the family as follows:

- Assume a sitting position.
- Insert a lubricated 22- to 28-F catheter into the stoma.
- Expect resistance after inserting the tube approximately 2 in.; this is the location of the valve that controls the retention of liquid stool or urine.
- Gently advance the catheter through the valve at the end of exhalation, while coughing, or while bearing down as if to pass stool.
- Lower the external end of the catheter at least 12 in. below the stoma.
- Direct the end of the catheter into a container or toilet as stool or urine begins to flow.
- Allow at least 5 to 10 minutes for complete emptying.
- Remove the catheter and clean it with warm soapy water.
- Place the clean catheter in a sealable plastic bag until its next use.
- Cover the stoma with a gauze square or a large bandage.
- If the catheter becomes plugged with stool or mucus:
  - Bear down as if to have a bowel movement.
  - Rotate the catheter tip inside the stoma.
  - Milk the catheter.
  - If these are not successful, remove the catheter, rinse it, and try again.
  - Notify the physician if these efforts do not result in drainage.
- Never wait longer than 6 hours without obtaining drainage.

With regulation, a client with a sigmoid colostomy may not need to wear an appliance. The colostomy irrigation helps to train the bowel to eliminate formed stool following the irrigation. Once the client has eliminated the stool, he or she will expel no more until the next irrigation. This mimics the pattern of natural bowel elimination for most people. Because of the predictability of bowel elimination, some clients with a sigmoid colostomy feel it is unnecessary to wear an appliance.

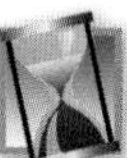

Gerontologic Considerations

■ Musculoskeletal disorders, such as arthritis of the hands, may interfere with an older person's ability to care for an ostomy appliance or perform colostomy irrigations. An occupational or enterostomal therapist can offer suggestions for promoting self-care.

Stop, Think, and Respond Box 31-4

Discuss the various ways an ostomy affects the lives of clients.

NURSING IMPLICATIONS

While assessing and caring for clients with altered bowel elimination, the nurse may identify one or more of the following nursing diagnoses:

- Constipation
- Risk for Constipation
- Perceived Constipation
- Diarrhea
- Bowel Incontinence
- Toileting Self-Care Deficit
- Situational Low Self-Esteem

Nursing Care Plan 31-1 reflects the nursing process as it applies to a client with constipation. NANDA-I defines constipation (2012, p. 203) as "a decrease in normal frequency of defecation accompanied by difficult or incomplete passage of stool and/or passage of excessively hard, dry stool."

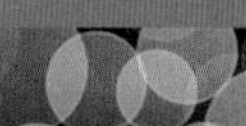

NURSING CARE PLAN 31-1 Constipation

Assessment

- Note the frequency, amount, and texture of the expelled stool.
- Ask the client about the effort required to eliminate stool.
- Inquire as to whether the client feels that he or she empties the bowel during stool elimination and if there is any discomfort in the rectal area.
- Auscultate bowel sounds daily.
- Palpate the abdomen to determine if there is any distention.
- Determine if any of the client's medications are constipating.
- Ask the client about measures he or she uses to promote bowel elimination and their frequency.
- Ask the client to describe his or her daily intake of fluid and food, including types of beverages and foods commonly eaten.
- Explore lifestyle patterns that may interfere with bowel elimination such as a lack of privacy or lengthy travel that interferes with accessing a toilet when there is a need to eliminate stool.
- Note if any physical problems may compromise bowel elimination such as impaired physical mobility or dementia.

Nursing Diagnosis. **Constipation** related to inadequate dietary habits as manifested by a distended abdomen; hypoactive bowel sounds in all four quadrants; and client's statement: "I've got a problem. I haven't had a bowel movement in 4 days even though I've felt like I need to pass stool. I sit and strain but I only pass a small amount of hard stool. I used to have a problem now and then when I was a kid; but since I'm living alone it's getting to be very frequent. Maybe it's because I don't eat regularly and when I do, it's a lot of convenience food."

Expected Outcome. The client will have a bowel movement within 24 hours and will list three ways to improve the regularity of bowel elimination by 10/25.

Interventions	Rationales
Give an oil retention enema as ordered for p.r.n. administration.	This type of enema lubricates the bowel and softens the stool for easier expulsion.
Give prescribed laxative at bedtime 10/23 if no bowel movement has occurred.	Laxatives facilitate bowel elimination in various ways; some common mechanisms of action include increasing intestinal peristalsis, irritating the bowel, and attracting water into the large intestine.
Encourage drinking at least 8–10 glasses of fluid per day; offer prune juice or apple juice.	Oral fluid promotes hydration and avoids dry stool; prune juice has a laxative effect; apple juice contains pectin, which also adds bulk to the stool.
Instruct about high-fiber foods, and that their intake should be gradually increased as tolerated until the desired effect is achieved.	Intestinal fiber adds bulk by pulling water into stool; a bulky soft stool distends the rectum and promotes the urge to defecate.

(continued)

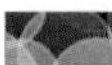

NURSING CARE PLAN 31-1 **Constipation (continued)**

Evaluation of Expected Outcomes

- The client eliminated moderate amount of brown-formed stool approximately 6 hours following the administration of the oil retention enema.
- The client identified a minimum goal of consuming eight 8-oz glasses of fluid daily.
- The client can name sources of fiber such as wheat bran, whole wheat bread, whole grain cereal, fresh fruits and vegetables, dried peas and beans, and nuts.
- The client stated that increasing active exercise for a total of 30 minutes each day either all at once or divided and performed several times during the day promotes bowel elimination.

CRITICAL THINKING EXERCISE

1. When inserting a rectal suppository, the nurse feels a hard mass of stool. What actions should be taken next?

2. What are some possible consequences of chronic constipation?

3. Formulate suggestions to promote bowel continence among older adults with impaired cognition such as those with Alzheimer's disease.

4. What nursing actions are appropriate when peristomal skin appears red and excoriated?

NCLEX-STYLE REVIEW QUESTIONS

1. When a client tells the nurse that he or she cannot have a bowel movement without taking a daily laxative, what information is essential for the nurse to explain?

1. The chronic use of laxatives impairs natural bowel tone.
2. Stool softeners are likely to be less harsh.
3. Daily enemas are more preferable than laxatives.
4. Dilating the anal sphincter may aid bowel elimination.

2. Which of the following assessments is the best indication that a client has a fecal impaction?

1. The client passes liquid stool frequently.
2. The client has extremely offending bad breath.
3. The client requests medication for a headache.
4. The client has not been eating well lately.

3. Before inserting a rectal tube, which of the following nursing measures is most helpful for eliminating intestinal gas?

1. Ambulate the client in the hall.
2. Provide a carbonated beverage.
3. Restrict the intake of solid food.
4. Administer a narcotic analgesic.

4. During the administration of a cleansing soapsuds enema, a client experiences cramping and has the urge to defecate. Which is the best nursing action to take at this time?

1. Quickly finish instilling the remaining solution.
2. Tell the client to hold his or her breath and bear down.
3. Briefly stop the administration of the enema solution.
4. Withdraw the tip of the enema tubing from the rectum.

5. When the nurse assesses the stoma of a client with an ostomy, what is the expected normal appearance?

1. Pale pink
2. Bright red
3. Dark tan
4. Dusky blue

SKILL 31-1 Inserting a Rectal Tube

Suggested Action	Reason for Action
ASSESSMENT	
Check the medical orders.	Ensures collaboration between nursing activities and the medical treatment.
Use two methods to identify the client.	Supports the principles of safety recommended by The Joint Commission.
Inspect the abdomen, auscultate bowel sounds, and gently palpate for distention and fullness.	Provides baseline data for future comparisons.
Determine how much the client understands the procedure.	Provides an opportunity for health teaching.
PLANNING	
Obtain a 22- to 32-F catheter and lubricant.	Ensures proper size and easy insertion.
IMPLEMENTATION	
Wash your hands or perform an alcohol-based hand rub (see Chap. 10); don gloves.	Reduces the transmission of microorganisms.
Pull the privacy curtain.	Demonstrates respect for the client's dignity.
Place the client in a Sims' position.	Facilitates access to the rectum.
Lubricate the tip of the tube generously (Fig. A).	Eases insertion.

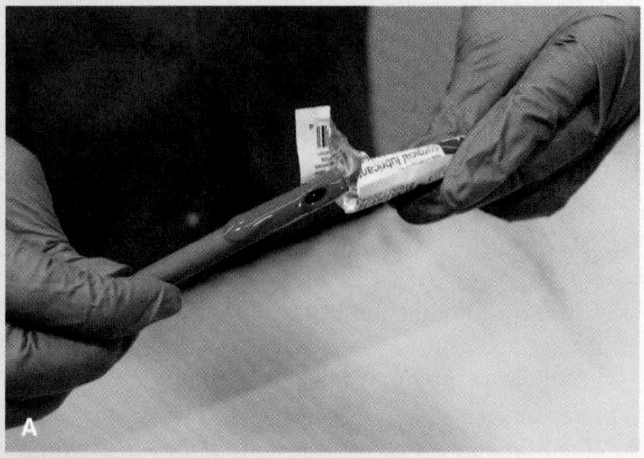

A

Lubricating the rectal tube.

Suggested Action	Reason for Action
Separate the buttocks well so that the anus is in plain view (Fig. B).	Helps visualize the insertion location.

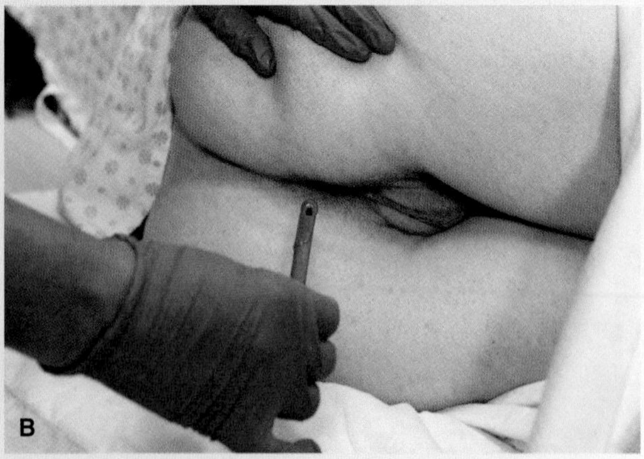

B

Separating the buttocks.

(continued)

Inserting a Rectal Tube (continued)

IMPLEMENTATION (CONTINUED)

Insert the tube 4–6 in. (10–15 cm) in an adult (Fig. C).

Places the distal tip above the sphincter muscles, stimulates peristalsis, and prevents displacement of the tube.

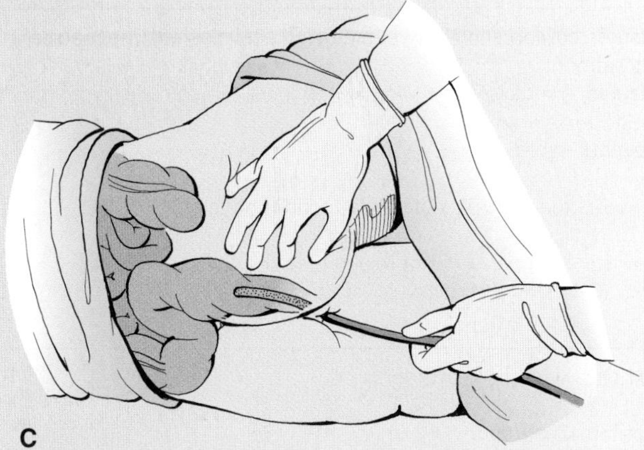

Inserting the rectal tube.

Enclose the free end of the tube within a clean, soft washcloth, disposable bed pad, or gauze square (Fig. D).

Provides a means for absorbing stool should it drain from the tube.

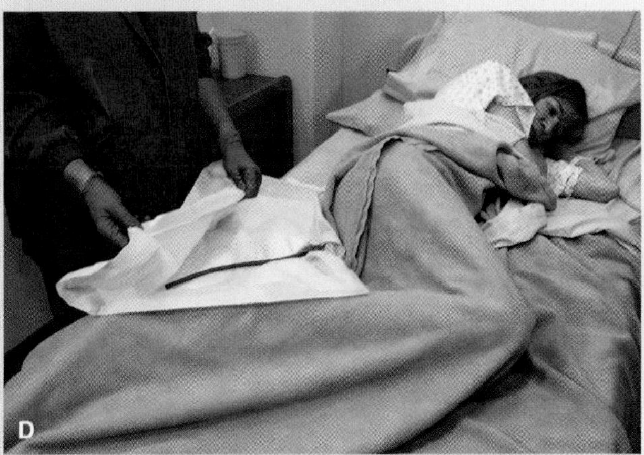

Enclosing the rectal tube.

Tape the tube to the buttocks or inner thigh.

Allows the client to ambulate or change positions without tube displacement.

Leave the rectal tube in place no longer than 20 minutes.

Reduces the risk for impairing the sphincter.

Reinsert the tube every 3–4 hours if discomfort returns.

Reinstitutes therapeutic management.

Evaluation

- Intestinal gas is eliminated.
- The client states symptoms are relieved.
- The client reports no ill effects.

Document

- Assessment data
- Intervention
- Length of time tube was in place
- Client response

SAMPLE DOCUMENTATION

Date and Time Abdomen round, firm, and tympanic. Bowel sounds present in all four quadrants, but difficult to hear because of distention. States, "I can't hardly stand the pain anymore." Ambulated without relief. 26-F straight catheter inserted into rectum for 20 minutes. Flatus expelled during tube insertion. Abdomen softer. ———— SIGNATURE/TITLE

SKILL 31-2 Inserting a Rectal Suppository

Suggested Action	Reason for Action
ASSESSMENT	
Check the medical orders.	Ensures collaboration between nursing activities and the medical treatment.
Compare the medication administration record (MAR) with the written medical order.	Ensures accuracy.
Read and compare the label on the suppository with the MAR at least three times—before, during, and after preparing the drug.	Prevents errors.
Use two methods to identify the client.	Supports the principles of safety recommended by The Joint Commission.
Determine how much the client understands the purpose and technique for administering a suppository.	Provides an opportunity for health teaching.
PLANNING	
Prepare to administer the suppository according to the time prescribed by the physician.	Complies with medical orders.
Obtain clean gloves and lubricant.	Facilitates insertion.
IMPLEMENTATION	
Wash your hands or perform an alcohol-based hand rub (see Chap. 10).	Reduces the transmission of microorganisms.
Read the name on the client's identification band.	Prevents errors.
Pull the privacy curtain.	Demonstrates respect for the client's modesty and dignity.
Place the client in a Sims' position.	Facilitates access to the rectum.
Drape the client to expose only the buttocks.	Ensures modesty and dignity.
Don gloves.	Reduces the transmission of microorganisms and complies with standard precautions.
Lubricate the suppository and index finger of the dominant hand and separate the buttocks so that the anus is in plain view (Fig. A).	Reduces friction and tissue trauma and enhances visualization.

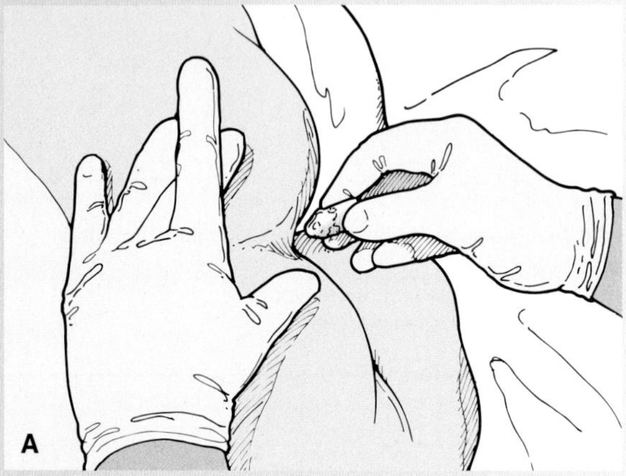

A

The lubricated suppository and insertion finger.

(continued)

Inserting a Rectal Suppository (continued)

Suggested Action	Reason for Action
IMPLEMENTATION (CONTINUED)	
Instruct the client to take several slow, deep breaths. Introduce the suppository, tapered end first, beyond the internal sphincter, about the distance of the finger (Fig. B).	Promotes muscle relaxation and places the suppository in the best location for achieving a local effect.

Rectum
Suppository
Rectal sphincter

B

Inserting the suppository.

Suggested Action	Reason for Action
Avoid placing the suppository within stool.	Reduces effectiveness.
Wipe excess lubricant from around the anus with a paper tissue.	Promotes comfort.
Tell the client to try to retain the suppository for at least 15 minutes.	Enhances effectiveness.
Suggest contracting the gluteal muscles if there is a premature urge to expel the suppository.	Tightens the anal sphincters.
Ask the client to wait to flush the toilet until the stool has been inspected.	Provides an opportunity for evaluating the drug's effectiveness.
Remove your gloves and wash your hands.	Reduces the transmission of microorganisms.

Evaluation
- The client retains the suppository for 15 minutes.
- Bowel elimination occurs.

Document
- Drug, dose, route, and time (see Chap. 32)
- Outcome of drug administration

SAMPLE DOCUMENTATION

Date and Time Bisacodyl (Dulcolax) suppository inserted within rectum. Lg. brown-formed stool expelled.
SIGNATURE/TITLE

SKILL 31-3 Administering a Cleansing Enema

Suggested Action	Reason for Action
ASSESSMENT	
Check the medical orders for the type of enema and prescribed solution.	Ensures collaboration between nursing activities and the medical treatment.
Check the date of the client's last bowel movement.	Helps to determine the need to check for an impaction or the basis for realistic expected outcomes.
Use two methods to identify the client.	Supports the principles of safety recommended by The Joint Commission.

(continued)

Administering a Cleansing Enema (continued)

ASSESSMENT (CONTINUED)

Action	Rationale
Wash hands or perform an alcohol-based hand rub (see Chap 10).	Reduces the transmission of microorganisms.
Auscultate bowel sounds.	Establishes the status of peristalsis.
Determine how much the client understands the procedure.	Provides an opportunity for health teaching.

PLANNING

Action	Rationale
Plan the location where the client will expel the enema solution and stool.	Determines if a bedpan is necessary.
Obtain the appropriate equipment including an enema set, solution, an absorbent pad, lubricant, a bath blanket, and gloves.	Facilitates organization and efficient time management.
Plan to perform the procedure according to the time specified by the physician or when it is most appropriate during client care.	Demonstrates collaboration and participation of the client in decision making.
Prepare the solution and equipment in the utility room.	Provides access to supplies.
Warm the solution to approximately 105°–110°F (40°–43°C).	Promotes comfort and safety.
Clamp the tubing on the enema set.	Prevents the loss of fluid.
Fill the container with the specified solution.	Provides the mechanism for cleansing the bowel.

IMPLEMENTATION

Action	Rationale
Pull the privacy curtain.	Demonstrates respect for the client's dignity.
Place the client in a Sims' position.	Facilitates access to the rectum.
Drape the client, exposing the buttocks, and place a waterproof pad under the hips (Fig. A).	Preserves modesty and protects bed linen.

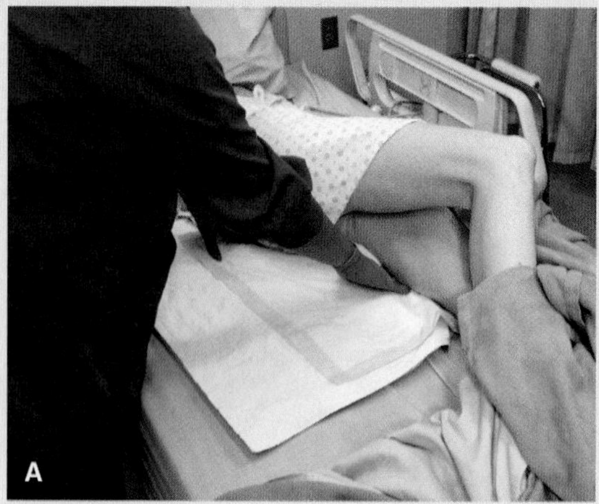

Draping for an enema.

Action	Rationale
Don gloves.	Reduces the transmission of microorganisms and complies with standard precautions.
Place (or hang) the solution container so that it is 12–20 in. (30–50 cm) above the level of the client's anus.	Facilitates gravity flow.
Open the clamp and fill the tubing with solution (Fig. B). Reclamp.	Purges air from the tubing.

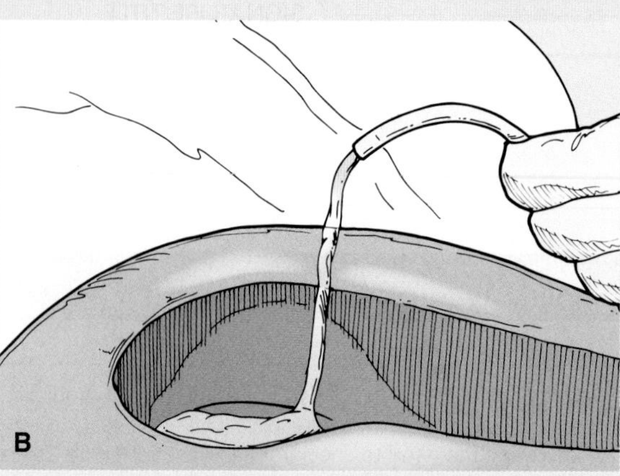

Purging air.

(continued)

Administering a Cleansing Enema (continued)

IMPLEMENTATION (CONTINUED)

Action	Rationale
Lubricate the tip of the tube generously (Fig. C).	Eases insertion.
C — Lubricating the tube.	
Separate the buttocks well so that the anus is in plain view.	Helps to visualize insertion.
Insert the tube 3–4 in. (7–10 cm) in an adult.	Places the distal tip above the sphincters.
Direct the tubing at an angle pointing toward the umbilicus (Fig. D).	Follows the contour of the rectum.
D — The direction for tube insertion.	
Hold the tube in place with one hand (Fig. E).	Avoids displacement.
E — Holding the tube in place.	

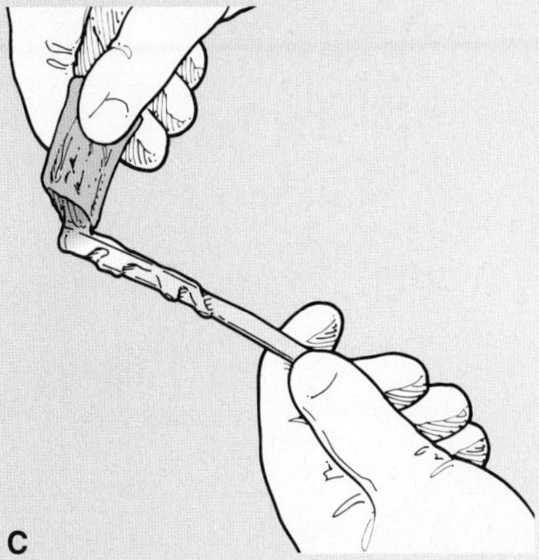

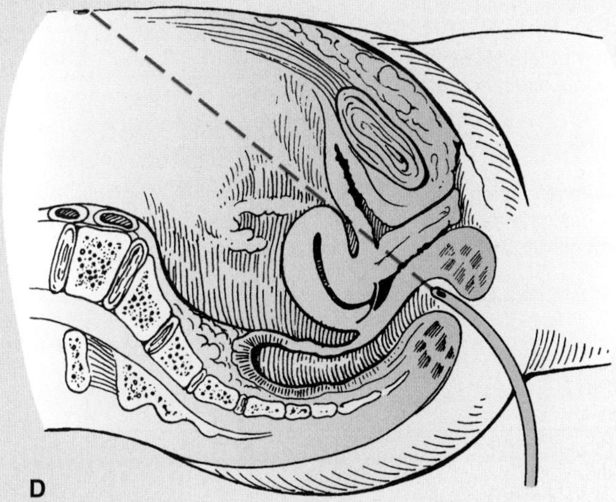

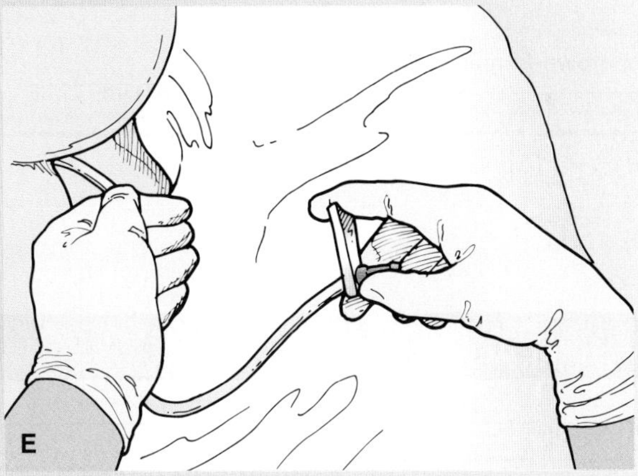

(continued)

Administering a Cleansing Enema (continued)

Suggested Action	Reason for Action
IMPLEMENTATION (CONTINUED)	
Release the clamp.	Promotes instillation.
Instill the solution gradually over 5–10 minutes (Fig. F).	Fills the rectum.

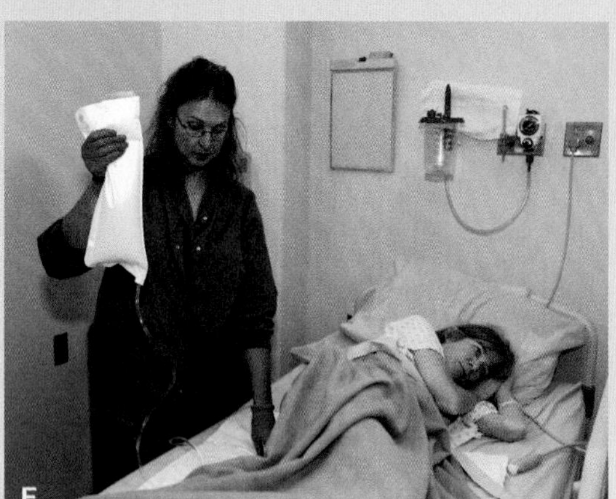

Instilling the enema solution.

Suggested Action	Reason for Action
Clamp the tube for a brief period while the client takes deep breaths and contracts the anal sphincters if cramping occurs.	Avoids further stimulation.
Resume instillation when the cramping is relieved.	Facilitates effectiveness.
Clamp and remove the tubing after sufficient solution has been instilled or the client states that he or she cannot retain more.	Completes the procedure.
Encourage the client to retain the solution for 5–15 minutes.	Promotes effectiveness.
Hold the enema tubing in one hand and pull a glove over the inserting end of the tubing.	Prevents direct contact.
Remove and discard the remaining glove and dispose of the enema equipment.	Follows the principles of medical asepsis.
Assist the client to sit while eliminating the solution and stool.	Aids in defecation.
Examine the expelled solution.	Provides data for evaluating the effectiveness of the procedure.
Clean and dry the client; help him or her to a comfortable position.	Demonstrates concern for the client's well-being.

Evaluation

- A sufficient amount of solution is instilled.
- A comparable amount of solution is expelled.
- The client eliminates stool.

Document

- Type of enema solution
- Volume instilled
- Outcome of procedure

SAMPLE DOCUMENTATION

Date and Time 1,000 mL tap water enema administered. Lg. amt of brown-formed stool expelled.

SIGNATURE/TITLE

SKILL 31-4 Changing an Ostomy Appliance

Suggested Action	Reason for Action
ASSESSMENT	
Wash hands or perform an alcohol-based hand rub (see Chap. 10).	Reduces the transmission of microorganisms and complies with standard precautions.
Use two methods to identify the client.	Supports the principles of safety recommended by The Joint Commission.

(continued)

Changing an Ostomy Appliance (continued)

ASSESSMENT (CONTINUED)	
Inspect the faceplate, pouch, and peristomal skin.	Determines the necessity for changing the appliance and provides data about the condition of the stoma and the surrounding skin.
Determine how much the client understands about stomal care and changing an ostomy appliance.	Provides an opportunity for health teaching; prepares the client for assuming self-care.
PLANNING	
Obtain replacement equipment, supplies for removing the adhesive (eg, the manufacturer's recommended solvent if appropriate), and products for skin care.	Facilitates organization and efficient time management.
Plan to replace the appliance immediately if the client has localized symptoms.	Prevents complications.
Schedule an appliance change for an asymptomatic client before a meal.	Coincides with a time when the gastrocolic reflex is less active.
Plan to empty the pouch just before the appliance will be changed.	Prevents soiling.
IMPLEMENTATION	
Pull the privacy curtain.	Demonstrates respect for the client's dignity.
Place the client in a supine or dorsal recumbent position.	Facilitates access to the stoma.
Wash your hands or perform an alcohol-based hand rub; don gloves.	Reduces the transmission of microorganisms; complies with standard precautions.
Unfasten the pouch and discard it in a lined receptacle or waterproof container.	Facilitates access to the faceplate.
Gently peel the faceplate from the skin (Fig. A).	Prevents skin trauma.

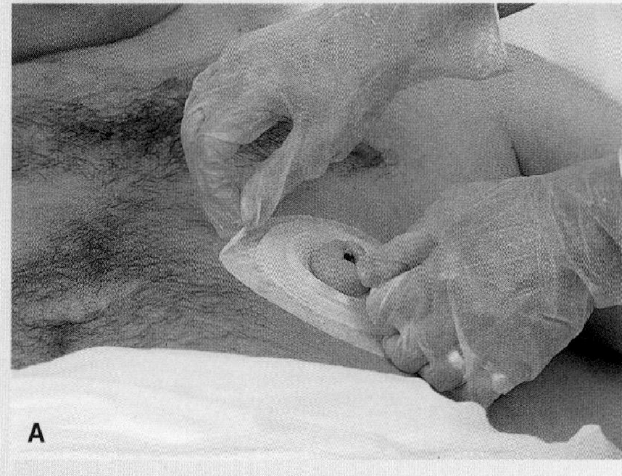

A Removing the faceplate. (Photo by B. Proud.)

Wash the peristomal area with water or mild soapy water using a soft washcloth or gauze square.	Cleans mucus and stool from the skin.
Suggest that the client shower or bathe at this time.	Provides an opportunity for daily hygiene and will not affect the exposed stoma.
After or instead of bathing, pat the peristomal skin dry.	Promotes the potential for adhesion when the faceplate is applied.
Measure the stoma using a stomal guide (Fig. B).	Determines the size of the stomal opening in the faceplate.

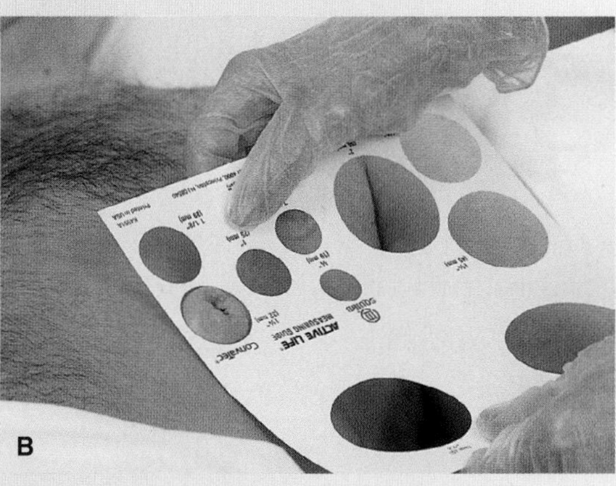

B Measuring the stoma. (Photo by B. Proud.)

(continued)

Changing an Ostomy Appliance (continued)

IMPLEMENTATION (CONTINUED)

Trim the opening in the faceplate to the measured diameter plus approximately ⅛ to ¼ inch larger (Fig. C).

Avoids pinching of or pressure on the stoma and causing circulatory impairment.

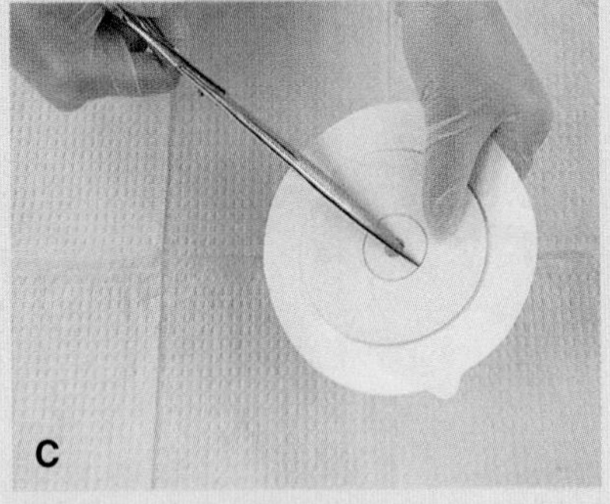

Trimming the stomal opening. (Photo by B. Proud.)

Attach a new pouch to the ring of the faceplate (Fig. D).

Avoids pushing the pouch into place after the faceplate has been applied.

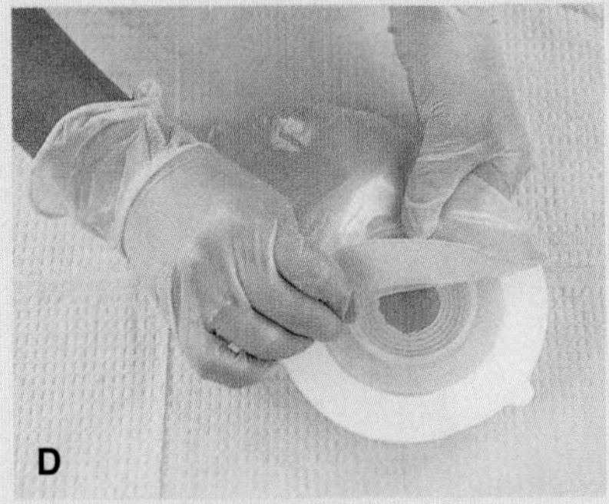

Attaching the pouch. (Photo by B. Proud.)

Fold and clamp the bottom of the pouch (Fig. E).

Seals the pouch so leaking will not occur.

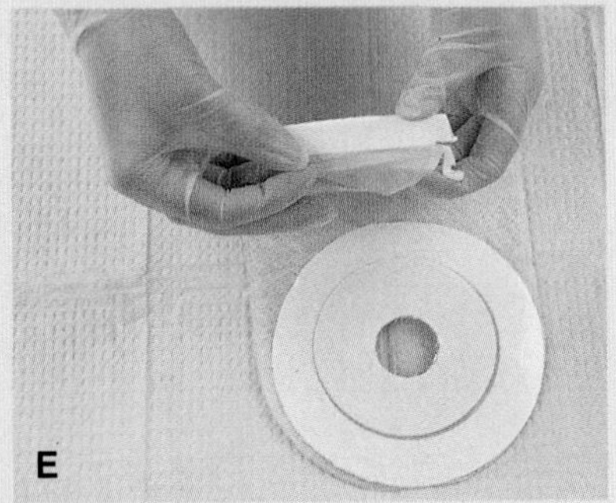

Sealing the pouch. (Photo by B. Proud.)

Peel the backing from the adhesive on the faceplate (Fig. F).

Prepares the appliance for application.

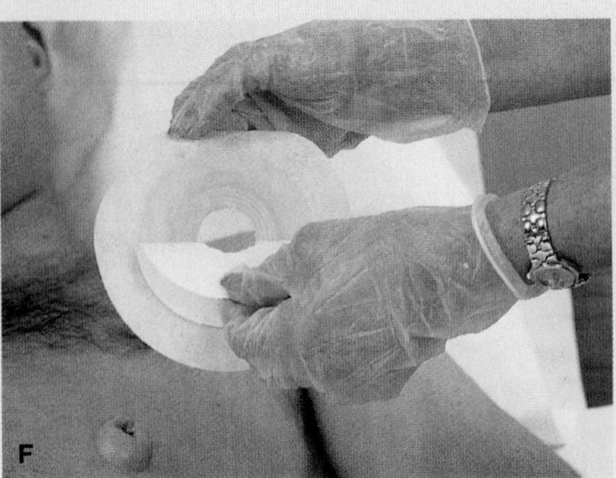

Removing the adhesive backing. (Photo by B. Proud.)

(continued)

Changing an Ostomy Appliance (continued)

Suggested Action	Reason for Action
IMPLEMENTATION (CONTINUED)	
Have the client stand or lie flat.	Keeps the skin taut and avoids wrinkles.
Position the opening over the stoma and press into place from the center outward (Fig. G).	Prevents air gaps and skin wrinkles.
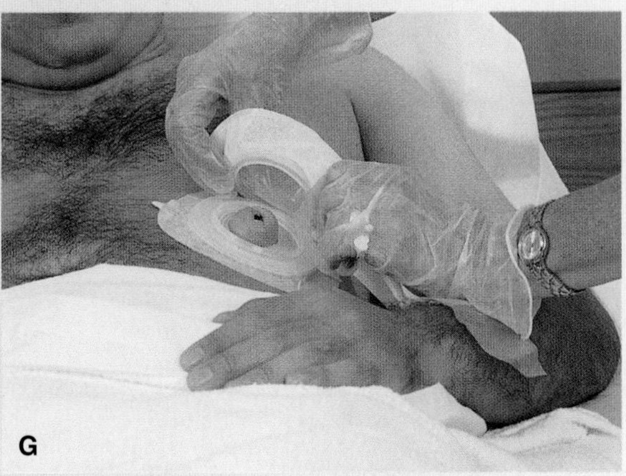	Attaching the appliance. (Photo by B. Proud.)
Perform hand hygiene after removing gloves.	Removes transient microorganisms.

Evaluation

- The stoma appears pink and moist.
- The skin is clean, dry, and intact with no evidence of redness, irritation, or excoriation.
- The new appliance adheres to the skin without wrinkles or gaps.

Document

- Assessment data
- Peristomal care
- Application of new appliance

SAMPLE DOCUMENTATION

Date and Time Ostomy appliance removed. Peristomal skin cleansed with soapy water and patted dry. Stoma is pink and moist. Peristomal skin is intact and painless. New appliance applied over stoma.

—————————— SIGNATURE/TITLE

SKILL 31-5 Irrigating a Colostomy

Suggested Action	Reason for Action
ASSESSMENT	
Check the medical orders to verify the written order and type of solution to use.	Ensures collaboration between nursing activities and the medical treatment.
Use two methods to identify the client.	Supports the principles of safety recommended by The Joint Commission.
Determine how much the client understands about colostomy irrigation.	Provides an opportunity for health teaching; prepares the client to assume self-care.

(continued)

Irrigating a Colostomy (continued)

PLANNING	
Obtain an irrigating bag and sleeve, lubricant, and a belt (Fig. A). A bedpan will be needed if the client is confined to the bed.	Promotes organization and efficient time management.

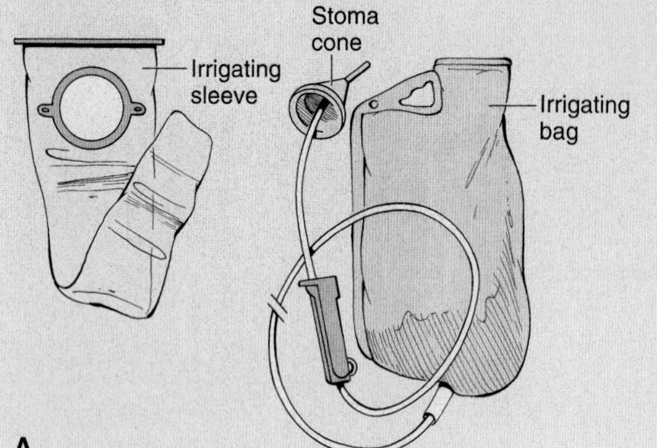

Irrigating the sleeve and bag.

Prepare the irrigating bag with solution in the same way as for an enema set (see Skill 31-3).	Provides the mechanism for cleansing the bowel.
Unclamp the tubing and fill it with solution.	Purges air from the tubing.
IMPLEMENTATION	
Place the client in a sitting position in bed, in a chair in front or beside the toilet, or on the toilet itself.	Facilitates collecting drainage.
Place absorbent pads or towels on the client's lap.	Prevents soiling of linen or clothing.
Hang the container approximately 12 in. (30 cm) above the stoma.	Facilitates gravity flow.
Wash your hands or perform an alcohol-based hand rub; don gloves.	Reduces the transmission of microorganisms; complies with standard precautions.
Empty and remove the pouch from the faceplate if the client is wearing one.	Provides access to the stoma.
Secure the sleeve over the stoma and fasten it around the client with an elastic belt (Fig. B).	Provides a pathway for drainage.

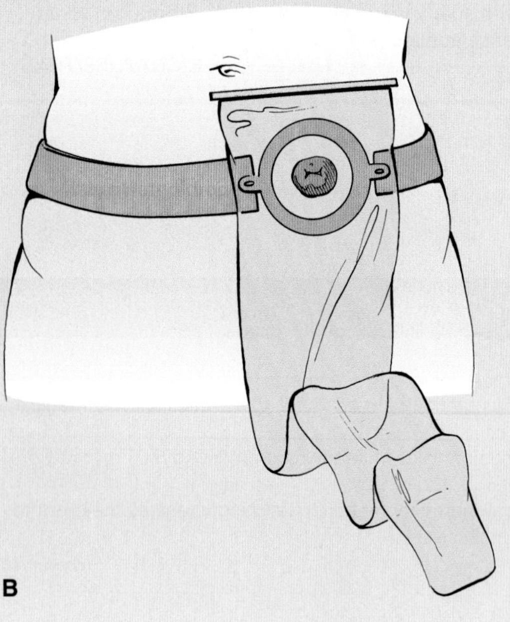

Positioning the irrigation sleeve.

(continued)

Irrigating a Colostomy (continued)

IMPLEMENTATION (CONTINUED)

Action	Rationale
Place the lower end of the sleeve into the toilet, commode, or bedpan (Fig. C).	Collects drainage.

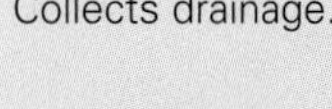

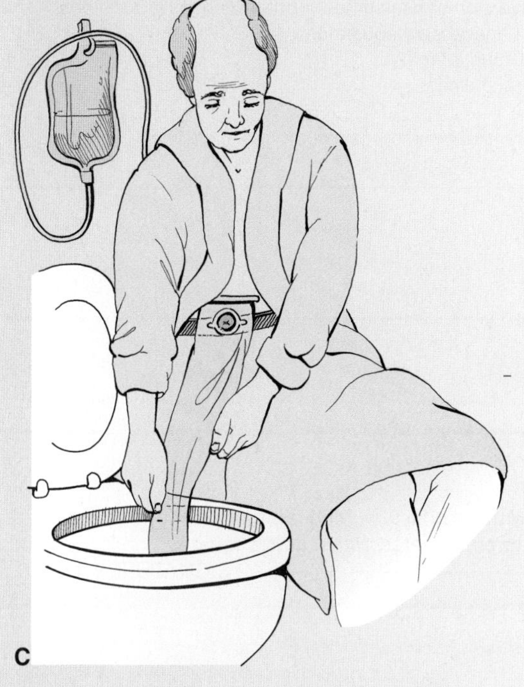

C Placing the distal end of the sleeve.

Action	Rationale
Lubricate the cone at the end of the irrigating bag.	Facilitates insertion.
Open the top of the irrigating sleeve.	Provides access to the stoma.
Insert the cone into the stoma (Fig. D).	Dilates the stoma and provides a means for instilling fluid.

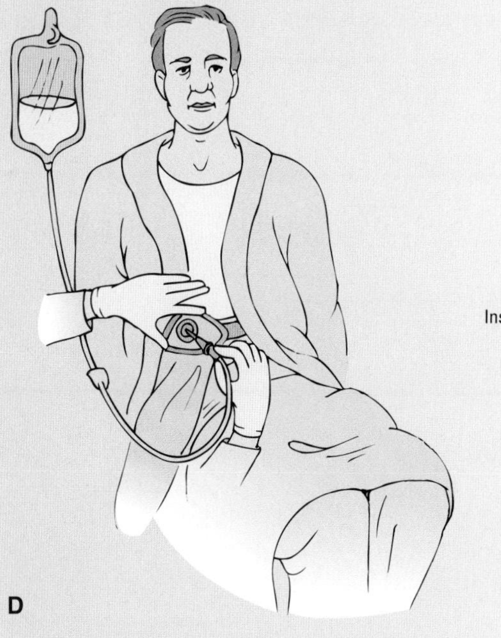

D Inserting the irrigation cone.

Action	Rationale
Hold the cone in place and release the clamp on the tubing.	Prevents expulsion of the cone and initiates the instillation.
Clamp the tubing and wait if cramping occurs.	Interrupts the instillation while the bowel adjusts.
Release the clamp and continue once the discomfort disappears.	Resumes instilling the fluid without discomfort to the client.

(continued)

Irrigating a Colostomy (continued)

IMPLEMENTATION (CONTINUED)

Clamp the tubing and remove the cone when the irrigating solution has been instilled.	Discontinues the administration of solution.
Close the top of the irrigating sleeve.	Keeps drainage in a downward direction.
Give the client reading materials or hygiene supplies.	Provides diversion or uses time for other productive activities.
Remove the belt and sleeve when the draining has stopped.	Eliminates unnecessary equipment.
Clean the stoma and pat it dry.	Maintains tissue integrity.
If client is wearing an appliance, place a clean pouch over the stoma or cover the stoma temporarily with a gauze square.	Collects fecal drainage.
Repeat hand hygiene measures after removing gloves.	Removes transient microorganisms.

Evaluation

- A sufficient amount of solution is instilled.
- A comparable amount of solution is expelled.
- Stool is eliminated.

Document

- Type of irrigation solution
- Volume instilled
- Outcome of procedure

SAMPLE DOCUMENTATION

Date and Time Colostomy irrigated with 500 mL of tap water. Instilled without difficulty. Mod. amt. of semiformed stool expelled with solution. Stoma cleansed with water and dried. Covered with a gauze square.
——————————————— SIGNATURE/TITLE

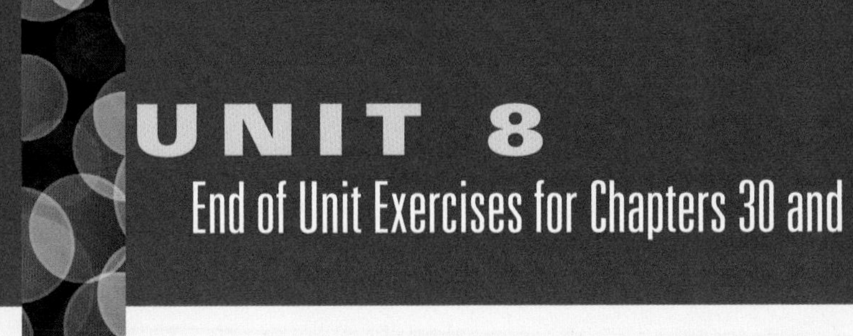

UNIT 8
End of Unit Exercises for Chapters 30 and 31

Section I: Reviewing What You've Learned

Activity A: *Fill in the blanks by choosing the correct word from the options given in parentheses.*

1. ________________ means greater than normal urinary volume. (Anuria, Oliguria, Polyuria)
2. Hypertonic enema solutions are available in commercially prepared disposable containers that hold approximately ________________ mL of solution. (60, 120, 180)
3. ________________ constipation results from medical treatment. (Iatrogenic, Pseudo, Secondary)
4. A ________________ is a bedside seatlike container used for the elimination of body waste. (bedpan, commode, urinal)

Activity B: *Mark each statement as either T (True) or F (False). Correct any false statements.*

1. T___F___ Catheterization is the insertion of a hollow tube inside the bladder.
2. T___F___ The urinary meatus is the opening to the urethra.
3. T___F___ A straight catheter is an indwelling catheter left in place for a period of time.
4. T___F___ Vegetables such as cabbage and cucumbers are known to prevent intestinal gas.

Activity C: *Write the correct term for each description below.*

1. Urine containing blood ________________
2. Skin around the stoma ________________
3. The rhythmic contraction of intestinal smooth muscle that facilitates defecation ________________
4. Chemical injury to the skin resulting from enzymes present in stool ________________

Activity D: *1. Match the terms related to defecation and ostomy in Column A with their explanations in Column B.*

Column A	Column B
1. ________________ Gastrocolic reflex	A. Entrance to a surgically created opening to an organ of elimination
2. ________________ Anal sphincter	B. Closing the glottis and contracting the pelvic and abdominal muscles to increase abdominal pressure
3. ________________ Stoma	C. Accelerated intestinal peristalsis that usually occurs during or after eating
4. ________________ Valsalva maneuver	D. Ring-shaped band of muscles

Activity E: *1. Differentiate between fecal impaction and fecal incontinence based on the categories given below.*

	Fecal Impaction	Fecal Incontinence
Definition		
Causes		
Symptoms		

Activity F: *Consider the following figures.*

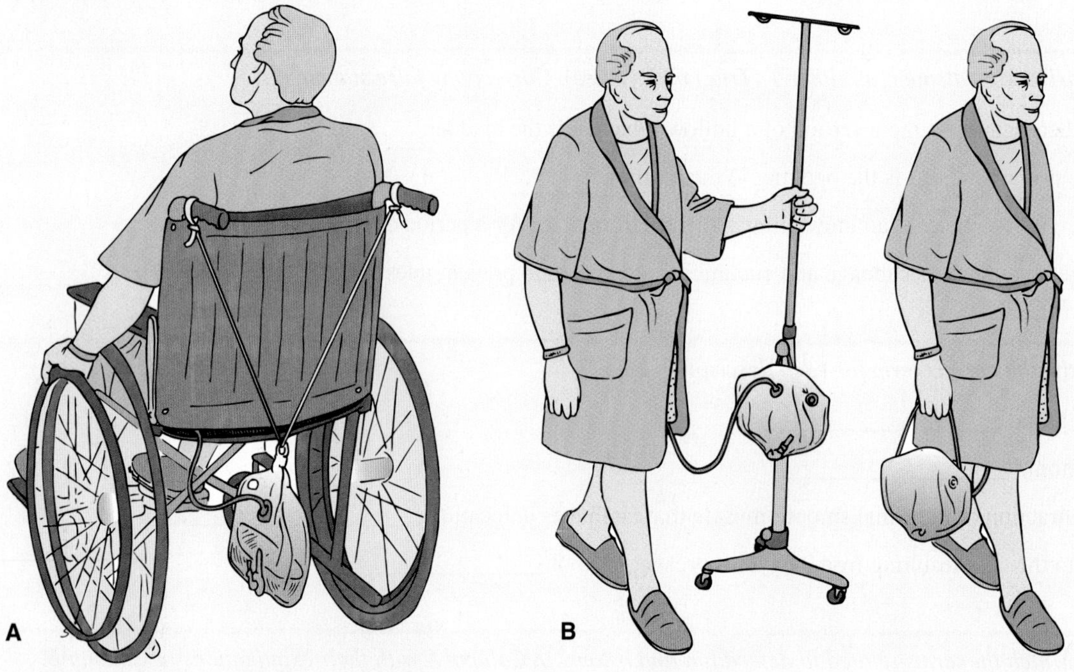

1. Identify what is shown in the figures.
2. Explain the techniques in the figures.

Activity G: *A catheter is removed when it needs to be replaced or when its use can be discontinued. Write in the boxes provided below the correct sequence for removing a Foley catheter.*

1. Empty the balloon by aspirating the fluid with a syringe.
2. Measure the volume of each voiding for the next 8 to 10 hours.
3. Wash hands and put on clean gloves.
4. Inspect the catheter and discard it, if it appears to be intact.
5. Gently pull the catheter to the point where it exits from the meatus.
6. Clean the urinary meatus.

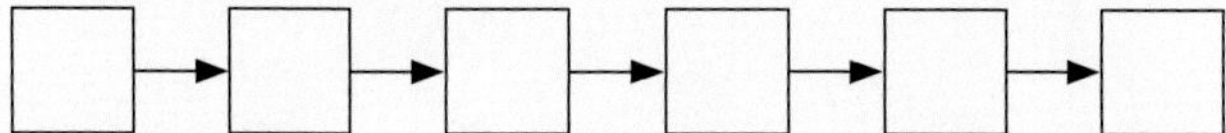

Activity H: *Answer the following questions.*

1. What are the four physical characteristics of urine?

2. What are the uses of a urinary catheter?

3. What are the two components of a bowel elimination assessment?

4. What are the various signs and symptoms of constipation?

5. What are the potential problems of using condom catheters?

Section II: Applying Your Knowledge

Activity I: *Give rationales for the following questions.*

1. Why is the first voided specimen of the day preferred as a urine sample?

2. Why is urination during the night considered unusual?

3. Why is it important for the nurse to be cautious when administering large-volume enemas to clients?

4. Why is tap water used when administering an enema?

Activity J: *Answer the following questions focusing on nursing roles and responsibilities.*

1. A nurse is caring for a client with urinary incontinence. What nursing diagnoses might be applicable in this situation?

2. A middle-aged client has an indwelling retention catheter. What nursing care is appropriate for this client?

3. A nurse is caring for a client with a colostomy. What are the steps in performing a colostomy irrigation?

4. A nurse is caring for a client with constipation.
   a. What are two interventions used to promote bowel elimination for a client with constipation?

   b. How should the nurse administer a commercially prepared, disposable container of hypertonic enema solution?

Activity K: *Consider the following questions. Discuss them with your instructor or peers.*

1. A nurse is caring for an elderly client with urinary incontinence who has an indwelling catheter.
   a. What possible problems could occur in this client?
   b. Describe the appropriate nursing care for this client.
2. A middle-aged client who is scheduled to undergo a colostomy is concerned about how the surgery and its outcomes will affect his everyday life.
   a. How can the nurse prepare the client physically and emotionally for managing the ostomy independently?
   b. How can the nurse prepare the family who may need to assist with the care of the client with an ostomy after discharge?

Section III: Getting Ready for NCLEX

Activity L: *Answer the following questions.*

1. A client who is paralyzed from the waist down is experiencing spontaneous loss of urine. How should the nurse document this client's condition?
   a. Reflex incontinence
   b. Stress incontinence
   c. Functional incontinence
   d. Urge incontinence
2. A nurse is teaching a client to perform a Credé's maneuver as part of urinary continence training. Which of the following instructions should the nurse tell the client regarding this maneuver?
   a. Massage or tap the skin lightly above the pubic area.
   b. Bend forward and apply hand pressure over the bladder.
   c. Relax the urinary sphincter in response to physical stimulation.
   d. Contract and relax the muscles alternately for 10 seconds.
3. An elderly client with a musculoskeletal disorder cannot elevate the hips. The nurse is using a fracture pan to collect the client's urine and stool. What interventions should the nurse follow when using a nonmetallic fracture pan? Select all that apply.
   a. Warm the bedpan with warm running water.
   b. Palpate the client's lower abdomen.
   c. Place soiled tissue in the fracture pan.
   d. Slip the fracture pan just beneath the buttocks.
   e. Raise the head of the client's bed.
4. A client at the health care facility reports a frequent desire to defecate but has been passing liquid stool in small quantities for 2 days. What interventions should the nurse follow when removing a fecal impaction? Select all that apply.
   a. Ask the client to contract the gluteal muscles.
   b. Instruct the client to breathe slowly and deeply.
   c. Place the client in the Sims' position.
   d. Use a lubricated gloved forefinger to break up the mass of stool.
   e. Provide periods of rest until the mass is removed.

5. Which of the following statements accurately describes a nursing action involved in draining accumulated urine or stool from a continent ileostomy?
   a. Keep the external end of the catheter at the level of the stoma.
   b. Leave the stoma uncovered at all times.
   c. Clean the removed catheter with cold soapy water.
   d. Expect resistance after inserting the tube approximately 2 inches.

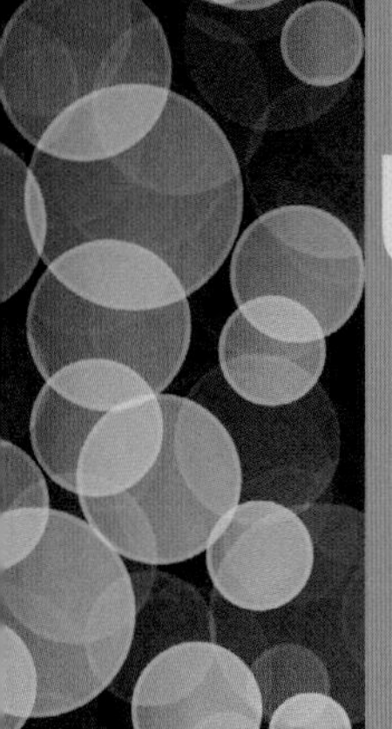

UNIT 9
Medication Administration

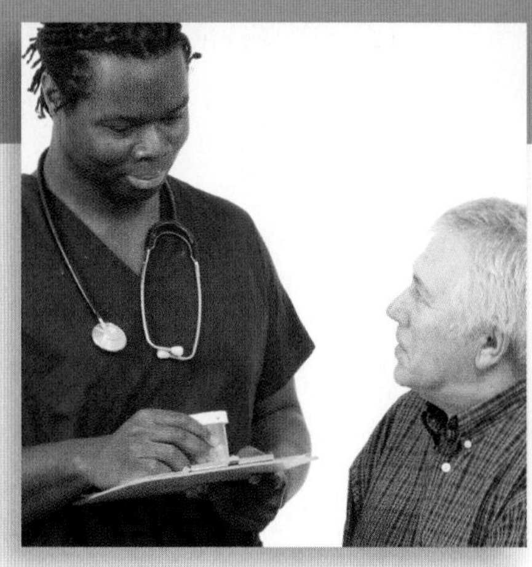

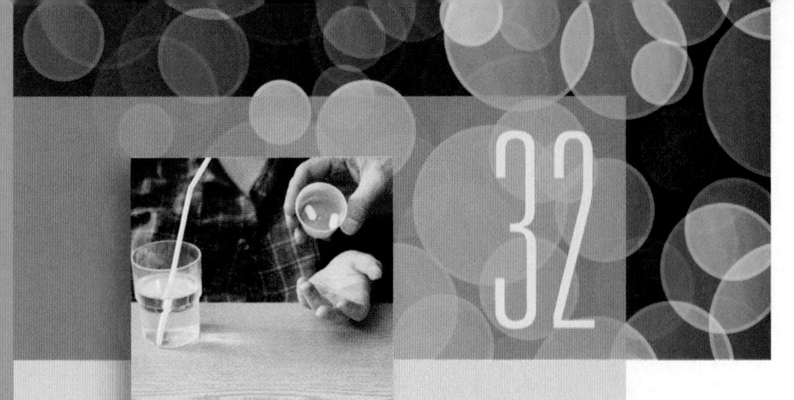

32 Oral Medications

Words To Know

barcode medication administration system
dose
drug diversion
enteric-coated tablet
generic name
individual supply
medication administration record
medication order
medications
oral route
over-the-counter medication
polypharmacy
route of administration
scored tablet
stock supply
sustained release
trade name
unit dose supply
xerostomia

Learning Objectives

On completion of this chapter, the reader should be able to:

1. Define the term *medication*.
2. Name seven components of a drug order.
3. Explain the difference between trade and generic drug names.
4. Name four common routes for administration.
5. Describe the oral route and two general forms of medication administered this way.
6. Explain the purpose of a medication record.
7. Name three ways that drugs are supplied.
8. Discuss two nursing responsibilities that apply to the administration of narcotics.
9. Name the five rights of medication administration.
10. Give the formula for calculating a drug dose.
11. Discuss at least one guideline that applies to the safe administration of medications.
12. Discuss one point to stress when teaching clients about taking medications.
13. Explain the circumstances involved in giving oral medications by an enteral tube and one commonly associated problem.
14. Describe three appropriate actions in the event of a medication error.

One of the nurse's most important responsibilities is the administration of **medications** (chemical substances that change body function). This chapter emphasizes the safe preparation and administration of medications, particularly those given by the oral route. This chapter uses the terms *medications* and *drugs* synonymously; information on specific drugs can be found in pharmacology texts or in drug reference manuals.

MEDICATION ORDERS

A **medication order** lists the drug name and directions for its administration. Usually, physicians or dentists write a medication order. Other medical personnel, such as a physician's assistant or an advanced practice nurse, also can write medication orders if legally designated to do so by state statutes. Medication orders written on the client's medical record are used here for the purposes of discussion.

Components of a Medication Order

All medication orders must have seven components:

1. The client's name
2. The date and time the order is written
3. The drug name
4. The dose to be administered
5. The route of administration
6. The frequency of administration
7. The signature of the person ordering the drug

If any one of these components is absent, the nurse must withhold the drug until he or she has obtained the missing information. Medication errors are serious. *Nurses never implement a questionable medication order until after consulting with the person who has written the order.*

Drug Name

Each drug has a **trade name** (the name by which a pharmaceutical company identifies its drug). A trade name is sometimes called a brand or proprietary name. A drug's trade name is generally capitalized and followed by an R within a circle, as in ®.

Drugs also have a **generic name** (a chemical name not protected by a company's trademark), which is written in lowercase letters. For example, Demerol® is a trade name used by Winthrop Pharmaceuticals for the generically named drug meperidine hydrochloride.

The Joint Commission (2010) cautions health care providers such as physicians, nurses, and pharmacists that there are many look-alike and sound-alike drug names. Everyone involved in prescribing and administering medications should refer to a list that identifies commonly confused drug names. The list should be updated at least yearly. Knowing the purpose for the drug's administration also may help in ensuring that the appropriate drug has been prescribed.

Drug Dose

The **dose** means the amount of drug to administer and is prescribed using the metric system. Some drugs are also prescribed in units, milliunits, international units, and milliequivalents (mEq), a unique measurement primarily used for chemical compounds such as potassium chloride.

For the purposes of safety, The Joint Commission (2010) mandates that apothecary measurements, an antiquated system of drug dosing, is now subject to exclusion. This safety measure was brought about because apothecary abbreviations were frequently misread, misinterpreted, and confused with metric-system abbreviations. Refer to Table 32-1 for "Do Not Use" abbreviations in prescribed medications that The Joint Commission has established.

For home use, drug dosages are converted to household measurements that are more easily interpreted by nonprofessionals.

Route of Administration

The **route of administration** means how the drug is given, which may be by an oral, topical, inhalant, or parenteral route (Table 32-2). Topical and inhalant routes of administration are discussed in Chapter 33; parenteral administration is described in Chapters 34 and 35.

TABLE 32-1 The Joint Commission's Official "Do Not Use" List of Abbreviations

DO NOT USE	POTENTIAL PROBLEM	USE INSTEAD
U (unit)	Mistaken for "0" (zero), the number "4" (four), or "cc" (see below)	Write "unit"
IU (International Unit)	Mistaken for IV (intravenous) or the number 10 (ten)	Write "International Unit"
Q.D., QD, q.d., qd (daily)	Mistaken for each other	Write "daily"
Q.O.D., QOD, q.o.d, qod (every other day)	Period after the Q mistaken for "I" and the "O" mistaken for "I"	Write "every other day"
Trailing zero (X.0 mg) in any medication order or medication-related documentation	Decimal point is missed	Write X mg
Lack of leading zero (.X mg)	Decimal point is missed	Write 0.X mg
MS	Can mean morphine sulfate or magnesium sulfate	Write "morphine sulfate" or "magnesium sulfate"
For possible future inclusion in the Official "Do Not Use" List		
> (greater than)	Misinterpreted as the number "7" (seven) or the letter "L"	Write "greater than"
< (less than)	Confused with "greater than"	Write "less than"
Abbreviations for drug names	Misinterpreted because of similar abbreviations for multiple drugs	Write drug names in full
Apothecary units	Unfamiliar to many practitioners; confused with metric units	Use metric units
@	Mistaken for the number "2" (two)	Write "at"
cc (cubic centimeter)	Mistaken for U (units) when poorly written	Write "mL" or "milliliters"
µg (microgram)	Mistaken for mg (milligrams), resulting in 1,000-fold overdose	Write "mcg" or "micrograms"

Adapted from The Official "Do Not Use" List (2010). Available at http://www.jointcommission.org/

TABLE 32-2 Routes of Drug Administration

ROUTE	METHOD OF ADMINISTRATION
Oral	Swallowing Instillation through an enteral tube
Topical	Application to skin or mucous membrane
Inhalant	Aerosol
Parenteral	Injection

The **oral route** (the administration of drugs by swallowing or instillation through an enteral tube) facilitates drug absorption through the gastrointestinal tract. It is the most common route for medication administration because it is safer, more economical, and more comfortable than others. Medications administered by the oral route come in both solid and liquid forms.

Solid medications include tablets and capsules. A **scored tablet** (a solid drug manufactured with a groove in the center) is convenient when only part of a tablet is needed. **Enteric-coated tablets** (a solid drug covered with a substance that dissolves beyond the stomach) are manufactured for drugs that cause irritation of the stomach. Enteric-coated tablets are never cut, crushed, or chewed because when the integrity of the coating is impaired, the drug dissolves prematurely in gastric secretions. Some capsules also contain beads or pellets of drugs for **sustained release** (a drug that dissolves at timed intervals). Sustained release capsules are never crushed: doing so affects the rate of drug absorption.

Liquid forms of oral drugs include syrups, elixirs, and suspensions. Nurses measure and administer liquid medications in calibrated cups, droppers, or syringes, or with a dosing spoon (Fig. 32-1).

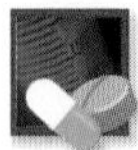

Pharmacologic Considerations

- **Polypharmacy** (the administration of multiple medications to the same person) increases the risk for drug interactions and adverse medication reactions. Older people taking more than one medication are more likely to develop mental changes as an early and common sign of adverse effects. In fact, medications are the most common physiologic cause of mental changes in older adults. Therefore, any change in an older client's mental status must be reported, with an evaluation of the potential causative factors.
- Diminished kidney and liver function increases the concentration of many drugs. Increased proportions of body water and fat and decreased proportion of lean tissue affect the concentration of some medications. Decreased blood albumin levels increase the active drug components for protein-bound medications. Decreased gastric acidity reduces or delays absorption of some drugs. Urinary changes influence medications excreted through the kidneys. Information regarding the metabolism of each medication should be considered for anyone with decreased renal, hepatic, gastrointestinal, or circulatory function.

Frequency of Administration

The frequency of drug administration refers to how often and how regularly the medication is to be given. Frequency of administration is written using standard abbreviations of Latin origin. Some common examples include the following:

- Stat—immediately
- b.i.d.—twice a day
- t.i.d.—three times a day
- q.i.d.—four times a day
- q.h.—hourly
- q4h—every 4 hours
- p.r.n.—as needed

Chapter 9 and Appendix B list other common abbreviations.

When the medication order is implemented, drug administration is scheduled according to the prescribed frequency. The health agency sets a predetermined timetable for drug administrations; hours of administration may vary among agencies. For example, if a physician orders a q.i.d. (four times a day) administration of a medication, it may be scheduled for administration at 8 a.m., noon, 4 p.m., and 8 p.m.; at 10 a.m., 2 p.m., 6 p.m., and 10 p.m.; or at 6 a.m., noon, 6 p.m., and midnight.

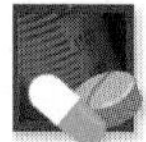

Pharmacologic Considerations

- The prescribing health care provider may be able to simplify a complex medication regimen by prescribing a longer-acting drug to decrease the frequency of administration or a medication combination to decrease the number of pills the client must take at one time.

Verbal and Telephone Orders

Verbal orders are instructions for client care that are given during face-to-face conversations. Telephone orders are obtained from a physician during a telephone conversation.

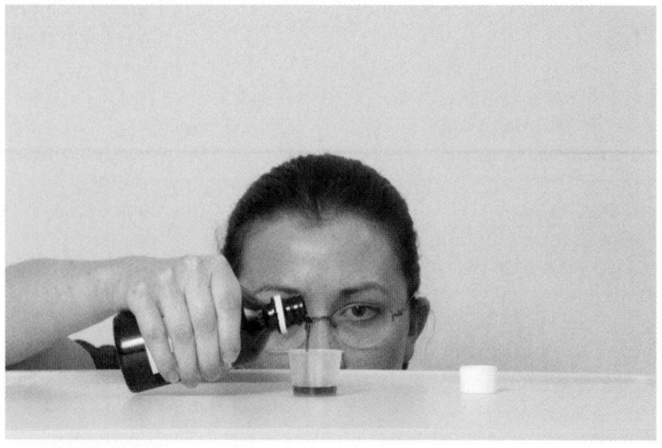

FIGURE 32-1 Measuring liquid medication with a calibrated cup held at eye level. (Photo by B. Proud.)

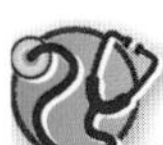

NURSING GUIDELINES 32-1

Taking Telephone Orders

- Have a second nurse listen simultaneously on an extension. *A second nurse serves as a witness to the communication.*
- Record the drug order directly on the client's medical record. *A written recording avoids errors in memory.*
- Repeat the written information back to the prescriber. *Repetition clarifies understanding.*
- Make sure the order includes the essential components. *Doing so complies with standards for care.*
- Clarify any drug names that sound similar, such as Celebrex and Cerebrex, or Nicobid and Nitro-Bid. *Checking avoids medication errors.*
- Spell or repeat numbers that could be misinterpreted, such as 15 (one, five) and 50 (five, zero). *This step avoids medication errors.*
- Use the abbreviation "T.O." at the end of the order. *This abbreviation indicates the order is a telephone order.*
- Write the prescriber's name and cosign with your name and title. *These steps comply with legal standards and demonstrate accountability for the communication.*

Both types of orders are more likely to result in misinterpretation than are written orders. If a prescriber is physically present, it is appropriate to ask tactfully that the order be handwritten. When obtaining phone orders, it is important to repeat the dosages of drugs and to spell drug names for confirmation of accuracy. Some nurses ask a second nurse to listen to a telephone order on an extension (see Nursing Guidelines 32-1). The person who prescribed the medication must sign the verbal or telephone order within 48 hours or according to the agency's policy.

Documentation in the Medication Administration Record

Once the nurse has obtained the medication order, he or she transcribes it to the **medication administration record** (MAR; agency form used to document drug administration). Use of the MAR ensures timely and safe medication administration. Some agencies use a form on which nurses transcribe the drug order by hand; others use a computer-generated form (Fig. 32-2). Regardless of the type, all MARs provide a space for documenting when a drug is given, along with a place for the signature, title, and initials of each nurse who administers a medication. The current MAR is usually kept separate from the client's medical record, but it eventually becomes a permanent part of it.

METHODS OF SUPPLYING MEDICATIONS

After transcribing the medication order to the MAR, the nurse requests the drug from the pharmacy with either a paper or a facsimile (fax) transmission request. Drugs are supplied, or dispensed, in three major ways. An **individual supply** is a container with enough of the prescribed drug for several days or weeks, which is common in long-term care facilities such as nursing homes (Fig. 32-3). A **unit dose supply** (a self-contained packet that holds one tablet or capsule) is most common in acute care hospitals that stock drugs for individual clients several times in 1 day (Fig. 32-4). A **stock supply** (stored drugs) remains on the nursing unit for use in an emergency so that a nurse can give a drug without delay.

Some facilities use automated medication-dispensing systems (Fig. 32-5). These systems usually contain frequently used medications for that unit, any as-needed (p.r.n.) medications, controlled drugs, and emergency medications. The nurse accesses the system by using a personal password and then selects the appropriate choice from a computerized menu. This type of system automatically keeps a record of dispensed medications and records the password, user name, and title. To avoid **drug diversion**—a term used by the U.S. Drug Enforcement Administration (DEA) when referring to the theft or possession of drugs—usually controlled substances, prescribed for someone else, the user's password should never be shared with anyone.

Storing Medications

Each health agency has one area for storing drugs. Some agencies keep medications in a mobile cart; others store them in a medication room. Each client has a separate drawer or cubicle to hold his or her prescribed medications. Regardless of their location, the supply of medications remains locked until the drugs are administered.

Accounting for Narcotics

Narcotics are controlled substances, meaning that federal laws regulate their possession and administration. Health agencies keep narcotics in a double-locked drawer, a box, a room in the nursing unit, or in an automated medication dispensing system. Because narcotics usually are delivered by stock supply, nurses are responsible for an accurate account of their use. They keep a record of each narcotic used from the stock supply. Any controlled substance that is wasted in whole or in part must be co-signed by a witness.

Nurses count narcotics regularly, usually at each change of shift. One nurse counts the number in the supply, while another checks the record of their administration or amounts that have been wasted. Both counts must agree with inconsistencies accounted for as soon as possible.

MEDICATION ADMINISTRATION

Safety is the main concern in medication administration. Taking various precautions before, during, and after

MEDICATION ADMINISTRATION RECORD

PAGE 1

SHIFT	FULL NAME/TITLE	INITIAL
0701 - 1500		
0701 - 1500		
0701 - 1500		
1501 - 2300		
1501 - 2300		
1501 - 2300		
2301 - 0700		
2301 - 0700		

01/02/11 00010 PHARMACY/CHART
TESTDP DON'T DISC AGE: 041
00000000107 DEMPSEY. JAMES
ACCT #: 000000108 ADMIT DATE 12/31/10
DIAG.: ASTHMA-EXACERBATED BY PNEUMONIA
ALL: CODEINE TETRACYCLINE

	1501 01/02/11 THRU 1500 DATE 01/03/11	1501 - 2300 / 0701 - 1500	2301 - 0700 / 1501 - 2300	0701 - 1500 / 2301 - 0700	COMMENTS
1	(01016) 01/01/11 1800 SOLU-CORTEF 100 MG/2ML-HYDROCORT DOSE: 100 MG. IP Q6H IP RATE = 500 MG. OVER 1 MIN. ABBOTT	1800	0000 0600	1200	
2	(03090) 12/31/10 0900 ACETAMINOPHEN EXTRA ST.CAP DOSE: 1 PO DAILY TYLENOL			0900	
3	(04841) 01/01/11 0900 TENORMIN TAB. 50 MG. DOSE: 50 MG. PO DAILY			0900	
4	(03096) 01/01/11 0900 LANOXIN (DIGOXIN) TAB. 0.25 MG. DOSE: 0.25 MG. PO DAILY			0900	
5	(00543) 01/01/11 1800 BRETHINE AMP. 1 MG./ML. 1 ML. DOSE: 0.25MG SC Q6H (TERBUTALINE)	1800	0000 0600	1200	
6					
7					
8					
9					
10					
11					
12					
13					

TESTDP DON'T DIS 00000000107 DEMPSEY. JAMES THRU 1500 01/03/11

FIGURE 32-2 A computer-generated medication administration record (MAR).

each administration reduces the potential for medication errors. Some precautions include ensuring the five rights of medication administration, calculating drug dosages accurately, preparing medications carefully, and recording their administration.

Applying the Five Rights

To safeguard against medication errors, nurses follow the five rights of medication administration (Fig. 32-6). Some nurses have added a sixth right, the right to refuse. Every rational adult client has the right to refuse medication. If this

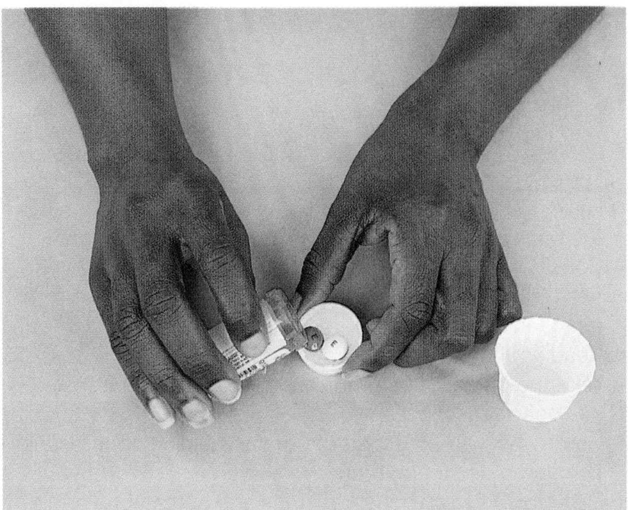

FIGURE 32-3 Medication from an individual supply. (Photo by B. Proud.)

happens, the nurse identifies the reason why he or she did not administer the drug, circles the scheduled time on the MAR, and reports the situation to the prescriber.

In an effort to reduce medication errors, some hospitals are using a **barcode medication administration system**, a point of care software that verifies the name of the medication, the administration time, the dosage, the drug form, and the client for whom the drug is prescribed; that is, the five rights to ensure accuracy by scanning a barcode on the drug's unopened package and identification band on the client. The software also documents the name and title of the nurse who administers the medication by scanning a barcode on the nurse's employee badge.

Calculating Dosages

One of the major nursing responsibilities, and one of the five rights, is preparing the dose accurately. Preparing an accurate dose sometimes requires the nurse to convert doses into metric and household equivalents. Once the prescribed and supplied amounts are in the same measurements and system of measurement, the quantity for administration can be easily calculated using a standard formula (Box 32-1) (see Nursing Guidelines 32-2).

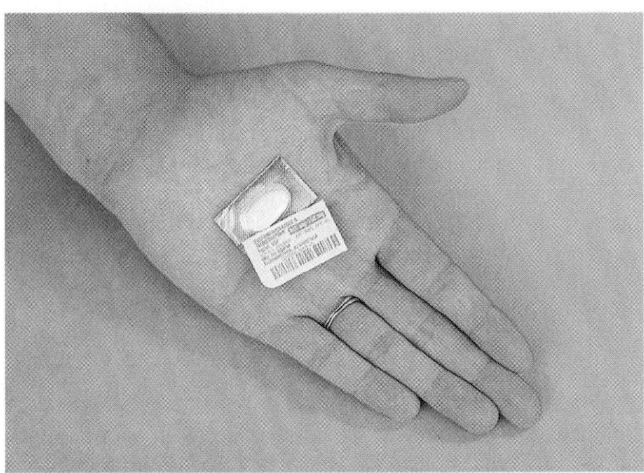

FIGURE 32-4 Unit dose medications. (Photo by B. Proud.)

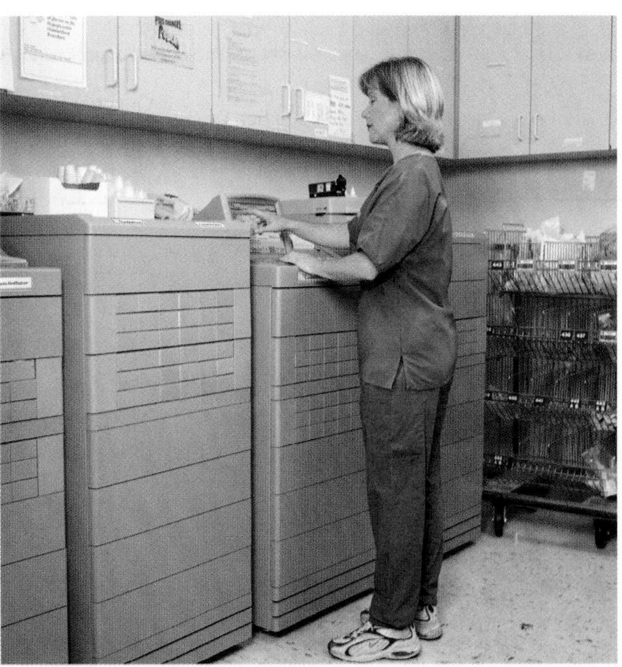

FIGURE 32-5 An automated medication dispensing system.

Administering Oral Medications

Nurses prepare and bring oral medications to the client in a paper or a plastic cup (Skill 32-1). The nurse administers only those medications that he or she has personally prepared; *never administer medications prepared by another nurse.* Once at the bedside, it is also important for the nurse to remain with the client while he or she takes medications.

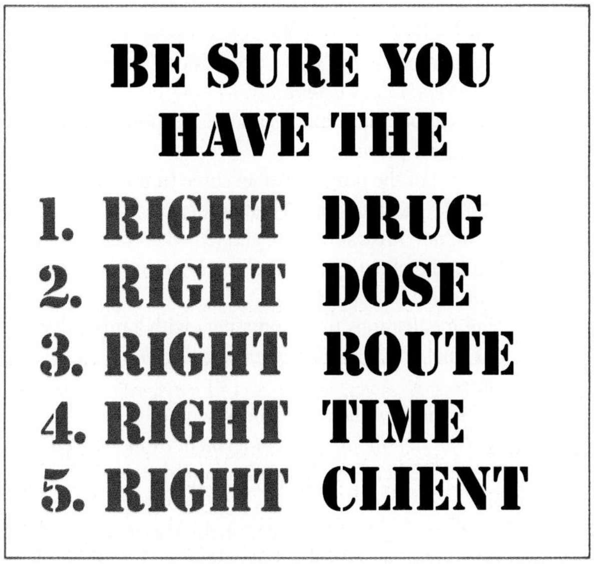

BE SURE YOU HAVE THE

1. **RIGHT DRUG**
2. **RIGHT DOSE**
3. **RIGHT ROUTE**
4. **RIGHT TIME**
5. **RIGHT CLIENT**

FIGURE 32-6 The five rights of medication administration.

BOX 32-1 Drug Calculation Formula

$$\frac{D}{H} \times Q = \frac{\text{Desired dose}}{\text{Dose on hand (supplied dose)}} \times \text{Quantity}$$
$$= \text{Amount to administer}$$

Example

Drug order: Tetracycline 500 mg (desired dose) by mouth q.i.d.
Dose supplied: 250 mg (*dose on hand*) per 5 mL (*quantity*)

$$\text{Calculation: } \frac{500 \text{ mg}}{250 \text{ mg}} \times 5 \text{ mL} = 10 \text{ mL}$$

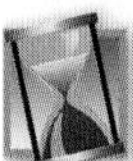

Gerontologic Considerations

■ Older people who have had cerebrovascular accidents (or strokes) or who are experiencing middle-to-late stages of dementia may have impaired swallowing. Speech therapists are helpful in evaluating swallowing difficulties (dysphagia) and recommending safe and effective methods of administering oral medications.

■ Some older adults have diminished salivary gland secretions and develop **xerostomia** (dry mouth). Offering a sip of water before administering medications or mixing oral medications with some soft food (such as applesauce) may prevent medication from adhering to the tongue and, thus, facilitate administration.

If a client is not on the unit at the time of medication administration, the nurse returns the medications to the medication cart or room. Leaving medications unattended may result in their loss or accidental ingestion by someone else.

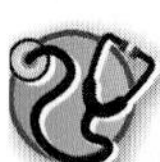

NURSING GUIDELINES 32-2

Preparing Medications Safely

- Prepare medications under well-lit conditions. *Light improves the ability to read labels accurately.*
- Work alone without interruptions and distractions. *This promotes concentration.*
- Check the label of the drug container three times: (1) when reaching for the medication, (2) just before placing the medication into an administration cup, and (3) when returning the medication to the client's drawer. *Checking ensures attention to important information.*
- Avoid using medications from containers with a missing or obliterated label. *This eliminates speculating on the drug name or dose.*
- Return medications with dubious or obscured labels to the pharmacy. *This step facilitates replacement or new labeling.*
- Never transfer medications from one container to another. *Such transfers could lead to mismatching contents.*
- Check the expiration dates on liquid medications. *Doing so ensures administration at desired potency.*
- Inspect the medication and reject any that appear to be decomposing. *These steps promote appropriate absorption.*

Client and Family Teaching 32-1
Taking Medications

The nurse teaches the client and the family as follows:

- Inform the prescriber of all other drugs that you are currently taking.
- Have prescriptions filled at the same pharmacy so that the pharmacist can spot any potential drug interactions.
- Consider asking for a new prescription to be partially filled. This provides an opportunity to evaluate the drug's effect and side effects before purchasing the full amount.
- Read and follow the label directions carefully.
- Take the prescription medication for the full time that it has been prescribed.
- Check with the prescriber before combining nonprescription and prescription drugs.
- Dispose of old prescription drugs and outdated over-the-counter medications; they tend to disintegrate or change in potency.
- Consult with the prescriber if a drug does not relieve symptoms or causes additional discomfort.
- Ask the prescriber or pharmacist whether it is appropriate to take specific medications with food or on an empty stomach.
- Drink a liberal amount of water or other fluids each day to assist with the appropriate absorption and elimination of drugs.
- Do not take drugs prescribed for someone else, even if your symptoms are similar.
- Wear a Medic-Alert tag if you are taking prescription drugs on a regular and long-term basis.
- Use a pill organizer if you have trouble remembering whether you took a medication.

Many opportunities exist for teaching when administering medications. Teaching is especially important before discharge because the client often receives prescriptions for oral medications. Providing health teaching helps to ensure that clients administer their own medications safely and remain compliant. Compliance means that the client follows instructions for medication administration. Even clients who purchase **over-the-counter medications** (nonprescription drugs) may benefit from instruction (see Client and Family Teaching 32-1).

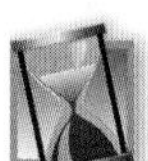

Gerontologic Considerations

■ If an older person has difficulty comprehending information about medication routines, include a second responsible person in the discharge instructions to ensure client safety. A referral for skilled nursing visits is appropriate for homebound older adults who need additional instructions about medication routines after discharge.

■ Older people should be taught to carry in their wallet or purse a current list of all their medications, dosages, times of administration, and names of the prescribing provider. Should an older client be found wandering or unconscious, an evaluation for possible medication adverse effects can happen more quickly if he or she has such information readily available.

■ Older people should use eyeglasses or hearing aids as needed to optimize their learning conditions. Other important considerations for the teaching–learning environment are adequate nonglare lighting and little, if any, background noise.

■ An evaluation of comprehension may be best done by having the older person repeat instructions after they are provided. Reinforce verbal instructions with written instructions at the older person's reading level. A copier may be used to enlarge instructions for clients with visual impairments. Written instructions are particularly important for clients with hearing impairments. They provide a reference for older adults with difficulty recalling or comprehending information. In addition, written instructions serve as a point of reference for caregivers who may assist with medication administration.

■ Older adults who have problems with manual dexterity or strength may request that pharmacists use nonchild-proof caps on their prescription containers.

■ Clients with visual impairments may benefit from methods of identifying their medication containers other than reading labels. Suggestions include using rubber bands or textured materials on certain containers or using bright colors to mark the labels. Many simple-to-use medication management systems, sometimes called pill organizers, are available. Often, a family member is helpful in setting up weekly medication management systems. For example, a family member may set out the medications in specially designed containers weekly. This method enables others to monitor patterns and the adherence to the medication regimen and may be especially helpful when working with older people experiencing memory impairments.

■ Older adults with insurance coverage for prescription payments may find it easier and more economical to have prescriptions filled every 3 months. It may also be more economical to purchase prescriptions by mail or Internet if the insurance provider approves this option.

■ Encourage older adults to question the primary health care provider about prescribing generic forms of medication for cost savings.

Stop, Think, and Respond Box 32-1

What actions are appropriate if a client cannot swallow medications prescribed by the oral route?

Administering Oral Medications by Enteral Tube

When a client cannot swallow oral medications, they can be instilled by enteral tube (Skill 32-2). Because the lumen of a tube is smaller than the esophagus, special techniques may be required to avoid obstruction (see Nursing Guidelines 32-3).

Nurses use slightly different techniques for administering medications through an enteral tube than they do for tubes used for decompression or nourishment (see Chap. 29). They may give medications through gastric tubes used for decompression (eg, suctioning; see Chap. 29). After administering the drug, the nurse clamps or plugs the tube for at least 30 minutes to prevent removing the drug before it leaves the stomach.

Nurses can give medications while a client is receiving tube feedings, but they instill the medications separately—that is, they do not add the medications to the formula. This is done for two reasons. First, some drugs may physically interact with the components in the formula, causing it to curdle or otherwise change its consistency. Also, a slow infusion would alter the rate of absorption of the drug.

Documentation

If the nurse is not using a barcode medication system that documents drug administration immediately and automatically, the nurse should document medication administration manually on the MAR, the client's chart, or both as soon as possible (Fig. 32-7). Timely documentation prevents medication errors: if the nurse does not record the dose, another nurse may assume that the client has not received the medication and may give a second dose.

If a nurse withholds a medication, he or she documents its omission according to agency policy. A common method of such documentation is to circle the time of administration and initial the entry. The nurse may document the reason for the omission in a comment section on the MAR or elsewhere in the client's medical record.

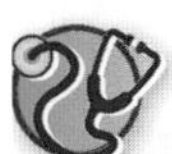

NURSING GUIDELINES 32-3

Preparing Medications for Enteral Tube Administration

- Use the liquid form of the drug whenever possible. *It promotes tube patency.*
- Add 15–60 mL of water to thick liquid medications. *Water dilutes the medication and facilitates instillation.*
- Pulverize tablets except those that are enteric coated. *Pulverizing creates small granules that may instill more readily.*
- Open the shell of a capsule to release the powdered drug. *This step facilitates mixing into a liquid form.*
- Avoid crushing sustained-release pellets. *Keeping them whole ensures their sequential rate of absorption.*
- Mix each drug separately with at least 15–30 mL of water. *Water provides a medium and dilute volume for administration.*
- Use warm water when mixing powdered drugs. *It promotes dissolving the solid form.*
- Pierce the end of a sealed gelatin capsule and squeeze out the liquid medication, or aspirate it with a needle and syringe. *These measures facilitate access to the medication.*
- As an alternative, soak a soft gelatin capsule in 15–30 mL of warm water for approximately 1 hour. *Soaking dissolves the gelatin seal.*
- Avoid administering bulk-forming laxatives through an enteral tube. *Such laxatives could obstruct the tube.*
- Interrupt a tube feeding for 15–30 minutes before and after administration of a drug that should be given on an empty stomach. *Doing so facilitates the drug's therapeutic action or its absorption.*
- Clamp a nasogastric tube that is being used to suction gastric secretions for 30 minutes after administering medication. *Keeping the tubing temporarily clamped allows time for the medication to move beyond the stomach and be absorbed.*

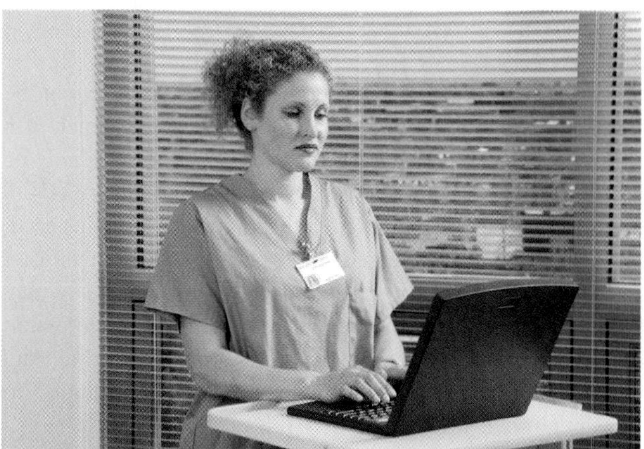

FIGURE 32-7 Documentation of the medication administration is an important nursing requirement. (Photo by B. Proud.)

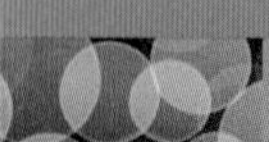

Stop, Think, and Respond Box 32-2

Give reasons to administer medications through a gastric or intestinal tube rather than having the client swallow them.

Medication Errors

Medication errors happen too often. When errors occur, nurses have an ethical and legal responsibility to report them to maintain the client's safety.

As soon as he or she recognizes an error, the nurse checks the client's condition and reports the mistake to the prescriber and the supervising nurse immediately. Health care agencies have a form for reporting medication errors called an incident sheet, or accident sheet (see Chap. 3). The incident sheet is neither a part of the client's permanent record nor does the nurse make any reference in the chart to the fact that he or she has completed an incident sheet.

NURSING IMPLICATIONS

Whenever nursing care involves the administration of medications, one or more of the following nursing diagnoses may be applicable:

- Deficient Knowledge; Readiness for Enhanced Knowledge
- Risk for Aspiration
- Ineffective Therapeutic Regimen Management
- Ineffective Self-Help Management
- Noncompliance

Nursing Care Plan 32-1 shows how nurses can follow the steps in the nursing process to manage the care of a client with the nursing diagnosis of Noncompliance, defined by NANDA-I (2012, p. 400) as "the person's or caregiver's behavior is fully or partially nonadherent and may lead to clinically ineffective or partially ineffective outcomes."

NURSING CARE PLAN 32-1 Noncompliance

Assessment

- Check whether the client is returning for scheduled appointments with the prescribing physician or health care provider.
- Assess the current status of the client's health problem to determine whether the response to the prescribed plan of care is that which is expected.
- Ask to examine the client's containers of medications.
- Review the labels attached to prescription medications.
- Have the client identify the number of pills or capsules per dose, the frequency of self-administration, and time of the last dose.
- Determine by the dates on the containers and the number of medications in the container(s) whether the client is using or partially using medication.
- Encourage the client to relate problems encountered with self-administration of medications such as intolerance of side effects, an inability to pay for refills, a belief that the medication is ineffective, difficulty remembering the dosing schedule, and trouble opening the containers.

Nursing Diagnosis. **Noncompliance** related to an inaccurate belief regarding the use and benefit of prescribed medication therapy as manifested by pulse rate of 94 at rest, BP of 178/94 in R arm while sitting, dyspnea following coronary bypass surgery, and the statement, "I didn't get my prescriptions filled last week. I wasn't having any chest pain and I figured the surgery fixed my heart."

Expected Outcome. The client will (1) explain the purpose of prescribed medications and possible consequences if they are not taken and (2) resume taking prescribed medications within 24 hours (3/7).

Interventions	Rationales
Provide the client with the following information: • The purpose for the prescribed beta-blocker and diuretic medications is to reduce the work of the heart. • The diuretic helps to lower blood pressure, so the heart does not have to pump as much circulating blood and can eject the blood from the heart more easily. • Easing the work of the heart reduces the potential for recurring chest pain, a subsequent myocardial infarction (heart attack), or congestive heart failure.	Health teaching helps clarify the rationale for medication therapy and promotes compliance.

(continued)

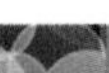

NURSING CARE PLAN 32-1 Noncompliance (continued)

Interventions	Rationales
Have the client rephrase explanations for drug therapy in his own words.	Rephrasing provides evidence that the client has understood the nurse's explanation.
Note the client's level of understanding.	Doing so indicates whether or not the nurse needs to clarify misinformation.
Acknowledge when the client's explanation is accurate or re-explain information that continues to be misunderstood.	These measures reinforce learning.
Go over the schedule of medication administration with the client.	Reviewing the schedule helps the client to plan a routine for self-administration.
Suggest that the client discuss any deviations in medication schedule or dosage with the physician.	This offers an alternative if the client feels a need to alter or discontinue self-administration.

Evaluation of Expected Outcomes

- The client correctly paraphrased information regarding drug therapy.
- The client states, "I know people take nitroglycerin for heart problems, but I didn't know how important these other drugs are. I'd rather take some pills than to have to go back to the hospital again."
- The client plans to have prescriptions filled before returning home following the office visit.
- The client indicates that he will take one beta-blocker each morning if his heart rate is at least 60 beats per minute and one diuretic tablet every other day, which correlates with the dosing regimen.
- The client is scheduled for another office check-up in 1 month. He states, "I'll be sure to call if I think there's a reason I can't take my medications."

CRITICAL THINKING EXERCISES

1. The nurse is administering medications to a client. The client says, "I've never taken that little yellow pill before." What actions are appropriate next?
2. A client who lives alone says, "You have to be a genius to keep all these pills straight." How could you help this client organize her medication regimen?
3. What action(s) are appropriate if a barcode medication administration system sounds an alert to a problem during the process of administering medication to a client?
4. What response would be appropriate if a nurse of long-standing asked you to document being a witness to a wasted controlled substance medication you did not observe?

NCLEX-STYLE REVIEW QUESTIONS

1. When a nurse checks the medication administration record (MAR) and reads "diphenoxylate hydrochloride, 5 mg p.o. q.i.d.", how many times a day will he or she administer the drug?
    1. Once a day
    2. Every other day
    3. Three times a day
    4. Four times a day
2. If a physician orders 250 mg of a drug, and it is supplied in 500-mg scored tablets, which of the following nursing actions is best?
    1. Ask the pharmacist to provide 250-mg tablets instead.
    2. Consult the physician about the prescribed dose.
    3. Give the client half of the 500-mg tablet.
    4. Check whether the drug is manufactured in a smaller dose.
3. Which action is best when a nurse brings medication to a room for a client named Anna Jones, but the client in that room is not wearing an identification bracelet?
    1. The nurse asks the client, "Are you Anna Jones?"
    2. The nurse asks the client, "What is your name?"
    3. The nurse asks a nursing assistant to identify the client.
    4. The nurse asks the client, "What medications do you take?"
4. When a nurse observes that a client has difficulty swallowing a capsule of medication, which action is best?
    1. Soak the capsule in water until soft.
    2. Tell the client to chew the capsule.
    3. Empty the capsule in the client's mouth.
    4. Offer the client water before giving the capsule.
5. Which of the following techniques is incorrect when administering oral medication through a nasogastric tube used to administer a tube feeding?
    1. Crush the medication finely and mix it with 30 mL of warm water.
    2. Flush the nasogastric tube with 30 mL of water before instilling the drug.
    3. Add the liquefied medication to the bag of tube-feeding formula.
    4. Flush the nasogastric tube with 30 mL of water after instilling the drug.

SKILL 32-1 Administering Oral Medications

Suggested Action	Reason for Action
ASSESSMENT	
Compare the medication administration record (MAR) with the written medical order.	Prevents medication errors.
Review the client's drug, allergy, and medical history.	Avoids potential complications.
Consult a current drug reference concerning the drug's action, side effects, contraindications, and administration information.	Ensures appropriate administration based on a thorough knowledge base.
PLANNING	
Plan to administer medications within 30–60 min of their scheduled time.	Demonstrates a timely administration and compliance with the medical order.
Allow sufficient time to prepare the medications in a location with minimal distractions.	Promotes safe preparation of drugs.
Make sure that there is a sufficient supply of paper and plastic medication cups.	Facilitates organization and efficient time management.
Chill oily medications.	Reduces their unpleasant odor and improves palatability.
IMPLEMENTATION	
Wash your hands or perform an alcohol-based hand rub (see Chap. 10).	Removes colonizing microorganisms.
Read and compare the label on the drug with the MAR at least three times—before, during, and after preparing the drug (Fig. A).	Ensures that the *right drug* is given at the *right time* by the *right route.*
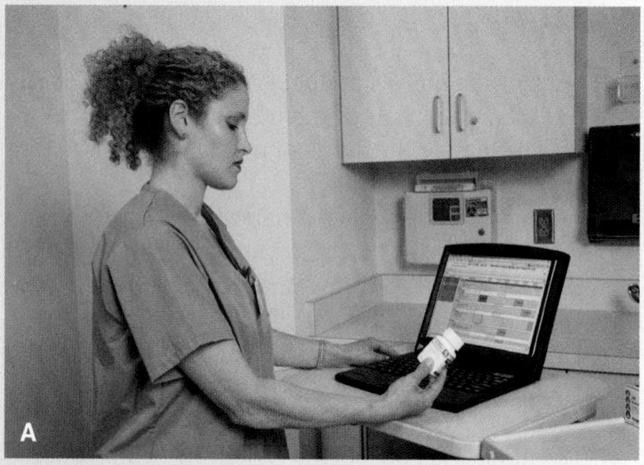 A	Comparing the drug label and the medication administration record (MAR). (Photo by B. Proud.)
Calculate doses.	Complies with the medical order and ensures that the *right dose* is given.
Place medications or unit dose packets within a paper or plastic cup without touching the medication itself.	Supports principles of asepsis.
Keep drugs that require special assessments or special administration techniques in a separate cup.	Helps identify drugs that require special nursing actions.
Pour liquids with the drug label toward the palm of the hand.	Prevents liquid from running onto the label.
Hold the cup for liquid medications at eye level when pouring.	Facilitates accurate measurement.
Prepare a supply of soft-textured food such as applesauce or pudding, according to the client's individual needs.	Facilitates the administration for clients with impaired swallowing.
Help the client to a sitting position.	Facilitates swallowing and prevents aspiration.

(continued)

Administering Oral Medications (continued)

IMPLEMENTATION (CONTINUED)

Identify the client using at least two methods, for example, checking the wristband and asking the client's name (Fig. B). — Ensures that medications are given to the *right client; complies with the National Patient Safety Goals.*

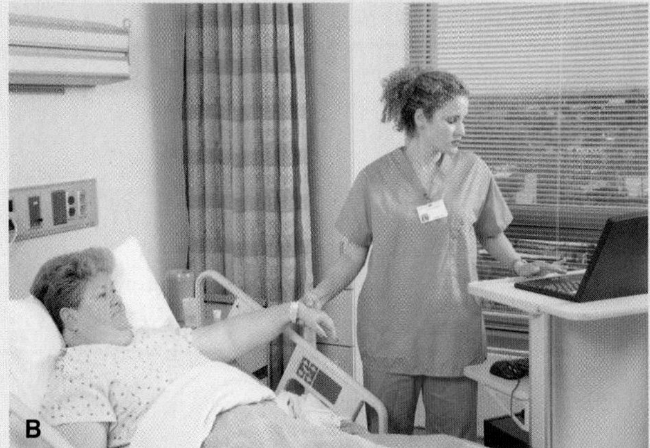

Checking the identification band. (Photo by B. Proud.)

Offer a cup of water with solid forms of oral medications (Fig. C). — Water moistens mucous membranes and prevents medication from sticking.

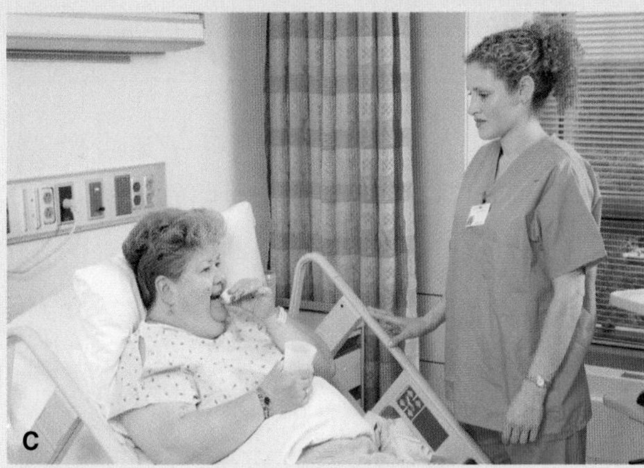

Offering the patient medication and water. (Photo by B. Proud.)

Advise the client to take medications one at a time or in amounts easily swallowed. — Prevents choking.

Encourage the client to keep his or her head in a neutral position or one of slight flexion, rather than hyperextending the neck (Fig. D). — Protects the airway.

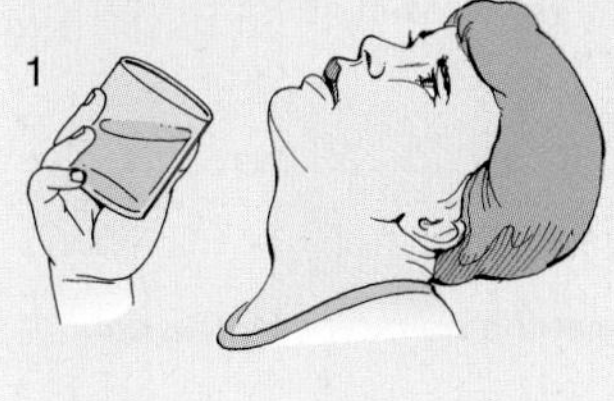

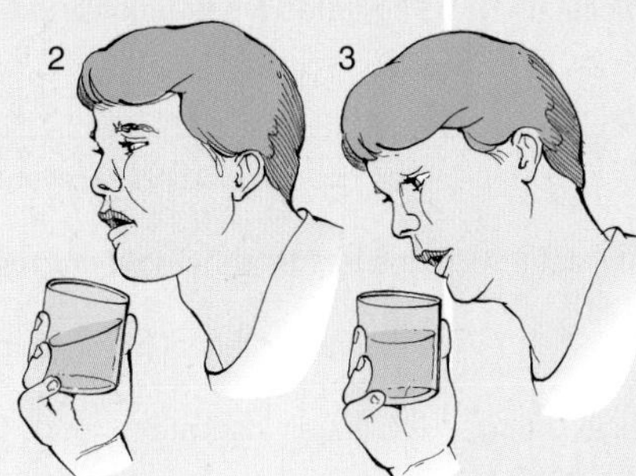

D

(1) Inappropriate neck position; and (2–3) appropriate neck positions.

Remain with the client until he or she has swallowed the medications. — Ensures the appropriate administration.

Restore the client to a position of comfort and safety. — Shows concern for the client's well-being.

Record the volume of fluid consumed on the intake and output record. — Demonstrates responsibility for accurate fluid assessment.

Record the administration of the medication. — Prevents medication errors.

Assess the client in 30 min for desired and undesired drug effects. — Aids in evaluating the client's response and the effect of drug therapy.

(continued)

Administering Oral Medications (continued)

Evaluation

- The five rights are upheld.
- The client experiences no choking or aspiration.
- The client exhibits a therapeutic response to the medication.
- The client demonstrates minimal or absent side effects.

Document

- Preassessment data, if indicated
- Date, time, drug, dose, route, signature, title, and initials (usually on the MAR)
- Evidence of client's response, if it can be determined

SAMPLE DOCUMENTATION

Date and Time Temp. 103.8°F. Tylenol tabs ii given by mouth for relief of fever. Fever reduced to 103°F 30 minutes later.
——————————————— SIGNATURE/TITLE

SKILL 32-2 Administering Medications Through an Enteral Tube

Suggested Action	Reason for Action
ASSESSMENT	
Check the medication administration record (MAR) and compare the information with the written medical order.	Prevents medication errors.
Review the client's drug, allergy, and medical history.	Avoids potential complications.
Consult a current drug reference concerning the drug's action, side effects, contraindications, and administration information.	Ensures the appropriate administration based on a thorough knowledge base.
Verify the location of the tube by auscultating instilled air or aspirating secretions.	Ensures airway protection and proper tube placement.
Compare the length of the external tube with its measurement at the time of insertion.	Determines whether the tube has migrated.
Inspect the client's mouth and throat.	Determines whether the tube has been displaced and is coiled at the back of the throat.
PLANNING	
Plan to administer medications within 30–60 min of the scheduled time.	Demonstrates timely administration and compliance with the medical order.
Separate and clamp or plug a feeding tube for 15–30 min if the drug will interact with food.	Ensures that the stomach will be relatively empty.
Allow sufficient time to prepare the medications in a location with minimal distractions.	Promotes the safe preparation of drugs.
Make sure that there is a sufficient supply of plastic medication cups.	Facilitates organization and efficient time management.
IMPLEMENTATION	
Wash your hands or perform an alcohol-based hand rub (see Chap. 10).	Removes colonizing microorganisms.
Read and compare the label on the drug with the MAR at least three times—before, during, and after preparing the drug.	Ensures that the *right drug* is given at the *right time* by the *right route.*
Prepare each drug separately.	Prevents potential physical changes when some drugs are combined.
Take the cups containing diluted medications to the bedside, along with water for flushing, a 30–50-mL syringe, a towel or disposable pad, and clean gloves.	Facilitates installation.
Identify the client using at least two methods, for example, checking the wristband and asking the client's name.	Ensures that medications are given to the *right client; complies with the National Patient Safety Goals.*

(continued)

Administering Medications Through an Enteral Tube (continued)

IMPLEMENTATION (CONTINUED)

Help the client into a Fowler's position.	Prevents gastric reflux.
Don clean gloves.	Prevents contact with body fluids.
Insert the syringe into the tube and instill 15–30 mL of water by gravity (Fig. A).	Flushes and reduces the surface tension of the tube.

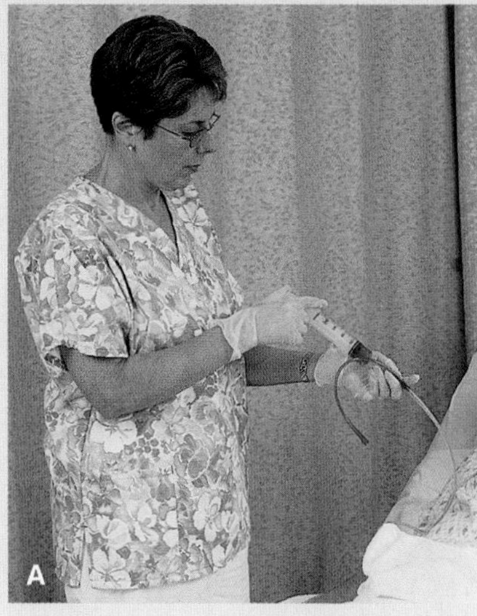

Instilling the medication. (Photo by B. Proud.)

Add the diluted medication to the syringe as it becomes nearly empty.	Prevents instilling air.
Apply gentle pressure with the plunger or bulb of a syringe if the medication fails to instill easily.	Provides positive pressure.
Flush with at least 5 mL of water between each instillation of medication and as much as 30 mL after instilling all the medications.	Prevents drug interactions and obstruction of the tube; fully instills all the prescribed drug.
Pinch the tube as the syringe empties.	Prevents distending the stomach with air; maintains patency of the tube.
Clamp or plug the tube for 30 min before reconnecting a tube to the suction (Fig. B).	Prevents removing the medication after it has been instilled.

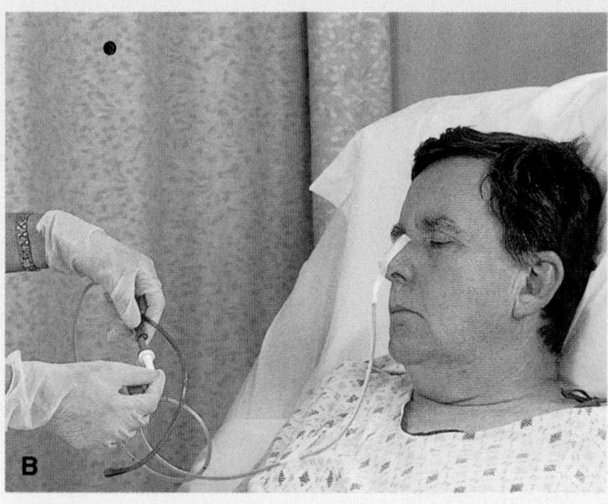

Plugging a gastric tube. (Photo by B. Proud.)

Connect a tube used for nourishment immediately if the medication and formula will not interact.	Facilitates the primary purpose of the enteral tube.
Keep the head of the bed elevated for at least 30 min.	Reduces the potential for aspiration.

(continued)

Administering Medications Through an Enteral Tube (continued)

Evaluation

- The tube placement is verified.
- The five rights are upheld.
- The medications instill freely and are flushed afterward.
- The client experiences no abdominal distention, nausea, vomiting, or other undesirable effects.
- The tube remains patent.

Document

- Preadministration assessment data
- Medication administration on the MAR
- Volume of fluid instilled with the medication as well as for flushing the tube on the bedside intake and output record
- Response of the client

SAMPLE DOCUMENTATION

Date and Time Placement of NG tube verified by auscultation. No evidence of tube migration. Medications administered (see MAR) per NG tube. Flushed with 30 mL after instilling medications. Tube clamped at this time. No evidence of nausea or distention. —————— SIGNATURE/TITLE

Topical and Inhalant Medications

Words To Know

aerosol
buccal application
cutaneous application
dry powder inhaler
inhalant route
inhalers
inunction
metered-dose inhaler
nebulizer
ophthalmic application
otic application
paste
rebound effect
skin patches
spacer
sublingual application
topical route
transdermal application

Learning Objectives

On completion of this chapter, the reader should be able to:

1. Explain how topical medications are administered and commonly applied.
2. Give three examples of an inunction.
3. Name two forms of drugs applied by the transdermal route and principles to follow when applying a skin patch.
4. Describe where eye medications are applied.
5. Explain how the administration of ear medications differs for adults and children.
6. Explain the rebound effect that accompanies the administration of nasal decongestants.
7. Describe the difference between sublingual and buccal administration.
8. Name a common reason for vaginal applications.
9. Give the form of medication used most often for rectal administration.
10. Explain why inhalation is a good route for medication administration.
11. Name two types of inhalers and alternatives for administering inhaled medications.

Drugs are administered by routes other than oral (see Chap. 32). This chapter describes the techniques used to administer drugs by the topical and inhalant routes.

TOPICAL ROUTE

Drugs given by the **topical route** (the administration of medications to the skin or mucous membranes) can be applied externally or internally (Table 33-1). Topically applied drugs have a local or systemic effect. Many are administered to achieve a direct effect on the tissue to which they are applied.

Cutaneous Applications

Cutaneous applications are drugs rubbed into or placed in contact with the skin. They include inunctions and transdermal patches and pastes.

Inunction Application

An **inunction** is a medication incorporated into an agent (eg, ointment, oil, lotion, cream) that is administered by rubbing it into the skin.

TABLE 33-1 Topical Medications

ROUTES	LOCATION	VEHICLE	EXAMPLES
Cutaneous	Skin	Ointment	hydrocortisone (Cortaid)
	Skin	Cream	benzocaine (Lanacane)
	Scalp	Liquid	permethrin (Nix)
	Skin	Lotion	Lubriderm[a]
	Skin	Patch	estrogen (Estraderm)
	Skin	Paste	nitroglycerin (Nitrol)
	Oral mucous membrane	Gel	benzocaine (Anbesol)
Ophthalmic	In the eye	Drops	timolol (Timoptic)
		Ointment	polymyxin, neomycin, bacitracin (Neosporin)
Otic	In the ear	Drops	hydrocortisone, neomycin, polymyxin (Cortisporin Otic)
		Irrigation	carbamide peroxide (Debrox)
Nasal	In the nose	Spray	oxymetazoline (Afrin)
		Drops	oxymetazoline (Neo-Synephrine)
Sublingual	Under the tongue	Tablet	nitroglycerin (Nitrostat)
		Spray	nitroglycerin (Nitrolingual)
Buccal	Between the cheek and gum	Tablet	nitroglycerin (Nitrogard)
		Lozenge	Cepacol[a]
Vaginal	In the vagina	Douche	povidone iodine (Massengill medicated douche)
		Cream	clotrimazole (Gyne-Lotrimin)
		Suppository	fluconazole (Monistat)
Rectal	To or within rectum	Irrigation	sodium phosphate (Fleet Enema)
		Suppository	bisacodyl (Dulcolax)
		Ointment	hydrocortisone (Anusol)

[a]Indicates a nonprescription item that is a combination of ingredients.

Alert clients may self-administer an inunction after receiving proper instruction. In that situation, the nurse teaches proper application techniques and checks that the client has applied the medication appropriately and as often as prescribed. For clients who cannot apply their own inunctions, the nurse does so (see Nursing Guidelines 33-1).

Transdermal Applications

Drugs incorporated into patches or pastes are administered as **transdermal applications** (the method of applying a drug on the skin and allowing it to become passively absorbed). After application, the drug migrates through the skin and eventually is absorbed into the bloodstream.

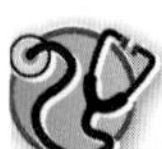

NURSING GUIDELINES 33-1

Applying an Inunction

- Wash your hands or perform an alcohol-based hand rub (see Chap. 10). *Hand hygiene removes colonizing microorganisms.*
- Check the identity of the client. *Doing so prevents administering the medication to the wrong person.*
- Don clean gloves if your skin or that of the client is not intact. *Gloves provide a barrier to pathogens.*
- Cleanse the area of application with soap and water. *Clean skin promotes absorption.*
- Warm the inunction if it will be applied to a sensitive area of the skin by holding it temporarily in your hands or placing the sealed container in warm water. *Warmth promotes comfort.*
- Shake the contents of liquid inunctions. *Shaking mixes the contents uniformly.*
- Apply the inunction to the skin with the fingertips, a cotton ball, or a gauze square. *Correct application distributes the substance over a wide area.*
- Rub the inunction into the skin. *Rubbing promotes absorption.*
- Apply local heat to the area if desired (see Chap. 28). *Heat dilates peripheral blood vessels and speeds absorption.*

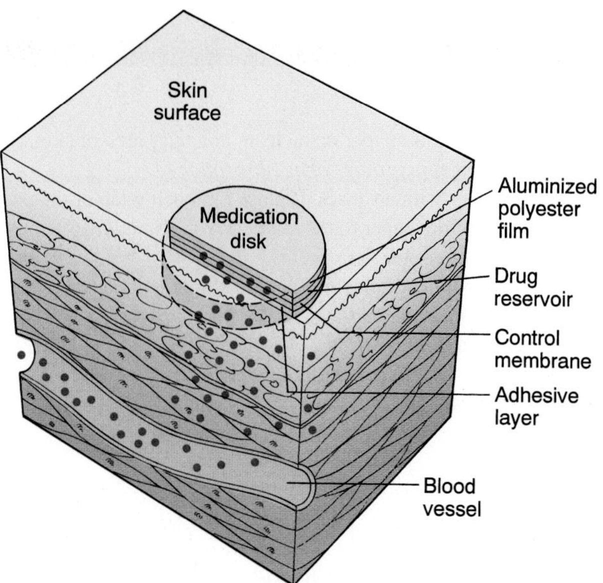

FIGURE 33-1 The pathway of absorption from a transdermal skin patch.

Skin Patches

Skin patches are drugs bonded to an adhesive bandage and applied to the skin (Fig. 33-1).

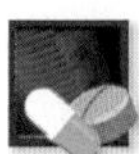

Pharmacologic Considerations

- Several drugs are now prepared in patch form, including nitroglycerin (used to dilate the coronary arteries), scopolamine (used to relieve motion sickness), and estrogen (a hormone used to treat menopausal symptoms), and potent pain medications (fentanyl). Nicotine withdrawal therapy and contraceptive drugs also are available as skin patches.
- A severe headache, hypotension, and flushing are side effects associated with nitroglycerin. If side effects occur, consult the physician, who may recommend removal of the transdermal application.
- Clients who are prescribed nitroglycerin in any form should not concurrently take a drug for erectile dysfunction because the combination may contribute to hypotension due to the combined vasodilation effect.
- A transdermal nitroglycerin patch is usually worn for 12 to 14 hours and then removed for 10 hours to facilitate the drug's continued effectiveness.

Skin patches are applied to any skin area with adequate circulation. Most patches are applied to parts of the upper body such as the chest, shoulders, and upper arms. Small patches can be applied behind the ear. Each time a new patch is applied, it is placed in a slightly different location. Clipping extremely hairy skin areas before an application may help adhesion.

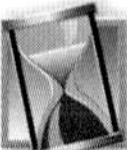

Gerontologic Considerations

- The onset of drug action may be atypical when administering topical medications to older adults because of their diminished subcutaneous fat, which leads to a more rapid absorption of topical medications.

After application of the patch, it may take approximately 30 minutes for the drug to reach a therapeutic level. Thereafter, the patch provides a continuous supply of medication. In fact, the drug may still be active for up to 30 minutes after removal of the patch. It is always best to date and initial a patch so that others can determine when it was applied. The older patch is removed when a new patch is applied.

Drug Paste

A **paste** contains a drug within a thick base and is applied to but not rubbed into the skin. Nitroglycerin can be applied as a paste. Although sometimes the product is referred to as an ointment, the term is a misnomer because the skin is not massaged once the drug is applied (see Nursing Guidelines 33-2 and Fig. 33-2).

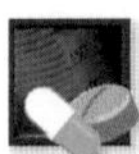

Pharmacologic Considerations

- Nitroglycerin paste (an ointment) has a shorter duration of action than that supplied in a transdermal patch. Consequently, it must be applied more frequently to provide a sustained effect.
- When discontinuing transdermal nitroglycerin, the dose should be decreased gradually rather than stopping it abruptly to prevent the resumption of symptoms such as chest pain.

Ophthalmic Applications

An **ophthalmic application** is a method of applying drugs onto the mucous membrane of one or both eyes (described in Skill 33-1). The mucous membrane of the eyes is called the *conjunctiva.* It lines the inner eyelids and the anterior surface of the *sclera* (Fig. 33-3).

Ophthalmic medications are supplied either in liquid form and instilled as drops, or as ointments applied along the lower lid margin. Blinking, rather than rubbing, distributes the drug over the surface of the eye. The eye is a delicate structure susceptible to infection and injury, just like any other tissue. Therefore, nurses take care to keep the applicator tip of the medication container sterile.

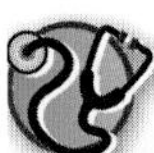

NURSING GUIDELINES 33-2

Applying Nitroglycerin Paste

- Wash your hands or perform an alcohol-based hand rub (see Chap. 10). *Hand hygiene removes colonizing microorganisms.*
- Check the identity of the client. *Doing so prevents administering the medication to the wrong person.*
- Squeeze a ribbon of paste from the tube onto an application paper (see Fig. 33-2). *This complies with the medication order, which usually specifies the dose in inches.*
- Fold the paper or use a wooden applicator to spread the paste over approximately a 2.25 × 3.5 in. (5.6 × 8.8 cm) area of the paper. *These techniques facilitate distributing the drug over a wide area for quick absorption.*
- Do not touch the paste with your bare fingers. *Touching the paste could cause self-absorption of the drug.*
- Place the application paper on a clean, nonhairy area of skin. *Such a placement facilitates drug absorption.*
- Cover the paper with a square of plastic kitchen wrap or tape all the edges of the paper to the skin. *This seals the drug between the paper and the skin.*
- Remove one application before applying another and remove any residue remaining on the skin. *Careful application prevents excessive drug levels.*
- Rotate the sites of medication placement. *Site rotation reduces the potential for skin irritation.*

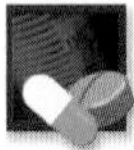

Pharmacologic Considerations

■ Some people have difficulty instilling eye medications independently. Devices are available that can diminish the frequency of instillation or can facilitate administration. For example, one type of medication for glaucoma is inserted inside the lower eyelid, requiring administration only every 7 days. Sight centers, which provide assistive devices for people with visual impairment, are a good resource for other devices that facilitate the instillation of eye drops.
■ Clients who require complex ophthalmic medication regimens that involve the instillation of one or more types of drops up to four times daily may collaborate with the prescribing practitioner about longer acting medications that may decrease the frequency of medication routines.
■ When more than one eye medication is prescribed, it is best to wait 5 minutes between instillation of eye drops.
■ Eye medications can have adverse systemic effects and can interact with other medications, herbal supplements, or both.

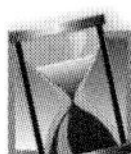

Gerontologic Considerations

■ Some older adults use two or more types of eye medications once or several times daily. If the tops of the eye medications are not color-coded, suggest ways to color-code the containers to help distinguish the different medications.

Stop, Think, and Respond Box 33-1

What actions should the nurse take if the tip of the ophthalmic medication becomes contaminated?

Otic Applications

An **otic application** is a drug instilled in the outer ear. It is usually administered to moisten impacted cerumen or to instill medications to treat a local bacterial or fungal infection.

When instilling ear medication, the nurse first manipulates the ear to straighten the auditory canal. The technique varies depending on whether the client is a young child (the nurse pulls the ear down and back) or an adult (the nurse pulls the ear up and back; see Chap. 13).

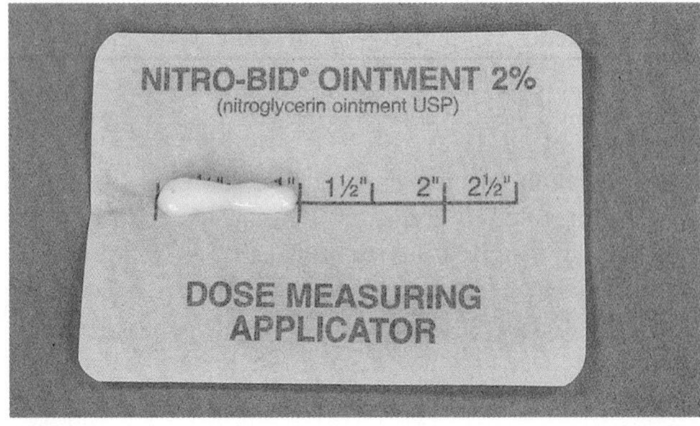

FIGURE 33-2 A paste and applicator paper. (Photo by B. Proud.)

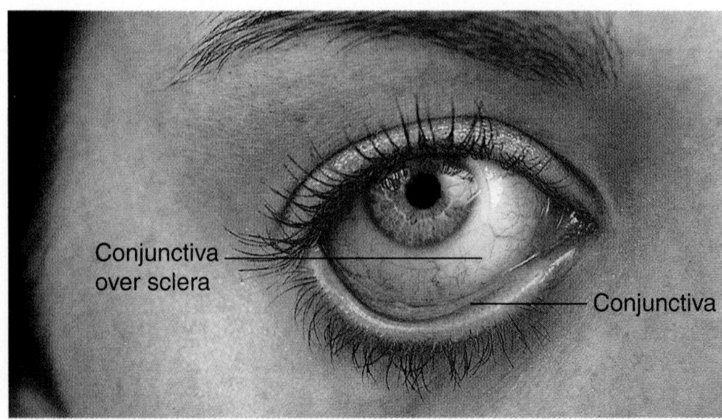

FIGURE 33-3 Ophthalmic application sites. (Photo by B. Proud.)

Tilting the client's head away, the nurse instills the prescribed number of drops of medication within the ear. The client remains in this position briefly as the solution travels toward the eardrum. The nurse can place a small cotton ball loosely in the ear to absorb excess medication. If a bilateral administration is prescribed, the nurse waits at least 15 minutes before instilling medication in the opposite ear. Briefly postponing the application within the second ear avoids displacing the initially instilled medication when repositioning the client.

Nasal Applications

Topical medications are dropped or sprayed within the nose (Skill 33-2). A proper instillation is important to avoid displacing the medication into nearby structures such as the back of the throat. Adults often self-administer their own nasal medications, but sometimes nurses must assist older adults and children.

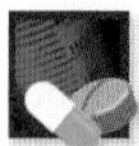

Pharmacologic Considerations

- Nurses warn clients who use over-the-counter decongestant nasal sprays that if they use the medication too frequently or administer more than the recommended amount, a **rebound effect** (swelling of the nasal mucosa within a short time of drug administration) can occur. Clients can avoid a rebound effect by following label directions or by using nasal sprays containing only normal saline solution.
- A prolonged use of topical nasal decongestants can cause irritation of the nares (American Academy of Family Physicians, 2005).

Sublingual and Buccal Applications

A tablet given by **sublingual application** (a drug placed under the tongue) is left to dissolve slowly and becomes absorbed by the rich blood supply in the area. Some drugs in spray form also are administered sublingually. A **buccal application** (a drug placed against the mucous membranes of the inner cheek) is another method of drug administration.

When giving sublingual or buccal administrations, nurses instruct clients not to chew or swallow the medication. Eating and smoking also are contraindicated during the brief time needed for a solid medication to dissolve.

Vaginal Applications

Topical vaginal applications are used most often to treat local infections, which are common and usually result from the colonization of vaginal tissue by microorganisms abundant in stool (eg, yeasts). The microorganisms usually get transferred during bowel elimination if the client wipes stool from the rectal area toward (not away from) the vagina. Symptoms of a yeast infection include intense vaginal itching and a white, cheese-like vaginal discharge.

Several nonprescription drugs useful in treating vaginal yeast infections are available in suppository, dissolvable tablet, and cream form. Early and appropriate self-treatment restores normal tissue integrity. Providing clients with instructions about how to administer vaginal medications for the most effective action may be helpful (see Client and Family Teaching 33-1 and Fig. 33-4).

If the client cannot self-administer a vaginal medication, the nurse wears gloves to avoid contact with secretions. After removing the gloves, hand washing or an alcohol-based hand rub is critical. The same advice holds true for rectal applications.

Client and Family Teaching 33-1 Administering Medications Vaginally

The nurse teaches the client as follows:

- Obtain a form of medication based on personal preference; all come with a vaginal applicator.
- Plan to instill the medication before going to bed so that it can be retained for a prolonged period.
- Empty the bladder just before inserting the medication.
- Place the drug in the applicator (see Fig. 33-4A).
- Lubricate the applicator tip with a water-soluble lubricant such as K-Y Jelly.
- Lie down, bend your knees, and spread your legs.
- Separate the labia and insert the applicator into the vagina to the length recommended in the package directions, usually 2–4 in. (5–10 cm) (see Fig. 33-4B).
- Depress the plunger once it reaches the proper distance within the vagina to insert the medication.
- Remove the applicator and place it on a clean tissue.
- Apply a sanitary pad if you prefer.
- Remain recumbent for at least 10–30 minutes.
- Discard the applicator if it is disposable. Wash a reusable applicator with soap and water when you wash your hands.
- Consult a physician if symptoms persist.

Rectal Applications

Drugs administered rectally are usually in the form of suppositories (see Chap. 31); however, creams and ointments also may be prescribed. The technique for using a rectal applicator is similar to that for using a vaginal applicator.

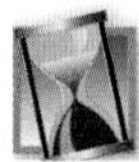

Gerontologic Considerations

- Some older clients have difficulty reaching areas of the body to which topical drugs are applied. For example, arthritis may interfere with applying medication within the vagina or rectum, or to skin lesions on the lower extremities.

INHALANT ROUTE

The **inhalant route** administers drugs to the lower airways. This method of medication administration is effective because the lungs provide an extensive area from which the circulatory system can quickly absorb the drug.

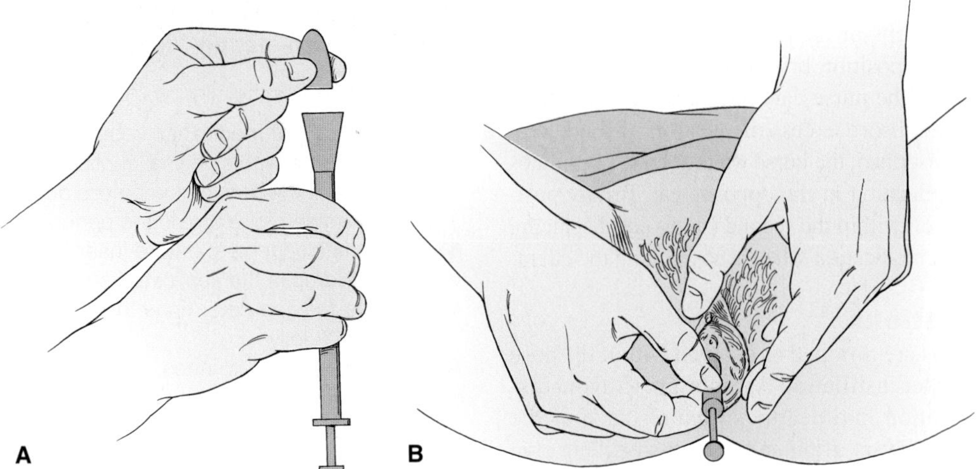

FIGURE 33-4 Administering drugs vaginally. **A.** Placing the drug in the applicator. **B.** Inserting the applicator with the drug.

A simple method of administering inhaled medications is through an inhaler. **Inhalers** are handheld devices for delivering medication into the respiratory passages. They consist of a container of medication and a holder with a mouthpiece through which the drug is inhaled.

There are two types of inhalers: (1) a **dry powder inhaler** holds a reservoir of pulverized drug and a carrier substance, and (2) a **metered-dose inhaler** that delivers aerosolized medication, which is a liquid drug forced through a narrow channel via a chemical propellant (Fig. 33-5).

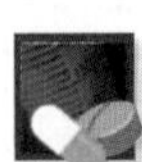

Pharmacologic Considerations

- Traditionally, metered-dose inhalers have been propelled with chloroflurocarbons, which contribute to environmental pollution. Current global regulations require them to be reformulated to contain non-ozone-depleting substances.

Dry powder inhalers depend on the client's inspiratory effort to deliver the medication into the lungs. If the inspiratory effort is ineffective, the dose of the drug is reduced. A metered-dose inhaler contains medication under pressure within a canister. The canister is placed into a holder containing a mouthpiece; when the container is compressed, a measured volume (the metered dose) of aerosolized drug is released. Clients who use metered-dose inhalers do not always do so correctly. As a result, they may swallow, rather than inhale, much of the medication. As a result, their respiratory symptoms may not be relieved (see Client and Family Teaching 33-2 and Fig. 33-6).

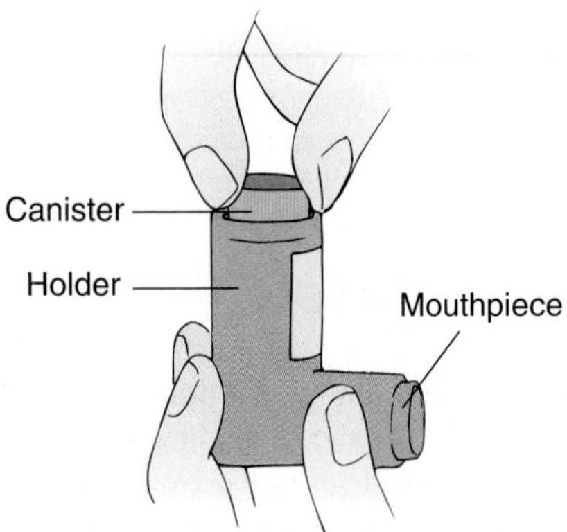

FIGURE 33-5 The parts of metered-dose inhaler.

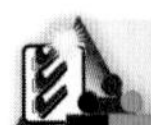

Client and Family Teaching 33-2
Using a Metered-Dose Inhaler

The nurse teaches the client and the family as follows:

- Insert the canister into the holder.
- Shake the canister to distribute the drug in the pressurized chamber.
- Remove the cap from the mouthpiece.
- Tilt your head back slightly and exhale slowly through pursed lips.
- Open your mouth and place the inhaler 1–2 in. away (see Fig. 33-6). If you have difficulty with this method, place the inhaler in your mouth and close your lips around the mouthpiece.
- Press down on the canister once to release the medication.
- As the medication is released, breathe in slowly through your mouth for approximately 3–5 seconds.
- Hold your breath for 10 seconds to let the medication reach your lungs.
- Exhale slowly through pursed lips.
- Wait 1 full minute before doing another inhalation if more than one is ordered.
- Clean the inhaler (holder and mouthpiece) daily by rinsing it in warm water and weekly with mild soap and water. Allow the inhaler to air dry. Have another inhaler available to use while the first is drying.
- Check the amount of medication in the canister by floating it in a bowl of water; the higher the canister floats, the less medication it contains.
- Obtain a refill of inhalant medication when the current canister shows signs of becoming empty.

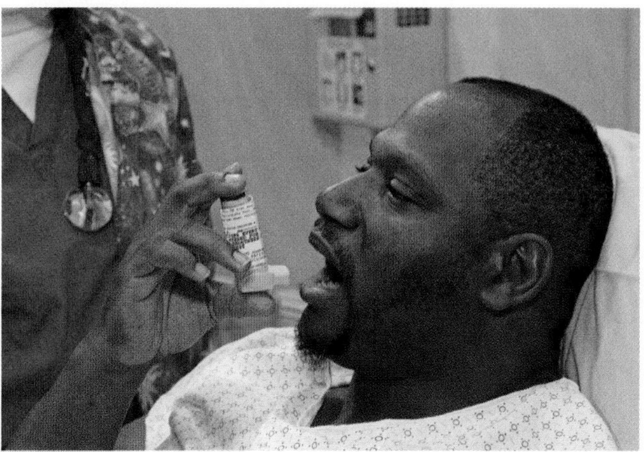

FIGURE 33-6 A metered-dose inhaler can be used by holding the mouthpiece 1 to 2 in. away prior to depressing the canister and inhaling, or the mouthpiece can be placed in the mouth and sealed by the lips prior to administering the drug.

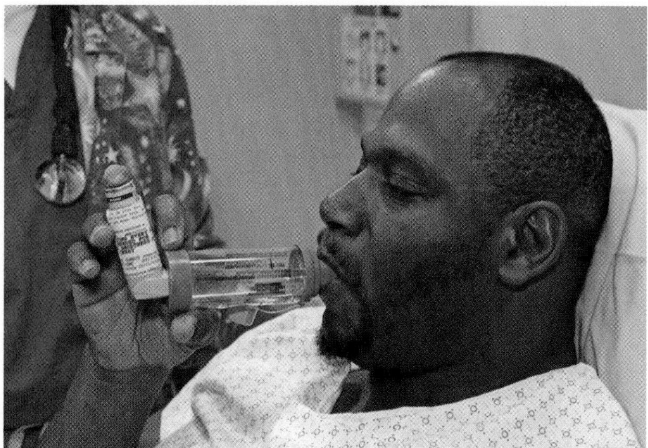

FIGURE 33-7 Using a metered-dose inhaler with a spacer.

Some clients find that the inhaled drug leaves an unpleasant aftertaste. Gargling with salt water may diminish this. Drug residue may accumulate in the mouthpiece; therefore, the client should rinse the mouthpiece in warm water after use.

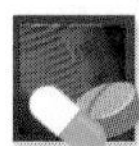

Pharmacologic Considerations

- Sometimes, two inhalers containing different drugs are prescribed. During teaching sessions, it is important to educate how and when each drug is used, and the anticipated action. For example, one drug may act to expand the bronchioles and would improve the overall outcome to be administered before a medication that loosens secretions. Providing simple written instructions with each medication is also helpful.

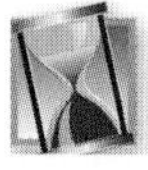

Gerontologic Considerations

- Monitoring the heart rate and blood pressure of older adults who use inhaled bronchodilators is important because these medications commonly cause tachycardia and hypertension. Either or both of these effects increases the risks for complications, especially in older adults with an underlying cardiovascular disease.

Clients who have problems coordinating their breathing with the use of an inhaler may not receive the full dose of **aerosol.** A **spacer** (a chamber attached to an inhaler; Fig. 33-7) can be helpful in this situation. Spacers provide a reservoir for the aerosol medication. As the client takes additional breaths, he or she continues to inhale the medication held in the reservoir. This tends to maximize drug absorption because it prevents drug loss. Some clients also find that prolonging inhalation of the drug reduces side effects such as tachycardia or tremulousness.

Some clients, such as infants, young children, and older adults, who have difficulty coordinating inspiration with the use of a hand held inhaler, may use a nebulizer as an alternative to administering an inhalant. A **nebulizer,** sometimes called a "breathing machine," is a device that converts liquid medication to an aerosol using compressed air. The aerosol is inhaled through a mouthpiece or a face mask over 10 to 20 minutes until the mist is no longer visible (Fig. 33-8). The components of the nebulizer are cleaned after each use with soapy water and a small brush. After rinsing the cleaned parts, they are allowed to air dry before storing them in a closed container.

NURSING IMPLICATIONS

When administering topical or inhalant drugs, nurses often assess and take steps to maintain the integrity of the skin and mucous membranes. Health teaching may be important to prevent improper self-administration. Applicable nursing diagnoses may include the following:

- Deficient Knowledge; Readiness for Enhanced Knowledge
- Ineffective Self-Help Management
- Impaired Gas Exchange
- Impaired Skin Integrity
- Impaired Tissue Integrity
- Ineffective Breathing Patterns

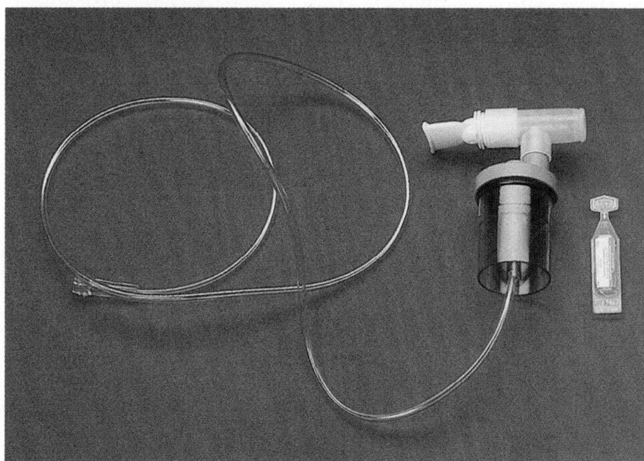

FIGURE 33-8 A nebulizer consists of a cup to which liquid medication is added, a mouthpiece, and tubing that connects to an electric or a battery-operated source for compressed air.

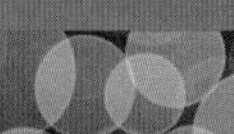

NURSING CARE PLAN 33-1 Ineffective Breathing Patterns

Assessment

- Count the client's respiratory rate for a full minute.
- Observe the client's pattern of respirations such as effort, nasal or mouth breathing, position used to enhance breathing, and use of accessory muscles.
- Establish if the client feels comfortable or anxious with regard to breathing.
- Measure the client's hemoglobin saturation with a pulse oximeter.
- Determine techniques the client uses to restore quiet, effortless breathing.

Nursing Diagnosis. **Ineffective Breathing Patterns** related to an improper technique using metered-dose inhaler to manage shortness of breath and mild hypoxemia associated with underlying lung disease as manifested by the client's statement, "I struggle to breathe and my chest gets tight even though I use the inhaler my doctor gave me 2 days ago."

Expected Outcome. The client's breathing pattern will be effective as evidenced by quiet, effortless breathing at a respiratory rate between 16 and 28 breaths per minute with the correct use of the metered-dose inhaler.

Interventions	Rationales
Re-demonstrate the correct use of a metered-dose inhaler.	Visual and verbal techniques enhance learning.
Observe the client's technique when using the metered-dose inhaler at least four times after demonstration.	Observation provides a means for evaluating the client's level of understanding.
Monitor the client's SpO_2 with a pulse oximeter before and after the use of the metered-dose inhaler.	Results will help to evaluate the client's technique using a metered-dose inhaler and the drug's effectiveness.

Evaluation of Expected Outcomes

- The client is shown how to use a metered-dose inhaler.
- The client has been observed to perform the technique appropriately with each of the two puffs from the inhaler.
- Breathing changes from 32 breaths per minute with effort and an SpO_2 of 88% to 28 quiet breaths per minute and an SpO_2 of 90% within 15 minutes of using the inhaler.

Nursing Care Plan 33-1 shows how nurses use the steps of the nursing process when managing the care of a client with the diagnosis of Ineffective Breathing Patterns, defined in the NANDA-I taxonomy (2012, p. 233) as "inspiration and/or expiration that does not provide adequate ventilation."

CRITICAL THINKING EXERCISES

1. Before discharge from the hospital, a client who has had a heart attack says, "You nurses always put my nitroglycerin patches on my back. How can I do that when I have to do it myself?" How would you respond?
2. How might you help a client who is legally blind and lives alone identify two different containers of eye medication?
3. How can a nurse prevent eye drops from rolling down a client's cheek?
4. What questions would be important to ask if a client's symptoms persist after being treated for a vaginal infection with a regimen of self-administered medication?

NCLEX-STYLE REVIEW QUESTIONS

1. Which body position is best for the nurse to identify when teaching a client how to self-administer nose drops?
   1. Bend the head forward
   2. Push the nose laterally
   3. Tilt the head backward
   4. Open the mouth wide
2. Which instruction is best when teaching a client about inserting vaginal medication?
   1. Place the applicator just inside the vaginal opening.
   2. Insert the applicator while sitting on the toilet.
   3. Instill the medication just before retiring for sleep.
   4. Don disposable gloves before applying the drug.
3. What is the best technique for the nurse to use when instilling eye drops?
   1. Drop the medication onto the cornea.
   2. Drop the medication at the inner canthus.
   3. Drop the medication at the outer canthus.
   4. Drop the medication in the conjunctival sac.
4. What is the most appropriate nursing action before instilling ear drops?
   1. Ensure that the medication is room temperature.
   2. Refrigerate the medication for 30 minutes.
   3. Clean the outer surface of the dropper.
   4. Fill the dropper with no more than 1 mL.
5. After instilling medication within an ear, what instruction is most appropriate for the nurse to give to the client?
   1. Remain in position for at least 5 minutes.
   2. Pack a cotton pledget tightly in the ear.
   3. Do not blow your nose for at least 1 hour.
   4. Avoid drinking very warm or cold beverages.

SKILL 33-1 Instilling Eye Medications

Suggested Action	Reason for Action
ASSESSMENT	
Compare the medication administration record (MAR) with the written medical order.	Prevents medication errors.
Review the client's drug, allergy, and medical history.	Avoids potential complications.
Consult a current drug reference concerning the drug's action, side effects, contraindications, and administration information.	Ensures appropriate administration based on a thorough knowledge base.
PLANNING	
Plan to administer medications within 30–60 min of their scheduled time.	Demonstrates timely administration and compliance with the medical order.
Allow sufficient time to prepare medications in a location with minimal distractions.	Promotes the safe preparation of drugs.
Warm eye drops and ointments by holding the container between the hands if they have not been stored at room temperature.	Promotes comfort.
Read and compare the label on the drug with the MAR at least three times—before, during, and after preparing the drug.	Ensures that the *right drug* is given at the *right time* by the *right route*.
IMPLEMENTATION	
Wash your hands or perform an alcohol-based hand rub (see Chap. 10).	Removes colonizing microorganisms.
Identify the client using at least two methods, for example, checking the wristband and asking the client's name.	Ensures that medications are given to the *right client;* complies with the National Patient Safety Goals.
Position the client supine or sitting with the head tilted back and slightly to the side into which the medication will be instilled.	Prevents the drug from passing into the nasolacrimal duct or being blinked onto the cheek.
Don clean gloves.	Acts as a barrier to pathogens in body fluids.
Clean the lids and lashes if they contain debris. Use a cotton ball or tissue moistened with water.	Promotes comfort and maximizes the potential for absorption.
Wipe the eye from the corner by the nose, called the "inner canthus," toward the corner near the temple, called the "outer canthus."	Moves debris away from the nasolacrimal duct.
Instruct the client to look toward the ceiling.	Prevents looking directly at the applicator, which usually causes a blinking reflex as it comes close to the eye.
Make a pouch in the lower lid by pulling the skin downward over the bony orbit.	Provides a natural reservoir for depositing liquid medication.
Move the container of medication from below the client's line of vision or from the side of the eye.	Prevents a blink reflex.
Steady the container above the location for instillation without touching the eye surface.	Prevents injury.
Instill the prescribed number of drops into the appropriate eye within the conjunctival pouch (Fig. A).	Complies with the medical order by administering the *right dose.*

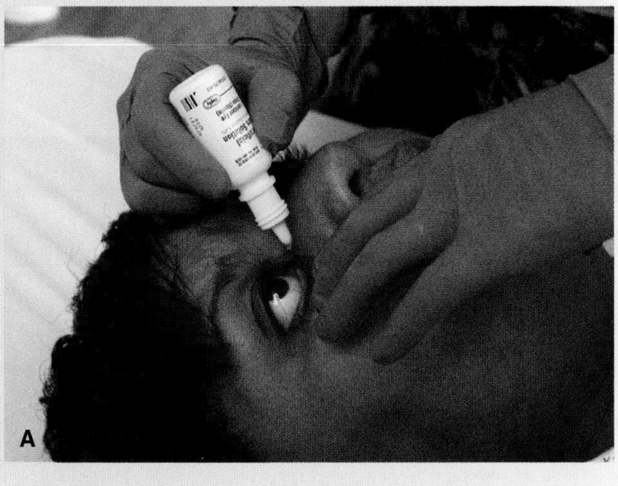

A

Instilling eye drops.

(continued)

Instilling Eye Medications (continued)

Suggested Action	Reason for Action
IMPLEMENTATION (CONTINUED)	
If using ointment, squeeze a ribbon onto the lower lid margin (Fig. B).	Applies the ointment to the conjunctiva.

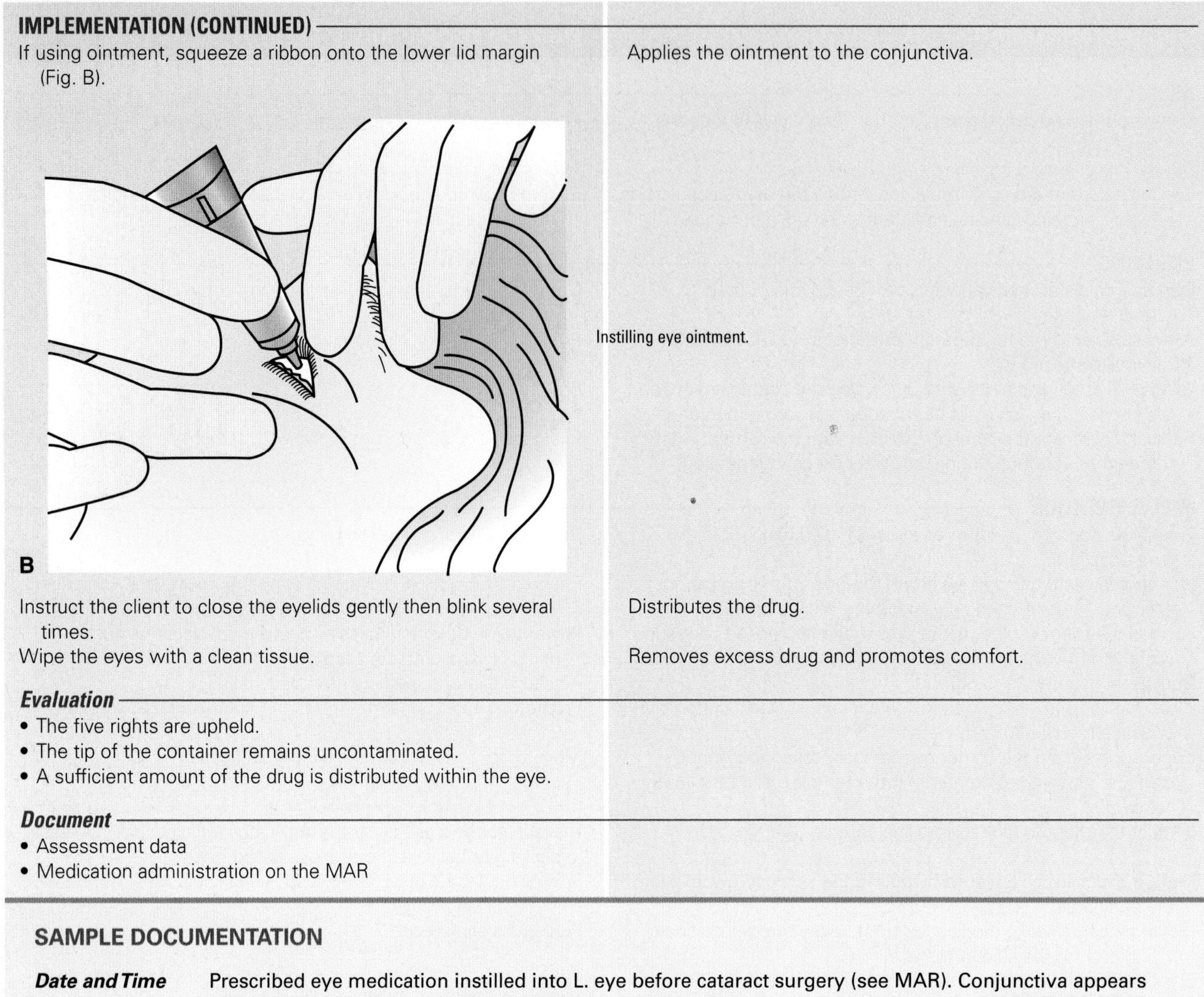

Instilling eye ointment.

Suggested Action	Reason for Action
Instruct the client to close the eyelids gently then blink several times.	Distributes the drug.
Wipe the eyes with a clean tissue.	Removes excess drug and promotes comfort.

Evaluation

- The five rights are upheld.
- The tip of the container remains uncontaminated.
- A sufficient amount of the drug is distributed within the eye.

Document

- Assessment data
- Medication administration on the MAR

SAMPLE DOCUMENTATION

Date and Time Prescribed eye medication instilled into L. eye before cataract surgery (see MAR). Conjunctiva appears pink and intact. Lens is opaque. Eyelashes have been clipped. ——————— SIGNATURE/TITLE

SKILL 33-2 Administering Nasal Medications

Suggested Action	Reason for Action
ASSESSMENT	
Compare the medication administration record (MAR) with the written medical order.	Prevents medication errors.
Review the client's drug, allergy, and medical history.	Avoids potential complications.
Consult a current drug reference concerning the drug's action, side effects, contraindications, and administration information.	Ensures appropriate administration based on a thorough knowledge of the drug.
PLANNING	
Plan to administer medications within 30–60 min of their scheduled time.	Demonstrates timely administration and compliance with the medical order.
Allow sufficient time to prepare the medications in a location with minimal distractions.	Promotes the safe preparation of drugs.

(continued)

Administering Nasal Medications (continued)

PLANNING (CONTINUED)	
Read and compare the label on the drug with the MAR at least three times—before, during, and after preparing the drug.	Ensures that the *right drug* is given at the *right time* by the *right route.*
IMPLEMENTATION	
Wash your hands or perform an alcohol-based hand rub (see Chap. 10).	Removes colonizing microorganisms.
Identify the client using at least two methods, for example, checking the wristband and asking the client's name	Ensures that medications are given to the *right client;* complies with the National Patient Safety Goals.
Help the client to a sitting or lying position with his or her head tilted backward or to the side if the drug needs to reach one or the other sinuses.	Facilitates depositing the drug where its effect is desired.
Place a rolled towel or pillow beneath the neck if the client cannot sit.	Provides support and aids in positioning.
Remove the cap from the liquid medication to which a dropper usually is attached.	Provides a means for administering the drug.
Aim the tip of the dropper toward the nasal passage and squeeze the rubber portion of the cap to administer the number of drops prescribed (Fig. A).	Deposits the drug within the nose rather than into the throat and ensures administering the *right dose.*

A

Instilling nasal medication.

Instruct the client to breathe through the mouth as the drops are instilled.	Prevents inhaling large droplets.
If the drug is in a spray form, place the tip of the container just inside the nostril.	Confines the spray within the nasal passage.
Occlude the opposite nostril.	Administers medication to one and then the other nasal passage.
Instruct the client to inhale as the container is squeezed.	Distributes the aerosol.
Repeat in the opposite nostril.	Deposits the drug bilaterally for maximum effect.
Advise the client to remain in position for approximately 5 min.	Promotes local absorption.
Recap the container and replace it where the medications are stored.	Supports the principles of asepsis and demonstrates responsibility for the client's property.

Evaluation

- The five rights are upheld.
- A sufficient amount of the drug is distributed within the nose.
- The client reports decreased nasal congestion.

Document

- Assessment data
- Medication administration on the MAR

SAMPLE DOCUMENTATION

Date and Time Indicates nasal passages are congested. Observed to be breathing through the mouth. Nasal medication administered (see MAR). States symptoms are relieved. ———————— SIGNATURE/TITLE

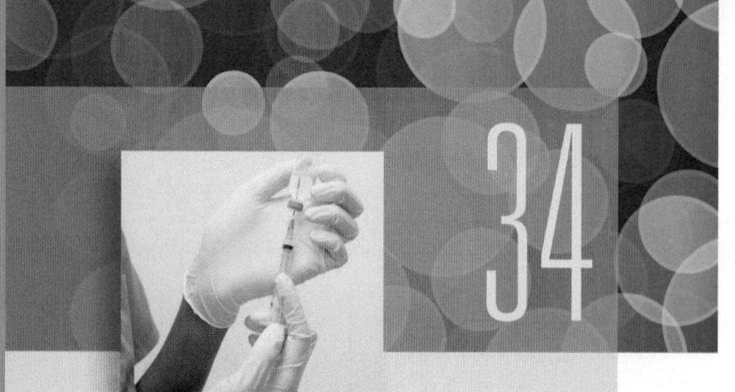

34 Parenteral Medications

Words To Know

ampule
barrel
deltoid site
dorsogluteal site
gauge
induration
insulin syringe
intradermal injection
intramuscular injection
intravenous injection
lipoatrophy
lipohypertrophy
parenteral route
plunger
prefilled cartridge
reconstitution
rectus femoris site
scoop method
shaft
subcutaneous injection
tip
tuberculin syringe
vastus lateralis site
ventrogluteal site
vial
wheal
Z-track technique

Learning Objectives

On completion of this chapter, the reader should be able to:

1. Name three parts of a syringe.
2. List five factors to consider when selecting a syringe and needle.
3. Explain the rationale for redesigning conventional syringes and needles.
4. Name three ways that pharmaceutical companies prepare parenteral drugs.
5. Discuss an appropriate action before combining two drugs in a single syringe.
6. List four injection routes.
7. Identify common sites for intradermal, subcutaneous, and intramuscular injections.
8. Name a type of syringe commonly used to administer an intradermal, subcutaneous, and intramuscular injection.
9. Describe the angles of entry for intradermal, subcutaneous, and intramuscular injections.
10. Discuss why most insulin combinations must be administered within 15 minutes of being mixed.
11. Describe two techniques for preventing bruising when administering heparin subcutaneously.

The **parenteral route** means a route of drug administration other than oral or through the gastrointestinal tract. This term is commonly used when referring to medications given by injection. This chapter discusses techniques for administering injections. The preparation and administration of injections follow the principles of asepsis and infection control.

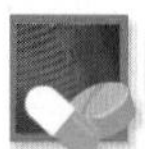

Pharmacologic Considerations

- Age-related changes and possible chronic diseases may impair the older person's ability to absorb and metabolize medications. A lower dose of parenteral medications may be indicated to prevent adverse effects.
- An assessment of an adverse drug effect should be considered when any change in mental status or behavior coincides with the administration of a new medication, regardless of the route of administration.

PARENTERAL ADMINISTRATION EQUIPMENT

The major equipment used to administer parenteral drugs consists of a syringe and a needle. Numerous types of syringes and needles are available.

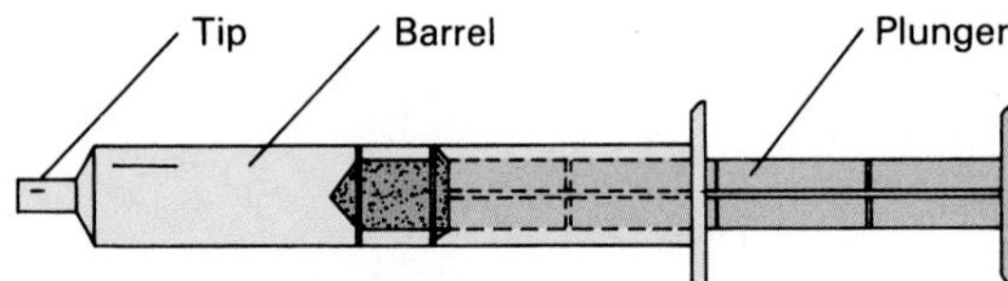

FIGURE 34-1 The parts of a syringe.

Syringes

All syringes contain a **barrel** (the part of the syringe that holds the medication), a **plunger** (the part of the syringe within the barrel that moves back and forth to withdraw and instill the medication), and a **tip** or hub (the part of the syringe to which the needle is attached; Fig. 34-1). Syringes are calibrated in milliliters (mL) or cubic centimeters (cc), and units (U).

Some syringes may still identify calibrations in minims (m), a measurement that is no longer used. When drugs are administered parenterally, syringes that hold 1 mL, or its equivalent in units, and up to 3 to 5 mL are used most commonly.

Needles

Needles are supplied in various lengths and gauges. The **shaft** (the length of the needle) depends on the depth to which the medication will be instilled. Needle lengths vary from approximately ½ to 2½ in. The tip of the shaft is beveled, or slanted, to pierce the skin more easily (see Skill 16-3, Starting an Intravenous Infusion). Filter needles that provide a barrier for glass particles are available when withdrawing medication from a glass ampule. Ampules are discussed later in this chapter.

The needle **gauge** (diameter) refers to its width. For most injections, 18- to 27-gauge needles are used; the smaller the number, the larger the diameter. For example, an 18-gauge needle is wider than a 27-gauge needle. A wider diameter provides a larger lumen, or opening, through which drugs are administered into the tissue.

Several factors are considered when selecting a syringe and needle:

- The type of medication
- The depth of tissue
- The volume of prescribed drug
- The viscosity of the drug
- The size of the client

Table 34-1 lists common sizes of syringes and needles used for various types of injections.

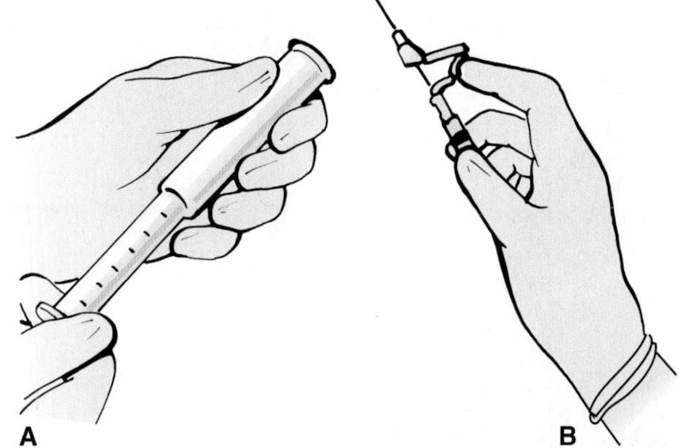

FIGURE 34-2 Safety injection devices. **A.** A syringe with a circular sleeve that covers the needle. **B.** A syringe with an articulated levered shield that glides over the needle after it is used.

Modified Safety Injection Equipment

Conventional syringes and needles are being redesigned to avoid needlestick injuries and, thus, to reduce the risk of acquiring a blood-borne viral disease such as hepatitis or AIDS. Currently, there are three different safety injection devices: (1) those with plastic shields that cover the needle after its use (Fig. 34-2), (2) those with needles that retract into the syringe, and (3) gas-pressured devices that inject medications without needles. Most health agencies already are using one or several types of modified equipment to enclose or cover the needle. Some syringes contain blunt substitutes for needles that can pierce laser-cut rubber ports. Twenty-one states now require safety needles or needleless devices for administering medications and withdrawing bodily fluids since California enacted legislation for using safer needles in 1998 (National Institute for Occupational Safety and Health, 2009).

If modified safety injection devices are not available, two techniques are used with standard equipment to prevent needlestick injuries. *Before administering an injection,* the protective cap covering a needle is replaced by using the **scoop method** (the technique of threading the needle within the cap without touching the cap itself; Fig. 34-3). *After administering an injection,* the needle is left uncapped and deposited in the nearest biohazard container, which is usually at the client's bedside.

Should an accidental injury occur, health care workers should follow these recommendations:

- Report the injury to a supervisor.
- Document the injury in writing.

TABLE 34-1 Common Sizes of Syringes and Needles

TYPE OF INJECTION	SIZES OF SYRINGES	SIZES OF NEEDLES
Intradermal (tuberculin)	1 mL calibrated in 0.01 mL or in minims	25, 26, or 27 gauge, ½- to ⅝-in.
Subcutaneous	1, 2, 2.5, or 3 mL calibrated in 0.1 mL	23, 25, or 26 gauge, ½- or ⅝-in.
Insulin, given subcutaneously	1 mL calibrated in units	25, 2, or 27 gauge, ½- or ⅝-in.
Intramuscular	3 or 5 mL calibrated in 0.2 mL	20, 21, 22, or 23 gauge, 1½- or 2-in.

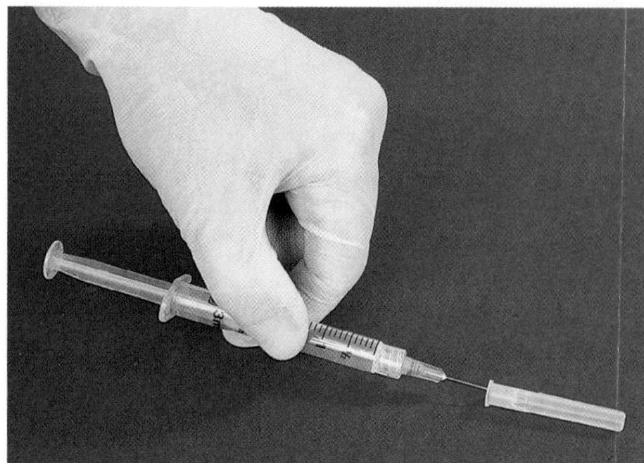

FIGURE 34-3 The scoop method for covering a needle. (Photo by B. Proud.)

- Identify the client if possible.
- Obtain HIV and hepatitis B virus client status results, if it is legal to do so.
- Obtain counseling on the potential for infection.
- Receive the most appropriate postexposure drug treatment prophylaxis.
- Be tested for the presence of antibodies at appropriate intervals.
- Monitor for potential symptoms and obtain a medical follow-up.

DRUG PREPARATION

Drug preparation involves withdrawing medication from an ampule or vial or assembling a prefilled syringe cartridge (Fig. 34-4).

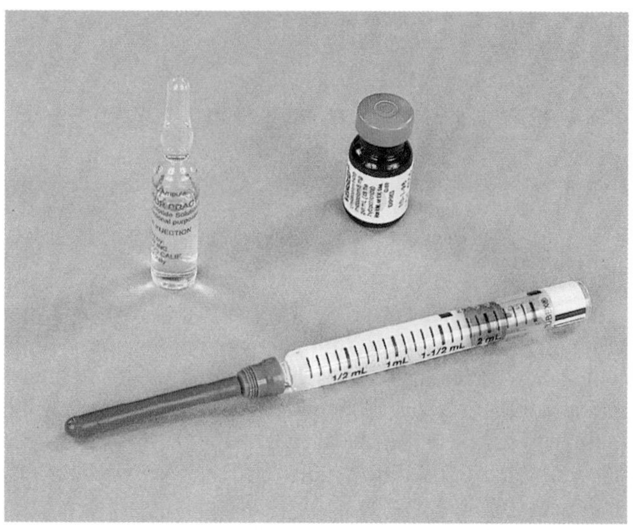

FIGURE 34-4 An ampule, a vial, and a prefilled cartridge. (Photo by B. Proud.)

Ampules

An **ampule** (a sealed glass drug container) must be broken to withdraw the medication (see Nursing Guidelines 34-1 and Fig. 34-5).

Vials

A **vial** (a glass or plastic container of parenteral medication with a self-sealing rubber stopper) must be pierced with a needle or a needleless adapter to remove medication. The amount of drug in a vial may be enough for one or multiple doses. Any unused drug is dated before it is stored for future use (see Nursing Guidelines 34-2 and Fig. 34-6).

Usually, drugs in vials are in liquid form, but sometimes they are supplied as powders that must be dissolved. **Reconstitution** (the process of adding liquid, known as diluent,

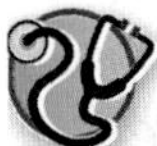

NURSING GUIDELINES 34-1

Withdrawing Medication from an Ampule

- Select an appropriate syringe and filter needle. *Proper equipment ensures appropriate drug administration and prevents aspirating glass particles within the barrel of the syringe.*
- Tap the top of the ampule. *Tapping distributes all the medication to the lower portion of the ampule.*
- Protect your thumb and fingers with a gauze square or alcohol swab. *These devices reduce the potential for injury.*
- Snap the neck of the ampule away from your body. *Doing so avoids accidental injury.*
- Insert the filter needle into the ampule. Avoid touching the outside of the ampule. *These methods ensure sterility of the needle.*
- Invert the ampule (see Fig. 34-5). *Inversion facilitates withdrawing the medication.*
- Pull back on the plunger. *This step fills the syringe.*
- Remove the needle from the ampule when the volume has been withdrawn. *This prepares for drug administration.*
- Tap the barrel of the syringe near the hub. *Tapping moves air toward the needle.*
- Push carefully on the plunger. *Pushing expels air or excess medication.*
- Empty the unused portion of medication from the syringe. *Doing so prevents illegal drug use.*
- Discard the glass ampule in a puncture-resistant container. *Proper disposal prevents accidental injury.*
- Remove the filter needle and attach a sterile needle for administering the injection. *These techniques prevent injecting glass particles into the client.*
- Scoop the needle within its protective cap or extend a guard that recesses the needle. *These measures reduce the risk of a needlestick injury.*

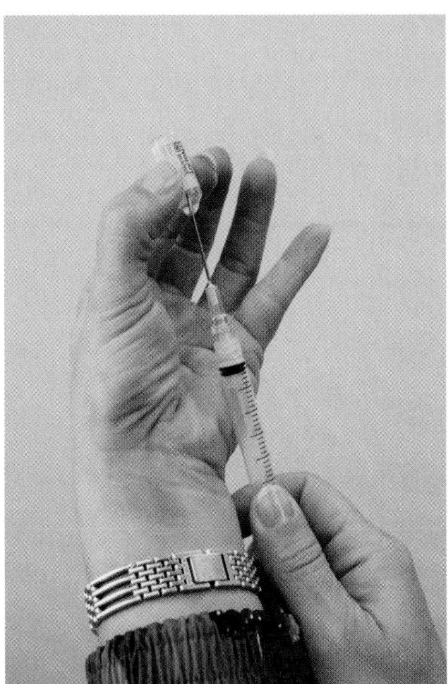

FIGURE 34-5 Withdrawing the drug from an ampule.

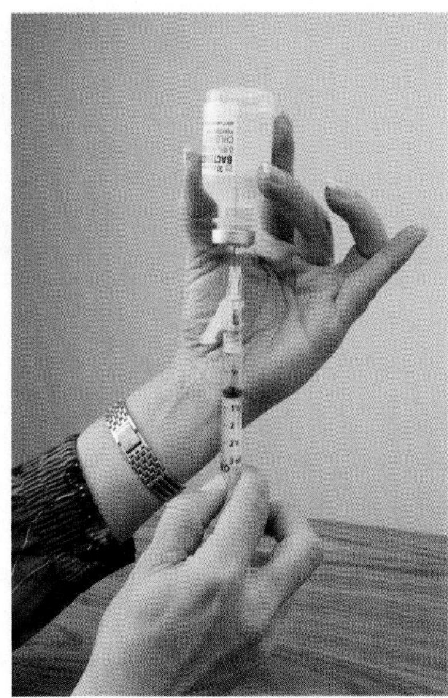

FIGURE 34-6 Withdrawing the drug from a vial.

to a powdered substance) is done before administering the drug parenterally. Common diluents for injectable drugs are sterile water or sterile normal saline. Reconstituting a drug just before it is needed ensures maximum potency. When reconstitution is necessary, the drug label lists the following:

- The type of diluent to use
- The amount of diluent to add
- The dosage per volume after reconstitution
- Directions for storing the drug

If the medication will be used for more than one administration, the preparer writes the date and time on the vial label and initials it. In some cases, when the directions provide several options in diluent volumes, the preparer also writes the amount on the vial.

Prefilled Cartridges

Pharmaceutical companies supply some drugs in a **prefilled cartridge** (a sealed glass cylinder of parenteral medication). The cartridge comes with an attached needle. The cylinder is made so that it fits in a specially designed syringe (Fig. 34-7).

Combining Medications in One Syringe

Sometimes it is necessary or appropriate to combine more than one drug in a single syringe. Exact amounts must be withdrawn from each drug container because once the drugs are in the barrel of the syringe, there is no way to expel one without expelling some of the other (see section on Mixing

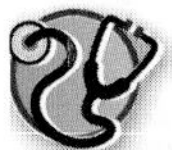

NURSING GUIDELINES 34-2

Withdrawing Medication from a Vial

- Select an appropriate syringe and needle. *The correct equipment ensures appropriate drug administration.*
- Remove the metal cover from the rubber stopper. *This step facilitates inserting the needle or needleless adaptor.*
- Clean a preopened vial with an alcohol swab. *Alcohol swabs remove colonizing microorganisms.*
- Fill the syringe with a volume of air equal to the volume that will be withdrawn from the vial. *This step provides a means for increasing pressure within the vial.*
- Pierce the rubber stopper with the needle or tip of a needleless syringe and instill the air. *Doing so facilitates the withdrawal of the drug.*
- Invert the vial, hold, and brace it while pulling on the plunger (see Fig. 34-6). *This step locates medication near the tip of the needle or needleless adaptor to facilitate its withdrawal.*
- Remove the needle or adaptor when the desired volume has entered the barrel of the syringe. *Doing so leaves the remaining drug for additional administrations.*
- If the medication is a controlled substance such as a narcotic, aspirate the entire contents from the vial. *Full aspiration prevents illegal drug use.*
- Discard any excess medication; if the drug is a narcotic, have someone witness this action. *These measures comply with federal laws to prevent illegal drug use.*
- Cover the needle or needleless adaptor and care for the used supplies as described in the guidelines for withdrawing from an ampule. *Nurses follow aseptic and safety principles.*
- Date and initial the vial if the remaining drug will be used in the near future. *Doing so supports the principles of asepsis.*

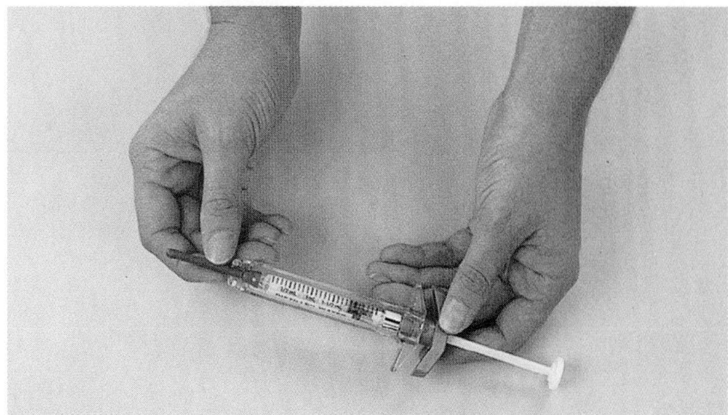

FIGURE 34-7 Inserting a prefilled cartridge. (Photo by B. Proud.)

Insulins). Before mixing any drugs, however, the nurse consults a drug reference or compatibility chart because some drugs interact chemically when combined. The chemical reaction often causes formation of a precipitate.

INJECTION ROUTES

There are four injection routes for parenteral administration: **intradermal injections** (injections between the layers of the skin), **subcutaneous injections** (injections beneath the skin but above the muscle), **intramuscular injections** (injections in muscle tissue), and **intravenous injections** (injections instilled into veins; Fig. 34-8). Each site requires a slightly different injection technique. Intravenous medication administration is discussed in Chapter 35.

Intradermal Injections

Intradermal injections are commonly used for diagnostic purposes. Examples include tuberculin tests and allergy testing. Small volumes, usually 0.01 to 0.05 mL, are injected because of the small tissue space.

Injection Sites

A common site for an intradermal injection is the inner aspect of the forearm. Other areas that may be used are the back and upper chest.

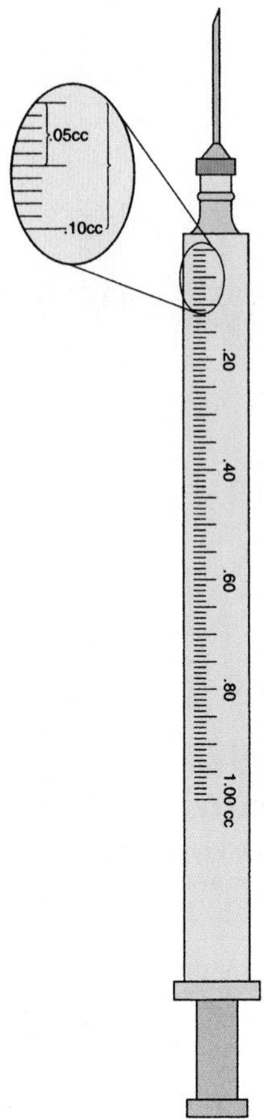

FIGURE 34-9 A tuberculin syringe.

Injection Equipment

A **tuberculin syringe** holds 1 mL of fluid and is calibrated in 0.01-mL increments (Fig. 34-9). It is used to administer intradermal injections. A 25- to 27-gauge needle measuring a half-inch in length is commonly used when administering an intradermal injection.

Injection Technique

When giving an intradermal injection, the nurse instills the medication shallowly at a 10- to 15-degree angle of entry (Skill 34-1).

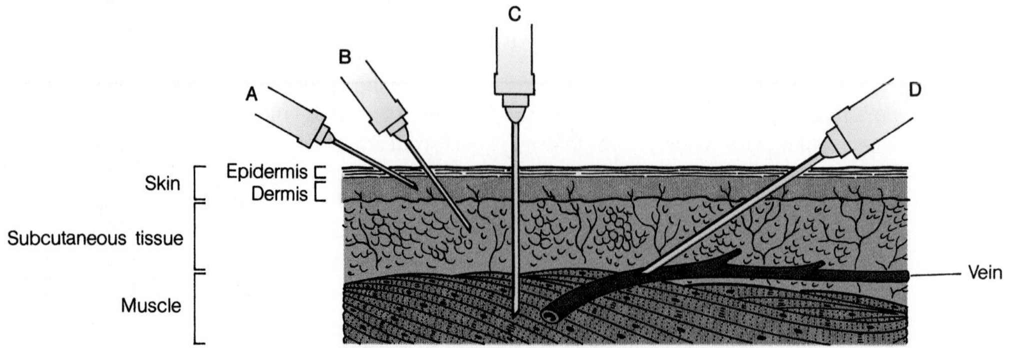

FIGURE 34-8 Injection routes: intradermal (**A**), subcutaneous (**B**), intramuscular and subcutaneous in other than thin persons (**C**), and intravenous (**D**).

Stop, Think, and Respond Box 34-1

What actions are appropriate if the client shows signs of an allergic reaction to an agent given intradermally?

Subcutaneous Injections

A subcutaneous injection is administered more deeply than an intradermal injection. Medication is instilled between the skin and muscle and absorbed fairly rapidly: the medication usually begins acting within 15 to 30 minutes of administration. The volume of a subcutaneous injection is usually up to 1 mL. The subcutaneous route is commonly used to administer insulin and heparin.

Injection Sites

The preferred site for giving a subcutaneous injection of insulin and heparin is the abdomen. When using the abdomen, avoid a 2-in. central area around the umbilicus. Additional or alternative injection sites for insulin are the outer back area of the upper arm, where it is fleshier, and the outer areas of the thigh and upper buttocks. Subcutaneous injection sites are shown in Figure 34-10.

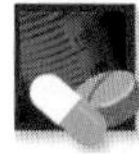

Pharmacologic Considerations

- Insulin is absorbed at a more consistent rate from one injection to the next when the abdominal site is used. Exercising an arm or leg after an injection can increase blood flow and hasten insulin absorption from those areas (Diabetes Self-Management, 2006).

Rotating within one injection site, preferably the abdomen, is recommended rather than rotating to a different area with each injection (American Diabetes Association, 2007). Injection sites are rotated a finger's width apart (about 1 in.) from a previous site to avoid repeatedly injecting into the same area in a short amount of time. Rotating sites avoids tissue injury. The rate of drug absorption at various subcutaneous sites from fastest to slowest is the abdomen, arms, thighs, and upper buttocks.

Injection Equipment

Equipment used for a subcutaneous injection may depend on the type of medication prescribed. Insulin is prepared in an **insulin syringe** (see section on Administering Insulin).

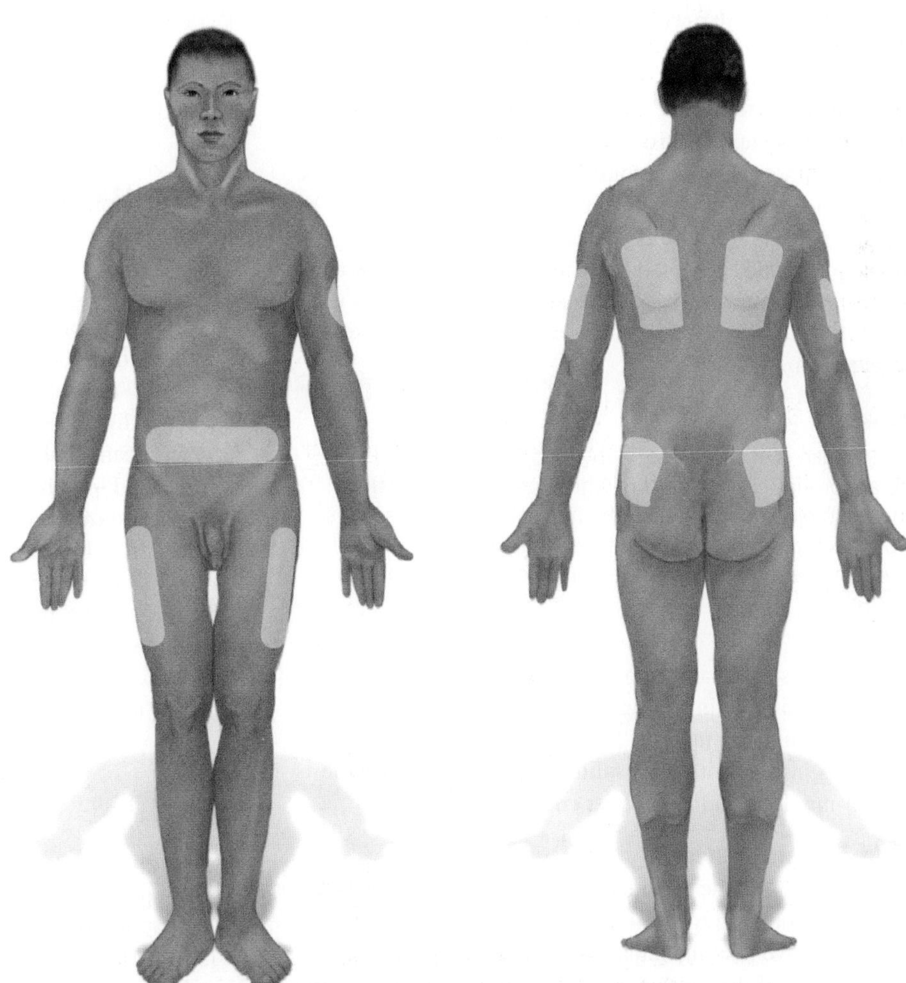

FIGURE 34-10 Subcutaneous injection sites.

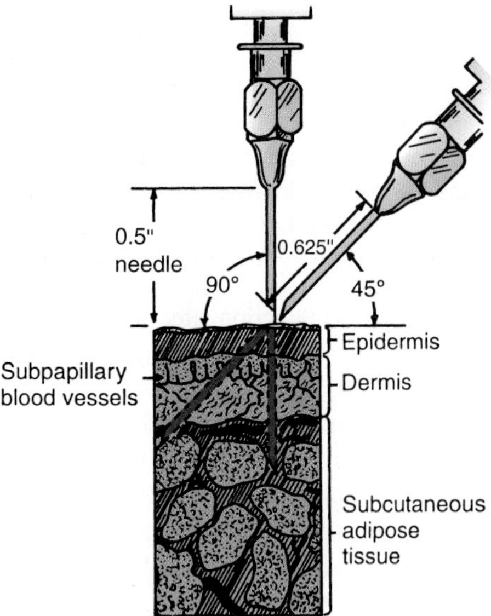

FIGURE 34-11 Angles and needle lengths for subcutaneous injections.

Heparin is prepared in a tuberculin syringe, or it may be supplied in a prefilled cartridge. A 25-gauge needle is used most often because medications administered subcutaneously usually are not viscous. Needle lengths may vary from ½ to ⅝ in.

Injection Technique

To reach subcutaneous tissue in a normal-sized or obese person who has a 2-in. tissue fold when it is bunched, the nurse inserts the needle at a 90-degree angle. For thin clients who have a 1-in. fold of tissue, the nurse inserts the needle at a 45-degree angle (Fig. 34-11). Skill 34-2 describes the technique for administering a subcutaneous injection.

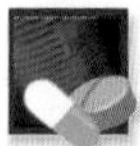

Pharmacologic Considerations

- If insulin is injected too deeply and reaches the muscle, its absorption is accelerated, which increases the risk of lowering blood sugar below the normal range. If insulin is not injected deeply enough, it may leak from the site, thus reducing its effectiveness (Becton, Dickinson, & Company, 2008).

The tissue usually is bunched between the thumb and fingers before administering the injection to avoid instilling insulin within the muscle. Bunching is unnecessary when injecting insulin with an insulin pen because the needle is only 5-mm long and unlikely to enter a muscle.

Administering Insulin

Insulin is a hormone required by some clients with diabetes. The most common route of administration is by subcutaneous or intravenous injection. Injectable insulin is supplied and prescribed in a dosage strength called units (U); a special syringe called an insulin syringe (a syringe calibrated in units) is used. Various insulin syringes hold volumes of 0.3, 0.5, and 1 mL. The standard dosage strength of insulin is 100 U/mL. Typically, low-dose insulin syringes are used to deliver insulin dosages of 30 to 50 U or less. A standard insulin syringe can administer up to 100 U of insulin (Fig. 34-12).

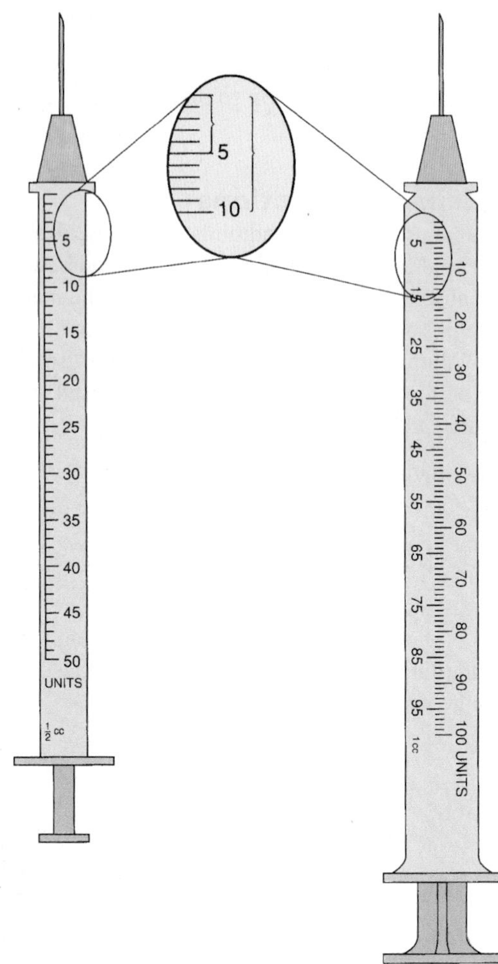

FIGURE 34-12 Low-dose and standard insulin syringes.

Prefilled pen-like devices that facilitate the repeated administration of insulin through a special pen needle are also available. Depending on the manufacturer, insulin pens can be adjusted to provide insulin in doses from 0.5 to 80 U by dialing the prescribed amount on the pen. The pen generally holds 1 mL (100 U) of insulin. Only the needle is changed with each injection. The insulin in prefilled pens is stable for up to 30 days.

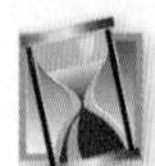

Gerontologic Considerations

- Older clients with diabetes often have visual problems interfering with their ability to fill their own syringe. They are candidates for using an insulin pen or a loading gauge that prevents filling a syringe with more than the prescribed dose. Sight centers are a good resource for obtaining assistive devices to facilitate self-administration of insulin.

■ Older adults learning to administer insulin may benefit from a referral for skilled nursing or diabetic health education following discharge. Health insurance companies sometimes reimburse such services.

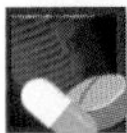

Pharmacologic Considerations

■ Containers of insulin are refrigerated *until they are opened;* thereafter, they are stored at room temperature.

■ Some experts recommend leaving the needle in place following the injection of insulin for 5 to 10 seconds to ensure that all the insulin is within the injection site and will not be lost due to leakage from the skin (Samuels, 2009; Wolfe, 2006).

■ The needle on an insulin pen should be removed immediately after use. If left in place, air bubbles may enter the syringe and reduce the next dose.

Clients who require insulin receive one or more daily injections. Over time, the injection sites tend to undergo changes that interfere with insulin absorption. To avoid **lipoatrophy** (the breakdown of subcutaneous fat at the site of repeated insulin injections) and **lipohypertrophy** (the thickening of subcutaneous fat at the site of repeated insulin injections), the sites are rotated each time an injection is administered.

Stop, Think, and Respond Box 34-2

In addition to documenting the site of an insulin injection, discuss additional techniques for ensuring a rotation of sites with each subsequent injection.

Preparing Insulin

Types of insulin vary in their onset, peak effect, and duration of action. The nurse must read the vial labels carefully because they look similar.

Some preparations of insulin contain an additive that delays its absorption. Insulin and the additive tend to separate on standing. Therefore, when preparing other than rapid-acting and short-acting insulin or the long-acting insulin glargine (Lantus), the nurse rotates the vial between the palms to redistribute the additive and insulin before filling the syringe.

Mixing Insulins

When mixed together, insulins tend to bind and become equilibrated. This means that the unique characteristics of each are offset by those of the other. For this reason, most types of insulin are combined just before administration. When injected within 15 minutes of being combined, they act as if they had been injected separately. Rapid-acting insulin and short-acting insulin, which are additive free, are often combined with an intermediate-acting insulin. The long-acting insulin, glargine, is never mixed with any other type of insulin (see Nursing Guidelines 34-3 and Fig. 34-13).

Pharmaceutical companies provide some combinations of insulin premixed in a single vial. Novolin 70/30 contains 70% of an intermediate-acting insulin and 30% of a short-acting insulin. Humulin 50/50 contains equal amounts of intermediate-acting and short-acting insulin. Commercially premixed insulins are stable and can be administered without concern for time after withdrawal from the vial.

Administering Heparin

Heparin is an anticoagulant drug, meaning that it prolongs the time it takes for blood to clot. Heparin frequently is administered subcutaneously as well as intravenously. Its

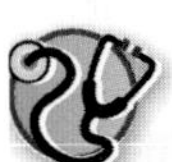

NURSING GUIDELINES 34-3

Mixing Insulins

- Roll the vial of insulin containing an additive between the palms. *Rolling between the palms mixes the insulin without damaging the protein molecules.*
- Cleanse the rubber stoppers of both vials of insulin. *Cleaning removes colonizing microorganisms.*
- Instill an amount of air equal to the volume that will be withdrawn from the vial containing the insulin with the additive. Do not insert the needle into the insulin itself (see Fig. 34-13A, B). *These measures avoid coating the needle.*
- Withdraw the needle and use the same syringe to repeat the previous step, but this time invert and withdraw the prescribed number of additive-free insulin units (see Fig. 34-13C). *Clear insulin is always placed in the syringe before adding the cloudy insulin to avoid altering the additive-free insulin within the vial.*
- Ask another nurse to check the label on the insulin and the number of units in the syringe. *An additional check helps to prevent a medication error.*
- Swab the rubber stopper of the other vial and pierce it with the needle of the partially filled syringe. *This step facilitates withdrawing the other type of insulin.*
- Withdraw the specified number of units from the vial containing the insulin with the additive. *Doing so prepares the full prescribed dose.*
- Ask another nurse to check the label on the insulin and the number of units in the syringe. *This step prevents a medication error.*
- Administer within 15 minutes of mixing. *Prompt administration avoids equilibration.*

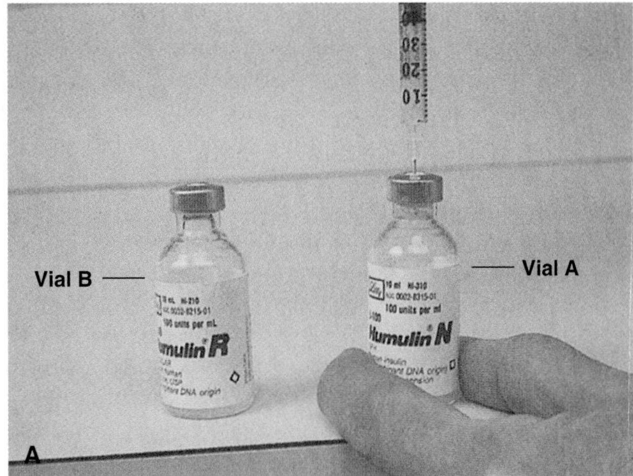

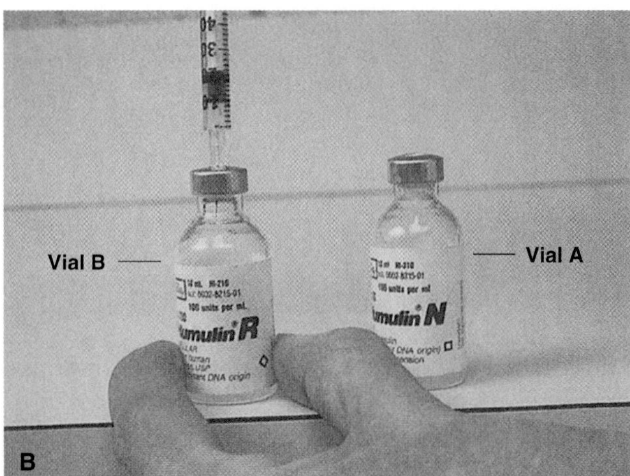

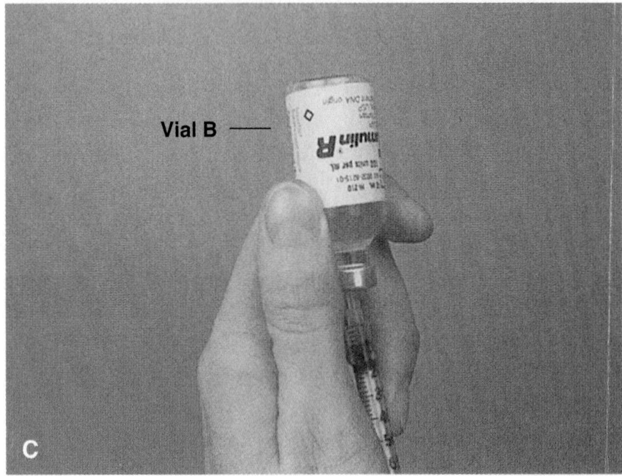

FIGURE 34-13 Mixing insulin. **A.** Instilling air into a vial with additive insulin. **B.** Instilling air into the additive free insulin. **C.** Withdrawing from an additive-free insulin vial.

unique characteristics require special techniques when using the subcutaneous route for administration.

Heparin is supplied in multiple-dose vials or prefilled cartridges. The dosages are very small volumes that may require a tuberculin syringe to ensure accuracy. The nurse removes the needle after withdrawal of the drug from a multidose vial and replaces it with another before administration.

Certain modifications are necessary for the prevention of bruising in the area of the injection. The nurse changes the needle after filling the syringe with the dose of heparin, that is, before injecting the client. He or she rotates the sites with each injection to avoid a previous area where there has been local bleeding. The nurse does not aspirate the plunger once the needle is in place. Massaging the site is contraindicated because this can increase the tendency for local bleeding.

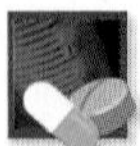

Pharmacologic Considerations

- The dose of unfractionated (standard) heparin may change on a daily or even hourly basis depending on the route of administration. The dose is determined after reporting laboratory test results of the client's partial thromboplastin time to the physician.
- Some clients are prescribed one of several low-molecular weight heparins (LMWH) such as enoxaparin (Lovenox). LMWH has the advantage of being prescribed in a consistent daily dose with no or fewer required anticoagulation blood tests, less risk for side effects than standard heparin, and it can be self-administered outside the hospital.

Intramuscular Injections

An intramuscular injection is the administration of up to 3 mL of medication into one muscle or muscle group. Because deep muscles have few nerve endings, irritating medications commonly are given intramuscularly. Except for medications injected directly into the bloodstream, absorption from an intramuscular injection occurs more rapidly than from the other parenteral routes. Injections should not be administered into limbs that are paralyzed, inactive, or affected by poor circulation. If an older client has had a mastectomy or has a vascular site for hemodialysis, the arm on the affected side should be avoided, if possible.

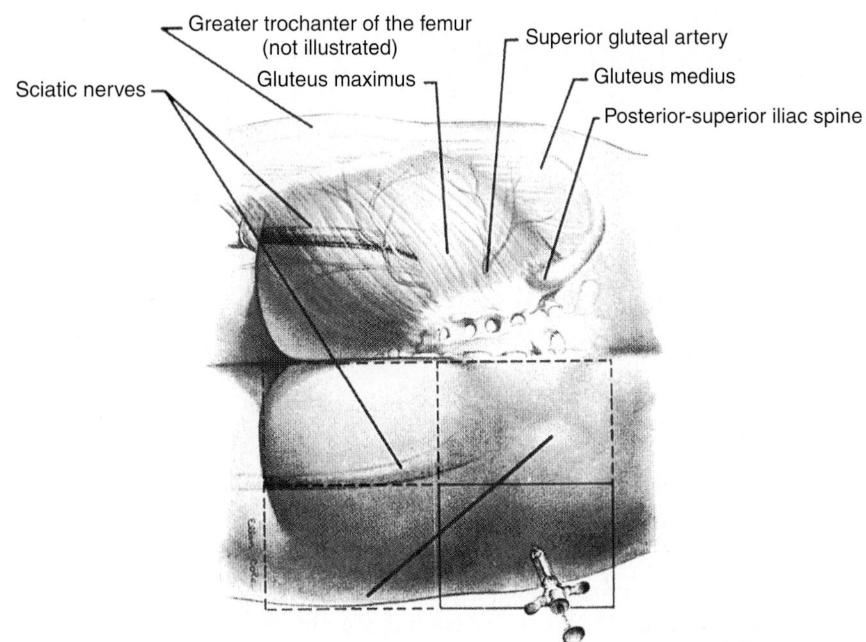

FIGURE 34-14 The dorsogluteal site. (Courtesy of Wyeth Laboratories, Philadelphia, PA.)

Injection Sites

The five common intramuscular injection sites are named for the muscles into which the medications are injected: the dorsogluteal, the ventrogluteal, the vastus lateralis, the rectus femoris, and the deltoid.

Dorsogluteal Site

The **dorsogluteal site** is the upper outer quadrant of the buttocks. The primary muscle in this site is the gluteus maximus, which is large and therefore can hold a fair amount of injected medication with minimal postinjection discomfort. This site is avoided in clients younger than 3 years of age because this muscle is not yet sufficiently developed.

If the dorsogluteal site is not identified correctly, damage to the sciatic nerve with subsequent paralysis of the leg can result. To locate the appropriate landmarks, perform the following (Fig. 34-14):

- Divide the buttock into four imaginary quadrants.
- Palpate the posterior iliac spine and the greater trochanter.
- Draw an imaginary diagonal line between the two landmarks.
- Insert the needle superiorly and laterally to the midpoint of the diagonal line.

Ventrogluteal Site

The **ventrogluteal site** uses the gluteus medius and gluteus minimus muscles in the hip for injection. This site has several advantages over the dorsogluteal site: it has no large nerves or blood vessels, and it is usually less fatty and

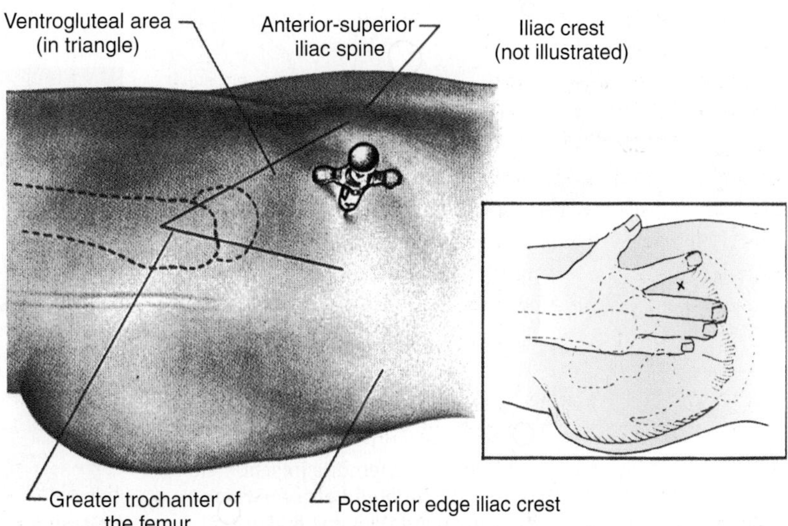

FIGURE 34-15 The ventrogluteal site. (Courtesy of Wyeth Laboratories, Philadelphia, PA.)

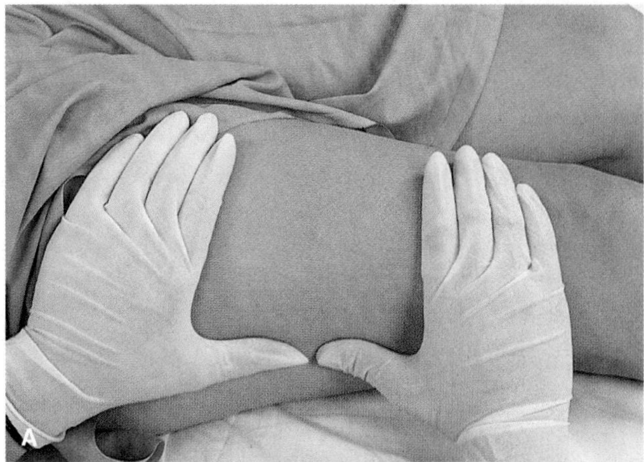

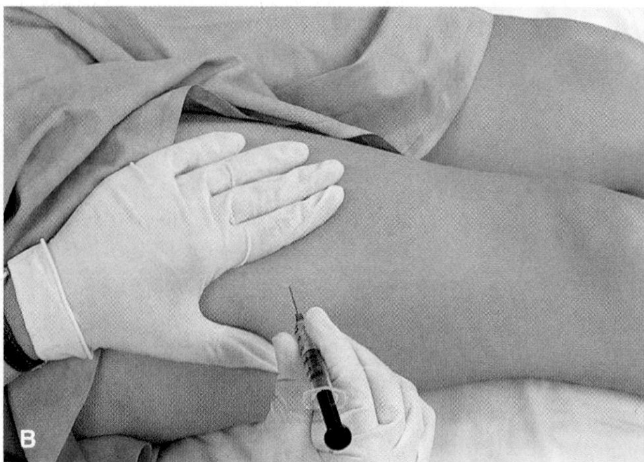

FIGURE 34-16 **A.** Locating the vastus lateralis muscle. **B.** Spreading the skin at the vastus lateralis site and darting the tissue. (Photo by B. Proud.)

cleaner because fecal contamination is rare at this site. This is the favored injection site for adults, but it is also safe for use in children. Its main disadvantage is that there is only a small area for administering the injection (Hunt, 2008).

To locate the ventrogluteal site:

- Place the palm of the hand on the greater trochanter and the index finger on the anterior-superior iliac spine (Fig. 34-15).
- Move the middle finger away from the index finger as far as possible along the iliac crest.
- Inject into the center of the triangle formed by the index finger, the middle finger, and the iliac crest.

Vastus Lateralis Site

The **vastus lateralis site** uses the vastus lateralis muscle—one of the muscles in the quadriceps group of the outer thigh. Large nerves and blood vessels usually are absent in this area, which makes it safer. It is a particularly desirable site for administering injections to infants and small children and clients who are thin or debilitated with poorly developed gluteal muscles.

The nurse locates the vastus lateralis site by placing one hand above the knee and one hand just below the greater trochanter at the top of the thigh. He or she then inserts the needle into the lateral area of the thigh (Fig. 34-16).

Rectus Femoris Site

The **rectus femoris site** is in the anterior aspect of the thigh. This site may be used for infants. The nurse places an injection in this site in the middle third of the thigh, with the client sitting or supine (Fig. 34-17).

Deltoid Site

The **deltoid site,** in the lateral aspect of the upper arm (Fig. 34-18), is the least used intramuscular injection site because it is a smaller muscle than the others. It is used only for adults because the muscle is not sufficiently developed in infants and children. Because of its small capacity,

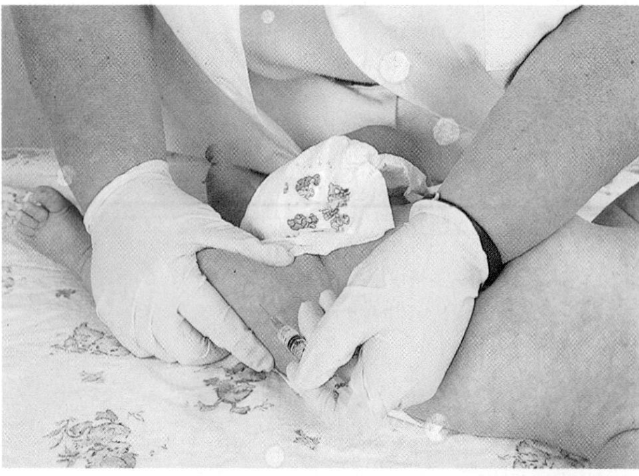

FIGURE 34-17 The location of the rectus femoris injection site. (Craven, R.F., & Hirnle, C.J. [2009]. *Fundamentals of nursing* [6th ed., p 530]. Philadelphia: Lippincott Williams & Wilkins.)

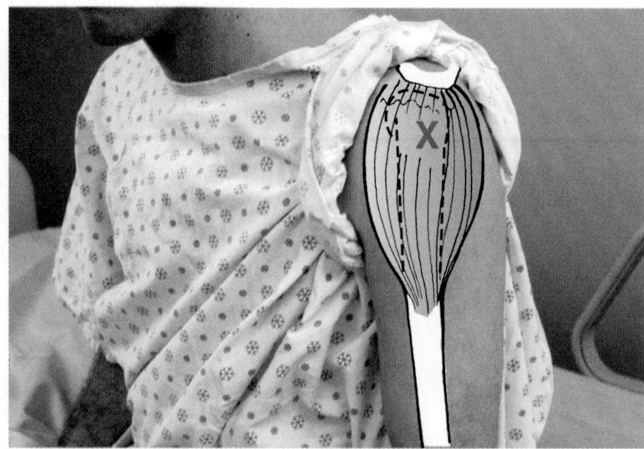

FIGURE 34-18 The deltoid site.

intramuscular injections into this site are limited to 1 mL of solution.

There is a risk of damaging the radial nerve and artery if the deltoid site is not well identified. To use this site safely:

- Have the client lie down, sit, or stand with the shoulder well exposed.
- Palpate the lower edge of the acromion process.
- Draw an imaginary line at the axilla.
- Inject in the area between these two landmarks.

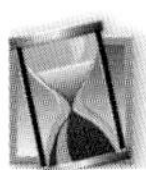

Gerontologic Considerations

■ Selection and identification of injection site landmarks may be difficult when working with older adults experiencing dementia or musculoskeletal deformities such as contractures. Assistance from a second person to maintain the required position for an injection may be helpful. An explanation of what will be done is always indicated before the intervention. The second person may be able to assist with providing comfort.
■ If an older person has decreased subcutaneous fat, pinching the muscular tissue together may be needed to avoid striking bone when administering an intramuscular injection.
■ The deltoid or ventrogluteal muscles may be the preferred intramuscular sites for older adults experiencing impaired mobility. The dorsogluteal site should be avoided because of the risk for damage to the sciatic nerve with diminished musculature.

Injection Equipment

Generally, 3- to 5-mL syringes are used to administer medications by the intramuscular route. A 22-gauge needle that is 1½ to 2 in. long is usually adequate for depositing medication in most sites.

Injection Technique

When administering intramuscular injections, nurses use a 90-degree angle for piercing the skin (Skill 34-3). Nurses may administer drugs that may be irritating to the upper levels of tissue by the **Z-track technique** (a technique for manipulating the tissue to seal a medication, especially an irritant, in the muscle). Sometimes called the zigzag technique, the maneuver resembles the letter Z (see Nursing Guidelines 34-4 and Fig. 34-19).

Nurses can give any intramuscular injection by the Z-track technique. Clients report slightly less pain during and the next day after a Z-track injection compared with the usual intramuscular injection technique.

Stop, Think, and Respond Box 34-3

What could occur if parenteral medication intended for the intramuscular route is instilled into a blood vessel? How could this be prevented?

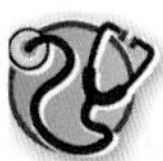

NURSING GUIDELINES 34-4

Giving an Injection by the Z-Track Technique

- Fill the syringe with the prepared drug and then change the needle. *This measure prevents tissue contact with the irritating drug.*
- Attach a needle at least 1½ to 2 in. long. *The correct needle length helps to deposit the drug deep within the muscle.*
- Add a 0.2-mL bubble of air in the syringe. *Air flushes all the medication from the syringe during the injection.*
- Select a large muscular injection site such as the ventrogluteal site. *A large site provides a location with the capacity for depositing and absorbing the drug.*
- Wash your hands and don gloves. *These measures reduce the transmission of microorganisms.*
- Use the side of the hand to pull the tissue laterally about 1 in. (2.5 cm) until the tissue is taut (see Fig. 34-19A). *Taut tissue creates the mechanism for sealing the drug within the muscle.*
- Insert the needle at a 90-degree angle while continuing to hold the tissue laterally. *Correct placement directs the tip of the needle well within the muscle.*
- Steady the barrel of the syringe with the fingers and use the thumb to manipulate the plunger (see Fig. 34-19B). *These measures avoid releasing the tissue held taut by the nondominant hand.*
- Aspirate for a blood return. *Doing so determines whether or not the needle is in a blood vessel.*
- Instill the medication by depressing the plunger with the thumb. *This measure deposits the medication into the muscle.*
- Wait 10 seconds with the needle still in place and the skin held taut. *This duration provides time to distribute the medication in a larger area.*
- Withdraw the needle and immediately release the taut skin. *Doing so creates a diagonal path that prevents leaking into the subcutaneous and dermal layers of tissue* (see Fig. 34-19C).
- Apply pressure, but do not massage the site. *This ensures that the medication remains sealed.*
- Discard the syringe without recapping the needle. *Proper disposal reduces the potential for a needlestick injury.*
- Remove gloves and wash your hands or perform an alcohol-based hand rub. *These measures reduce the transmission of microorganisms.*
- Document the medication administration. *Proper recording maintains a current record of client care.*

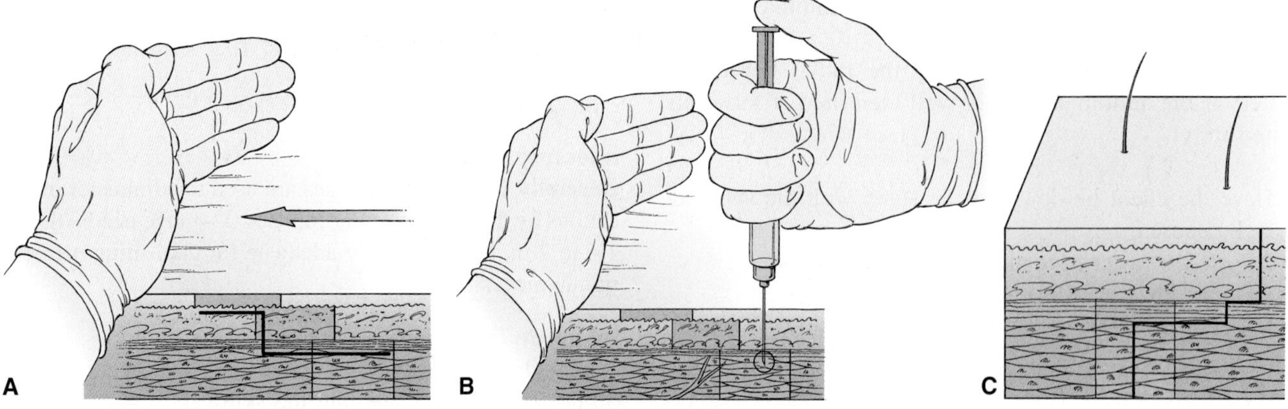

FIGURE 34-19 A. Stretching the tissue laterally. **B.** Manipulating the plunger. **C.** An interrupted pathway to the sealed medication.

REDUCING INJECTION DISCOMFORT

All injections cause discomfort, and some cause more than others. The nurse can use the following alternative techniques to reduce discomfort associated with injections:

- Use the smallest gauge needle that is appropriate.
- Change the needle before administering a drug that is irritating to tissue.
- Select a site that is free of irritation.
- Rotate injection sites.
- Numb the skin with an ice pack before the injection.
- Insert and withdraw the needle without hesitation.
- Instill the medication slowly and steadily.
- Use the Z-track technique for intramuscular injections.
- Apply pressure to the site during needle withdrawal.
- Massage the site afterward, if appropriate.

The client also can assist in minimizing the pain associated with injections. Instructions commonly focus on positioning and relaxation techniques (see Client and Family Teaching 34-1).

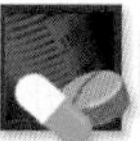

Pharmacologic Considerations

■ A few products are available that produce anesthesia when applied to the skin or mucous membranes. One example is eutectic mixture of local anesthetic (EMLA), which reduces or eliminates the local discomfort of invasive procedures that pierce the skin. It can take 60 to 120 minutes after application for EMLA cream to take effect. These time constraints make EMLA impractical for most situations when time is of the essence in administering an injection.

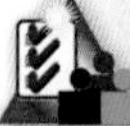

Client and Family Teaching 34-1
Reducing Injection Discomfort

The nurse teaches the client and the family as follows:

- Lie prone and point the toes inward when receiving an injection into the dorsogluteal site.
- Perform deep breathing and other relaxation techniques before receiving an injection.
- Avoid watching when the injection is given.
- Ambulate or move the extremity where the injection was given as much as possible.

NURSING IMPLICATIONS

Nurses who administer parenteral medications may identify nursing diagnoses as follows:

- Acute Pain
- Anxiety
- Fear
- Risk for Trauma
- Deficient Knowledge
- Risk for Ineffective Self-Health Management

Nursing Care Plan 34-1 demonstrates the nursing process for a client with the nursing diagnosis Risk for Ineffective Self-Health Management, defined in the NANDA-I taxonomy (2012, p. 161) as "a pattern of regulating and integrating into daily living a program for treatment of illness and its sequelae that is unsatisfactory for meeting specific health goals."

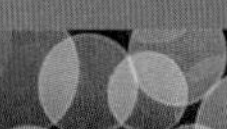

NURSING CARE PLAN 34-1 Risk for Ineffective Self-Health Management

Assessment

- Determine the client's desire to learn about his or her illness.
- Assess the client's ability and interest in managing the disorder.
- Review the client's history for evidence that complications developed from mismanagement of his or her disorder.
- Consider the complexity of self-care skills necessary after the client is discharged.
- Identify any problems that may pose a barrier to carrying out a regimen of self-care (eg, dementia, physical weakness, pain, diminished self-confidence).
- Explore any health beliefs that may cause conflict in achieving the goals of therapy.
- Inquire about the client's financial resources for complying with the health care regimen.
- Observe the client's network of significant others and their potential for providing physical and emotional support.
- Evaluate the client's level of understanding of ongoing health teaching throughout the period of nursing care.

Nursing Diagnosis. **Risk for Ineffective Self-Health Management** related to confusion concerning techniques for balancing insulin therapy and dietary intake.

Expected Outcome. The client will describe the need to eat food within 30 minutes of an insulin injection and ways to raise blood glucose levels if symptoms of hypoglycemia develop.

Interventions	Rationales
Review onset, peak, and duration of Humulin N insulin each morning when administering the client's dose of insulin.	The repetition of information enhances learning.
Emphasize that breakfast is required within 30 minutes of injecting the prescribed dose of insulin.	Demonstrating a regular pattern between administering insulin and eating food shortly afterward reinforces learning.
Assist the client with testing his or her own blood glucose level before and 2 hours after meals.	Testing capillary blood glucose provides objective evidence of the relationship between blood glucose levels before and after eating.
Review the signs and symptoms of low blood glucose level; ask client to recall as many signs and symptoms as possible.	Providing information and testing the client's ability to accurately recall the information measure the client's learning.
Give the client a list of foods or beverages that can raise blood glucose levels when signs or symptoms of low blood glucose level occur.	Identifying techniques for resolving the problem of low blood glucose levels provides the client with options for managing self-care.

Evaluation of Expected Outcomes

- Client noted time of insulin administration at 0730 and delivery of breakfast at 0745.
- Client stated, "I will eat a meal within a half hour of giving myself my morning insulin."
- Client observed that blood glucose level was 98 mg/dL before eating breakfast and increased to 122 mg/dL 2 hours later.
- Client named grape juice, orange juice, regular soft drinks, and LifeSavers as foods or beverages to consume if she experienced symptoms of low blood glucose levels.

CRITICAL THINKING EXERCISES

1. How does administration of an intramuscular injection differ for a 3-year-old client versus a 33-year-old client?
2. You are to administer an intramuscular injection to a 76-year-old client. What factors are important to consider before choosing the equipment and injection site?
3. What information would be appropriate for the nurse to provide to a client who repeatedly administers insulin in nearly the exact same location with each injection?
4. What techniques might a nurse use to avoid injecting into a muscle when giving a thin client a subcutaneous injection?

NCLEX-STYLE REVIEW QUESTIONS

1. The nurse chooses to inject a prescribed intramuscular medication into the dorsogluteal site. If the nurse selects the site correctly, in what location is the injection administered?
   1. Hip
   2. Arm
   3. Thigh
   4. Buttock

2. What is a technique that helps reduce discomfort when giving an intramuscular injection into the dorsogluteal site?
   1. Have the client point the toes inward.
   2. Have the client tighten the gluteal muscles.
   3. Have the client cross the legs at the ankles.
   4. Have the client flex the knees.
3. Just before inserting the needle into the muscle using the Z-track technique, in which direction is the nurse correct in pulling the tissue at the injection site?
   1. Laterally
   2. Diagonally
   3. Downward
   4. Upward
4. When administering an intradermal tuberculin skin test, which angle of needle insertion is correct?
   1. 180-degree angle
   2. 90-degree angle
   3. 45-degree angle
   4. 10-degree angle
5. Which of the following actions best indicates that the client needs more practice to combine two insulins, short- and intermediate-acting, before discharge?
   1. The client rolls the vial of intermediate-acting insulin to mix it with its additive.
   2. The client instills air into the short-acting and intermediate-acting insulin vials.
   3. The client instills intermediate-acting insulin into the vial of short-acting insulin.
   4. The client inverts each vial before withdrawing the specified amount of insulin.

SKILL 34-1 Administering Intradermal Injections

Suggested Action	Reason for Action
ASSESSMENT	
Check the medical orders.	Collaborates the nursing activities with the medical treatment.
Compare the medication administration record (MAR) with the written medical order.	Ensures accuracy.
Read and compare the label on the drug with the MAR at least three times—before, during, and after preparing the drug.	Prevents errors.
Check for any documented allergies to food or drugs.	Ensures safety.
Determine how much the client understands about the purpose and technique for administering the injection.	Provides an opportunity for health teaching.
PLANNING	
Prepare to administer the injection according to the schedule prescribed.	Complies with medical orders.
Obtain clean gloves, a tuberculin syringe, the appropriate needle, and alcohol swabs.	Facilitates drug preparation and administration.
Prepare the syringe with the medication.	Fills the syringe with the appropriate volume.
IMPLEMENTATION	
Wash your hands or perform an alcohol-based hand rub (see Chap. 10); don gloves.	Reduces the transmission of microorganisms.
Identify the client using at least two methods; for example, checking the wristband and asking the client's name.	Ensures that medications are given to the *right client;* complies with the National Patient Safety Goals.
Pull the privacy curtain.	Demonstrates respect for the client's dignity.
Select an area on the inner aspect of the forearm, approximately a hand's breadth above the client's wrist.	Provides a convenient and easy location for accessing intradermal tissue.
Cleanse the area with an alcohol swab using a circular motion outward from the site where the needle will pierce the skin.	Removes microorganisms following the principles of asepsis.
Allow the skin to dry.	Reduces tissue irritation.
Hold the client's arm and stretch the skin taut.	Helps to control the placement of the needle.
Hold the syringe almost parallel to the skin at a 10- to 15-degree angle with the bevel pointing upward.[a] Then insert the needle about ⅛ in. (Fig. A).	Facilitates delivering the drug between the layers of the skin and advances the needle to the desired depth.

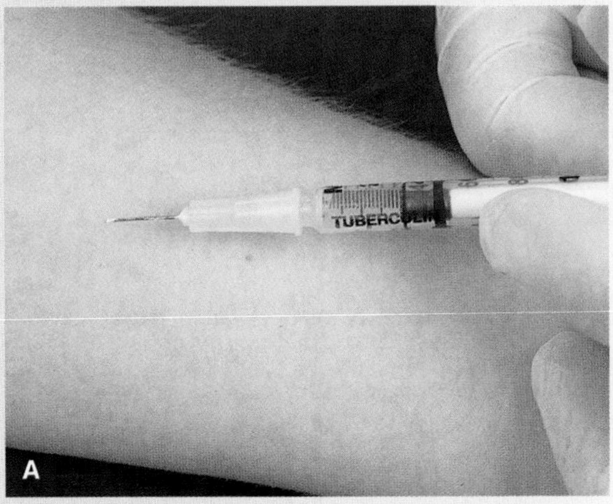

A

Entering the skin. (Photo by B. Proud.)

(continued)

Administering Intradermal Injections (continued)

IMPLEMENTATION (CONTINUED)

Push the plunger of the syringe and watch for a small **wheal** (elevated circle) to appear (Fig. B). — Verifies the correct injection of the drug.

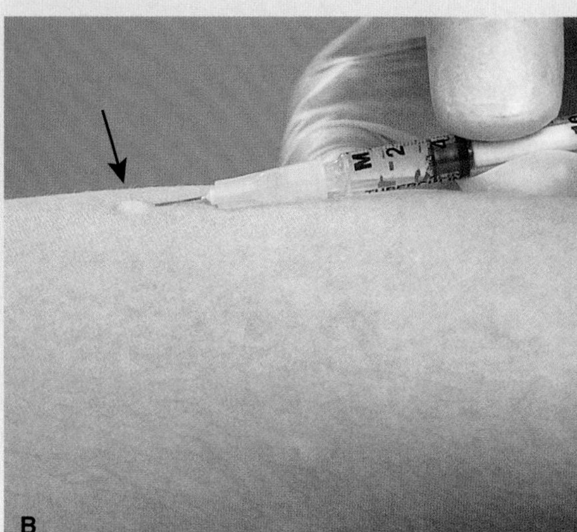

Forming a wheal. (Photo by B. Proud.)

Withdraw the needle at the same angle at which it was inserted. — Minimizes tissue trauma and discomfort.

Do not massage the area after removing the needle. — Prevents interfering with test results.

Deposit the uncapped needle and syringe in a puncture-resistant container. — Prevents injury.

Remove gloves and perform hand hygiene. — Reduces the risk for the transmission of microorganisms.

Observe the client's condition for at least the first 30 minutes after performing an allergy test. — Ensures that emergency treatment can be quickly administered.

Observe the area for signs of a local reaction at standard intervals such as 24 and 48 hours after the injection. — Determines the extent to which the client responds to the injected substance.

Evaluation

- The injection is administered.
- The client remains free of any untoward effects.

Document

- The date, time, drug, dose, route, and specific site
- Client response

SAMPLE DOCUMENTATION

Date and Time Tuberculin skin test administered intradermally in L. forearm with no immediate untoward effects. Instructed to return in 48 hours for inspection of site. ——— SIGNATURE/TITLE

[a]One study of a small sample of new learners showed inserting the bevel down decreased bleeding from the site, avoided squirting the solution into the air, facilitated forming a bleb, and increased the comfort level of clients (Howard et al., 1997).

SKILL 34-2 Administering Subcutaneous Injections

Suggested Action	Reason for Action
ASSESSMENT	
Check the medical orders.	Collaborates the nursing activities with the medical treatment.
Compare the medication administration record (MAR) with the written medical order.	Ensures accuracy.
Read and compare the label on the drug with the MAR at least three times—before, during, and after preparing the drug.	Prevents errors.
Check for any documented allergies to food or drugs.	Ensures safety.
Determine where the last injection was given to ensure site rotation.	Prevents tissue injury.
Determine how much the client understands about the purpose and technique for administering the injection.	Provides an opportunity for health teaching.
Inspect the potential injection site for signs of bruising, swelling, redness, warmth, or tenderness.	Indicates injured tissue areas to avoid.
PLANNING	
Prepare to administer the injection according to the schedule prescribed.	Complies with medical orders.
Obtain clean gloves, the appropriate syringe and needle, and alcohol swabs.	Facilitates drug preparation and administration.
Prepare the syringe with the medication.	Fills the syringe with the appropriate volume.
Add 0.1–0.2 mL of air to the syringe.	Flushes all the medication from the syringe at the time of the injection.
IMPLEMENTATION	
Wash your hands or perform an alcohol-based hand rub (see Chap. 10); don gloves.	Reduces the transmission of microorganisms.
Identify the client using at least two methods; for example, checking the wristband and asking the client's name.	Ensures that medications are given to the *right client;* complies with the National Patient Safety Goals.
Pull the privacy curtain.	Demonstrates respect for the client's dignity.
Select and prepare an appropriate site by cleansing it with an alcohol swab.	Removes colonizing microorganisms.
Allow the skin to dry.	Reduces tissue irritation.
Bunch the skin.	Facilitates placement in the subcutaneous level of tissue.
Pierce the skin at a 45-degree (Fig. A) or 90-degree (Fig. B) angle of entry.	Facilitates placement in the subcutaneous level of tissue according to the length of the needle used and the client's body composition.

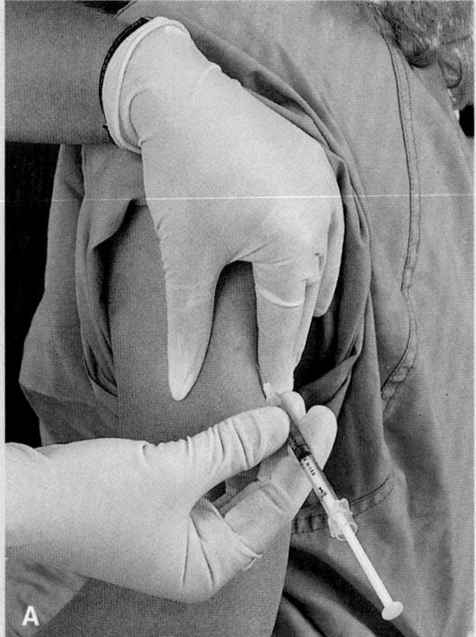

Entering the tissue at a 45-degree angle. (Photo by B. Proud.)

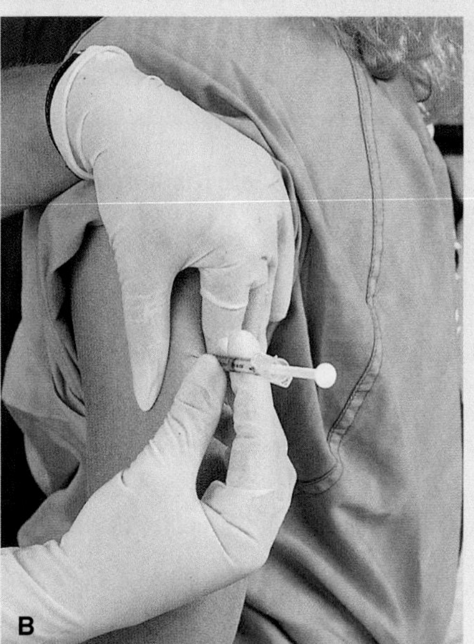

Entering the tissue at a 90-degree angle. (Photo by B. Proud.)

(continued)

Administering Subcutaneous Injections (continued)

Suggested Action	Reason for Action
IMPLEMENTATION (CONTINUED)	
Release the tissue once the needle is inserted; use the hand to support the syringe at its hub.	Steadies the syringe.
Do not aspirate.	Subcutaneous tissue does not contain major blood vessels, which negates the need to aspirate, a standard that once was common practice (Kohn, 2009).
Inject the medication 5 seconds after the needle has been embedded within the tissue by pushing on the plunger.	Ensures complete delivery of the insulin.
Withdraw the needle quickly while applying pressure against the medication site.	Controls bleeding.
Massage the site, unless contraindicated.	Promotes absorption and relieves discomfort.
Deposit the uncapped needle and syringe in a puncture-resistant container.	Prevents injury.
Remove gloves; perform hand hygiene.	Reduces the transmission of microorganisms.
Assess the client's condition at least 30 minutes after giving the injection.	Aids in evaluating the drug's effectiveness.

Evaluation

- The injection is administered.
- The client experiences no untoward effects.

Document

- The date, time, drug, dose, route, and specific site
- Site assessment data
- Client's response

SAMPLE DOCUMENTATION[a]

Date and Time 10 U of regular insulin administered subcutaneously in 3-o'clock position in abdomen. Site appears free of redness, swelling, warmth, tenderness, and bruising. Alert and oriented 30 minutes after injection. —— SIGNATURE/TITLE

[a]The administration of drugs usually is documented on the MAR.

SKILL 34-3 Administering Intramuscular Injections

Suggested Action	Reason for Action
ASSESSMENT	
Check the medical orders.	Collaborates the nursing activities with the medical treatment.
Compare the medication administration record (MAR) with the written medical order.	Ensures accuracy.
Read and compare the label on the drug with the MAR at least three times—before, during, and after preparing the drug.	Prevents errors.
Check for any documented drug allergies.	Ensures safety.
Determine where the last injection was given.	Prevents tissue injury.
Determine how much the client understands about the purpose and technique for administering the injection.	Provides an opportunity for health teaching.
Inspect the potential injection site for signs of bruising, swelling, redness, warmth, tenderness, or **induration** (hardness).	Indicates tissue injury.
PLANNING	
Prepare to administer the injection according to the schedule prescribed.	Complies with medical orders.
Obtain clean gloves, the appropriate syringe and needle, and alcohol swabs.	Facilitates drug preparation and administration.
Prepare the syringe with the medication.	Fills the syringe with the appropriate volume.
Add 0.2 mL of air to the syringe.	Flushes all the medication from the syringe at the time of the injection.

(continued)

Administering Intramuscular Injections (continued)

IMPLEMENTATION

Wash your hands or perform an alcohol-based hand rub (see Chap. 10); don gloves.	Reduces the transmission of microorganisms.
Identify the client using at least two methods; for example, checking the wristband and asking the client's name.	Ensures that medications are given to the *right client;* complies with the National Patient Safety Goals.
Pull the privacy curtain.	Demonstrates respect for the client's dignity.
Select and prepare an appropriate site by cleansing it with an alcohol swab.	Removes colonizing microorganisms.
Allow the skin to dry.	Reduces tissue irritation.
Spread the tissue taut.	Facilitates placement in the muscle.
Hold the syringe like a dart and pierce the skin at a 90-degree angle (Fig. A).	Reduces discomfort.

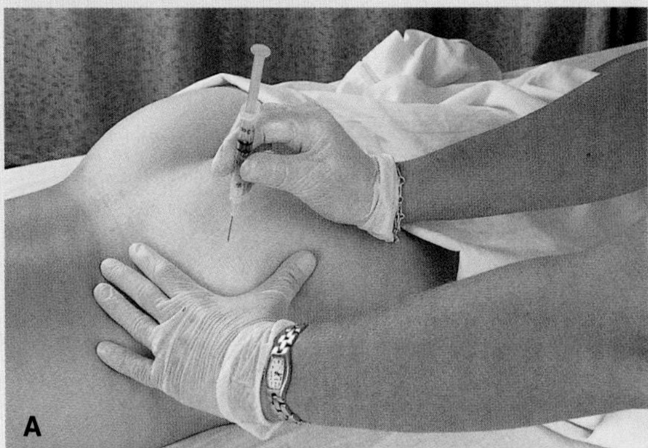

Holding syringe like a dart. (Photo by B. Proud.)

Steady the syringe and aspirate to observe for blood.	Determines whether the needle is in a blood vessel; muscular tissue is more vascular than subcutaneous tissue.
Instill the drug if no blood is apparent.	Deposits the drug into the muscle.
Withdraw the needle quickly at the same angle it was inserted while applying pressure against the site (Fig. B).	Reduces discomfort and controls bleeding.

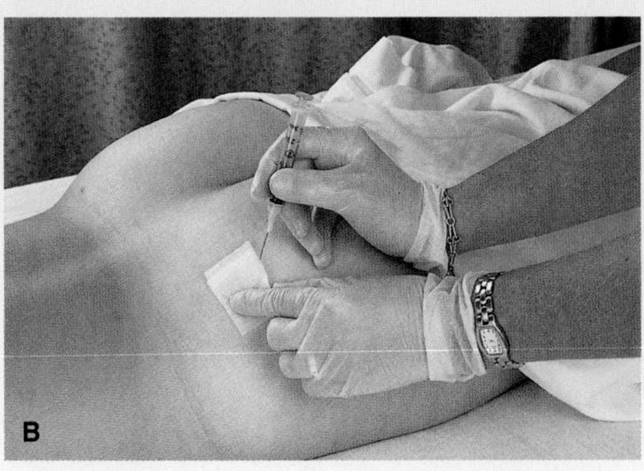

Withdrawing the needle. (Photo by B. Proud.)

(continued)

Administering Intramuscular Injections (continued)

IMPLEMENTATION (CONTINUED)

Massage the injection site with the alcohol swab unless contraindicated (Fig. C). — Distributes the medication and reduces discomfort.

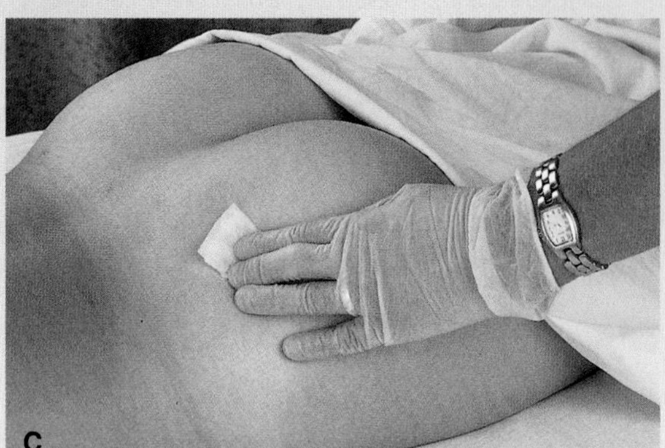

Massaging the site. (Photo by B. Proud.)

Deposit the uncapped needle and syringe in a puncture-resistant container. — Prevents injury.

Remove gloves; perform hand hygiene. — Reduces the transmission of microorganisms.

Assess the client's condition at least 30 minutes after giving the injection. — Aids in evaluating the drug's effectiveness.

Evaluation

- The injection is administered.
- The client experiences no untoward effects.

Document

- The date, time, drug, dose, route, and specific site
- Site assessment data
- Client's response

SAMPLE DOCUMENTATION[a]

Date and Time Demerol 50 mg given IM into R. dorsogluteal site for pain rated as No. 8 on a scale of 0–10. No signs of irritation at the site. Rates pain at No. 5 30 min. after injection. ———— SIGNATURE/TITLE

[a]The administration of drugs usually is documented on the MAR; p.r.n. drugs may be documented both in the nurse's notes and in the MAR.

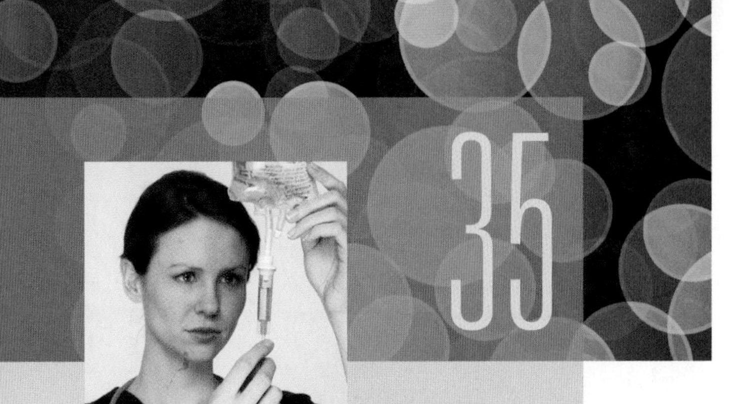

35 Intravenous Medications

Words To Know

antineoplastic drugs
bolus administration
central venous catheter
continuous infusion
intermittent infusion
intravenous route
port
secondary infusion
volume-control set

Learning Objectives

On completion of this chapter, the reader should be able to:

1. Name two types of veins into which intravenous medications are administered.
2. Describe at least three appropriate situations for administering intravenous medications.
3. Name two ways by which intravenous medications are administered.
4. Describe one method for giving bolus administrations of intravenous medications.
5. Describe two methods for administering medicated solutions intermittently.
6. Explain the technique for administering a piggyback infusion.
7. Discuss two purposes for using a volume-control set.
8. Describe a central venous catheter.
9. Name three types of central venous catheters.
10. Discuss two techniques for protecting oneself when administering antineoplastic drugs.

Administering intravenous (IV) solutions (see Chap. 16) is considered a form of IV medication administration. The focus of this chapter, however, is on the methods for administering IV drugs, not fluid replacement solutions, and the techniques for using various venous access devices.

The **intravenous route** (a drug administration through peripheral and central veins) provides an immediate effect. Consequently, this route of drug administration is the most dangerous. Drugs given in this manner cannot be retrieved once they have been delivered. Hence, only specially qualified nurses are permitted to administer IV medications. Those responsible for IV medication administration must use extreme caution in preparation and instillation.

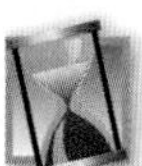

Gerontologic Considerations

- Older adults are often reluctant to ask questions of health care professionals. Therefore, it is imperative that nurses explain the purpose and potential side effects for each drug administered, especially by the IV route.
- A portion of many drugs is bound to protein in the blood. The portion not bound is called free drug, the physiologically active form. Older adults tend to have more free drug in proportion to bound drug because of diminished protein components in their blood and may, therefore, experience an increased effect from the drug.

■ Older adults tend to metabolize and excrete drugs at a slower rate. This factor may predispose them to toxic effects from an accumulation of medications. This toxicity may occur more rapidly when the drug is administered IV. Adjustments may be needed in the amount or frequency of dosing. Older adults require frequent and comprehensive assessments during and after IV medication administration.

INTRAVENOUS MEDICATION ADMINISTRATION

Despite its risks, IV administration given either continuously or intermittently is the route chosen when:

- A quick response is needed during an emergency.
- Clients have disorders (eg, serious burns) that affect the absorption or metabolism of drugs.
- Blood levels of drugs need to be maintained at a consistent therapeutic level such as when treating infections caused by drug-resistant pathogens or providing pain relief.
- It is in the client's interest to avoid the discomfort of repeated intramuscular injections.
- A mechanism is needed to administer drug therapy over a prolonged period, as with cancer.

Continuous Administration

A **continuous infusion** (an instillation of a parenteral drug over several hours), also called a continuous drip, involves adding medication to a large volume (500 to 1,000 mL) of IV solution (Skill 35-1). Drugs may be added to a new container of IV solution or to an existing infusion if there is a sufficient volume to dilute the drug. After the medication is added, the solution is administered by gravity infusion or, more commonly, with an electronic infusion device such as a controller or pump (see Chap. 16).

Stop, Think, and Respond Box 35-1

What are some advantages of administering an IV medication by a continuous infusion?

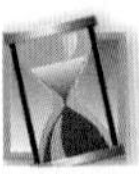

Gerontologic Considerations

■ Older adults with dementia often experience more confusion and disorientation with an acute illness. An assessment of confused older adults is required to ensure the safe administration of IV medications and maintenance of the IV insertion site to ensure that the venipuncture device is not displaced.

Intermittent Administration

Intermittent infusion is a short-term (from minutes up to 1 hour), parenteral administration of medication. Intermittent infusions are administered in three ways: bolus administrations, secondary administrations, and those in which a volume-control set is used.

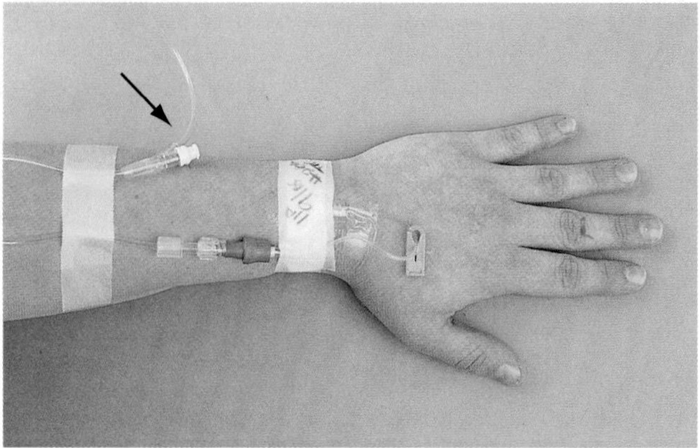

FIGURE 35-1 An intravenous port. (Photo by B. Proud.)

Bolus Administration

The term *bolus* refers to a substance given all at one time. A **bolus administration** (an undiluted or a diluted medication given into a vein in 1 or more minutes) sometimes is described as a drug given by an IV push. Although the term "push" is used, the medication is administered at the rate specified in a drug reference or at a rate of 1 mL per minute if no information is available.

Bolus administrations are given in one of two ways: through a port in an existing IV line or through a medication lock (see Chap. 16).

Using an IV Port

A **port** (a sealed opening) extends from the IV tubing (Fig. 35-1). The seal is made of latex or another substance that can be pierced with a needle or needleless adapter (see Nursing Guidelines 35-1 and Fig. 35-2).

Because the entire dose is administered quickly, a bolus administration has the greatest potential for causing life-threatening changes should a drug reaction occur. If the client's condition changes for any reason, the administration is ceased immediately, and emergency measures are taken to protect the client's safety.

Using a Medication Lock

A medication lock is also called a saline or heparin lock or an intermittent infusion device. The insertion and technique for maintaining the patency of a medication lock are described in Chapter 16.

Briefly, a medication lock is a plug that, when inserted into the end of a IV catheter, allows for instant access to the venous system. One of its best features is that it eliminates the need for a continuous, and sometimes unnecessary, administration of IV fluid.

Instilling IV medication through a lock is similar to the routine for keeping it patent (see Skill 16-7). The technique varies depending on whether the agency's policy

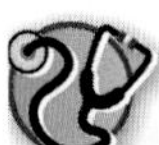

NURSING GUIDELINES 35-1

Administering Medications Through an Intravenous Port

- Prepare the medication in a syringe. *This provides a means for accessing the port.*
- Check the client's identity using at least two methods; for example, checking the wristband and asking the client's name. *Ensures that medications are given to the right client; complies with the National Patient Safety Goals.*
- Locate the port nearest the IV insertion site. *This location provides the most rapid placement of medication in the circulatory system.*
- Swab the port with an alcohol sponge (see Fig. 35-2A). *Alcohol swabbing removes colonizing microorganisms.*
- Pierce the port with the needle or a needleless adapter (see Fig. 35-2B). *Piercing provides access to inside the tubing.*
- Pinch the tubing above the access port (see Fig. 35-2C). *Pinching temporarily stops the flow of the IV fluid.*
- Pull back on the plunger of the syringe. *Pulling back creates negative pressure.*
- Observe for blood in the tubing near the IV catheter or insertion device. *Blood validates that the IV catheter is in the vein.*
- Gently instill a few tenths of a milliliter of medication. *This amount initiates the bolus administration.*
- Release the tubing. *Releasing allows some IV fluid to flow.*
- Continue the pattern of pinching the tubing, instilling a small amount of drug, and releasing the tubing until the medication has been administered over the specified period. *This method delivers the drug gradually and keeps the catheter or venous insertion device patent when medication is not being instilled. Pinching the tubing while instilling the drug ensures the administration of the drug to the client rather than backfilling the tubing.*

is to maintain patency with a 0.9% normal saline solution or heparin. The trend is to use saline.

Nurses use the mnemonic SAS or SASH as a guide to the steps involved in administering IV medication into a lock. SAS stands for flush with **s**aline, **a**dminister the drug, flush again with **s**aline; SASH refers to flush with **s**aline, **a**dminister the drug, flush again with **s**aline, instill **h**eparin (see Nursing Guidelines 35-2 and Fig. 35-3).

To maintain patency, nurses usually flush medication locks after each use with saline or heparin or every 8 to 12 hours

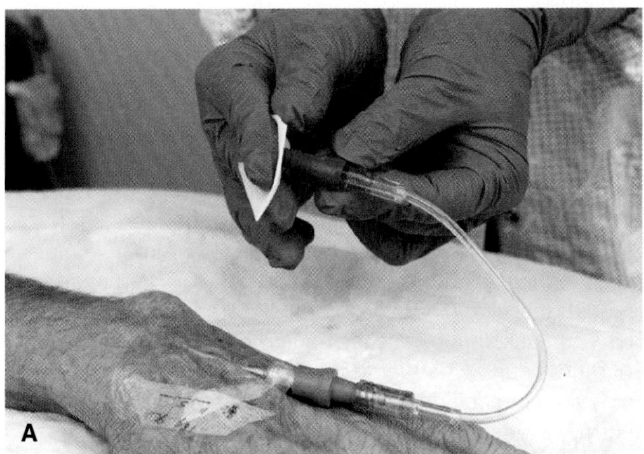

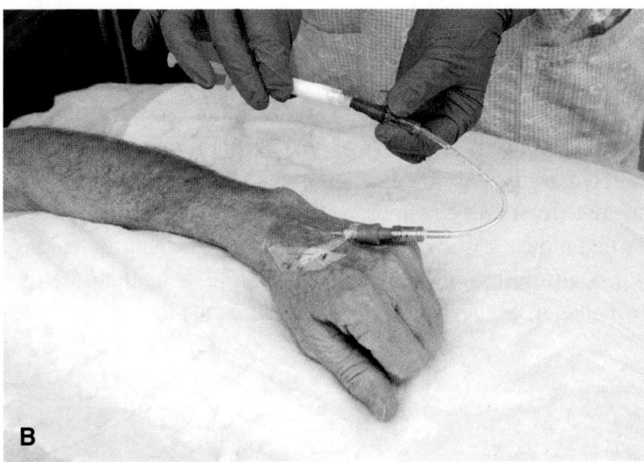

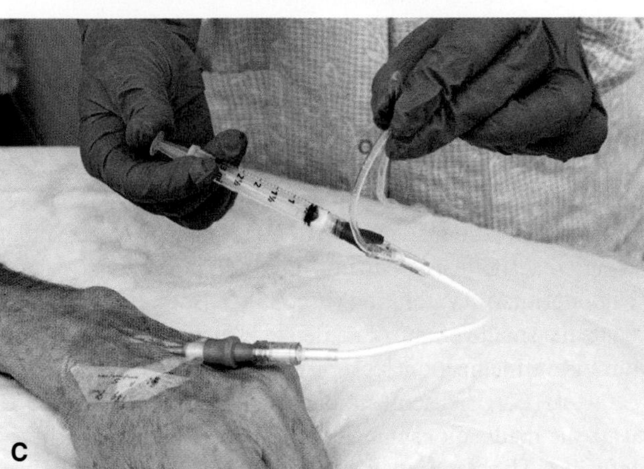

FIGURE 35-2 A. Swabbing the injection port on an infusing intravenous tubing. **B.** Inserting the syringe into the injection port. **C.** Clamping the tubing above the injection port.

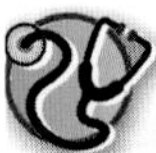

NURSING GUIDELINES 35-2

Administering Medications Through a Lock

- Prepare three syringes, two with at least 1 mL of sterile normal saline and one with the prescribed medication. *This preparation facilitates flushing the lock before and after medication administration.*
- Prepare a fourth syringe with heparin (10 U/mL), if it is the agency's policy to use it. *Heparin maintains patency by interfering with clot formation.*
- Label all the syringes in some way such as attaching pieces of tape with the letters "S" and "H." *Labels can help to identify the contents of syringes.*
- Check the client's identity using at least two methods; for example, checking the wristband and asking the client's name. *Ensures that medications are given to the right client; complies with the National Patient Safety Goals.*
- Wipe the medication port with an alcohol swab. *Alcohol swabs remove colonizing microorganisms.*
- Insert the needle or needleless device from the syringe containing saline through the "bull's eye" of the rubber seal on the medication lock (see Fig. 35-3). *Such insertion provides the least resistance when introducing the needle or needleless device.*
- Hold the lock and pull back on the plunger of the syringe. *Doing so stabilizes the lock while aspirating for blood.*
- Observe for blood in the tubing where the tubing connects to the venous catheter or in the barrel of the syringe. *Blood verifies that the lock is still patent and in the vein (depending on the gauge of the needle, blood return may not always be observed).*
- Instill the saline (the first "S" in the mnemonic). *Saline clears the lock and the venous access device.*
- Remove the syringe when empty, wipe the tip of the lock, and insert the syringe containing the drug. *These steps facilitate administering the medication.*
- Gently and gradually administer the medication over the specified time period (the letter "A" in the mnemonic). *Following recommendations from an authoritative source ensures safety.*
- Remove the syringe when it is empty, wipe the lock again, insert the second syringe with saline, and instill the fluid (the second "S" in the mnemonic). *This pushes the medication that remains in the lock into the venous system and fills the lock with saline.*
- Begin to withdraw the syringe while instilling the last of the fluid in the syringe. *Doing so prevents drawing blood, which may clot, into the lumen of the IV catheter and ensures future patency.*
- Wipe, insert, and instill the heparin (the "H" in the mnemonic), if that is agency policy, using the same technique for withdrawal as with the final flush with saline. *Heparin maintains patency using an anticoagulant.*
- Deposit all uncapped syringes in the nearest puncture-resistant biohazard container. *Proper disposal prevents needlestick injuries.*

if the lock has been unused. The flushing technique is the same except only one syringe of flush solution is required.

Nurses change medication locks when changing the IV site or at least every 72 hours. If the nurse cannot verify patency by obtaining a blood return, and if there is resistance or leaking when administering the flush solution, she or he removes the IV catheter, changes the site, and replaces the lock.

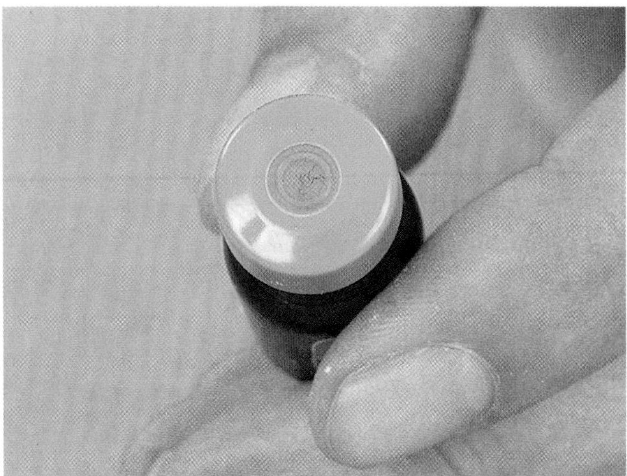

FIGURE 35-3 The bull's eye on a medication lock. (Photo by B. Proud.)

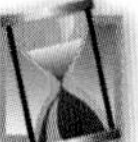

Gerontologic Considerations

- Older adults comprise the largest age group of clients cared for in acute and long-term health care facilities. The administration of IV medications is quite common in older clients. Increasing the emphasis on early discharges may require teaching older adults, family caregivers, or both how to flush venous access equipment.
- Older adults who are discharged with a medication lock may require additional time for repeated practice due to normal age-related problems such as decreased visual acuity and manual dexterity, or for a referral for skilled nursing care.

Secondary Infusions

A **secondary infusion** is the administration of a parenteral drug that has been diluted in a small volume of IV solution, usually 50 to 100 mL, over 30 to 60 minutes. It also is called a piggyback infusion because it is administered in tandem with a primary IV solution (Fig. 35-4). Both are misnomers when the small volume of medicated solution is administered through a medication lock or the port of a central venous catheter (CVC; discussed later). When administered this way, the medications are actually independent of a primary infusion. There are also instances when small volumes of

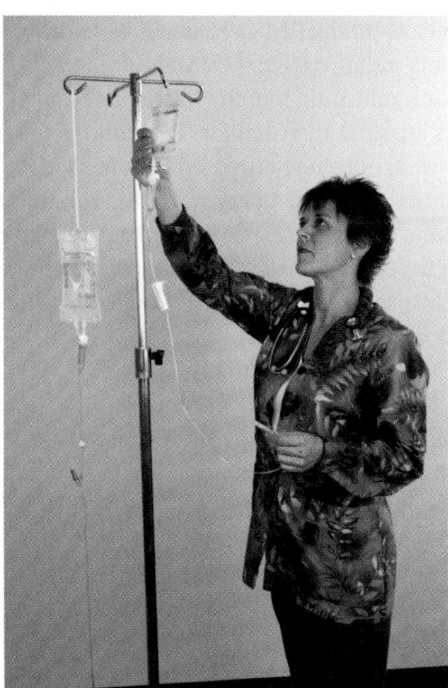

FIGURE 35-4 A piggyback arrangement.

medicated solution are given simultaneously with a primary infusion. This method involves using dual types of electronic infusion devices. Skill 35-2 describes how nurses administer secondary infusions by gravity in tandem with a currently infusing primary solution.

> **Stop, Think, and Respond Box 35-2**
>
> *Other than using a drug reference book, whom or what might you consult to determine the compatibility of two drugs that will infuse through the same IV tubing?*

Volume-Control Set

A **volume-control set** is a chamber in IV tubing that holds a portion of the solution from a larger container (Fig. 35-5). It is known by various commercial names such as Volutrol, Soluset, and Buretrol. A volume-control set is used to administer IV medication in a small volume of solution at intermittent intervals and to avoid accidentally overloading the circulatory system. The volume-control set essentially substitutes for the separate secondary container of solution, therefore eliminating the need for additional fluid.

When caring for clients who are at risk for or manifest signs of fluid excess, it is appropriate to consult the physician and pharmacy department about using a volume-control set to administer intermittent IV medications (Skill 35-3).

> **Stop, Think, and Respond Box 35-3**
>
> *Why might the administration of IV medications and fluid with a volume-control set be preferable to a secondary or continuous infusion when the client is an infant or small child?*

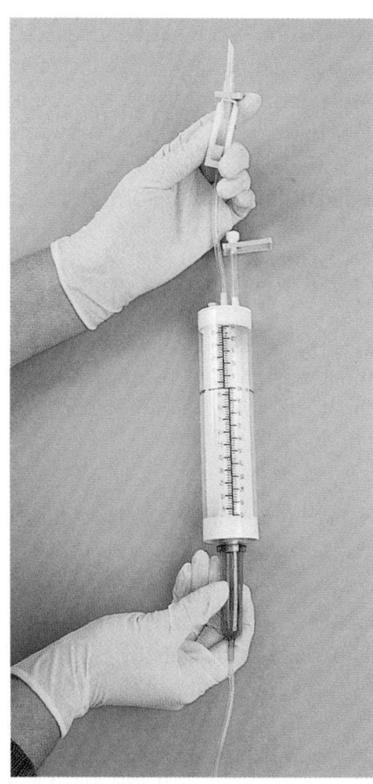

FIGURE 35-5 A volume-control set. (Photo by B. Proud.)

CENTRAL VENOUS CATHETERS

A **central venous catheter** (a venous access device that extends to the superior vena cava) provides a means of administering parenteral medication in a large volume of blood. A CVC is used when:

- Clients require long-term IV fluid or medication administration.
- IV medications are irritating to peripheral veins.
- It is difficult to insert or maintain a peripherally inserted venous catheter.

CVCs have single or multiple lumens (Fig. 35-6). With multiple lumens, incompatible substances or more than one

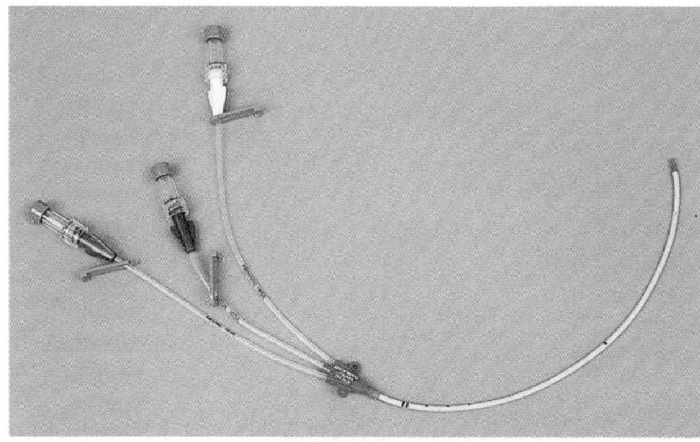

FIGURE 35-6 A triple-lumen central venous catheter. (Photo by B. Proud.)

solution or drug can be given simultaneously. Each infuses through a separate channel and exits the catheter at a different location near the heart. Thus, the drugs or solutions never interact. When a lumen is used only intermittently, it is capped with a medication lock. The unused lumen is kept patent by scheduled flushes with normal saline or heparin.

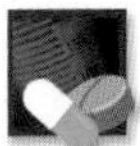

Pharmacologic Considerations

■ Heparin 100 U/mL is the usual strength used for flushing a CVC. As with all medications, be sure to read the label on the supplied flush solution three times because the commonly available strength is 10 U/mL.

There are three types of CVCs: percutaneous, tunneled, and implanted.

Nontunneled Percutaneous Catheters

A nontunneled percutaneous catheter is inserted through the skin in a peripheral vein (eg, the basilic, cephalic, jugular, or subclavian vein) with the distal end terminating in the superior vena cava; see Chap. 16) (Fig. 35-7). Nurses who are certified may insert a peripherally inserted central catheter (PICC) line. Nontunneled percutaneous catheters are used when clients require short-term fluid therapy, parenteral nutrition, or medication therapy lasting a few days or weeks.

PICCs are safer than catheters inserted in the subclavian or jugular veins because there is a reduced potential for a pneumothorax (punctured pleura resulting in the collapse of a lung) at the time of insertion. Catheter-related complications such as venous thrombosis (clot formation), and bacteremia (bacterial infection in the bloodstream) are inherent risks when CVCs are used.

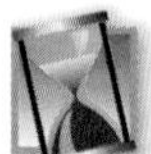

Gerontologic Considerations

■ The veins of older adults tend to be quite fragile. Inserting a percutaneous central venous line is often better than risking the trauma of repeated attempts at restarting or changing peripheral IV sites.

Tunneled Catheters

Tunneled catheters are inserted into a central vein with part of the catheter secured in the subcutaneous tissue. The end of the catheter exits from the skin lateral to the xiphoid process

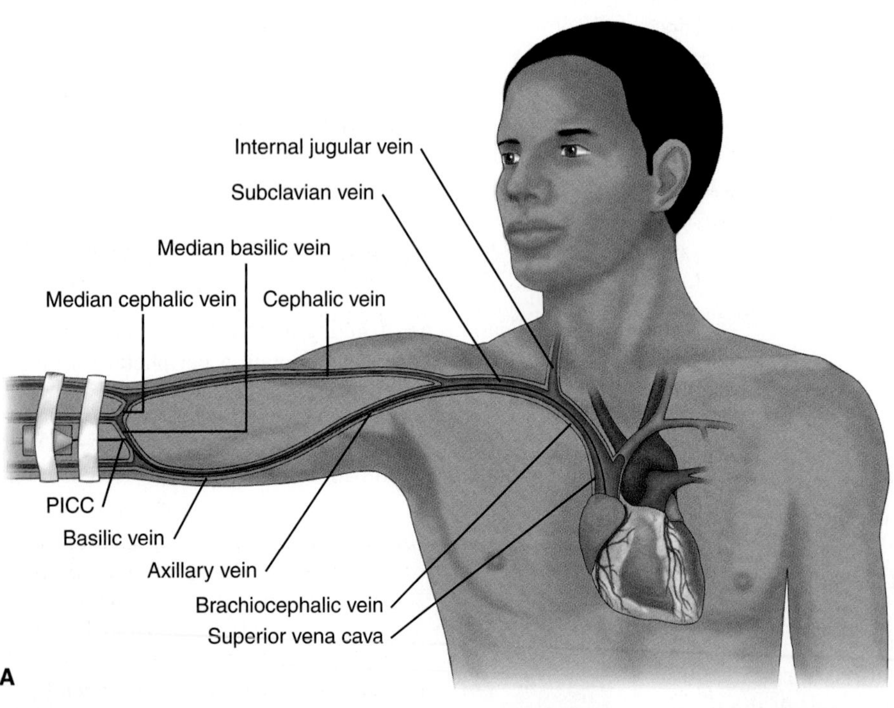

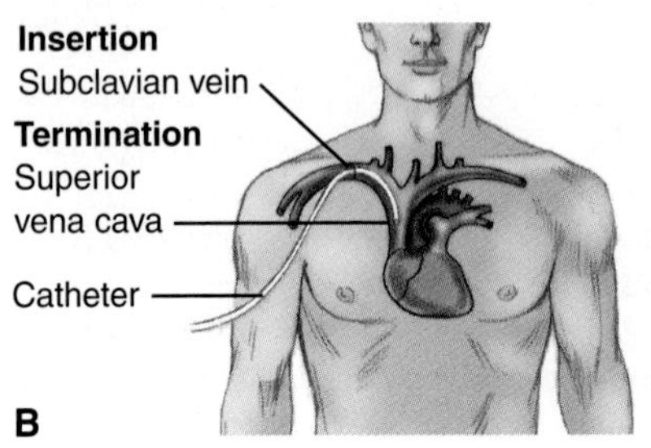

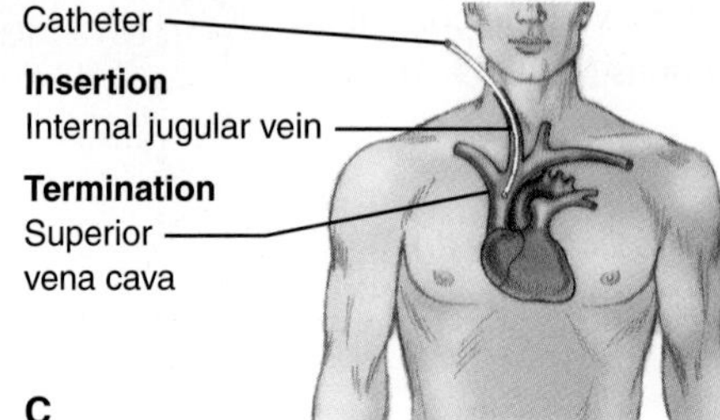

FIGURE 35-7 **A.** The location of a peripherally inserted central catheter (PICC). **B.** The location of a percutaneous catheter inserted in the subclavian vein. **C.** The location of a percutaneous catheter inserted in the jugular vein.

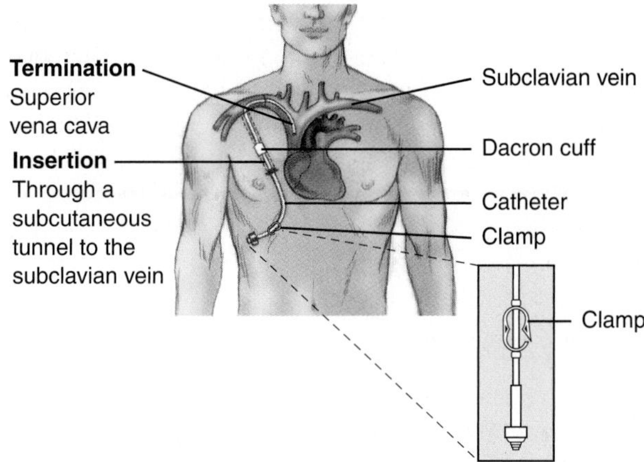

FIGURE 35-8 A tunneled catheter.

(Fig. 35-8). Tunneled catheters are used when the client requires extended therapy. Tunneling helps to stabilize the catheter and also reduces the potential for infection because an internal cuff acts as a barrier against migrating microorganisms. Some examples of tunneled catheters are the Hickman, Broviac, and Groshong catheters.

Implanted Catheters

An implanted catheter (eg, the Porta-Cath) is sealed beneath the skin (Fig. 35-9) and provides the greatest protection against infection because it is totally confined internally without any exposed external portion.

Implanted catheters have a self-sealing port pierced through the skin with a special needle when administering IV medications or solutions. To reduce skin discomfort, a local anesthetic is first applied topically. Implanted ports can sustain approximately 2,000 punctures; thus, the catheter can remain in place for several years, barring complications. A dressing is applied only when the port is pierced and the catheter is being used. Implanted catheters remain patent with a periodic flushing with heparin.

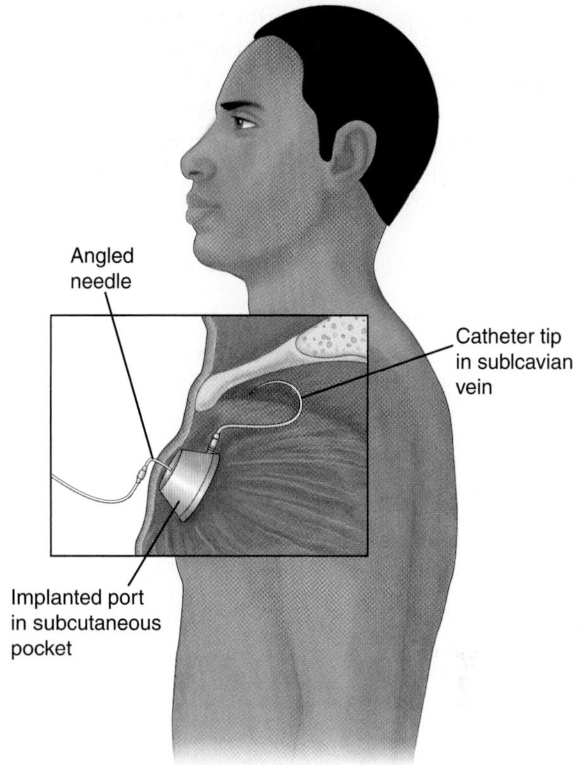

FIGURE 35-9 The placement of an implanted catheter with access via a port and angled needle.

Medication Administration Using a Central Venous Catheter

IV medications may be instilled through any type of CVC. Continuous or intermittent infusions may be used (see Nursing Guidelines 35-3 and Fig. 35-10).

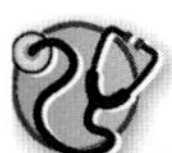

NURSING GUIDELINES 35-3

Using a Central Venous Catheter

- Prepare the IV solution, tubing, and drug using the steps for administering a continuous or secondary infusion. *Preparation principles are similar.*
- Prepare a syringe with 3–5 mL of sterile normal saline solution. *Saline facilitates clearing the catheter of heparin if used to maintain patency; a larger volume displaces the current fluid within the lumen of the catheter.*
- Release the clamp, if there is one, on the exposed section of the catheter. *Releasing the clamp facilitates flushing the catheter.*
- Swab the sealed port at the end of the catheter with alcohol. *Alcohol swabbing removes colonizing microorganisms.*
- Insert the syringe containing the saline into the port and instill the flush solution (see Fig. 35-10). *Piercing clears the catheter of previous flush solution.*
- Swab again and insert the needle, the recessed needle, or the needleless adapter that connects to the prepared IV medication through the port. *Doing so provides access to the circulatory system.*
- Tape the connection. *Taping prevents displacement.*
- Release the clamp on the tubing and regulate the rate of infusion. *These steps administer the medication according to the prescribed rate.*
- Remove the needle or adapter from the port when the medicated solution has instilled. *Removal terminates the current use of the catheter.*
- Flush the catheter with saline or heparin or both according to agency protocol. *Flushing maintains catheter patency.*
- Reclamp the catheter. *Reclamping prevents complications such as air embolism (see Chap. 16).*

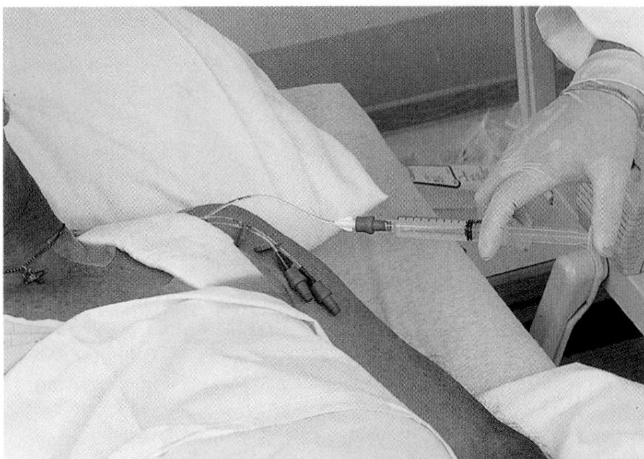

FIGURE 35-10 Flushing the lumen. (Photo by B. Proud.)

Antineoplastic drugs (medications used to destroy or slow the growth of malignant cells) also are commonly referred to as chemotherapy or just chemo. CVCs often are used to administer antineoplastic drugs to clients with cancer.

Antineoplastic agents are toxic to both normal and abnormal cells. These drugs can even cause adverse effects in the pharmacists who mix them and in the nurses who administer them. Caregivers can absorb antineoplastic drugs through skin contact, inhalation of tiny fluid droplets or dust particles on which the droplets fall, or oral absorption of drug residue during hand-to-mouth contact. When transferred to the caregiver, these drugs can cause headaches, nausea, dizziness, and burning or itching of the skin. Long-term exposure can lead to changes in fast-growing body cells, including sperm, ova, or fetal tissue. It is important, therefore, that nurses use safety measures when administering these drugs and avoid exposure and contact with hazardous materials.

In most cases, these drugs are reconstituted or diluted with sterile IV solutions in the pharmacy. The pharmacist wears protective clothing when preparing the drugs under a vertical flow containment hood or biologic safety cabinet (Fig. 35-11). The pharmacist usually attaches a special label to warn nurses to take special precautions during drug administration.

Common recommendations for avoiding self-contamination with antineoplastic drugs include the following:

- Cover the drug preparation area with a disposable paper pad, which will absorb small drug spills.
- Wear a long-sleeved, cuffed, low-permeability gown with a closed front.
- Wear one or two pairs of surgical latex, *nonpowdered* gloves to reduce the potential for skin contact and inhalation of drug powder.
- Cover the cuffs of the gown with the cuffs of the gloves.
- Wear a mask or respirator and goggles if there is a potential for aerosolization or drug splash.
- Pour 70% alcohol over any drug spill to inactivate the drug.

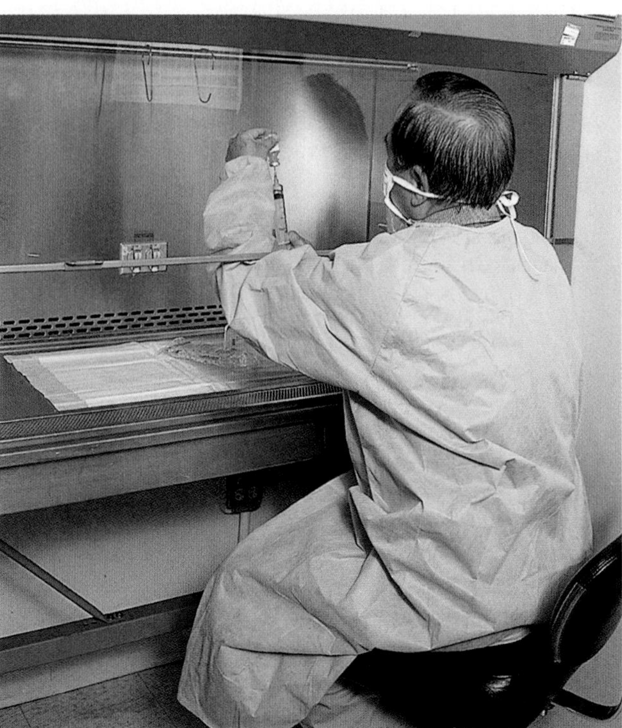

FIGURE 35-11 A pharmacy preparation of antineoplastic drugs using self-protective garments and equipment. (Photo by B. Proud.)

- Clean the spill area with detergent and water at least three times, and then rinse with clean water.
- Dispose of all substances that contain drug material in a biohazard container.
- Perform scrupulous hand washing after removing gloves.

NURSING IMPLICATIONS

Although the administration of all parenteral drugs involves specialized skills, the administration of IV medications in general and antineoplastic drugs in particular requires extreme caution. Nurses may identify the following nursing diagnoses:

- Anxiety
- Risk for Infection
- Fear
- Excess Fluid Volume
- Risk for Injury
- Ineffective Protection

Nursing Care Plan 35-1 demonstrates the nursing process as applied to a client with the nursing diagnosis Ineffective Protection, defined in the 2012 NANDA-I taxonomy (p. 160) as "a decrease in the ability to guard self from internal or external threats such as illness or injury." This diagnosis may be associated with the undesirable consequences of antineoplastic medication therapy; an example might be deficient immunity or a decreased ability to control bleeding.

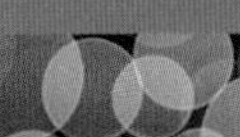

NURSING CARE PLAN 35-1 Ineffective Protection

Assessment

- Review laboratory findings for evidence of decreased mature white blood cells, reduced platelets, insufficient erythrocytes and hemoglobin, or the potential for prolonged clotting.
- Read the client's history for information indicating a bleeding disorder from an acquired or inherited condition in which a clotting factor is missing.
- Analyze the client's weight in relation to height or calculate body mass index (BMI) for evidence of inadequate nutrition.
- Refer to the client's medical record for current diagnoses such as cancer, alcohol or other forms of substance abuse, and immune-related disorders.
- Determine if the client is undergoing therapeutic management of disorders with drugs that suppress bone marrow function, cause immunosuppression, or interfere with clot formation.

Nursing Diagnosis. **Ineffective Protection** related to a debilitated state and a tendency to bleed secondary to chemotherapy for Hodgkin's lymphoma as manifested by enlarged cervical and axillary lymph nodes, complete blood count that reveals thrombocytopenia, and the client's statement: "I haven't been eating much. It's difficult to swallow; as a result I'm losing weight and feeling very weak."

Expected Outcome. The client will maintain effective protection from bleeding as evidenced by minimal blood loss, platelet count within a normal range, and negative occult blood tests on urine and stool throughout the hospital stay.

Interventions	Rationales
Monitor platelet count from a specimen drawn from CVC.	Platelets play a role in blood clotting; the normal range of platelets is 150,000–250,000/mm^3.
Report platelet counts below normal and expect that chemotherapy will be withheld if count is less than 100,000/mm^3.	The nurse informs the physician of data that put the client at risk for complications; withholding a chemotherapeutic drug that suppresses bone marrow function protects the client by avoiding a further decline in platelets.
Assess skin for bruising and the catheter site for bleeding, and test urine and stool for occult blood every day.	Physical assessments provide data that indicate evidence of blood loss and decreased clotting ability.
Consult the physician if he or she inadvertently prescribes aspirin, products containing salicylates, or other types of drugs that interfere with clotting.	Questioning an order for a medication that interferes with clotting protects the client from factors that increase the risk for bleeding.
Use a soft-bristle toothbrush or foam swabs for mouth care.	These devices avoid oral and dental trauma that can result in blood loss.
Apply pressure for at least 3 minutes to control bleeding at an injection site if parenteral medications must be given by a route other than through the CVC.	Direct pressure helps to control bleeding.

Evaluation of Expected Outcomes

- Platelet count remains in low normal range or higher.
- There is no evidence of bleeding from CVC insertion site.
- No bruises are noted on the skin.
- Urine and stool test negative for occult blood.
- There is no evidence of active bleeding from gums after mouth care with soft-bristled toothbrush.

CRITICAL THINKING EXERCISES

1. Discuss the advantages and disadvantages of giving IV medications to older adults.
2. When preparing to administer an IV medication through an IV port or lock, you find no blood return on aspiration. Discuss the significance of this finding and appropriate actions.
3. If the volume of an IV medication is 4 mL by bolus administration, but there is no published recommended period of time for its administration, how long should the nurse allow when instilling the drug?
4. Why do many oncology departments have a policy of excluding the employment of nurses who are currently pregnant?

NCLEX-STYLE REVIEW QUESTIONS

1. Which of the following actions is essential before a nurse administers an IV medication by bolus (IV push) through a port of an infusing solution that also contains a medication?
   1. Dilute the bolus drug in a small volume of solution.
   2. Check that the bolus and the infusing drugs are compatible.
   3. Stop the infusing solution for approximately 3 minutes.
   4. Flush the port with 5 mL of sterile normal saline.

2. When the nurse instills a medication intravenously by bolus administration (IV push), which technique is correct for determining that the IV catheter is within the vein?
   1. The nurse increases the rate of infusion and looks for edema at the site.
   2. The nurse inspects the site looking for redness along the course of the vein.
   3. The nurse palpates the area of the infusion to note a difference in temperature.
   4. The nurse pulls back on the plunger of the syringe and looks for a blood return.
3. What does the nurse instill first before administering an IV medication through a peripherally inserted intermittent infusion device (medication lock)?
   1. Sterile bacteriostatic water
   2. Sterile normal saline
   3. Sterile isopropyl alcohol
   4. Sterile hydrogen peroxide
4. What is the best answer the nurse can provide when a client asks why the physician recommended inserting an implanted CVC for administering cancer medications?
   1. An implanted catheter has the lowest incidence of infection.
   2. An implanted catheter is best for short-term use.
   3. An implanted catheter will never need to be removed.
   4. An implanted catheter is easy to cover with a dressing.
5. Which of the following techniques is best for avoiding self-contamination with IV antineoplastic drugs?
   1. Stay at least 5 ft away from a client receiving an infusion of an antineoplastic drug.
   2. Wear a high efficiency air filter respirator while in the area where an antineoplastic drug is being given.
   3. Perform meticulous hand washing for about 5 minutes after handling a container of antineoplastic drugs.
   4. Don two pairs of nonpowdered gloves when preparing to administer the antineoplastic drug.

SKILL 35-1 Administering IV Medication by Continuous Infusion

ASSESSMENT

Suggested Action	Reason for Action
Check the medical orders.	Collaborates nursing activities with medical treatment.
Compare the medication administration record (MAR) with the written medical order.	Ensures accuracy.
Read the label on the drug and compare it with the MAR (see Fig. A).	Prevents errors.

A

Comparing the drug label with the medication administration record (Photo by B. Proud.)

Suggested Action	Reason for Action
Make sure the drug label indicates that it is for IV use.	Prevents injuring the client.
Check for any documented drug allergies.	Ensures safety.
Review the drug action and side effects.	Promotes safe client care.
Consult a compatibility chart or drug reference.	Determines if the solution and drug are known to interact when mixed.
Determine how much the client understands about the purpose and technique for administering the medication.	Provides an opportunity for health teaching.
Perform assessments that will provide a basis for evaluating the drug's effectiveness.	Provides a baseline for future comparisons.
Inspect the current infusion site for swelling, redness, and tenderness.	Determines if a site change is needed.

PLANNING

Suggested Action	Reason for Action
Prepare the medication, taking care to read the medication label at least three times.	Avoids medication errors.
Have a second nurse double check your drug calculations.	Ensures accuracy.

IMPLEMENTATION

Suggested Action	Reason for Action
Wash your hands or perform an alcohol-based hand rub (see Chap. 10).	Reduces the transmission of microorganisms.
Identify the client using at least two methods; for example, checking the wristband and asking the client's name (see Fig. B).	Ensures that medications are given to the *right client;* complies with the National Patient Safety Goals.

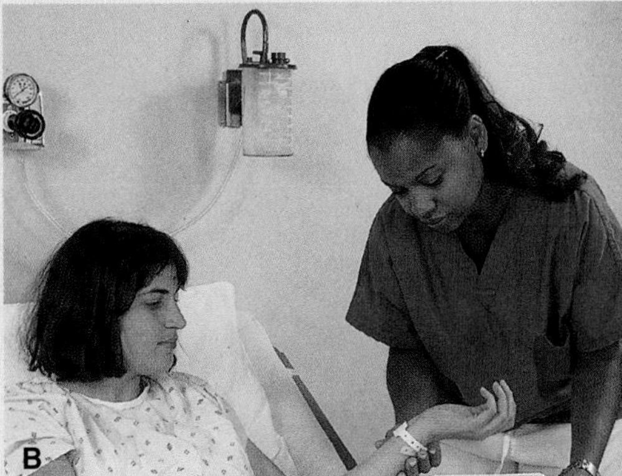

Checking the client's identification band. (Photo by B. Proud.)

(continued)

Administering Intravenous Medication by Continuous Infusion (continued)

IMPLEMENTATI ON (CONTINUED)

Clamp or stop the current infusion of fluid.	Prevents administering a concentrated amount of medication while it is being added to the solution.
Swab the appropriate port on the container of IV fluid (see Fig. C).	Removes colonizing microorganisms.

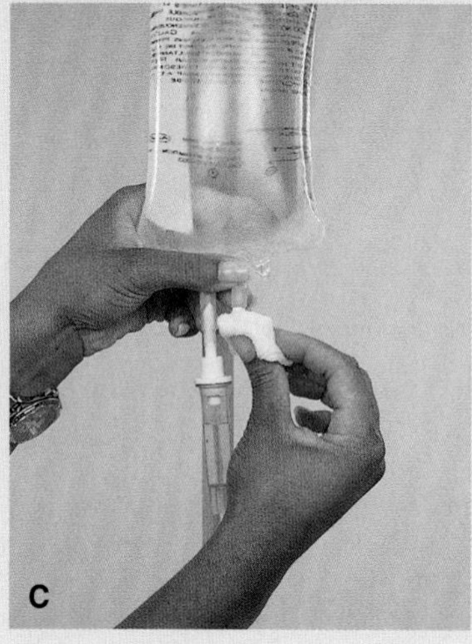

Swabbing the port on the container. (Photo by B. Proud.)

Instill the medication through the port into the full container of infusing fluid (see Fig. D).	Promotes the dilution of concentrated additive.

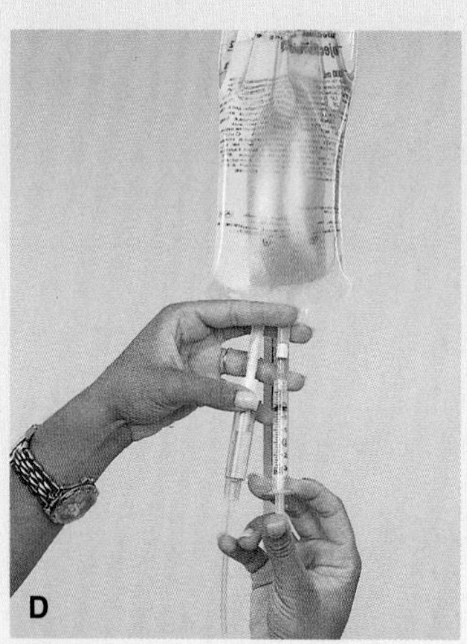

Instilling the medication. (Photo by B. Proud.)

Lower the bag and gently rotate it back and forth.	Distributes the medication equally throughout the fluid.
Suspend the solution and release the clamp.	Facilitates infusion.

(continued)

Administering Intravenous Medication by Continuous Infusion (continued)

IMPLEMENTATION (CONTINUED)

Regulate the rate of flow by using the roller clamp or programming the rate on the electronic infusion device (see Fig. E).

Promotes a continuous infusion at the prescribed rate.

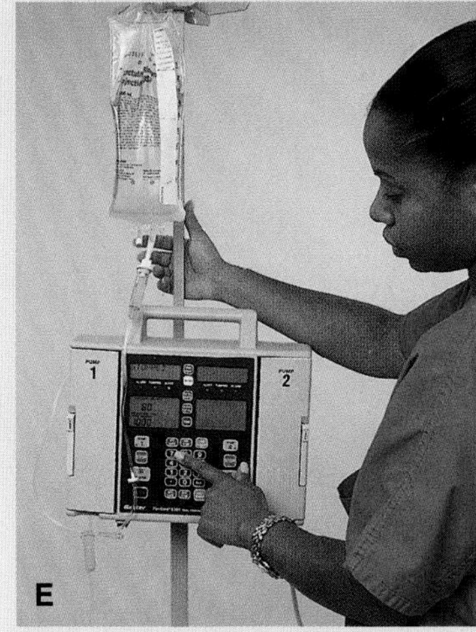

Programming the rate. (Photo by B. Proud.)

Attach a label to the container of fluid identifying the drug, its dose, the time it was added, and your initials (see Fig. F).

Provides information for others and demonstrates accountability for nursing actions.

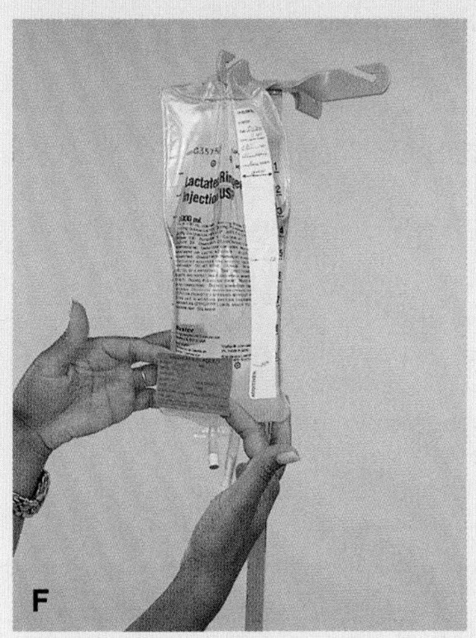

Attaching the drug label. (Photo by B. Proud.)

Record the medication administration in the MAR.

Documents the nursing care; avoids medication errors.

Check the client and the progress of the infusion at least hourly.

Promotes early intervention for complications.

Evaluation

- Medication instills at a prescribed rate.
- Client remains free of any adverse effects.

Document

- Client and site assessment data
- The date, time, drug, dose, and initials
- Solution to which the drug has been added
- Client's response

SAMPLE DOCUMENTATION[a]

Date and Time IV infusing in L. forearm. No tenderness, swelling, or redness observed. KCl 20 mEq added to 1,000 mL of D5/W. IV infusing at 125 mL/h. Heart rate is regular and ranges between 65 and 75 bpm.
———————————————————— SIGNATURE/TITLE

[a]The administration of drugs usually is documented on the MAR.

SKILL 35-2 Administering an Intermittent Secondary Infusion

Suggested Action	Reason for Action
ASSESSMENT	
Check the medical orders.	Collaborates nursing activities with the medical treatment
Compare the medication administration record (MAR) with the written medical order.	Ensures accuracy.
Read the label on the medicated solution and compare it with the MAR.	Prevents errors.
Check for any documented drug allergies.	Ensures safety.
Inspect the current infusion site for swelling, redness, and tenderness.	Determines if a site change is needed.
Review the drug action and side effects.	Promotes safe client care.
Consult a compatibility chart or drug reference.	Determines if the drug in the secondary solution may interact when mixed with the solution in the primary tubing.
Determine how much the client understands about the purpose and technique for administering the medication.	Provides an opportunity for health teaching.
Perform assessments that will provide a basis for evaluating the drug's effectiveness.	Provides a baseline for future comparisons.
PLANNING	
Plan to administer the secondary infusion within 30–60 minutes of the scheduled time for drug administration established by the agency.	Complies with agency policy.
Remove a refrigerated secondary solution at least 30 minutes before administration.	Warms the solution slightly to promote comfort during instillation.
Check the drop factor on the package of secondary (short) IV tubing and calculate the rate for infusion (see Chap. 16).	Ensures that the secondary infusion will be instilled within the specified time.
Have a second nurse double check your calculations for the rate of infusion.	Ensures accuracy.
Attach the tubing to the solution (see Skill 15-2), fill the drip chamber, and purge the air from the tubing.	Prepares the medicated solution for administration.
Attach a needle, a recessed needle, or a needleless adapter.	Facilitates accessing the port while minimizing the risk for needle-stick injury.
IMPLEMENTATION	
Wash your hands or perform an alcohol-based hand rub (see Chap. 10).	Reduces the transmission of microorganisms.
Identify the client using at least two methods; for example, checking the wristband and asking the client's name.	Ensures that medications are given to the *right client;* complies with the National Patient Safety Goals.
Hang the secondary solution on the IV pole or standard.	Prepares the solution for administration.
Lower the container of primary solution approximately 10 in. (25 cm) below the height of the secondary solution using a plastic or metal hanger.	Positions the secondary solution to instill under greater hydrostatic pressure.
Wipe the *uppermost port* on the primary tubing with an alcohol swab.	Removes colonized microorganisms.
Insert the needle or modified adapter within the port.	Provides access to the venous system.
Lock the connection.	Prevents separation from the port.
Release the roller clamp on the secondary solution.	Initiates the infusion.
Regulate the rate of flow by counting the drip rate and adjusting the roller clamp or by programming an electronic infusion device.	Establishes the maintenance rate of flow to instill the solution in the time specified.
Clamp the tubing when the solution has instilled.	Prevents backfilling with the primary solution.
Rehang the primary container of solution and readjust the rate of flow.	Continues the fluid replacement therapy at its appropriate rate.
Leave the secondary tubing in place within the port if another secondary infusion of the same medication is scheduled again within the next 24 hours.	Controls health care costs without jeopardizing client safety; different tubing, however, is used if other drugs are administered as secondary infusions.

(continued)

Administering an Intermittent Secondary Infusion (continued)

Evaluation

- The secondary infusion instills at the prescribed rate.
- The client remains free of any adverse effects.

Document

- Client and site assessment data
- The date, time, drug, dose, and initials
- Client's response

SAMPLE DOCUMENTATION[a]

Date and Time IV infusing in L. forearm. No tenderness, swelling, or redness observed. Vancomycin 1 g administered in 100 mL of NSS as a secondary infusion over 60 minutes without signs of a reaction. ———— SIGNATURE/TITLE

[a]The administration of drugs usually is documented on the MAR.

SKILL 35-3 Using a Volume-Control Set

Suggested Action	Reason for Action
ASSESSMENT	
Check the medical orders.	Collaborates nursing activities with medical treatment.
Compare the medication administration record (MAR) with the written medical order.	Ensures accuracy.
Review the drug action and side effects.	Promotes safe client care.
Consult a compatibility chart or drug reference.	Determines if the medication interacts when diluted with the IV solution.
Read the label on the medication and compare it with the MAR.	Prevents errors.
Check for any documented drug allergies.	Ensures safety.
Assess the client's fluid status (see Chap. 16) and perform other assessments that will provide a basis for evaluating the drug's effectiveness.	Provides a baseline for future comparisons.
Inspect the current infusion site for swelling, redness, and tenderness.	Determines if a site change is needed.
Determine how much the client understands about the purpose and technique for administering the medication.	Provides an opportunity for health teaching.
PLANNING	
Plan to administer the medication within 30–60 minutes of the scheduled time for drug administration established by the agency.	Complies with agency policy.
Obtain a volume-control set.	Provides the means for instilling an intermittent infusion.
Determine the drop factor on the volume-control set and calculate the rate of infusion.	Differs, in some instances, from the drop size on IV tubing.
Have a second nurse double check your calculations for the rate of infusion.	Ensures accuracy.
IMPLEMENTATION	
Wash your hands or perform an alcohol-based hand rub (see Chap. 10).	Reduces the transmission of microorganisms.
Identify the client using at least two methods; for example, checking the wristband and asking the client's name.	Ensures that medications are given to the *right client;* complies with the National Patient Safety Goals.

(continued)

Using a Volume-Control Set (continued)

IMPLEMENTATION (CONTINUED)

Close all the clamps on the volume-control set and insert the spike into the IV solution (see Fig. A).

Prepares the equipment for medication administration.

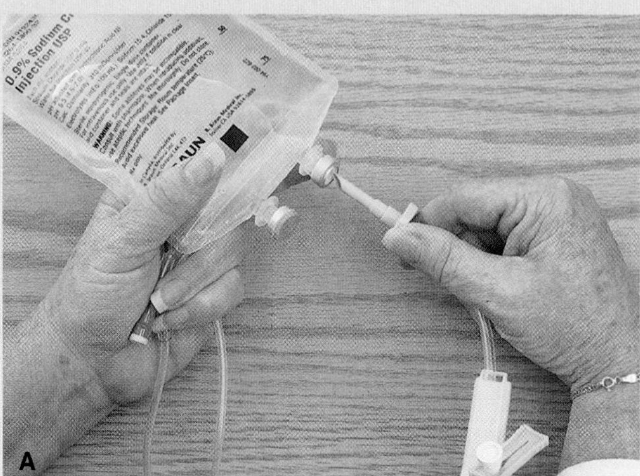

Inserting the spike. (Photo by B. Proud.)

Seal the air vent located to the side of the spike on the volume-control set if the solution is in a plastic bag; if the container is glass, leave the air vent open.

Facilitates the administration of fluid from collapsible or noncollapsible containers.

Release the clamp above the fluid chamber.

Permits fluid to enter the calibrated container.

Fill the calibrated chamber with approximately 30 mL of IV solution and retighten the clamp.

Provides a small volume with which to fill the drip chamber and purge air from the distal tubing.

Squeeze and release the drip chamber until it is half full (see Fig. B). Note: *For volume-control sets with a membrane filter, the clamp below the drip chamber must be open when the drip chamber is filled or the set will be damaged.*

Fills the drip chamber with fluid.

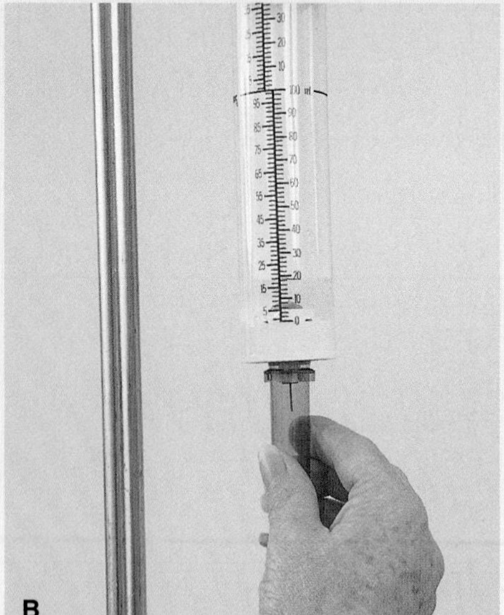

Squeezing the drip chamber. (Photo by B. Proud.)

Open the lower clamp until the tubing is filled with fluid; then reclamp.

Purges air from the tubing.

Open the clamp above the calibrated container, fill the chamber with the desired volume of fluid, and reclamp.

Provides diluent for the medication.

Swab the injection port on the calibrated container.

Removes colonizing microorganisms.

(continued)

Using a Volume-Control Set (continued)

IMPLEMENTATION (CONTINUED)

Action	Rationale
Instill the prepared medication (see Fig. C).	Prepares the drug for administration.

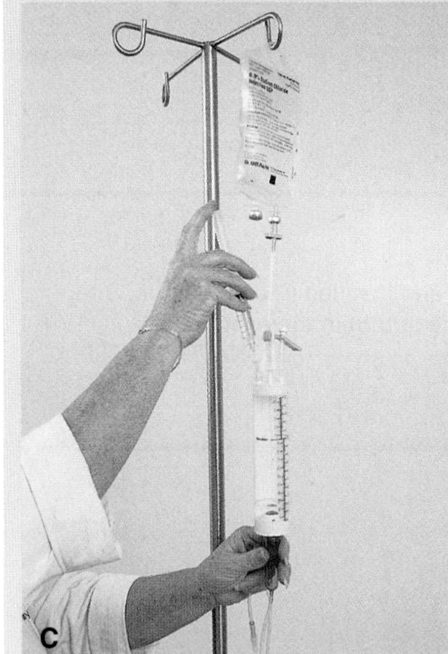

Instilling the medication. (Photo by B. Proud.)

Action	Rationale
Rotate the fluid chamber back and forth.	Mixes the drug throughout the fluid.
Connect the tubing to the client's IV catheter.	Completes the circuit for administering an IV medication.
Release the lower clamp and regulate the drip rate.	Continues the administration of fluid replacement.
Add a label to the fluid chamber identifying the name of the drug, dose, time it was added, and your initials (see Fig. D).	Provides information for other health professionals.

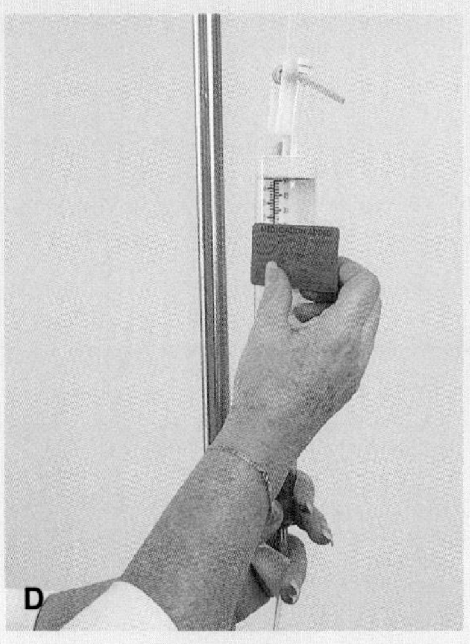

Attaching a drug label. (Photo by B. Proud.)

Action	Rationale
Return before the time the medication is due to finish instilling.	Facilitates further fluid therapy.
Release the upper clamp when the fluid chamber is empty and refill it with the next hour's worth of fluid.	Continues the administration of fluid replacement.
Readjust the rate if necessary.	Accommodates for differences between the rates for medication and fluid administration.
Remove the drug label from the fluid chamber.	No longer applies after the medication is instilled.

(continued)

Using a Volume-Control Set (continued)

Evaluation

- The medicated solution instills within the specified period.
- The client experiences no adverse effects.

Document

- Client and site assessment data
- The date, time, drug, dose, and initials
- Solution to which drug has been added
- Client's response

SAMPLE DOCUMENTATION[a]

Date and Time Azactam 1 g added to 100 mL of D5/W within volume-control chamber and instilled IV over 60 min. Site is neither irritated, tender, nor swollen. Lungs sound clear. 100 mL urine output in the past hour.
———————————— SIGNATURE/TITLE

[a]The administration of drugs usually is documented on the MAR.

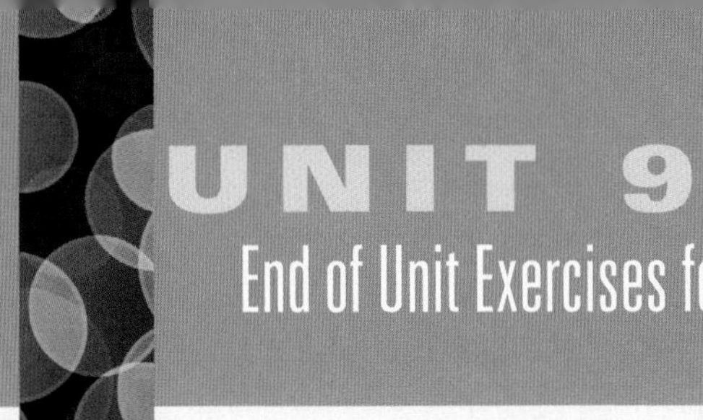

UNIT 9

End of Unit Exercises for Chapters 32, 33, 34, and 35

Section I: Reviewing What You've Learned

Activity A: *Fill in the blanks by choosing the correct word from the options given in parentheses.*

1. Drugs have a ________________ name, which is the chemical name and is not protected by a company's trademark. (brand, generic, proprietary)
2. The application of a drug to the skin or mucous membrane is an example of the ________________ route of drug administration. (inhalant, parental, topical)
3. ________________ application is the method of applying a drug on the skin and allowing it to be passively absorbed. (Cutaneous, Inunction, Transdermal)
4. ________________ is a drug used to dilate the coronary arteries. (Estrogen, Nitroglycerin, Scopolamine)
5. The part of the syringe that holds the medication is called the ________________. (barrel, plunger, tip)
6. With a/an ________________ injection, a drug is administered parenterally between the layers of the skin. (intradermal, intravenous, subcutaneous)
7. An undiluted medication given quickly into a vein is called a ________________ administration. (bolus, piggyback, soluset)
8. ________________ catheters are inserted into a central vein, with part of the catheter secured in the subcutaneous tissue. (Implanted, Percutaneous, Tunneled)

Activity B: *Mark each statement as either T (True) or F (False). Correct any false statements.*

1. T____F____ Drugs that dissolve at timed intervals are called sustained-release medications.
2. T____F____ A scored tablet is a solid drug manufactured with a groove in the center.
3. T____F____ The nurse asks the client to swallow the drug during sublingual or buccal administration.
4. T____F____ Needle lengths vary from approximately 2½ to 3½ inches.
5. T____F____ Lipoatrophy is an accumulation of subcutaneous fat at the site of repeated insulin injections.
6. T____F____ Volume-control set infusions require connecting a second bag of intravenous solution to a primary infusing solution.
7. T____F____ Hickman and Broviac catheters are examples of implanted catheters.

Activity C: *Write the correct term for each description below.*

1. Chemical substances that change body function ________________
2. The term given to drugs covered with a substance that dissolves beyond the stomach ________________
3. Swelling of the nasal mucosa that accompanies the overuse of nasal decongestants ________________
4. The chamber attached to an inhaler ________________
5. The process of adding a diluent to a powdered drug before parenteral administration ________________
6. Medications used to destroy or slow the growth of malignant cells ________________

Activity D: *1. Match the terms related to intramuscular injection sites in Column A with their explanations in Column B.*

Column A		Column B
1. ________________	Dorsogluteal site	A. Muscles in the quadriceps group of the outer thigh
2. ________________	Ventrogluteal site	B. Lateral aspect of the upper arm
3. ________________	Vastus lateralis site	C. Anterior aspect of the thigh
4. ________________	Rectus femoris site	D. Upper outer quadrant of the buttock
5. ________________	Deltoid site	E. Medius and minimus muscles in the hip

2. Match the terms related to intravenous medications in Column A with their explanations in Column B.

Column A		Column B
1. ________________	Central venous catheter	A. Instillation of parenteral drug over several hours
2. ________________	Intravenous route	B. Instillation of parenteral drug over several minutes up to 1 hour
3. ________________	Continuous administration	C. A device that extends to the superior vena cava
4. ________________	Intermittent administration	D. Drug administration via peripheral veins

Activity E: *1. Differentiate between turbo and metered-dose inhalers based on the categories given below.*

	Turbo Inhaler	Metered-Dose Inhaler
Description		
Method of Medication Delivery		
Ease of Use		

2. Differentiate between tunneled and percutaneous catheters based on the categories given below.

	Tunneled Catheters	Percutaneous Catheters
Method of Insertion		
Uses		

Activity F: *Consider the following figure.*

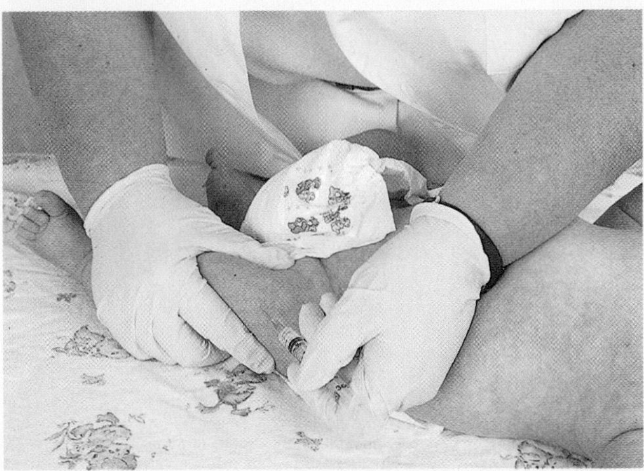

1. Identify what is shown in the figure.
2. Explain the technique being used.

Activity G: *When administering topical drugs, the nurse takes steps to maintain the integrity of the skin and mucous membranes. Write in the boxes provided below the correct sequence for topical vaginal administration.*

1. Depress the plunger once it reaches the proper distance within the vagina.
2. Insert the applicator into the vagina to the length recommended in the package directions.
3. Apply a sanitary pad and ask the client to remain recumbent for at least 10 to 30 minutes.
4. Place the drug in the applicator and apply lubricant to the tip.
5. Remove the applicator and place it on a clean tissue.
6. Have the client empty the bladder before inserting the medication.

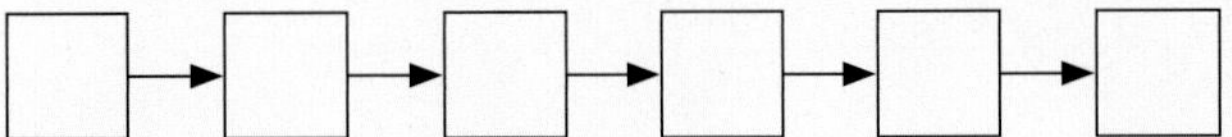

Activity H: *Answer the following questions.*

1. What are the seven components of a medication order?

2. What is the purpose of a medication administration record?

3. What is an inunction application?

4. What are ophthalmic applications?

5. What are five factors to consider when selecting a syringe and needle?

6. What are prefilled cartridges?

7. When are intravenous administrations appropriate for clients?

8. What are the advantages of using a medication lock?

Section II: Applying Your Knowledge

Activity I: *Give rationales for the following questions.*

1. Why are enteric-coated tablets never cut, crushed, or chewed?

2. When are metric doses converted to household measurements?

3. Why are certain drugs administered by application to the skin?

4. Why should extremely hairy areas be clipped before applying skin patches?

5. Why is an 18-gauge needle wider than a 27-gauge needle?

6. Why are conventional syringes and needles being redesigned?

7. Why is the intravenous route of drug administration considered the most dangerous?

8. Why do some central venous catheters have multiple lumens?

Activity J: *Answer the following questions focusing on nursing roles and responsibilities.*

1. A physician has listed drug names and directions for administering them in a client's medication order. The nurse, while transcribing the medication order, observes that the drug order is incomplete.

   a. What immediate actions should the nurse perform in this situation?

   b. What are the five rights of medication administration?

2. A nurse is caring for an adult client recovering from an appendectomy who is experiencing postoperative pain and discomfort. The physician provides telephone instructions for follow-up care to the nurse. What steps should the nurse take when receiving telephone orders from the physician?

3. A client undergoing nicotine withdrawal therapy has been ordered medication in the form of skin patches. How should these skin patches be applied?

4. A physician has prescribed otic application of neomycin for a client with severe itching in his ear.
   a. How will the nurse instill this application?
   b. How does administration of otic drugs differ for adults and children?

5. A client with diabetes has been prescribed a combination of regular and intermediate-acting insulin.
   a. What interventions should the nurse follow when mixing insulins?
   b. What actions should the nurse take if needlestick injuries occur?

6. A nurse is preparing to give a client an intramuscular injection at the dorsogluteal site.
   a. What process will the nurse follow to identify an appropriate landmark?
   b. What damage could result if the nurse does not identify the dorsogluteal site correctly?

7. A physician has prescribed a bolus drug administration for a client. What interventions should the nurse perform when using a medication lock?

Activity K: *Consider the following questions. Discuss them with your instructor or peers.*

1. A nurse is caring for a teenager who has been prescribed antibiotics.
   a. What actions can the nurse take if the client cannot swallow the drugs?
   b. Can the nurse use intestinal or gastric tubes to administer medications to the client?
2. A physician has prescribed timolol (Timoptic) for a client with glaucoma.
   a. What care should the nurse take when administering an ophthalmic application?
   b. What should the nurse do if the applicator tip becomes contaminated?
3. What actions should a nurse take if a client shows signs of an allergic reaction to a drug given parenterally?
4. A nurse is caring for a client with severe burns for whom the physician has prescribed pain medication by the intravenous route. What is a possible rationale for administering pain medication by this route?

Section III: Getting Ready for NCLEX

Activity L: *Answer the following questions.*

1. A nurse is caring for a client whose medication administration record reads amoxicillin t.i.d. How often should the nurse administer this drug?
   a. Three times a day
   b. Every 3 hours
   c. Every 3rd day
   d. For 3 days
2. Which of the following interventions should the nurse perform when administering liquid oral medications?
   a. Pour liquids with the drug label toward the palm of the hand.
   b. Leave the medication cup on a side table if the client is absent.
   c. Offer a cup of water along with the medication.
   d. Ask the client to hyperextend the neck when taking the drug.
3. What instructions should the nurse provide when teaching a client to use a metered-dose inhaler? Select all that apply.
   a. Shake the canister prior to use.
   b. Exhale quickly through open lips.
   c. Float the canister in a water bowl.
   d. Inhale while depressing the canister.
   e. Ask the client to hold his or her breath for 20 seconds.
4. What is the most accurate instruction the nurse can provide when teaching a client how to use prescribed nasal medication?
   a. Place a rolled towel or pillow beneath the neck before administration.
   b. Place the tip of the container in front of the nostril.
   c. Ensure that both the nostrils are open during administration.
   d. Remain in position for 1 full minute after administration.
5. What important considerations should the nurse keep in mind when using the Z-track technique to inject medications? Select all that apply.
   a. Use the Z-track technique only in the deltoid muscles.
   b. Massage the injection site after Z-track administration.
   c. Insert the needle, aspirate, and inject the medication.
   d. Select a large muscular site for injection.
   e. Withdraw the needle and immediately release the taut skin.
6. A nurse is preparing to perform a subcutaneous injection. What important measures should the nurse take when drawing up this medication from an ampule?
   a. Hold the ampule at an angle of 45 degrees from the body.
   b. Avoid tapping the top of the ampule.
   c. Insert the filter needle along the rim of the ampule.
   d. Snap off the ampule's neck away from the body.

7. A nurse is caring for a client with a malignant tumor who has been prescribed antineoplastic drugs. Which of the following measures should the nurse take to avoid self-contamination with antineoplastic drugs?
   a. Wear one or two pairs of nonpowdered surgical gloves.
   b. Pour 10% alcohol over every drug spill.
   c. Wear a short-sleeved gown with a closed front.
   d. Clean the spilled drug area with water.

8. A nurse is caring for a client receiving a piggyback infusion along with a primary intravenous solution. What action should the nurse perform when administering the secondary infusion?
   a. Remove a refrigerated secondary solution 10 minutes before the infusion.
   b. Administer the secondary infusion at the same rate as that of the primary infusion.
   c. Set the height of the secondary solution 10 inches below the primary solution.
   d. Wipe the uppermost port of the primary tubing with an alcohol swab.

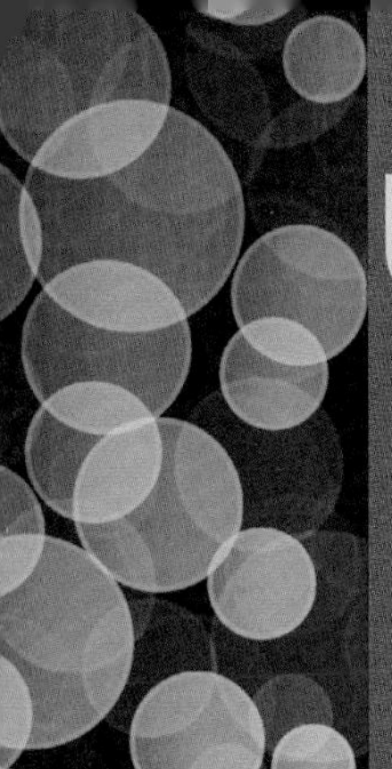

UNIT 10
Intervening in Emergency Situations

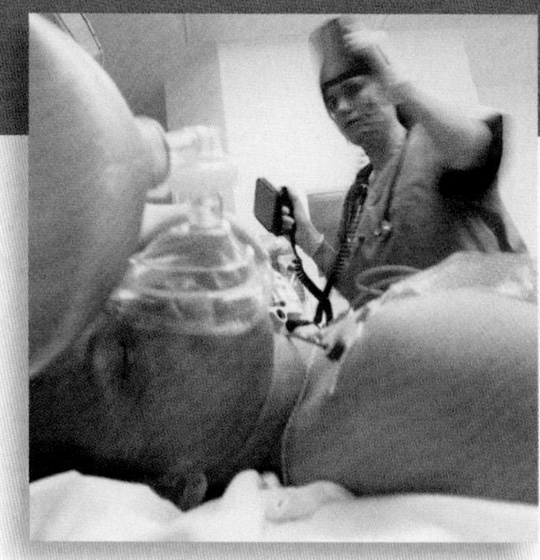

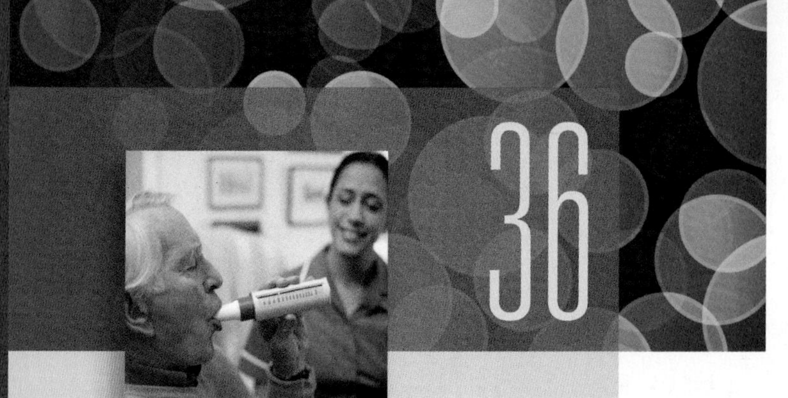

36 Airway Management

Words To Know

airway
airway management
chest physiotherapy
inhalation therapy
mucus
nasopharyngeal suctioning
nasotracheal suctioning
oral airway
oral suctioning
oropharyngeal suctioning
percussion
postural drainage
sputum
suctioning
tracheostomy
tracheostomy care
tracheostomy tube
vibration

Learning Objectives

On completion of this chapter, the reader should be able to:

1. Define airway management.
2. Identify the structural components of the airway.
3. Discuss four natural mechanisms that protect the airway.
4. Explain the methods nurses use to help maintain the natural airway.
5. Name two techniques for liquefying respiratory secretions.
6. Explain the three techniques of chest physiotherapy.
7. Describe at least three suctioning techniques used to clear secretions from the airway.
8. Discuss two indications for inserting an artificial airway.
9. Name two examples of artificial airways.
10. Identify three components of tracheostomy care.

The primary function of the respiratory system is to permit ventilation (the movement of air in and out of the lungs) for an appropriate exchange of oxygen and carbon dioxide at the cellular level (see Chap. 21). A clear **airway** (the collective system of tubes in the upper and lower respiratory tracts) is necessary for adequate ventilation. Many factors can jeopardize airway patency:

- An increased volume of **mucus** (a mixture of water, mucin, white blood cells, electrolytes, and cells that have been shed through the natural process of tissue replacement)
- Thick mucus
- Fatigue or weakness
- A decreased level of consciousness
- An ineffective cough
- An impaired airway

Consequently, nurses sometimes need to assist clients with measures that support or replace their own natural efforts. This chapter focuses on **airway management**, or those essential nursing skills that maintain natural or artificial airways for compromised clients.

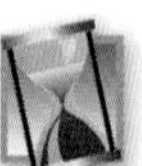

Gerontologic Considerations

■ Conditions affecting the respiratory system are among the most common life-threatening disorders that older adults experience. The severity of chronic pulmonary diseases increases with age.
■ Many older adults with pathologic pulmonary changes have a history of smoking cigarettes since their youth, working in occupations

where they inhaled pollutants that affected their lungs, or living for an extended time in industrial areas known for toxic emissions.

■ Inquiring about a current history of coughing, determining how long the cough has been present, and observing and describing any sputum are important when assessing older adults.

■ If not relieved quickly, a persistent, dry cough may consume the older adult's energy and result in fatigue.

THE AIRWAY

The upper airway consists of the nose and pharynx, which is subdivided into the nasopharynx, oropharynx, and laryngopharynx. The lower airway consists of the trachea, bronchi, bronchioles, and alveoli. Gases travel through these structures to and from the blood (Fig. 36-1).

Certain structures protect the airway from a wide variety of inhaled substances. These structures include the epiglottis, tracheal cartilage, mucous membrane, and cilia. The *epiglottis* is a protrusion of flexible cartilage above the larynx. It acts as a lid that closes during swallowing, helping to direct fluid and food toward the esophagus rather than the respiratory tract. The rings of *tracheal cartilage* ensure that the trachea, the portion of the airway beneath the larynx, remains open. The *mucous membrane*, a type of tissue from which mucus is secreted, lines the respiratory passages. The sticky mucus traps particulate matter. Hair-like projections called cilia beat debris that collects in the lower airway upward (Fig. 36-2).

Various mechanisms keep the airway open. For example, sneezing or blowing the nose can clear debris there. Coughing, expectoration, or swallowing clears **sputum** (mucus raised to the level of the upper airways).

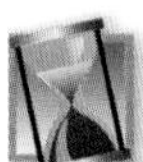

Gerontologic Considerations

■ Reduced air exchange and a reduced efficiency in ventilation are the primary age-related changes affecting the older adult's respiratory system.

■ The muscular structures of the larynx tend to atrophy with age, which can affect the ability to clear the airway.

■ Usually, the bases of the older adult's lungs receive less ventilation, contributing to the retention of secretions, decreased air exchange, and compromised ventilation. Respiratory cilia become less efficient with age, predisposing older adults to a high incidence of pneumonia.

■ Diminished strength of accessory muscles for respiration, an increased rigidity of the chest wall, and a diminished cough reflex make it difficult for older adults to cough productively and effectively.

■ Older adults with difficulty swallowing (dysphagia), often associated with strokes or middle and late stages of dementia, are more vulnerable to aspiration pneumonia. An evaluation of the dysphagia is important for implementing appropriate interventions to prevent aspiration.

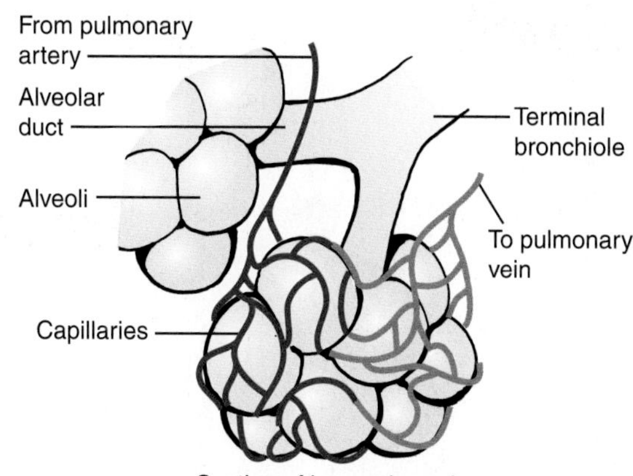

FIGURE 36-1 The airway and related structures.

NATURAL AIRWAY MANAGEMENT

The most common methods of maintaining the natural airway are keeping respiratory secretions liquefied, promoting their mobilization and expectoration with chest physiotherapy, and mechanically clearing mucus from the airway by suctioning.

Liquefying Secretions

The body continuously produces mucus. The volume of water in mucus affects its *viscosity*, or thickness. *Hydration*, the process of providing adequate fluid intake, tends to keep mucous membranes moist and mucus thin. A thin consistency promotes expectoration (see Chap. 16). An essential nursing activity is ensuring that clients are well hydrated.

In addition, nurses may assist with **inhalation therapy** (respiratory treatments that provide a mixture of oxygen, humidification, and aerosolized medications directly to the lungs). The aerosol is delivered through a mask or a handheld mouthpiece (Fig. 36-3; also see Chap. 33). Aerosol therapy

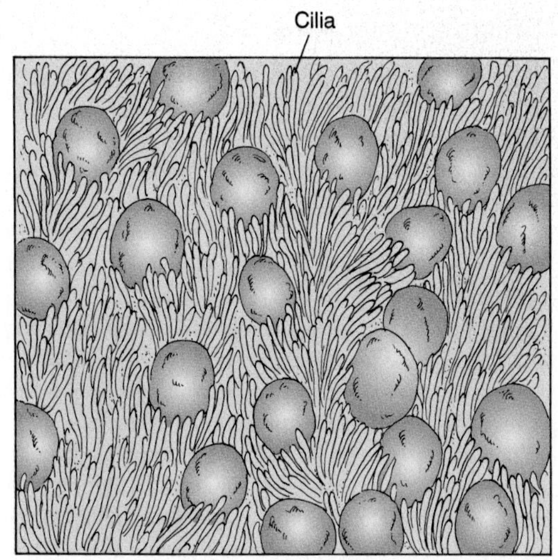

FIGURE 36-2 The cilia and mucus-producing cells.

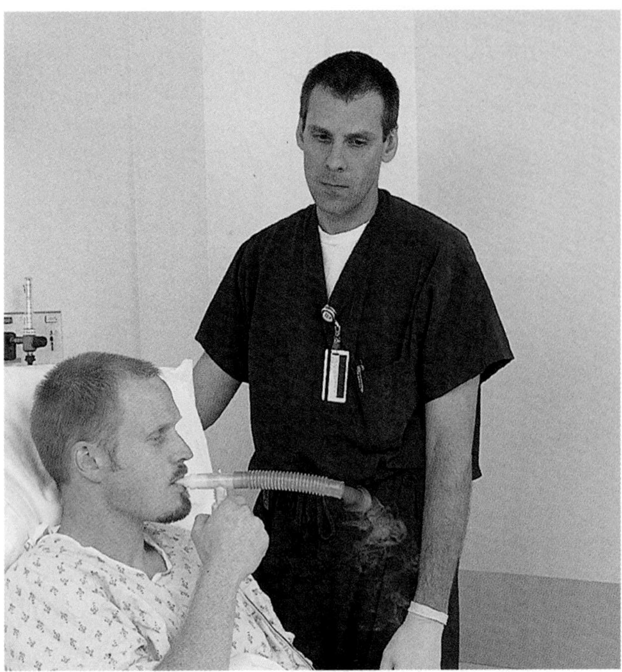

FIGURE 36-3 Aerosol therapy. (Photo by B. Proud.)

improves breathing, encourages spontaneous coughing, and helps clients to raise sputum for diagnostic purposes (see Nursing Guidelines 36-1).

Mobilizing Secretions

To help clients mobilize secretions from distal airways, health care professionals often use **chest physiotherapy** (techniques including postural drainage, percussion, and vibration). Chest physiotherapy usually is indicated for clients with chronic respiratory diseases who have difficulty coughing or raising thick mucus.

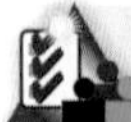

Client and Family Teaching 36-1
Performing Postural Drainage

The nurse teaches the client and family as follows:

- Plan to perform postural drainage two to four times daily (eg, before meals and at bedtime).
- Administer the prescribed inhalant medications (see Chap. 33) before performing postural drainage.
- Have paper tissues and waterproof container nearby for collecting expectorated sputum.
- Position yourself to drain the appropriate lung areas.
- Cough and expectorate secretions that drain into the upper airway.
- Remain in each prescribed position for 15–30 minutes (no longer than 45 minutes).
- Resume a comfortable position after expectorating the usual volume of sputum or if you become tired, feel lightheaded, or have a rapid pulse rate, difficulty breathing, or chest pain.

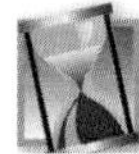

Gerontologic Considerations

- Deep-breathing exercises may improve an older adult's ability to eliminate respiratory secretions.

Postural Drainage

Postural drainage is a positioning technique that promotes the drainage of secretions from various lobes or segments of the lungs with the use of gravity (Fig. 36-4). In most hospitals, respiratory therapists are responsible for postural drainage. In long-term care facilities and home health care, however, nurses may teach clients and families to perform this technique (see Client and Family Teaching 36-1). Combining postural drainage with percussion and vibration enhances overall effectiveness.

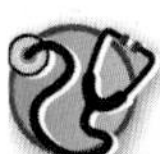

NURSING GUIDELINES 36-1

Collecting a Sputum Specimen

- Plan to collect a sputum specimen just after the client awakens or after an aerosol treatment. *This timing allows for a collection when more mucus is available or is in a thinner state.*
- Obtain a sterile sputum specimen cup. *Sterility prevents contamination of the specimen.*
- Help the client to a sitting position. *Sitting provides for an increased volume of inspired air and more forceful coughing to expel mucus.*
- Encourage the client to rinse the mouth with tap water. *Tap water removes some microorganisms and food residue.*
- Explain that the desired specimen should be from deep within the respiratory passages, not saliva from within the mouth. *The correct instruction helps to prevent inconclusive or invalid test results.*
- Instruct the client to take several deep breaths, attempt a forceful cough, and expectorate into the specimen container. *These measures help to mobilize secretions from the lower airway.*
- Collect at least a 1- to 3-mL (nearly a half teaspoon) specimen. *This quantity is sufficient for analysis.*
- Wear gloves and cover and enclose the specimen container in a clear plastic bag. *These steps reduce the potential for the transmission of microorganisms.*
- Offer oral hygiene. *It promotes comfort and well-being.*
- Attach a label and laboratory request form to the specimen. *Doing so ensures the correct specimen identification and test procedure.*
- Take the specimen to the laboratory immediately. *Prompt delivery facilitates a timely and accurate analysis of the specimen.*
- Document in the client's medical record the appearance of the specimen and its delivery to the laboratory. *Such recording provides assessment data and information about the disposition of the specimen.*

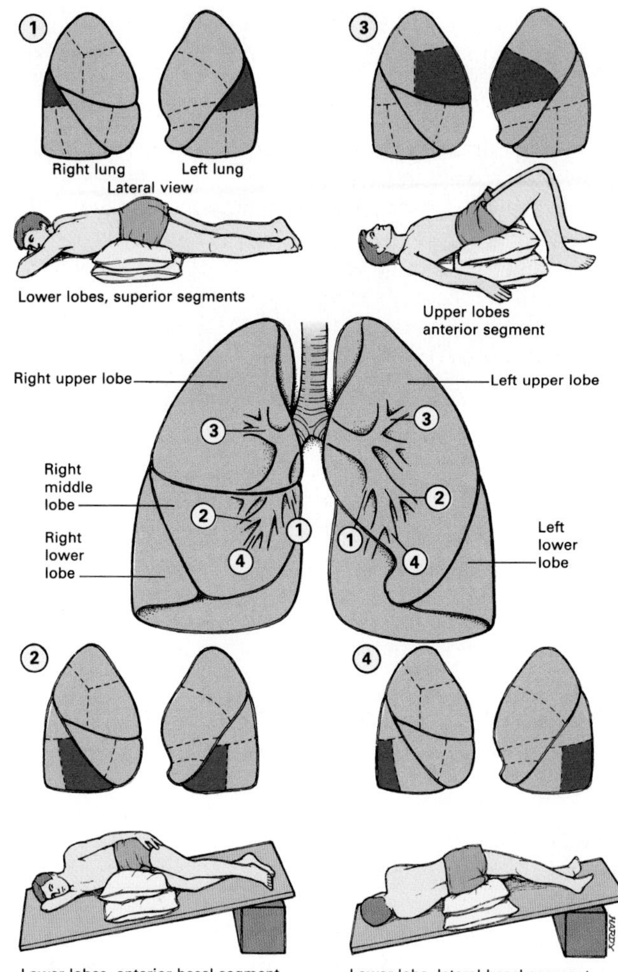

FIGURE 36-4 The lung segments and corresponding postural drainage positions. (Rosdahl, C. [2007]. *Textbook of basic nursing*, 9th ed. Philadelphia: Lippincott Williams & Wilkins.)

Percussion

Percussion (the rhythmic striking of the chest wall) helps to dislodge respiratory secretions that adhere to the bronchial walls. To perform percussion, the nurse cups the hands, keeping the fingers and thumb together, as if carrying water. He or she then applies the cupped hands to the client's chest as if trapping air between them and the thoracic wall (Fig. 36-5). The nurse performs percussion for 3 to 5 minutes in each postural drainage position, taking care to avoid striking the breasts of female clients and any areas of chest injury or bone disease.

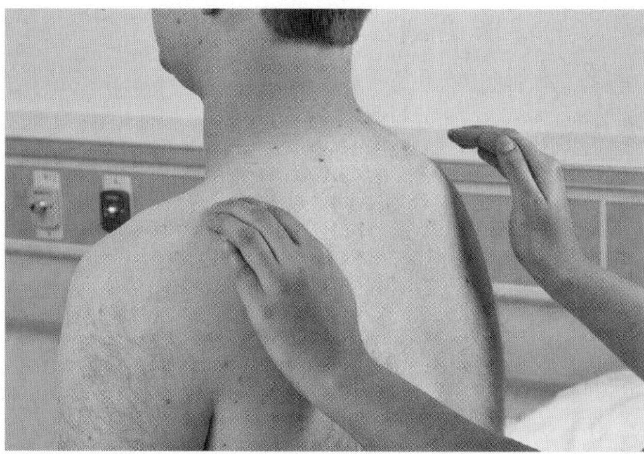

FIGURE 36-5 Performing percussion.

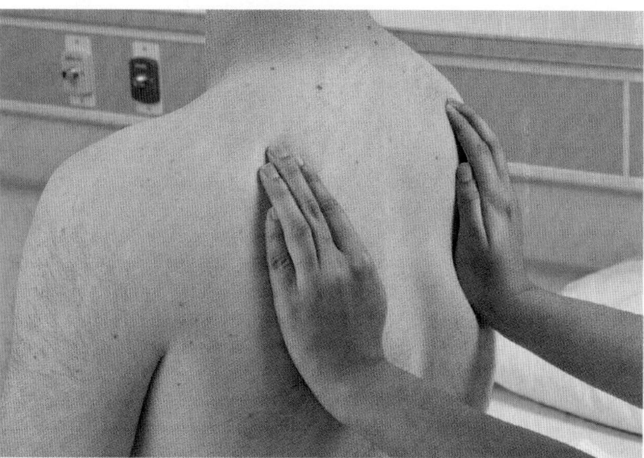

FIGURE 36-6 Performing vibration.

Vibration

Vibration uses the palms of the hands to shake underlying tissue and loosen retained secretions. The nurse positions the hands on the client's chest or back during inhalation and then vibrates them as the client exhales to increase the intensity of expiration (Fig. 36-6). Vibration is used with or as an alternative to percussion, especially for frail clients.

Suctioning Secretions

Suctioning relies on negative (vacuum) pressure to remove liquid secretions with a catheter. The amount of negative pressure varies depending on the client and the type of suction equipment (Table 36-1). Nurses may suction the upper airway, lower airway, or both. In all cases, they suction the airway from the nose or mouth (Skill 36-1).

Nasopharyngeal suctioning (removing secretions from the throat through a nasally inserted catheter) is more common than **nasotracheal suctioning** (removing secretions from the upper portion of the lower airway through a nasally inserted catheter). A nasopharyngeal airway, sometimes called a trumpet (Fig. 36-7), can be used to protect the nostril if frequent suctioning is necessary. An alternative method is **oropharyngeal suctioning** (removing secretions

TABLE 36-1 Variations in Suction Pressure

AGE	WALL SUCTION	PORTABLE SUCTION MACHINE
Adults	100–140 mm Hg	10–15 mm Hg
Children	95–100 mm Hg	5–10 mm Hg
Infants	50–95 mm Hg	2–5 mm Hg

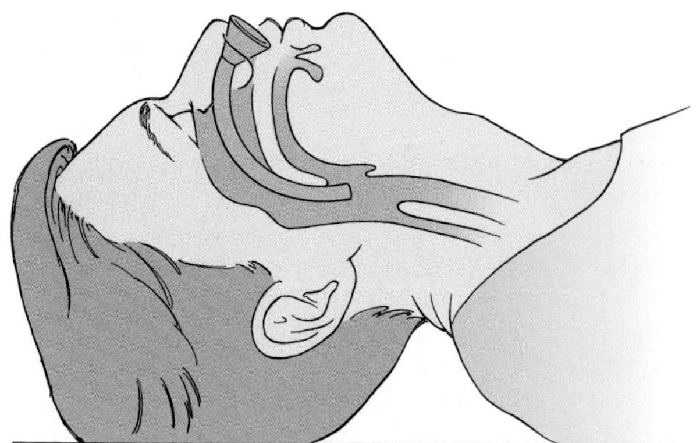

FIGURE 36-7 The placement of a nasopharyngeal trumpet.

from the throat through an orally inserted catheter). Nurses perform **oral suctioning** (removing secretions from the mouth) with a suctioning device called a Yankauer-tip or tonsil-tip catheter (Fig. 36-8).

Stop, Think, and Respond Box 36-1

In addition to an SpO_2 less than 90%, what signs or symptoms does a person with hypoxia manifest?

ARTIFICIAL AIRWAY MANAGEMENT

Clients at risk for airway obstruction or who require long-term mechanical ventilation are candidates for an artificial airway. Two common types are an oral airway and a tracheostomy tube.

Oral Airway

An **oral airway** is a curved device that keeps a relaxed tongue positioned forward within the mouth, preventing the tongue from obstructing the upper airway (Fig. 36-9). It is most commonly used in clients who are unconscious and cannot protect their own airway, such as those recovering from general anesthesia or a seizure. Nurses insert oral airways, which usually are in place for a brief time only (see Nursing Guidelines 36-2).

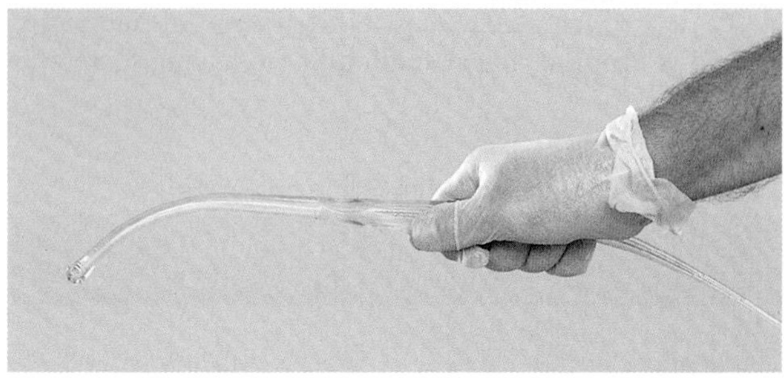

FIGURE 36-8 A Yankauer-tip suction device for oral suctioning. (Photo by B. Proud.)

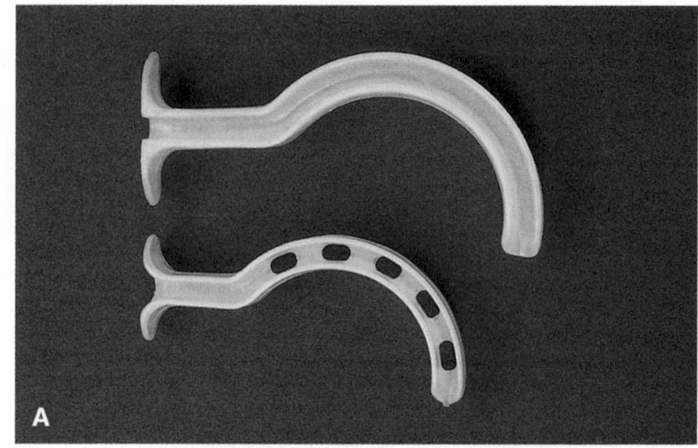

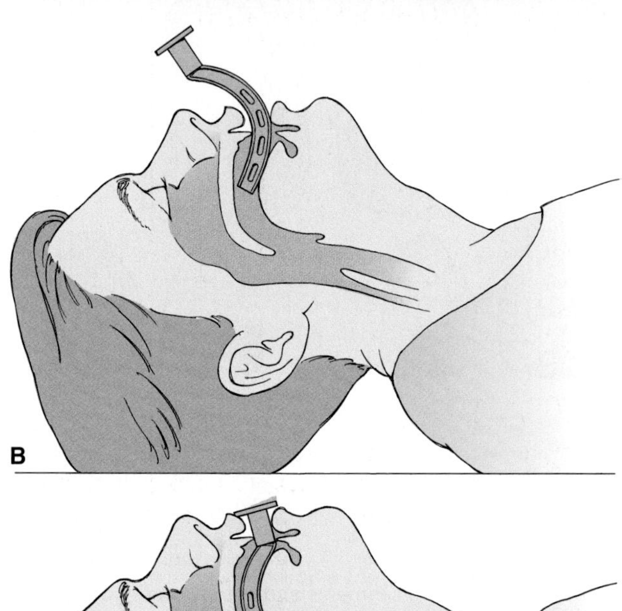

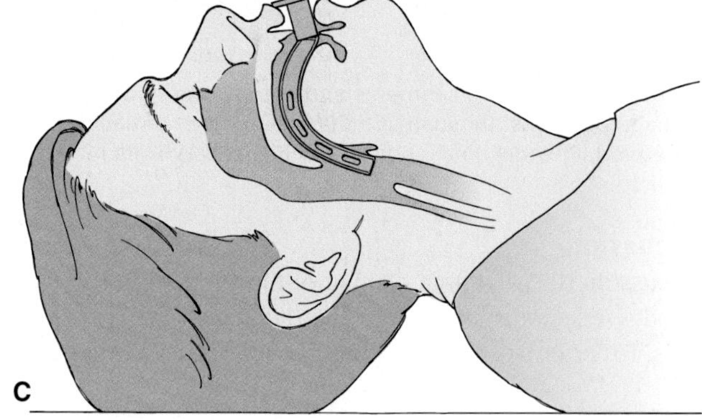

FIGURE 36-9 A. Examples of oral airways. **B.** The initial insertion position. **C.** The final position after rotation.

Tracheostomy

Clients who are less stable, have an upper airway obstruction, or who require prolonged mechanical ventilation and oxygenation are more likely to be candidates for a **tracheostomy** (a surgically created opening into the trachea). A tube is inserted through the opening to maintain the airway and provide a new route for ventilation.

Tracheostomy Tube

A **tracheostomy tube** (a curved, hollow plastic tube) is also called a cannula. Some devices have an inner and an outer cannula. Tracheostomy tubes also may have a balloon cuff

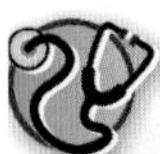

NURSING GUIDELINES 36-2

Inserting an Oral Airway

- Gather the following supplies: various sizes of oral airways (most adults can accommodate an 80-mm airway), gloves, a tongue blade, and suction equipment. *Gathering equipment promotes organization and efficient time management.*
- Place the airway on the outside of the client's cheek so that the front portion is parallel with the front teeth. Note whether or not the back of the airway reaches the angle of the jaw. *Assessment determines the appropriate size to use. (An airway that is too short will be ineffective. An airway that is too long will depress the epiglottis, increasing the risk of airway obstruction.)*
- Wash your hands or perform an alcohol-based hand rub (see Chap. 10); don clean gloves. *These measures reduce the transmission of microorganisms.*
- Explain the procedure to the client. *Instruction provides information that even unconscious clients may comprehend, despite being unable to respond verbally.*
- Perform oral suctioning if necessary. *Doing so clears saliva from the mouth and prevents aspiration.*
- Position the client supine with the neck hyperextended unless contraindicated. *This position opens the airway and facilitates insertion.*
- Open the client's mouth using a gloved finger and thumb or a tongue blade. *Doing so prevents injury to the teeth during insertion.*
- Hold the airway so that the curved tip points upward toward the roof of the mouth (see Fig. 36-9B) or the side of the cheek. Insert it about halfway. *Such placement prevents pushing the tongue into the pharynx during insertion.*
- Rotate the airway over the top of the tongue and continue inserting it until the front flange is flush with the lips (see Fig. 36-9C). *This ensures that the artificial airway follows the natural curve of the upper airway.*
- Assess breathing. *Checking breathing validates that the natural airway is patent.*
- Remove the airway every 4 hours, provide oral hygiene, and clean and reinsert the airway. *Hygiene and cleaning remove transient bacteria and promote the integrity of the oral mucosa.*
- As the client's level of consciousness improves, many clients extubate themselves independently.

(Fig. 36-10); when inflated, the cuff seals the upper airway to prevent aspiration of oral fluids and to provide more efficient ventilation. During insertion of a tracheostomy tube, an obturator, a curved guide, is used. Once the tube is in place, the obturator is removed.

Because a tracheostomy tube is below the level of the larynx, clients usually cannot speak. Communication may involve writing or reading the client's lips. Being unable to call for help is frightening; therefore, the nurse should check these clients frequently and respond immediately when they signal.

Stop, Think, and Respond Box 36-2

Discuss the physical and psychological effects a client with a tracheostomy may develop as a consequence of being unable to speak.

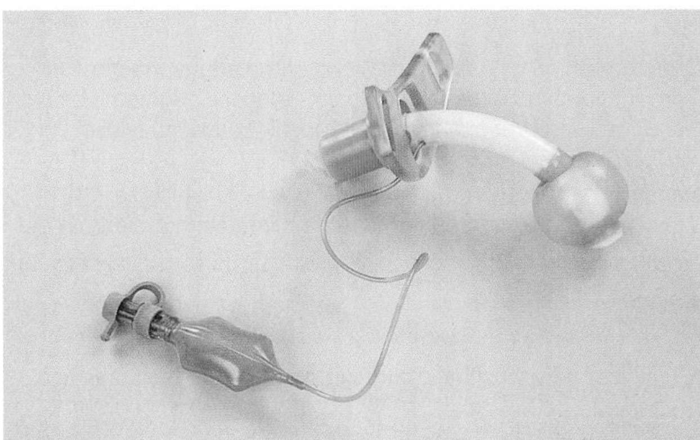

FIGURE 36-10 A cuffed tracheostomy tube. (Photo by B. Proud.)

Tracheostomy Suctioning

Most clients with a tracheostomy require frequent suctioning. Although they can cough, the force of the cough may be ineffective in completely clearing the airway, or the cough may be inadequate to clear the volume of respiratory secretions. Therefore, suctioning is necessary when secretions are copious.

Tracheostomy suctioning is similar to nasotracheal suctioning except that catheter insertion is through the tracheostomy tube rather than the nose (Fig. 36-11). When suctioning a tracheostomy, the nurse inserts the catheter a shorter distance (approximately 4 to 5 in. [10 to 12.5 cm] or until resistance is felt) because the tube already lies in the trachea. The

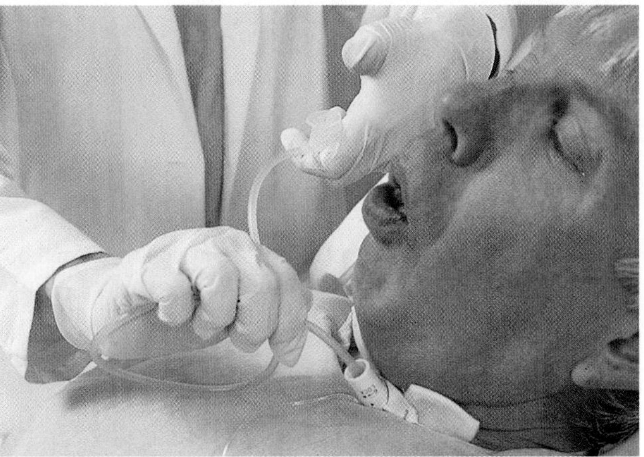

FIGURE 36-11 Suctioning through a tracheostomy tube. (Courtesy of Swedish Hospital Medical Center.)

resistance is caused by contact between the catheter tip and the carina, the ridge at the lower end of the tracheal cartilage where the main bronchi are located. The nurse then raises the catheter about 0.5 in. (1.25 cm) and applies suction.

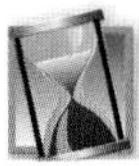

Gerontologic Considerations

■ Older adults are at increased risk for cardiac dysrhythmias during suctioning because many have preexisting hypoxemia from illnesses and age-related changes in ventilation.

Tracheostomy Care

Tracheostomy care means cleaning the skin around the stoma, changing the dressing, and cleaning the inner cannula (Skill 36-2). Nurses perform tracheostomy care at least every 8 hours or as often as clients need to keep the secretions from becoming dried, then narrowing or occluding the airway. They may do tracheal suctioning separately from or at the same time as tracheostomy care.

NURSING IMPLICATIONS

Maintaining an open and patent airway is a priority for nursing care. Lack of oxygen for more than 4 to 6 minutes can result in death or permanent brain damage. Therefore, it is essential to identify nursing diagnoses that apply to respiratory problems and to plan care accordingly for clients at risk. Some possible nursing diagnoses include the following:

- Ineffective Airway Clearance
- Impaired Gas Exchange
- Risk for Infection
- Impaired Spontaneous Ventilation
- Anxiety
- Deficient Knowledge

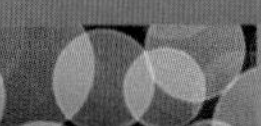

NURSING CARE PLAN 36-1 Ineffective Airway Clearance

Assessment

- Observe characteristics of the client's breathing and ability to cough forcefully.
- Inspect the sputum for evidence of a viscid consistency.
- Auscultate the lungs to detect adventitious breath sounds suggestive of retained secretions.
- Assess vital signs to detect manifestations of impaired oxygenation.
- Review the client's medical record for conditions that may alter the ability to protect and clear the airway, such as a decreased level of consciousness, unusual weakness or easy fatigability, moderate-to-severe pain, and a surgical incision about the thorax or abdomen.
- Note if the client's fluid intake is adequate.

Nursing Diagnosis. **Ineffective Airway Clearance** related to retained secretions as manifested by weak and persistent cough without raising sputum, rapid and shallow respirations, use of accessory muscles, inspiratory gurgles heard in distal right upper lobe both anteriorly and posteriorly, and history of smoking two packs of cigarettes a day.

Expected Outcome. The client's airway will be effectively cleared as evidenced by raising sputum sufficiently to keep lung sounds clear by 12/4.

Interventions	Rationales
Auscultate the lungs every shift and before and after coughing or other respiratory therapy.	Auscultation provides data indicating the presence or absence of retained respiratory secretions.
Elevate the head of the bed at all times.	The Fowler's position helps to provide maximum room for lung expansion.
Maintain 2,000–3,000 mL fluid intake of client's choice (avoid milk) for 24 hours.	Keeping the client well hydrated helps thin respiratory mucus.
Instruct client to take three deep breaths in through the nose and out the mouth, lean forward, and cough forcefully. Repeat every 1–2 hours while the client is awake.	Deep breathing dilates the airways, stimulates surfactant production, and expands the lung surface. Coughing loosens and forces secretions into the bronchi (Carpenito-Moyet, 2005).
Perform oral/pharyngeal suctioning if secretions are loose but the client does not expectorate them.	Negative pressure produces a pulling effect, which can remove mucoid secretions that the client cannot clear independently.

Evaluation of Expected Outcomes

- Client is instructed on deep breathing and the coughing technique.
- Client can raise tenacious, purulent sputum after breathing and coughing.
- Lungs sound less congested.

Nursing Care Plan 36-1 shows how the nursing process applies to a client with the nursing diagnosis of Ineffective Airway Clearance, defined in the 2012 NANDA-I taxonomy (p. 421) as the "inability to clear secretions or obstructions from the respiratory tract to maintain a clear airway."

CRITICAL THINKING EXERCISE

1. What suggestions would you offer an individual to discourage him or her from continuing to smoke cigarettes?
2. What pulmonary diseases are likely to be diagnosed by examining a sputum specimen, and what nursing actions facilitate an accurate examination of the collected specimen?
3. Why do body positions that place the head lower than the chest facilitate the expectoration of pulmonary secretions?
4. Discuss ways to relieve the anxiety of a client with a tracheostomy who needs frequent suctioning but fears he or she will be unable to obtain assistance when needed.

NCLEX-STYLE REVIEW QUESTIONS

1. Besides describing the characteristics of a client's cough, what other information is most important to document?
   1. The client's family history of respiratory disease
   2. A current assessment of the client's vital signs
   3. The appearance of the respiratory secretions
   4. The types of self-treatments that the client is using
2. If all the following nursing measures are possible, which helps most when planning to obtain a sputum specimen?
   1. Provide the client with a generous fluid intake.
   2. Assist the client to change positions regularly.
   3. Ask the dietitian to send a high-protein diet.
   4. Ensure that the client has sufficient rest periods.
3. What time of the day is it best for the nurse to attempt to obtain a sputum specimen?
   1. Before bedtime
   2. After a meal
   3. Between meals
   4. Upon awakening
4. When suctioning a client with a tracheostomy tube, when is the best time to occlude the vent on the suction catheter?
   1. When inserting the catheter
   2. When inside the inner cannula
   3. When withdrawing the catheter
   4. When the client begins coughing
5. When suctioning the airway of a client with a tracheostomy, the nurse applies suction for no longer than how long?
   1. 5 to 7 seconds
   2. 10 to 15 seconds
   3. 15 to 20 seconds
   4. 20 to 30 seconds

SKILL 36-1 Suctioning the Airway

Suggested Action	Reason for Action
ASSESSMENT	
Assess the client's lung sounds, respiratory effort, and oxygen saturation level.	Determines the need for suctioning.
Determine how much the client understands about suctioning the airway.	Provides an opportunity for health teaching.
Inspect the nose to determine which nostril is more patent.	Eases insertion of the catheter.
PLANNING	
Consider using a face shield and wearing a cover gown in addition to gloves when suctioning a client.	The nurse can choose to wear a face shield and cover gown as part of standard precautions.
Obtain a suction kit. All kits contain a basin and one or two sterile gloves. Some also contain a sterile suction catheter.	Promotes organization and efficient time management.
If the kit does not include a catheter, select one that will not occlude the nostril; usually a 12–18 F catheter is appropriate for adults.	Promotes comfort and reduces the potential for injury.
Obtain a flask of sterile normal saline and a suction machine if a wall outlet is unavailable.	Provides items that are not prepackaged.
Attach the suction canister to the wall outlet or plug a portable suction machine into an electrical outlet.	Provides a source for negative pressure.
Connect the suction tubing to the canister.	Provides a means for connecting the canister to the suction catheter.
Turn on the suction machine, occlude the suction tubing, and adjust the pressure gauge to the desired amount.	Ensures safe pressure during suctioning.
Open the container of saline.	Reduces the risk for later contamination.
IMPLEMENTATION	
Pull the privacy curtains.	Demonstrates respect for the client.
Elevate the head of the bed unless contraindicated.	Aids in ventilation.
Wash your hands or perform an alcohol-based hand rub (see Chap. 10).	Reduces the transmission of microorganisms.
Preoxygenate the client for 1–2 minutes until the SpO_2 is maintained at 95%–100%.	Reduces the risk for hypoxemia.
Open the suction kit without contaminating the contents.	Follows the principles of asepsis.
Don sterile glove(s). If the kit provides only one, don a clean glove on the nondominant hand and then don the sterile glove on the dominant hand.	Prevents the transmission of microorganisms.
Pour sterile normal saline into the basin with your nondominant hand.	Prepares the solution for wetting and rinsing the suction catheter.
Consider the nondominant hand contaminated.	Follows principles of asepsis.
Pick up the suction catheter with your sterile (dominant) hand and connect it to the suction tubing (Fig. A).	Completes the circuit for applying suction.

A

Connecting the catheter. (Photo by B. Proud.)

(continued)

Suctioning the Airway (continued)

IMPLEMENTATION (CONTINUED)

Place the catheter tip in the saline and occlude the vent (Fig. B). — Wets the outer and inner surfaces of the catheter, which reduces friction and facilitates insertion.

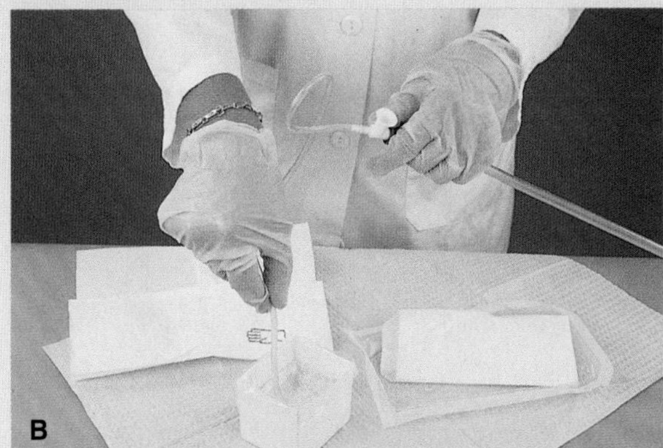

Wetting the catheter. (Photo by B. Proud.)

Insert the catheter without applying suction along the floor of the nose or side of the mouth (Fig. C). — Reduces the potential for sneezing or gagging.

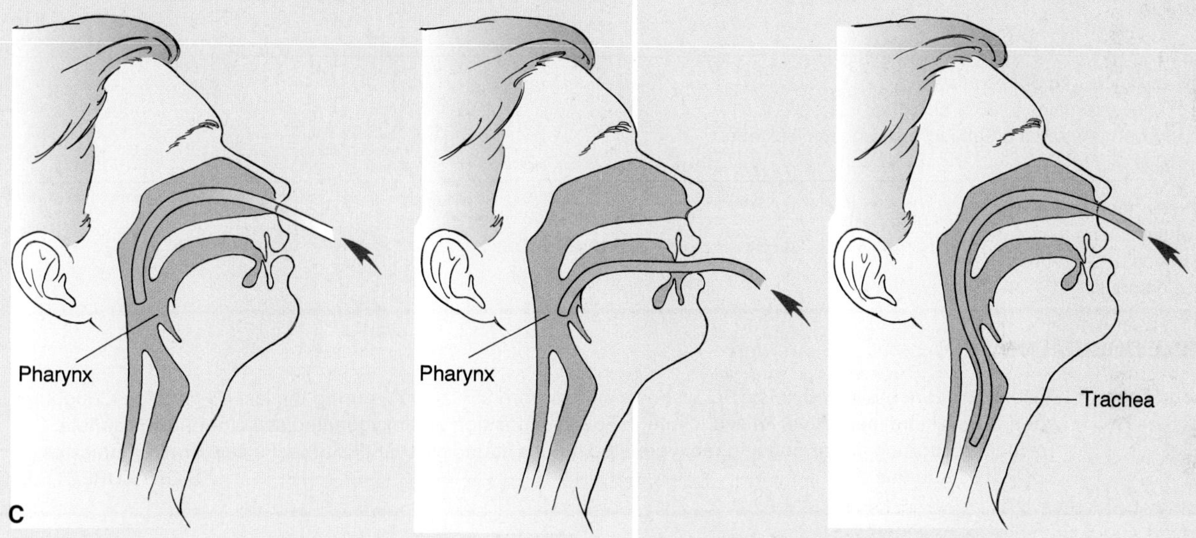

Catheter placement: nasopharyngeal (*left*), oropharyngeal (*center*), and nasotracheal (*right*).

Advance the catheter 5–6 in. (12.5–15 cm) in the nose or 3–4 in. (7.5–10 cm) in the mouth. — Places the distal tip in the pharynx.

For tracheal suctioning, wait until the client takes a breath and then advance the tubing 8–10 in. (20–25 cm). — Eases insertion below the larynx.

Encourage the client to cough if coughing does not occur spontaneously. — Breaks up mucus and raises secretions.

Occlude the air vent and rotate the catheter as it is withdrawn. — Maximizes the effectiveness of suctioning.

Complete the process in no more than 15 seconds from insertion to removal of the catheter, occluding the vent no longer than 10 seconds. — Prevents hypoxemia.

Rinse secretions from the catheter by inserting its tip in the basin of saline and applying suction. — Flushes the mucus from the inner lumen.

Provide 2–3 minutes of rest while the client continues to breathe oxygen. — Reoxygenates the blood.

Suction again if necessary. — Bases decision on individual assessment data.

(continued)

Suctioning the Airway (continued)

IMPLEMENTATION (CONTINUED)

Remove the gloves to enclose the suction catheter in an inverted glove (Fig. D).	Encloses the soiled catheter, reducing the transmission of microorganisms.

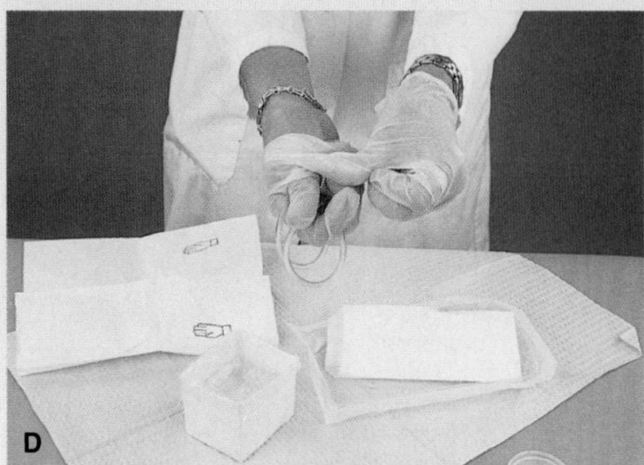

Enclosing the catheter. (Photo by B. Proud.)

Discard suction kit, catheter, and gloves in a lined waste receptacle.	Follows principles of asepsis.

Evaluation

- The airway is cleared of secretions.
- The SpO_2 level remains at 95% or higher.
- The client demonstrates breathing that requires less effort.

Document

- Preassessment data
- Type of suctioning performed
- Appearance of secretions
- Client's response

SAMPLE DOCUMENTATION

Date and Time Respirations are moist and noisy. SpO_2 shows a drop from 95% to 90% during the last 15 minutes. Coughing effort is weak and ineffective. Raised to a high Fowler's position and oxygenated at 4 L per nasal cannula. Tracheal suctioning performed and reoxygenated. Lungs sound clear at this time. Pulse oximeter indicates SpO_2 at 95% at this time. ——— SIGNATURE/TITLE

SKILL 36-2 Providing Tracheostomy Care

Suggested Action	Reason for Action
ASSESSMENT	
Check the nursing care plan to determine the schedule for providing tracheostomy care.	Provides continuity of care.
Review the client's record for documentation concerning previous tracheostomy care.	Provides a data base for comparison.
Assess the condition of the dressing and the skin around the tracheostomy tube.	Determines the need for a dressing change and skin care.
Determine the client's understanding of tracheostomy care.	Provides an opportunity for health teaching.

(continued)

Providing Tracheostomy Care (continued)

PLANNING

Consult with the client on an appropriate time for tracheostomy care if only routine care is needed.	Demonstrates respect for the client's right to participate in decisions.
Consider using a face shield and wearing a cover gown in addition to gloves when suctioning a client.	The nurse can choose to wear a face shield and cover gown as part of standard precautions.
Obtain a container of hydrogen peroxide and a flask of normal saline. Remove the cap from each container.	Provides items that are not prepackaged and prevents the contamination of one gloved hand later in the procedure.

IMPLEMENTATION

Wash your hands or perform an alcohol-based hand rub (see Chap. 10).	Removes colonizing microorganisms.
Raise the bed to an appropriate height.	Prevents back strain.
Place the client in a supine or low Fowler's position.	Facilitates access to the tracheostomy tube.
Don a clean glove; remove the soiled stomal dressing and discard it, glove and all, in a lined waste receptacle.	Follows the principles of asepsis.
Wash your hands or perform an alcohol-based hand rub again.	Reduces the transmission of microorganisms.
Open the tracheostomy kit, taking care not to contaminate its contents.	Provides access to and maintains the sterility of supplies.
Don sterile gloves.	Prevents transferring microorganisms to the lower airway.
Add equal parts of sterile normal saline and sterile hydrogen peroxide to one basin and sterile normal saline to the other (Fig. A).	The diluted hydrogen peroxide cleans mucoid secretions; the sterile normal saline rinses the peroxide solution from the skin and inner cannula.

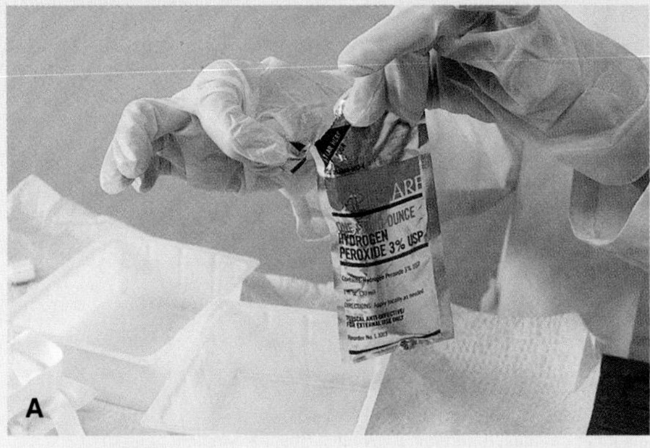

Adding the cleaning solutions. (Courtesy of Swedish Hospital Medical Center.)

Unlock the inner cannula (using one hand, which is now considered contaminated) by turning it counterclockwise; deposit it in the basin with the hydrogen peroxide and saline solution (Fig. B).	Loosens protein secretions and reduces colonizing microorganisms.

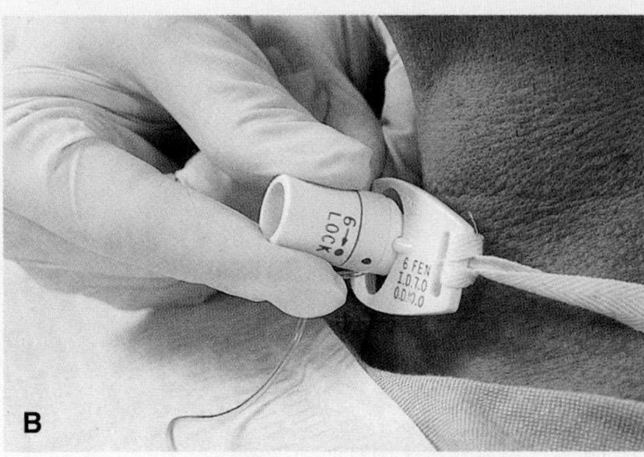

Removing the inner cannula. (Courtesy of Swedish Hospital Medical Center.)

(continued)

Providing Tracheostomy Care (continued)

IMPLEMENTATION (CONTINUED)

Clean the inside and outside of a plastic cannula with pipe cleaners; use pipe cleaners or a soft brush for a metal cannula (Fig. C).

Removes gross debris; pipe cleaners are less likely to scratch a plastic cannula.

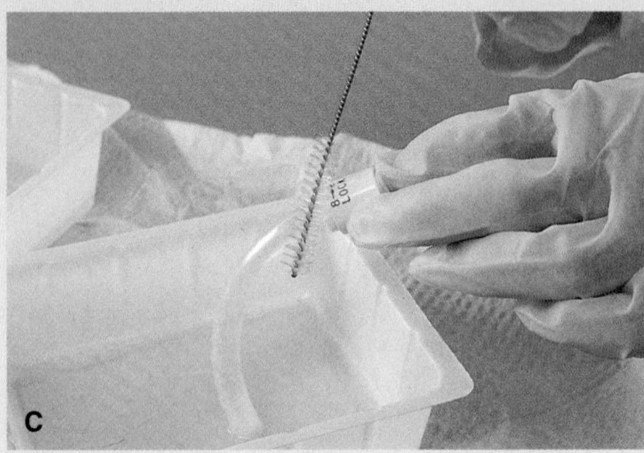

C Cleaning the inner cannula. (Courtesy of Swedish Hospital Medical Center.)

Deposit contaminated supplies in a lined or waterproof waste receptacle.

Reduces the potential for contaminating sterile supplies.

Rinse the cleaned cannula in the basin of normal saline.

Removes remnants of hydrogen peroxide.

Tap the rinsed cannula against the edge of the basin and wipe the excess solution with a gauze square.

Removes large droplets of fluid.

Replace the inner cannula and turn it clockwise within the outer cannula (Fig. D).

Secures the inner cannula.

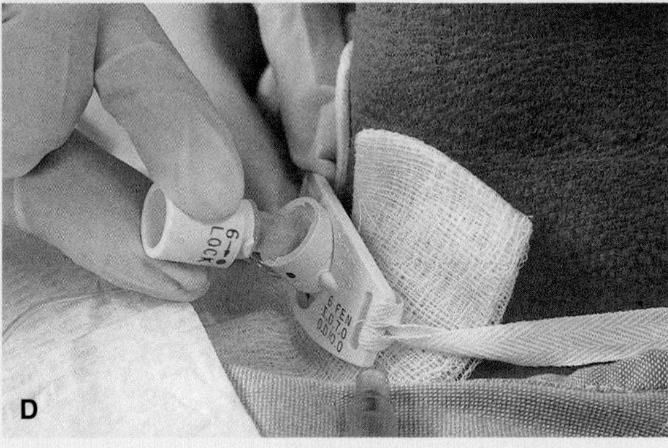

D Replacing the inner cannula. (Courtesy of Swedish Hospital Medical Center.)

Clean around the stoma with an applicator moistened with the diluted peroxide (Fig. E).

Never go back over an area once you have cleaned it.

Removes secretions and colonizing microorganisms from the tracheal opening.

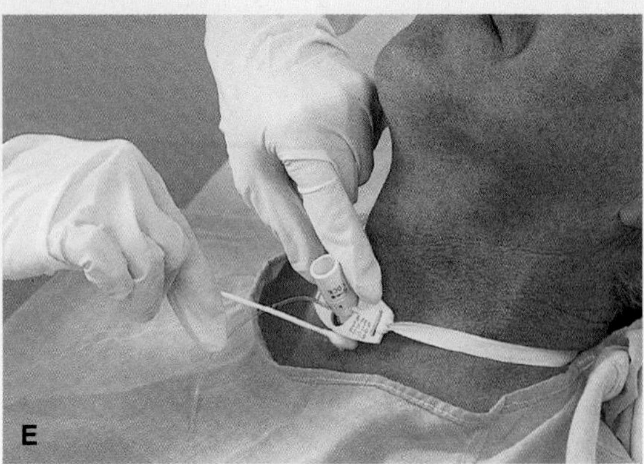

E Cleaning the stoma. (Courtesy of Swedish Hospital Medical Center.)

(continued)

Providing Tracheostomy Care (continued)

IMPLEMENTATION (CONTINUED)

Action	Rationale
Wipe the same area in the same manner with another applicator moistened with saline.	Removes hydrogen peroxide from the skin.
Place the sterile stomal dressing beneath the flanges and outer cannula of the tracheostomy tube (Fig. F).	Absorbs secretions and keeps the stomal area clean.

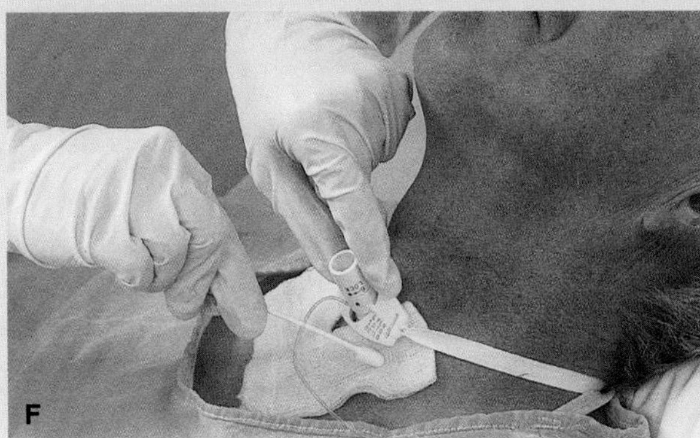

Applying the stomal dressing. (Photo by B. Proud.)

Action	Rationale
Change the tracheostomy ties by threading them through the slits of each flange of the tracheostomy tube and tying them in place (Fig. G).	Holds the tracheostomy tube in place.

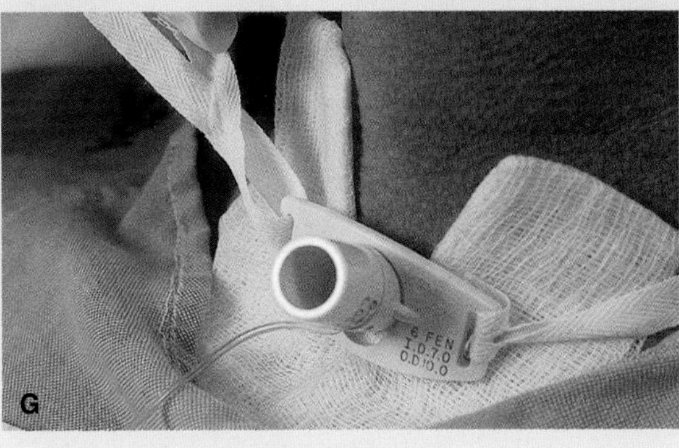

Securing the tracheostomy ties. (Courtesy of Swedish Hospital Medical Center.)

Action	Rationale
Wait to remove the previous ties until after the new ones are secure, if working alone. Otherwise, have an assistant stabilize the tracheostomy tube while you cut the soiled ties and apply the new ties.	Prevents accidental extubation.
Tie the two ends snugly, but not tightly, at the side of the neck. Make sure there is room to insert your little finger within the ties before securing the ends.	Prevents skin impairment.
Discard all soiled supplies, remove your gloves, and wash your hands or perform an alcohol-based hand rub.	Follows the principles of asepsis.
Return the client to a safe and comfortable position.	Demonstrates concern for the client's well-being.
Restore a means that the client can use to signal for assistance (eg, call button, bell).	Facilitates meeting the client's needs in emergencies and nonemergencies.

(continued)

Providing Tracheostomy Care (continued)

Evaluation

- The tracheostomy tube remains patent.
- The stomal opening is clean and without evidence of infection.
- The dressing is clean and dry.
- The skin around the neck is intact.

Document

- Preassessment data
- Procedure as it was performed
- Appearance of skin and secretions
- Client's response

SAMPLE DOCUMENTATION

Date and Time Respirations are quiet and effortless. Routine tracheostomy care provided. Moderate amount of clear mucus removed from inner cannula during cleaning. Stomal skin is pink, but there is no redness, tenderness, swelling, or purulent drainage. Neck skin is intact; skin color is comparable to surrounding areas. ——— SIGNATURE/TITLE

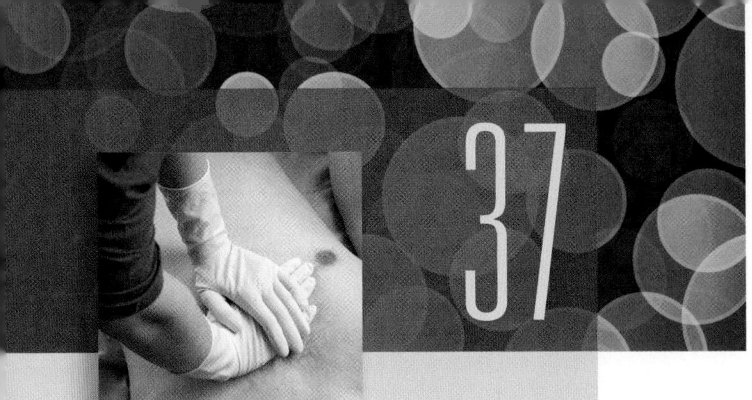

37 Resuscitation

Words To Know

asystole
automated external defibrillator
cardiac arrest
cardiopulmonary resuscitation
Chain of Survival
code
head-tilt/chin-lift technique
Heimlich maneuver
jaw-thrust maneuver
recovery position
rescue breathing
resuscitation team
subdiaphragmatic thrust
ventricular fibrillation

Learning Objectives

On completion of this chapter, the reader should be able to:

1. Explain why an airway obstruction is life threatening, and give at least three signs of an airway obstruction.
2. Describe appropriate actions if a client has a partial airway obstruction.
3. Explain the purpose of the Heimlich maneuver and describe the circumstances for using subdiaphragmatic and chest thrusts.
4. Identify the recommended action for relieving an airway obstruction in an infant and in an unconscious person.
5. List the five steps in the Chain of Survival.
6. Explain cardiopulmonary resuscitation (CPR) and its associated Circulation, Airway, Breathing (CAB).
7. Describe the purpose of chest compression.
8. Name two techniques for opening the airway and list three ways a trained rescuer administers rescue breathing.
9. Discuss the appropriate use of an automated external defibrillator (AED).
10. Name at least three criteria used in the decision to discontinue resuscitation efforts.

Nurses are often the first to respond to pulmonary or cardiac emergencies. The information in this chapter reflects the American Heart Association's (AHA) International CPR and Emergency Cardiovascular Care (ECC) Guidelines of 2010 for performing basic life-support techniques.

AIRWAY OBSTRUCTION

The upper airway, can become occluded for various reasons (Box 37-1). Sometimes, the airway swells because of injury; in such cases, the client may need an artificial airway to promote and sustain breathing (see Chap. 36). A bolus of food or some other foreign object may cause mechanical airway obstruction. Regardless of the cause, airway obstruction compromises air exchange and subsequent oxygenation of cells and tissues. For this reason, unrelieved airway obstruction will lead to a loss of consciousness, and, eventually, death.

Stop, Think, and Respond Box 37-1

Discuss circumstances in which a person is at high risk for mechanical airway obstruction.

BOX 37-1 Common Causes of Airway Obstruction

- Compromised swallowing
- Aspiration of vomitus
- Insufficient chewing
- Consuming large pieces of food
- Laughing or talking while chewing
- Eating when intoxicated
- Inhaling foreign objects from the mouth

Identifying Signs of Airway Obstruction

Signs of airway obstruction (Box 37-2) generally occur while the person is eating. The victim immediately may grasp his or her throat with the hands (Fig. 37-1) and make aggressive efforts to cough and breathe. He or she may make a high-pitched sound while inhaling. The face initially reddens then becomes pale or blue.

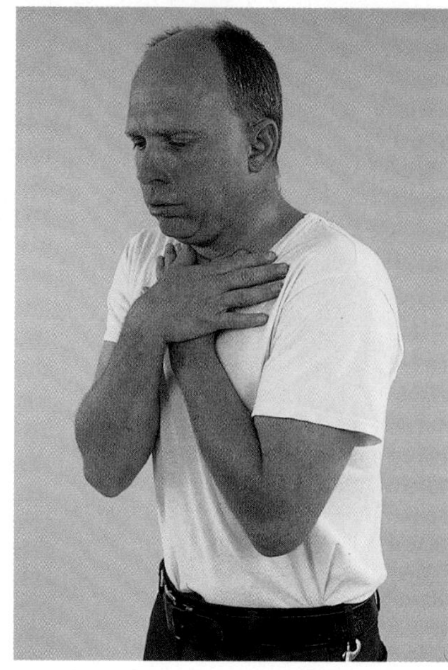

FIGURE 37-1 The universal sign for choking. (Photo by B. Proud.)

Relieving an Obstruction

If the victim can speak or cough, he or she is exchanging some air, which indicates only a partial obstruction. Because infants cannot talk or make the universal choking sign, the ability to cry is the best evidence of partial obstruction in this age group. Other than encouraging and supporting the victim, a partial obstruction requires no additional resuscitation efforts.

If the victim's independent efforts to relieve a partial obstruction are unsuccessful or if the situation worsens, activating the emergency medical system is appropriate. In the hospital, staff members do this by calling a **code** (summoning personnel trained in advanced life support techniques). In the community, people can obtain assistance by dialing 911 or another emergency number.

If an obstruction becomes complete, immediate action is necessary to dislodge the obstruction. When the victim is *conscious*, the **Heimlich maneuver** (the method for relieving a mechanical airway obstruction) is appropriate. It involves the use of **subdiaphragmatic thrusts** (pressure to the abdomen) or chest thrusts. The victim's age determines how these thrusts should be performed.

BOX 37-2 Signs of a Partial or Complete Airway Obstruction

- Coughing or gagging while eating
- Audibly wheezing
- Persistently attempting to clear throat
- Making hoarse or wet vocal sounds
- Resisting efforts to be fed
- Being unable to speak
- Holding throat
- Being unable to breathe
- Exhibiting cyanosis

- For infants (children younger than 1 year of age), the rescuer supports the baby over his or her forearm. Holding the infant prone with the head downward, the rescuer uses the heel of one hand to administer five back slaps between the shoulder blades (Fig. 37-2A). The rescuer turns the infant supine and uses two fingers to give five chest thrusts at approximately one per second to the middle of the breastbone, just below the nipple line (see Fig. 37-2B). He or she repeatedly alternates five back blows and chest thrusts until the object is dislodged or the infant fails to respond. The rescuer does not use finger sweeps unless he or she can see the obstructing object. If the infant becomes unconscious, the rescuer performs CPR (described later).
- For all people older than 1 year of age, the rescuer gives a series of five quick subdiaphragmatic (abdominal) upward thrusts slightly above the navel to increase intrathoracic pressure equivalent to a cough (Fig. 37-3). The rescuer opens the victim's airway with the head-tilt/chin-lift maneuver (described later) and continues administering upward thrusts if initial efforts are not successful. He or she avoids blind finger sweeps unless the object in the airway is visible. If the person becomes unconscious, the rescuer supports the victim to the floor, activates the emergency response system, and begins performing CPR (described later). The victim's mouth is checked for any visible object when each attempt at ventilation is made.

When the victim is *unconscious*, the AHA recommends the use of basic CPR (described later in this chapter), using chest compressions rather than abdominal thrusts. Chest compressions in CPR creates enough pressure in unconscious victims to eject a foreign body from the airway (Berg et al., 2010; Salati, 2006).

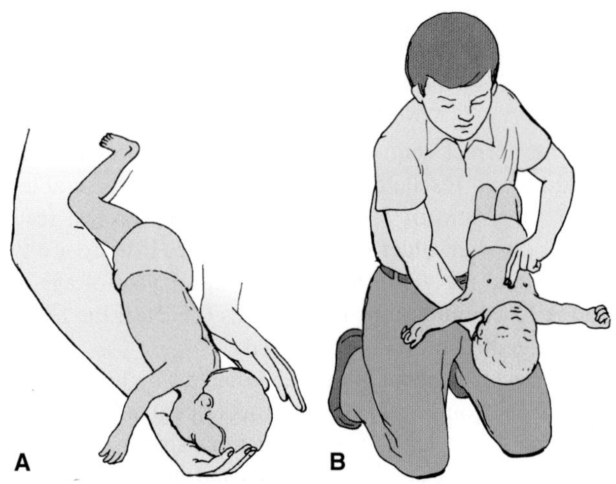

FIGURE 37-2 Assisting an infant with an obstruction. **A.** Giving back blows. **B.** Delivering chest thrusts.

CHAIN OF SURVIVAL

If a person's unresponsiveness may be the result of **cardiac arrest** (the cessation of heart contraction or a life-sustaining heart rhythm), rescuers implement a five-step intervention process known as the **Chain of Survival**. The steps involve (1) immediate recognition and access of emergency services, (2) early CPR with a focus on compressions, (3) rapid defibrillation if appropriate, (4) effective advanced life support, and (5) integrated postcardiac arrest care. Survival rates following cardiac arrest depend greatly on the speed with which rescuers initiate the Chain of Survival. The faster the steps occur, the better the victim's chances. Outcomes are best when rescuers perform these steps rapidly.

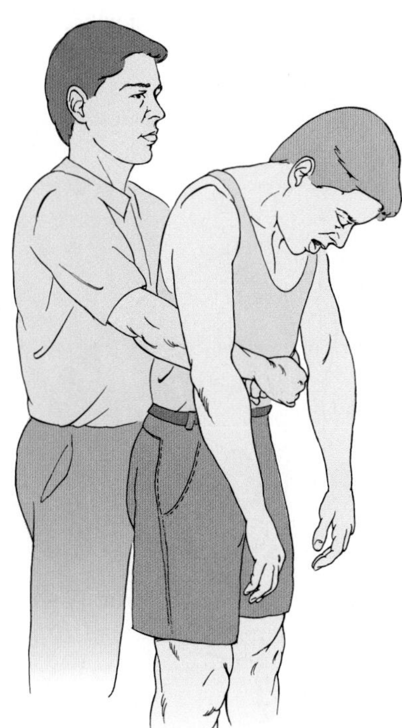
FIGURE 37-3 Giving subdiaphragmatic thrusts.

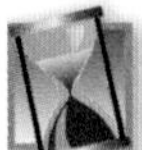
Gerontologic Considerations

- Congress legislated a person's right to refuse medical treatment in 1990. All states implemented the Patient Self-Determination Act in 1991. This act recognizes that the client, not the health care provider, is the ultimate authority in making decisions related to life-sustaining treatments.
- Federal law mandates that all health care institutions that participate in Medicare and Medicaid provide information about the Patient Self-Determination Act as it applies to establishing an advance directive or living will.
- Older adults may need very clear and pertinent descriptions of various treatments and measures for resuscitation addressed in advance directives. An older adult's advance directive should specify exactly the type of resuscitation he or she wishes. For example, some clients approve the use of emergency drugs but refuse mechanical ventilation.
- When possible, it is important to allow several days for older adults to consider advance directives before they sign legal documents. They may benefit from consulting trusted members of their religious affiliation or trusted medical authorities. Also, discussing the implications of advance directives as they apply to various settings is important. For example, if a person at home has an advance directive prohibiting resuscitation, family members and caregivers need to understand that it may not be appropriate to call 911 or begin basic life-support procedures.
- Nurses are responsible for ascertaining whether an older client has an existing advance directive and ensuring that the directions continue to reflect the client's wishes.
- Family caregivers, particularly those designated as having health care powers of attorney, should be included in discussions about resuscitation efforts. A helpful booklet, *Hard Choices for Loving People: CPR, Artificial Feeding, Comfort Measures Only and the Elderly Patient* by Hank Dunn, is available at http://www.hardchoices.com.
- Some older adults fear that if they specify that they do not wish to be resuscitated, they will receive less-than-appropriate care and treatment of their illness. The client's record must contain his or her resuscitation status. If no information is documented, CPR is administered in any life-threatening situation regardless of the client's age.
- Advance directives are to be reviewed periodically (at least annually and whenever a major change occurs in the older adult's health status) and updated according to the current situation and living arrangement. For example, if an older adult is in a long-term care institutional setting, the staff needs specific directives about when to send him or her to an emergency room. Similarly, in home care situations, caregivers need very specific guidelines about what course of action to take under various circumstances.
- Older adults need to be informed that they may change their mind about advance directives and instructions for resuscitation at any time. All changes must be communicated to the physician, and a written copy should be stored in a safe location.

Early Recognition and Access of Emergency Services

With the victim in a supine position on a dry, firm surface, a quick assessment taking no more than 10 seconds is performed to determine unresponsiveness and the absence of normal breathing. Responsiveness is determined by shouting and shaking the victim. If the victim appears lifeless or is not breathing normally, it is essential to activate the emergency medical response system, whether outside or within a health care facility. This can be done by a bystander or second rescuer as well. In most locations, emergency medical assistance is obtained by dialing 911 and providing information to a central phone operator. The person making the call gives the following facts:

- The address where assistance is needed
- A description of the situation
- The victim's current condition
- What actions have been taken

Emergency medical technicians or paramedics are then dispatched to the scene. If the emergency involves someone within a health care agency, the **resuscitation team** (a group of people who have been trained and certified in advanced cardiac life-support [ACLS] techniques) is alerted by notifying the switchboard operator that assistance is needed and the location of the emergency.

Early Cardiopulmonary Resuscitation

Resuscitation must proceed with CAB (circulation, airway, breathing if the rescuer is a trained health provider, or hands-only chest compressions if untrained in defibrillation) or **cardiopulmonary resuscitation** (CPR), a technique used to restore circulation and breathing.

Promoting Circulation

Circulation is achieved by performing chest compressions. Chest compression promotes circulation in one of two ways. Squeezing the heart between the sternum and the vertebrae increases pressure in the ventricles, which is thought to push blood into the pulmonary arteries and aorta. Chest compressions also are thought to increase pressure in thoracic blood vessels, promoting systemic blood flow. For chest compressions to be effective, the rescuer must deliver them hard and fast. Thirty chest compressions should be administered initially before attempting to open the airway and give rescue breaths. The chest of an adult victim should be depressed to at least 2 in. at a rate of 100 times per minute, a pace that compares to the beat in the Bee Gees' disco song, "Stayin' Alive."

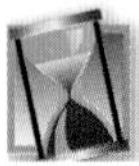

Gerontologic Considerations

- In the performance of chest compressions, older adults are at a greater risk for fractured ribs because of the increased likelihood of osteoporosis. Similarly, those with vascular disease may not receive adequate blood perfusion of the brain during CPR, and they may experience brain damage as a result.
- Older adults who take a daily dose of aspirin or some other anticoagulant drug are more apt to bleed internally during chest compressions.

The correct sequence is 30 chest compressions followed by two rescue breaths for rescuers who are able to do so, or a ratio of 30:2 (whether by one or two rescuers) for children older than 1 year of age. If there are two rescuers and the victim is younger than 1 year of age, the ratio is 15 compressions to 2 breaths (15:2); if the rescuer is alone, a 30:2 ratio is maintained.

Correct placement of the hands and the body is essential during chest compressions. The rescuer puts the heel of one hand over the lower half of the victim's sternum but above the xiphoid process and the other hand on top, then interlocking or extending his or her fingers. The rescuer positions his or her body over the hands to deliver a straight downward motion with each compression and allowing the chest wall to recoil afterwards (Fig. 37-4). The hands remain in contact with the chest, and the elbows stay locked to avoid rocking back and forth over the victim. Table 37-1 lists variations in rescue breathing and chest compressions to accommodate anatomic differences and the physiologic needs of various age groups.

Basic CPR is not interrupted for more than 10 seconds except when:

- There is a pulse and the victim resumes breathing.
- The rescuer becomes exhausted.
- The victim's condition deteriorates despite resuscitation efforts.
- There is written evidence that resuscitation is contrary to the victim's wishes.
- ACLS measures such as defibrillation are administered.

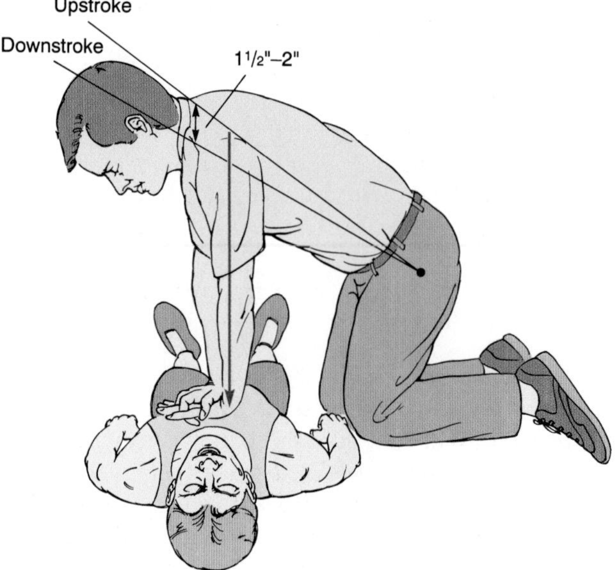

FIGURE 37-4 The correct hand and body position.

TABLE 37-1 Differences in CPR Among Infants, Children, and Adults

TECHNIQUE	INFANT (UP TO 1 YEAR OF AGE)	CHILD (1–8 YEARS)	ADULT (OVER 8 YEARS OF AGE)
Compressions			
Location	In the midline, one finger width below the nipples	Center of the chest between the nipples	Center of the chest between the nipples
Hand use	Two thumbs with the hands encircling the chest for two rescuers or two fingers on the breastbone if alone	Heel of one hand with second hand on top, or heel of one hand only	Two hands; heel of one hand with other hand on top
Rate	100/min	100/min	100/min
Depth	At least one-third the depth of the chest, about 1½ in.	At least one-third the depth of the chest, about 2 in.	2 in. or more
Rescue Breaths			
Compressions only when rescuer is untrained or trained but not proficient			
Ratio of compressions to ventilation until advanced airway is in place	30:2 (one rescuer) 15:2 (two rescuers)	30:2 (one rescuer) 15:2 (two rescuers)	30:2 (one or two rescuers)
Duration	1 second with visible rise in chest	1 second with visible rise in chest	1 second with visible rise in chest

Opening the Airway

In the absence of head or neck trauma and taking care not to twist the spine in case there is unidentified trauma, a rescuer can use the **head-tilt/chin-lift technique** (a method of choice for opening the airway; Fig. 37-5A) or the **jaw-thrust maneuver** (an alternative method for opening the airway by grasping the lower jaw and lifting it while tilting the head backward; Fig. 37-5B). The jaw-thrust maneuver is not recommended for lay rescuers because it is difficult to perform safely and may cause injury to the spine. When the airway is opened, rescuers remove any foreign material that is visible within the victim's mouth.

After opening the airway, the presence of spontaneous breathing can be determined, but minimizing hands-off time is essential. Rescuers observe for the rising and falling of the chest and listen and feel for air escaping from the nose or mouth. A breathing victim is placed in the **recovery position** (a side-lying position that helps to maintain an open airway and prevent aspiration of fluid). If breathing is not restored within 10 seconds, the victim remains supine and CPR is continued.

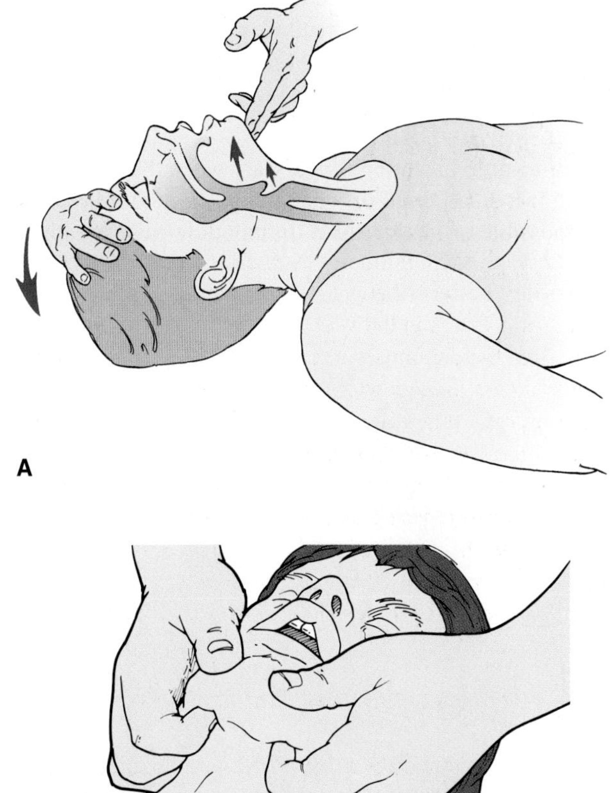

FIGURE 37-5 Techniques to open the airway. **A.** The head-tilt/chin-lift technique. **B.** The jaw-thrust technique.

Performing Rescue Breathing

Rescuers who are health professionals perform **rescue breathing** (the process of ventilating the lungs) through the victim's mouth, nose, or stoma. They should use a one-way valve mask or other protective face shield if available. These devices theoretically reduce the potential for acquiring infectious diseases (eg, hepatitis, AIDS); however, the lack of a barrier device should not interfere with attempting rescue breathing.

Because many lay bystanders are unwilling to perform mouth-to-mouth ventilation because of fears of disease transmission, continuous chest compressions alone are better than totally avoiding efforts at resuscitation. Continuous chest compressions by laypersons produce similar survival when compared with those who receive rescue breathing combined with chest compressions (Cone, 2010; Bobrow et al., 2010).

When the rescuer is trained, each rescue breath should last 1 second and should cause the chest to rise visibly. Rescue breathing continues at the rate of two breaths for every 30 compressions for an adult for one or two rescuers; for children or infants, the rate is two breaths for every 30 compressions for a single trained rescuer or two breaths for every 15 compressions when administered by two trained rescuers. Once an advanced airway is in place, rescue breathing is administered at a rate of 8 to 10 breaths per minute for infants, children, and adults without a pause in chest compressions.

Mouth-to-Mouth Breathing

In mouth-to-mouth breathing, a rescuer seals the victim's nose, uses his or her mouth to cover the victim's mouth, and blows air into the victim (Fig. 37-6). Giving a breath that lasts a full second reduces the potential for distending the esophagus and stomach, which may promote regurgitation and aspiration. If breathing is not restored, the victim remains supine, an advanced airway is placed, and rescue breathing continues at the rate of one breath every 6 to 8 seconds without interrupting chest compressions.

Mouth-to-Nose Breathing

Mouth-to-nose breathing is necessary when the victim is an infant or a small child or when mouth-to-mouth breathing is impossible or unsuccessful. In mouth-to-nose breathing, the rescuer closes the victim's mouth and blows air into the nose.

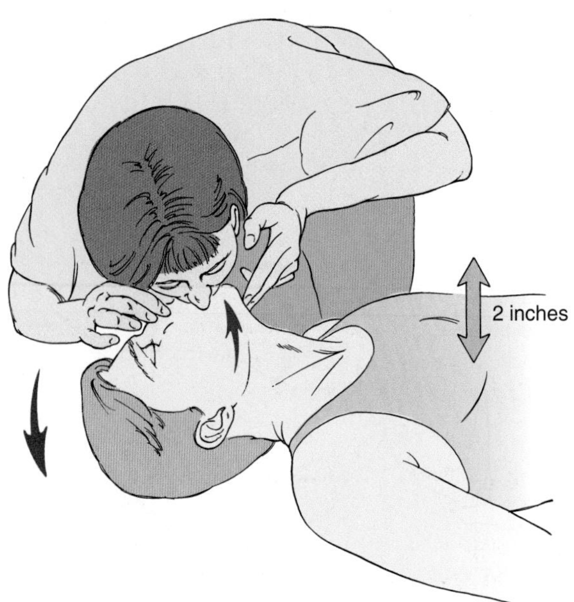

FIGURE 37-6 Mouth-to-mouth rescue breathing.

Mouth-to-Stoma Breathing

The rescuer can give rescue breathing to a client with a laryngectomy by sealing his or her mouth over the victim's stoma. Because the upper airway is essentially a blind pathway, the nose does not require sealing.

For clients with a tracheostomy tube, rescue breathing is through the tube with the mouth or a one-way valve mask. If the tracheostomy tube does not have an inflated cuff, the rescuer must seal the victim's nose.

Early Defibrillation

If there is no circulation, breathing or movement after five cycles of cardiac compressions and rescue breathing, an AED is attached without exceeding a 10-second interruption in CPR. An **automated external defibrillator** (AED) is a portable, battery-operated device that analyzes heart rhythms and delivers an electrical shock to restore a functional heartbeat. With the exception of newborns, defibrillation is performed as soon as possible in victims experiencing **ventricular fibrillation**, an ineffective heart rhythm (Fig. 37-7). In children from 1 to 8 years of age or who weigh less than 55 lb, the AED must be capable of delivering a pediatric shockable dose using cables that reduce the amount of energy directed at the heart (Schiammarella & Stoppler, 2007).

Ideally, an AED is used as rapidly as possible. Survival rates after cardiac arrest decrease significantly with every minute that defibrillation is delayed. **Asystole**, the absence of any heart rhythm, quickly follows ventricular fibrillation. Outcomes are best when defibrillation occurs within 3 minutes of chest compressions (Berg et al., 2010; Link et al., 2010).

AEDs are located in many public access locations, such as schools, airports, and police stations. Once obtained, the user turns on the AED, so that he or she can observe its monitor screen. Most AEDs have pictorial instructions and the capacity to provide voice instructions.

Attaching the Electrode Pads

The rescuer attaches the preconnected electrode pads to the victim's skin (Fig. 37-8). If the monitor displays an error message, it may be because the victim's skin is diaphoretic or extremely hairy, which interferes with effective contact. The rescuer can wipe the skin with a towel, shave or clip chest hair, and apply a second set of electrode pads.

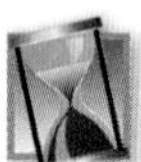

Gerontologic Considerations

- If a person has an implanted defibrillator or a pacemaker evidenced by a hard object beneath the skin with an overlying scar, the AED pad must be placed at least 1 in. to the side of the implanted device.

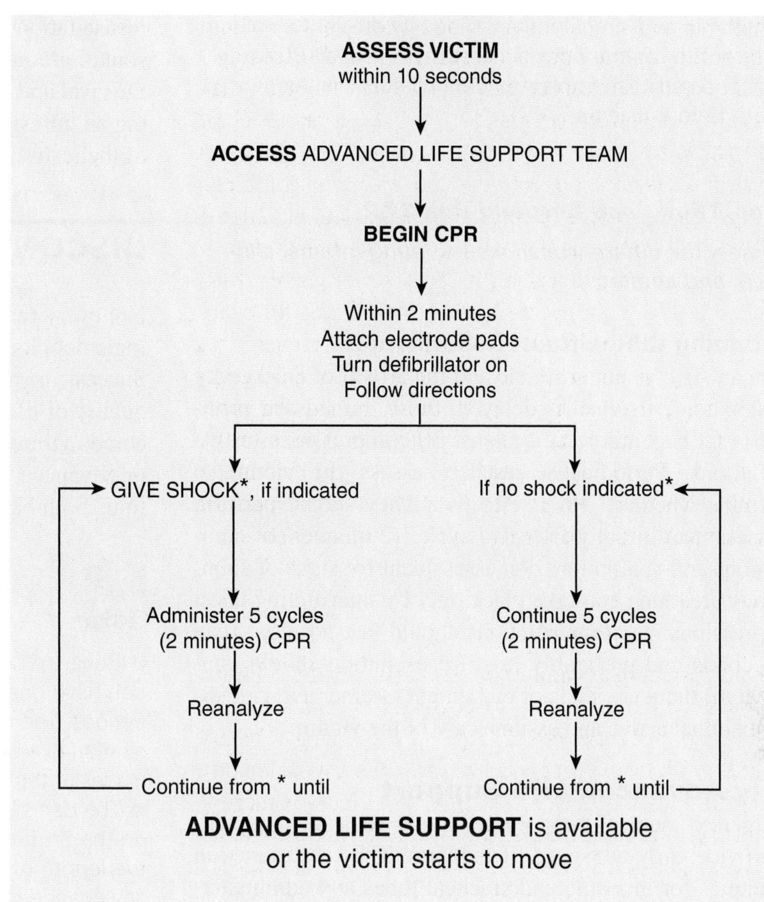

FIGURE 37-7 An algorithm for resuscitation.

Analyzing the Rhythm

When the electrode pads are in place and the victim is motionless, the rescuer presses an analyze button on the AED or the process occurs automatically. After 5 to 15 seconds, the AED provides a message indicating that the victim needs "shock" or "no shock."

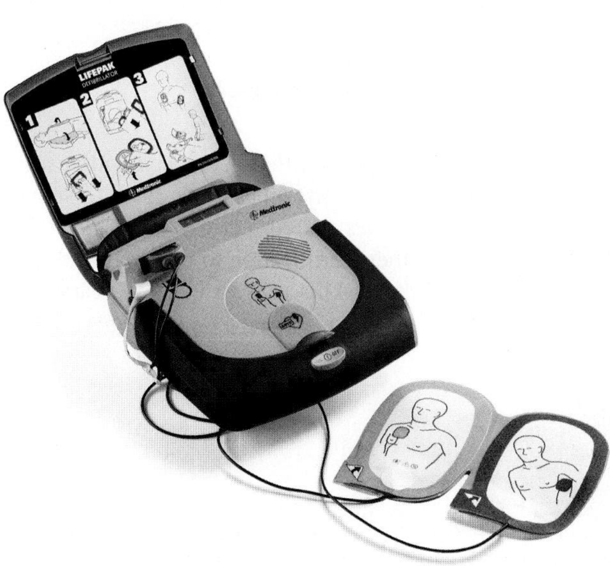

FIGURE 37-8 An automated external defibrillator (AED). (Courtesy of Medtronic, Inc.)

Administering a Shock

When the AED indicates "shock," the rescuer looks to make sure that no one is touching the victim. Saying "clear" or "everybody clear" in a loud voice is recommended before pressing the shock button. The AED discharges the shock, which is confirmed by the victim's sudden muscle contraction. CPR resumes immediately after the shock and continues for five cycles (approximately 2 minutes) before analyzing the rhythm again with the AED. The rescuer then facilitates another analysis of the rhythm and waits for the next message to shock or not shock. The rescuer repeats the shock, if indicated, then 2 minutes of CPR, and then the analysis steps again and again until either the AED gives a "no shock" message, the victim begins to move, or personnel with ACLS skills arrive to assist.

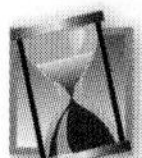

Gerontologic Considerations

- Some older adults with a history of chronic, life-threatening dysrhythmias who are unresponsive to drug therapy have an automatic internal cardiac defibrillator surgically inserted within their chest. The device senses the dysrhythmia and almost instantaneously delivers an electrical current to restore normal heart rhythm. Wait 30 to 60 seconds after an implanted defibrillator finishes giving a shock before using an AED.

Stop, Think, and Respond Box 37-2

Review the differences in resuscitating infants, children, and adults.

Continuing CPR without Defibrillation

When an AED is not available and the arrival of emergency resuscitation personnel is delayed, those trained and proficient in CPR continue at a rate of 30 compressions to two ventilations. Periodically, rescuers assess the victim to determine whether CPR is effective. They should perform an assessment initially after five cycles (2 minutes) of compressions and ventilations. An assessment for signs of spontaneous breathing can take place only by interrupting chest compressions; such interruptions should last no more than 10 seconds and preferably less. Resuscitation should continue until there are signs of movement or emergency medical personnel arrive and assume care of the victim.

Early Advanced Life Support

Emergency medical support personnel such as paramedics provide early advanced life support. They are trained in techniques for inserting endotracheal tubes and administering supplemental oxygen. They also carry an AED as part of their resuscitative equipment and can administer defibrillation if a public access defibrillator is unavailable. Paramedics administer emergency medications that can improve the potential for resuscitation before and during the transport of the victim to a hospital's emergency department.

RECOVERY

When there is evidence of circulation and breathing, rescuers place the victim in a recovery position (Fig. 37-9). If an AED has been used, the electrodes remain in place. Rescuers continue to monitor the victim and stand prepared to reactivate the defibrillator if the victim's condition worsens again.

Once the victim is stable, rescuers evaluate their interventions and operation of the AED for quality assurance. Internal self-evaluation provides a means to improve similar resuscitation efforts in the future. Health care facility personnel are admonished to follow the steps in the Chain of Survival and use an AED as soon as possible when discovering an unresponsive client rather than waiting for the arrival of the resuscitation team.

DISCONTINUING RESUSCITATION

Not every resuscitation attempt is successful. Severe neurologic deficits often result even when a victim's life is saved. Success is measured more appropriately by the victim's quality of life rather than its quantity. Therefore, there often comes a time, in the absence of a "Do Not Resuscitate" order or advanced directive, when a team must decide to discontinue both basic and advanced life-support efforts.

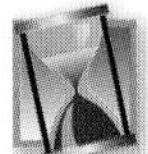

Gerontologic Considerations

- Because no clear-cut guidelines for suspending resuscitation have been established, efforts may extend for long periods. The decision in a health care facility to stop resuscitation is a medical judgment made by the physician or leader of the code.
- The decision to stop resuscitation efforts often is based on the time that elapsed before resuscitation was begun, the length of time that resuscitation has continued without any change in the victim's condition, the age and diagnosis of the victim, and objective data such as arterial blood gas results and electrolyte studies. Regardless of the basis for the decision, it is not made lightly, and those involved in an unsuccessful code need support from their colleagues. It has been noted that family presence during resuscitation has positive psychological value regardless of the outcome. It is also important that a staff member supports the observers throughout the experience as well as afterward.

NURSING IMPLICATIONS

Nurses have several responsibilities associated with resuscitation. They must learn to perform basic cardiac life-support measures, which includes the correct use of an AED, and they must maintain their certification to do so. If nurses do not use or refresh these skills at least every 2 years, their

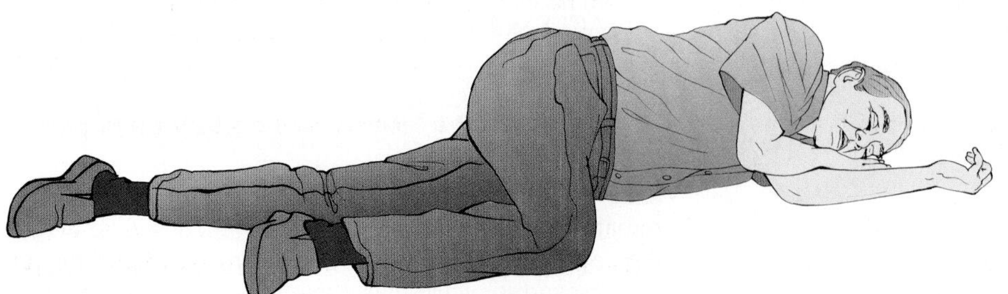

FIGURE 37-9 The recovery position.

abilities may be less than adequate. They also must support and participate in efforts to teach lay people, both adults and children, how to perform CPR and carry out the Chain of Survival. Nurses must discuss advance directives (see Chap. 3) with all clients regardless of the reason for admission to a health care agency. Honoring the client's right to participate in the decision-making process is important.

The following nursing diagnoses may be relevant in a resuscitation situation:

- Ineffective Airway Clearance
- Impaired Spontaneous Ventilation
- Impaired Gas Exchange
- Decreased Cardiac Output
- Ineffective Cardiopulmonary Tissue Perfusion
- Ineffective Cerebral Tissue Perfusion
- Ineffective Renal Tissue Perfusion
- Decisional Conflict

Nursing Care Plan 37-1 shows how nurses can use the steps in the nursing process for a client with Impaired Spontaneous Ventilation, defined in the NANDA-I taxonomy (2012, p. 239) as "decreased energy reserves (that) result in an individual's inability to maintain breathing adequate to support life."

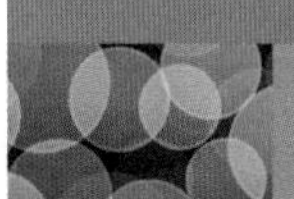

NURSING CARE PLAN 37-1 Risk for Inability to Sustain Spontaneous Ventilation

Assessment

- Monitor respiratory rate and breathing pattern.
- Observe for tachypnea, bradypnea, and periods of apnea.
- Note signs of respiratory distress such as the use of accessory muscles, sitting upright, nasal flaring, restlessness, and cyanosis.
- Ask the client if he or she is choking or look for the universal sign of the hand to the throat.
- Check for tachycardia.
- Apply a pulse oximeter and note the SpO_2 level.
- Obtain and analyze the findings of an arterial blood gas.
- Determine if the client has received medication that causes respiratory depression.
- Check the cause for high- or low-pressure alarms on a mechanical ventilator; it could be malfunctioning.
- Assess the client's level of consciousness and responsiveness.
- Determine if there is an absence of breathing, coughing, and movement.

Nursing Diagnosis. **Risk for Inability to Sustain Spontaneous Ventilation** related to progressive respiratory muscle weakness secondary to amyotrophic lateral sclerosis (Lou Gehrig's disease) as manifested by shallow respirations of 32 per minute; SpO_2 of 85% with oxygen at 6 L per Venturi mask; difficulty talking and swallowing; resuscitation by paramedics who responded to the family's 911 call for assistance; and statement, "It has been more and more difficult for me to breathe. My doctor told me that's the usual outcome from this disease."

Expected Outcome. The client will breathe spontaneously at a ventilation rate to sustain life.

Interventions	Rationales
Monitor SpO_2 with pulse oximeter at all times.	The pulse oximeter measures the amount of oxygen bound to hemoglobin; sustained SpO_2 levels of <90% indicate a need for supplemental oxygen. An SpO_2 level of 80% equals an approximate PaO_2 of 45 mm Hg. This finding indicates moderate-to-severe hypoxemia and the need for mechanical ventilation.
Administer oxygen at 45% using a Venturi mask.	A Venturi mask delivers the exact amount of prescribed oxygen; 45% oxygen is slightly double the amount of oxygen in room air; supplemental oxygen helps to relieve hypoxemia.
Maintain the client in a Fowler's position.	It facilitates chest expansion by lowering abdominal organs away from the diaphragm, thus increasing the potential for a greater volume of inspired air.
Replace the Venturi mask with a non-rebreather mask if SpO_2 falls below 80%.	A non-rebreather mask can deliver 90%–100% oxygen until the client can receive ventilation assistance.
Obtain arterial blood gas when SpO_2 is sustained below 80% for more than 10 min.	An arterial blood gas identifies several important measurements, such as pH of the blood, PaO_2, $PaCO_2$, and HCO_3. Findings will facilitate the subsequent medical management of the client.
Follow the Chain of Survival if respiratory or cardiac arrest occurs.	The Chain of Survival has the greatest potential for resuscitating a lifeless person.

Evaluation of Expected Outcomes

- Client continues to breathe spontaneously.
- The client's SpO_2 is 90% with 45% oxygen via a Venturi mask.

CRITICAL THINKING EXERCISE

1. Arrange the following adult resuscitation steps in the correct sequence: activate the emergency medical system; open the airway; administer chest compressions at a rate of 100 per minute; assess responsiveness and presence of breathing; attach an automated external defibrillator and follow instructions; give cardiopulmonary resuscitation for 2 minutes and reanalyze heart rhythm; combine compressions with ventilations at a rate of 30:2.
2. Explain the reason chest compressions are now initially preferable before administering two quick breaths upon finding someone who is unresponsive and not breathing normally.
3. Give a reason for the de-emphasis on checking a pulse as a method for determining heart contractions on individuals who are unresponsive.
4. What criteria are used to determine if rescue breathing is being delivered effectively?

NCLEX-STYLE REVIEW QUESTIONS

1. A nurse is managing care for all the following clients. For whom would the nurse most anticipate an airway obstruction?
   1. Client A, who has had a cerebral vascular accident (stroke)
   2. Client B, who has had a full mouth extraction of teeth
   3. Client C, who has had a biopsy of a tongue lesion
   4. Client D, who has had facial cosmetic surgery
2. Which of the following should the nurse instruct parents of a 6-month-old child to avoid when purchasing a toy because of the risk for accidental choking?
   1. A teething ring with gel filling
   2. A stuffed animal with button eyes
   3. A mobile with suspended objects
   4. A ball measuring 5″ in diameter
3. Which of the following is the best evidence that the nurse should implement the Heimlich maneuver to relieve an airway obstruction in a conscious person?
   1. Forceful coughing
   2. Attempts to clear throat
   3. Inability to speak
   4. Audible wheezing
4. When a person is in cardiac arrest, which is the first step the nurse takes in the Chain of Survival?
   1. Early cardiopulmonary resuscitation
   2. Early cardiac defibrillation
   3. Early activation of emergency services
   4. Early advanced life support
5. Before administering the shock from an automated external defibrillator (AED), which of the following actions should the nurse take?
   1. Place the victim in the recovery position.
   2. Loosen the victim's belt.
   3. Shout, "Everybody clear."
   4. Give three rescue breaths.

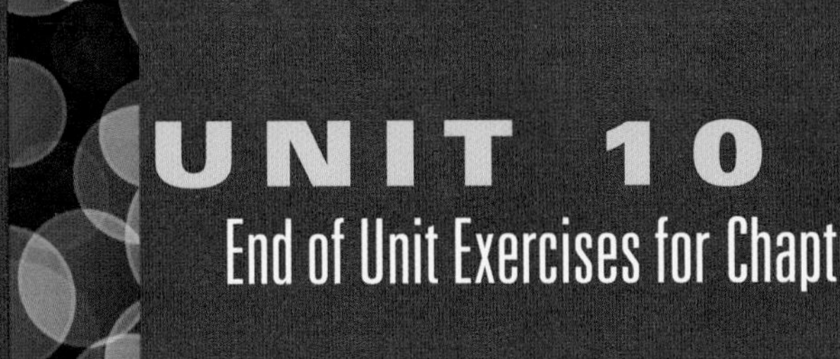

UNIT 10
End of Unit Exercises for Chapters 36 and 37

Section I: Reviewing What You've Learned

Activity A: *Fill in the blanks by choosing the correct word from the options given in parentheses.*

1. The lower airway contains the ________________. (alveoli, laryngopharynx, oropharynx)
2. Removing secretions from the upper portion of the lower airway through a nasally inserted catheter is called ________________ suctioning. (nasopharyngeal, nasotracheal, oropharyngeal)
3. Health professionals use the ________________ artery to assess circulation in infants. (brachial, carotid, femoral)
4. The CAB of cardiopulmonary resuscitation are ________________ airway, and breathing. (circulation, congestion, cyanosis)

Activity B: *Mark each statement as either T (True) or F (False). Correct any false statements.*

1. T____F____ Nurses perform nasotracheal suctioning with a device called the Yankauer tip.
2. T____F____ Tracheal cartilage is a protrusion of flexible cartilage above the larynx.
3. T____F____ The jaw-thrust maneuver helps to remove any foreign material within the client's mouth.

Activity C: *Write the correct term for each description below.*

1. The collective system of tubes in the upper and lower respiratory tracts ________________
2. A surgically created opening in the trachea ________________
3. In a hospital, the summoning of personnel trained in advanced life-support techniques ________________
4. A side-lying position in resuscitation that helps a breathing person maintain an open airway and prevent aspiration of fluid ________________

Activity D: *Match the terms related to resuscitation in Column A with their explanations in Column B.*

Column A		Column B
1. ________________	Heimlich maneuver	A. Using techniques to restore breathing and circulation
2. ________________	Subdiaphragmatic thrusts	B. Ventilating the lungs
3. ________________	Cardiopulmonary resuscitation	C. The preferred method for opening the airway
4. ________________	Head-tilt/chin-lift technique	D. Relieving a mechanical airway obstruction
5. ________________	Rescue breathing	E. Applying pressure to the abdomen

Activity E: *Differentiate between mouth-to-mouth breathing and mouth-to-stoma breathing based on the categories given below.*

	Mouth-to-Mouth Breathing	Mouth-to-Stoma Breathing
Technique		
Sealing of the Client's Nose		

Activity F: *Consider the following figure.*

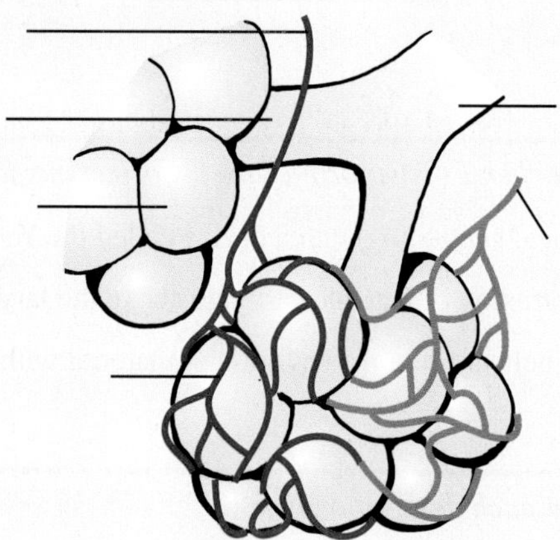

1. Identify and label the figure.
2. What is the function of these structures?

Activity G: *Cardiac arrest may lead to unresponsiveness. Rescuers implement a five-step survival process known as the Chain of Survival. Write in the boxes provided below the correct sequence of the chain of survival.*

1. Effective advanced life support
2. Integrated post-cardiac arrest care
3. Early cardiopulmonary resuscitation with a focus on compressions
4. Immediate recognition and access to emergency services
5. Rapid defibrillation

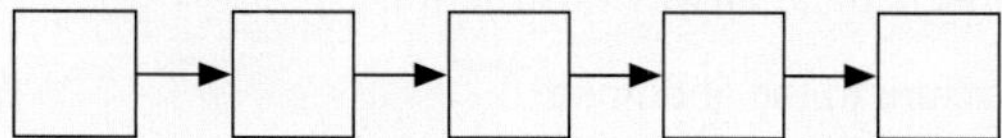

Activity H: *Answer the following questions.*

1. What four natural mechanisms protect the airway?

2. What conditions may result in the need to insert an artificial airway?

3. What are various signs of a partial and complete airway obstruction?

4. For how long and for what reasons can basic cardiopulmonary resuscitation be interrupted?

Section II: Applying Your Knowledge

Activity I: *Give rationales for the following questions.*

1. Why it is important for the nurse to frequently assess clients who have a tracheostomy?

2. Why should nurses ensure adequate hydration in clients with a severe cough?

3. Why is a one-way valve mask used for rescue breathing?

4. In what cases would a monitor display an error message during the attachment of an AED's electrode pad?

Activity J: *Answer the following questions focusing on nursing roles and responsibilities.*

1. A physician has asked a nurse to perform chest physiotherapy using percussion and vibration techniques for a client with a chronic respiratory disorder.
   a. What interventions should the nurse perform during the percussion technique?

   b. What interventions should the nurse perform during the vibration technique?

2. Describe instructions that a nurse should provide when teaching postural drainage to a client with thick mucus and the family.

3. An 8-year-old client develops an obstructed airway.
   a. What immediate steps should the nurse take to relieve the client's obstruction?

   b. What should the nurse do if the child is unconscious?

Activity K: *Consider the following questions. Discuss them with your instructor or peers.*

1. A 9-month-old infant accidentally inhales a button used for an eye on a toy.
   a. How is clearing the airway for an infant different than clearing the airway of an adult?
   b. What suggestions should the nurse impart to the client's family to prevent such a situation?

Section III: Getting Ready for NCLEX

Activity L: *Answer the following questions.*

1. A nurse is to obtain a sputum specimen from a client who has been receiving aerosol treatments for a respiratory disease. Which of the following should the nurse do when collecting the sputum specimen?
   a. Tell the client to avoid rinsing the mouth before the specimen collection.
   b. Instruct the client to attempt a forceful cough and expectorate.
   c. Obtain the sputum specimen before an aerosol treatment.
   d. Obtain saliva from within the mouth.

2. A nurse is caring for a client with a weak and persistent cough. Which intervention should the nurse follow when caring for this client?
   a. Maintain 2,000 to 3,000 mL fluid intake for 24 hours.
   b. Instruct the client to breathe through the mouth.
   c. Ensure that the client is supine at all times.
   d. Provide the client with warm milk 3 to 4 times a day.
3. A client has undergone a tracheotomy for an upper airway obstruction. Which intervention should the nurse perform when providing tracheostomy care for this client?
   a. Remove the inner cannula and place it in a saline solution.
   b. Clean the area around the stoma with diluted peroxide.
   c. Blow-dry the cannula after cleaning it with a saline solution.
   d. Remove the used ties before applying new ties.
4. A triage nurse is examining an unresponsive 6-year-old child. When performing CPR, which of the following should the nurse do?
   a. Apply compression in the midline one finger width below the nipples.
   b. Compress using two thumbs with the hands encircling the chest.
   c. Place the heel of the hand at the center of the chest between the nipples.
   d. Provide one breath every 5 seconds at the rate of 10 breaths per minute.
5. A nurse is caring for a client with impaired ventilation. Which intervention should the nurse perform for this client?
   a. Administer oxygen at 20% using a Venturi mask.
   b. Ensure that the client is supine at all times.
   c. Replace the Venturi mask with a non-rebreather mask if SpO_2 is 90%.
   d. Continually monitor the client's SpO_2 with a pulse oximeter.

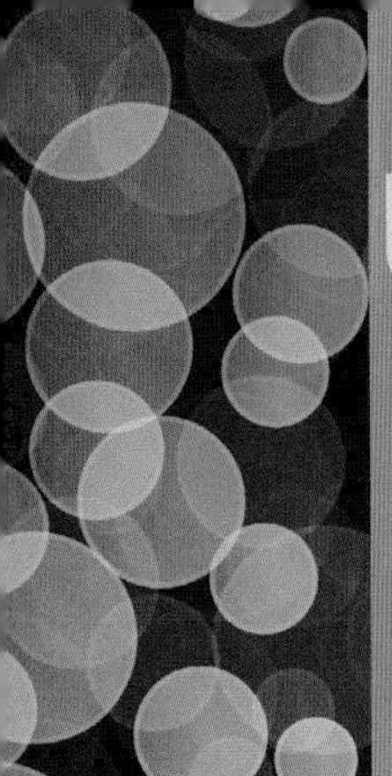

UNIT 11
Caring for the Terminally Ill

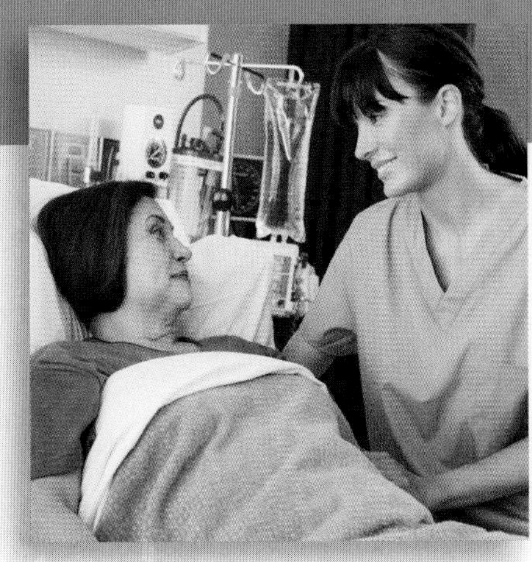

38 End-of-Life Care

Words To Know

acceptance
anger
anticipatory grieving
autopsy
bargaining
brain death
coroner
death certificate
denial
depression
dying with dignity
grief response
grief work
grieving
hospice
morgue
mortician
multiple organ failure
paranormal experiences
pathologic grief
postmortem care
respite care
shroud
terminal illness
waiting for permission phenomenon

Learning Objectives

On completion of this chapter, the reader should be able to:

1. Define terminal illness.
2. Name the five stages of dying.
3. Describe two methods by which nurses can promote the acceptance of death in dying clients.
4. Define respite care.
5. Discuss the philosophy of hospice care.
6. List at least five aspects of terminal care.
7. Name at least five signs of multiple organ failure.
8. Explain why a discussion of organ donation must take place as expeditiously as possible following a client's death.
9. Name three components of postmortem care.
10. Discuss the benefit of grieving and one sign that grief is being resolved.

In the United States, life expectancy continues to lengthen each year (Fig. 38-1). Nevertheless, death remains a certainty for all people; the only unknowns are when, where, and how it will occur.

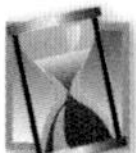

Gerontologic Considerations

■ Older adults may read obituaries and death notices in the newspaper daily in an effort to keep up with acquaintances. Families may view this activity as potentially depressing, but it may actually be an effective coping mechanism in helping to develop a peaceful and accepting attitude toward death.

Nurses and other health care personnel probably are more involved than any other group with people who experience impending death. This chapter deals with aspects of caring for terminally ill clients and the grieving experience for all those involved in the dying process.

TERMINAL ILLNESS AND CARE

A **terminal illness** means a condition from which recovery is beyond a reasonable expectation. Such a diagnosis is devastating news. On learning that death is imminent, clients tend to experience several stages as they process the information.

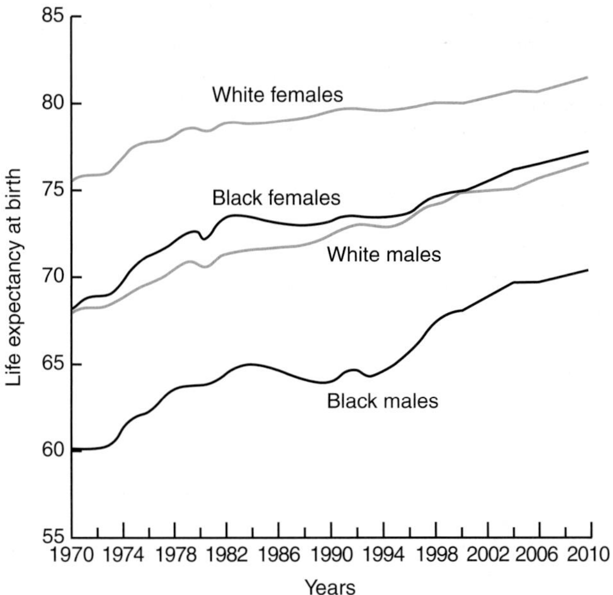

FIGURE 38-1 Life expectancy in the United States, 1970–2010.

Stages of Dying

Dr. Elisabeth Kübler-Ross (1969), an authority on dying, described stages through which many terminally ill clients progress. These are denial, anger, bargaining, depression, and acceptance (Table 38-1). These stages may occur in a progressive fashion, or a person can move back and forth through the stages. There is no specific time period for the rate of progression, duration, or completion of the stages.

Denial

Denial, the psychological defense mechanism by which a person refuses to believe certain information, helps people to cope initially with the reality of death. Terminally ill clients may first refuse to believe that their diagnosis is accurate. They may speculate that test results are wrong or that their reports have been confused with those of others.

Anger

Anger (the emotional response to feeling victimized) occurs because there is no way to retaliate against fate. Clients often displace their anger onto nurses, physicians, family members, even God. They may express anger in less-than-obvious ways; for example, by complaining about care or overreacting to even the slightest annoyances.

TABLE 38-1 Stages of Dying

STAGE	TYPICAL EMOTIONAL RESPONSE	TYPICAL COMMENT
First stage	Denial	"No, not me"
Second stage	Anger	"Why me?"
Third stage	Bargaining	"Yes, me, but if only..."
Fourth stage	Depression	"Yes, me."
Fifth stage	Acceptance	"I am ready."

Bargaining

Bargaining, a psychological mechanism for delaying the inevitable, involves a process of negotiation, usually with God or some other higher power. Usually, dying clients have come to terms with their death, but want to extend their lives temporarily until some significant event takes place (eg, a child's wedding).

Depression

Depression (a sad mood) indicates the realization that death will come sooner rather than later. The sad mood is a result of confronting potential losses.

Acceptance

Acceptance (an attitude of complacency) occurs after clients have dealt with their losses and completed unfinished business. Kübler-Ross describes unfinished business in two ways. Literally, it refers to completing legal and financial matters to provide the best security for survivors. It also refers to addressing social and spiritual matters, such as saying goodbye to loved ones and making peace with God. It is as important for dying clients as it is for their families to say, "Thank you for. . ." and "I'm sorry for. . ."

After tying up all loose ends, dying clients feel prepared to die. Some even happily anticipate death, viewing it as a bridge to a better dimension.

Promoting Acceptance

Nurses can help clients to pass from one stage to another by providing emotional support and by supporting the client's choices concerning terminal care. Facilitating the client's directives helps to maintain the client's personal dignity and locus of control.

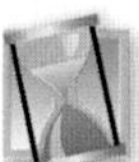

Gerontologic Considerations

- Include all older adults, as well as others who are dying, in as many aspects of care as possible. The emphasis is on maintaining self-esteem and personal dignity.
- Clients of all ages may feel that the use of machines and equipment designed to maintain life support threatens their dignity.
- Death is a very individualized experience that is highly influenced by prior experiences, cultural practices, and level of personal development. Many older adults are realistically aware of their pending and inevitable death. Often, they are relieved when health care providers are comfortable discussing death with them. Older adults may benefit from counseling regarding their own death and dying, especially if they have a history of accepting help in coping with challenging issues.

Emotional Support

Emotional support is always part of nursing care; however, it may be more necessary for dying clients than in any other situation. Sometimes a dying client simply wants an opportunity to express his or her feelings and verbally work through

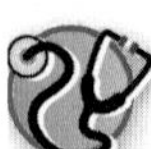

NURSING GUIDELINES 38-1

Helping Dying Clients Cope

- Accept the client's behavior, no matter what it is. *Doing so demonstrates respect for individuality.*
- Provide opportunities for the client to express feelings freely. *Giving such opportunities demonstrates an attention to meeting individual needs.*
- Try to understand the client's feelings. *Understanding reinforces the client's uniqueness.*
- Use statements with broad openings such as "It must be difficult for you" and "Do you want to talk about it?" *Such language encourages communication and allows the client to choose the topic or manner of response.*

emotions. Nurses can act as a nonjudgmental sounding board in such instances (see Nursing Guidelines 38-1).

In addition to being available for conversation, nurses provide emotional support to dying clients by acknowledging them as unique and worthwhile. **Dying with dignity** means the process by which the nurse cares for dying clients with respect, no matter what their emotional, physical, or cognitive state. This process reflects the concepts stated in the Dying Patient's Bill of Rights (Box 38-1).

BOX 38-1 The Dying Person's Bill of Rights

- I have the right to be treated as a living human being until I die.
- I have the right to maintain a sense of hopefulness, however changing its focus may be.
- I have the right to be cared for by those who can maintain a sense of hopefulness, however changing this might be.
- I have the right to express my feelings and emotions about my approaching death in my own way.
- I have the right to participate in decisions concerning my care.
- I have the right to expect continuing medical and nursing attention even though "cure" goals must be changed to "comfort" goals.
- I have the right not to die alone.
- I have the right to be free from pain.
- I have the right to have my questions answered honestly.
- I have the right not to be deceived.
- I have the right to have help from and for my family in accepting my death.
- I have the right to die in peace and dignity.
- I have the right to retain my individuality and not be judged for my decisions which may be contrary to beliefs of others.
- I have the right to discuss and enlarge my religious and/or spiritual experiences, whatever these may mean to others.
- I have the right to expect that the sanctity of the human body will be respected after death.
- I have the right to be cared for by caring, sensitive, knowledgeable people who will attempt to understand my needs and will be able to gain some satisfaction in helping me face my death.

From Barbus AJ. The Dying Person's Bill of Rights. © 1975, American Journal of Nursing Company. Reprinted with permission from the *American Journal of Nursing,* January 1975;75(1):99.

Arrangements for Care

Respecting the rights of dying clients includes helping them to choose how and where they want to receive terminal care. Clients may find it comforting to prepare an advance directive (see Chap. 3). Many also appreciate learning about available settings for care. In general, clients have four choices: home care, hospice care (which may be the same as home care), residential care, and acute care.

Home Care

Many clients with a terminal illness remain at home (Fig. 38-2). They may travel to and from a hospital or clinic for brief treatments, tests, and medical evaluations. Nurses may help to coordinate community services, secure home equipment, and arrange for home nursing visits.

Because the major burden of home care often falls on a spouse, family member, or significant other, nurses who care for home-bound clients periodically assess the toll this burden takes on the primary caregiver. The focus of support may shift back and forth from the client to the caregiver. **Respite care** (relief for the caregiver by a surrogate) is important because it gives the caregiver an opportunity to enjoy brief periods away from home. Nurses can encourage the caregiver to identify relatives or friends who will volunteer relief time with the client. If no one is available, nurses can refer the caregiver to services through a home health care agency or hospice care.

Hospice Care

The term **hospice** is used to indicate both a facility for providing the care of terminally ill clients and the concept of such care itself. The word originally derives from a place of refuge for travelers. Today's hospice movement is modeled after facilities established by Dr. Cicely Saunders in England in the late 1960s; the movement spread to the United States in

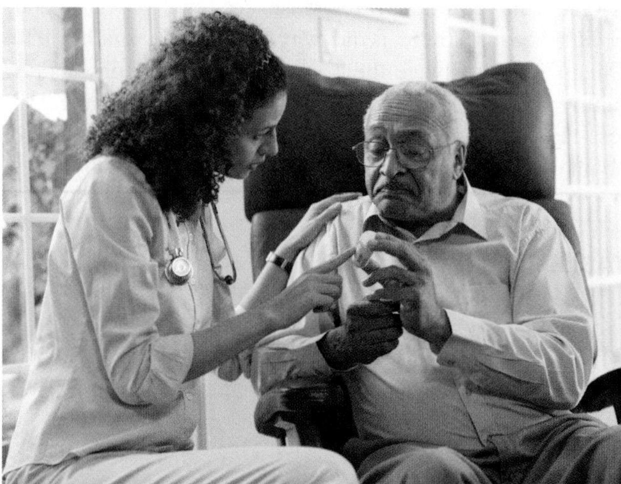

FIGURE 38-2 Home care.

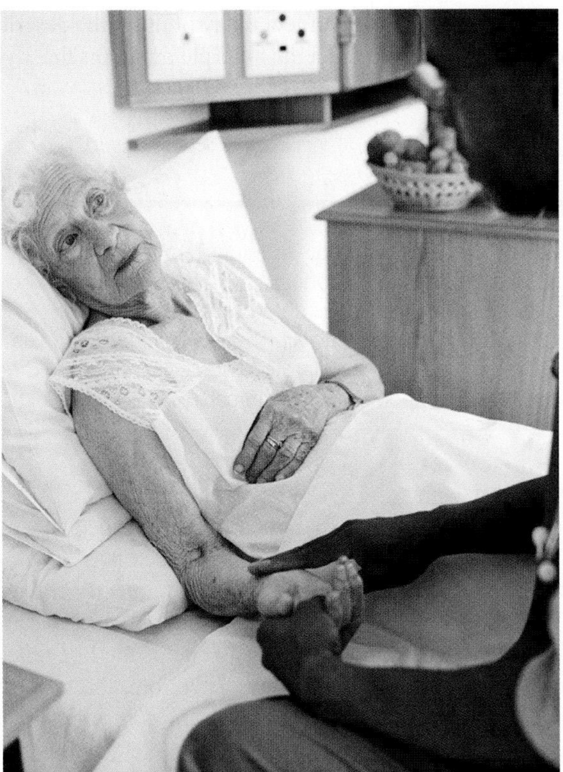

FIGURE 38-3 A hospice patient and nurse.

BOX 38-2 Medicare Home Hospice Benefits[a]

- Hospice nurse and physician on-call 24 hours a day/7 days a week
- Hospice aide and homemaker services
- Medications for symptom control or pain relief[b]
- Medical supplies and equipment
- Physical therapy, occupational therapy, and speech-language pathology services
- Social work and counseling services for the client and caregivers
- Dietary counseling services
- Short-term respite care[b]
- Short-term inpatient care for pain and symptom management
- Grief and loss counseling for client and family
- Any other Medicare-covered services needed to manage pain and other symptoms as recommended by the hospice team

[a]Medicare will pay for hospice care if all the following requirements are met: (1) the terminal illness is certified by physician; (2) the client elects the hospice benefit; and (3) the hospice program is Medicare-certified.

[b]There may be a small copayment.

Source: U.S. Department of Health and Human Services. (2010). Medicare hospice benefits. Publication 02154. http://www.medicare.gov/publications/pubs/pdf02154.pdf

the 1970s. The National Hospice Organization, now known as the National Hospice and Palliative Care Organization, was formed in 1978. Its goals are providing relief from distressing symptoms, easing pain, and enhancing quality of life. In 1982, the US Congress adopted the Medicare Hospice Benefits program to provide funds for hospice care (Hall, 2003). Hospice care involves helping clients to live their final days in comfort, with dignity, and in a caring environment (Fig. 38-3).

Eligibility for Hospice Care. In general, clients with 6 months or less to live as certified by a physician are accepted for hospice care in the United States. If a client survives beyond 6 months, he or she continues to receive care as long as the physician certifies that the client continues to meet hospice criteria. While receiving hospice care, the client can "transfer to another hospice program, but may not be discharged because of inability to pay, high cost of treatment, 'high-tech' palliative care ordered by the physician, or 'difficult' behavior" (Hall, 2007, p. 5).

Hospice Services. Most hospice clients receive care in their own homes. A multidisciplinary team of hospice professionals and volunteers supports care given by the family (Box 38-2). Hospice organizations also provide support programs for family members and significant others. They offer individual and group counseling both during and after the client's death to help survivors cope with grief.

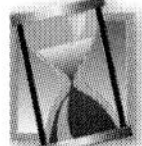

Gerontologic Considerations

- Older adults with chronic illnesses, such as dementia, and their family may benefit from the hospice approach to care and available support services. Often, families and older adults are relieved when providers discuss hospice care so they can be involved in choices about the type of care they receive.

Terminating Hospice Care. According to Hall (2007), hospice services can be terminated in one of two ways: (1) when the client withdraws for any reason to receive treatment not covered in the hospice plan of care or (2) when the client no longer meets the Medicare criteria. Once Medicare Hospice Benefits are discontinued, the client forfeits the remaining days of the benefit period; however, he or she can reapply for benefits if circumstances change.

Residential Care. Residential care is a form of intermediate care. Nursing homes or long-term care facilities are the usual settings for this type of subacute care. These facilities provide around-the-clock nursing care for clients who cannot live independently (Fig. 38-4). Family members have peace of mind knowing that their loved one is receiving care, and they enjoy the opportunity to visit as much as possible. Such care, however, is costly. Once clients have exhausted their savings, programs such as Medicaid may pay their expenses.

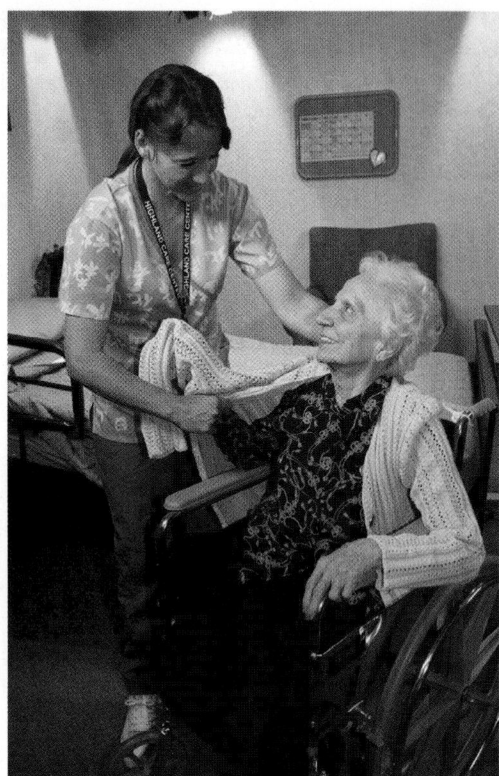

FIGURE 38-4 Residential care.

Acute Care. A client needs acute care, with its sophisticated technology and labor-intensive treatment, if his or her condition is unstable (Fig. 38-5). This form of care is the most expensive. Expenses for acute care provided in the hours, days, or weeks before a client's death can be significant.

Providing Terminal Care

Throughout a terminal illness and immediately before a client's death, nurses meet his or her basic physical needs for hydration, nourishment, elimination, hygiene, positioning, and comfort. Nurses implement many of the skills described throughout this text to meet the multiple problems that dying clients experience.

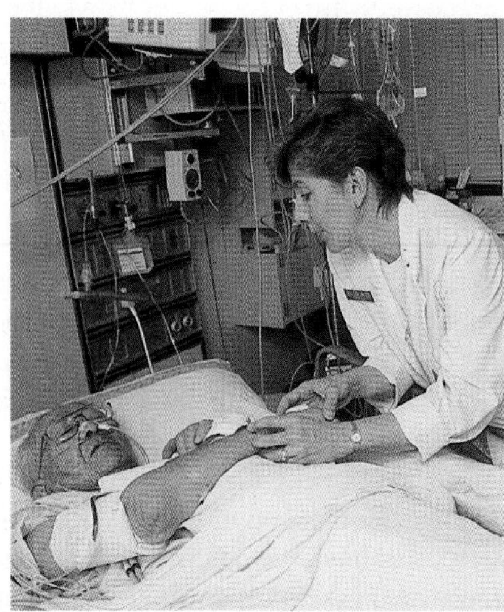

FIGURE 38-5 Acute care.

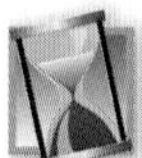

Gerontologic Considerations

■ Many older adults and other adults with foresight prepare advance directives concerning their health care and identify a person with a durable power of health care at the same time they prepare a will. These advance directives must be reviewed and updated periodically and should be accessible to all those involved in care.

Hydration

Hydration involves the maintenance of an adequate fluid volume. If the client's swallowing reflex remains intact, the nurse offers water and other beverages frequently. As swallowing becomes impaired, the client is at risk for aspiration, followed by pneumonia. Sucking is one of the last reflexes to disappear as death approaches. Therefore, the nurse can provide a moist cloth or wrapped ice cubes for the client to suck. Eventually, the client may need intravenous fluids.

Nourishment

Some terminally ill clients have little interest in eating. The effort may be too exhausting, or nausea and vomiting may result in inadequate consumption of food. Poor nutrition leads to weakness, infection, and other complications, such as pressure sores. Consequently, the client may need tube feedings or total parenteral nutrition to maintain nutritional and fluid intake.

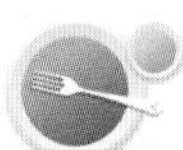

Nutrition Notes

■ Clients who are dying should not be made to feel guilty for not wanting to eat or drink. Nutritionists recommend comfort measures such as relieving a dry mouth with oral hygiene measures and artificial saliva, providing humidified air, and offering hard candies (Servodidio & Steed, 2007).

Elimination

Some terminally ill clients are incontinent of urine and stool; others experience urinary retention and constipation. All these conditions are uncomfortable. A physician may order cleansing enemas or suppositories. Catheterization also may be necessary. Skin care becomes particularly important for incontinent clients because urine and stool left in contact with the skin contribute to skin breakdown and produce foul odors.

Hygiene

The dignity of clients is related largely to their personal appearance. Therefore, nurses strive to keep dying clients clean, well groomed, and free of unpleasant odors.

Frequent mouth care may be necessary. Suctioning helps to remove mucus and saliva that the client cannot swallow or expectorate. A lateral position keeps the mouth and throat free of accumulating secretions. The lips may need periodic lubrication because they may become dried from mouth breathing or the administration of oxygen.

Positioning

The lateral position helps to prevent choking and aspiration. Nevertheless, the nurse changes the client's position at least every 2 hours (as for any other client) to promote comfort and circulation.

Comfort

Relieving pain may be the most challenging problem when caring for dying clients. The goal is to keep clients free from pain but not to dull consciousness, suppress respirations, or inhibit the ability to communicate.

Most clients initially receive non-narcotics for pain; later, the physician may change the drug order to a combination of a non-narcotic and narcotic analgesic or, eventually, a potent narcotic. He or she also may change the route from oral to parenteral or transdermal (refer to Chap. 20).

Analgesia may be more effective when the client receives the drug on a routine schedule. Giving pain medication regularly, such as every 4 hours or by continuous release through a transdermal patch rather than on an as-needed (p.r.n.) basis maintains a consistent level of pain relief. The dosage will probably need to be increased because of drug tolerance (see Chap. 20).

Fear of addiction should not interfere with efforts to relieve pain. The frequency of addiction in previously non-drug-abusing clients is rare (National Cancer Institute, 2008; McCaffery et al., 1990). Unfortunately, nurses and physicians often misinterpret increased requests for pain medication as evidence of addiction. In reality, an increased desire for pain medication may be the result of the development of drug tolerance or an increase in pain related to disease progression.

Clients develop tolerance to the pain-relieving property of analgesic drugs; however, clients who are tolerant to opioids concomitantly develop resistance to respiratory depression, a common side effect of narcotic analgesics (Hall, 2007; McCaffery & Beebe, 1989). Sedation generally precedes respiratory depression. Therefore, as long as the client is alert, the potential for respiratory depression is minimized. Narcotic antagonists can be given for severe respiratory depression, should it develop, but the dosage must be reduced to avoid producing withdrawal symptoms and eliminating the desired analgesic state. Constipation may be a more common consequence of continuous narcotic analgesia.

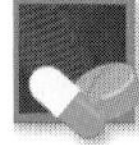

Pharmacologic Considerations

- Evaluating the use of antidepressants and other therapies for adults who are seriously depressed often is appropriate. Older adults have the highest rate of suicide as well as the highest rate of completed suicides in proportion to unsuccessful attempts. Health care professionals need to assess the client's suicide risk and implement appropriate precautions.

Family Involvement

Family members may appreciate involvement in the client's care because they often feel helpless. Involvement tends to maintain family bonds and helps survivors to cope with future grief. Many welcome the opportunity to assist. Nevertheless, nurses should not burden family members with major responsibilities.

Some terminally ill clients forestall dying when they feel that their loved ones are not yet prepared to deal with their death. This has been described as the **waiting for permission phenomenon**, because death often occurs shortly after a significant family member communicates that he or she is strong enough and ready to "let go." Nurses must support family members at this time because family members may feel as though they have given up and let down their loved one.

Approaching Death

As death nears, the client exhibits signs indicating a decrease then, ultimately, a cessation of function. As these signs appear, the nurse informs the client's family that death is approaching.

Multiple Organ Failure

The signs of approaching death are the result of **multiple organ failure** (a condition in which two or more organ systems gradually cease to function), which directly relates to the quality of cellular oxygenation. When the supply of oxygen begins to fall below levels required to sustain life, cells, followed by tissues and organs, begin to deteriorate. The cardiovascular, pulmonary, hepatic, and renal systems are most vulnerable to failure.

As they cease to function, cells release their intracellular chemicals. Preexisting hypoxia is first complicated by a localized rather then a generalized inflammatory response (see Chap. 28) that causes the signs of multiple organ failure, heralding approaching death (Table 38-2). This process may take place gradually over hours or days.

Family Notification

As the client shows signs of approaching death, the nurse must make the family aware that the end is near. The nurse informs the physician first, however. See Nursing Guidelines 38-2.

If death has already occurred, the physician is responsible for contacting the family and releasing that information. Sometimes, the physician delays the news until he or she can talk with the family in person to avoid precipitating acts such as suicide or contributing to a traffic accident.

TABLE 38-2 Signs of Multiple Organ Failure

ORGAN	SIGNS
Heart	• Hypotension • Irregular, weak, and rapid pulse • Cold, clammy, and mottled skin
Liver	• Internal bleeding • Edema • Jaundice • Impaired digestion, distention, anorexia, nausea, and vomiting
Lungs	• Dyspnea • Accumulation of fluid ("death rattle")
Kidneys	• Oliguria • Anuria • Pruritus (itching skin)
Brain	• Fever • Confusion and disorientation • Hypoesthesia (reduced sensation) • Hyporeflexia (reduced reflexes) • Stupor • Coma

TABLE 38-3 Age Criteria for Organ Donation

ORGAN	AGE RANGE
Kidney	6 months–55 years
Liver	<50 years
Heart	<40 years
Pancreas	2–50 years
Corneas	Any age
Skin	15–74 years

Guidelines established by the Organ Procurement Agency of Michigan, Ann Arbor, MI.

Meeting Relatives

To promote a smooth transition, relatives of the dying client are met by the nurse who informed them. If that is not possible, another support person is designated.

On arrival, the nurse shows family members to a private room or area or takes them directly to the client's bedside, depending on their wishes. Privacy allows people the freedom to express feelings without social inhibitions. People have different ways of expressing grief. Some weep and sob uncontrollably; others do not. Nurses remember that those with less outward signs of grief may be feeling sorrow that is just as strong as those who cry and grieve openly.

It is important that nurses remain objective and supportive when there are cultural differences surrounding a death. For example, Native American Lakota Sioux females wail loudly while the males sing mourning songs at the bedside. Buddhists and Hindu from Indian cultures maintain a calm presence and chant to promote the client's passage into *nirvana*, a state of being free from suffering (Servodidio & Steed, 2007). Similarly, people from Bali, whose religion is a combination of Hinduism, Buddhism, and Islamic concepts mixed with ancient beliefs and customs, control the demonstration of emotions in the belief that their gods will not hear prayers that are offered hysterically.

Discussing Organ Donation

Virtually anyone, from the very young to older adults, may be an organ donor. If the donor is younger than 18 years of age, he or she must sign a donor card, along with the parents or legal guardian. Age requirements and organ acceptance are determined on an individual basis at the time of organ procurement (Table 38-3).

Some people have the foresight to communicate whether they are interested in organ donation; others do not. In either case, if the dying or dead client meets the donation criteria, the possibility of harvesting organs is considered.

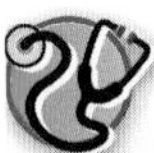

NURSING GUIDELINES 38-2

Summoning the Family of a Dying Client

- Plan to notify the family in a timely manner. *Prompt attention allows the family to be with the client at death.*
- Check the client's medical record for the next of kin or a responsible party. *Doing so ensures that the nurse notifies someone significantly involved in the client's well-being.*
- Identify yourself by name, title, and location. *Identification provides more personal communication.*
- Ask for the family member by name. *Doing so ensures that you communicate information to the appropriate person.*
- Speak in a calm and controlled voice. *Doing so conveys a serious, competent demeanor.*
- Use short sentences to provide small bits of information. *This technique helps the listener to process and comprehend the news.*
- Explain that the client's condition is deteriorating. *This explanation clarifies the purpose for the call.*
- Pause after giving the most important information. *A pause allows the family member to respond.*
- Give brief answers to questions. Emphasize the level of care that the client is receiving. *Such responses reinforce that the client is receiving appropriate care.*
- Urge family members to come as soon as possible. *This ensures that the people most important to the client are there at death.*
- Document the time, the person to whom you communicated the information, and the message. *Appropriate documentation provides a permanent record.*

Organ donation may or may not be discussed with the next of kin based on the 2006 revision of the Uniform Anatomical Gift Act (UAGA). The UAGA, which has been adopted by almost all states, stipulates that (1) if a dying or deceased person has a document identifying an intention to donate organs or has expressly refused organ donation, the next of kin or someone with a power of attorney for health care need not be involved; (2) if no documentation of intent is available, consent for organ donation on behalf of the client can be sought; (3) without a signed refusal, life support may not be withdrawn until the potential for organ donation is determined even if doing so contradicts a person's advanced directives because life support that has the potential to save lives overrides the desire to withhold or withdraw life support (Verheijde et al., 2007).

Involving the next of kin or the person with a power of attorney for health care concerning organ donation is generally a courtesy even when it is not absolutely required. This is done delicately by an organ procurement officer. This person is trained in techniques for sensitively requesting organ donations from family members grieving the death of a loved one. The health care agency selects the person who will solicit organ donations. Typically, the facility's transplant coordinator is the organ procurement officer.

Solicitation for organ donation cannot be delayed; some organs, such as the heart and lungs, must be harvested within a few hours to ensure a successful transplant. In some cases, the client is kept on life support prior to removing organs. To protect the health care facility from any legal consequences, permission may be obtained in writing (Fig. 38-6).

Confirming Death

Death is generally determined on the basis that breathing and circulation have ceased. In most cases, when these criteria are met, there is no question that the person is dead. Legally, a physician is responsible for pronouncing a client dead, but in a few states, nurses are authorized to do so.

Brain Death

In some situations involving irreversible brain damage, a mechanical ventilator can sustain breathing and circulation that continues reflexively. In 1968, the Ad Hoc Committee of the Harvard Medical School released a report on the definition of **brain death**, a condition in which there is an irreversible loss of function of the whole brain, including the brainstem. Their recommendations served as the basis for the Uniform Definition of Death Act drafted by the National Conference of Commissioners on Uniform State Laws and approved by the American Medical Association and American Bar Association in 1980.

Consequently, an irreversible cessation of circulatory and respiratory functions or a cessation of all brain functions is now considered the most incontestable criterion for establishing whether a person is dead or alive. Although more than 30 different sets of criteria for determining brain death have appeared in the medical literature since 1978, the following standards commonly are used as guidelines to ensure that brain activity is assessed consistently and accurately. Irreversible brain death is considered to be present if, in the absence of hypothermia, central nervous system depressants, or conditions that may simulate brain death, there is

- Unreceptiveness and unresponsiveness to even intense painful stimuli.
- No movement or spontaneous respiration after being disconnected for 8 minutes from a mechanical ventilator.
- $PaCO_2$ greater than or equal to 60 mm Hg (in the absence of metabolic alkalosis) after being preoxygenated with 100% oxygen.
- Complete absence of central and deep tendon reflexes.
- Flat electroencephalogram for at least 10 minutes or confirmation of neurologic inactivity using other standard neuroimaging techniques.
- No change in clinical findings on a second assessment 6, 12, or 24 hours later (Byrne, 1999; Sullivan et al., 1999). The time frame relates to each state's medical standard.

Once death is confirmed, the physician issues a death certificate and obtains written permission for an autopsy if one is desirable.

Death Certificate

A **death certificate** (a legal document attesting that the person named on the form has been found dead) also indicates the presumptive cause of the person's death. Death certificates are sent to local health departments that use the information to compile mortality statistics. The statistics are important in identifying trends, needs, and problems in the fields of health and medicine.

The **mortician** (the person who prepares the body for burial or cremation) is responsible for filing the death certificate with the proper authorities. The death certificate also carries the mortician's signature and, in some states, his or her license number.

Permission for Autopsy

An **autopsy** is an examination of the organs and tissues of a human body after death. It is not necessary after all deaths, but it is useful for determining more conclusively the cause of death. The findings may affect the medical care of blood relatives who may be at risk for a similar disorder, or the results may contribute to medical science. It is usually the physician's responsibility to obtain permission for an autopsy.

A **coroner** (the person legally designated to investigate deaths that may not be the result of natural causes) has the authority to order an autopsy. The coroner, who may or may not be a physician, does not need permission from the next of kin to do so. In general, a coroner orders an autopsy if the death involved a crime, was of a suspicious nature, or occurred without any recent medical consultation.

OPAM

Organ Procurement Agency of Michigan

Subsidiary Of
TRANSPLANTATION SOCIETY OF MICHIGAN
2203 Platt Road, Ann Arbor, Michigan 48104

1-800-482-4881 (313) 973-1577 Detroit—464-7988

ANATOMICAL GIFT DONATION STATEMENT

I understand that in the present state of medical practice, several organs and tissues are being removed from persons who have died unexpectedly, and are being used for transplantation to living persons or for medical or scientific research. I understand that organs are removed after my relative has died, and before the organs suffer any damage, (usually within eight [8] hours) and that this gift authorizes all examinations of the body which are necessary to assure the medical acceptability of the gift.

I appreciate the benefits that come from organ donation and also understand the criteria used in determining death in the case of decedent. I am the surviving:

(1) _____ Spouse
(2) _____ Adult son or daughter
(3) _____ Mother or Father
(4) _____ Adult brother or sister
(5) _____ Guardian of the patient at the time of death
(6) _____ Other person authorized or obligated to dispose of the body

____
Relationship

Relatives or persons in a class before my class are not available to sign this form (or have already signed such a form). I have no knowledge that during his or her lifetime the decedent, _______________, was opposed to or said things against making an anatomical gift or organ donation such as the one described below. I do not know of any relative or person in a class before mine who is opposed to this gift, nor do I know of any person in the same class as myself who is opposed to this gift.

I hereby make the following anatomical gift from the body of _____________________:

( ) Any needed organs or parts, or
( ) Only the following organs or parts:

____
(Please specify the organ(s) or part(s)

The specified organ(s) and/or part(s) may be used for any of the purposes allowed by law, i.e. transplantation, therapy, medical research and education.

WITNESSES:

_____________________ _____________________
Name

_____________________ _____________________
Relation

____
Date

FIGURE 38-6 An organ procurement form.

Performing Postmortem Care

Postmortem care (care of the body after death) involves cleaning and preparing the body to enhance its appearance during viewing at the funeral home, ensuring proper identification, and releasing the body to mortuary personnel (Skill 38-1).

Stop, Think, and Respond Box 38-1

Discuss nursing activities that demonstrate dignity and respect for the dead person's body.

GRIEVING

Grieving means the process of feeling acute sorrow over a loss. It is a painful experience, but it helps survivors to resolve the loss. Some people experience **anticipatory grieving**, or grieving that begins before the loss occurs. The longer people have to anticipate a loss, the sooner they eventually resolve it. **Grief work** (activities involved in grieving) includes participating in the burial rituals common to a culture. Although such rituals differ, the **grief response** (the psychological and physical phenomena experienced by those grieving) is universal. Psychological reactions commonly are identified as the stages of grief:

- Shock and disbelief: the refusal to accept that a loved one is about to die or has died
- Developing awareness: the physical and emotional responses such as feeling sick, sad, empty, or angry
- Restitution period: a recognition of the loss
- Idealization: an exaggeration of the good qualities of the deceased

Some survivors have **paranormal experiences** (experiences outside scientific explanation), such as seeing, hearing, or feeling the continued presence of the deceased.

Survivors feel physical symptoms more acutely immediately after the death of a loved one. Some grieving people report symptoms such as anorexia, tightness in the chest and throat, difficulty breathing, lack of strength, and sleep disturbances. No identifiable pathologic state other than grief can explain these symptoms.

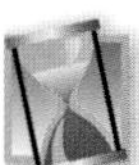

Gerontologic Considerations

■ Research has shown that some people develop life-threatening illnesses and die within 6 months of the death of a spouse. Encouraging older adults who have experienced the death of a close friend or family member to express feelings associated with grieving is important. Referrals for individual counseling or grief support groups are appropriate.

Pathologic Grief

In **pathologic grief**, also called dysfunctional grief, a person cannot accept someone's death. Sometimes, people manifest pathologic grief by bizarre or morbid behaviors. For example, survivors may keep the possessions of a deceased loved one exactly as they were at the time of death for a prolonged period. Others may attempt to contact the deceased through séances. In rare instances, survivors may keep a corpse in the home for an extended period after death.

Resolution of Grief

Mourning takes longer for some than for others; there is no standard length of time for "normal" grieving. One sign that a person is resolving his or her grief is an ability to talk about the dead person without becoming emotionally overwhelmed. Another sign is that the grieving person describes the good and bad qualities of the deceased.

NURSING IMPLICATIONS

Nurses who care for dying clients, their family members, and their friends may identify many different nursing diagnoses:

- Acute (or Chronic) Pain
- Fear
- Spiritual Distress
- Social Isolation
- Ineffective Role Performance
- Interrupted Family Processes
- Ineffective Coping
- Disabled Family Coping
- Decisional Conflict
- Hopelessness
- Powerlessness
- Grieving
- Complicated Grieving
- Caregiver Role Strain
- Death Anxiety
- Chronic Sorrow

Nursing Care Plan 38-1 applies the nursing process to the care of a client with a diagnosis of Hopelessness, defined in NANDA-I's 2012 taxonomy (p. 279) as a "subjective state in which an individual sees limited or no alternatives or personal choices available and is unable to mobilize energy on (his or her) own behalf." Lynda Carpenito-Moyet (2009) further explains, "Hopelessness differs from powerlessness in that a hopeless person sees no solution to his problem and/or way to achieve what is desired, even if he has control of his life. A powerless person, on the other hand, may see an alternative or answer to the problem, yet be unable to do anything about it because of lack of control and resources."

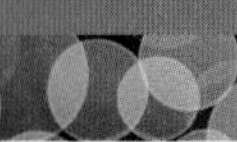

NURSING CARE PLAN 38-1 Hopelessness

Assessment

- Monitor the client's physical manifestations such as loss of appetite, weight loss, fatigue, and sleep disturbances.
- Observe behavioral manifestations such as reduced motivation, passivity, neglect of hygiene, withdrawal, reduced verbal interaction, and disinterest in the future.
- Observe emotional manifestations such as feelings of helplessness, apathy, sadness, defeat, and abandonment.
- Observe cognitive manifestations such as suicidal ideation, decreased attention and concentration, illogical thinking, decreased ability to process or integrate information, and fixation on loss(es).
- Listen for verbal cues that suggest despair, resignation, and surrender.

Nursing Diagnosis. **Hopelessness** related to psychological distress over the development of HIV-related complication (*Pneumocystis carinii* pneumonia) as manifested by little eye contact during interaction, staring out of window, and the statement, "It doesn't matter what's done or not done anymore. One of these days you won't be able to stop the infections," and partner's statement, "I'm afraid he'll just stop eating and taking his medications."

Expected Outcome. The client will regain hope as evidenced by identifying interest in one future-related activity or achievement by the time of transfer to home health care service.

Interventions	Rationales
Reinforce at appropriate times that drug therapy can cure the pneumonia and control the primary illness indefinitely.	Remaining compliant with HIV drug therapy reduces the potential for drug resistance and extends survival.
Share normal as well as abnormal findings after periodic physical examinations or laboratory tests.	Sharing positive information may encourage the client to believe in the likelihood for an improved health status.
Explore the goals the client hoped to accomplish before the illness.	Assisting with reminiscence may motivate the client toward future-related activities.
Ask the client to identify goals that could be realistically accomplished in the next 6–12 months.	Focusing on short-term goals offers an alternative to defeat that the client may feel over accomplishing unrealistic long-term goals.
Encourage the client to develop a plan for accomplishing one future-related goal.	Developing a plan provides a tool for accomplishing goals.

Evaluation of Expected Outcomes

- The client lists evidence that the current health problem is resolving, such as clearer lung sounds and slight weight gain.
- The client discusses various literary works that he has published and was working on prior to this illness.
- The client describes plans to contact a publisher who was interested in a collection of his poems.

CRITICAL THINKING EXERCISES

1. Does being maintained on life-support equipment contradict the right to die in peace and dignity (see the Dying Person's Bill of Rights)?
2. Select a right from the Dying Person's Bill of Rights and explain how it might be violated. How can nurses protect this right?
3. What qualities would be helpful for someone who is an organ procurement officer?
4. How is grieving an unexpected death different than grieving the death of a person suffering from a prolonged illness or disorder?

NCLEX-STYLE REVIEW QUESTIONS

1. When the nurse cares for a client with no hope of recovery, which of the following is the most conclusive criterion for declaring the person brain dead?
   1. A lack of response to verbal stimulation
   2. Urine output less than 100 mL/24 hours
   3. No spontaneous respiratory efforts
   4. Unequal pupils in response to light

2. Place the stages of dying in their usual sequence as identified by Dr. Elisabeth Kübler-Ross. Use all the options.
   1. Depression
   2. Anger
   3. Acceptance
   4. Denial
   5. Bargaining
3. If a terminally ill client made the following statements to a nurse, which is the best evidence that the client is in the bargaining stage?
   1. "There must be some mistake in the pathology report."
   2. "If I can just live until my son graduates, I won't ask for anything else."
   3. "I don't know why I would deserve to die at such a young age."
   4. "I hope my death comes quickly; I'm ready to go."
4. When a terminally ill client refuses to eat or drink, what nursing measures can be independently implemented? Select all that apply.
   1. Inserting a nasogastric feeding tube
   2. Providing frequent oral hygiene measures
   3. Humidifying the room air
   4. Offering hard candies periodically
   5. Administering intravenous fluids
5. When a client has died, under what circumstance can health care professionals proceed with the protocol for harvesting organs for transplantation?
   1. The deceased client has a document indicating his or her desire to be an organ donor.
   2. The nursing supervisor believes the deceased has suitable organs for transplantation.
   3. The deceased client's next of kin gives permission to harvest the organs.
   4. The physician has declared and documented the client's time of death.

SKILL 38-1 Performing Postmortem Care

Suggested Action	Reason for Action
ASSESSMENT	
Determine that the client is dead by assessing breathing and circulation.	Confirms that the client is lifeless in all but cases in which life support equipment is used.
Determine if the physician and family have been notified.	Establishes the chain of communication.
Notify the nursing supervisor and switchboard of the client's death.	Makes others aware of a change in the client's status.
Check the medical record for the name of the mortuary where the body will be taken.	Facilitates collaboration.
PLANNING	
Inform mortuary personnel that the family has chosen them to manage the burial.	Communicates a need for services.
Ask when to expect mortuary personnel.	Facilitates efficient time management.
Contact any individuals involved in organ procurement.	Promotes the timely harvesting of organs.
Obtain a postmortem kit or supplies for cleaning, wrapping, and identifying the body if there will be a delay in transport to a mortuary.	Promotes organization when preparing a body that will be temporarily held in the **morgue** (an area where bodies of dead persons are temporarily held or examined).
IMPLEMENTATION	
Pull the curtains around the bed.	Ensures privacy.
Don gloves.	Follows standard precautions.
Place the body supine with the arms extended at the sides or folded over the abdomen.	Prevents skin discoloration in areas that will be visible in a casket.
Remove all medical equipment[a] such as intravenous catheters, urinary catheters, and dressings.	Eliminates unnecessary equipment.
Remove hairpins or clips.	Prevents accidental trauma to the face.
Close the eyelids.	Ensures that eyes will close when the body is prepared.
Replace or keep dentures in the mouth.	Maintains the natural contour of the face.
Place a small rolled towel beneath the chin to close the mouth.	Promotes a natural appearance.
Cleanse secretions and drainage from the skin.	Ensures the delivery of a hygienic body.
Apply one or more disposable pads between the legs and under the buttocks.	Absorbs urine or stool should they escape.
Attach an identification tag to the ankle or wrist; pad the wrist first if it is used.	Facilitates the accurate identification of the body; prevents damage to tissue that will be visible.
Wrap the body in a paper **shroud** (a covering for the body); cover the body with a sheet.	Demonstrates respect for the dignity of the deceased person.
Tidy the bedside area; dispose of soiled equipment.	Follows the principles of medical asepsis.
Remove gloves and wash your hands.	Removes colonizing microorganisms.
Leave the room and close the door, or transport the body to the morgue (Fig. A).	Provides a temporary location for the body until mortuary personnel arrive.

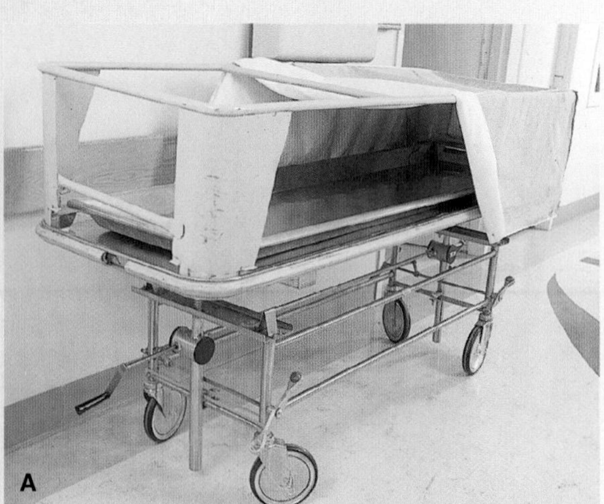

A morgue cart. (Photo by B. Proud.)

(continued)

Performing Postmortem Care (continued)

IMPLEMENTATION (CONTINUED)

Action	Rationale
Make an inventory of valuables and send them to an administrative office for placement in a safe.	Ensures the safekeeping and accountability for valuables until a family member can claim them.
Notify housekeeping after the body is removed from the room.	Facilitates cleaning and the preparation for another admission.

Evaluation

- The body is cleaned and prepared appropriately.
- The body is transferred to mortuary personnel.

Document

- Assessments that indicate the client is dead
- Time of death
- People notified of death
- Care of the body
- Time body is transported to the morgue or transferred to mortuary personnel

SAMPLE DOCUMENTATION

Date and Time No breathing noted and no pulse at 1400. Dr. Williams notified at 1415. Dr. Williams pronounced death and called client's wife. Foster's Funeral Home notified. Mortuary personnel unavailable until 1800. Postmortem care provided. Body transported to morgue after wife and children departed.

———————— SIGNATURE/TITLE

[a]Except in coroner's cases.

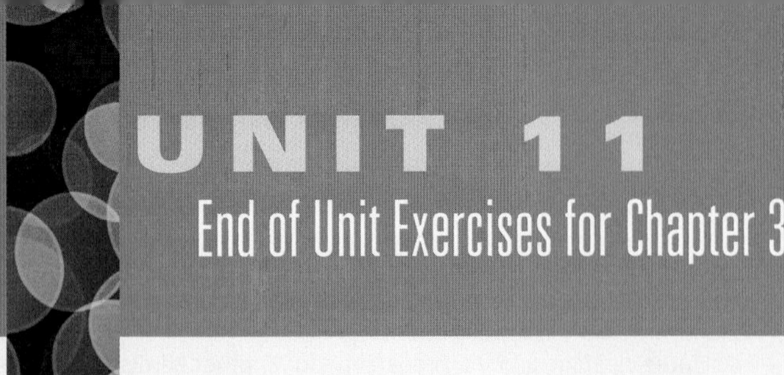

UNIT 11
End of Unit Exercises for Chapter 38

Section I: Reviewing What You've Learned

Activity A: *Fill in the blanks by choosing the correct word from the options given in parentheses.*

1. ________________ involves a process of negotiation, usually with God or some higher power, in an attempt to delay the inevitability of death. (Bargaining, Denial, Depression)
2. ________________ care provides around-the-clock nursing care for clients who cannot live independently. (Hospice, Residential, Respite)
3. The ability to ________________ is one of the last reflexes to disappear as death approaches. (hear, smell, suck)

Activity B: *Mark each statement as either T (True) or F (False). Correct any false statements.*

1. T____F____ Diarrhea may be a common consequence of continuous narcotic analgesia.
2. T____F____ An autopsy is the examination of human organs and tissues to treat a disease.

Activity C: *Write the correct term for each description below.*

1. A person legally designated to investigate an unnatural death ________________
2. A legal document attesting that the person named on the form is deceased ________________
3. A condition in which two or more organ systems gradually cease to function ________________

Activity D: *Match the terms related to grieving in Column A with their explanations in Column B.*

Column A	Column B
1. ________________ Anticipatory grief	A. Activities involved in grieving
2. ________________ Pathologic grief	B. Psychological and physical experiences while grieving
3. ________________ Grief work	C. Inability to accept someone's death
4. ________________ Grief response	D. Feeling sad before someone's death

Activity E: *Differentiate between home care and residential care based on the categories given below.*

	Home Care	Residential Care
Role of Nurses		
Delivery of Care		

Activity F: *Dr. Elisabeth Kübler-Ross described stages through which terminally ill clients progress. Write in the boxes provided below the usual sequence of typical comments during the stages of dying.*

1. "Why me?"
2. "Yes, me."
3. "Yes, me, but if only . . ."
4. "I am ready."
5. "No, not me."

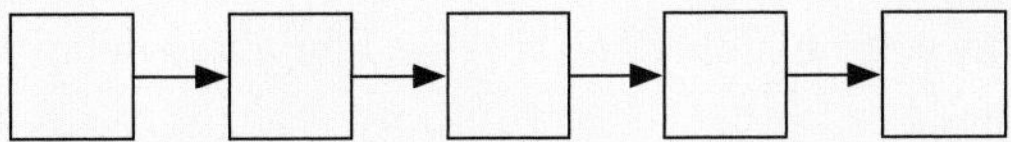

Activity G: *Answer the following questions.*

1. What classifies an illness as terminal?

2. When can hospice care be terminated?

Section II: Applying Your Knowledge

Activity H: *Give rationales for the following questions.*

1. Why is skin care important for terminally ill, incontinent clients?

2. Why do the lips of terminally ill clients need periodic lubrication?

3. Why are death certificates sent to the local health department?

Activity I: *Answer the following questions focusing on nursing roles and responsibilities.*

1. What are two methods that nurses can use to promote an acceptance of death in dying clients? What interventions can nurses use to provide emotional support to these clients?

2. A nurse is caring for a client in the last stages of terminal brain cancer. What nursing diagnoses might apply for this client and his or her family members?

3. A nurse is caring for a dying client.
   a. What nursing actions are appropriate related to the client's hygiene and nourishment?

   b. How can the nurse ensure that the client receives adequate fluids?

Activity J: *Consider the following questions. Discuss them with your instructor or peers.*

1. A nurse is providing postmortem care for an elderly client who has died of cancer. How can the nurse demonstrate dignity and respect for the client's body?
2. A nurse is caring for a client who is unresponsive to even painful stimuli, cannot breathe independently, and has completely absent central and deep tendon reflexes. The physician has confirmed that the client is brain dead.
   a. What should the nurse do if the family asks to discontinue life support systems for the client?
   b. What information should the nurse provide to the family about the legal implications of their request?

Section III: Getting Ready For NCLEX

Activity K: *Answer the following questions.*

1. A nurse at an extended care facility is caring for a client with cancer and a limited prognosis for long-term survival. Which of the following interventions is most appropriate when caring for this client?
   a. Share information, such as trends in vital signs, with the client.
   b. Ask the client to identify goals that could be accomplished in 24 months.
   c. Encourage the client to seek alternative forms of treatment.
   d. Ask the client not to dwell on old memories and goals previously established.
2. A nurse is caring for a client who had medical equipment attached to her at the time of death. What measures will the nurse implement when providing postmortem care of the client's body? Select all that apply.
   a. Obtain supplies for cleaning and wrapping the body.
   b. Keep all the medical equipment attached to the body.
   c. Contact individuals involved in organ procurement.
   d. Ask for the approximate arrival time of the mortuary personnel.
   e. Remove the disposable pads from between the legs.
3. When caring for a dying client, which of the following are appropriate for procuring organ or tissue donations? Select all that apply.
   a. Determine the dying client's wishes concerning organ and tissue donation.
   b. Obtain permission from the next of kin as the client nears death.
   c. Inform the mortician to remove specific organs when preparing the body.
   d. Contact the pathologist in charge of performing autopsies.
   e. Enlist the assistance of an organ procurement coordinator.
4. A nurse is caring for a stuporous and cold client who has developed mottled skin. Failure of which of the following body parts could have led to this condition?
   a. Brain and heart
   b. Liver and kidney
   c. Pancreas and stomach
   d. Intestine and bladder

References and Suggested Readings

Adams, L. A., Shephard, N., Caruso, R. A., et al. (2009). Putting evidence into practice: Evidence-based interventions to prevent and manage anorexia. *Clinical Journal of Oncology Nursing, 13*(1), 95–102.

Administration on Aging. (2008). *A profile of older Americans: 2008.* Accessed January 20, 2010, from http://www.aoa.gov/AoARoot/Aging_Statistics/Profile/2008/16.aspx

Advice, P. R. N. (2006). Home health care: A new job for plastic wrap. *Nursing, 36*(2), 12.

Agency for Healthcare Research and Quality. (2004). *Hospital nurse staffing and quality of care.* Retrieved September, 2009, from http://www.ahrq.gov/research/nursestaffing/nursestaff.htm

Aiken, L., Clark, S. P., Sloan, D. M., et al. (2008). Effects of hospital care environment on patient mortality and nurse outcomes. *Journal of Nursing Administration, 38*(5), 223–229.

Aiken, T. D. (2004). *Legal, ethical, and political issues in nursing.* Philadelphia: F. A. Davis.

Al Naami, M., & Afzal, M. F. (2006). *Alcohol based hand rub vs. traditional surgical scrub and the risk of wound infection: A randomized controlled trial.* Accessed January 16, 2010, from http://faculty.ksu.edu.sa/19985/Alcohol%20based%20hand%20rub%20vs%20traditional%surgical.ppt

Alfaro-LeFevre, R. (2009). *Applying nursing process: A tool for critical thinking* (7th ed.). Philadelphia: Lippincott Williams & Wilkins.

Alford, D. M. (2006a). Legal issues in gerontological nursing; standards of care. *Journal of Gerontological Nursing, 32*(3), 9–12.

Alford, D. M. (2006b). Legal issues in gerontological nursing; what are the hot topics? *Journal of Gerontological Nursing, 32*(1), 8–9.

Allen, G. (2005). Evidence for practice. Use of conscious sedation for upper gastrointestinal endoscopy. *Association of periOperative Registered Nurses (AORN) journal, 81*(2), 427–428.

Allibone, L. (2005). Respiratory care. Principles for inserting and managing chest drains. *Nursing Times, 101*(42), 45–49.

Amatayakul, M. (2009). Measuring meaningful use: The healthcare industry is abuzz with questions about what it means to demonstrate "meaningful use" of electronic health record (HER) technology to be eligible for federal stimulus incentives. *Healthcare Financial Management, 63*(23), 100–101.

Amella, E. J., Grant, A. P., & Mulloy, C. (2007). Eating behavior in persons with moderate to late-stage dementia: Assessment and interventions. *Journal of the American Psychiatric Nurses Association, 13*(6), 360–367.

American Academy of Family Physicians. (2005). *Vasomotor rhinitis.* Accessed August 12, 2010, from http://www.aafp.org/afp/2005/0915/1057.html

American Academy of Orthopaedic Surgeons. (2007). *Care of casts and splints.* Accessed May 12, 2010, from http://orthoinfo.aaos.org/topic=a00095

American Academy of Orthopedic Surgeons. (2007). *How to use crutches, canes, and walkers.* Accessed May 18, 2010, from http://orthoinfo.aaos.org/topic.cfm?topic=a00181

American Agency for Healthcare Research and Quality; U.S. Preventive Services Task Force. (2009). *Screening for breast cancer.* Accessed February 1, 2010, from http://www.ahrq.gov/clinic/USpstf/uspsbrca.htm

American Association of Colleges of Nursing. (2005). *Nurse Reinvestment Act at a glance.* Retrieved September 2, 2009, 2006 from http://www.aacn.nche.edu/media/nraataglance.htm

American Association of Retired Persons. (2005). *Profile of older Americans: 2005.* Accessed January 20, 2010, from http://assets.aarp.org/rgcenter/general/profile_2005.pdf

American Cancer Society. (2009). *American Cancer Society guidelines for the early detection of cancer.* Accessed February 1, 2010, from http://www.cancer.org/docroot/PED/content/ped_2_3x_ACS_Cancer_Detection_Guidelines_36.asp

American Cancer Society. (2009). *American Cancer Society responds to changes in USPSTF mammography guidelines.* Accessed February 1, 2010, from http://www.cancer.org/docroot/MED/content/MED_2_1x_American_Cancer_Society_Responds_to_Changes_to_USPSTF_Mammography_Guidelines.asp

American Cancer Society. (2009). *Can breast cancer be found early?* Accessed February 1, 2010, from http://www.cancer.org/docroot/cri/content/cri_2_4_3x_can_breast_cancer_be_found_early_5.asp

American Cancer Society. (2009). *Cervical cancer: Prevention and early detection.* Accessed February 8, 2010, from http://www.cancer.org/docroot/CRI/content/CRI_2_6x_cervical_cancer_prevention_and_early_detection_8.asp

American Chronic Pain Association. (2004). *Americans living with pain survey.* Accessed March 22, 2010, from http://www.theacpa.org/documents/surveyresults.pdf

American College of Sports Medicine. (2003). *ACSM guidelines for healthy aerobic activity.* Retrieved January 23, 2007, from http://www.acsm.org/health+fitness/index.htm

American College of Surgeons. (2002). *Statement on ensuring correct patient, correct site, and correct procedure.* Accessed May 26, 2010, from http://www.facs.org/fellows_info/statements/st-41.html

American Congress of Obstetricians and Gynecologists. (2009). *Education pamphlet AP085—The Pap test.* Accessed February 8, 2010, from http://www.acog.org/publications/patient_education/bp085.cfm

American Diabetes Association. (2007). *Insulin administration.* Accessed August 18, 2010, from http://care.diabetesjournals.org/content/26/suppl_1/s121.full

American Diabetes Association. (2008). Standards of medical care in diabetes. Clinical practice recommendations. *Diabetes Care, 31,* Suppl. 1, S12–S54.

American Diabetes Association. (2010). *Checking your blood glucose.* Accessed February 10, 2010, from http://www.diabetes.org/living-with-diabetes/treatment-and-care/blood-glucose-control/checking-your-blood-glucose.html

American Dietetic Association. (2009). *Position of the American Dietetic Association: Vegetarian diets.* Accessed February 16, 2010, from http://www.vrg.org/nutrition/2009_ADA_position_paper.pdf

American Heart Association. (2010a). *Trans fats.* Accessed February 15, 2010, from http://www.americanheart.org/presenter.jhtml?identifier=3045792

American Heart Association. (2010b). *Vegetarian diets.* Accessed February 16, 2010, from http://www.americanheart.org/presenter.jhtml?identifier=4777

American Institutes for Research. (2009). *Technical report and data file user's manual for 2003 National Assessment of Adult Literacy.* Accessed December 31, 2009, from http://nces.ed.gov/pubsinfo.asp?pubid=2009476

American Nurses Association. (1998). *Standards of clinical nursing practice* (2nd ed.). Washington, DC: Author.

American Nurses Association. (2010). *Nursing: A social policy statement* (3rd ed.). Kansas City, MO: Author.

American Nurses Association. (2003). *Position statement on elimination of manual patient handling to prevent work-related musculoskeletal disorders.* Accessed April 19, 2010, from http://www.unap.org/files/Safe%20Patient%20Handling%20-%20ANA%20position.pdf

American Obesity Association. (2005). *Morbid obesity.* Accessed April 23, 2010, from http://obesity1.tempdomainname.com/subs/fastfacts/morbidobesity.shtml

American Pain Society. (2005a). APS position statement on the use of placebos in pain management. *The Journal of Pain, 6*(4), 215–217.

American Pain Society. (2005b). *Guideline for the management of cancer pain.* Glenview, IL: Author.

American Pain Society. (2005c). *Improving quality of acute and cancer pain management.* Glenview, IL: Author.

American Pain Society. (2008). *Principles of analgesic use in the treatment of acute pain and cancer pain* (6th ed.). Glenview, IL: Author.

American Psychiatric Association. (2000). Insomnia, primary. In *Diagnostic and statistical manual of mental disorders* (4th ed., text revision). Washington, DC: Author.

American recovery and reinvestment act includes funding for nursing education. (2009). Accessed January 5, 2012, from http://allnurses.com/nursing-news/american-recovery-reinvestment-372032.html

American Red Cross. (2011). *Blood donor requirements.* Accessed February 9, 2011, from http://www.bloodbook.com/donr-requir.html

American Society of Anesthesiologists. (1999). *Practice guidelines for preoperative fasting and the use of pharmacologic agents to reduce the risk of pulmonary aspiration: Application to healthy patients undergoing elective procedures.* Accessed May 26, 2010, from http://www.asahq.org/publicationsAndServices/NPO.pdf

American Society on Aging, & American Society of Consultant Pharmacists Foundation. (2006). *Improving medication adherence in older adults.* Accessed January 20, 2010, from http://www.adultmeducation.com

Amerine, E., & Keirsey, M. (2006a). How should you respond to constipation? Learn solutions to this common problem among hospitalized patients. *Nursing, 36*(10), 64hn1–64hn4.

Amerine, E., & Keirsey, M. (2006b). Managing acute diarrhea. *Nursing, 36*(9), 64hn1–64hn2, 64hn4.

Anderson, J. (2006). *Safe patient lifting legislation makes progress.* Accessed April 21, 2010, from http://www.ergoweb.com/news/detail.cfm?print?=on&id=1661

Anderson, J., Langemo, D., Hanson, D., et al. (2007). Wound & skin care. What you can learn from a comprehensive skin assessment. *Nursing, 37*(4), 65–66.

Andrews, J. D. (2005). *Cultural, ethnic, and religious reference manual for health care providers* (3rd ed.). Winston-Salem, NC: JAMARDA Resources.

Andrews, M. M., & Boyle, J. S. (2011). *Transcultural concepts in nursing care* (6th ed.). Philadelphia: Lippincott Williams & Wilkins.

Arbique, J. (2006). *Fingernail length and microbes; relationship between nail length and microbe yield.* Accessed January 14, 2010, from http://microbiology.suite101.com/article.cfm/fingernail_length_and_microbes

Armstrong, J., & Mitchell, E. (2008). Comprehensive nursing assessing in the care of older people. *Nursing Older People, 20*(1), 36–40.

Aschenbrenner, D. S. (2009). Drug watch. Unsafe injection practices put patients at risk. *American Journal of Nursing, 109*(7), 45–46.

Association of Perioperative Registered Nurses. (2008). *Recommended practices for preoperative patient skin antisepsis.* Accessed May 24, 2010, from http://www.aorn.org/docs/assets/956D86EC-9983-6D4F-67A54D9500767E9F/RP_skinprep_pub%20com_10_12_07.pdf

Association of Perioperative Registered Nurses. (2007). *Standard, recommended practices and Guidelines.* Denver, CO: AORN.

Association of Reproductive Health Professionals. (2004). *The periodic well-woman visit.* Accessed February 8, 2010, from http://arhp.power-point-generator.com/presentations/Periodic%20Well%20Woman%Visit.ppt

Austgen, L., & Bowen, R. (2009). *Brown adipose tissue.* Accessed January 25, 2010, from http://www.vivo.colostate.edu/hbooks/pathophys/misc_topics/brownfat.html

Banschbach, S. K. (2008). Recommitting your practice to patient safety. *Association of periOperative Nurses (AORN) Journal, 88*(6), 887–888.

Baranoski, S. (2008a). Wound & skin care. Choosing a wound dressing, part 1. *Nursing, 38*(1), 60–61.

Baranoski, S. (2008b). Wound & skin care. Choosing a wound dressing, part 2. *Nursing, 38*(2), 14–15.

Baranoski, S., & Ayello, E. (2008c). *Wound care essentials: Practice principles* (2nd ed.). Philadelphia: Lippincott Williams & Wilkins.

Barclay, L., & Murata, P. (2009). *World Health Organization issues guidelines on hand hygiene in healthcare.* Accessed May 17, 2009, from http://cme.medscape.com/viewarticle/702403/

Barnhart, K. T., Davidson, B., Kellogg-Spadt, S., et al. (2010). *Roundtable discussion. How do you begin the discussion of vaginal delivery of medications with patients?* Accessed August 12, 2010, from http://cme.medscape.com/viewarticle/504375_6

Beattie, S., & Asch-Goodkin, J. (2006). Back to basics with O_2 therapy. *RN, 69*(9), 37–40.

Beattie, S., & Roman, L. M. (2007). Bedside emergency. Respiratory distress. *RN, 70*(7), 34–39.

Beaulieu, L., & Freeman, M. (2009). Nursing shortcuts can shortcut safety. *Nursing, 39*(12), 16–17.

Becton, Dickinson and Company. (2008). *Insulin injection "at-a-glance"*. Accessed August 18, 2010, from http://bd.com/resource.aspx?IDX=11314

Becton, Dickinson and Company. (2009). *Good insulin injection practices*. Accessed August 18, 2010, from http://www.diabeteshealth.com/read/2009/12/18/6486/good-insulin-injection-practices/

Benbow, M. (2009). Dressing application and removal. *Practice Nurse, 37*(10), 21–22, 24–27.

Bennett, B. (2008a). *Three seconds: The first impression.* Accessed December, 2009, from http://www.yeartosuccess.com/y2s/blog/VIEW/00000009/00000093/Three-Seconds-The-First-Impression.html

Bennett, B. (2008b). *Reading body language*. Accessed December, 2009, from http://www.yeartosuccess.com/y2s/blog/VIEW/00000009/00000097/Reading-Body-Language.html

Berg, R. A., Hemphill, R., Abella, B. S., et al. (2010). *Part 5: Adult basic life support: 2010 American Heart Association Guidelines for Cardiopulmonary Resuscitation and Emergency Cardiovascular Care*. http://circ.ahajournals.org/cgi/content/full/122/18_suppl_3/S686

Bergstrom, N., Horn, S. D., Smout, R. J., et al. (2005). The national pressure ulcer long-term care study: Outcomes of pressure ulcer treatments in long-term care. *Journal of the American Geriatrics Society, 53*(10), 1721–1729.

Beyea, S. C. (2009). Patient safety first. Essential reading for every perioperative clinician. *Association of periOperative Nurses (AORN) Journal, 89*(4), 763–765.

Bickley, L. S. (2008). *Bates' guide to physical examination and history taking*. Philadelphia: Lippincott Williams & Wilkins.

Bisanz, A. (2007). Chronic constipation. *American Journal of Nursing (Hospital Extra), 107*(4), 72B–72D, 72F–72H.

Bland, M., Gaines, B., & Law, E. (2007). Are we still doing the right thing? An evidence-based review of the management of constipation. *Oncology Nursing Forum, 34*(2), 24–27.

Bloom, H. G., Ahmed, I., Alessi, C. A., et al. (2009). Evidence-based recommendations for the assessment and management of sleep disorders in older persons. *Journal of the American Geriatrics Society, 57*(5), 761–789.

Bobrow, B. J., Spaite, D. W., Berg, R. A., et al. (2010). Chest compression-only CPR by lay rescuers and survival from out-of-hospital cardiac arrest. *Journal of the American Medical Association, 304*(13), 1447–1454.

Bolek, B. (2006). Strictly clinical. Facing cranial nerve assessment. *American Nurse Today, 1*(2), 21–22.

Bott, M. J., Gajewski, B., Lee, R., et al. (2007). Care planning efficiency for nursing facilities. *Nursing Economica, 25*(2), 85–94.

Boulanger, C., & Toghill, M. (2009). How to measure and record vital signs to ensure detection of deteriorating patients. *Nursing Times, 105*(47), 10–12.

Boyce, J. M., & Pittet, D. (2002). Guideline for hand hygiene in health-care settings. Recommendations of the Healthcare Control Practice Advisory Committee and the HICPAC/SHEA/APIC/IDSA Hand Hygiene Task Force [Electronic version]. *Morbidity & Mortality Weekly Report, 51*(RR16), 1–44.

Boyd, R., Leigh, B., & Stuart, P. (2005). *Capillary versus venous bedside glucose estimations.* Accessed February 12, 2010, from http://emj.bmj.com/content/22/3/177.abstract

Boyle, M. E. (2008). Optimizing the treatment of type 2 diabetes using current and future insulin technologies. *MedSurg Nursing, 17*(6), 383–390.

Bradley, R. (2007). Improving respiratory assessment skills. *Journal of Nurse Practitioners, 3*(4), 276–277.

Bradley, S. F. (2005). Double, double, toil and trouble: Infections still spreading in long-term care facilities. *Infection Control and Hospital Epidemiology, 26*(3), 227–230.

Brenner, I., & Marsella, A. (2008–2009) Factors influencing exercise participation by clients in long-term care. *The Journal of the Gerontological Nursing Association, 32*(4), 5–11.

Brooke, P. S. (2009). Legal questions. *Nursing, 39*(6), 15–16.

Brown, J. L., & Krause, R. S. (2005). *Cast care.* Accessed May 12, 2010, from http://www.emedicinehealth.com/cast_care/article_em.htm

Brownfield, E. (2004). *Measuring blood pressure in legs*. Accessed January 28, 2010, from http://www.medscape.com/viewarticle/471829

Bruccoliere, T. (2000). How to make patient teaching stick. *RN, 63*(2), 34–36.

Bryant, H. (2007). Dehydration in older people: Assessment and management. *Emergency Nurse, 15*(4), 22–26.

Burch, J. (2006). Caring for the older ostomate: An update. *Nursing & Residential Care, 8*(3), 117–118, 120.

Bureau of Labor Statistics. (2009). *Occupational injuries and illnesses by selected characteristics news release*. Accessed April 21, 2010, from http://www.bls.gov/news.release/archives/osh2_12042009.htm

Bureau of Labor Statistics, & U.S. Department of Labor. (2007a). *Occupational outlook handbook, 2008–2009 edition, Licensed practical and licensed vocational nurses.* Accessed September, 2009, from http://www.bls.gov/oco/ocos102.htm

Byrne, P. A. (1999). *Brain death. Euthanasia: Imposed death.* St. Paul, MN: Human Life Alliance of Minnesota Education Fund.

Calianno, C., & Jakubek, P. (2006a). Wound & skin care. Wound bed preparation: Laying the foundation for treating chronic wounds, part 1. *Nursing, 36*(2), 70–71.

Calianno, C., & Jakubek, P. (2006b). Wound & skin care. Wound bed preparation: The key to success for chronic wounds, part II. *Nursing, 36*(3), 76–77.

Carpenito-Moyet, L. J. (2005). *Understanding the nursing process*. Philadelphia: Lippincott Williams & Wilkins.

Carpenito-Moyet, L. J. (2008). *Nursing care plans and documentation* (5th ed.). Philadelphia: Lippincott Williams & Wilkins.

Carpenito-Moyet, L. J. (2009). *Nursing diagnosis: Application to clinical practice* (13th ed.). Philadelphia: Lippincott Williams & Wilkins.

Cassel, B. G., Parkers, V., Poon, R., et al. (2008). Quality improvement: Best practices and long-term indwelling urinary catheters. *The Journal of the Gerontological Nursing Association, 32*(1), 13–17.

Cassey, M. Z. (2007). Building a case for using technology: Health literacy and patient education. *Nursing Economics, 25*(3), 186–188.

Centers for Disease Control and Prevention. (2005). Guidelines for preventing the transmission of *Mycobacterium tuberculosis* in healthcare settings. *Morbidity and Mortality Weekly Report, 54*(RR17), 1–141.

Centers for Disease Control and Prevention. (2007). *2007 Guidelines for isolation precautions: Prevention transmission of infectious agents in healthcare settings.* http://www.cdc.gov/ncidod/dhqp/pdf/isolation2007.pdf

Centers for Disease Control and Prevention. (2008a). *Alcohol-attributable deaths and years of potential life lost among American Indians and Alaska Natives—United States, 2001–2005.* Accessed and Retrieved November, 2009, from http://www.cdc.gov/mmwr/preview/mmwrhtml/mm5734a3.htm

Centers for Disease Control and Prevention. (2008b). *Sterilization & disinfection in healthcare Facilities, 2008.* Accessed January 15, 2010, from http://www.cdc.gov/ncidod/dhqp/pdf/guidelines/Disinfection_Nov_2008.pdf

Centers for Disease Control and Prevention. (2008c). *Surgical Site Infection (SSI).* Accessed May 24, 2010, from http://www.cdc.gov/ncidod/dhqp/FAQ_SSI.html

Centers for Disease Control and Prevention. (2009a). *Cover your cough.* Accessed April 12, 2010, from http://www.cdc.gov/flu/protect/covercough.htm

Centers for Disease Control and Prevention. (2009b). *Falls among older adults: An overview.* Accessed March 17, 2010, from http://www.cdc.gov/HomeandRecreationalSafety/falls/adultfalls.html

Centers for Disease Control and Prevention. (2009c). *Guideline for prevention of catheter-associated urinary tract infections.* Accessed June 28, 2010, from http://www.cdc.gov.hicpac/pdf/CAUTI/CAUTIguideline2009final.pdf

Centers for Disease Control and Prevention. (2009d). *The Tuskegee timeline.* Accessed November, 2009, from http://www.cdc.gov/tuskegee/timeline.htm

Centers for Disease Control and Prevention. (2009e). *What you should know about using facemasks and respirators during a flu epidemic.* Accessed January 15, 2010, from http://www.cdc.gov/features/masksrespirators/

Centers for Disease Control and Prevention. (2010). *Target heart rate and estimated maximum heart rate.* Accessed April 27, 2010, from http://www.cdc.gov/physicalactivity/everyone/measuring/heartrate.html

Chadha, A. (2009). Assessing the skin. *Practice Nurse, 38*(7), 43–48.

Chaloner, C. (2007). Ethics in nursing: The way forward. *Nursing Standard, 21*(38), 40–41.

Chan, E. A., Chung, J. W. Y., & Wong, T. K. S. (2008). Learning from the severe acute respiratory syndrome (SARS) epidemic. *Journal of Clinical Nursing, 17*(8), 1023–1034.

Chart Smart. Documenting gastric lavage. (2009). *Nursing, 39*(7), 60.

Cheyne, D. (2005). We must be alert to the warning signs of stress. *Nursing Standard, 20*(10), 72.

Childers, M. K. (2009). *Botulinum toxin in pain management.* Accessed March 24, 2010, from http://emedicine.medscape.com/article/3255574-overview

Chronic wound care: Many suffer during dressing changes. (2008). *Nursing, 38*(9), 24.

Clark, A. P., John, L. D., & Clark, A. P. (2006). Legal and ethical. Nosocomial infections and bath water: Any cause for concern? *The Journal of Advanced Nursing Practice, 20*(3), 119–123.

Clarkson, A. (2007). Dressing remedies: A concept for improving access to and use of dressings in nursing homes. *Journal of Wound Care, 16*(1), 11–13.

Classen, J. (2009). Verification: A golden opportunity… "A case of mistaken identity: Staff input on patient ID errors". *Nursing Management, 40*(8), 8.

Clinical case: Drug therapy affecting the kidney and body fluid composition part 1: Diuretic agents. (2005). *Journal of Practical Nursing, 55*(2), 10–17.

Cluett, J. (2008). *Taking care of your cast.* Accessed May 12, 2010, from http://orthopedics.about.com/od/castsfracturtreatments/p/casts.htm

Cohen, H., & Shastay, A. D. (2008). Getting to the root of medication errors. *Nursing, 38*(12), 39–49.

Cohen, S. A. (2009). A review of demographic and infrastructural factors and potential solutions to the physician and nursing shortage predicted to impact the growing US elderly population. *Journal of Public Health Management and Practice, 15*(4), 352–363.

Cohen, S., & Herbert, T. (1996). Health psychology: Psychological factors and physical disease from the perspective of human psychoneuroimmunology. *Annual Review of Psychology, 47,* 113–142.

Cohn, C. S., & Cushing, M. M. (2009). Oxygen therapeutics: Perfluorocarbons and blood substitute safety. *Critical Care Clinics, 25*(2), 399–414.

Collopy, K. T., & Friese, G. (2010). Hospice and DNR. *EMS Magazine, 39*(8), 52–57.

Cone, D. C. (2010). Compression-only CPR: Pushing science forward. *Journal of the American Medical Association, 304*(13), 1493–1495.

Cook, L., Castrogiovanni, A., David, D., et al. (2008). Patient education documentation: Is it being done? *MedSurg Nursing, 17*(5), 306–310.

Cooper, G. (2005). *Blueprint orthopedics.* Philadelphia: Lippincott Williams & Wilkins.

Copstead-Kirkhorn, L. C., & Banasik, J. L. (2010). *Pathophysiology, biological and behavioral perspectives* (4th ed.). Philadelphia: W.B. Saunders.

Cornforth, T. (2006). *Easy tips for accurate Pap smears. What should I do before my Pap smear?* Accessed February 11, 2010, from http://womenshealth.about.com/qt/papsmeartip.htm

Cornforth, T. (2009). *Understanding your Pap smear results.* Accessed February 11, 2010, from http://womenshealth.about.com/cs/papsmears/a/papsmearresults.htm

Cornforth, T. (2010a). *What happens during an annual Pap test and pelvic exam?* Accessed February 11, 2010, from http://womenshealth.about.com/od/gynecologicalhealthissues/a/gyn101_4.htm

Cornforth, T. (2010b). *What is the bimanual exam during my pelvic exam?* Accessed February 11, 2010, from http://womenshealth.about.com/od/gynecologicalhealthissues/a/gyn101_5.htm

Coughlin, A. M., & Parchinsky, C. (2006). Go with the flow of chest tube therapy. *Nursing, 36*(3), 36–42.

Cousins, N. (1979). *Anatomy of an illness as perceived by the patient.* New York: Norton.

Cowan, T. (2009). Singing the praises of tissue viability. *Journal of Wound Care, 18*(11), 445.

Cranton, E. M. (2007). *Introduction to hyperbaric oxygen therapy.* Accessed April 1, 2010, from http://www.drcranton.com/hyperbar.htm

Cranwell-Bruce, L. (2009). Antiemetic drugs. *MedSurg Nursing, 18*(5), 309–314

deAguilar-Nascimento, J. E., & Dock-Nascimento, D. B. (2010). *Reducing preoperative fasting time: A trend based on evidence.* Accessed May 26, 2010, from http://www.wjgnet.com/1948-9366/pdf/v2/i3/57.pdf

deCastro, A.B. (2004). "Handle with Care®": The American Nurses Association's campaign to address work-related musculoskeletal disorders. *Online Journal of Issues in Nursing, 9*(3), Manuscript 2. Accessed April 20, 2010, from http://www.nursingworld.org/MainMenuCategories/ANAMarketplace/ANAPeriodicals/OJIN/TableofContents/Volume92004/No3Sept04/HandleWithCare.aspx

Delahanty, K. M., & Myers, F. E. III. (2007). Nursing 2007 infection control survey report. *Nursing, 37*(6), 28–38.

Delahanty, K. M., & Myers, F. E. III. (2009). I.V. infection control survey report. *Nursing, 39*(12), 24–32.

Department of Health and Human Services, & Centers for Medicare & Medicaid Services. (2009). *Medicare prescription drug plan premiums to increase slightly Medicare beneficiaries may need to enroll in new plans.* Accessed September, 2009, from http://www.cms.hhs.gov/apps/media/press/release.asp?Counter=3494&intNumPerPage=10&checkDate=&checkKey=2&srchType=2&numDays=0srchOpt=0srchData=prescription+plans+keywordType=All&chkNewsType=1%2C+2%2C+3%2C+4%2C+5&intPage=showall=1+pYear=&year=)&des=cboOrder=date

Department of the Interior, Bureau of Indian Affairs. (2009). *What we do.* Accessed November, 2009, from http://www.bia.gov/WhatWeDo/index.htm

Diabetes Self-Management. (2006). *Injection site rotation.* Accessed August 18, 2010, from http://www.diabetesselfmanagement.com/Articles/Diabetes-Definitions/injection_site_rotation/

Dietz, D., & Gates, J. (2010). Wound & skin care. Basic ostomy management, part 1. *Nursing, 40*(2), 61–62.

Donahue, M. P. (1985). *Nursing: The Finest Art.* St. Louis, MO: Mosby.

Drug news. Medication safety: Nurses work around bar-code safeguards. *Nursing, 38*(9), 17.

Dudek, S. G. (2009). *Nutrition essentials for nursing practice* (6th ed.). Philadelphia: Lippincott Williams & Wilkins.

Duggan, C., Watkins, J. B., & Walker, W. A. (2008). *Nutrition in Pediatrics* (4th ed.). Shelton, CT: People's Medical Publishing House.

Dulak, S. B., & Metules, T. (2005). Hands-on help: Removing chest tubes. *RN (Acute Care Focus), 68*(8), 28ac1–28ac4.

Durai, R., Venkatraman, R., & Ng, P. C. (2009). Nasogastric tubes. 2: Risks and guidance on avoiding and dealing with complications. *Nursing Times, 105*(17), 14–16.

Ecklund, M. M., & Ecklund, C. R. (2007). How to recognize and respond to hypovolemic shock: What to do when you patient's fluid bottoms out. *American Nurse Today, 2*(4), 28–31.

Education-Portal.com. (2007). *Grim illiteracy statistics indicate Americans have a reading problem.* Accessed December 31, 2009, from http://education-portal.com/articles/Grim_Illiteracy_Statistics_Indicate_Americans_Have_a_Reading_Problem.html

Edwards, S. L. (1999). Update. Hypothermia. *Professional Nurse, 14*(4), 253, 255–258.

Eliopoulos, C. (2009). *Gerontological nursing* (7th ed.). Philadelphia: Lippincott Williams & Wilkins.

Ellis, J. R., & Bentz, P. M. (2007). *Modules for basic nursing skills* (7th ed.). Philadelphia: Lippincott Williams & Wilkins.

Ellis, K. C. (2008). Keeping asthma at bay: The latest evidence-based guidelines highlight ways to help patients control the disorder. *American Nurse Today, 3*(2), 20–26.

Ervin, R. B. (2009). *Prevalence of metabolic syndrome among adults 20 years of age and over, by sex, age, race, and ethnicity, and body mass index: United States, 2003–2006.* Accessed February 15, 2010, from http://www.cdc.gov/nchs/data/nhsr/nhsr013.pdf

Erwin-Toth, P., Stricker, J. L., & van Rijswijk, L. (2010). Peristomal skin complications. *American Journal of Nursing, 110*(2), 43–48.

Evans, M. M., Evans, M., Lashinski, K., et al. (2009). Clinical do's & don'ts. Assessing the abdomen. *Nursing, 39*(11), 12.

Fakih, M. G., Dueweke, C., Meisner, S., et al. (2008). Effect of nurse-led multidisciplinary rounds on reducing the unnecessary use of urinary catheterization in hospitalized patients. *Infection Control and Hospital Epidemiology, 29*(9), 815–819.

Falkinham, J. O. (2007). Growth in catheter biofilms and antibiotic resistance of *Mycobacterium avium. Journal of Medical Microbiology, 56,* 250–254.

Finerty, E. A. (2008). Did you say "measles"? *American Journal of Nursing, 108*(12), 27–29.

Fingeld-Connett, D. (2008). Qualitative convergence of three nursing concepts: Art of nursing, presence, and caring. *Journal of Advanced Nursing, 63*(5), 527–535.

Finke, E., Light, J., & Kitko, L. (2008). A systematic review of the effectiveness of nurse communication with patients with complex communication needs with a focus on the use of augmentative and alternative communication. *Journal of Clinical Nursing, 17*(16), 2102–2115.

Finn, D. R., & Malani, P. N. (2009). Infection control in long-term care facilities: The need for engagement. *Journal of the American Geriatrics Society, 57*(3), 569–570.

Fischbach, F., & Dunning, M. B. (2008). *A manual of laboratory and diagnostic tests* (8th ed.). Philadelphia: Lippincott Williams & Wilkins.

Fisher, M. (2007). Resuscitation guidelines—managing change in practice. *Pediatric Intensive Care Nursing, 8*(1), 7–10.

Flori, L. (2007). Healthier aging. Don't throw in the towel: Tips for bathing a patient who has dementia. *Nursing, 37*(7), 22–23.

Fok, M., Stewart, R., Besset, A., et al. (2010). Incidence and persistence of sleep complaints in a community older population. *International Journal of Geriatric Psychiatry, 25*(1), 37–45.

Forbes, D. A. (2007). An exercise programme led to a slower decline in activities of daily living in nursing home patients with Alzheimer's disease. *Evidence-Based Nursing, 10*(3), 89.

Fowler, M. D. M., & American Nurses Association. (2010). *Guide to the code of ethics for nurses: Interpretation and application.* Silver Spring, MD: American Nurses Association.

Fowler, S. B., Sohler, P., & Zarillo, D. F. (2009). Bar-code technology for medication administration; medication errors and nurse satisfaction. *MedSurg Nursing, 18*(2), 103–109.

Fragala, G., Haiduven, D., Lloyd, J. L., et al. (2005). *Patient care ergonomics resource guide: Safe patient handing and movement.* Accessed April 20, 2010, from http://www.visn8.va.gov/patientsafetycenter/resfuide/ErgoGuidePtOne.pdf

Franklin, M. (2006). Using patient safety science to explore strategies for improving safety in intravenous medication administration. *Journal of the Association for Vascular Access, 11*(3), 157–160.

Frazer, C. A., Frazer, R. Q., & Byron, R. J. Jr. (2009). Prevent infections with good denture care. *Nursing, 39*(8), 50–53.

Fuller, F., & North, G. (2009). All that vomits is not the flu: Identifying and managing nausea and vomiting. *EMS Magazine, 38*(11), 52–56.

Galloway, M. (2010). Insertion and placement of central catheters in the oncology patient. *Seminars in Oncology Nursing, 26*(2) 102–112.

Gaunt, M. J., Johnston, J., & Davis, M. M. (2007). Safety monitor. Automated dispensing cabinets. *American Journal of Nursing, 107*(8), 27–28.

Gebel, E. (2010). *Insulin pens.* Accessed August 18, 2010, from http://forecast.diabetes.org/magazine/features/insulin-pens

Gemender, J. M., & Reising, D. L. (2007). Investigating nurses' dressing change techniques: Nursing research sheds light on when and why nurses use sterile instead of clean technique. *American Nurse Today, 2*(4): 53–55.

Getting patients back on their feet. (2005). *LPN2005, 1*(5): 35–53.

Giger, J. N., & Davidhizar, R. E. (2008). *Transcultural nursing: Assessment and intervention* (5th ed.). St. Louis, MO: Elsevier.

Gile, T. J. (2009). *Fingernails, food, and beards.* Accessed January 14, 2010, from http://blogs.hcpro.com/osha/2009/01/fingernails-food-and-beards/

Gilroy, N., & Howard, P. K. (2008). Compliance with hand hygiene guidelines. *Advanced Emergency Nursing Journal, 30*(3), 193–200.

Ginsberg, D. A., Phillips, S. F., Wallace, J., et al. (2007). Evaluating and managing constipation in the elderly. *Urologic Nursing, 27*(3), 191–201, 212.

Glassman, P. (2008). *Health literacy.* Accessed December 31, 2009, from http://nnlm.gov/outreach/consumer/hlthlit.html

Gleeson, M., & Timmins, F. (2005). A review of the use and clinical effectiveness of touch as a nursing intervention. *Clinical Effectiveness in Nursing, 9*(1/2), 69–77.

Godbout, J. P., & Glaser, R. (2006). Stress-induced immune dysregulation: Implications for wound healing, infectious disease and cancer. *Journal of Neuroimmune Pharmacology, 1*(4), 421–427.

Goldmann, D. (2006). System failure versus personal accountability—the case for clean hands. *The New England Journal of Medicine, 355*(2), 121–123.

Goodman, P., Murdaugh. C. L., Moneyham, L. D., et al. (2007). Role of decision-making in women's self-diagnosis and management of vaginitis. *Women's Health Care: A Practical Journal for Nurse Practitioners, 6*(2): 57–64.

Gorski, L. A. (2009). The peripheral intravenous catheter: An appropriate yet often overlooked choice for venous access. *Home Healthcare Nurse, 27*(2), 130–132.

Gozdan, M. J. (2009). Using technology to reduce medication errors. *Nursing, 39*(6), 57–58.

Gracyk, T. (2008). *The principle of double effect.* Retrieved September, 2009, from http://www.mnstate.edu/gracyk/courses/phil%20115/doubleEffect.htm

Grant, B., & Colello, S. (2009). Patient safety. Engaging the patient in handoff communication at the bedside. *Nursing, 39*(10), 22, 24.

Griffith, R. (2009). Managing fire safety in care homes. *Nursing & Residential Care, 11*(5), 249, 251–253, 255.

Habel, M. (2005). *Getting your message across: Patient teaching.* Accessed December 22, 2009, from http://www.patienteducationupdate.com/2005-05-01/article6.asp

Hadaway, L. (2008). Targeting therapy with central venous access devices. *Nursing, 38*(6), 34–41.

Hadaway, L., & Hinkle, J. L. (2006). Pharmacology update. Practical considerations in administering intravenous medications. *Journal of Neuroscience Nursing, 38*(2), 119–124.

Hall, E. T. (1959). *The silent language.* New York: Fawcett.

Hall, E. T. (1963). A system for the notation of proxemic behavior. *American Anthropologist, 65*(3), 1003–1026.

Hall, E. T. (1966). *The hidden dimension.* New York: Doubleday.

Hall, J. M. (2007). *Hospice and palliative care; right patient, right time, right place.* Accessed September 17, 2010, from http://www.ce.nurse.com/CE312-60/Hospice-and-Palliative-Care-Right-Patient-Right-Time-Right-Place/

Hampton, S. (2007). Care of a colostomy. *Journal of Community Nursing, 21*(9), 20, 22, 24.

Hand Hygiene Resource Center. (2009). *Improving hand hygiene practices in healthcare settings.* Accessed January 14, 2010, from http://www.handhygiene.org

Hard to swallow: Understanding dysphagia. (2008). *Nursing, 38*(3), 44–45.

Harris, C. A. (2008). COPD: Help your patients breathe easier. *RN, 71*(1), 21–27.

Harris, T. A. (2010). Inspiring change. Changing practice to reduce the use of urinary catheters. *Nursing, 40*(2), 18–20.

Hartmann, M., & McManus, J. G. (2005). *Crutches.* Accessed May 18, 2010, from http://www.emedicinehealth.com/crutches/article_em.htm

Harvard Medical School, Division of Sleep Medicine. (2007). *Changes in sleep with age.* Accessed March 10, 2010, from http://healthysleep.med.harvard.edu/healthy/sciene/variations/changes-in-sleep-with-age

Health Resources and Services Administration, & U.S. Department of Health and Human Services. (2005). *Nursing education in five states: 2005.* Accessed September, 2009, from http://bhpr.hrsa.gov/healthworkforce/reports/nurseed/intro.htm

Heenan, A. (2007). Alginates: An effective primary dressing for exuding wounds. *Nursing Standard, 22*(7): 53–54, 56, 58+.

Heisler, J. (2009). *Understanding and dealing with a fear of surgery.* Accessed May 26, 2010 http://surgery.about.com/od/ingandsurgery/ss/SurgeryAnxiety.htm

Hess, C. T. (2003). Wound and skin care. Managing a diabetic ulcer. *Nursing, 33*(7), 82–83.

Higgins, D. (2005). Oxygen therapy. *Nursing Times, 101*(4), 30–31.

Higgins, D. (2006). Removal of chest drains. *Nursing Times, 102*(13), 26–27.

Holer, S. E. (2004). Tips for better patient teaching. *Nursing, 34*(7), 32hn7–32hn8.

Holmes, T. H., & Rahe, R. H. (1967). The social readjustment rating scale. *Journal of Psychosomatic Research, 11*(8), 216.

Holzhauer, J. K., Reith, V., Sawin, K. J., et al. (2009). Evaluation of temporal artery thermometry in children 3–36 months old. *Journal of Specialists in Pediatric Nursing, 14*(4), 239–244.

Hoskins, A. B. (2006). *Occupational injuries, illnesses, and fatalities among nursing, psychiatric, and home health aides*, 1995–2004. Accessed April 21, 2010, from http://www.bls.gov/opub/cwc/sh20060628ar01pl.htm

Howard, A., Mercer, P., Nataraj, H. C., et al. (1997). Bevel-down superior to bevel-up in intradermal skin testing. *Annals of Allergy, Asthma, & Immunology, 78*(6), 594–596.

Howlett, M. S., Alexander, G. A., & Tsuchiya, B. (2010). Health care providers' attitudes regarding family presence during resuscitation of adults: An integrated review of the literature. *Clinical Nurse Specialist: The Journal for Advanced Nursing Practice, 24*(3), 161–174.

Huckabay, L. M. (2009). Clinical reasoned judgment and the nursing process. *Nursing Forum, 44*(2), 72–78.

Hughes, C. M., & Goldie, R. (2009). "I just take what I am given": Adherence and resident involvement in decision making on medicines in nursing homes for older people. *Drugs & Aging, 26*(6), 505–517.

Hughes, R. G., & Clancy, C. M. (2009). AHQR commentary. Nurses' role in patient safety. *Journal of Nursing Care Quality, 24*(1), 1–4.

Hunt, C. W., & King, J. E. (2008). Clinical queries. Which site is best for an I.M. injection? *Nursing, 38*(11), 62.

Hunter, S., Thompson, P., Langemo, D., et al. (2007). Wound & skin care. Understanding wound Dehiscence. *Nursing, 37*(9), 28, 30.

Huntley, A. (2009). Action stat. Transfusion reaction. *Nursing, 39*(1), 72.

In the know: New JCAHO documentation guidelines required nationwide. (2004). *Nursing, 34*(2) Travel Supplement, 2.

Irazusta, A., Gil, S. Ruiz, F., et al. (2006). Exercise, physical fitness, and dietary habits of first-year female nursing students. *Biological Research for Nursing, 7*(3), 175–186.

Ironside, P. M., Jeffries, P. R., & Martin, A. (2009). Fostering patient safety competencies using multiple-patient simulation experiences. *Nursing Outlook, 57*(6), 332–337.

Jevon, P. (2006a). Resuscitation skills—part one: The recovery position. *Nursing Times, 102*(25), 28–29.

Jevon, P. (2006b). Resuscitation skills—part two: Clearing the airway. *Nursing Times, 102*(26), 26–27.

Jevon, P. (2007). Respiratory procedures: Part 1—use of a non-rebreathing oxygen mask. *Nursing Times, 103*(32), 26–27.

Joanna Briggs Institute. (2007). *Preoperative hair removal to reduce surgical site infection*. Accessed May 24, 2010, from http://www.joannabriggs.edu/au/pdf/BPISEng_11_4.pdf

Johnson, K., Long, L. E., Tierney, C., et al. (2007). Evidence-based practice project: Subcutaneous aspiration. *Journal of Pediatric Nursing, 22*(2), 145.

Johnson, L. R., Barret, K. E., Gishan, F. K., et al. (2006). *Physiology of the gastrointestinal tract*. Miamisburg, OH: Reed Elsevier.

Johnson, M., & Martinson, M. (2007). *Efficacy of electrical nerve stimulation for chronic musculoskeletal pain: A meta-analysis of randomized controlled trials*. Accessed March 25, 2010, from http://www.globuscorporation.com/sciref/Efficacy%20of%20electrical%20nerve%20stimulation%20for%20chronic%20muscluloskeltal%20pain.pdf

The Joint Commission. (2009). *Measuring hand hygiene adherence: Overcoming the challenges*. Accessed January 15, 2010, from http://jointcommission.org/NR/donlyres/68B9CB2FB387666BCC/0/hh_monograph.pdf

The Joint Commission. (2010a). *2010 National Patient Safety Goals (NPDGs)*. Accessed August 2, 2010, from http://www.jointcommission.org/patientsafety/nationalpatientsafetygoals/

The Joint Commission. (2010b). *Official "Do Not Use" list of abbreviations*. Accessed August 2, 2010, from http://www.jointcommission.org/PatientSafety/DoNotUseList/

The Joint Commission. (2010c). *Updated universal protocol for preventing wrong site, wrong procedure, wrong person surgery*. Accessed May 26, 2010, from http://www.jointcommission.org/patientsafety/universalprotocol

Joint Commission on Accreditation of Healthcare Organizations. (2009). *Restraint/seclusion for hospitals that use the Joint Commission for deemed status purposes*. Accessed March 17, 2010, from http://www.jointcommission.org/AccreditationPrograms/Hospitals/Standards/09_FAQs/PC/Restraint+Seclusion+For+Hospitals+That+Use+The+Joint+Commission+For+Deemed+Status+Purposes.htm

Joint Commission on Accreditation of Healthcare Organizations. (2010). *Comprehensive accreditation for hospitals. The official handbook*. Oak Terrace, IL: Author.

Jones, L. (2009). The healing relationship. *Nursing Standard, 24*(3), 64.

Jones, M. L. (2008). Assessing and managing wound pain during dressing changes. *Nursing & Residential Care, 10*(7), 325, 327, 329–330.

Jordan, K., & Liu, H. (2009). Assessment of canes used by older people in senior living communities. *Clinical Nurse Specialist: The Journal for Advanced Nursing Practice, 23*(2), 95.

Josey, K. (2009). *How to make a nursing patient teaching plan*. Accessed December 28, 2009, from http://www.ehow.com/how_4587946_nursing-patient-teaching-plan.html

Joy, J. (2009). Patient safety first. Nurses: The patient's first-and perhaps last-line of defense. *Association of periOperative Nurses (AORN) Journal, 89*(6), 1133–1136.

Juvé Udina, M., Vallis-Miró, C., Carreño, et al. (2009). To return or to discard? Randomized trial on gastric residual volume management. *Intensive & Critical Care Nursing, 25*(5), 258–267.

Kaiser Family Foundation. (2009). *The medicare prescription drug benefit*. Accessed September 2009, from http://www.kff.org/medicare/#7044.09.cfm

Kayser-Jones, J. (2006). Preventable causes of dehydration: Nursing home residents are especially vulnerable. *American Journal of Nursing, 106*(6), 45.

Kelly, B. M., & Pangilinan, P. H. (2009). *Lower limb prosthetics*. Accessed May18, 2010, from http://www.emedicine.medscape.com/article/317358-overview

Kelly, C., & Riches, A. (2007). Respiratory nursing. Emergency oxygen for respiratory patients. *Nursing Times, 103*(45), 40–42.

Kelly, G. S. (1999). Nutritional and botanical interventions to assist with the adaptation. *Alternative Medicine Review: A Journal of Chemical Therapeutics, 4*(4), 249–265.

Kiss, P., De Meester, M., & Braeckman, L. (2008). Needlestick injuries in nursing homes: The prominent role of insulin pens. *Infection Control and Hospital Epidemiology, 29*(12), 1192–1194.

Kleiman, S., Frederickson, K., & Lundy, T. (2004). Using an eclectic model to educate students about cultural influences on the nurse–patient relationship. *Nursing Education Perspectives, 25*(5), 249–253.

Kohn, J. (2009). *Injection insulin—aspirate?* Accessed August 19, 2010, from http://www.myfreestyle.com/fs/d/en_US50.90:90/injection-insulin—aspirate

Kovach, T. (2003). *Choosing an alcohol hand sanitizer; expand hand wash compliance by breaking the chain of infection*. Accessed January 12, 2010, from http://www.infectioncontroltoday.com/articles/361feat4.html

Kraman, P. (2004). *Prescription drug diversion*. Accessed August 2, 2010, from http://www.csg.org/knowledgecenter/docs/TA0404DrugDiversion.pdf

Kübler-Ross, E. (1969). *On death and dying*. New York: Macmillan.

Kutner, M., Greenberg, E., Jin, Y., et al. (2006). *The Health Literacy of America's Adults: Results from the 2003 National Assessment of Adult Literacy (NCES 2006-483).*Washington, DC: National Center for Education Statistics, U.S. Department of Education.

Kyle, G. (2007). Bowel care: Part 1—Assessment of constipation. *Nursing Times, 103*(42), 26–27.

Laakso, K., Hartelius, L., & Idvall, M. (2009). Ventilator-supported communication: A case study of patient and staff experiences. *Journal of Medical Speech-Language Pathology, 17*(4), 153–164.

LaDuke, S. (2009). Playing it safe with bar code medication administration. *Nursing, 39*(5), 32–34.

Lambert, C. (2005). *Deep into sleep*. Accessed March 11, 2010, from http://harvardmagazine.com/2005/07/deep-into-sleep.html

Langham, G. E., Maheshwari, A., Contrera, K., et al. (2009). Noninvasive temperature monitoring in postanesthesia care units. *Anesthesiology, 111*(1), 90–96.

Larson, J. (2008). *Are LPN jobs moving outside the hospital?* Accessed September, 2009, from http://www.nursezone.com/nursing-news-events/more-news/Are-LPN-Jobs-Moving-Outside-the-Hospital_26658.aspx

Lattanzi-Licht, M., Mahoney, J., & Miller, G. (1998). *The hospice choice: In pursuit of a peaceful death.* New York: Simon & Schuster.

Laubach, G. (2010). Speaking up for older patients with hearing loss. *Nursing, 40*(1), 60–62.

Leach, M. J. (2008). Planning: A necessary step in clinical care. *Journal of Clinical Nursing, 17*(13), 1728–1734.

Learning retention pyramid (myth). (2009). Accessed December 29, 2009, from http://www.rememberanything.com/learning-retention-pyramid-myth/

Lessons from a guru: How relevant is Florence Nightingale's Notes on Nursing today? (2009). *Nursing Standard, 23*(19), 20–23.

Letvak, S., & Buck, R. (2008). Factors influencing work productivity and intent to stay in nursing. *Nursing Economics, 26*(3), 159–165.

Levy, J. H. (2010). *Blood substitutes: Hemoglobin-based oxygen carriers*. Accessed February 22, 2010, from http://www.asiaing.com/blood-substitutes-hemoglobin-based-oxygen-carriers.html

Lewthwaite, B. J. (2009). What do nurses know about postoperative nausea and vomiting? *MedSurg Nursing, 18*(2), 110–113.

Leyshon, J. (2007). Correct technique for using aerosol inhaler devices. *Nursing Standard, 21*(52), 38–40.

Link, M. S., Atkins, D. L., Passman, R. S., et al. (2010). *Part 6: CPR overview: 2010 American Heart Association Guidelines for Cardiopulmonary Resuscitation and Emergency Cardiovascular Care*. Accessed October 21, 2010, from http://circ.ahajournals.org/cgi/content/full/122/18_suppl_3/S706

Lippincott's Visual Encyclopedia of Clinical Skills. (2009). Philadelphia: Lippincott Williams & Wilkins.

Lipson, J. G., & Dibble, S. L. (2005). *Culture and clinical care.* San Francisco: UCSF Nursing Press.

Lomas, C. (2008). Falls risk reduction by boosting fluid intake. *Nursing Times, 104*(26), 9.

Lopez, R. P. (2009). Decision-making for acutely ill nursing home residents: Nurses in the middle. *Journal of Advanced Nursing, 65*(5), 1001–1009.

Lorentz, M. (2008). TELENURSING and home healthcare: The many facets of technology. *Home Healthcare Nurse: The Journal for the Home Care and Hospice Professional, 26*(4), 237–243.

Love, G. H. (2006). Clinical do's & don'ts. Administering an intradermal injection. *Nursing, 36*(6), 20.

Ludeman, K. (2007). Choosing the right vascular access device. *Nursing, 37*(9), 38–41.

Ludeman, K. (2008). I.V. essentials: Which vascular access device is right for your patient? *Nursing Made Incredibly Easy, 6*(4), 7, 9–11.

MacKeracher, D. (2004). *Making sense of adult learning* (2nd ed.). Toronto, ON: University of Toronto Press.

Malkin, B. (2009). The importance of patients' oral health and nurses' role in assessing and maintaining it. *Nursing Times, 105*(17), 19–23.

Malkin, B., & Berridge, P. (2009). Guidance on maintaining personal hygiene in nail care. *Nursing Standard, 23*(41), 35–38.

Marable, K., Shafer, L. E. T., Dizon, V., et al. (2009). Temporal artery scanning falls short as a secondary, noninvasive thermometry method for trauma patients. *Journal of Trauma Nursing, 16*(1), 41–47.

Mathes, M. (2004). Ethical decision making and nursing. *MedSurg Nursing, 13*(6), 429–431.

Mathes, M. (2005). Ethical decision making and nursing. *Dermatology Nursing, 17*(6), 444–447.

Mathus-Vliegen, E., Duflou, A., Spanier, M., et al. (2010). Nasoenteral feeding tube placement by nurses using an electromagnetic guidance system (with video). *Gastrointestinal Endoscopy, 71*(4), 728–736.

Mauk, K. L. (2005). Healthier aging: Caring for older adults. Keeping an older adult on her toes. *Nursing, 35*(1), 24.

Mayo Clinic Staff. (2009). *Slide show: How to choose and use a walker*. Accessed May 18, 2010, from http://www.mayoclinic.com/health/walker/HA00060

Mayo Clinic. (2009a). *Alzheimer's disease*. Accessed September 2009, from http://discoverysedge.mayo.edu/alzheimers_disease/index.cfm

Mayo Clinic. (2009b). *Belly fat in men. Why weight loss matters.* Accessed February 16, 2010, from http://www.mayoclinic.com/health/belly-fat/MC00054

Mayo Clinic. (2009c). *How you feel pain*. Accessed March 22, 2010, from http://www.mayoclinic.com/health/pain/pn0017

Mayo Clinic. (2009d). *Hyperbaric oxygen therapy*. Accessed April 1, 2010, from http://www.mayoclinic.com/health/hyperbaric-oxygen-therapy/MY00829

McAleer, M. (2006). Communicating effectively with deaf patients. *Nursing Standard, 20*(19), 51–54.

McCaffery, M. (1968). *Nursing practice theories related to cognition, bodily pain and main environment interactions*. Los Angeles: University of California, Los Angeles

McCaffery, M. (1997). Pain management handbook. *Nursing, 27*(4), 42–45.

McCaffery, M. (1999). Controlling pain. Understanding your patient's pain tolerance. *Nursing, 29*(12), 17.

McCaffery, M., & Beebe, A. (1999). *Pain clinical manual for nursing practice.* St. Louis, MO: Mosby.

McCaffery, M., & Ferrell, B. F. (1999). Opioids and pain management: What do nurses know? *Nursing, 29*(3), 48–52.

McCaffery, M., & Pasero, C. (1999). *Pain: Clinical manual* (2nd ed.). St. Louis, MO: Mosby.

McCaffery, M., Ferrell, B., O'Neill-Page, E., et al. (1990). Nurses' knowledge of opioid analgesic drugs and psychological dependence. *Cancer Nursing, 13*(1), 21–27.

McCoskey, K. L. (2007). Ergonomics and patient handling. *American Association of Occupational Health Nurses Journal, 55*(11), 454–462.

McGraw, C., & Drennan, V. (2009). Assisting older people with bathing. *Journal of Community Nursing, 23*(9), 12, 15–16.

McIntosh, A. E., & MacMillan, M. (2009). The attitudes of student and registered nurses to sleep promotion in hospitals. *International Journal of Nursing Practice, 15*(6), 560–565.

MD Anderson Cancer Center. (2009). *Botulinum toxin for the treatment of chronic pain syndromes*. Accessed March 24, 2010, from http://www.mdanderson.org/transcripts/botulinum-toxin-transcript.html

Medical News Today. (2007, December 3). New study finds temporal artery thermometers superior. Accessed January 25, 2010, from http://www.medicalnewstoday.com/articles/90410.php

Mentes, J. (2006). Oral hydration in older adults: Greater awareness is needed in preventing, recognizing, and treating dehydration. *American Journal of Nursing, 106*(6), 40–49.

Mercer, S. E. (2008). Practice corner. Role of the LPN in blood administration. *KBN Connection (Kentucky Board of Nursing), Fall*(17), 18.

Merrel, P., & Fisher, C. (2007). Fine-turning your feeding-tube insertion skills: What every nurse should know to make feeding-tube insertion safer. *American Nurse Today, 2*(8), 33–35.

Metules, T. J., & Bauer, J. (2007). Part 2. JCAHO's patient safety goals: Preventing med errors. *RN, 70*(1), 39–44.

Miller, C. A. (2011). *Nursing for wellness in older adults* (6th ed.). Philadelphia: Lippincott Williams & Wilkins.

Mitchell, P. R., & Grippando, G. M. (1993). *Nursing perspectives and issues* (5th ed.). New York: Delmar.

Moffitt, B. (2009). Untying the patient: Nurses following a vision of restraint-free/safe care. *Clinical Nurse Specialist: The Journal for Advanced Nursing Practice, 23*(2), 110–111.

Monitoring your adult patient with bedside pulse oximetry. (2008). *Nursing, 38*(9), 42–44.

Monturo, C., & Hook, K. (2009). From means to ends: Artificial nutrition and hydration. *Nursing Clinics of North America, 44*(4), 505–515.

Moore, E. E., Moore, F. A., & Fabian, T. C. (2009). Human polymerized hemoglobin for the treatment of hemorrhagic shock when blood is unavailable: The USA multicenter trial. *Journal of the American College of Surgeons, 208*(1), 1–13.

Morley, J. E. (2007). Weight loss in the nursing home. *Journal of the American Medical Directors Association, 8*(4), 201–204.

Moses, S. (2009). *Saline gauze dressing*. Accessed June 2, 2010, from http://www.fpnotebook.com/Surgery/Pharm/SlnGzDrsng.htm

Mottram, A. (2009). Therapeutic relationships in day surgery: A grounded theory study. *Journal of Clinical Nursing, 18*(20) 2830–2837.

Mundy, C. A. (2007). Innovative teaching strategies: Educating student nurses on vascular access management. *Journal of the Association for Vascular Access, 12*(4), 232–239.

Nadzam, D. M. (2009). Nurses' role in communication and patient safety. *Journal of Nursing Care Quality, 24*(3), 184–188.

Nakazawa, N. (2010). Infectious and thrombotic complications of central venous catheters. *Seminars in Oncology Nursing, 26*(2), 121–131.

NANDA International. (2012). *Nursing diagnoses: Definitions and classification*, 2012–2014. Oxford: Wiley-Blackwell.

National Cancer Institute. (2008). *Substance abuse issues in cancer. Risk of abuse and addiction in populations without drug abuse histories*. Accessed September 19, 2010, from http://www.cancer.gov/cancertopics/pdq/supportivecare/substanceabuse/HealthProfessional/page4/print

National Cancer Institute. (2009). *Pap test*. Accessed February 11, 2010, from http://www.cncer.gov/cancertopics/factsheet/Detection/Pap-test

National Cancer Institute. (2010). *Understanding cervical changes: A health guide for women*. Accessed February 11, 2010, from http://www.cancer.gov/cancertopcs/understandingcervical-changes

National Center for Complementary and Alternative Medicine. (2009). *Acupuncture for pain*. Accessed March 25, 2010, from http://ncam.nih.gov/health/acupuncture/acupuncture-for-pain.htm

National Council of State Boards of Nursing (2008). *NCLEX-PN Detailed Test Plan*. Accessed September, 2009, from http://www.ncsbn.org/2008_PN_Test_Plan_Web.pdf

National Council of State Boards of Nursing. (2005a). *Practical nurse scope of practice white paper*. Accessed September, 2009, from http://www.ncsbn.org/pdfs/Final_11_05_Practical_Nurse_Scope_Practice_White_Paper.pdf

National Council of State Boards of Nursing. (2005b). *Working with others: A position paper*. Accessed September, 2009, from http://www.ncsbn.org/Working_with_Others.pdf

National Council of State Boards of Nursing. (2005c). *Nursing regulation and the interpretation of nursing scopes of practice*. Retrieved September, 2009, from http://www.ncsbn.org/NursingReganandInterpretationofSop.pdf

National Council of State Boards of Nursing. (2009). *Quarterly examination statistics*. Accessed September 2009, from http://www.ncsbn.org/NCLEX_Stats_2008_Q4.pdf

National Heart, Lung, and Blood Institute. (2002). *Working meeting on blood pressure measurement*. Accessed January 27, 2010, from http://www.nhlbi.nih.gov/health/prof/heart/hbp/bpmeasu.htm

National Heart, Lung, and Blood Institute. (2004). *The seventh report of the Joint National Committee on Prevention, Detection, Evaluation, and Treatment of High Blood Pressure*. Accessed January 28, 2010, from http://www.nhlbi.nih.gov/guidelines/hypertension/jnc7full.htm

National Heart, Lung, and Blood Institute. (2006). *Your guide to lowering your blood pressure with DASH*. Accessed January 29, 2010, from http://www.nhlbi.nih.gov/health/public/heart/hbp/dash/new_dash.pdf

National Heart, Lung, Blood Institute. (2000). *The practical guide: Identification, evaluation, and treatment of overweight and obesity in adults*. Accessed February 16, 2010, from http://www.nhlbi.nih.gov/guidelines/obesity/prctgde.htm

National Institute for Occupational Safety and Health. (2008). *Respirators: Your TB defense*. Accessed January 14, 2010, from http://www.cdc.gov/niosh/docs/video/tb.html

National Institute for Occupational Safety and Health. (2009). *Overview of state needle safety legislation*. Accessed August 18, 2010, from http://www.cdc.gov/niosh/topics/bbp/ndl-law.html

National Institute of Allergy and Infectious Diseases. (2009). *Genes key to staph disease severity, drug resistance found hitchhiking together*. Accessed January 11, 2009, from http://www3.niaid.nih.gov/newsreleases/2009/staphgenes.htm

National Institute of Child Health and Human Development. (2006). *Questions and answers for professionals on infant sleeping position and SIDS*. Accessed April 21, 2010, from http://www.nichd.nih.gov/sids/sids_qa.cfm

National Institute of Diabetes and Digestive and Kidney Diseases. (2005). *Urinary tract infections in adults*. Accessed June 28, 2010, from http://kidney.niddk.nih.gov/kudiseases/pubs/utiadult/

National Institute of Neurological Disorders and Stroke. (2007). *Brain basics: Understanding sleep*. Retrieved June, 2007, from http://www.ninds.nih.gov/disorders/brain-basics/understanding_sleep.htm

National Institutes of Health. (2002). *National high blood pressure education program (NHBPEP)/National Heart, Lung, and Blood Institute (NHLBI) and American Heart Association (AHA), Working meeting on blood pressure measurement, Summary report*. Accessed January 28, 2010, from http://www.nhlbi.nih.gov/health/prof/heart/hbp/bpmeasu.pdf

National Institutes of Health. (2008). *Understanding adult obesity*. Accessed February 16, 2010, from http://win.niddk.nih.gov/publications/understanding.htm

National League for Nursing. (2008). *Nursing education research; Annual survey of schools of nursing academic year 2006–2007: Executive summary*. Accessed September, 2009, from http://www.nln.org/research/slides/index.htm

National Pressure Ulcer Advisory Panel. (2007). *Pressure ulcer stages revised by NPUAP*. Accessed June 4, 2010, from http://www.npuap.or/pr2.htm

National Sleep Foundation. (2009a). *2009 health and safety*. Accessed March 12, 2010, from http://www.sleepfoundation.org/article/sleep-america-polls/2009-health-and-safety

National Sleep Foundation. (2009b). *Aging and sleep—poll data*. Accessed March 9, 2010, from http://www.sleepfoundation.org/article/topics/aging-and-sleep-poll-data

Nazarko, L. (2007a). Assessing fluid intake. *Nursing Times, 103* (28), 10.

Nazarko, L. (2007b). Infection control: Policies and practice. *Nursing & Residential Care, 9*(8), 355–356, 358.

Neal-Boylan, L. (2007). Health assessment of the very old person at home. *Home Healthcare Nurse, 25*(6), 388–400.

Nelson, A. Baptiste, A. S. (2006). Update on evidence-based practices for safe patient handling and movement. *Orthopaedic Nursing, 25*(6), 367–368.

Nelson, R. (2009). Nursing shortage, or not? It comes down to location, location, location. *American Journal of Nursing, 109*(5), 21–24.

Newman, D. K. (2008). Internal and external urinary catheters: A primer for clinical practice. *Ostomy Wound Management, 54*(12), 18–20, 22–26, 28–35.

Nicholl, L. H. (2002). Heat in motion: Evaluating and managing temperature. *Nursing, 32*(5), Suppl, 1–12.

Nijs, K., deGraaf, C., van Staveren, W. A., et al. (2009). Malnutrition and mealtime ambiance in nursing homes. *Journal of the American Medical Directors Association, 10*(4), 226–229.

Norris, B. (2009). Human factors and safe patient care. *Journal of Nursing Management, 17*(2), 203–211.

Nuernberger, P. (1981). *Freedom from stress.* Honesdale, PA: The Himalayan International Institute of Yoga Science and Philosophy.

Nurses Quick Check: Skills (2005). Ambler, PA: Springhouse.

Nursing shortage expected to worsen through 2016. *RN, 72*(2), 15.

Odom-Forren, J. (2006). Preventing surgical site infections. *Nursing, 36*(6), 59–64.

Office of Disease Prevention and Health Promotion. (2009). *Healthy people 2020: The road ahead.* Accessed September, 2009, from http://healthypeople.gov/HP2020

Office of Management and Budget. (1997). *Revisions to the standards for classification of federal data on race and ethnicity.* Accessed November, 2009, from http://www.whitehouse.gov/omb/fedreg_1997standards/

Ogg, M. (2009). Clinical issues. Perioperative care of patients using transdermal medication patches. *Association of periOperative Registered Nurses (AORN) Journal, 90*(5), 756, 758–759.

Olsen, D. P. (2006). Ethical issues. Should RNs be forced to get the flu vaccine? Some facilities are mandating it, in an effort to protect patients. *American Journal of Nursing, 106*(10), 76–78.

Oncology Nursing Society. (2007). *The impact of the national nursing shortage on quality cancer care*. Accessed September, 2009, from http://www.ons.org/publications/positions/Nursing Shortage.shtml

Paragas, J. (2008). Keeping the beat with pulse oximetry. *Nursing, 38*(11), 56hn1–56hn2.

Paul-Cheadle, D. (2003). *A guide to hand-hygiene agents*. Retrieved June 18, 2003, from http://www.infectioncontroltoday.com/articles/361feat3.html

Payne, K. (2009). Ethics column: Working through an ethical dilemma. *Tennessee Nurse, 72*(2): 1–2.

Pelletier, K. M. (1977). *Mind as healer, mind as slayer*. New York: Delacorte and Delta.

Pelletier, K. M. (1995). *Sound mind–sound body: A new model for life-long health*. New York: Simon & Schuster.

Perkins, J., Youdelman, M., & Wong, D. (2003). *Ensuring linguistic access in health care settings: Legal rights and responsibilities.* Washington, DC: National Health Law Program.

Perry, J., Galloway, S., Bottorff, J., et al. (2005). Nurse–patient communication in dementia: Improving the odds. *Journal of Gerontological Nursing, 31*(4), 43–52.

Petechuk, D. (2006). *Organ transplantation*. Santa Barbara: Greenwood Publishing Group.

Pfeidler Enterprises. (2009). *Preoperative hair removal: Impact on surgical site infections*. Accessed May 24, 2010, from http://www.pfiedlerenterprises.com/1091/1091.pdf

Phaneuf, M. (2007). *Teaching in caregiving*. Accessed December 28, 2009, from http://www.infiressources.ca/fer/Depotdocument_anglais/Teaching-in-caregiving.pdf

Pickering, T. G., Hall, J. E., Appel, L. J., et al. (2005). *Recommendations for blood pressure measurement in humans and experimental animals. Part 1: Blood pressure measurement in humans: A statement for professions from the Subcommittee of professionals from the American Heart Association Council on High Blood Pressure Research.* Accessed January 28, 2010, from http://www.guideline.gov/summary/summary.aspx?ss=15&doc_id=6527&nbr=4093

Pilch, J. (1981). *Your invitation to full life.* Minneapolis, MN: Winston Press.

Pipe, T. B. (2007). Optimizing nursing care by integrating theory-driven evidence-based practice. *Journal of Nursing Care Quality, 22*(3), 234.

Pompei, F., & Pompei, M. (2004). *Non-invasive temporal artery thermometry: Physics, physiology, and clinical accuracy.* Accessed January 28, 2010, from http://www.exergen.com/medical/PDFs/Pompei_and_Pompei_SPIE%20paper_2.pdf

Porth, C. M., & Matfin, G. (2008). *Pathophysiology: Concepts of altered health states* (8th ed.). Philadelphia: Lippincott Williams & Wilkins.

Porth, C. M., & Matfin, G. (2011). *Essentials of pathophysiology: Concepts of altered health states* (3rd ed.). Philadelphia: Lippincott Williams & Wilkins.

Potera, C. (2009a). Infection control: Whose job is it? *American Journal of Nursing, 109*(4), 15.

Potera, C. (2009b). The nursing shortage: Bad news, good news. *American Journal of Nursing 109*(1), 22.

Pownall, M. (2007). Nurses' role in switching asthma patients to CFC-free inhalers. *Primary Health Care, 17*(2), 37–38.

Prahlow, J. A., Prahlow, T. J., Rakow, R. J., et al. (2009). Case study: Asphyxia caused by inspissated oral and nasopharyngeal secretions: One case shows the tragedy that can occur when oral care is neglected. *American Journal of Nursing, 109*(6), 38–43.

Pullen, R. L. Jr. (2007). Assessing skin lesions: Learn to identify the different types and document their characteristics. *Nursing, 37*(8), 44–45.

Pytel, C., Fielden, N. M., Meyer, K. H., et al. (2009). Nurse-patient/visitor communication in the emergency department. *Journal of Emergency Nursing, 35*(5), 406–411.

Rader, J., Barrick, A. L., Hoeffer, B., et al. (2006). The bathing of older adults with dementia: Easing the unnecessarily unpleasant aspects of assisted bathing. *American Journal of Nursing, 106*(4), 40–49.

Radwan, C. M. (2009). Clinical highlights. Brushing patients' teeth lowers risk of pneumonia. *RN, 72*(3), 19.

Regan, E. N., & Dallachiesa, L. (2009). How to care for a patient with a tracheostomy. *Nursing, 39*(8), 34–40.

Reuters News Service. (2005). *US death rates decline in four of six causes: Study*. Accessed September, 2009, from http://www.health-news.org/breaking/3413/us-death-rates-decline-in-four-of-six-causes-study.htm

Richardson, A., Crow, W., Coghill, E., et al. (2007). A comparison of sleep assessment tools by nurses and patients in critical care. *Journal of Clinical Nursing, 16*(9), 1660–1668.

Roan, S. (2005). *A new theory on a painful problem.* Accessed March 22, 2010, from http://www.azcentral.com/health/women/articles/0825fibromain-on.html

Roat, C. (2005). *Addressing language access issues in your practice: A toolkit for physicians and their staff.* San Francisco: California Academy of Family Physicians.

Roman, M., & Mercado, D. (2006). Clinical "how to". Review of chest tube use. *MedSurg Nursing, 15*(1), 41–43.

Roman, M., Thimothee, S., & Vidal, J. E. (2008). Arterial blood gases. *MedSurg Nursing, 17*(4), 268–269.

Rosenthal, K. (2007). Avoiding common perils of drug administration. *Nursing, 37*(4), 20–21.

Ross, H., & Lockhart, J. (2007). Keeping practical orthopaedic nursing skills alive: Developing a photographic traction guide. *Journal of Orthopaedic Nursing, 11*(1), 38–42.

Rowley, J. A. (2009). *Obstructive sleep apnea–hypopnea syndrome.* Accessed March 12, 2010, from http://emedicine.medscape.com/article/302773-overview

Rushing, J. (2004). Clinical do's and don'ts. How to administer a subcutaneous injection. *Nursing, 34*(6), 32.

Rushing, J. (2005). Protect your patient during abdominal paracentesis. *Nursing, 35*(8), 14.

Rushing, J. (2007a). Assisting with lumbar puncture. *Nursing, 37*(1), 23.

Rushing, J. (2007b). Obtaining a throat culture. *Nursing, 37*(2), 20.

Rushing, J. (2008). Clinical do's & don'ts. Administering an enoxaparin injection. *Nursing, 38*(3), 19.

Rushing, J. (2009a). Clinical do's & don'ts. Visual screening for scoliosis. *Nursing, 35*(5), 13.

Rushing, J. (2009b). Wrapping an ankle with an elastic compression bandage. *Nursing, 39*(12), 12.

Rushing, J., & Pullen, R. L. Jr. (2009). Clinical do's & don'ts. Assessing for dehydration in adults. *Nursing, 38*(4), 14.

Russo, C. A., & Elixhauser, A. (2006). *Statistical brief #6; hospitalizations in the elderly population, 2003.* Accessed January 20, 2010, from http://www.hcup-us.ahrq.gov/reports/statbriefs/sb6.jsp

Rutola, W. A., & Weber, D. J. (2001). *New disinfection and sterilization methods.* Accessed January 15, 2010, from http://www.cdc.gov.ncidod/eid/vol7no2/rutola.htm

Sabol, V. K., & Carlson, K. K. (2007). Diarrhea: Applying research to bedside practice. *AACN Advanced Critical Care, 18*(1), 32–44.

Sakakeenya-Zaal, K., & Zimmerman, P. G. (2007). Emergency pediatric orthopnea and total airway obstruction. *American Journal of Nursing, 107*(4), 40–43.

Salati, D. S. (2006). Photo guide: Responding to foreign-body airway obstruction. *Nursing, 36*(12), 50–51.

Samuels, T. M. (2009). *What is the proper way to give insulin shots?* Accessed August 18, 2010, from http://www.ehow.com/way_5719066-proper-way-give-insulin-shots-.html

Sandler, M. (2007). What the doctor ordered: Nurses have a key role to play in infection control. *Nursing Times, 103*(44), 13.

Scarpaci, L. T., Tsoukleris, M. G., & McPherson, M. L. (2007). Assessment of hospice nurses' technique in use of inhalers and nebulizers. *Journal of Palliative Medicine, 10*(3), 665–676.

Schaffer, E. (2007). *Preparing to use a prosthesis.* Accessed May 18, 2010, from http://www.merck.com/mmje/sec25/ch30788/ch30788c.html

Schaffer, E. (2007). *Prosthetic parts and options.* Accessed May 18, 2010, from http://www.merck.com/mmje/sec25/ch30788/ch30788b.html

Schiammarella, J., & Stoppler, M. C. (2007). *Automated external defibrillators.* Accessed October 21, 2010, from http://www.emedicinehealth.com/automated_external_defibrillators _aed/page7_em.htm

Schlenker, E., & Long, S. (2007). *Williams' essentials of nutrition and diet therapy* (9th ed.). St. Louis, MO: Elsevier Health Sciences.

Scroggins, L. M. (2008). The developmental processes for NANDA International Nursing Diagnoses. *International Journal of Nursing Terminologies and Classifications, 19*(2), 57–64.

Self-test. Physical exam challenges. (2005a). *Nursing, 35*(5), 73–75.

Self-test. Physical exam challenges, part 2. (2005b). *Nursing, 35*(6), 70–71.

Selye, H. (1956). *The stress of life.* New York: McGraw-Hill.

SerVaas, C. (2005). Clean your keyboard and wash your hands. *Medical Update, 31*(1), 51.

Servodidio, C., & Steed, M. (2007). *End-of-life issues.* Accessed September 17, 2010, from http://ce.nurse.com/ce257-60/EndofLife-Issues/

Sharpe, C. C. (2000). *Telenursing, nursing in cyberspace.* Santa Barbara: Greenwood Publishing Group.

Sheldon, L. K., Barrett, R., & Ellington, L. (2006). Difficult communication in nursing. *Journal of Nursing Scholarship, 38*(2), 141–147.

Shin, H. B., & Bruno, R. (2003). *Language use and English-speaking ability: 2000.* Accessed November, 2009, from http://www.census.gov/prod/2003pubs/c2kbr-29.pdf

Siskowski, C. (2010). *Family caregivers, doing double duty.* Accessed September 17, 2010, from http://ce.nurse.com/CE268-60/Family-Caregivers-Doing-Double-Duty

Skeletal traction and pin site care. (2008). Accessed May 12, 2010, from http://allnurses.com/nursing-student-assistance/skeletal-traction-pin-345327.html

Skiba, D. (2005). Emerging technology center: Do your students wiki? *Nursing Education Perspectives, 26*(2), 120–121.

Skiba, D. J., & Barton, A. J. (2006). Adapting your teaching to accommodate the net generation of learners. *The Online Journal of Issues in Nursing, 11*(2), Manuscript 4.

Smaldino, S., Lowther, D., & Russell, J. D. (2007). *Instructional media and technologies for learning* (9th ed.). New Jersey: Prentice-Hall.

Smeltzer, S. C., & Bare, B. G. (2010). *Brunner and Suddarth's textbook of medical-surgical nursing* (12th ed.). Philadelphia, Lippincott Williams & Wilkins.

Smith, J. M., & Lokhorst, D. B. (2009). *Infection control: Can nurses improve hand hygiene practices?* Accessed January 12, 2010, from http://www.juns.nursing.arizona.edu/Fall%202009/infection%20conrol.htm

Smyth, C. (2008). The Pittsburgh Sleep Quality Index. *American Journal of Nursing, 108*(5), 47.

Smyth, C. (2009). The Epworth Sleepiness Scale. *MedSurg Nursing, 18*(2), 134.

Smyth, C. A. (2008). How to try this: Evaluating sleep quality in older adults. *American Journal of Nursing, 108*(5), 42–43, 45–46, 48–51.

Snyder, L., & Moore, K. A. (2008). Wound basics: Types, treatment, and care. *RN Magazine, 71*(8): 32–37.

Springhouse. (2005). *Documentation in action.* Philadelphia: Lippincott Williams & Wilkins.

Springhouse. (2006). *Charting: An incredibly easy! pocket guide.* Philadelphia: Lippincott Williams & Wilkins.

Springhouse. (2007a). *Complete guide to documentation.* Philadelphia: Lippincott Williams & Wilkins.

Springhouse. (2007b). *Lippincott manual of nursing practice series: Documentation.* Philadelphia: Lippincott Williams & Wilkins.

Stanier, M. B. (2007). *It's a catastrophe! The fine art of catastrophizing.* Accessed October 2009, from http://www.inner-view.org/show Article.php?id-245

Stein, P. S., & Henry, R. G. (2009). Poor oral hygiene in long-term care: Nurses must provide better oral care to older adults and patients with severe disabilities. *American Journal of Nursing, 109*(6), 44–51.

Steris Corporation. (2006). *The liquid chemical sterilization story.* Accessed January 15, 2010, from http://www.csao.net/files/pdfs/Liquid%20Chemical%20Sterilization.pdf

Stickley, T., & Freshwater, D. (2006). The art of listening in the therapeutic relationship. *Mental Health Practice, 9*(5), 12–18.

Stitch, J. C., & Cassella, D. M. (2009). Getting inspired about oxygen delivery devices. *Nursing 39*(9), 51–54.

Straker, J. A., & Bailer, A. J. (2009). A review of the MDS Process in nursing homes. *Journal of Gerontological Nursing, 34*(10), 36–44.

Stranges, E., & Friedman, B. (2009). *Statistical brief #83; potentially preventable hospitalization rates declined for older adults, 2003–2007.* Accessed January 20, 2010, from http://www.hcup-us.ahrq.gov/reports/statbriefs/sb83.jsp

Strep test. The test. (2009). Accessed February 11, 2010, from http://www.labtestsonline.org/understanding/analytes/strep/test.htm

Substance Abuse and Mental Health Services Administration. (2007). *Fetal alcohol spectrum disorders among Native Americans.* Accessed November 2009, from http://download.ncadi.samhsa.gov/Prevline/pdfs/SMA06-4245.pdf

Sullivan, J., Seem, D. L., & Chabalewski, F. (1999). Determining brain death. *Critical Care Nurse, 19*(2), 37–46.

Survey calls for patient safety. (2008). *RN, 71*(12), 16.

Swann, J. (2005c). Enabling residents to enjoy showering. *Nursing & Residential Care, 7*(11), 516–518.

Swann, J. (2009a). Correct positioning: Reducing the risk of pressure damage. *Nursing & Residential Care, 11*(8), 415–417.

Swann, J. (2009b). Good positioning: The importance of posture. *Nursing & Residential Care, 11*(9), 467–469.

Sweetow, R. (2009a). Hearing aid delivery models: Part 1 of 2. *Audiology Today, 21*(5), 48–58.

Sweetow, R. (2009b). Hearing aid delivery models: Part 2 of 2. *Audiology Today, 21*(6), 32–37.

Taccone, P., Pesenti, A., Latini, R., et al. (2009). *Prone positioning in patients with moderate and severe acute respiratory distress syndrome.* Accessed April 21, 2010, from http://jama.ama-assn.org/cgi/content/abstract/302/18/1977

Tailored response: How does a nurse's appearance affect confidence in his or her performance and professionalism? (2006). *Nursing Standard, 20*(29), 26–27.

Talley, N. J., Lasch, K. L., & Baum, C. L. (2008). A gap in our understanding: Chronic constipation and its comorbid conditions. *Clinical Gastroenterology and Hepatology, 7*(1), 9–19.

Tanner, J. (2008). Surgical hand antisepsis: The evidence. *Journal of Perioperative Practice, 18*(8), 330–335.

Tele-nursing: Lifting the burden on emergency medical services. (2009). Retrieved September, 2009, from http://www.philadelphiacontroller.org/publications/audits/04_31_09_tele_nursing%20report.pdf

Thalheimer, W. (2006). *People remember 10%, 20% ... oh really?* Accessed December 29, 2009, from http://www.willatworklearning.com/2006/05/people_remember.html

Thieman, L. (2009). Each one reach one nurse. *Nursing, 39*(5), 6.

Thompson, P. D., Buchner, D., & Pina, I. L. (2003). Exercise and physical activity in the prevention and treatment of atherosclerotic cardiovascular disease. A statement for the Council on Clinical Cardiology (Subcommittee on Exercise, Rehabilitation, and Prevention) and the Council on Nutrition, Physical Activity, and Metabolism (Subcommittee on Physical Activity). *Circulation, 107*(24), 3109–3116.

Tideiksaar, R. (2010). *Falls in older people, prevention and management* (4th ed.). Baltimore: Health Professions Press.

Tomlinson, K. R., Golden, I. J., Mallory, J. L., et al. (2010). Family presence during adult resuscitation: A survey of emergency department registered nurses and staff attitudes. *Advanced Emergency Nursing Journal, 32*(1), 45–58.

Touhy, T. A., & Jett, K. (2010). *Ebersole and Hess' gerontologic nursing and healthy aging*, (3rd ed.). St. Louis, MO: Elsevier.

Travers, A. H., Rea, T. D., Bobrow, B. J., et al. (2010). *Part 4: CPR overview. 2010 American Heart Association Guidelines for Cardiopulmonary Resuscitation and Emergency Cardiovascular Care.* Accessed October 18, 2010, from http://circ.ahajournals.org/cgi/content/full/122/18_suppl_3/S676

Tubongbanua, N. (2005). Understanding pulse oximetry helps effective assessment. *Nursing Times, 101*(7), 37.

U.S. Census Bureau. (2008). *An older and more diverse nation by midcentury.* Accessed November, 2009, from http://www.census.gov/Press-Release/www/releases/archives/population/012496.html

U.S. Census Bureau. (2009). *Quick facts from the US Census Bureau.* Accessed November, 2009, from http://quickfacts.census.gov/qfd/states/04000.html

U.S. Department of Agriculture. (2008). *Dietary guidelines for Americans 2010.* Accessed February 28, 2011, from http://www.health.gov/dietaryguidelines/dga2010/DietaryGuidelines2010.pdf

U.S. Department of Health and Human Services. (2005). *HIPAA—general information.* Accessed January, 2010, from http://www.cms.hhs.gov/hipaaGenInfo/

U.S. Department of Health and Human Services. (2009). *The Secretary's Advisory Committee on National Health Promotion and Disease Prevention Objectives for 2020*. Accessed February 15, 2010, from http://www.healthypeople.gov/HP2020/advisory/

U.S. Department of Health and Human Services. (2010). *Medicare hospice benefits*. Accessed September 17, 2010, from http://www.medicare.gov/publications/pubs/pdf02154.pdf

U.S. Department of Labor. (2008). *Needlestick/sharps injuries*. Accessed February 24, 2010, from http://www.osha.gov/SLTC/etools/hospital/hazards/sharps/sharps.html

U.S. Food and Drug Administration. (2010). *Trans fat now listed with saturated fat and cholesterol on the nutrition facts label*. Accessed February 15, 2010, from http://www.fda.gov/Food/LabelingNutrition/ConsumerInformation/ucm109832.htm

Ufema, J. (2010). DNR orders: A dose of common sense. *Nursing, 40*(1), 68.

United States 107th Congress. (2002). *Mercury Reduction Act of 2002*. Accessed January 27, 2010, from http://thomas.loc.gov/cgibin/bdquery/z?d107:SN00351:AAAL&summ2=m&

United States 109th Congress. (2005). *Safe Communities and Safe Schools Mercury Reduction Act of 2005*. Accessed January 27, 2010, from http://frwebgate.access.gpo.gov/cgi-bin/getdoc.cgi?dbname=109_cong_bills&docid=f:h2391ih.txt.pdf

University of Arkansas, Pat Walker Health Center. (2007). *Crutches*. http://health.uark.edu/virtualbrochures/GeneralHealth/Crutches_kt_tags_DONE.pdf

Unlu, H., Sardan, Y. C., & Ulker, S. (2007). Comparison of sampling methods for urine cultures. *Journal of Nursing Scholarship, 39*(4), 325–229.

Updated guidelines for infectious diseases in ED New buzzwords: respiratory hygiene, cough etiquette. (2007). *Emergency Department Nursing, 10*(11), 125–126.

Valdez-Lowe, C., Ghareeb, S. A., & Artinian, N. T. (2009). Pulse oximetry in adults. *American Journal of Nursing, 109*(6), 52–60.

van den Bemt, P. M. L., Cussell, M. B. I., Overbeeke, P. W., et al. (2006). Quality improvement of oral medication administration in patients with enteral feeding tubes. *Quality & Safety in Health Care, 15*(1), 44–47.

Van Rijswijk, L. (2006). So many dressings, so little information: Choosing a treatment when evidence is limited or conflicting. *American Journal of Nursing, 106*(12), 66.

Vega, G. L., Adams-Huet, B., Peshock, R. et al. (2006). Influence of body fat content and distribution on variation in metabolic risk. *The Journal of Clinical Endocrinology and Metabolism, 91*(11), 4459–4466.

Verheijde, J. L., Rady, M. Y., & McGregor, J. L. (2007). *The United States Revised Uniform Anatomical Gift Act (2006): New challenges in balancing patient rights and physician responsibilities*. Accessed September 19, 2020, from http://www.ncbi.nlm.nih.gov/pmc/articles/PMC2001294/

Vigneau, C., Baudel, J., Guidet, B., et al. (2005). Sonography as an alternative to radiography for nasogastric feeding tube location. *Intensive Care Medicine, 31*(11), 1570–1572.

Wardell, D. (2010). What one thing could you change to improve patient safety? *Nursing Times, 106*(5), 9.

Washer, P. (2009). Talking with people from other cultures. *Independent Nurse, July.*

Watson, R. (2005). Pulling the plug on bath-time. *Nursing Older People, 16*(10), 44–45.

Weber. S. (2008). Ergonomics standards: An overview. *Nursing Management, 39*(7), 28–32.

Weitzel, T., Vollmer, C. M., Plunkett, D., et al. (2008). Doing it better. To cath or not to cath? *Nursing, 38*(2), 20–21.

Wheeler, T. (2009). Diagnosing common skin conditions in a care home. *Nursing & Residential Care, 11*(12), 600, 602–603.

White, B. A., Jablonski, R. A., & Falkenstern, S. K. (2009). *Diabetes in the nursing home*. http://annalsoflongtermcare.com/content/diabetes-nursing-home

Whitehead, S. (2004). *Blood on tap. Part 1: History in the making*. Accessed March 7, 2011, from http://www.emsworld.com/print/EMS-World/Blood-On-Tap-Part1-History-in-the-Making/1$2340

Whiteing, N. L. (2009). Skin assessment of patients at risk of pressure ulcers. *Nursing Standard, 24*(10), 40–44.

Whiting, M. (2008). *Evidence based research paper on wet to dry dressings*. Accessed June 2, 2010, from http://marlaynawhiting.efoliomn.com/vertical/Sites/%7B1BAD0AE1-8A3F-428C-80FACD96D4D1%7D/uploads/%7BF0E6FC48-6487-4D4C-9208-6C3EE6FC90A2%7D.DOCX

Winemaker, S. (2008). *Palliative care*. Accessed September 17, 2010, from http://www.alsont.ca/_media/File/.../Dr%20Winemaker%20Presentation.ppt

Wolfe, L. (2006). *Insulin therapy. How to inject insulin with a syringe or insulin pen*. Accessed August 18, 2010, from http://www.isletsofhope.com/diabetes/treatment/insulin_inject_1.html

Wong, B., Kennedy, M. S., & Jacobson, J. (2009). Safe-practice recommendations released. *American Journal of Nursing, 109*(6), 22.

Woo, A., Ranji, U., & Salganicoff, A. (2008). *Reducing medical errors*. Accessed March 15, 2010, from http://www.kaiseredu.org/topics_im.asp?id=137&parentID=70&imID=1

Woo, E. (2009). Device safety. Keep an eye out for contact lens problems. *Nursing, 39*(11), 66.

Woodrow, P. (2005). Recognizing and managing stress. *Nursing Older People, 17*(7), 31–32.

Woodrow, P. (2007). Caring for patients receiving oxygen therapy. *Nursing Older People, 19*(1):31–36.

Woodward, S. (2009). The inseparable link between nursing and patient safety. *Nursing Times, 105*(12), 26.

World Health Organization. (2005). *Protecting healthcare workers: Preventing needlestick injuries toolkit*. Accessed February 24, 2010, from http://www.who.int/occupational_health/activities/pnitoolkit/en/print.html

World Health Organization. (2009). *Appraising the WHO analgesic ladder on its 20th anniversary*. Accessed March 24, 2010, from http://whocancerpain.wisc.edu/?q=node/86

World Health Organization. (2010). *WHO's pain relief ladder*. Accessed March 24, 2010, from http://www.who.int.cancer/palliative/painladder/en/

Worth, T. (2008). Seeking real solutions to the nursing shortage: Increasing educational capacity gets at the root of the problem. *American Journal of Nursing, 108*(10), 21.

Worth, T. (2010). Nurses as sentinels for safety. *American Journal of Nursing, 110*(3), 19

Wright, S. (2005). Stress factor: How do you recognize that you are stressed. *Nursing Standard, 20*(3), 36–37.

Wysong, P. R., & Driver, E. (2009). Patients' perceptions of nurses' skill. *Critical Care Nurse, 29*(4), 24–38.

Yardley, W. (2009). *First death for Washington assisted-suicide law*. Retrieved September, 2009, from http://nytimes.com/2009/05/23/us/23suicide.html

Yokoyama, M., Xiaohui, S., Satoru, O., et al. (2004). Comparison of percutaneous electrical nerve stimulation with transcutaneous electrical nerve stimulation for long-term pain relief in patients with chronic back pain. *Anesthesia & Analgesia, 98*(6), 1552–1556.

Young, R. J., Chapman, M. J., Fraser, R., et al. (2005). A novel technique for post-pyloric feeding tube placement in critically ill patients: A pilot study. *Anesthesia and Intensive Care, 22*(2), 229–234.

Zerwekl, J., & Claborn, J. C. (2009). *Nursing Today: Transition and Trends* (6th ed.). St. Louis, MO: Saunders Elsevier.

Zomorodi, M., & Foley, B. J. (2009). The nature of advocacy vs. paternalism in nursing: Clarifying the "thin line". *Journal of Advanced Nursing, 65*(8), 1746–1756.

Zuelzer, H. B. (2009). Opportunities and challenges: Wound and skin alterations of obesity. *Bariatric Nursing & Surgical Patient Care, 4*(4), 283.

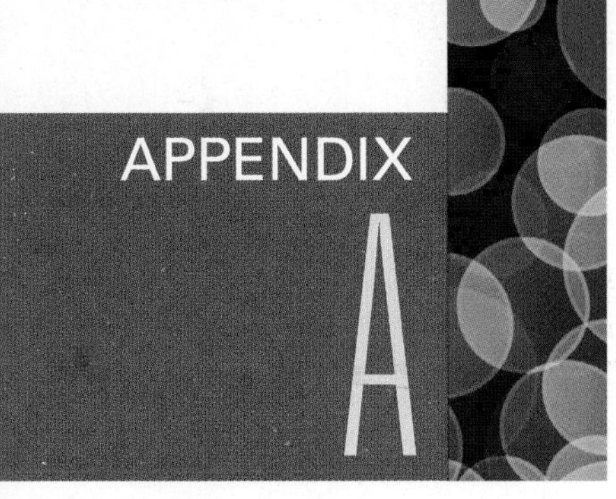

Chapter Summaries

CHAPTER 1

- The art of nursing declined in England with the exile of Catholic religious orders, forcing the government to assume responsibility for caring for the sick, aged, and infirm. Eventually, the state delegated this care to untrained and generally uninterested people of questionable character.
- Florence Nightingale changed the image of nursing by training nurses to care for the sick, selecting only those with upstanding character as potential nurses, improving the sanitary conditions within clients' environments, significantly reducing the morbidity and mortality rates of British soldiers, providing formal nursing classes separate from clinical experience, and arguing that nursing education should be a lifelong process.
- Training schools in the United States deviated from the pattern established by Nightingale. No criteria established which hospitals were to train nurses. Students staffed the hospitals without being paid. There was no uniformity in what was taught; students learned more by experience than by formal instruction. Nursing students were taught from a physician's perspective. Students were required to work and to live at the beck and call of the hospital administrator and after graduation students were left to seek employment elsewhere.
- In addition to employment within hospitals, early graduates of nursing programs met the health needs of poor immigrants by living among them in settlement houses in the ghettos of large cities, by serving as midwives for rural women who lacked medical care, and by caring for sick and wounded soldiers.
- What started as an art, passing on the skills of nursing from one practitioner to another, was soon augmented by science, a unique body of knowledge that made it possible to predict which nursing interventions would be most appropriate for producing desired outcomes, a process referred to as evidence-based practice.
- Most recently, nursing has become theory based, which means that nursing scholars are proposing what the process of nursing encompasses by explaining the relationship between four essential components: humans, health, environment, and nursing.
- One of the earliest definitions of nursing outlined the scope of practice as caring for the sick. More recently, the definition has been refined with the addition of the nurse's role in health promotion and independent practice.
- Those who wish to pursue a career in nursing may choose among a practical/vocational nursing program or a registered nursing program taught in a career center, hospital school, community or junior college, or university.
- The choice of nursing educational program depends on one's career goals, location of schools, costs involved, length of the program, reputation and success of graduates, flexibility in course scheduling, opportunities for part-time or full-time enrollment, and ease of articulation to the next level of education.
- Continuing education is necessary for contemporary nurses because it demonstrates personal accountability, promotes the public's trust, ensures competence in current nursing practice, and keeps the nurse abreast of how technology is affecting client care.
- Several trends are affecting health care. One of the major issues is the growing shortage of nurses. In addition, many people, such as older adults, minorities, and the poor, are not receiving adequate health care. The number of uninsured people is rising. Various cost-containment practices reduce access to tests, treatment, and services, increase ratios of clients per nurse in employment settings, and contribute to a higher acuity of clients in previously nonacute settings.
- To address the nursing shortage, the federal Nurse Reinvestment Act, renamed the American Recovery and Reinvestment Act and signed into law in 2009, authorizes loan repayment programs and scholarships; funding for public service announcements; career ladder programs; and grants for nurse retention, client safety enhancement, and gerontology. Nurses are proactively pursuing post-licensure education; training for advanced practice; cross-training; learning more about multicultural diversity; supporting national health insurance legislation; promoting community-based programs; emphasizing health promotion; referring clients with health problems for early treatment; coordinating nursing services across care settings; developing and implementing clinical pathways; participating in quality assurance; and focusing on geriatric populations.
- Regardless of educational background, all nurses use assessment, caring, counseling, and comforting skills in clinical practice.

CHAPTER 2

- The nursing process is an organized sequence of steps used to identify health problems and to manage client care.
- Characteristics of the nursing process are that it is within the legal scope of nursing practice, based on unique knowledge, planned, client centered, goal directed, prioritized, and dynamic.
- The steps in the nursing process are assessment, diagnosis, planning, implementation, and evaluation.
- Resources for data include the client, the client's family, medical records, and other health care workers.
- Data base assessments provide vast information about a client at the time of admission. Focus assessments, which are ongoing, expand the data base with additional information. Functional assessments, which are performed on a cyclical basis, provide a comprehensive appraisal of a client's physical, psychological, and social status to maintain current strengths and avoid potential decline.
- A nursing diagnosis is a health problem that nurses can treat independently. A collaborative problem is a physiologic complication that requires the skills and interventions of both nurses and physicians.
- A nursing diagnostic statement generally consists of three parts: the problem, the etiology for the problem, and the signs and symptoms or evidence for the problem.
- Setting priorities for care helps to maximize efficiency in minimal time.
- Short-term goals are those the nurse expects to accomplish in a few days to 1 week, usually when caring for clients in acute care settings (eg, hospitals). Long-term goals may take weeks to months to accomplish after discharge from the health care agency. They are identified when caring for clients with chronic problems who are receiving nursing care in a long-term health facility or through community health agencies or home health care.
- Methods of documentation include writing the problems, goals, and nursing orders by hand; individualizing a standardized or computer-generated care plan; or following an agency's written standards for care or clinical pathways.
- Nurses demonstrate implementation of the plan of care by correlating the written plan with nursing documentation in the medical record.
- When evaluating the client's progress, nursing orders are discontinued if the client has met the goal and the problem no longer exists. The nurse revises the care plan if the client has made progress but the goal remains unmet or if there has been no progress in reaching a desired outcome.
- Concept mapping (also known as care mapping) is a method of organizing information in a graphic or pictorial form. The process involves

drawing lines or arrows to link or correlate relationships within the map. This foundation provides a bridge for developing more complex skills like identifying nursing diagnoses, setting goals and expected outcomes, implementing nursing interventions, and evaluating the results of care.

CHAPTER 3

- The six types of laws are constitutional, statutory, administrative, common, criminal, and civil.
- Each state's nurse practice act defines the unique role of the nurse and differentiates it from that of other health care practitioners. Each state's board of nursing is the regulatory agency for managing its nurse practice act.
- Violations of civil laws include intentional and unintentional torts. In an intentional tort, a private citizen sues another for a deliberately aggressive act. In an unintentional tort, the lawsuit charges that harm resulted from a person's negligence even though he or she intended no harm.
- Negligence lawsuits allege that a person's actions, or lack thereof, caused harm. The defendant is held to a standard expected of any other reasonable person. In the case of malpractice, the plaintiff alleges that a professional's actions, or lack thereof, caused harm. The defendant is held to the standard expected of others with similar knowledge and education.
- Professional liability insurance is advantageous for nurses to obtain because (1) nurses are increasingly being named in medical lawsuits, (2) financial damages, when awarded, can be extremely high, and (3) it ensures having an attorney working on the nurse's behalf.
- A nurse's professional liability can be mitigated by laws such as a state's Good Samaritan Act, expiration of the statute of limitations, legal principles such as a client's assumption of risk, accurate and complete documentation, and aggressive risk management.
- Ethics refers to moral or philosophical principles that classify actions as right or wrong.
- A code of ethics is a written statement that describes ideal behavior for members of a particular discipline.
- There are two ethical theories: teleology and deontology. Teleology proposes that the best ethical decision is the one that will result in benefits for the majority of individuals. Deontology proposes that the basis for an ethical decision is simply whether the action is morally right or wrong.
- Six principles that form a foundation for ethical practice are beneficence, nonmaleficence, autonomy, veracity, fidelity, and justice.
- Some common ethical issues that nurses encounter in everyday practice include telling the truth, protecting clients' confidentiality, ensuring that clients' wishes for withholding and withdrawing treatment are followed, advocating for the nondiscriminatory allocation of scarce resources, and reporting incompetent or unethical practices.

CHAPTER 4

- The World Health Organization (WHO) defines health as "a state of complete physical, mental, and social well-being and not merely the absence of disease or infirmity."
- Values are the ideals that an individual believes are honorable attributes. Beliefs are concepts that individuals hold to be true.
- Most Americans believe that health is a resource, a right, and a personal responsibility.
- How "whole" or well a person feels is the sum of his or her physical, emotional, social, and spiritual health, a concept referred to as *holism*. Any change in one component, positive or negative, automatically creates repercussions in the others.
- There are five levels of human needs: physiologic (first level), safety and security (second level), love and belonging (third level), esteem and self-esteem (fourth level), and self-actualization (fifth level). By satisfying needs at each subsequent level, individuals can realize their maximum potential for health and well-being.
- Illness is a state of discomfort that results when a person's health becomes impaired through disease, stress, or an accident or injury.
- Morbidity refers to the incidence of a specific disease, disorder, or injury. Mortality refers to the death rate from a specific condition. An acute illness is one that comes on suddenly and lasts a short time. A chronic illness is one that comes on slowly and lasts a long time. A terminal illness is one in which there is no potential for cure. A primary illness is one that developed independently of another disease. Any subsequent disorder that develops from a preexisting condition is referred to as a secondary illness. Remission refers to the disappearance of the signs and symptoms associated with a particular disease. An exacerbation refers to the time when the disorder becomes reactivated or reverts from a chronic to an acute state. A hereditary condition is one acquired from the genetic codes of one or both parents. Congenital disorders are those that are present at birth but result from faulty embryonic development. An idiopathic illness's cause is unexplained.
- Primary care refers to the services provided by the first health care professional or agency an individual contacts. Secondary care pertains to the services to which primary caregivers refer clients for consultation and additional testing, such as a cardiac catheterization laboratory. Tertiary care takes place in a hospital where complex technology and specialists are available. Extended care involves meeting the health needs of clients who no longer require hospital care but who continue to need health services.
- Two programs that help to finance health care for the aged, disabled, and poor are Medicare and Medicaid.
- Methods for controlling escalating health care costs include a system of prospective payment known as the diagnosis-related group, managed care, health maintenance organizations, preferred provider organizations, and capitation.
- National health goals for 2020 include: (1) Attain high quality, longer lives free of preventable disease, disability, injury, and premature death; (2) achieve health equity, eliminate disparities, and improve the health of all groups; (3) create social and physical environments that promote good health for all; and (4) promote quality of life, healthy development, and healthy behaviors across all life stages.
- One of several patterns may be used when providing nursing care for clients. In functional nursing, each nurse on a unit is assigned specific tasks. The case method involves assigning one nurse to administer all the care a client needs for a designated period of time. In team nursing, many nursing personnel divide the client care and all work until everything is completed. Primary nursing is a method in which the admitting nurse assumes responsibility for planning client care and evaluating the progress of the client. In managed care, a nurse manager plans the nursing care of clients based on their illness or medical diagnosis and evaluates client progress so that each client is ready for discharge by the time designated by prospective payment systems.

CHAPTER 5

- Homeostasis refers to a relatively stable state of physiologic equilibrium.
- Physiologic, psychological, social, and spiritual stressors affect homeostasis.
- The philosophic concept of holism leads to two commonly held beliefs: both the mind and the body directly influence humans, and the relationship between the mind and the body has the potential for sustaining health as well as causing illness.
- Adaptation refers to how an organism responds to change. Successful adaptation is the key to maintaining and preserving homeostasis. Unsuccessful adaptation leads to illness and death.
- Adaptive changes occur through the cortex, which communicates with and through the reticular activating system, the hypothalamus, the autonomic nervous system, and the pituitary gland along with other endocrine glands under its control.
- The sympathetic nervous system, a division of the autonomic nervous system, accelerates the physiologic functions that ensure survival through strength or a rapid escape. The parasympathetic nervous system, a second division of the autonomic nervous system, inhibits physiologic stimulation, which restores homeostasis and provides an alternative mechanism for dealing with stressors.
- Stress involves the physiologic and behavioral reactions that occur when the body's equilibrium is disturbed.

- People vary in their response to stressors depending on the intensity and duration of the stressor, the number of stressors at one time, physical status, life experiences, coping strategies, social support system, and personal beliefs, attitudes, and values.
- The general adaptation syndrome, a physiologic stress response described by Hans Selye, consists of the alarm stage, stage of resistance, and stage of exhaustion. In most cases, the alarm stage and stage of resistance restore homeostasis. When the stage of resistance is prolonged, however, adaptive resources are overwhelmed and the person enters the stage of exhaustion, which is characterized by stress-related disorders and, in some cases, death.
- Stress-related disorders and their consequences are minimized at three levels. Primary prevention involves reducing the potential for a disorder. Secondary prevention involves public screening and early diagnosis. Tertiary prevention uses rehabilitation and aggressive management when a disorder develops.
- Psychological adaptation occurs through the use of coping mechanisms and coping strategies. Healthy use of coping mechanisms and coping strategies allows people to postpone the emotional effects of stress, permitting them to deal with reality eventually and gain emotional maturity. Unhealthy use of coping mechanisms tends to distort reality to such an extent that the person fails to see or correct his or her weaknesses. Nontherapeutic coping strategies provide temporary relief but eventually cause problems.
- Nursing care of clients under stress includes identifying stressors, assessing the client's response to stressors, eliminating or reducing stressors, preventing additional stressors, promoting adaptive responses, supporting coping strategies, maintaining a client's network of support, and implementing stress reduction and stress management techniques.
- Four methods for preventing, reducing, or eliminating a stress response include using stress reduction techniques such as providing adequate explanations in understandable language; implementing stress management interventions such as progressive relaxation; promoting the release of endorphins through massage, for example; and manipulating sensory stimuli as might be done with aromatherapy.

CHAPTER 6

- Culture refers to the values, beliefs, and practices of a particular group. Race refers to biologic variations such as skin color, hair texture, and eye shape. Ethnicity is the bond or kinship a person feels with his or her country of birth or place of ancestral origin.
- Two factors that interfere with perceiving others as individuals are stereotyping, which involves ascribing fixed beliefs about people based on some general characteristic, and ethnocentrism, the belief that one's own ethnicity is superior to all others.
- US culture is said to be Anglicized because many of the values, beliefs, and practices evolved from the early English settlers.
- Some examples of Anglo-American culture include speaking English; valuing work, time, and technology; holding parents responsible for the health care, behavior, and education of minor children; keeping government separate from religion; and seeking assistance from licensed individuals when health care is necessary.
- A subculture is a unique cultural group that coexists within the dominant culture. The four major US subcultures are African American, Latino, Asian American, and Native American.
- Subcultural groups differ from Anglo-Americans in one or more of the following ways: language, communication style, biologic and physiologic variations, prevalence of diseases, and health beliefs and practices.
- The four characteristics of culturally sensitive nursing care are data collection of a cultural nature, acceptance of each client as an individual, knowledge of health problems that affect particular cultural groups, and planning care within the client's health belief system to achieve the best health outcomes.
- Some ways that nurses can demonstrate cultural sensitivity include learning a second language, performing physical assessments and care according to the client's unique biologic differences, consulting each client as to his or her cultural preferences, arranging for modifications in diet and dress according to the client's customs, and allowing clients to continue relying on cultural health practices (if they are not harmful).

CHAPTER 7

- In a nurse–client relationship, nurses meet client needs by performing any or all of the following roles: caregiver, educator, collaborator, and delegator.
- The role of clients is to be actively involved in their care, to communicate, to ask questions, to assist in planning their care, and above all to retain as much independence as possible.
- Some principles underlying a therapeutic nurse–client relationship include treating each client as a unique person; respecting the client's feelings; striving to promote the client's physical, emotional, social, and spiritual well-being; encouraging the client to participate in problem solving and decision making; and accepting that a client has the potential for growth and change.
- A nurse–client relationship usually encompasses three phases: introductory, working, and termination.
- Communication involves sending and receiving messages between two or more people followed by feedback indicating that the information was understood or requires further clarification. Therapeutic communication refers to using words and gestures to accomplish a particular objective.
- Examples of therapeutic verbal communication techniques include questioning, reflecting, paraphrasing, sharing perceptions, and clarifying. Examples of nontherapeutic verbal communication techniques include giving false reassurance, using clichés, giving approval or disapproval, demanding an explanation, and giving advice.
- Some factors that may affect oral communication include language compatibility; verbal skills; hearing and visual acuity; motor functions involving the throat, tongue, and teeth; sensory distractions; and interpersonal attitudes.
- The four forms of nonverbal communication are kinesics (body language), paralanguage (vocal sounds), proxemics (how space is used in communication), and touch.
- Task-related touch involves the personal contact required when performing nursing procedures. Affective touch is used to demonstrate concern or affection.
- Affective touch is appropriate in many situations. Examples include caring for clients who are lonely, uncomfortable, near death, or anxious and those with sensory deprivation.

CHAPTER 8

- Health teaching is nursing activity that is mandated by state nurse practice acts, the Joint Commission (2010), which has made it a criterion for accreditation, and the professional position published in the American Nurses Association's Social Policy Statement.
- Client teaching generally focuses on combinations of the following subject areas: the plan of care, treatment and services; safe self-administration of medications; the pain assessment process and methods for pain management; directions and practice in using equipment for self-care; dietary instructions; rehabilitation program; available community resources; plan for medical follow-up; and signs of complications and actions to take.
- Benefits of client teaching include (1) reduced length of stay, (2) cost-effectiveness of health care, (3) better allocation of resources, (4) increased client satisfaction, and (5) decreased readmission rates.
- The three learning domains are the cognitive domain (information usually provided in oral or written forms), the affective domain (information that appeals to a person's feelings, beliefs, or values), and the psychomotor domain (learning by doing).
- Three age-related categories of learners are pedagogic (children), androgogic (young and middle-aged adults), and gerogogic (older adults).
- Examples of characteristics unique to gerogogic learners are that they are motivated to learn by a personal need, they may be experiencing degenerative physical changes, and they can draw on a vast repertoire of past experiences.
- Before teaching a client, the nurse assesses the client's learning style, age and development, capacity to learn (includes level of literacy, any sensory deficits, and cultural differences), ability to pay attention and concentrate, motivation, learning readiness, and learning needs.

CHAPTER 9

- Medical records are used as a permanent account of a person's health problems, care, and progress; to share information among health care personnel; as a resource for investigating the quality of care in an institution; to acquire and maintain Joint Commission accreditation; to obtain reimbursement for billed services and products; to conduct research; and as legal evidence in malpractice cases.
- Medical records generally contain an information sheet about the client, medical information, a plan of care, nursing documentation, medication administration records, and laboratory and diagnostic test results.
- Health care agencies may organize information in the medical record using a source-oriented or a problem-oriented format. Source-oriented records categorize information according to the source reporting it; problem-oriented records are organized according to the client's health problems, regardless of who does the documentation.
- Nurses may document information in the medical record using one of the following methods: narrative charting, SOAP charting, focus charting, PIE charting, charting by exception, and computerized charting.
- HIPAA legislation was enacted originally to protect health information communicated from one insurance company to another when a person changed employment. Recent revisions to that legislation now regulate methods for further ensuring the client's privacy in the workplace and security of data.
- Regardless of the charting style, all documentation in an acute health care agency includes ongoing assessment data, a plan of care, a record of the care provided, and the outcomes of the implemented care.
- Nurses use only agency-approved abbreviations when documenting information to promote clarity in communication among health professionals and to ensure accurate interpretation of the documented information if the chart is subpoenaed as legal evidence.
- Military time is based on a 24-hour clock. Time is indicated using a different four-digit number. After noon, the time is identified by adding 12 to each hour.
- Some principles of charting when it is hand-written include the following: ensure that the documentation form identifies the client; use a pen; print or write legibly; record the time of each entry; fill all the space on a line; use only approved abbreviations; describe information objectively, providing precise measurements when possible; avoid obliterating information; and sign each entry by name and title.
- Written forms of communication other than the medical record include the nursing care plan, nursing Kardex, checklists, and flow sheets.
- In addition to the written record, the health care team may exchange information during change of shift reports, client care assignments, team conferences, rounds, and telephone calls.

CHAPTER 10

- Microorganisms are living animals or plants visible only with a microscope.
- Some examples of microorganisms are bacteria, viruses, fungi, rickettsiae, protozoans, mycoplasmas, helminths, and prions.
- Nonpathogens are generally harmless microorganisms, whereas pathogens have a high potential for causing infections and contagious diseases. Resident microorganisms are generally nonpathogens that are always present on the skin. Transient microorganisms are generally pathogens that are more easily removed through hand hygiene. Aerobic microorganisms require oxygen for survival, whereas anaerobic microorganisms do not.
- Some microorganisms have ensured their survival by developing the capacity to form spores and resist antibiotic drug therapy.
- The components of the chain of infection are an infectious agent, a reservoir for growth and reproduction, an exit route from the reservoir, a mode of transmission, a port of entry, and a susceptible host.
- Several biologic defenses reduce susceptibility to infectious agents. Examples include intact skin and mucous membranes; reflexes such as sneezing, coughing, and vomiting; infection-fighting blood cells; enzymes such as lysozyme which is present in tears, saliva, and other secretions; the acidity of gastric acid; and antibodies.
- Nosocomial infections are those acquired by previously uninfected clients while they are being cared for in a health care facility.
- Asepsis refers to practices that decrease the numbers of infectious agents, their reservoirs, and vehicles for transmission.
- Medical asepsis involves practices that confine or reduce microorganisms. The most effective method of medical asepsis is hand hygiene, an essential nursing activity that must be performed repeatedly when caring for clients. Surgical asepsis involves measures that render supplies and equipment totally free of microorganisms and practices that avoid contamination during their use.
- Principles of medical asepsis include frequent handwashing or hand antisepsis and maintaining intact skin (the best methods for reducing the transmission of microorganisms); using personal protective equipment (gloves, gown, mask, goggles, and hair and shoe covers); and maintaining a clean environment.
- Surgical asepsis involves sterilization measures such as ultraviolet radiation, heat, or chemicals.
- Three of the principles of surgical asepsis are as follows: sterility is preserved by touching one sterile item with another sterile item; once a sterile item touches something that is not sterile, it is considered contaminated; and any partially unwrapped sterile package is considered contaminated.
- Nurses apply principles of surgical asepsis when they create a sterile field, add supplies or liquids to a sterile field, and don sterile gloves.

CHAPTER 11

- The process of admission involves obtaining authorization from a physician, obtaining billing information, completing nursing responsibilities such as orienting the client and obtaining a data base assessment, developing an initial plan for nursing care, and fulfilling medical responsibilities such as documenting the client's history and results of a physical examination.
- Some common reactions of newly admitted clients are anxiety, loneliness, potential for compromised privacy, and loss of identity.
- The discharge process consists of obtaining a written medical order for discharge, completing discharge instructions, notifying the business office, helping the client leave the agency, writing a summary of the discharge in the medical record, and requesting that the room be cleaned.
- Examples of the use of transfers in client care include moving a client from one level of care to another when his or her condition improves, worsens, or no longer meets the criteria initially established but still needs some type of attention.
- A transfer involves discharging a client from one unit or agency and admitting him or her to another without the client going home in the interim. A referral involves sending a client who will be discharged to another person or agency for special services.
- Nursing homes may provide skilled, intermediate, or basic care.
- To determine the level of care a client requires, federal law requires licensed extended care facilities to complete a Minimum Data Set assessment form on admission and every 3 months thereafter or whenever the client's condition changes.
- The demand for home health care services has increased due to limits on insurance reimbursement for hospital stays and the growing number of older adults in the population who need health care assistance.

CHAPTER 12

- Vital signs include temperature, pulse, respirations, and blood pressure. Pain is considered the fifth vital sign. Pain assessment, which is discussed in Chapter 20, is performed at least daily and whenever vital signs are taken.
- Shell temperature is the degree of warmth at the skin surface; core temperature is the degree of warmth near the center of the body where vital organs are located.
- Temperature is measured using the Celsius or Fahrenheit scale.
- The mouth, rectum, axilla, and ear are common sites for assessing body temperature; the temperature of the tympanic membrane in the ear and

behind the ear over the path of the temporal artery is the closest approximation of core temperature.

- Electronic, infrared, chemical, and digital thermometers are used to assess body temperature; glass mercury thermometers are no longer recommended for use because mercury is an environmental and human toxin.
- A fever exists when a client has a body temperature that exceeds 99.3°F (37.4°C). Hyperthermia is a life-threatening condition characterized by a body temperature that exceeds 105.8°F (40.6°C).
- A fever generally has four phases: prodromal, onset or invasion, stationary, and resolution or defervescence.
- A fever is accompanied by chills, flushed skin, irritability, and headache, as well as several other signs and symptoms.
- An infrared tympanic thermometer is the best assessment tool for measuring subnormal temperatures because other common clinical thermometers cannot accurately measure temperatures in hypothermic ranges and the blood flow in the mouth, rectum, and axilla is generally so low that measurements taken from these sites are inaccurate.
- Subnormal temperatures are accompanied by shivering, pale skin, listlessness, and impaired muscle coordination as well as several other signs and symptoms.
- A pulse assessment includes the rate per minute, rhythm, and volume.
- The radial artery is the most common pulse assessment site; however, similar data may be obtained by assessing the apical heart rate or the apical-radial rate or by using a Doppler ultrasound device.
- Respiration refers to the exchange of oxygen and carbon dioxide. Ventilation is the movement of air in and out of the chest. The rate of ventilation is assessed when obtaining vital signs.
- Some abnormal breathing characteristics that may be noted are tachypnea (rapid breathing), bradypnea (slow breathing), dyspnea (labored breathing), and apnea (absence of breathing).
- Blood pressure measurements reflect the ability of the arteries to stretch, the volume of circulating blood, and the amount of resistance the heart must overcome when it pumps blood.
- Systolic pressure is the pressure within the arterial system when the heart contracts. Diastolic pressure is the pressure within the arterial system when the heart relaxes and fills with blood.
- A stethoscope, an inflatable cuff, and a sphygmomanometer are usually required for measuring blood pressure.
- During an auscultated blood pressure assessment, five distinct sounds, called Korotkoff sounds, are heard. Phase I is characterized by faint tapping sounds; in phase II, the sounds are swishing; in phase III, the sounds are loud and crisp; in phase IV, the sound becomes suddenly muffled; and in phase V there is one last sound, followed by silence.
- Blood pressure may be measured with an electronic sphygmomanometer, which provides a digital display of the pressure measurements. The blood pressure also can be measured by palpating the brachial pulse while releasing the air from the cuff bladder, by using a Doppler stethoscope or an automated blood pressure machine, or taking the blood pressure at the thigh.

CHAPTER 13

- Physical assessments are performed to evaluate the client's current physical condition, to detect early signs of developing health problems, to establish a database for future comparisons, and to evaluate responses to medical and nursing interventions.
- There are four physical assessment techniques: inspection, percussion, palpation, and auscultation.
- Before performing a physical assessment, the nurse needs gloves, examination gown, cloth or paper drape, stethoscope, penlight, and tongue blade, as well as other assessment instruments for taking vital signs and weighing and measuring the client.
- The assessment environment should be near a restroom, private, warm, and adequately lit. There should be an adjustable examination table or bed.
- During an initial survey of a client, the nurse observes physical appearance, level of consciousness, body size, posture, gait, movement, use of ambulatory aids, and mood and emotional tone.
- Drapes during a physical examination protect the client's modesty and provide warmth.
- There are two approaches for data collection. The head-to-toe approach involves gathering data from the top of the body and then working toward the feet. The systems approach organizes data collection according to the functional systems of the body.
- The body may be divided into six general components when organizing data collection: the head and neck, the chest, the extremities, the abdomen, the genitalia, and the anus and rectum.
- Whenever an opportunity arises, nurses teach adult clients how to perform breast and testicular self-examinations.

CHAPTER 14

- An examination is a procedure that involves the physical inspection of body structures and evidence of their functions. A test involves the examination of body fluids or specimens.
- Whenever clients undergo special examinations and tests, the nurse is generally responsible for determining the client's understanding of the procedure, checking that the consent form is signed, following test preparation requirements or teaching outpatients how to prepare themselves, obtaining equipment and supplies, arranging the examination area, positioning and draping clients, assisting the examiner, providing clients with physical and emotional support, caring for specimens, and recording and reporting significant information.
- The five common examination positions are dorsal recumbent, Sims', lithotomy, knee–chest, and modified standing.
- A pelvic examination involves the inspection and palpation of the vagina and adjacent organs. This examination often includes the collection of secretions for a Pap test to identify any abnormal cells, levels of hormone activity, and identity of infectious microorganisms.
- Tests and examinations commonly involve the use of specimens, x-rays, endoscopes, radioactive substances, sound waves, and electrical activity.
- When determining how particular tests are performed, it is helpful to understand four word endings: -graphy, as in angiography, means to record an image; -scopy, as in bronchoscopy, means to look through a lensed instrument; -centesis, as in amniocentesis, means to puncture; and -metry, as in pelvimetry, means to measure with an instrument.
- Nurses often are called on to assist with sigmoidoscopy (inspecting the rectum and sigmoid section of the lower intestine with an endoscope), paracentesis (puncturing the skin and withdrawing fluid from the abdominal cavity), and lumbar puncture (inserting a needle between lumbar vertebrae in the spine but below the spinal cord itself); to collect a throat culture specimen; and to measure capillary blood glucose levels using a glucometer.
- When the client undergoing special examinations and tests is an older adult, the nurse faces special challenges such as preventing fatigue and dehydration, maintaining or adjusting current drug therapy and avoiding misinterpretation of laboratory test results that are based on norms for younger adults.

CHAPTER 15

- Nutrition is the process by which the body uses food. Malnutrition results from inadequate consumption of nutrients.
- The components of basic nutrition include adequate calories, proteins, carbohydrates, fats, vitamins, and minerals.
- Some factors that affect nutritional needs include age, height and weight, growth, activity, and health status.
- MyPlate from the United States Department of Agriculture is a guide for promoting a healthy daily intake of food.
- Nutrition labels must indicate the serving size in household measurements and the daily value for specific nutrients per serving. They must meet specified criteria if they make health-related claims for the product.
- Protein complementation is the practice of combining two or more plant protein sources to obtain all the essential amino acids required for healthy nutrition.
- Data that provide objective information about a person's nutritional status include anthropometric measurements, physical examination data, and results from laboratory tests.

- A diet history is the information obtained by asking a person to describe his or her eating habits and factors that may affect nutrition.
- Problems commonly identified after a nutritional assessment include weight problems, anorexia, nausea, vomiting, and stomach gas.
- If a nutritional problem is beyond the scope of independent nursing practice, the nurse consults with the physician. If the problem can be resolved through independent nursing measures, the nurse may proceed by collaborating with the dietitian, selecting appropriate nursing interventions, and continuing to monitor the client to evaluate the effectiveness of the nursing care plan.
- Common hospital diets are regular, light, soft, mechanical soft, full liquid, and clear liquid, and various therapeutic modifications to these diets.
- Nurses are generally responsible for ordering and canceling diets for clients, serving and collecting meal trays, helping clients to eat, and recording the percentage of food eaten.
- Nurses must know the type of diet prescribed for each client, the purpose for the diet, and its characteristics.
- Influences on the nutritional status of older adults include age-related physical changes, underlying medical conditions, adverse effects of medication therapy, functional impairments, psychosocial conditions, and socioeconomic and environmental barriers.

CHAPTER 16

- Body fluid is a mixture of water, chemicals called electrolytes and nonelectrolytes, and blood cells.
- Fluid and its components are distributed within each fluid compartment by means of osmosis, filtration, passive diffusion, facilitated diffusion, and active transport.
- The nurse assesses fluid volume status by measuring a client's intake and output, obtaining daily weights, obtaining vital signs, monitoring bowel elimination patterns and stool characteristics, observing the color of urine, and assessing skin turgor, the condition of the oral mucous membranes, lung sounds, and level of consciousness.
- Fluid volume is restored by treating the underlying disorder, increasing oral intake, administering IV fluid replacements, controlling fluid losses, or a combination of these measures.
- Fluid volume excess is reduced or eliminated by treating the underlying disorder, restricting or limiting oral fluids, reducing salt consumption, discontinuing IV fluid infusions or reducing the infusing volume, administering drugs that promote urine elimination, or a combination of these interventions.
- IV fluids are administered to maintain or restore fluid balance, maintain or replace electrolytes, administer water-soluble vitamins, provide calories, administer drugs, and replace blood and blood products.
- Crystalloid solutions are mixtures of water and substances such as salt and sugar that totally dissolve. Colloid solutions are mixtures of water and suspended, undissolved substances such as blood cells.
- An isotonic solution has the same concentration of dissolved substances as plasma; a hypotonic solution has fewer dissolved substances; and a hypertonic solution is more concentrated than plasma.
- When selecting tubing for administering IV solutions, the nurse must consider whether to use primary or secondary tubing and vented or unvented tubing, which drop size is most appropriate, and whether or not a filter is needed.
- IV fluids may be infused by gravity or with the assistance of an infusion device such as a pump or volumetric controller.
- When selecting a vein for venipuncture, the nurse gives priority to a vein in the nondominant hand or arm that is fairly straight, is larger than the needle or catheter gauge, is likely to be undisturbed by joint movement, and appears unimpaired by previous trauma or use.
- Complications of IV fluid therapy include infiltration, phlebitis, infection, circulatory overload, thrombus formation, pulmonary embolus, and air embolism.
- An intermittent venous access device is used in clients who require intermittent IV fluid or medication administration or for emergency access to the vascular system.
- When administering blood, the nurse assesses vital signs before and during the transfusion; uses no smaller than a 20-gauge needle or catheter, normal saline solution, and Y-set tubing; and infuses the blood within 4 hours or less.
- During a blood transfusion, the nurse monitors the client closely for incompatibility; febrile, septic, and allergic reactions; chilling; circulatory overload; and signs of hypocalcemia.
- Parenteral nutrition is a technique for providing nutrients, such as protein, carbohydrate, fat, vitamins, minerals, and trace elements, intravenously rather than orally.

CHAPTER 17

- Hygiene refers to practices that promote health through personal cleanliness.
- Hygiene practices that most people perform regularly include bathing, shaving, oral hygiene, hair care, and nail care.
- A partial bath is more appropriate for older adults than a daily tub bath or shower, because they do not perspire as much as young adults and soap tends to dry their skin.
- Towel and bag baths add lubrication to the skin; avoid friction to preserve skin integrity; reduce transmission of microorganisms from one part of the body to another; save time; provide more opportunity for self-care; and promote comfort because of the warmth of the liquid.
- Use of a safety razor is contraindicated for clients who have clotting disorders, those receiving anticoagulants and thrombolytics, and those who are depressed and suicidal.
- Most dentists recommend using a soft-bristled or electric toothbrush, tartar-control toothpaste with fluoride, and dental floss.
- The chief hazard in providing oral hygiene for unconscious clients is aspiration of liquid into the lungs. To prevent aspiration, nurses position unconscious clients on the side with the head lower than the body. They use oral suction equipment to remove liquid from the mouth.
- To prevent damage during cleaning, the nurse holds dentures over a plastic or towel-lined container and uses cold or tepid water.
- The nurse can detangle a client's hair by applying conditioner, using a wide-toothed comb, and combing from the end of the hair toward the scalp.
- The nurse consults the physician about nail care for clients with diabetes or poor circulation.
- Daily hygiene also includes cleaning and caring for visual or hearing devices such as eyeglasses, contact lenses, artificial eyes, or hearing aids.
- Clients who cannot insert and care for contact lenses may consider wearing eyeglasses, using a magnifying lens, or doing without while they are ill.
- The sound that a hearing aid produces may be altered as a result of dead or weak batteries, batteries that are not making full contact, corroded batteries, malposition within the ear, excessive volume, impacted cerumen, and dirty or damaged components.
- Infrared listening devices are an alternative to hearing aids. They convert sound into infrared light and then reconvert the light into sound through a receiver worn in a headset with earphones.

CHAPTER 18

- Comfort is a state in which a person is relieved of distress. Rest is a waking state characterized by reduced activity and mental stimulation. Sleep is a state of arousable unconsciousness.
- Some environmental factors that promote comfort, rest, and sleep are colorful walls and room decor, reduced noise, increased natural sunlight, and a comfortable climate.
- Standard furnishings in all client rooms are the bed, the overbed table, the bedside stand, and at least one chair.
- Sleep is a basic human need. Among other things, it reduces fatigue, stabilizes mood, increases protein synthesis, promotes cellular growth and repair, and improves the capacity for learning and memory storage.
- The two phases of sleep are nonrapid and rapid eye movement sleep. During nonrapid eye movement (NREM) sleep and its four subdivisions, the body is active but the brain is not. During rapid eye movement (REM) sleep, the body is physically inactive but the brain is highly active.
- As humans age, they sleep fewer hours and spend less time in REM sleep. Newborns spend 16 to 20 hours of each day sleeping, approximately half in the REM phase. Older adults require 7 to 9 hours of sleep and spend only 13% to 15% in the REM phase.

- Circadian rhythms, activity, the environment, motivation, emotions and moods, food and beverages, illness, and drugs can affect the amount and quality of sleep.
- Four major categories of drugs either promote or interfere with sleep. Sedatives and tranquilizers produce a relaxing and calming effect, hypnotics induce sleep, and stimulants excite structures in the brain, causing wakefulness.
- Sleep questionnaires, sleep diaries, polysomnographic evaluations, and the multiple sleep latency test are techniques used to assess sleep patterns.
- Sleep disorders fall into four major categories: insomnia (difficulty falling asleep or staying asleep, or early morning awakening), hypersomnias (conditions resulting in daytime sleepiness despite adequate nighttime sleep), sleep–wake cycle disturbances (resulting from desynchronized periods of sleeping and wakefulness), and parasomnias (associated with activities that cause arousal or partial arousal usually during transitions in NREM periods of sleep).
- Sleep is promoted by exercising regularly during the day; avoiding alcohol, nicotine, and caffeine; performing sleep rituals; going to bed and getting up at about the same time every day; and getting out of bed if sleep does not come easily and returning after some nonstimulating activity.
- To promote relaxation, which facilitates the onset of sleep, nurses assist clients with progressive relaxation exercises or provide a back massage.
- Older adults tend to have more difficulty falling asleep, they awaken more readily, and they spend less time in the deeper stages of sleep. This explains why some older adults feel tired even though they have slept an appropriate time.

CHAPTER 19

- The Joint Commission considers safety a priority when caring for clients by identifying National Patient Safety Goals. The purpose of these goals, is to help health care organizations obtain and retain their accreditation by demonstrating safe and effective care of the highest quality. Compliance and achievement of the patient safety goals is evidenced by a reduced number of deaths and injuries among those being cared for in health agencies. Current examples of these goals can be obtained at http://www.jointcommission.org/standards_information/npsgs.aspx.
- Accidental injuries vary according to the victim's stage of development. Because infants must rely on their caretakers, they are susceptible to falls. Poisonings are common among toddlers. School-aged children suffer play-related injuries, and adolescents are often the victims of sport-related injuries. Young adults commonly are involved in motor-vehicle accidents. Middle-aged adults suffer a variety of physical traumas such as back injuries. Falls are common among older adults.
- Environmental hazards often contribute to injuries and deaths from latex sensitization, burns, asphyxiation, electrical shock, poisoning, and falls.
- Measures to reduce latex sensitization include using nonlatex gloves and medical equipment, washing hands after removing latex gloves, and avoiding use of petroleum-based hand creams or lotions, which retain latex protein on the skin.
- Most fire plans incorporate four steps: rescue those in danger, sound an alarm, confine the fire, and extinguish the blaze.
- There are four classes of fire extinguishers. Class A extinguishers are used for paper, wood, and cloth fires. Class B extinguishers are used on fuels and flammable liquids. Class C extinguishers are used for electrical fires. Class ABC extinguishers can be used on any type of fire.
- Methods of preventing burns include installing and maintaining smoke detectors, developing and practicing a fire evacuation plan, and never going back into a burning building.
- Common causes of asphyxiation include smoke inhalation, carbon monoxide poisoning, and drowning.
- Measures to prevent drowning are wearing approved flotation devices, avoiding alcohol consumption when around water, and never swimming alone.
- Humans are susceptible to injury from electrical shock because the human body is predominately composed of water and electrolytes, which are good conductors of electrical current.
- Electrical shock may be prevented by using three-pronged grounded equipment, making sure all cover plates are intact, and replacing equipment with frayed electrical cords.
- Substances commonly implicated in poisonings include chemicals such as drugs, cleaning agents, paint solvents, heavy metals, cosmetics, and plants.
- Poisonings may be prevented by using childproof caps on medication bottles, installing latches on storage cupboards, and never transferring a toxic substance to a container generally associated with food.
- Although physical restraints prevent falls, they create concomitant risks for constipation, incontinence, infections such as pneumonia, pressure ulcers, and a progressive decline in the ability to perform activities of daily living.
- The overuse of physical restraints in health care facilities has led to the passage of legislation and accreditation standards regulating their use.
- Restraints are devices that restrict movement; restraint alternatives are protective and adaptive devices that clients can remove independently.
- Restraint use may be justified when clients have a history of previous falls or may experience life-threatening consequences, when there has been an unsatisfactory response to restraint alternatives, when clients are seriously impaired mentally or physically, or if their movement must be restricted during a life-threatening event.
- If an accident occurs, the nurse's first concerns are the safety of the client and the potential for allegations of malpractice.
- Older adults in general are prone to falling because they have gait and balance problems resulting from age-related changes, visual impairment, postural hypotension, and urinary urgency.

CHAPTER 20

- Pain is an unpleasant sensation usually associated with disease or injury. All clients should have access to the best pain relief that can safely be provided.
- The four phases of pain are transduction, transmission, perception, and modulation.
- The pain threshold is the point at which pain-transmitting neurochemicals reach the brain and cause conscious awareness known as pain perception. Pain tolerance is the amount of pain a person endures once the threshold has been reached.
- Endogenous opioids are naturally produced chemicals with morphine-like characteristics. It is believed that these chemicals bind to sites on the nerve cell's membrane, blocking the transmission of pain-producing neurotransmitters.
- The five general types of pain are cutaneous pain, visceral pain, neuropathic pain, acute pain, and chronic pain.
- Acute pain differs from chronic pain in its duration, etiology, and response to therapeutic measures.
- When performing a basic pain assessment, the nurse asks the client to describe the onset, quality, intensity, location, and duration of pain.
- Four commonly used pain-intensity assessment tools are a numeric scale, a word scale, a linear scale, and a picture scale like the Wong–Baker FACES Pain Rating Scale.
- A pain assessment is performed, at a minimum, on admission, whenever vital signs are assessed, once per shift when pain is an actual or potential problem, and before and after implementing a pain-management intervention.
- The physiologic basis for pain management involves interrupting pain-transmitting chemicals at the site of injury, altering pain transmission at the spinal cord, and blocking pain perception in the brain.
- Three categories of drugs used to manage pain are nonopioids, opioids, and adjuvant drugs. The injection of botulinum toxin is a fairly new method for treating painful skeletal muscle conditions and headaches.
- Rhizotomy and cordotomy are surgical pain-management techniques used when other methods are ineffective.
- Examples of nondrug/nonsurgical methods of pain management are educating clients about pain and its control and using imagery, meditation, distraction, relaxation, and interventions such as applications of heat and cold, transcutaneous electrical nerve stimulation, acupuncture and acupressure, percutaneous electrical nerve stimulation, biofeedback, and hypnosis.

- Clients often request frequent doses of pain-relieving medications because the dosage or schedule for administration is not controlling the pain.
- Addiction is "a pattern of compulsive drug use characterized by a continued craving for an opioid and the need to use the opioid for effects other than pain relief."
- The fear of addiction leads to inadequate pain management.
- A placebo is an inactive substance given as a substitute for an actual drug. The positive effect some clients have from placebos probably results from the trust they have in the physician or nurse.

CHAPTER 21

- Ventilation is the act of moving air in and out of the lungs. Respiration refers to the mechanisms by which oxygen is delivered to the cells.
- External respiration takes place through alveolar–capillary membranes. Internal respiration occurs at the cellular level via hemoglobin and body cells.
- The oxygenation status of clients can be determined at the bedside by performing focused physical assessments, monitoring ABGs, and using pulse oximetry.
- Five signs of inadequate oxygenation are restlessness, rapid breathing, rapid heart rate, sitting up to breathe, and using accessory muscles.
- Nurses can improve the oxygenation of clients by positioning clients with the head and chest elevated and teaching them to perform breathing exercises.
- When oxygen therapy is prescribed, a source for the oxygen, a flowmeter, an oxygen delivery device, and in some cases an oxygen analyzer or humidifier are all needed.
- Oxygen may be supplied through a wall outlet, in portable tanks, within a liquid oxygen unit, or with an oxygen concentrator.
- Most clients receive oxygen therapy through a nasal cannula, any one of several types of masks, or a face tent. Those who have had an opening created in their trachea may receive oxygen through a tracheostomy collar, T-piece, or transtracheal catheter.
- Whenever oxygen is administered, nurses must be concerned about two hazards: the potential for fire and oxygen toxicity.
- Water seal chest tube drainage and hyperbaric oxygen chambers are two therapeutic techniques related to oxygenation.
- Older adults have unique respiratory risk factors for several reasons. They often have age-related structural and functional changes that may compromise ventilation and respiration.

CHAPTER 22

- Infectious diseases, also called community-acquired, contagious, or communicable diseases, are spread from one person to another.
- An infection is a condition that results when microorganisms cause injury to their host. Colonization refers to a condition in which microorganisms are present but the host is not damaged and has no signs or symptoms.
- Infectious diseases usually follow five stages: incubation, prodromal, acute, convalescent, and resolution.
- Infection control measures are designed to curtail the spread of infectious diseases.
- The two major categories of infection control measures are standard precautions and transmission-based precautions.
- Standard precautions are measures for reducing the risk of microorganism transmission from both recognized and unrecognized sources of infection. Transmission-based precautions are measures to control the spread of infectious agents from clients known to be or suspected of being infected with pathogens.
- Standard precautions include hand hygiene; use of gloves, gown, mask, and eye protection or face shield; and safe injection practices depending on the nature of the client interaction and extent of anticipated blood, body fluid, or pathogen exposure.
- Transmission-based precautions are used to prevent spreading pathogens via air, droplets, or contact with clients or objects that contain infectious microorganisms.
- Airborne precautions are used to block very small pathogens that remain suspended in the air or are attached to dust particles. Droplet precautions are used to block larger pathogens contained within moist droplets. Contact precautions are used to block the transmission of pathogens by direct or indirect contact.
- Personal protective equipment is defined as garments that block the transfer of pathogens from a person, place, or object to oneself or others.
- When removing personal protective equipment, nurses perform an orderly sequence, accompanied by hand hygiene, to prevent self-contamination and transmission of pathogens to others.
- Double-bagging is an infection control measure for removing contaminated items such as trash or laundry from the client's environment. It involves placing one bag within another held by someone outside the client's room.
- Clients with infectious diseases often have decreased social interaction and sensory deprivation because they are confined to their room.
- To prevent infections, people should obtain appropriate immunizations; practice a healthy lifestyle such as eating the recommended number of servings from the MyPlate nutrition guidelines; and avoid sharing personal items such as washcloths and towels, razors, and cups.
- Symptoms of infectious disorders tend to be subtler in older adults.

CHAPTER 23

- When standing, keep the feet parallel and distribute weight equally on both feet to provide a broad base of support. When sitting, the buttocks and upper thighs are the base of support on the chair; both feet rest on the floor. Correct posture for lying down is the same as for standing but in the horizontal plane; body parts are in neutral position.
- Principles of correct body mechanics include the following: distribute gravity through the center of the body over a wide base of support; push, pull, or roll objects rather than lifting them; and hold objects close to the body.
- Ergonomics is a field of engineering science devoted to promoting comfort, performance, and health in the workplace by improving the design of the work environment and equipment that is used.
- Two examples of ergonomic recommendations are to use assistive devices when lifting or transporting heavy items and to use alternatives for tasks that require repetitive motions.
- Disuse syndrome is associated with weakness, atony, poor alignment, contractures, foot drop, impaired circulation, atelectasis, urinary tract infections, anorexia, and pressure sores.
- Common client positions are supine (on the back), lateral (on the side), lateral oblique (on the side with slight hip and knee flexion), prone (on the abdomen), Sims' (semiprone on the left side with the right knee drawn up toward the chest), and Fowler's (semisitting or sitting).
- Positioning devices include the following: adjustable bed—allows the position of the head and knees to be changed; pillows—provide support and elevate a body part; trochanter rolls—prevent legs from turning outward; hand rolls—maintain function of the hand and prevent contractures; and foot boards—keep the feet in normal walking position.
- Pressure-relieving devices include the following: siderails—help clients to change position; mattress overlays—reduce pressure and promote skin integrity; and cradle—keeps linen off client's feet or legs.
- Devices used to help transfer clients include a transfer handle, a transfer belt, a transfer board, and a mechanical lift.
- Guidelines to follow when transferring clients include the following: know the client's diagnosis, capabilities, weaknesses, and activity level; be realistic about how much you can safely lift; transfer clients across the shortest distance possible; solicit the client's help; and use smooth rather than jerky movements.

CHAPTER 24

- Regular exercise has many benefits including reduced blood pressure, blood glucose and blood lipid levels, tension, and depression and increased bone density.
- Fitness refers to a person's capacity to perform physical activities.
- Factors that interfere with fitness include chronic inactivity, concurrent health problems, impaired musculoskeletal function, obesity, advancing age, smoking, and high blood pressure.
- Several approaches can be used to determine a person's level of fitness. Two objective methods are a stress electrocardiogram and a submaximal fitness test such as a step test.

- Exercise, regardless of type, should be performed within the person's target heart rate, which is calculated by subtracting the person's age from 220 (maximum heart rate) and then multiplying that number by 60% (0.6) to 90% (0.9), based on the person's fitness level.
- Metabolic energy equivalent (MET) is the measure of energy and oxygen consumption that a person's cardiovascular system can support safely. When an exercise prescription is given, exercises are correlated with their MET value.
- Fitness exercises are physical activities that develop and maintain cardiorespiratory function, muscular strength, and endurance in healthy adults. Therapeutic exercises involve physical activities designed to prevent health-related complications from an established medical condition or its treatment or to restore lost physical functions.
- Isotonic exercise involves movement and work; an example is aerobic exercise. Isometric exercise refers to stationary activities performed against a resistive force; examples are body building and weight lifting.
- Active exercise is performed independently after proper instruction. Passive exercise is performed with the assistance of another person.
- Range-of-motion (ROM) exercise is a form of therapeutic exercise that moves joints in the directions they normally permit. ROM exercises can be active or passive. Two common reasons for performing them are to maintain joint mobility and flexibility, especially in inactive clients, and to evaluate the client's response to a therapeutic exercise program.
- Nurses encourage older adults to exercise by walking in shopping malls or joining social groups that include activities such as line dancing or ballroom dancing.

CHAPTER 25

- Immobilization is used to relieve pain and muscle spasm, support and align skeletal injuries, and restrict movement while injuries heal.
- Four types of splints include inflatable splints, traction splints, immobilizers, and molded splints.
- Slings are cloth devices used to elevate and support parts of the body. Braces are custom-made or custom-fitted devices designed to support weakened structures during activity.
- Casts are rigid molds used to immobilize an injured structure that has been restored to correct anatomic alignment. Casts are formed from plaster of Paris or fiberglass.
- Three types of casts are cylinder, body, and spica.
- Appropriate nursing care of clients with casts includes checking circulation, mobility, and sensation in the area of the cast; using the palms of the hands to handle a wet cast; elevating the casted extremity to reduce swelling; circling areas where blood has seeped through; and padding and reinforcing the cast edges to prevent skin breakdown.
- Most casts are removed with an electric cast cutter, an instrument that looks like a circular saw.
- Traction is the application of a pulling effect on a part of the skeletal system.
- Three types of traction are manual traction, skin traction, and skeletal traction.
- To be effective, traction must produce a pulling effect on the body, countertraction must be maintained, the pull of traction and the counterpull must be in exactly opposite directions, splints and slings must be suspended without interference, ropes must move freely through each pulley, the prescribed amount of weight must be applied, and the weights must hang free.
- An external fixator is used to stabilize fragments of broken bones during healing.
- Pin site care is essential for preventing infection because the insertion of pins impairs skin integrity and provides a port of entry for pathogens.

CHAPTER 26

- Activities that help to prepare clients for ambulation include performing isometric exercises with the lower limbs, strengthening the upper arms, dangling at the bedside, and using a tilt table.
- Two isometric exercises that tone and strengthen the lower extremities are quadriceps setting and gluteal setting.
- The upper arms are strengthened by a regimen of flexing and extending the arms and wrists, raising and lowering weights with the hands, squeezing a ball or spring grip, and performing modified hand push-ups while in a bed or chair.
- Clients dangle or are placed on a tilt table to normalize their blood pressure and help them adjust to being upright.
- Parallel bars and walking belts are devices used to assist clients with ambulation.
- Three types of ambulatory aids are canes, walkers, and crutches.
- Walkers are the most stable form of ambulatory aid. Straight canes are the least stable.
- Crutches should permit the client to stand upright with the shoulders relaxed, provide space for two fingers between the axilla and the axillary bar, and facilitate approximately 30 degrees of elbow flexion and slight hyperextension of the wrist.
- The four types of crutch-walking gaits are four-point, three-point (non-weight-bearing or partial weight-bearing), two-point, and swing-through.
- A temporary prosthesis facilitates early ambulation, promotes an intact body image, and controls stump swelling immediately after surgery.
- The permanent prosthesis is constructed when the surgical wound heals and the stump size is relatively stable.
- Components of permanent prostheses for BK amputees are a socket, a shank, and an ankle/foot system; AK prostheses also include a knee system and thigh socket.
- To apply a prosthetic limb, the client covers the stump with an optional nylon sheath over which one or more stump socks are applied. A nylon stocking is used to ease the sock-covered stump into the socket and is eventually removed. The client pumps the stump within the socket to expel air and create a vacuum seal. If the socket has supportive belts or slings, they are fastened when the stump is well seated in the socket.
- Older adults tend to acquire flexion of the spine as they get older; this may alter their center of gravity. They tend to compensate by flexing their hips and knees when walking and may have a swaying or shuffling gait.

CHAPTER 27

- Perioperative care refers to the nursing care that clients receive before, during, and after surgery.
- Perioperative care spans the preoperative, intraoperative, and postoperative periods.
- Inpatient surgery is performed on clients who remain in the hospital at least overnight. Outpatient surgery is performed on clients who return home the same day.
- Laser surgery, which can be performed on an outpatient basis, offers several advantages: it is cost-effective, requires smaller incisions, results in minimal blood loss, and produces less pain.
- Some clients choose to donate their own blood before surgery or ask specific donors to do so.
- Four major activities for nurses to complete during the immediate preoperative period are conducting a nursing assessment, providing preoperative teaching, preparing the skin, and completing the surgical checklist.
- Nurses teach preoperative clients how to perform deep breathing, coughing, and leg exercises.
- Surgical clients wear antiembolism stockings to prevent thrombi and emboli.
- Skin preparation involves cleansing the skin and in some cases hair removal when it is likely to interfere with the incision. The goal is to decrease transient and resident bacteria without compromising skin integrity.
- When hair removal is required, electric clippers, depilatory agents, or a safety razor may be used depending on agency policy and medical orders.
- On the preoperative checklist, the nurse verifies that the history and physical examination have been completed, the name of the procedure matches the one scheduled, the surgical consent form has been signed and witnessed, the client is wearing an identification bracelet, and all laboratory test results have been returned and reported if abnormal.
- The receiving room, the operating room, and the surgical waiting room are three areas in the surgical department used during the intraoperative period.

- During immediate postoperative care, nurses focus on monitoring the client for complications, preparing the client's room, and continuing assessments to detect developing problems.
- Common postoperative complications are airway obstruction, hemorrhage, pulmonary embolus, and shock.
- During recovery, a pneumatic compression device may be prescribed to promote circulation of venous blood and relocation of excess fluid into the lymphatic vessels.
- Discharge instructions for surgical clients include how to care for the incisional site, signs of complications to report, and how to self-administer prescription drugs.
- Older adults have unique surgical needs and problems. For example, the period of fluid restriction before surgery may be shortened for older adults to reduce their risk for dehydration and hypotension. In addition, the cardiac status of older adults must be monitored carefully after surgery because they may not be able to circulate or eliminate intravenous fluids given at standard rates.

CHAPTER 28

- A wound is damaged skin or soft tissue.
- Wound repair involves three sequential phases: inflammation, proliferation, and remodeling.
- Signs and symptoms classically associated with inflammation are swelling, redness, warmth, pain, and decreased function.
- Phagocytosis, a process that removes pathogens, coagulated blood, and cellular debris, is performed by white blood cells known as neutrophils and monocytes.
- The integrity of damaged skin and tissue is restored by resolution, regeneration, or scar formation.
- Wounds heal by first, second, or third intention.
- Two common types of wounds that require special care are pressure ulcers and surgical wounds.
- Some purposes for covering a wound with a dressing are keeping it clean, absorbing drainage, and controlling bleeding.
- A moist wound heals more quickly because new cells grow more rapidly in a wet environment.
- Open or closed drains are placed in or near a wound to remove blood and drainage.
- Sutures or staples hold the edges of an incision together.
- A bandage or binder helps to hold a dressing in place, especially when tape cannot be used or the dressing is extremely large; reduces pain by supporting the wound; or limits movement to promote healing.
- A T-binder is used to secure a dressing to the anus, perineum, or groin.
- Four methods used to debride nonliving tissue from a wound are sharp debridement, enzymatic debridement, autolytic debridement, and mechanical debridement. A wound irrigation is an example of mechanical debridement.
- An irrigation is used to flush debris from a wound or body area such as the eye, ear, or vagina.
- Heat is applied to promote circulation and speed healing; cold is used to prevent swelling and control bleeding.
- Methods for applying heat or cold include ice bags, compresses, soaks, and therapeutic baths.
- Five factors that place clients at risk for developing pressure ulcers are inactivity, immobility, malnutrition, dehydration, and incontinence.
- Techniques for preventing pressure ulcers include changing clients' positions every 1 to 2 hours, keeping the skin clean and dry, and preventing friction and shearing force on the skin.

CHAPTER 29

- Intubation refers to the insertion of a tube into a body structure.
- GI intubation is used to provide nourishment; administer medications; obtain diagnostic samples; remove poisons, gases, and secretions; and control bleeding.
- Four types of tubes used to intubate the GI system are orogastric, nasogastric, nasointestinal, and transabdominal tubes.
- Common assessments performed before inserting a tube nasally include determining the client's level of consciousness, the characteristics and location of bowel sounds, the structure and integrity of the nose, and the client's ability to swallow, cough, and gag.
- A NEX measurement helps to determine how far to insert a tube for stomach placement. It is the distance from the nose to the earlobe and then to the xiphoid process.
- Nurses check stomach placement of tubes by aspirating gastric fluid, auscultating the abdomen as they instill a bolus of air, and testing the pH of aspirated fluid.
- Nasointestinal feeding tubes differ from their nasogastric counterparts in that they are longer, narrower, and more flexible; their lubricant is bonded to the tube; they are frequently inserted with a stylet; and an x-ray is used to confirm their placement.
- Although transabdominal feeding tubes can be used for long periods, they are prone to leaking and causing skin impairment.
- Enteral nutrition refers to nourishing clients by means of the stomach or small intestine rather than the oral route.
- Four common schedules for administering tube feedings are bolus, intermittent, cyclic, and continuous.
- Nurses check gastric residual to determine if the rate or volume of feeding exceeds the client's physiologic capacity.
- Caring for clients with feeding tubes involves maintaining tube patency, clearing any obstructions, providing adequate hydration, dealing with common formula-related problems, and preparing clients for home care.
- Before discharge, nurses provide clients who will administer their own tube feedings at home with written instructions on ways to obtain equipment and formula, the amount and schedule for each feeding, guidelines for delaying a feeding, and skin or nose care.
- When assisting with the insertion of a tungsten-weighted tube, nurses are responsible for promoting and monitoring its movement into the intestine.

CHAPTER 30

- The urinary system is composed of the kidneys, ureters, bladder, and urethra. Collectively, these organs serve to produce urine, collect it, and excrete it from the body.
- Various factors affect urination, such as a person's neuromuscular development, the integrity of the spinal cord, the volume of fluid intake, fluid losses from other sources, and the amount and type of food consumed.
- The physical characteristics of urine include its volume, color, clarity, and odor.
- Nurses often collect voided urine specimens, clean-catch urine specimens, catheter specimens, and 24-hour urine specimens.
- Some common abnormal patterns of urinary elimination include anuria, oliguria, polyuria, nocturia, dysuria, and incontinence.
- Other than a conventional toilet, a person may eliminate urine in a commode, urinal, or bedpan.
- Continence training is the process used to restore the ability to empty the bladder at an appropriate time and place.
- The three general types of catheters are external, straight, and retention.
- When using a closed drainage system, it is important to avoid dependent loops in the tubing, and the collection bag must be kept below the level of the bladder.
- Catheter care is important because it helps to deter the growth and spread of colonizing pathogens.
- Catheters are irrigated to keep them patent, or free-flowing.
- Catheters may be irrigated using an open or closed system or continuously by way of a three-way catheter.
- A urinary diversion is a procedure in which one or both ureters are surgically implanted elsewhere.
- Skin impairment is a common problem in clients with a urostomy because they require frequent appliance changes, and the contact of urine with the skin causes skin irritation.

CHAPTER 31

- Defecation, the elimination of stool, occurs when peristalsis moves fecal waste toward the rectum and the rectum distends, creating an urge to relax the anal sphincters; this releases stool.

- Two components of a bowel elimination assessment include elimination patterns and stool characteristics.
- Constipation, fecal impaction, flatulence, diarrhea, and fecal incontinence are common alterations in bowel elimination.
- The four types of constipation are primary constipation (which nurses can treat independently), secondary constipation, iatrogenic constipation, and pseudoconstipation.
- When bowel elimination does not occur naturally, inserting a rectal suppository or administering an enema can promote defecation.
- Two categories of enemas are cleansing and oil retention.
- Cleansing enemas are administered by instilling tap water, normal saline, soap and water, and other solutions.
- Oil retention enemas are given to lubricate and soften dry stool.
- When caring for clients with intestinal ostomies, nursing activities are likely to include providing peristomal care, applying an ostomy appliance, draining a continent ileostomy, and irrigating a colostomy.

CHAPTER 32

- A medication is a chemical substance that changes body function.
- A complete drug order contains the date and time of the order; the name of the client; the name of the drug, its dose, route, and frequency of administration; and the signature or name of the writer.
- A drug's trade name is the name by which a pharmaceutical company identifies its drug. A drug's generic name is a chemical name that is not exclusively used by any drug company.
- Common routes of medication administration are oral, topical, inhalant, and parenteral.
- The oral route is used to administer drugs intended for absorption in the gastrointestinal tract. Oral medications can be instilled by enteral tube when clients cannot swallow them.
- A medication administration record (MAR) is a form used to document and ensure timely and safe drug administration.
- Methods of supplying drugs to nursing units include an individual supply, a supply of unit dose packets, and a stock supply.
- Nurses are responsible for keeping the supply of narcotic medications locked and maintaining an accurate record of their use.
- The five rights involve making sure that the right client receives the right drug, in the right dose, at the right time, and by the right route.
- Once nurses have converted drug doses to the same system of measurement and the same measurement within that system, they can calculate the amount to administer by dividing the desired dose by the dose on hand and then multiplying it by the quantity of the supply.
- The nurse checks drug labels three times before administering the medication.
- When teaching clients about taking medications, nurses advise them to inform each health care provider of all prescription and nonprescription drugs currently being taken.
- A common problem when administering drugs through an enteral tube is maintaining the tube's patency.
- If a medication error occurs, nurses must report it to the prescriber and supervisor, assess the client for ill effects, and document the situation on an incident report or accident sheet.

CHAPTER 33

- Topical medications are applied to the skin or mucous membranes.
- Common locations for topical medications are the skin, eye, ear, nose, mouth, vagina, and rectum.
- An inunction is a medication incorporated into a vehicle, or transporting agent, such as an ointment, oil, lotion, or cream.
- Skin patches and applications of paste are two methods for administering transdermal medications.
- Skin patches can be applied to any skin area with adequate circulation. Each time a new patch is applied, it is placed in a different location.
- Eye medications are applied onto the mucous membrane, or conjunctiva, of the eye, which lines the inner eyelids and the anterior surface of the sclera.
- The major difference in the technique for administering ear medications to adults and children is how the ear is manipulated to straighten the auditory canal.
- The rebound effect is a phenomenon characterized by rapid swelling of the nasal mucosa. It is likely when clients chronically administer more than the recommended amount of nasal decongestant or use the drug too frequently.
- For sublingual administration, the drug is placed under the tongue. For buccal administration, the medication is placed in contact with the mucous membrane of the cheek.
- Vaginal applications are used most often to treat local infections.
- Drugs administered rectally usually are in the form of suppositories.
- The inhalant route is used for medication administration because the lungs provide an extensive area of tissue from which drugs may be absorbed.
- Drugs are commonly inhaled using dry powder inhalers or metered-dose inhalers. A dry powder inhaler delivers a burst of pulverized drug and a carrier substance at the time of inhalation. A metered-dose inhaler releases a measured volume of aerosolized drug when its canister is compressed.
- For clients who have difficulty mastering the use of an inhaler, a spacer provides a reservoir for aerosol medication that can be inhaled beyond the time of the initial breath. As an alternative, a nebulizer that converts liquid inhalant medication to an aerosol using compressed air that is subsequently inhaled through a mouthpiece or face mask over 10 to 20 minutes may be used.

CHAPTER 34

- Three parts of a syringe are the barrel, plunger, and tip, which is sometimes called the hub.
- When selecting a syringe and needle, the nurse considers the type of medication, depth of tissue, volume of prescribed drug, viscosity of the drug, and size of the client.
- Conventional syringes and needles are being redesigned to reduce the potential for needlestick injuries and transmission of blood-borne pathogens.
- Pharmaceutical companies supply drugs for parenteral administration in ampules, vials, and prefilled cartridges.
- Before combining two drugs in a single syringe, it is important to consult a drug reference or a compatibility chart to determine whether or not a chemical interaction may occur.
- Nurses use any of four parenteral injection routes: intradermal, subcutaneous, intramuscular, and intravenous.
- A common site for an intradermal injection is the inner forearm; subcutaneous injections are commonly given in the thigh, arm, or abdomen; intramuscular injections are given in the buttocks, hip, thigh, or arm.
- An intradermal injection is given with a tuberculin syringe. Insulin is administered subcutaneously with an insulin syringe. Intramuscular injections are usually given with a syringe that holds a volume up to 3 mL.
- For an intradermal injection, the needle is inserted at a 10- to 15-degree angle. For a subcutaneous injection, a 45- or 90-degree angle is used, depending on the client's size. For an intramuscular injection, a 90-degree angle is used.
- When two separate insulins are combined, they must be administered within 15 minutes to avoid equilibration (the loss of each insulin's unique characteristics).
- To prevent bruising when heparin is administered, the nurse avoids aspirating with the plunger and massaging the site afterward.

CHAPTER 35

- IV medications can be given into peripheral or central veins.
- The IV route is appropriate when a quick response is needed during an emergency, when clients have disorders that affect the absorption or metabolism of drugs, and when blood levels of drugs need to be maintained at a consistent therapeutic level.
- IV medications can be administered continuously or intermittently.
- Two methods for administering a bolus of IV medication are via a port on the IV tubing and via a medication lock.
- IV medication solutions may be administered intermittently using secondary (piggyback) infusions or a volume-control set.
- A piggyback solution is a small volume of diluted medication that is connected to and positioned higher than the primary solution.

- A volume-control set is used to administer IV medication in a small volume of solution at intermittent intervals to avoid overloading the circulatory system.
- A central venous catheter is a venous access device that extends to the superior vena cava or right atrium.
- The three general types of central venous catheters are percutaneous, tunneled, and implanted.
- When administering antineoplastic drugs, the nurse should wear a cover gown, one or two pairs of gloves, and a disposable or respirator mask to protect against contact with or inhalation of the medication.

CHAPTER 36

- Airway management refers to skills that nurses use to maintain natural or artificial airways for compromised clients.
- Structures of the airway are the nose, pharynx, trachea, bronchi, bronchioles, and alveoli.
- The airway serves as the collective system of tubes in the upper and lower respiratory tract through which gases travel during their passage to and from the blood.
- Structures to protect the airway include the epiglottis, which seals the airway when swallowing food and fluids; the rings of tracheal cartilage, which keep the trachea from collapsing; the mucous membrane, which traps particulate matter; and the cilia, which beat debris upward in the airway so that it can be coughed, expectorated, or swallowed.
- Methods of airway management include liquefying secretions, mobilizing secretions to promote their expectoration with chest physiotherapy, and mechanically suctioning mucus from the airway.
- When suctioning the airway, nurses use one of several approaches: nasopharyngeal, nasotracheal, oropharyngeal, oral, and tracheal suctioning.
- Artificial airways are used when clients are at risk for airway obstruction or when long-term mechanical ventilation is necessary.
- Two examples of artificial airways are an oral airway and a tracheostomy tube.
- Tracheostomy care includes cleaning the skin around the stoma, changing the dressing, and cleaning the inner cannula.

CHAPTER 37

- Airway obstruction is life-threatening because it interferes with ventilation and subsequently deprives cells and tissues of oxygen.
- Signs of airway obstruction include grasping the throat with the hands, making aggressive efforts to cough and breathe, and producing a high-pitched sound while inhaling.
- In cases of partial airway obstruction, appropriate actions include encouraging and supporting the victim's efforts to clear the obstruction independently and preparing to call for emergency assistance if the victim's condition worsens.
- The Heimlich maneuver is the technique used to relieve a complete airway obstruction by performing a series of subdiaphragmatic thrusts or chest thrusts on conscious victims.
- Subdiaphragmatic thrusts are appropriate for almost all adults and children beyond infancy. Chest thrusts are appropriate for infants less than 1 year old, obese adults, and women in advanced pregnancy.
- To dislodge an object from an infant's airway, the rescuer delivers a series of back blows followed by a series of chest thrusts.
- When a person with an airway obstruction becomes unconscious, rescuers perform basic cardiopulmonary resuscitation (CPR) rather than the Heimlich maneuver because chest compressions create enough pressure in unconscious victims to eject a foreign body from the airway.
- The Chain of Survival is a series of five steps that improves the outcome of resuscitating a person in cardiac arrest. The steps are (1) immediate recognition and access of emergency services; (2) early CPR, techniques used to restore circulation and breathing with a focus on compressions to circulate blood quickly and systemically; (3) rapid defibrillation, if appropriate; (4) effective advanced life support; and (5) integrated post-cardiac arrest care.
- Early cardiopulmonary resuscitation must proceed with CAB (Circulation, Airway, Breathing) if the rescuer is a trained health provider or hands-only chest compressions if untrained in cardiopulmonary resuscitation.
- The CAB of resuscitation involves administering chest compressions hard and fast, opening the airway to assess for the presence of spontaneous breathing, and performing rescue breathing.
- Rescuers can safely open a victim's airway under most circumstances by using the head tilt/chin lift technique or the jaw-thrust maneuver.
- Methods of administering rescue breathing are mouth-to-mouth, mouth-to-nose, and mouth-to-stoma.
- An automated external defibrillator is a portable, battery-operated device that analyzes heart rhythm and can deliver a series of electrical shocks to resuscitate a person who is lifeless or experiencing a lethal dysrhythmia. Ideally, an AED is used within 5 minutes of resuscitation efforts outside the hospital and within 2 minutes of resuscitation efforts within a health care facility.
- The decision to stop resuscitation efforts often is based on the time that elapsed before resuscitation began, the length of time that resuscitation has continued without any change in the victim's condition, and the age and diagnosis of the victim.

CHAPTER 38

- A terminal illness is one from which recovery is beyond reasonable expectation.
- The five stages of dying, as described by Dr. Elisabeth Kübler-Ross, are denial, anger, bargaining, depression, and acceptance.
- Nurses can promote acceptance by providing emotional support to dying clients and helping them to arrange their care.
- Respite care provides temporary relief for caregivers of dying loved ones.
- Hospice care involves helping clients to live their final days in comfort, with dignity, and in a caring environment.
- Some aspects that nurses address when providing terminal care are hydration, nourishment, elimination, hygiene, positioning, and comfort.
- Many terminal illnesses result in death from multiple organ failure. Signs of multiple organ failure include hypotension, rapid heart rate, difficulty breathing, cold and mottled skin, and decreased urinary output.
- When the criteria for organ donation are met, permission for organ removal must be obtained in a timely manner to ensure a successful transplant.
- Criteria used to confirm that a client has died include cessation of breathing and heart beat and absence of whole brain function.
- Postmortem care involves cleaning the body, ensuring proper identification, and releasing the body to mortuary personnel.
- Although grieving is painful, it promotes resolution of the loss.
- One sign that a person is resolving his or her grief is that he or she can talk about the deceased person without becoming emotionally overwhelmed.

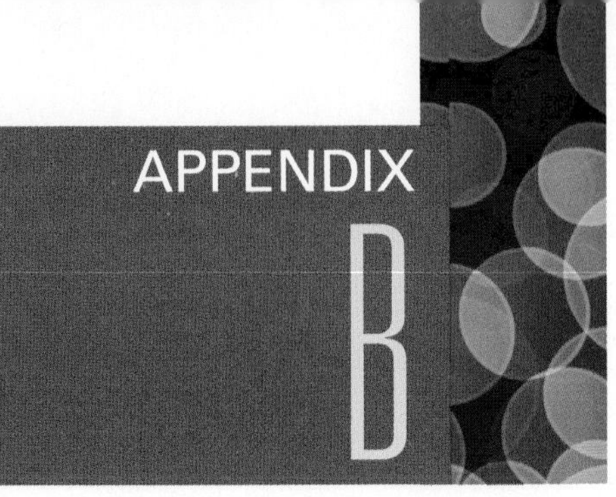

Commonly Used Abbreviations and Acronyms

SYMBOL

°	degree
<	less than
≤	equal to or less than
>	more than
≥	equal to or more than
±	plus or minus

WORDS

ADL	activities of daily living
AHCPR	Agency for Health Care Policy and Research
AIDS	acquired immune deficiency syndrome
AMA	against medical advice; *also* American Medical Association
ANA	American Nurses Association
BP	blood pressure
bpm	beats per minute
cal	calorie
CBC	complete blood count
CDC	Centers for Disease Control and Prevention
CHO	carbohydrate
CO_2	carbon dioxide
CPR	cardiopulmonary resuscitation
CT	computed tomography (also CAT)
CVC	central venous catheter
dL	deciliter (100 mL)
ECG	electrocardiogram (also EKG)
EEG	electroencephalogram
EMG	electromyography
EOMs	extraocular movements
g	gram
GI	gastrointestinal
HIV	human immunodeficiency virus
I&O	intake and output
ICN	International Council of Nurses
IM	intramuscular
IV	intravenous
IVP	IV push
IVPB	IV piggyback
JCAHO	Joint Commission on Accreditation of Healthcare Organizations; now known as the Joint Commission
kcal	kilocalorie
kg	kilogram (1,000 g)
L	liter
LPN	licensed practical nurse (also LVN, licensed vocational nurse)
MAR	medication administration record
mEq	milliequivalent
mg	milligram (one-thousandth g)
mL	milliliter (one-thousandth L)
mm Hg	millimeters of mercury
mph	miles per hour
MRI	magnetic resonance imaging
NANDA	North American Nursing Diagnosis Association
NAPNES	National Association for Practical Nurse Education and Service
NCLEX-PN	National Council Licensure Examination for Practical Nurses
NCLEX-RN	National Council Licensure Examination for Registered Nurses
NEX	nose, earlobe, xiphoid process
NKA	no known allergies
NLN	National League for Nursing
NPO	nil per os, nothing by mouth
NREM	nonrapid eye movement (sleep phase)
NSS	normal saline solution
NWB	non–weight-bearing
O_2	oxygen
OTC	over the counter (eg, nonprescription)
PACU	postanesthesia care unit
$PaCO_2$	partial pressure of carbon dioxide; that which is dissolved in plasma
PaO_2	partial pressure of oxygen; that which is dissolved in plasma
PCA	patient-controlled analgesia
PEG	percutaneous endoscopic gastrostomy
PEJ	percutaneous endoscopic jejunostomy
PERRLA	pupils equally round and react to light and accommodation
PET	positron emission tomography
pH	degree of acidity or alkalinity
PICC	peripherally inserted central catheter
PPN	peripheral parenteral nutrition
PWB	partial weight bearing
QA	quality assurance
RBC	red blood cell
REM	rapid eye movement (sleep phase)
RN	registered nurse
R/O	rule out; either confirm or eliminate
ROM	range of motion
SAD	seasonal affective disorder
SaO_2	oxygen saturation; percent of hemoglobin molecules saturated with oxygen
SNF	skilled nursing facility
SSE	soap suds enema
TPN	total parenteral nutrition
TPR	temperature, pulse, and respirations
WBC	white blood cell
WHO	World Health Organization

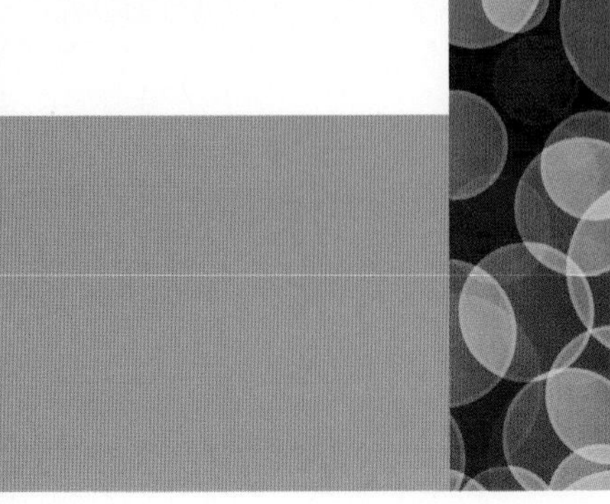

Glossary of Key Terms

A

ABO system method by which blood is identified as one of four blood types: A, B, AB, or O

Abdominal circumference indirect measurement of fatty (adipose) tissue that is distributed in and about the viscera of the abdomen

Acceptance attitude of complacency; last stage of dying, according to Dr. Kübler-Ross

Accommodation pupil constriction when looking at an object close by and dilation when looking at an object in the distance

Active exercise therapeutic activity performed independently

Active listening demonstrating full attention to what is being said; hearing both the content being communicated and the unspoken message

Active transport process of chemical distribution that requires an energy source

Activities of daily living acts that people normally do every day

Actual diagnosis problem that currently exists

Acultural nursing care care that lacks concern for cultural differences

Acupressure technique that involves tissue compression to reduce pain

Acupuncture pain-management technique in which long, thin needles are inserted into the skin

Acute illness one that comes on suddenly and lasts a short time

Acute pain discomfort of short duration

Adaptation manner in which an organism responds to change

Adjuvants drugs that assist in accomplishing the desired effect of a primary drug

Administrative laws legal provisions through which federal, state, and local agencies maintain self-regulation

Admission entering a health care agency for nursing care and medical or surgical treatment

Advance directive written statement identifying a competent person's wishes concerning terminal care

Advanced practice specialized areas of nursing expertise, such as nurse practitioner and nurse midwifery

Aerobic bacteria microorganisms that require oxygen to live

Aerobic exercise rhythmically moving all parts of the body at a moderate to slow speed without hindering the ability to breathe

Aerosol mist

Afebrile absence of a fever

Affective domain learning by appealing to a person's feelings, beliefs, or values

Affective touch touching that demonstrates concern or affection

African Americans those whose ancestral origin is Africa

Afterload force against which the heart pumps when ejecting blood

Ageism form of negative stereotypical thinking about older adults

Air embolism bubble of air in the vascular system

Airborne precautions infection control measures that reduce the risk for transmitting pathogens that remain infectious over long distances when suspended in the air

Airway collective system of tubes in the upper and lower respiratory tract

Airway management skills that maintain the patency of natural or artificial airways

Alarm stage the immediate physiologic response to a stressor

Alignment proper relation of one part to another

Allocation of scarce resources process of deciding how to distribute limited life-saving equipment or procedures

Allodynia exaggerated pain response due to increased sensitivity to stimuli such as air currents, pressure of clothing, and vibration

Alternative medical therapy treatment outside the mainstream of traditional medicine

Ambulatory electrocardiogram continuous recording of heart rate and rhythm during normal activity

Ampule sealed glass container for a drug

Anaerobic bacteria microorganisms that exist without oxygen

Analgesic pain-relieving drug

Anal sphincters ring-shaped bands of muscles in the anus

Anatomic position standing with arms at the sides and palms forward

Androgogy principles of teaching adult learners

Anecdotal record personal, handwritten account of an incident

Anesthesiologist physician who administers chemical agents that temporarily eliminate sensation and pain

Anesthetist nurse specialist who administers anesthesia under the direction of a physician

Anger emotional response to feeling victimized

Anglo-Americans people who trace their ancestry to the United Kingdom or Western Europe

Anions electrolytes with a negative charge

Ankylosis permanent loss of joint movement

Anorexia loss of appetite

Anorexia nervosa eating disorder characterized by an obsession for thinness that is achieved through self-starvation

Anthropometric data measurements of body size and composition

Anticipatory grieving grieving that begins before a loss actually occurs

Antiembolism stockings elastic stockings

Antimicrobial agents chemicals that limit the number of infectious microorganisms by destroying them or suppressing their growth

Antineoplastic drugs medications used to destroy or slow the growth of malignant cells

Antipyretics drugs that reduce fever

Antiseptics chemicals such as alcohol that inhibit the growth of, but do not kill, microorganisms

Anuria absence of urine, or up to a 100-mL volume in 24 hours
Apical heart rate number of ventricular contractions per minute
Apical-radial rate number of sounds heard at the apex of the heart and the rate of the radial pulse during the same period
Apnea absence of breathing
Appliance collection bag over a stoma
Aquathermia pad electrical heating or cooling device
Arrhythmia irregular pattern of heartbeats
Art ability to perform an act skillfully
Arterial blood gas laboratory test using blood from an artery
Asepsis practices that decrease or eliminate infectious agents, their reservoirs, and vehicles for transmission
Aseptic techniques measures that reduce or eliminate microorganisms
Asian Americans people who come from China, Japan, Korea, the Philippines, Thailand, Indochina, and Vietnam
Asphyxiation inability to breathe
Assault act in which there is a threat or attempt to do bodily harm
Assessment systematic collection of information
Assessment skills acts that involve collecting data
Asystole absence of heart rhythm
Atelectasis airless, collapsed lung areas
Audiometry measurement of hearing acuity at various sound frequencies
Auditors inspectors who examine client records
Auscultation listening to body sounds
Auscultatory gap period during which sound disappears and then reappears when taking a blood pressure measurement
Autologous transfusion self-donated blood
Automated external defibrillator device that delivers an electrical charge to the heart
Automated monitoring devices equipment that allows the simultaneous collection of multiple vital sign data
Autopsy postmortem examination
Axillary crutches standard type of crutches

B

Bag bath technique for bathing that involves the use of 8 to 10 premoistened, warmed, disposable cloths contained in a plastic bag
Balance steady position
Bandage strip or roll of cloth
Barcode medication administration system point of care software that verifies that the name of the medication, administration time, dosage, drug form, and client for whom the drug is prescribed are accurate by scanning a barcode on the drug and identification band on the client
Bargaining psychological mechanism for delaying the inevitable
Bariatric client person who is severely overweight with a body mass index (BMI) of 30 to 39.9 or morbidly obese with a BMI over 40
Barrel part of a syringe that holds the medication
Base of support area on which an object rests
Basic care facility agency that provides extended custodial care
Battery unauthorized physical contact
Bed bath washing with a basin of water at the bedside
Bed board rigid structure placed under a mattress
Bedpan seat-like container for elimination
Beliefs concepts that a person holds to be true
Beneficial disclosure an exemption whereby an agency can release private health information without a client's prior authorization
Bilingual able to speak a second language
Binder cloth covering applied to a body part such as the abdomen or breast
Biofeedback technique in which the client learns to control or alter a physiologic phenomenon
Biologic defense mechanisms methods that prevent microorganisms from causing an infectious disorder
Bivalved cast cast that is cut into two lengthwise pieces
Blood pressure force exerted by blood in the arteries
Blood substitutes fluids that when transfused carry and distribute oxygen to cells, tissues, and organs; also known as oxygen therapeutics
Board of nursing regulatory agency that manages the provisions of a state's nurse practice act
Body cast form of a cylinder cast that encircles the trunk of the body instead of an extremity
Body composition amount of body tissue that is lean versus fat
Body mass index numeric data used to compare a person's size in relation to norms for the adult population
Body mechanics efficient use of the musculoskeletal system
Body systems approach collection of data according to the functional systems of the body
Bolus larger dose of a drug administered initially or when pain is intense
Bolus administration undiluted or diluted medication given into a vein in one or more minutes of time
Bolus feeding instillation of liquid nourishment four to six times a day in less than 30 minutes
Braces custom-made or custom-fitted devices designed to support weakened structures
Bradycardia a pulse rate less than 60 beats per minute (bpm) in an adult
Bradypnea slower-than-normal respiratory rate at rest
Breakthrough pain acute pain that occasionally develops in those who have chronic pain
Bridge dental device that replaces one or several teeth
Bruxism grinding of the teeth
Buccal application drug placement against the mucous membranes of the inner cheek

C

Cachexia general wasting of body tissue
Calorie amount of heat that raises the temperature of 1 gram of water by 1°C
Cane hand-held ambulatory device made of wood or aluminum with a rubber tip
Capillary action movement of a liquid at the point of contact with a solid
Capillary refill time time duration for blood to resume flowing in the base of the nail beds
Capitation strategy for controlling health care costs by paying a fixed amount per member
Carbohydrates nutrients that contain molecules of carbon, hydrogen, and oxygen
Cardiac arrest cessation of heart contraction or life-sustaining heart rhythm
Cardiac ischemia impaired blood flow to the heart
Cardiac output volume of blood ejected from the left ventricle per minute
Cardiopulmonary resuscitation techniques used to restore circulation and breathing for lifeless victims
Caregiver one who performs health-related activities that a sick person cannot perform independently

Caries dental cavities

Caring skills nursing interventions that restore or maintain a person's health

Carriers asymptomatic clients or animals who harbor pathogens but do not show evidence of an infectious disease

Case method pattern in which one nurse manages a client's care for a designated period

Cast rigid mold around a body part

Cataplexy sudden loss of muscle tone, triggered by an emotional change such as laughing or anger

Catastrophize choosing to focus on all the potentially negative outcomes that may result from stressors

Catheter care hygiene measures used to keep the meatus and adjacent area of the catheter clean

Catheter irrigation flushing the lumen of a catheter

Catheterization act of applying or inserting a hollow tube

Cations electrolytes with a positive charge

Cellulose undigestible fiber in the stems, skin, and leaves of fruits and vegetables

Center of gravity point at which the mass of an object is centered

Centigrade scale scale that uses 0°C as the temperature at which water freezes and 100°C as the point at which it boils

Central venous catheter venous access device that extends to the superior vena cava

Certified interpreter translator who is certified by a professional organization through rigorous testing based on appropriate and consistent criteria

Cerumen ear wax

Cervical collar foam or rigid splint around the neck

Chain of infection sequence that enables the spread of disease-producing microorganisms

Chain of Survival intervention and rescue process including (1) immediate recognition and access of emergency services; (2) early CPR with a focus on compressions; (3) rapid defibrillation, if appropriate; (4) effective advanced life support; and (5) integrated post-cardiac arrest care

Change of shift report discussion between a nurse from the shift that is ending and personnel coming on duty

Chart binder or folder that enables the orderly collection, storage, and safekeeping of a client's medical records

Charting process of entering information

Charting by exception documentation method in which only abnormal assessment findings or care that deviates from the standard is charted

Checklist form of documentation in which the nurse indicates with a check mark or initials that routine care has been performed

Chemical restraint sedative medication that is not a standard treatment or dosage for the client's condition that is used to manage a violent or self-destructive client's behavior or freedom of movement

Chest physiotherapy techniques for mobilizing pulmonary secretions

Chronic illness one that comes on slowly and lasts a long time

Chronic pain discomfort that lasts longer than 6 months

Circadian rhythm phenomena that cycle on a 24-hour basis

Circulatory overload severely compromised heart function

Civil laws statutes that protect the personal freedoms and rights of individuals

Clean-catch specimen voided sample of urine that is considered sterile

Climate control mechanisms for maintaining temperature, humidity, and ventilation

Clinical pathways standardized multidisciplinary plans for a specific diagnosis or procedure that identify specific aspects of care to be performed during a designated length of stay

Clinical resume summary of previous care

Clinical thermometers instruments used to measure body temperature

Closed drainage system device used to collect urine from a catheter

Closed wound one in which there is no opening in the skin or mucous membrane

Code summoning personnel to administer advanced life support techniques

Code of ethics statements describing ideal behavior

Code status manner in which nurses or health care personnel must manage the care of a client during cardiac or respiratory arrest

Cognitive domain style of processing information by listening or reading facts and descriptions

Cold spot area with little or no radionuclide concentration

Collaborative problem physiologic complication whose treatment requires both nurse- and physician-prescribed interventions

Collaborator one who works with others to achieve a common goal

Collagen protein substance that is tough and inelastic

Colloidal osmotic pressure force for attracting water

Colloids undissolved protein substances

Colloid solutions water and molecules of suspended substances, such as blood cells, and blood products such as albumin

Colonization condition in which microorganisms are present but the host manifests no signs or symptoms of infection

Colostomy opening to some portion of the colon

Comfort state in which a person is relieved of distress

Comforting skills interventions that provide stability and security during a health crisis

Commode portable chair used for elimination

Common law decisions based on prior cases of a similar nature

Communicable diseases infectious diseases that can be transmitted to other people

Communication exchange of information

Community-acquired infections infectious diseases that can be transmitted to other people

Compartment syndrome complication following the application of a cast caused by pressure due to swelling within inelastic fascia that surrounds muscles

Complete proteins those that contain all of the essential amino acids

Compresses moist cloths that may be warm or cool

Computed tomography form of roentgenography that shows planes of tissue

Computerized charting documenting client information electronically

Concept mapping organizing information in a graphic or pictorial form

Concurrent disinfection measures that keep the client environment clean on a daily basis

Confidentiality safeguarding a client's health information from public disclosure

Congenital disorder disorder present at birth that results from faulty embryonic development

Conscious sedation state in which clients are sedated, relaxed, and emotionally comfortable, but not unconscious

Consensual response brisk, equal, and simultaneous constriction of both pupils when one eye and then the other are stimulated with light

Constipation condition in which dry, hard stool is difficult to pass

Contact precautions infection control measures used to block the transmission of pathogens by skin-to-skin contact with an infected or colonized person or touching a contaminated intermediate object in the client's environment

Contagious diseases infectious diseases that can be transmitted to other people

Continence training process of restoring control of urination

Continent ostomy surgically created opening in which liquid stool or urine is removed by siphoning

Continuity of care uninterrupted client care despite the change in caregivers

Continuous feeding instillation of liquid nutrition without interruption

Continuous infusion parenteral instillation over several hours

Continuous irrigation ongoing instillation of solution

Continuous passive motion machine electrical device that exercises joints

Continuous quality improvement process of promoting care that reflects established agency standards

Contractures permanently shortened muscles that resist stretching

Contrast medium substance that adds density to a body organ or cavity, such as barium sulfate or iodine

Controlled substances drugs whose prescription and dispensing are regulated by federal law because they have the potential for abuse

Coping mechanisms unconscious tactics used to protect the psyche

Coping strategies stress-reduction activities selected on a conscious level

Cordotomy surgical interruption of pain pathways in the spinal cord

Core temperature warmth at the center of the body

Coroner person legally designated to investigate deaths that may not be the result of natural causes

Counseling skills interventions that include communicating with clients, actively listening to the exchange of information, offering pertinent health teaching, and providing emotional support

CPAP mask device that maintains positive pressure in the airway throughout the respiratory cycle

Credé maneuver act of bending forward and applying hand pressure over the bladder to stimulate urination

Criminal laws penal codes that protect citizens from persons who are a threat to the public good

Critical thinking process of objective reasoning; analyzing facts to reach a valid conclusion

Cross-trained ability to assume a non-nursing job position, depending on the census or levels of client acuity on any given day

Crutches ambulatory aid, generally in pairs, constructed of wood or aluminum

Crutch palsy weakening of forearm, wrist, and hand muscles because of nerve impairment in the axilla caused by incorrectly fitted crutches or poor posture

Crystalloid solution water and other uniformly dissolved crystals, such as salt and sugar

Cultural shock bewilderment over behavior that is culturally atypical

Culturally sensitive nursing care care that is respectful of and is compatible with each client's culture

Culture (1) values, beliefs, and practices of a particular group; (2) incubation of microorganisms

Cutaneous application drug administration by rubbing medication into or placing it in contact with the skin

Cutaneous pain discomfort that originates at the skin level

Cutaneous triggering the act of lightly massaging or tapping the skin above the pubic area to stimulate urination

Cuticles thin edge of skin at the base of the nail

Cyclic feeding continuous instillation of liquid nourishment for 8 to 12 hours

Cylinder cast rigid mold that encircles an arm or leg

D

Dangling sitting on the edge of a bed

Data base assessment initial information about the client's physical, emotional, social, and spiritual health

Deaf unable to hear well enough to process information

Death certificate legal document confirming a person's death

Debridement removal of dead tissue

Decompression removal of gas and secretions from the stomach or bowel

Defamation act in which untrue information harms a person's reputation

Defecation bowel elimination

Defendant person charged with violating the law

Dehydration fluid deficit in both extracellular and intracellular compartments

Delegator one who assigns a task to someone

Deltoid site injection area in the lateral upper arm

Denial psychological defense mechanism in which a person refuses to believe that certain information is true

Dentures artificial teeth

Deontology ethical study based on duty or moral obligations

Depilatory agent chemical that removes hair

Depression sad mood

Diagnosis identification of health-related problems

Diagnostic examination procedure that involves physical inspection of body structures and evidence of their function

Diagnostic-related group classification system used to group clients with similar diagnoses

Diaphragmatic breathing breathing that promotes the use of the diaphragm rather than upper chest muscles

Diarrhea urgent passage of watery stools

Diastolic pressure pressure in the arterial system when the heart relaxes and fills with blood

Diet history assessment technique used to obtain facts about a person's eating habits and factors that affect nutrition

Directed donors relatives and friends who donate blood for a client

Discharge termination of care from a health care agency

Discharge instructions directions for managing self-care and medical follow-up

Discharge planning predetermining a client's post-discharge needs and coordinating the use of appropriate community resources to provide a continuum of care

Disinfectants chemicals that destroy active microorganisms but not spores

Distraction intentional diversion of attention
Disuse syndrome signs and symptoms that result from inactivity
Diversity differences among groups of people
Documenting process of entering information
Doppler stethoscope device that helps detect sounds created by the velocity of blood moving through a blood vessel
Dorsal recumbent position reclining posture with the knees bent, hips rotated outward, and feet flat
Dorsogluteal site injection area in the upper outer quadrant of the buttocks
Dose amount of drug
Double-bagging infection control measure in which one bag of contaminated items, such as trash or laundry, is placed within another, keeping the outer surface of the second bag clean
Double charting repetitious entry of the same information in the medical record
Douche procedure for cleansing the vaginal canal
Drains tubes that provide a means for removing blood and drainage from a wound
Drape sheet of soft cloth or paper
Drawdown effect cooling of the ear when it comes in contact with a thermometer probe
Dressing cover over a wound
Drop factor number of drops per milliliter in intravenous tubing
Droplet precautions measures that block transmission of infectious pathogens within moist droplets larger than 5 microns that are present in respiratory secretions or mucous membranes
Drowning situation in which fluid occupies the airway and interferes with ventilation
Drug diversion obtaining a drug through illicit methods such as theft from a person for whom the drug has been prescribed, "doctor shopping," purchase from illegal internet pharmacies, prescription forgery, or unnecessary prescriptions from less than ethical physicians
Drug tolerance diminished effect of a drug at its usual dosage range
Dry powder inhaler device containing a reservoir of pulverized drug and a carrier substance that relies on the client's inspiratory effort to deliver the drug into the lungs
Dumping syndrome cluster of symptoms resulting from the rapid deposition of calorie-dense nourishment into the small intestine
Durable power of attorney for healthcare proxy for making medical decisions when a client becomes incompetent or incapacitated and cannot make decisions independently
Duty obligation to provide care for a person claiming injury or harm
Dying with dignity treating a terminally ill person with respect regardless of his or her emotional, physical, or cognitive state
Dysphagia difficult swallowing
Dyspnea difficult or labored breathing
Dysrhythmia irregular pattern of heartbeats
Dysuria difficult or uncomfortable voiding

E

Echography soft tissue examination that uses sound waves in ranges beyond human hearing
Edema excessive fluid in tissue
Educator one who provides information
Electrical shock discharge of electricity through the body
Electrocardiography examination of the electrical activity in the heart
Electrochemical neutrality balance of cations with anions
Electroencephalography examination of the energy emitted by the brain
Electrolytes chemical compounds, such as sodium and chloride, that are dissolved, absorbed, and distributed in body fluid and possess an electrical charge
Electromyography examination of the energy produced by stimulated muscles
Emaciation excessive leanness
Emancipated minor adolescent living independent of parents or guardians and supporting himself or herself
Emboli moving clots
Emesis substance that is vomited
Empathy intuitive awareness of what the client is experiencing
Emulsion mixture of two liquids, one of which is insoluble in the other
Endogenous opioids naturally produced morphine-like chemicals
Endorphins natural body chemicals that produce effects similar to those of opiate drugs such as morphine
Endoscopy visual examination of internal structures
Enema introduction of a solution into the rectum
Energy capacity to do work
Enteral nutrition nourishment provided via the stomach or small intestine rather than via the oral route
Enteric-coated tablet tablet covered with a substance that does not dissolve until it is past the stomach
Enterostomal therapist a nurse certified in caring for ostomies and related skin problems
Environmental hazards potentially dangerous conditions in the physical surroundings
Environmental psychologist specialist who studies how the environment affects behavior
Equianalgesic dose oral dose that provides the same level of pain relief as a parenteral dose
Ergonomics field of engineering science devoted to promoting comfort, performance, and health in the workplace
Eructation belching
Essential amino acids protein components that must be obtained from food because they cannot be synthesized by the body
Ethical dilemma choice between two undesirable alternatives
Ethics moral or philosophical principles
Ethnicity bond or kinship a person feels with his or her country of birth or place of ancestral origin
Ethnocentrism belief that one's own ethnicity is superior to all others
Evaluation process of determining whether a goal has been reached
Evidence-based practice scientific knowledge used to predict nursing interventions most likely to produce a desired outcome
Exacerbation reactivation of a disorder, or one that reverts from a chronic to an acute state
Excoriation chemical skin injury
Exercise purposeful physical activity
Exit route means by which microorganisms escape from their original reservoir
Expiration exhalation; breathing out
Extended care services that meet the health needs of clients who no longer require acute hospital care
Extended care facility health care agency that provides long-term care

External catheter device applied to the skin that collects urine

External fixator metal device inserted into and through one or more bones

Extracellular fluid fluid outside cells

Extraocular movements eye movements controlled by several pairs of eye muscles

F

Face tent device that provides oxygen in an area around the nose and mouth

Facilitated diffusion process in which certain dissolved substances require the assistance of a carrier molecule to pass from one side of a semipermeable membrane to the other

Fahrenheit scale scale that uses 32°F as the temperature at which water freezes and 212°F as the point at which it boils

False imprisonment interference with a person's freedom to move about at will without legal authority to do so

Fat nutrient that contains molecules composed of glycerol and fatty acids called glycerides

Fat-soluble vitamins those carried and stored in fat; vitamins A, D, E, and K

Febrile elevated body temperature

Fecal impaction condition in which it is impossible to pass feces voluntarily

Fecal incontinence inability to control the elimination of stool

Feces stool

Feedback loop mechanism that turns hormone production off and on

Felony serious criminal offense

Fenestrated drape one with an open circle at its center

Fever body temperature that exceeds 99.3°F (37.4°C)

Fifth vital sign client's pain assessment that is checked and documented, in addition to his or her temperature, pulse, respirations, and blood pressure

Filtration process that regulates the movement of water and substances from a compartment where the pressure is high to one where the pressure is lower

Fingerspelling in sign language, alphabetical substitute for words that have no sign

Finger sweep insertion of the index finger into the mouth along the inside of the cheek and deeply into the throat to the base of the tongue

Fire plan procedure followed if there is a fire

First-intention healing reparative process when wound edges are directly next to one another

Fitness capacity to exercise

Fitness exercise physical activity performed by healthy adults

Flatulence accumulation of intestinal gas

Flatus gas formed in the intestine and released from the rectum

Fight or flight response physiologic process used to attack a stressor in an effort to overcome the danger it represents, or flee from the stressor to escape its threat

Flow sheet form of documentation that contains sections for recording frequently repeated assessment data

Flowmeter gauge used to regulate the number of liters of oxygen delivered to the client

Fluid imbalance condition in which the body's water is not in proper volume or location in the body

Fluoroscopy form of radiography that displays an image in real time

Focus assessment information that provides more details about specific problems

Focus charting modified form of SOAP charting

Folk medicine health practices unique to a particular group of people

Fomites nonliving reservoirs of pathogens

Foot drop permanent dysfunctional position caused by shortening of the calf muscles and lengthening of the opposing muscles on the anterior leg

Forced coughing coughing that is purposely produced

Forearm crutches crutches with an arm cuff but no axillary bar

Fowler's position upright seated position

Fraction of inspired oxygen portion of oxygen in relation to total inspired gas

Frenulum structure that attaches the undersurface of the tongue to the fleshy portion of the mouth

Frequency need to urinate often

Functional assessment determining a person's ability to perform self-care task

Functional braces braces that provide stability for a joint

Functional mobility alignment that maintains the potential for movement and ambulation

Functional nursing pattern in which each nurse on a unit is assigned specific tasks

Functional position position that promotes continued use and mobility

Functionally illiterate possessing minimal literacy skills

G

Gastric reflux reverse flow of gastric contents

Gastric residual volume of liquid remaining in the stomach

Gastrocolic reflex increased peristaltic activity

Gastrostomy tube, G-tube transabdominal tube located in the stomach

Gauge diameter

Gavage provision of nourishment

General adaptation syndrome collective physiologic processes that occur in response to a stressor

Generalization supposition that a person shares cultural characteristics with others of a similar background

Generic name chemical drug name that is not protected by a manufacturer's trademark

Gerogogy techniques that enhance learning among older adults

Gingivitis inflammation of the gums

Glucometer instrument that measures the amount of glucose in capillary blood

Gluteal setting contraction and relaxation of the gluteus muscles to strengthen and tone them

Goal expected or desired outcome

Good Samaritan laws legal immunity for passersby who provide emergency first aid to accident victims

Gram staining process of adding dye to a microscopic specimen

Granulation tissue combination of new blood vessels, fibroblasts, and epithelial cells

Gravity force that pulls objects toward the center of the earth

Grief response psychological and physical phenomena experienced by those who grieve

Grief work activities involved in grieving

Grieving process of feeling acute sorrow over a loss

H

Hand antisepsis removal and destruction of transient microorganisms from the hands

Hand hygiene methods for removing surface contaminants on the skin

Handwashing aseptic practice that involves scrubbing the hands with plain soap or detergent, water, and friction

Hard of hearing state of having limited hearing, in which communication is nonetheless possible

Head tilt/chin lift technique preferred method for opening the airway

Head-to-toe approach gathering data from the top of the body to the feet

Health state of complete physical, mental, and social well-being; not merely the absence of disease or infirmity

Health care system network of available health services

Health literacy degree to which individuals have the capacity to obtain, process, and understand basic health information and services needed to make appropriate health decisions

Health maintenance organizations corporations that charge members preset, fixed, yearly fees in exchange for providing health care

Hearing acuity ability to hear and to discriminate sound

Heimlich maneuver method for removing a mechanical airway obstruction

Hereditary condition disorder acquired from the genetic codes of one or both parents

Holism philosophical concept of interrelatedness

Home health care in-home health care provided by an employee of a home health agency

Homeostasis relatively stable state of physiologic equilibrium

Hospice facility for or concept addressing the care of terminally ill clients

Hot spot area where radionuclide is intensely concentrated

Human needs factors that motivate behavior

Humidifier device that produces small water droplets

Humidity amount of moisture in the air

Hydrostatic pressure pressure exerted against a membrane

Hydrotherapy therapeutic use of water

Hygiene personal cleanliness practices that promote health

Hyperalgesia amplified pain experience

Hyperbaric oxygen therapy delivery of 100% oxygen at three times the normal atmospheric pressure in an airtight chamber

Hypercarbia excessive levels of carbon dioxide in the blood

Hyperendemic infections infections that are considered highly dangerous in all age groups

Hypersomnia sleep disorder characterized by feeling sleepy despite getting a normal amount of sleep

Hypersomnolence excessive sleeping

Hypertension high blood pressure

Hyperthermia excessively high core temperature

Hypertonic solution solution that is more concentrated than body fluid

Hyperventilation rapid or deep breathing, or both

Hypervolemia higher-than-normal volume of water in the intravascular fluid compartment

Hypnogogic hallucinations dream-like auditory or visual experiences while dozing or falling asleep

Hypnosis therapeutic technique in which a person enters a trance-like state

Hypnotic agent that produces sleep

Hypoalbuminemia deficit of albumin in the blood

Hypopnea hypoventilation

Hypotension low blood pressure

Hypothalamus temperature-regulating structure in the brain

Hypothalamus-pituitary-adrenal (HPA) axis pathway of physiologic communication among the central nervous, endocrine, and immune systems

Hypothermia core body temperature less than 95°F (35°C)

Hypotonic solution one that contains fewer dissolved substances than normally found in plasma

Hypoventilation diminished breathing

Hypovolemia low volume in the extracellular fluid compartments

Hypoxemia insufficient oxygen in arterial blood

Hypoxia inadequate oxygen at the cellular level

I

Idiopathic illness one in which the cause is unexplained

Ileostomy surgically created opening to the ileum

Illiterate unable to read or write

Illness state of being unwell

Imagery using the mind to visualize an experience

Immobilizers commercial splints made from cloth and foam

Implementation carrying out a plan of care

Incentive spirometry technique for deep breathing using a calibrated device

Incident report written account of an unusual event involving a client, employee, or visitor that has the potential for being injurious

Incomplete proteins those that contain some, but not all, of the essential amino acids

Incontinence inability to control either urinary or bowel elimination

Individual supply single container of drugs with several days' worth of doses

Induration area of hardness

Infection condition that results when microorganisms cause injury to a host

Infection control precautions physical measures designed to curtail the spread of infectious diseases

Infectious diseases diseases spread from one person to another

Infiltration escape of intravenous fluid into the tissue

Inflammation physiologic defense that occurs immediately after tissue injury

Inflatable splints immobilizing devices that become rigid when filled with air

Informed consent permission that a person gives after having the risks, benefits, and alternatives explained

Infusion pump device that uses pressure to infuse solutions

Inhalant route drug administration into the lower airways

Inhalation therapy respiratory treatments that provide a mixture of oxygen, humidification, and aerosolized medication

Inhalers hand-held devices for delivering medication to the respiratory passages

Inpatient surgery operative procedures performed on persons admitted to a hospital and expected to remain for a period of time

Insomnia sleep disorder involving early awakening or difficulty falling asleep or staying asleep

Inspection purposeful observation

Inspiration inhalation; breathing in

Insulin syringe syringe that is calibrated in units and holds a volume of 0.5 to 1 mL of medication

Intake and output record of a client's fluid intake and fluid loss over a 24-hour period
Integrated delivery system network that provides a full range of healthcare services in a highly coordinated, cost-effective manner
Integument covering, the skin
Intentional tort lawsuit in which a plaintiff charges that a defendant committed a deliberately aggressive act
Intermediate care facility agency that provides health-related care and services to people who, because of their mental or physical condition, require institutional care but not 24-hour nursing care
Intermittent feeding gradual instillation of liquid nourishment four to six times a day
Intermittent infusion parenteral administration of medication over a relatively short period
Intermittent venous access device sealed chamber that provides a means for administering intravenous medications or solutions on a periodic basis
Interstitial fluid fluid in tissue space between and around cells
Intestinal decompression removal of gas and intestinal contents
Intimate space distance within 6 in. of a person
Intracellular fluid fluid inside cells
Intractable pain pain unresponsive to methods of pain management
Intradermal injection parenteral drug administration between the layers of the skin
Intramuscular injection parenteral drug administration into the muscle
Intraoperative period time when a client undergoes surgery
Intraspinal analgesia method of relieving pain by instilling a narcotic or local anesthetic via a catheter into the subarachnoid or epidural space of the spinal cord
Intravascular fluid watery plasma, or serum, portion of blood
Intravenous fluids solutions infused into a client's vein
Intravenous injection parenteral drug administration into a vein
Intravenous route drug administration via peripheral and central veins
Introductory phase period of getting acquainted
Intubation placement of a tube into a structure of the body
Inunction medication incorporated into an agent, such as an ointment, oil, lotion, or cream
Invasion of privacy failure to leave people and their property alone
Ions substances that carry either a positive or a negative electrical charge
Irrigation technique for flushing debris
Isometric exercise stationary exercises that are generally performed against a resistive force
Isotonic exercise activity that involves movement and work
Isotonic solution solution that contains the same concentration of dissolved substances as normally found in plasma

J

Jaeger chart visual assessment tool with small print
Jaw-thrust maneuver alternative method for opening the airway
Jejunostomy tube; J-tube transabdominal tube that leads to the jejunum of the small intestine
Jet lag emotional and physical changes experienced when arriving in a different time zone

K

Kardex quick reference for current information about the client and the client's care
Kegel exercises isometric exercises to improve the ability to retain urine within the bladder
Kilocalories 1,000 calories, or the amount of heat that raises the temperature of 1 kg of water by 1°C
Kinesics body language
Knee-chest position position in which the client rests on the knees and chest
Korotkoff sounds sounds that result from the vibrations of blood in the arterial wall or changes in blood flow

L

Laboratory test procedure that involves the examination of body fluids or specimens
Lateral oblique position variation of a side-lying position
Lateral position side-lying position
Latex-safe environment room stocked with latex-free equipment and wiped clean of glove powder
Latex sensitivity allergic response to the proteins in latex
Latinos people who trace their ethnic origin to South America
Lavage wash out; remove poisonous substances
Laws rules of conduct established and enforced by the government of a society
Leukocytes white blood cells
Leukocytosis increased production of white blood cells
Liability insurance contract between a person or corporation and a company who is willing to provide legal services and financial assistance when a policyholder is involved in a malpractice lawsuit
Libel damaging statement that is written and read by others
Limited English proficiency (LEP) inability to speak, read, write, or understand English at a level that permits effective interaction
Line of gravity imaginary vertical line that passes through the center of gravity
Lipoatrophy breakdown of subcutaneous fat at the site of repeated insulin injections
Lipohypertrophy thickening of subcutaneous fat at insulin injection sites
Lipoproteins combinations of fats and proteins
Liquid oxygen unit device that converts cooled liquid oxygen to a gas by passing it through heated coils
Literacy ability to read and write
Lithotomy position reclining posture with the feet in metal supports called stirrups
Living will a person's advance, written directive identifying medical interventions to use or not to use in cases of terminal condition, irreversible coma, or vegetative state with no hope of recovery
Loading dose larger dose of a drug administered initially or when pain is intense
Long-term goals desirable outcomes that take weeks or months to accomplish
Lumbar puncture procedure that involves insertion of a needle between lumbar vertebrae in the spine but below the spinal cord itself
Lumen channel

M

Macrophages white blood cells that consume cellular debris
Macroshock harmless distribution of low-amperage electricity over a large area of the body

Magnetic resonance imaging diagnostic tool used to identify disorders that affect structures in the body without performing surgery; a magnetic field excites hydrogen atoms within the body creating a radio signal that is converted into an image on a computer monitor

Malingerer someone who pretends to be sick or in pain

Malnutrition condition resulting from a lack of proper nutrients in the diet

Malpractice professional negligence

Managed care organizations private insurers who carefully plan and closely supervise distribution of their clients' health care services

Managed care practices cost-containment strategies used to plan and coordinate a client's care to avoid delays, unnecessary services, or overuse of expensive resources

Manual traction pulling on the body using a person's hands and muscular strength

Massage stroking the skin

Mattress overlay layer of foam or other devices placed on top of the mattress

Maximum heart rate highest limit for heart rate during exercise

Medicaid state-administered program designed to meet the needs of low-income residents

Medical asepsis practices that confine or reduce the numbers of microorganisms

Medical records written collection of information about a person's health problems, the care provided by health practitioners, and the progress of the client

Medicare federal program that finances health care costs of persons who are 65 years and older, permanently disabled workers and their dependents, and people with end-stage renal disease

Medication administration record agency form used to document drug administration

Medication order directions for administering a drug

Medications chemical substances that change body function

Meditation concentrating on a word or idea that promotes tranquility

Megadoses amounts exceeding those considered adequate for health

Melatonin hormone that induces drowsiness and sleep

Mental status assessment technique for determining the level of a client's cognitive functioning

Metabolic energy equivalent measure of energy and oxygen consumption during exercise

Metabolic rate use of calories for sustaining body functions

Metered-dose inhaler canister that contains medication under pressure

Microabrasions tiny cuts in the skin that provide an entrance for microorganisms

Microorganisms living animals or plants visible only with a microscope

Microshock low-voltage but high-amperage electricity

Microsleep unintentional sleep lasting 20 to 30 seconds

Midarm circumference measurement used to assess skeletal muscle mass

Military time time based on a 24-hour clock

Minerals noncaloric substances in food that are essential to all cells

Minimum disclosure portions or isolated pieces of information necessary for an immediate purpose

Minority people who differ from the majority in cultural characteristics like language, physical characteristics such as skin color, or both

Misdemeanor minor criminal offense

Mode of transmission manner in which infectious microorganisms move to another location

Modified standing position position in which the upper half of the body leans forward

Modulation last phase of pain impulse transmission when the brain interacts downward with spinal nerves to alter a pain experience

Molded splints orthotic devices made of rigid material

Montgomery straps strips of tape with eyelets

Morbidity incidence of a specific disease, disorder, or injury

Morgue area where dead bodies are temporarily held or examined

Mortality incidence of deaths

Mortician person who prepares the body for burial or cremation

Mucus substance that keeps mucous membranes moist

Multicultural diversity unique characteristics of ethnic groups

Multiple organ failure condition in which two or more organ systems gradually cease to function

Multiple sleep latency test assessment of daytime sleepiness

Muscle spasms sudden, forceful, involuntary muscle contractions

MyPlate color-coded diagram showing percentages of food that should be consumed each day

N

N95 respirator device that is individually fitted to each caregiver and can filter particles 1 micron in size, with a filter efficiency of 95% or more, provided it fits the face snugly

Narcolepsy sleep disorder characterized by the sudden onset of daytime sleep, a short NREM period before the first REM phase, and pathologic manifestations of REM sleep

Narrative charting style of documentation generally used in source-oriented records

Nasal cannula hollow tube with prongs that are placed into the client's nostrils for delivering oxygen

Nasal catheter tube for delivering oxygen that is inserted through the nose into the posterior nasal pharynx

Nasogastric intubation insertion of a tube through the nose into the stomach

Nasogastric tube tube that is placed in the nose and advanced to the stomach

Nasointestinal intubation insertion of a tube through the nose to the intestine

Nasointestinal tube tube inserted through the nose for distal placement below the stomach

Nasopharyngeal suctioning removal of secretions from the throat through a nasally inserted catheter

Nasotracheal suctioning removal of secretions from the trachea through a nasally inserted catheter

National Patient Safety Goals objectives designed to reduce the incidence of injuries to those being cared for in health agencies

Native Americans Indian nations found in North America, including the Eskimos and Aleuts

Nausea feeling that usually precedes vomiting

Nebulizer device that converts liquid inhalant medication to an aerosol using compressed air

Necrotic tissue nonliving tissue

Needleless systems equipment that eliminates the need for needles

Negligence harm that results because a person did not act reasonably

Neuropathic pain pain with atypical characteristics
Neurotransmitters chemical messengers synthesized in neurons
Neutral position limb that is turned neither toward nor away from the body's midline
NEX measurement distance from the nose to the earlobe to the xiphoid process
Nociceptors nerve receptors that transmit pain impulses
Nocturia nighttime urination
Nocturnal enuresis bedwetting
Nocturnal polysomnography technique used to obtain physiologic data during nighttime sleep
Nonelectrolytes chemical compounds that remain bound together when dissolved in solution
Nonessential amino acids protein components manufactured in the body
Nonopioids nonnarcotic drugs
Nonpathogens harmless and beneficial microorganisms
Nonrebreather mask oxygen delivery device in which all the exhaled air leaves the mask rather than partially entering the reservoir bag
Nonverbal communication exchange of information without using spoken or written words
Normal flora microorganisms that reside in and on humans
Nosocomial infections infections acquired while a person is being cared for in a hospital or other health care agency
Nuclear medicine department unit responsible for radionuclide imaging
Nurse-managed care pattern in which a nurse manager plans the nursing care of clients based on their illness or medical diagnosis
Nurse practice act statute that legally defines the unique role of the nurse and differentiates it from that of other health care practitioners, such as physicians
Nursing care plan written list of the client's problems, goals, and nursing orders for client care
Nursing diagnosis health problem that can be prevented, reduced, or resolved through independent nursing measures
Nursing orders directions for a client's nursing care
Nursing process organized sequence of problem-solving steps: assessment, diagnosis, planning, implementation, and evaluation
Nursing skills activities unique to the practice of nursing
Nursing team personnel who care for clients directly
Nursing theory proposal of what is involved in the process of nursing
Nutrition process by which the body uses food

O

Obesity condition in which a person's body mass index exceeds 30 or the triceps skinfold measurement exceeds 15 mm
Objective data facts that are observable and measurable
Occupied bed changing linen while the client remains in bed
Offsets predictive mathematical conversions
Oliguria urine output of less than 400 mL per 24 hours
Open wound wound in which the surface of the skin or mucous membrane is no longer intact
Ophthalmic application method of applying drugs onto the mucous membrane of one or both eyes
Ophthalmologist medical doctor who treats eye disorders
Opioids narcotic drugs; synthetic narcotics
Opportunistic infections disorders caused by nonpathogens that occur in people with compromised health
Optometrist person who prescribes corrective vision lenses
Oral airway curved device that keeps the tongue positioned forward within the mouth
Oral hygiene practices used to clean the mouth, especially the teeth
Oral route drug administration by swallowing or instillation through an enteral tube
Oral suctioning removal of secretions from the mouth
Orientation helping a person to become familiar with a new environment
Orogastric intubation insertion of a tube through the mouth into the stomach
Orogastric tube tube that is inserted from the mouth into the stomach
Oropharyngeal suctioning removal of secretions from the throat through a catheter inserted through the mouth
Orthopnea breathing that is facilitated by sitting up or standing
Orthopneic position seated position with the arms supported on pillows or the arm rests of a chair
Orthoses orthopedic devices that support or align a body part and prevent or correct deformities
Orthostatic hypotension sudden but temporary drop in blood pressure when rising from a reclining or seated position
Osmosis process that regulates the distribution of water
Ostomy surgically created opening
Otic application drug instillation in the outer ear
Outpatient surgery operative procedures from which clients recover and return home on the same day
Over-the-counter medication nonprescription drug
Oxygen analyzer device that measures the percentage of oxygen a client is receiving
Oxygen concentrator machine that collects and concentrates oxygen from room air and stores it for client use
Oxygen tent clear plastic enclosure that provides cooled, humidified oxygen
Oxygen therapeutics fluids that when transfused carry and distribute oxygen to cells, tissues, and organs; also known as blood substitutes
Oxygen therapy therapeutic intervention for administering more oxygen than exists in the atmosphere
Oxygen toxicity lung damage that develops when oxygen concentrations of more than 50% are administered for longer than 48 to 72 hours

P

Pack commercial device for applying moist heat
Pain unpleasant sensation usually associated with disease or injury
Pain management techniques for preventing, reducing, or relieving pain
Pain threshold point at which sufficient pain-transmitting neurochemicals reach the brain to cause awareness of discomfort
Pain tolerance amount of pain a person endures once the pain threshold is surpassed
Palpation lightly touching the body or applying pressure
Palpitation awareness of one's own heart contraction without having to feel the pulse
Pap test screening test that detects abnormal cervical cells, the status of reproductive hormone activity, or the presence of normal or infectious microorganisms in the uterus or vagina

Paracentesis procedure for withdrawing fluid from the abdominal cavity

Paralanguage vocal sounds that are not actually words

Parallel bars double row of stationary bars

Paranormal experiences those outside scientific explanation

Parasomnia condition associated with activities that cause arousal or partial arousal, usually during transitions in NREM periods of sleep

Parenteral nutrition nutrients, such as proteins, carbohydrate, fat, vitamins, minerals, and trace elements, which are administered intravenously

Parenteral route route of drug administration other than oral or through the gastrointestinal tract; administration by injection

Partial bath washing only the areas of the body that are subject to the greatest soiling or that are sources of body odor

Partial rebreather mask oxygen delivery device through which a client inhales a mixture of atmospheric air, oxygen from its source, and oxygen contained in a reservoir bag

Passive diffusion physiologic process in which dissolved substances, such as electrolytes and gases, move from an area of higher concentration to one of lower concentration through a semipermeable membrane

Passive exercise therapeutic activity performed with assistance

Paste vehicle that contains a drug in a viscous base

Pathogens microorganisms that cause illness

Pathologic grief condition in which a person cannot accept someone's death

Patient-controlled analgesia intervention that allows clients to self-administer pain medication

Pedagogy the science of teaching children or those with cognitive ability comparable to children

Pelvic examination physical inspection of the vagina and cervix, with palpation of the uterus and ovaries

Perception conscious experience of discomfort

Percussion (1) striking or tapping a part of the body; (2) type of chest physiotherapy performed by rhythmically striking the chest wall

Percutaneous electrical nerve stimulation pain management technique involving a combination of acupuncture needles and transcutaneous electrical nerve stimulation

Percutaneous endoscopic gastrostomy (PEG) tube transabdominal tube inserted into the stomach under endoscopic guidance

Percutaneous endoscopic jejunostomy (PEJ) tube tube that is passed through a PEG tube into the jejunum

Perineal care techniques used for cleansing the perineum

Periodontal disease condition that results in destruction of the tooth-supporting structures and jawbone

Perioperative care care that clients receive before, during, and after surgery

Peripheral parenteral nutrition isotonic or hypotonic intravenous nutrient solution instilled in a vein distant from the heart

Peristalsis rhythmic contractions of gastrointestinal smooth muscle

Peristomal skin skin around a stoma

Persistent vegetative state condition in which there is no cognitive function or capacity to experience emotions

Personal protective equipment garments that block the transfer of pathogens from one person, place, or object to oneself or others

Personal space distance of 6 in. to 4 ft

Petals strips of adhesive tape or moleskin applied to the rough edges of a cast for the purpose of reducing skin irritation

Phagocytosis process in which white blood cells consume cellular debris

Phlebitis inflammation of a vein

Photoperiod number of daylight hours

Phototherapy technique for suppressing melatonin by stimulating light receptors in the eye

Physical assessment systematic examination of body structures

Physical restraint method of immobilization that reduces the ability of a client to freely move his or her arms, legs, body, or head

PIE charting method of recording the client's progress under the headings of problem, intervention, and evaluation

Piloerection contraction of arrector pili muscles in skin follicles

Pin site location where pins, wires, or tongs enter or exit the skin

Placebo inactive substance or treatment measure that charades as one that is legitimate

Plaintiff person who claims injury

Planning process of prioritizing nursing diagnoses and collaborative problems, identifying measurable goals or outcomes, selecting appropriate interventions, and documenting the plan for care

Plaque substance composed of mucin and other gritty substances that deposits on teeth

Platform crutches crutches that support the forearm

Plume vaporized tissue, carbon, and water released during laser surgery

Plunger part of a syringe inside the barrel that moves back and forth to withdraw and instill medication

Pneumatic compression device machine that promotes circulation of venous blood and the movement of excess fluid into the lymphatic vessels

Pneumonia lung infection

Podiatrist person with special training in caring for feet

Poisoning injury caused by the ingestion, inhalation, or absorption of a toxic substance

Polypharmacy administration of multiple drugs to the same person

Polyuria larger-than-normal urinary volume

Port sealed opening

Port of entry site where microorganisms find their way onto or into a host

Positron emission tomography radionuclide scanning with the layered analysis of tomography

Possible diagnosis problem that may be present, but more information is needed to rule out or confirm its existence

Postanesthesia care unit area in the surgical department where clients are intensively monitored

Postmortem care care of the body after death

Postoperative care nursing care after surgery

Postoperative period interval that begins after surgery is completed

Postural drainage positioning technique that facilitates drainage of secretions from the lungs

Postural hypotension sudden but temporary drop in blood pressure when rising from a reclining or seated position

Posture position of the body, or the way in which it is held

Potential diagnosis problem a client is at risk for developing

Powered Air Purifying Respirator alternative device for a caregiver who has not been fitted for an N95 respirator; works by blowing atmospheric air through belt-mounted, air-purifying canisters to the facepiece via a flexible tube

Preferred provider organizations agents for health insurance companies that control health care costs on the basis of competition
Prefilled cartridge sealed glass cylinder of parenteral medication with a preattached needle
Preload volume of blood that fills the heart and stretches the heart muscle fibers during its resting phase
Preoperative checklist form that identifies the status of essential presurgical activities
Preoperative period time that starts when the client is informed that surgery is necessary and ends when he or she is transported to the operating room
Pressure ulcer wound caused by prolonged capillary compression sufficient to impair circulation to the skin and underlying tissue
Primary care first health care worker or agency to assess a person with a health need
Primary illness one that develops independently of any other disease
Primary nursing pattern in which the admitting nurse assumes responsibility for planning client care and evaluating the progress of the client
Problem-oriented records records organized according to the client's health problems
Primary prevention actions used to eliminate the potential for illness before it occurs
Progressive care units units for clients who were once in critical condition but have recovered sufficiently to require less intensive nursing care
Progressive relaxation therapeutic exercise whereby a person actively contracts and then relaxes muscle groups
Projectile vomiting vomiting that occurs with great force
Proliferation period during which new cells fill and seal a wound
Prone position position in which the client lies on the abdomen
Prophylactic braces braces used to prevent or reduce the severity of a joint injury
Prosthetic limb substitute for an arm or leg
Prosthetist person who constructs prosthetic limbs
Protein nutrient composed of amino acids; chemical compounds made up of nitrogen, carbon, hydrogen, and oxygen
Protein complementation combining plant sources of protein
Proxemics relation of space to communication
Psychomotor domain learning by doing
Public space distance of 12 ft or more
Pulmonary embolus blood clot that travels to the lung
Pulse wave-like sensation that can be palpated in a peripheral artery
Pulse deficit difference between the apical and radial pulse rates
Pulse oximetry noninvasive, transcutaneous technique for periodically or continuously monitoring the oxygen saturation of blood
Pulse pressure difference between systolic and diastolic blood pressure measurements
Pulse rate number of peripheral arterial pulsations palpated in a minute
Pulse rhythm pattern of the pulsations and pauses between them
Pulse volume quality of the pulsations that are felt
Pursed-lip breathing form of controlled ventilation in which the expiration phase of breathing is consciously prolonged
Purulent drainage white- or green-tinged fluid
Pyrexia fever

Q

Quadriceps setting isometric exercise in which a client alternately tenses and relaxes the quadriceps muscles
Quality assurance process of promoting care that reflects established agency standards

R

Race biologic variations
Radiography diagnostic procedures that use x-rays
Radionuclides elements whose molecular structures are altered to produce radiation
Range-of-motion exercises therapeutic activity in which joints are moved
Rebound effect swelling of the nasal mucosa within a short time of inhaled decongestant drug administration
Receiving room presurgical holding area
Reciprocity licensure based on evidence of having met licensing criteria in another state
Reconstitution process of adding liquid to a powdered substance
Recording process of writing information
Recovery index guide for determining a person's fitness level
Recovery position side-lying position that helps to maintain an open airway and prevent aspiration of liquids
Rectus femoris site injection area in the anterior thigh
Referral process of sending someone to another person or agency for special services
Referred pain discomfort perceived in an area of the body away from the site of origin
Regeneration cell duplication
Regurgitation bringing stomach contents to the throat and mouth without the effort of vomiting
Rehabilitative braces braces that allow protected motion of an injured joint that has been treated surgically
Relationship association between two people
Relative humidity ratio between the amount of moisture in the air and the greatest amount of water vapor the air can hold at a given temperature
Relaxation technique for releasing muscle tension and quieting the mind
Remission disappearance of signs and symptoms associated with a particular disease
Remodeling period during which a wound undergoes changes and maturation
Repetitive strain injuries disorders that result from cumulative trauma to musculoskeletal structures
Rescue breathing process of ventilating a nonbreathing victim's lungs
Reservoir place where microbes grow and reproduce providing a haven for sustaining microbial survival
Resident microorganisms generally nonpathogens that are constantly present on the skin
Residual urine urine that remains in the bladder after voiding
Resolution process by which damaged cells recover and reestablish their normal function
Respiration exchange of oxygen and carbon dioxide
Respiratory hygiene/cough etiquette infection control measures used when there are signs of illness suggesting an undiagnosed transmissible respiratory infection
Respiratory rate number of ventilations per minute
Respite care relief for a caregiver

Rest waking state characterized by reduced activity and reduced mental stimulation

Restless legs syndrome movement, typically in the legs, but occasionally in the arms or other body parts, to relieve disturbing skin sensations

Restraint alternatives protective or adaptive devices that promote client safety and postural support, but which the client can release independently

Restraints devices or chemicals that restrict movement or access to one's body

Resuscitation team group of people trained and certified in advanced cardiac life support (ACLS) techniques

Retching act of vomiting without producing vomitus

Retention catheter urinary tube that is left in place for a period of time

Retention enema solution held temporarily in the large intestine

Reversal drugs medications that counteract the effects of those used for conscious sedation

Rh factor protein surface marker on red blood cells

Rhizotomy surgical sectioning of a nerve root close to the spinal cord

Rinne test assessment technique for comparing air versus bone conduction of sound

Risk management process of identifying and reducing the costs of anticipated losses

Roentgenography general term for procedures that use x-rays

Rounds visits to clients on an individual basis or as a group

Route of administration oral, topical, inhalant, or parenteral route where a drug is administered

S

Safe injection practices infection control measures that prevent the transmission of blood borne pathogens through the use of aseptic techniques involving the preparation and administration of parenteral medications

Safety measures that prevent accidents or unintentional injuries

Saturated fats lipids that contain as much hydrogen as their molecular structure can hold

Scar formation replacement of damaged cells with fibrous tissue

Science body of knowledge unique to a particular subject

Scoop method technique for threading the needle of a syringe into the cap without touching the cap itself

Scored tablet tablet with a groove in its center

Secondary care health services to which primary caregivers refer clients for consultation and additional testing

Secondary illness disorder that develops from a preexisting condition

Secondary infusion administration of a diluted intravenous drug at the same time a solution is infusing, or intermittently with an infusing solution

Secondary prevention actions used to screen for risk factors that provide a means for early diagnosis of disease

Second-intention healing reparative process when wound edges are widely separated

Sedative drug that produces a relaxing and calming effect

Sensory manipulation using sensory stimuli to alter moods, feelings, and physiologic responses

Sepsis potentially fatal systemic infection

Sequelae consequences of a disease or its treatment

Serous drainage leaking plasma

Set point optimal body temperature

Shaft long portion of a needle

Shearing force exerted against the surface and layers of the skin as tissues slide in opposite but parallel directions

Shearing force effect that moves layers of tissue in opposite directions

Shell temperature warmth at the skin surface

Short-term goals outcomes that can be met in a few days to a week

Shroud covering for a dead body

Signing shortened term for American Sign Language communication

Signs objective data; information that is observable and measurable

Silence intentionally withholding verbal comments

Simple mask device for administering oxygen that fits over the nose and mouth

Sims' position lying on the left side with the chest leaning forward, the right knee bent toward the head, the right arm forward, and the left arm extended behind the body

Sitz bath soak of the perianal area

Skeletal traction pull exerted directly on the skeletal system by attaching wires, pins, or tongs into or through a bone

Skilled nursing facility nursing home that provides 24-hour nursing care under the direction of a registered nurse

Skin patches drugs that are bonded to an adhesive bandage

Skin tear shallow break in the skin

Skin traction pulling effect on the skeletal system by applying devices to the skin

Slander character attack uttered in the presence of others

Sleep state of arousable unconsciousness

Sleep apnea/hypopnea syndrome sleep disorder in which the sleeper stops breathing or the breathing slows for 10 seconds or longer, five or more times per hour

Sleep diary daily account of sleeping and waking activities

Sleep paralysis inability to move for a few minutes just before falling asleep or awakening

Sleep rituals habitual activities performed before retiring

Sleep-wake cycle disturbance condition that results from a sleep schedule that involves daytime sleeping

Sling cloth device used to elevate, cradle, and support parts of the body

Slough dead tissue on a wound surface that is moist, stringy, yellow tan, gray, or green

Smelling acuity ability to smell and identify odors

Snellen eye chart tool for assessing far vision

Soak procedure in which a part of the body is submerged in fluid

SOAP charting documentation style more likely to be used in a problem-oriented record

Social space distance of 4 to 12 ft

Somatic pain discomfort generated from deeper connective tissue

Somnambulism sleepwalking

Sordes dried crusts around the mouth containing mucus, microorganisms, and epithelial cells shed from the oral mucous membrane

Source-oriented records records organized according to the source of information

Spacer chamber that is attached to an inhaler

Specimens samples of tissue or body fluids

Speculum metal or plastic instrument for widening the vagina or other body cavity

Sphygmomanometer device for measuring blood pressure

Spica cast rigid mold that encircles one or both arms or legs and the chest or trunk

Spinal tap procedure that involves insertion of a needle between lumbar vertebrae in the spine but below the spinal cord itself

Splint device that immobilizes and protects an injured part of the body

Spore temporarily inactive microbial life form

Sputum mucus raised to the level of the upper airways

Stage of exhaustion the last phase in the general adaptation syndrome that develops when one or more adaptive or resistive mechanisms can no longer protect a person experiencing a stressor

Stage of resistance second phase in the general adaptation syndrome characterized by physiologic changes designed to restore homeostasis

Standard precautions infection control measures for reducing the risk of transmission among all clients, regardless of suspected or confirmed infection status

Standards for care policies that ensure quality client care

Staples wide metal clips

Stasis lack of movement

Statute of limitations designated amount of time within which a person can file a lawsuit

Statutory laws laws enacted by federal, state, or local legislatures

Stent tube that keeps a channel open

Stepdown units units for clients who were once in critical condition but have recovered sufficiently to require less intensive nursing care

Step test submaximal fitness test involving a timed stepping activity

Stereotypes fixed attitudes about all people who share a common characteristic

Sterile field work area free of microorganisms

Sterile technique practices that avoid contaminating microbe-free items

Sterilization physical and chemical techniques that destroy all microorganisms, including spores

Stertorous breathing noisy ventilation

Stethoscope instrument that carries sound to the ears

Stimulants drugs that excite structures in the brain

Stock supply drugs kept in a nursing unit for use in an emergency

Stoma entrance to a surgically created opening

Straight catheter urine drainage tube that is inserted but not left in place

Strength power to perform

Stress physiologic and behavioral reactions that occur in response to disequilibrium

Stress electrocardiogram test of electrical conduction through the heart during maximal activity

Stress management techniques therapeutic activities used to reestablish balance between the sympathetic and parasympathetic nervous systems

Stress-reduction techniques methods that promote physiologic comfort and emotional well-being

Stress-related disorders diseases that result from prolonged stimulation of the autonomic nervous and endocrine systems

Stressors changes that have the potential for disturbing equilibrium

Stridor harsh, high-pitched sound heard on inspiration when there is laryngeal obstruction

Stylet metal guidewire

Subcultures unique cultural groups that coexist within the dominant culture

Subcutaneous injection parenteral drug administration beneath the skin but above the muscle

Subdiaphragmatic thrust pressure to the abdomen

Subjective data information that only the client feels and can describe

Sublingual application placement of a drug under the tongue

Submaximal fitness test exercise test that does not stress a person to exhaustion

Substituted judgment court belief that a client would issue consent if he or she had the capacity to do so

Suctioning technique for removing liquid secretions with a catheter

Suffering emotional component of pain

Sump tubes tubes that contain a double lumen

Sundown syndrome onset of disorientation as the sun sets

Sunrise syndrome early morning confusion

Supine position position in which the person lies on the back

Suppository medicated oval or cone-shaped mass

Surfactant lipoprotein produced by cells in the alveoli that promotes elasticity of the lungs and enhances gas diffusion

Surgical asepsis measures that render supplies and equipment totally free of microorganisms

Surgical hand antisepsis medically aseptic hand hygiene procedure that is performed prior to the nurse's donning sterile gloves and garments in an operative or obstetrical procedure

Surgical waiting area room where family and friends await information about the surgical client

Susceptible host one whose biologic defense mechanisms are weakened in some way

Sustained release drug that dissolves at timed intervals

Sutures knotted ties that hold an incision together

Sympathy feeling as emotionally distraught as the client

Symptoms subjective data; that which only the client can identify

Syndrome diagnosis cluster of problems that is present due to an event or situation

Systolic pressure pressure in the arterial system when the heart contracts

T

Tachycardia heart rate between 100 and 150 beats per minute (bpm) at rest

Tachypnea rapid respiratory rate

Tamponade controlling gastric bleeding with internal pressure via a tube

Target heart rate goal for heart rate during exercise

Tartar hardened plaque

Task-oriented touch personal contact that is required when performing nursing procedures

Team nursing pattern in which nursing personnel divide the clients into groups and complete their care together

Telehome care visiting clients electronically in their home for the purpose of seeing and communicating in real time

Telehealth services technology that facilitates the transmission of health assessment and monitoring data with audio, video, and Internet-based devices

Telephonic interpreting language translation via telephone

Teleology ethical theory based on final outcomes

Temperature translation conversion of tympanic temperature into an oral, rectal, or core temperature

Tension pneumothorax extreme air pressure in the lung when there is no avenue for its escape
Terminal disinfection measures used to clean the client environment after discharge
Terminal illness illness with no potential for cure
Terminating phase ending of a nurse–client relationship when there is mutual agreement that the client's immediate health problems have improved
Tertiary care health services provided at hospitals or medical centers that offer specialists and complex technology
Tertiary prevention actions that minimize the consequences of a disorder through aggressive rehabilitation or appropriate management of the disease
Theory opinion, belief, or view that explains a process
Therapeutic baths baths performed for other than hygiene purposes
Therapeutic exercise activity performed by people with health risks or those being treated for a health problem
Therapeutic relationship association between people whose objective is to achieve a higher state of health
Therapeutic verbal communication using words and gestures to accomplish a particular objective
Thermal burn skin injury caused by flames, hot liquids, or steam
Thermister temperature sensor
Thermistor catheter heat-sensing device at the tip of an internally placed tube
Thermogenesis heat production
Thermoregulation ability to maintain stable body temperature
Third-intention healing reparative process when a wound is widely separated and later brought together with some type of closure material
Third-spacing movement of intravascular fluid to nonvascular fluid compartments, where it becomes trapped and useless
Thrombophlebitis inflammation of a vein caused by a thrombus
Thrombus stationary blood clot
Thrombus formation development of a stationary blood clot
Tidaling rhythmic rise and fall of water in a chest tube drainage system
Tilt table device that raises client from a supine to a standing position
Tip part of a syringe to which the needle is attached
Tone ability of muscles to respond when stimulated
Topical route drug administration to the skin or mucous membranes
Tort litigation in which one person asserts that an injury, which may be physical, emotional, or financial, occurred as a consequence of another's actions or failure to act
Total parenteral nutrition hypertonic solution of nutrients designed to meet almost all the caloric and nutritional needs of clients
Total quality improvement process of promoting care that reflects established agency standards
Touch tactile stimulus produced by making personal contact with another person or an object
Towel bath technique for bathing in which a single large towel is used to cover and wash a client
T-piece device that fits securely onto a tracheostomy tube or endotracheal tube
Tracheostomy surgically created opening into the trachea
Tracheostomy care hygiene and maintenance of a tracheostomy and tracheostomy tube
Tracheostomy collar device that delivers oxygen near an artificial opening in the neck
Tracheostomy tube curved, hollow plastic tube in the trachea
Traction pulling on a part of the skeletal system
Traction splints metal devices that immobilize and pull on muscles that are in a state of contraction
Trade name name by which a pharmaceutical company identifies its drug
Traditional time time based on two 12-hour revolutions on a clock
Training effect heart rate and consequently pulse rate become consistently lower than average with regular exercise
Tranquilizer drug that produce a relaxing and calming effect
Transabdominal tubes tubes placed through the abdominal wall
Transcultural nursing providing nursing care in the context of another's culture
Transcutaneous electrical nerve stimulation medically prescribed pain management technique that delivers bursts of electricity to the skin and underlying nerves
Transdermal application method of applying a drug on the skin and allowing it to become passively absorbed
Transducer instrument that receives and transmits biophysical energy
Transduction conversion of chemical information at the cellular level into electrical impulses that move toward the spinal cord
Trans fats unsaturated, hydrogenated fats
Transfer (1) discharging a client from one unit or agency and immediately admitting him or her to another; (2) moving a client from place to place
Transfer summary written review of the client's previous care
Transient microorganisms pathogens picked up during brief contact with contaminated reservoirs
Transitional care unit area for clients initially in a critical or unstable condition, but sufficiently recovered to require less intensive nursing care
Transmission phase during which stimuli move from the peripheral nervous system toward the brain
Transmission-based precautions measures for controlling the spread of highly transmissible or epidemiologically important infectious agents from clients when the known or suspected route(s) of transmission is (are) not completely interrupted using standard precautions alone
Transtracheal catheter hollow tube inserted into the trachea to deliver oxygen
Trauma injury
Truth telling ethical principle proposing that all clients have the right to receive complete and accurate information
Tuberculin syringe syringe that holds 1 mL of fluid and is calibrated in 0.01-mL increments
Turgor resiliency of the skin
Twenty-four-hour specimen collection of all the urine produced in a full 24-hour period

U

Ultrasonography soft tissue examination that uses sound waves in ranges beyond human hearing
Undermining erosion of tissue from underneath intact skin at a wound edge
Unintentional tort situation that results in an injury, although the person responsible did not mean to cause harm
Unit dose self-contained packet that holds one tablet or capsule
Universal donor person with Type O blood

Universal recipient person with Type AB blood
Unoccupied bed changing the linen when the bed is empty
Unsaturated fats lipids that are missing some hydrogen
Urgency strong feeling that urine must be eliminated quickly
Urinal cylindrical container for collecting urine
Urinary diversion procedure in which one or both ureters are surgically implanted elsewhere
Urinary elimination process of releasing excess fluid and metabolic wastes
Urinary retention condition in which urine is produced but is not released from the bladder
Urine fluid in the bladder
Urostomy urinary diversion that discharges urine from an opening on the abdomen

V

Valsalva maneuver act of closing the glottis and contracting the pelvic and abdominal muscles to increase abdominal pressure
Values ideals that a person believes are important
Vastus lateralis site injection area in the outer thigh
Vegan person who relies exclusively on plant sources for protein
Vegetarian person who restricts consumption of animal food sources
Venipuncture accessing the venous system by piercing a vein with a needle
Ventilation (1) movement of air in and out of the lungs; (2) movement of air in the environment
Ventricular fibrillation life-threatening dysrhythmia in which the heart muscle quivers and cannot contract sufficiently to circulate blood
Ventrogluteal site injection area in the hip
Venturi mask oxygen delivery device that mixes a precise amount of oxygen and atmospheric air
Verbal communication communication that uses words
Vial glass or plastic container of parenteral medication with a self-sealing rubber stopper
Vibration type of chest physiotherapy used to loosen retained secretions
Video interpreting communication in which a person signs in a remote location yet is visible to the health team member and client and vice versa
Viral load number of viral copies
Visceral pain discomfort arising from internal organs
Visual acuity ability to see both far and near
Visual field examination assessment of peripheral vision and continuity in the visual field
Vital signs body temperature, pulse rate, respiratory rate, and blood pressure
Vitamins chemical substances that are necessary in minute amounts for normal growth, maintenance of health, and functioning of the body
Voided specimen freshly urinated sample of urine
Voiding reflex spontaneous relaxation of the urinary sphincter in response to physical stimulation
Volume-control set chamber in intravenous tubing that holds a portion from a larger volume of intravenous solution
Volumetric controller electronic infusion device that instills intravenous solutions by gravity
Vomiting loss of stomach contents through the mouth
Vomitus substance that is vomited

W

Waiting-for-permission phenomenon a terminally ill client's forestalling of death when he or she feels that loved ones are not yet prepared to deal with the client's death
Walk-a-mile test fitness test that measures the time it takes a person to walk a mile
Walker ambulatory aid constructed of curved aluminum bars that form a three-sided enclosure, with four legs for support
Walking belt safety device applied around the client's waist used to provide ambulatory support and assistance
Water-seal chest tube drainage technique for evacuating air or blood from the pleural cavity
Water-soluble vitamins vitamins present and carried in body water; B complex and vitamin C
Webcam video camera that allows viewing via the Internet
Weber test assessment technique for determining equality or disparity of bone-conducted sound
Wellness full and balanced integration of all aspects of health
Wellness diagnosis situation in which a healthy person obtains nursing assistance to maintain his or her health or perform at a higher level
Wheal elevated circle on the skin
Whistle-blowing reporting incompetent or unethical practices
Whitecoat hypertension condition in which the blood pressure is elevated when taken by a health care worker but is normal at other times
Window square of plaster removed from a cast that provides an area for inspecting or treating underlying tissue.
Working phase period during which the nurse and the client plan the client's care and put the plan into action
Wound damaged skin or soft tissue

X

Xerostomia dry mouth

Z

Z-track technique injection method that prevents medication from leaking outside the muscle

Index

Note: Page numbers followed by f indicate figures; those followed by t indicate tables; those followed by b indicate box; and those followed by d indicate display text.

C

E

F

O

Q

R

U